Miller's Basics of
ANESTHESIA

EIGHTH EDITION

Manuel C. Pardo, Jr., MD

Professor and Vice Chair for Education
Department of Anesthesia and Perioperative Care
University of California, San Francisco
San Francisco, California

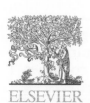

ELSEVIER

Elsevier

1600 John F. Kennedy Blvd.
Ste 1800
Philadelphia, PA 19103-2899

MILLER'S BASICS OF ANESTHESIA, EIGHTH EDITION

ISBN: 978-0-323796774

Notice

Previous editions copyrighted 2018, 2011, 2007, 2000, 1994, 1989, 1984.

Content Strategist: Kayla Wolfe
Content Development Specialist: Ann R. Anderson
Publishing Services Manager: Shereen Jameel
Project Manager: Beula Christopher
Design Direction: Ryan Cook

Printed in India.

Last digit is the print number: 9 8 7 6 5 4 3 2 1

To my wife, Susan, and daughter, Allison, for their support and encouragement while I was working on this book throughout the pandemic; to Dr. Ronald D. Miller for his mentorship, especially regarding textbooks; and to all students of this wondrous specialty of anesthesiology.

Manuel C. Pardo, Jr.

CONTRIBUTORS

Basem B. Abdelmalak, MD, FASA, SAMBA-F
Professor of Anesthesiology
Departments of General Anesthesiology and Outcomes Research
Anesthesiology Institute
Cleveland Clinic
Cleveland, Ohio

Christopher R. Abrecht, MD
Assistant Professor
Department of Anesthesia and Perioperative Care
Division of Pain Medicine
University of California, San Francisco
San Francisco, California

Meredith C.B. Adams, MD, MS
Assistant Professor
Department of Anesthesiology
Wake Forest Baptist Health
Winston-Salem, North Carolina

Ashish Agrawal, MD
Assistant Professor
Department of Anesthesia and Perioperative Care
University of California, San Francisco
San Francisco, California

Dean B. Andropoulos, MD, MHCM
Anesthesiologist-in-Chief
Anesthesiology, Perioperative and Pain Medicine
Texas Children's Hospital;
Professor and Vice Chair for Clinical Affairs
  Anesthesiology
Baylor College of Medicine
Houston, Texas

Charles B. Berde, MD, PhD
Senior Associate in Perioperative Anesthesia
Department of Anesthesiology, Critical Care, and Pain Medicine
Boston Children's Hospital;
Professor of Anesthesia and Pediatrics
Harvard Medical School
Boston, Massachusetts

Laura Berenstain, MD, FASA
Adjunct Professor of Clinical Anesthesiology
University of Cincinnati College of Medicine;
Division of Pediatric Cardiac Anesthesia
Cincinnati Children's Hospital Medical Center
Cincinnati, Ohio

Jeanna D. Blitz, MD
Associate Professor of Anesthesiology
Duke University School of Medicine;
Department of Anesthesiology
Duke University Medical Center
Durham, North Carolina

Michael P. Bokoch, MD, PhD
Assistant Professor
Department of Anesthesia and Perioperative Care
University of California, San Francisco
San Francisco, California

Emilee Borgmeier, MD
Assistant Professor of Anesthesiology
Department of Anesthesiology
University of Utah
Salt Lake City, Utah

Joanna Bouez, MD
Clinical Fellow
Department of Anesthesiology
Toronto Western Hospital, University Health Network
University of Toronto
Toronto, Ontario, Canada

Matthias R. Braehler, MD, PhD
Professor
Department of Anesthesia and Perioperative Care
University of California, San Francisco
San Francisco, California

Kristine E.W. Breyer, MD
Associate Professor
Department of Anesthesia and Perioperative Care
University of California, San Francisco
San Francisco, California

Richard Brull, MD, FRCPC
Professor
Department of Anesthesia
University of Toronto;
Evelyn Bateman Cara Operations Chair in Ambulatory
*   Anesthesia and Women's Health*
Women's College Hospital;
Staff Anesthesiologist
Toronto Western Hospital and Women's College Hospital
Toronto, Ontario, Canada

Joyce Chang, MD
Associate Professor
Department of Anesthesia and Perioperative Care
University of California, San Francisco
San Francisco, California

Tyler Seth Chernin, MD
Associate Professor
Department of Anesthesia and Perioperative Care
University of California, San Francisco
San Francisco, California

Catherine Chiu, MD
Fellow
Department of Anesthesia and Perioperative Care
University of California, San Francisco
San Francisco, California

Frances Chung, MBBS, FRCPC
Professor
Department of Anesthesiology
Toronto Western Hospital, University Health Network
University of Toronto
Toronto, Ontario, Canada

Hemra Cil, MD
Assistant Professor
Department of Anesthesia and Perioperative Care
University of California, San Francisco
San Francisco, California

Neal H. Cohen, MD, MPH, MS
Professor Emeritus
Anesthesia and Perioperative Care and Medicine
UCSF School of Medicine;
Vice Dean
UCSF School of Medicine
San Francisco, California

Heather A. Columbano, MD
Assistant Professor
Department of Anesthesiology
Wake Forest Baptist Health
Winston-Salem, North Carolina

Daniel Charles Cook, MD
Assistant Professor of Anesthesiology
Weill Cornell Medicine
New York, New York

Wilson Cui, MD, PhD
Associate Professor
Department of Anesthesia and Perioperative Care
University of California, San Francisco
San Francisco, California

Ryan Paul Davis, MD
Clinical Assistant Professor
Department of Anesthesiology
University of Michigan
Ann Arbor, Michigan

Andrew J. Deacon, B Biomed Sci (Hons), MBBS, FANZCA
Staff Specialist
Department of Anaesthesia and Pain Medicine
The Canberra Hospital
Garran, Australia

Anne L. Donovan, MD
Associate Clinical Professor
Department of Anesthesia and Perioperative Care
Division of Critical Care Medicine
University of California, San Francisco
San Francisco, California

Talmage D. Egan, BA, MD
Professor and Chair
Anesthesiology
University of Utah School of Medicine
Salt Lake City, Utah

John Feiner, MD
Professor
Department of Anesthesia and Perioperative Care
University of California, San Francisco
San Francisco, California

Alana Flexman, MD, MBA(C), FRCPC
Clinical Associate Professor
Department of Anesthesiology, Pharmacology and Therapeutics
The University of British Columbia
Vancouver, Canada

David Furgiuele, MD, FASA
Assistant Professor and Associate Director of Anesthesiology Service
New York University Langone Orthopedic Hospital
New York University Langone Health,
Department of Anesthesiology, Perioperative Care, and Pain Medicine
New York University Grossman School of Medicine
New York, New York

Seema Gandhi, MD
Clinical Professor
Department of Anesthesia and Perioperative Care
University of California, San Francisco
San Francisco, California

Steven Gayer, MD, MBA
Professor of Anesthesiology and Ophthalmology
Anesthesiology
University of Miami Miller School of Medicine
Miami, Florida

Sarah Gebauer, BA, MD
Anesthesiologist
Elk River Anesthesia Associates;
Chair, Perioperative Service Line
Yampa Valley Medical Center
Steamboat Springs, Colorado

David B. Glick, MD, MBA
Professor,
Section Chief, Multispecialty Adult Anesthesia
Anesthesia and Critical Care
University of Chicago
Chicago, Illinois

Erin A. Gottlieb, MD, MHCM
Associate Professor
Surgery and Perioperative Care
The University of Texas at Austin Dell Medical School;
Chief of Pediatric Cardiac Anesthesiology
Dell Children's Medical Center
Austin, Texas

Andrew T. Gray, MD, PhD
Professor
Department of Anesthesia and Perioperative Care
University of California, San Francisco
San Francisco, California

Hugh C. Hemmings, Jr., MD, PhD
Professor and Chair of Anesthesiology
Professor of Pharmacology
Senior Associate Dean for Research
Weill Cornell Medicine;
Anesthesiologist-in-Chief
NewYork-Presbyterian Hospital/Weill Cornell Medical Center
New York, New York

David W. Hewson, BSc (Hons), MBBS, PGCert Ed, FHEA, FRCA, PhD
Consultant Anaesthetist
Department of Anaesthesia and Critical Care
Nottingham University Hospitals NHS Trust;
Honorary Assistant Professor
Academic Unit of Injury, Inflammation and Recovery Science
University of Nottingham
Nottingham, United Kingdom

Lindsey L. Huddleston, MD
Associate Clinical Professor
Department of Anesthesia and Perioperative Care
University of California, San Francisco
San Francisco, California

Robert W. Hurley, MD, PhD
Professor of Anesthesiology, Neurobiology and Anatomy
Associate Dean
Wake Forest University School of Medicine;
Executive Director, Pain Shared Service Line
Atrium Health—Wake Forest Baptist
Winston Salem, North Carolina

Andrew Infosino, MD
Health Sciences Clinical Professor
Department of Anesthesia and Perioperative Care,
Health Sciences Clinical Professor
Department of Pediatrics
UCSF Benioff Children's Hospital
San Francisco, California

Ken B. Johnson, MD, MS
Professor
Department of Anesthesiology
University of Utah
Salt Lake City, Utah

Tae Kyun Kim, MD, PhD
Professor
Department of Anesthesia and Pain Medicine
Pusan National University Hospital
Seo-gu, Busan, South Korea

Anjali Koka, MD
Associate in Perioperative Anesthesia
Department of Anesthesiology, Critical Care, and Pain Medicine
Boston Children's Hospital;
Instructor of Anesthesia
Harvard Medical School
Boston, Massachusetts

Benn Lancman, MBBS, MHumFac, FANZCA
Specialist Anaesthesiologist
Department of Anaesthesia and Perioperative Medicine,
Trauma Consultant
Department of Surgery
Alfred Health;
Specialist Anaesthetist
Department of Anaesthesia, Perioperative and Pain Medicine
Peter Mac Callum Cancer Centre
Melbourne, Victoria, Australia

Chanhung Z. Lee, MD, PhD
Professor
Department of Anesthesia and Perioperative Care
University of California, San Francisco
San Francisco, California

Matthieu Legrand, MD, PhD
Professor
Department of Anesthesia and Perioperative Care
Division of Critical Care Medicine
University of California, San Francisco
San Francisco, California

Cynthia A. Lien, MD
Professor and Chair of Anesthesiology
Medical College of Wisconsin
Milwaukee, Wisconsin

Maytinee Lilaonitkul, MBBS, BSc, MRCP, FRCA
Assistant Clinical Professor
Department of Anesthesia and Perioperative Care
University of California, San Francisco
San Francisco, California

Linda L. Liu, MD
Professor
Department of Anesthesia and Perioperative Care
University of California, San Francisco
San Francisco, California

Alan J.R. Macfarlane, BSc (Hons), MBChB, MRCP, FRCA
Consultant Anaesthetist
Department of Anaesthesia
Glasgow Royal Infirmary;
Honorary Professor
Anaesthesia, Critical Care and Pain Medicine
University of Glasgow
Glasgow, United Kingdom

Vinod Malhotra, MBBS, MD, FACA
Professor and Senior Executive Advisor to the Chair
Anesthesiology,
Professor of Anesthesiology in Clinical Urology
Urology,
Weill Cornell Medicine–NewYork-Presbyterian Hospital
New York, New York

Solmaz Poorsattar Manuel, MD
Associate Clinical Professor
Department of Anesthesia and Perioperative Care
University of California, San Francisco
San Francisco, California

Mitchell H. Marshall, MD, FASA
Clinical Professor
Department of Anesthesiology, Perioperative Care, and Pain Medicine
New York University Grossman School of Medicine;
Chief of Anesthesiology
NYU Langone Orthopedic Hospital
New York, New York

Mary Ellen McCann, MD, MPH
Senior Associate in Anaesthesia
Department of Anesthesiology, Critical Care, and Pain Medicine
Boston Children's Hospital;
Associate Professor of Anaesthesia
Department of Anaesthesia
Harvard Medical School
Boston, Massachusetts

Grace C. McCarthy, MD
Assistant Professor
Department of Anesthesiology
Duke University Health System;
Staff Anesthesiologist
Veterans Affairs Health System
Durham, North Carolina

Matthew D. McEvoy, MD
Professor of Anesthesiology and Surgery
Vanderbilt University School of Medicine;
Vice Chair for Perioperative Medicine
Department of Anesthesiology
Vanderbilt University Medical Center
Nashville, Tennessee

Lingzhong Meng, MD
Endowed Professor and Chair
Department of Anesthesiology
The First Affiliated Hospital
Zhejiang University School of Medicine
Hangzhou, Zhejiang, China

Ronald D. Miller, MD, MS
Professor Emeritus
Department of Anesthesia and Perioperative Care
University of California, San Francisco
San Francisco, California

Ilan Mizrahi, MD
Instructor
Department of Anaesthesia
Harvard Medical School;
Staff Anesthesiologist
Department of Anesthesia, Critical Care, and Pain Medicine
Massachusetts General Hospital
Boston, Massachusetts

Shinju Obara, MD
Associate Professor
Fukushima Medical University Hospital, School of Medicine;
Deputy Director
Surgical Operation Department, and Center for Pain Management,
Department of Anesthesiology
Fukushima Medical University Hospital
Hikarigaoka, Fukushima City, Japan

Howard D. Palte, MBChB, FCA(SA)
Professor
Department of Anesthesiology
University of Miami
Miami, Florida

Anup Pamnani, MD
Assistant Professor of Anesthesiology
Department of Anesthesiology
Weill Cornell Medical College
New York, New York

Anil K. Panigrahi, MD, PhD
Clinical Associate Professor
Department of Anesthesiology, Perioperative and Pain Medicine and Department of Pathology
Division of Transfusion Medicine
Stanford University School of Medicine
Stanford, California

Manuel C. Pardo, Jr., MD, FASA
Professor and Vice Chair for Education
Department of Anesthesia and Perioperative Care
University of California, San Francisco
San Francisco, California

Sophia P. Poorsattar, MD
Assistant Clinical Professor
Department of Anesthesiology and Perioperative Medicine
UCLA David Geffen School of Medicine
Los Angeles, California

Mark D. Rollins, MD, PhD
Professor
Department of Anesthesiology and Perioperative Medicine
Mayo Clinic
Rochester, Minnesota

Andrew D. Rosenberg, MD, FASA
Professor and Dorothy Reaves Spatz MD
Chair, Department of Anesthesiology, Perioperative Care, and Pain Medicine
NYU Langone Medical Center
NYU Grossman School of Medicine
New York, New York

Ann Cai Shah, MD
Assistant Clinical Professor
Department of Anesthesia and Perioperative Care
University of California, San Francisco
San Francisco, California

David Shimabukuro, MDCM
Professor
Department of Anesthesia and Perioperative Care
University of California, San Francisco
San Francisco, California

Mandeep Singh, MBBS, MD, MSc, FRCPC
Assistant Professor
Department of Anesthesiology
Toronto Western Hospital, University Health Network
University of Toronto
Toronto, Ontario, Canada

Jina Sinskey, MD, FASA
Associate Professor
Department of Anesthesia and Perioperative Care
University of California, San Francisco
San Francisco, California

Peter D. Slinger, MD, FRCPC
Professor
Department of Anesthesia
University of Toronto
Toronto, Ontario, Canada

Wendy Smith, MD
Assistant Clinical Professor
Department of Anesthesia and Perioperative Care
University of California, San Francisco
San Francisco, California

Sulpicio G. Soriano, MD
Professor of Anesthesia
Harvard Medical School;
Endowed Chair in Pediatric Neuroanesthesia
Boston Children's Hospital
Boston, Massachusetts

Randolph H. Steadman, MD, MS
Chair
Department of Anesthesiology and Critical Care
Houston Methodist Hospital
Houston, Texas

Erica J. Stein, MD
Professor
Department of Anesthesiology
The Ohio State University
Columbus, Ohio

Marc P. Steurer, MD, MHA, DESA
Professor and Associate Chair of Finance
Department of Anesthesia and Perioperative Care
UCSF School of Medicine;
Associate Chief
Anesthesia and Perioperative Care
Zuckerberg San Francisco General Hospital;
San Francisco, California

Po-Yi Paul Su, MD
Assistant Professor
Department of Anesthesia and Perioperative Care
University of California, San Francisco
San Francisco, California

Kristina R. Sullivan, MD
Professor
Department of Anesthesia and Perioperative Care
University of California, San Francisco
San Francisco, California

Annemarie Thompson, MD
Professor
Anesthesiology and Medicine
Duke University
Durham, North Carolina

Chihiro Toda, MD
Staff Anesthesiologist
Department of General Anesthesiology
Cleveland Clinic
Cleveland, Ohio

Kevin K. Tremper, PhD, MD
Professor
Department of Anesthesiology
University of Michigan
Ann Arbor, Michigan

Avery Tung, MD
Professor
Department of Anesthesia and Critical Care
University of Chicago Medicine
Chicago, Illinois

Christine M. Warrick, MD
Assistant Professor
Department of Anesthesiology
University of Utah
Salt Lake City, Utah

Stephen D. Weston, MD
Associate Clinical Professor
Department of Anesthesia and Perioperative Care
University of California, San Francisco
San Francisco, California

Victor W. Xia, MD
Professor
Department of Anesthesiology
University of California, Los Angeles
Los Angeles, California

Edward N. Yap, MD
Senior Physician
Department of Anesthesia
The Permanente Medical Group, South San Francisco;
Assistant Professor
Department of Anesthesia and Perioperative Care
University of California, San Francisco
San Francisco, California

PREFACE

Basics of Anesthesia was first published in 1984 with the editorial leadership of Robert K. Stoelting and Ronald D. Miller. Their goal was to provide a concise source of information for the entire community of anesthesia learners, including students, residents, fellows, and other trainees. This eighth edition—the first without Dr. Miller as an editor—continues the pursuit of that goal while acknowledging how the specialty has evolved. The total number of chapters (49) is two fewer than the prior edition. Separate chapters on topics such as congenital heart disease and awareness were removed, but these subjects are now covered in other chapters. New chapters focus on clinician well-being, point-of-care ultrasound, perioperative medicine, and the environmental impact of anesthetics. The title "basics" belies the fact that chapters have more references than prior editions, consistent with the growth in knowledge and scholarly publications in the field.

This eighth edition is the first to be called *Miller's Basics of Anesthesia*, in recognition of Dr. Miller's leadership of the book throughout his career. It was an honor to collaborate with Dr. Miller on the sixth and seventh editions of this book, and I look forward to the challenge of maintaining its excellence as a learning resource.

I am thankful to the authors who contributed to this edition—an international group that includes over 35 new authors. My experience with the pandemic has only increased the gratitude I feel for all who contributed despite the impact on our personal and professional lives. Finally, I would like to acknowledge our publisher, Elsevier, and the dedication of their staff, including publisher Sarah Barth, senior content strategist Kayla Wolfe, senior content development specialist Ann Ruzycka Anderson, and senior project manager Beula Christopher—I appreciated our many Zoom calls to keep the book on track for publication.

Manuel C. Pardo, Jr.

FOREWORD

As an anesthesia resident at the University of California, San Francisco (UCSF), the first edition of *Basics of Anesthesia*, edited by Robert K. Stoelting and Ronald D. Miller, was my first textbook of anesthesia. My fellow residents and I used *Basics of Anesthesia* (which we fondly called "Baby Miller" or "Miller Light") as a concise source of foundational knowledge in our field, supplemented by more in-depth reading in the multivolume textbook *Anesthesia*, also edited by Dr. Miller.

Since then, under Dr. Miller's editorial leadership, both *Basics of Anesthesia* and *Anesthesia* have been regularly revised with the same goals. *Basics of Anesthesia* is oriented to the community of new anesthesia learners, while *Anesthesia's* intention is to be the most complete and thorough resource on the global scope and practice of contemporary anesthesiology.

In 2004, the sixth edition of *Anesthesia* was named *Miller's Anesthesia* in recognition of Dr. Miller's stewardship of the book. It is entirely fitting that this eighth edition of *Basics of Anesthesia* is now titled *Miller's Basics of Anesthesia*. Dr. Miller served as a coeditor for all seven prior editions—the first five with Dr. Stoelting and the last two with Dr. Manuel C. Pardo, Jr., who continues as the sole editor for this edition. The objective of *Miller's Basics of Anesthesia* remains the same: to provide updated and concise information for the entire anesthesia community. I encourage all learners of anesthesia to read and enjoy this book, including those new to the field as well as experienced clinicians who want to refresh and expand their knowledge of the specialty.

Michael A. Gropper, MD, PhD
Professor and Chair
Department of Anesthesia and
Perioperative Care
University of California, San Francisco
San Francisco, California

CONTENTS

Contents

INTRODUCTION

SCOPE OF ANESTHESIA PRACTICE

Manuel C. Pardo, Jr., Neal H. Cohen

ANESTHESIOLOGY AS A MULTIDISCIPLINARY SPECIALTY

PERIOPERATIVE PATIENT CARE

ANESTHESIA WORKFORCE

TRAINING AND CERTIFICATION IN ANESTHESIOLOGY

QUALITY AND SAFETY

VALUE-BASED CARE

FUTURE OF ANESTHESIA CARE

Surgery preceded the development of anesthesia as a medical specialty, with significant implications. Surgery has been performed for thousands of years. Archaeologists have discovered human skulls from prehistoric times with evidence of trephination, a surgical procedure involving drilling or scraping a hole in the skull to expose the brain. However, the brutality of surgery without anesthesia limited the types of surgery that could be performed and the disease processes that could be treated. Advances in surgery could only be accomplished as a result of improved ability to relieve pain during a procedure and manage the physiologic changes taking place both during surgery and thereafter. The first use of an anesthetic agent occurred in 1842 when the use of ether as a surgical anesthetic was administered by Crawford Long in Georgia. Although acknowledged as the first anesthetic administered to a human, it was not documented until Dr. Long published his experience in 1849. The first public demonstration of administration of ether anesthesia was provided by dentist William T.G. Morton at Massachusetts General Hospital on October 16, 1846. Since this initial administration of an inhaled anesthetic to reduce pain during a surgical procedure, the specialty of anesthesiology has advanced beyond the surgical suite to encompass the entire course of perioperative care in addition to associated subspecialties, including pain medicine, critical care medicine, palliative care, and sleep medicine.

ANESTHESIOLOGY AS A MULTIDISCIPLINARY SPECIALTY

Although anesthesia is understood to encompass administration of medications to facilitate surgical procedures, as the specialty has evolved, the scope of practice and expertise expected of an anesthesiologist have been formally defined by the American Board of Anesthesiology (ABA), a member of the American Board of Medical

---

Box 1.1 American Board of Anesthesiology Definition of Anesthesiology

The ABA defines anesthesiology as the practice of medicine dealing with but not limited to:

1. Assessment of, consultation for, and preparation of patients for anesthesia.
2. Relief and prevention of pain during and after surgical, obstetric, therapeutic, and diagnostic procedures.
3. Monitoring and maintenance of normal physiology during the perioperative or periprocedural period.
4. Management of critically ill patients.
5. Diagnosis and treatment of acute, chronic, and cancer-related pain.
6. Management of hospice and palliative care.
7. Clinical management and teaching of cardiac, pulmonary, and neurologic resuscitation.
8. Evaluation of respiratory function and application of respiratory therapy.
9. Conduct of clinical, translational, and basic science research.
10. Supervision, teaching, and evaluation of performance of both medical and allied health personnel involved in perioperative or periprocedural care, hospice and palliative care, critical care, and pain management.
11. Administrative involvement in health care facilities and organizations and medical schools as appropriate to our mission.

From Policy Book 2021. Raleigh: The American Board of Anesthesiology.

Specialties (ABMS) (Box 1.1). The ABA establishes and maintains criteria for board certification in anesthesiology and for subspecialty certification or special qualifications in the United States. Similar professional certification boards exist in many other countries. Currently, formal subspecialty certification is offered in anesthesiology and a number of subspecialties by the ABA, including critical care medicine (also see Chapter 41), pain medicine (also see Chapters 40 and 44), hospice and palliative medicine (also see Chapter 47), sleep medicine (also see Chapter 48), pediatric anesthesiology (also see Chapter 34), and neurocritical care (also see Chapter 30). Other ABMS boards also provide subspecialty qualifications in some of the same subspecialties, allowing providers to collaborate in the care of complex patients requiring specialized services.

The American Society of Anesthesiologists (ASA), founded in 1905 as the Long Island Society of Anesthetists, is the largest professional society for anesthesiologists. The ASA has over 100 committees and editorial boards dedicated to all anesthesia subspecialties and aspects of anesthesia practice. In addition to supporting the practice of anesthesiology and its subspecialties, the ASA advocates on behalf of anesthesiologists with other organizations, including Centers for Medicare & Medicaid Services (CMS), other medical specialties, hospital organizations, and payors. The International Anesthesia Research Society (IARS) and subspecialty societies also provide support for advancing clinical care and research in anesthesia and its subspecialties, reflecting the multidisciplinary growth of anesthesiology (Table 1.1).

PERIOPERATIVE PATIENT CARE

Although the specialty of anesthesiology began in the operating room, the scope of anesthesia practice has evolved as anesthesiologists and surgeons recognized that management of each patient before, during, and after surgery improved outcomes and quality of care. The preoperative evaluation of patients has become critical to the preparation for anesthesia and surgical management. For selected patients, perioperative management for those with underlying medical conditions has also improved outcomes and quality of care.[1] Similarly, postoperative assessment and management related to sequelae of anesthesia is an important component of perioperative care.

Based on this broader definition of anesthesia care, new drugs, monitoring capabilities, and documented improved outcomes in the surgical suite, anesthesia care has expanded to many locations within the health care system, including hospital-based locations, freestanding ambulatory care centers, and office practices (Table 1.2). Several other factors are contributing to the evolution of anesthesiology practice, including the advances in anesthesia care allowing patients with significant comorbidities to undergo complex procedures; the extremes of age of the surgical patient, including the expanding elderly population (also see Chapter 35); increasing importance of quality, safety, and value of health care delivery (also see Chapter 46); changing composition and expectations of the anesthesia workforce; increasing fragmentation of perioperative care with multiple handoffs and transitions of care; and changing payment methods for physicians that increasingly emphasize value-based approaches.[2]

In addition to the factors that affect the clinical practice of anesthesiology, anesthesiologists have assumed broader roles in health system leadership, including perioperative medical directors, chief quality officers, and other administrative and leadership positions related to both perioperative care and broader health system management.[3]

ANESTHESIA WORKFORCE

Anesthesia care is provided by physician anesthesiologists and other providers with various levels of training both in the United States and throughout the world. In the United States the anesthesia workforce includes physician anesthesiologists, certified registered nurse anesthetists (CRNAs), and anesthesia assistants (AAs). Although each state has different

Table 1.1	Selected Anesthesiology Professional Societies	
Society	**Year Founded**	**Mission**
American Society of Anesthesiologists (ASA)	1905	Advancing the practice and securing the future. Strategic pillars include advocacy, educational resources, leadership and professional development, member engagement, quality and practice advancement, research, and scientific discovery.
International Anesthesia Research Society (IARS)	1922	To encourage, stimulate, and fund ongoing anesthesia-related research projects that will enhance and advance the specialty and to disseminate current, state-of-the-art, basic, and clinical research data in all areas of clinical anesthesia, including perioperative medicine, critical care, and pain management.
World Federation of Societies of Anaesthesiologists (WFSA)	1955	To unite anesthesiologists around the world to improve patient care and access to safe anesthesia and perioperative medicine.
Society for Obstetric Anesthesia and Perinatology (SOAP)	1968	To advance and advocate for the health of pregnant women and their babies through research, education, and best practices in obstetric anesthesia care.
Society for Neuroscience in Anesthesiology and Critical Care (SNACC)	1973	Organization dedicated to the neurologically impaired patient.
International Association for the Study of Pain (IASP)	1974	IASP brings together scientists, clinicians, health care providers, and policy makers to stimulate and support the study of pain and to translate that knowledge into improved pain relief worldwide.
American Society of Regional Anesthesia (ASRA)	1975	To advance the science and practice of regional anesthesia and pain medicine to improve patient outcomes through research, education, and advocacy.
Society for Education in Anesthesia (SEA)	1985	Support, enrich, and advance anesthesia education and those who teach.
Society for Ambulatory Anesthesia (SAMBA)	1985	To be the resource for providers who practice in settings outside of hospital-based operating rooms.
Society for Pediatric Anesthesia (SPA)	1986	SPA advances the safety and quality of anesthesia care, perioperative care, and pain management in children by educating clinicians; supporting research; and fostering collaboration among clinicians, patient families, and professional organizations worldwide.
Society of Critical Care Anesthesiologists (SOCCA)	1987	Dedicated to the support and development of anesthesiologists who care for critically ill patients of all types.
Society for Technology in Anesthesia (STA)	1988	To improve the quality of patient care by improving technology and its application.
Society of Cardiovascular Anesthesiologists (SCA)	1989	International organization of physicians that promotes excellence in patient care through education and research in perioperative care for patients undergoing cardiothoracic and vascular procedures.
International Society for Anaesthetic Pharmacology (ISAP)	1990	Dedicated to teaching and research about clinical pharmacology in anesthesia, with particular reference to anesthetic drugs.
Society for Airway Management (SAM)	1995	Dedicated to the practice, teaching, and scientific advancements of the field of airway management.
Society of Anesthesia and Sleep Medicine (SASM)	2011	To advance standards of care for clinical problems shared by anesthesiology and sleep medicine, including perioperative management of sleep-disordered breathing, and to promote interdisciplinary communication, education, and research in matters common to anesthesia and sleep.
Trauma Anesthesiology Society	2014	To advance the art and science of trauma anesthesiology and all related fields through education and research.

| **Table 1.2** | Locations of Anesthesia Care |

Hospital					Outpatient		
Operating Room	Nonoperating Room Location	Preoperative Unit Regional Anesthesia Service Postanesthesia Care Unit	Intensive Care Unit	Hospital Ward - Acute Pain Service - Perioperative Medicine Service - Palliative Care Service - POCUS Service (including TEE/TTE)	Ambulatory Surgery Center	Preoperative Evaluation Clinic	Pain Medicine Clinic

POCUS, Point-of-care ultrasound; *TEE*, transesophageal echocardiography; *TTE*, transthoracic echocardiography.

requirements for delivery of care, scope of practice, and supervision, and some states have allowed CRNAs independent practice, most states currently require nonphysician anesthesia providers to be supervised by a physician. Those states that license AAs require that they be directly supervised by a physician. Dental anesthesia is provided by a physician anesthesiologist or a dentist who has received specialty training in anesthesia care. A 2017 global survey reported that the United States had 67,000 physician anesthesiologists, 49,000 nurse anesthesia providers, and 1960 nonphysician/nonnurse providers.[4]

The "care team" model that includes CRNAs and physician anesthesiologists is the most common practice model in most states. For most U.S. anesthesia groups, the working relationship between physician anesthesiologists and CRNAs is highly collaborative, benefiting patients by providing a coordinated approach to clinical management and immediate availability of a provider with the skills and background required to address emergencies or unforeseen clinical problems. In other countries anesthesia care is provided in a variety of different models. For most European and Asian countries, anesthesia services are provided exclusively by physician anesthesiologists or other physicians with additional training in anesthesiology. In other countries with limited numbers of physicians to provide all aspects of clinical management, alternative models are required to meet the clinical needs of the surgical patient populations. In some cases, depending on clinical needs and regulatory issues, other providers—often with limited formal educational experiences—deliver anesthesia services.

As a result of the expansion of surgical services and need for anesthesia care in nonoperating room environments, the breadth of anesthesia services has expanded dramatically over the past decade. Each of the surgical subspecialties prefers having a dedicated pool of subspecialty trained anesthesiologists; at the same time, the roles for other anesthesia subspecialists in critical care, pain medicine, preoperative management programs, and palliative care and sleep medicine have created significant workforce challenges. Despite the increasing need for anesthesia providers, the United States has had only a modest growth in the number of anesthesia providers; the demand for anesthesia services far exceeds the current supply. The Association of American Medical Colleges (AAMC) commissions annual reports to project future supply and demand for U.S. physicians. A 2021 AAMC report predicts that by 2034 the demand for physicians in the "Other Specialties" category, which includes anesthesiologists and seven other specialties, will exceed supply by 10,300 to 35,600, even with growth in advanced practice providers.[5] The main drivers of the increased physician demand include both population growth (approximately 10% growth during this time) and aging of the population (proportion of the population aged 65 or older is estimated to grow by 42%). CRNA programs have expanded to address the increasing need; in states that license AA programs these programs have also had increasing enrollment. Despite the increase in nonphysician anesthesia providers, the number of providers is not keeping pace with the increasing clinical demands.

The models of anesthesia practice have also changed considerably, as has the relationship with health systems and anesthesia practices.[2] Many community practices have consolidated, often through acquisition into regional and national anesthesia or multispecialty groups. In some parts of the country physicians, including anesthesiologists, have become employees of medical foundations or are directly employed by hospitals. Most academic practices are managed within the academic departments with varying financial models for managing both professional and technical fees with the academic health system. Although the primary motivation for some of these new business models is financial, the most critical value to the integrated models of care is the ability of the physicians, anesthesiologists and their medical colleagues, and the health systems to optimize clinical care, reduce complications, and more effectively manage resources. In addition, payors, including Medicare and private payors, are transitioning to "value-based" care, so this collaboration has been critical.

TRAINING AND CERTIFICATION IN ANESTHESIOLOGY

Training of anesthesia providers is based on background education, clinical knowledge and experience, and scope of practice. As a result, the training of anesthesia providers in the United States differs for physician anesthesiologists, CRNAs, and certified anesthesiologist assistants (CAAs).

For U.S. physician anesthesiologists, training in anesthesiology consists of 4 years of supervised experience in an approved program after the degree of Doctor of Medicine or Doctor of Osteopathy has been obtained. The first year of postgraduate training consists of education in the fundamental clinical skills of medicine. The second, third, and fourth postgraduate years (clinical anesthesia years 1 to 3) are spent learning about all aspects of clinical anesthesia, including subspecialty experience in obstetric anesthesia, pediatric anesthesia, cardiothoracic anesthesia, neuroanesthesia, preoperative medicine, postanesthesia care, regional anesthesia, and pain management. In addition to these subspecialty experiences, 4 months of training in critical care medicine is required as part of this core curriculum. The ABA is responsible for initial certification after completion of a training program accredited by the Accreditation Council for Graduate Medical Education (ACGME), in addition to subspecialty certification and maintenance of certification. The duration and structure of anesthesiology education differ in other countries, although most countries require 4 years or more of training in anesthesia care, often including critical care medicine within the core curriculum.[4]

The admission requirements for training as a CRNA include a bachelor's degree, registration as a professional nurse in the United States or its territories, and at least 1 year of full-time equivalent experience as a critical care registered nurse. Nurse anesthesia programs are accredited by the Council on Accreditation of Nurse Anesthesia Educational Programs (COA). All accredited nurse anesthesia programs offered master's-level

education by late 1998; by 2022 all programs must offer doctoral degrees.[6] The minimum duration of a master's-level program is 24 months of full-time study (or its part-time equivalent), whereas the curriculum for a practice-oriented doctoral degree is typically a minimum of 36 months of full-time study. After completion of an accredited program, a CRNA is eligible to take the National Certification Examination of the National Board of Certification and Recertification for Nurse Anesthetists.

AA education programs require that students have a bachelor's degree and premedical course work. After receiving 27 months of master's degree–level education in an accredited program, they are eligible for the Certifying Examination for Anesthesiologist Assistants, administered by the National Commission for Certification of Anesthesiologist Assistants (NCCAA) in collaboration with the National Board of Medical Examiners (NBME). CAAs must practice under the supervision of a physician anesthesiologist as part of the anesthesia care team model. Currently, CAAs may practice in 18 U.S. jurisdictions.

QUALITY AND SAFETY

For many years, clinical anesthesia practice has been recognized as a model for quality and safety in medicine. The 1999 Institute of Medicine (now the National Academy of Medicine) report, "To Err Is Human," specifically identified anesthesia as "an area in which very impressive improvements in safety have been made."[7] The ASA has been a leader within organized medicine in the development and implementation of formal, published standards of practice. ASA standards, practice guidelines, practice advisories, and alerts have significantly influenced how anesthesia is practiced in the United States.[8] Anesthesiologists have also formed patient safety–focused societies, such as the Anesthesia Patient Safety Foundation (APSF), an independent nonprofit corporation begun in 1985 with the vision "that no patient shall be harmed by anesthesia." The APSF is supported by the ASA and corporate sponsors, with members that include physician anesthesiologists, nurse anesthetists, manufacturers of equipment and drugs, engineers, and insurers. The APSF Newsletter is dedicated solely to safety and has become one of the most widely circulated anesthesia publications in the world.[9] The APSF has highlighted diverse issues such as anesthesia machine checkout, opioid-induced respiratory depression, residual neuromuscular blockade, postoperative visual loss, emergency manual use, and COVID-19 airway management. In 2018 the APSF board of directors generated a list of the top perioperative patient safety priorities; these priorities are reviewed on an annual basis. The 2021 top patient safety priorities are listed in Box 1.2. Although these

---

Box 1.2 APSF 2021 Perioperative Patient Safety Priorities

1. Culture of safety, inclusion, and diversity
2. Teamwork, collegial communication, and multidisciplinary collaboration
3. Preventing, detecting, and determining pathogenesis and mitigating clinical deterioration in the perioperative period
4. Safety in nonoperating room locations such as endoscopy, cardiac catheterization, and interventional radiology suites
5. Perioperative delirium, cognitive dysfunction, and brain health
6. Prevention and mitigation of opioid-related harm in surgical patients
7. Medication safety
8. Emerging infectious diseases (including but not limited to COVID-19), including patient management, guideline development, equipment modification, and determination of operative risk
9. Clinician safety: occupational health and wellness
10. Airway management difficulties, skills, and equipment

APSF, Anesthesia Patient Safety Foundation.
From APSF Newsletter. 2021;36(2):53.

---

advances in patient safety are significant, clinical challenges and complications still occur. Anesthesiology practices must maintain robust quality assessment and improvement programs to continue the leadership role of the specialty in advancing patient care. Many of the advances in perioperative care made by anesthesiologists have emphasized outcomes during a surgical procedure to reduce intraoperative adverse events. To continue to improve patient safety and quality of care will require more focused assessment of the entire perioperative period, including identifying postoperative outcomes for which anesthesia management might have contributed and developing strategies to minimize the likelihood of these adverse events prospectively, including the potential need for readmission.

VALUE-BASED CARE

U.S. health care spending continues to grow, reaching $4.1 trillion in 2020, approximately $12,530 per person, this represents 19.7% of the gross domestic product.[10] The high cost of health care has been challenging for clinicians and health systems to manage. As a result of the increasing costs of care, often without evidence of improved outcome, government (Medicare and Medicaid) and private insurance companies have implemented various types of alternative payment models (APMs) designed to incentivize "value." For these payment models, value is defined as outcome (or quality) divided by cost. A more complete description of quality includes six domains

identified by the Institute of Medicine: safety, efficacy, patient-centered, timely, efficient, and equitable.[11] Table 1.3 lists some drivers of value-based health care.[12] In a value-based payment model services are compensated based on improved patient health outcomes rather than specific services provided.

The value-based payment models, particularly for perioperative surgical services, have significant implications for anesthesia practices. A variety of approaches have been used to improve quality and value and create opportunities for providers to benefit from efforts to optimize care and reduce costs. Medicare has implemented the Merit-Based Incentive Payment System (MIPS) requiring anesthesia practices to report quality measures as part of the Quality Payment Program (QPP) from which payments will be adjusted based on performance. Although the MIPS program continues to be refined, the transition to a payment model for anesthesia services that is at least partly based on quality metrics will continue to have financial impact on anesthesia practices.

In addition to the MIPS program and other merit-based payment models, APMs that provide payment to all providers and a health system for a course of care are transforming how care is provided and requiring those participating in care to document their value. For anesthesia practices, the APMs have significant implications and provide opportunities for practices to assume a greater role in perioperative care, to manage costs, and to improve quality, all of which can allow the practices to receive financial benefit based on the value provided. Most important, the APMs represent a significant opportunity to expand the scope of practice across the continuum of the perioperative period to optimize management, reduce costs, and improve patient safety. Some examples in which anesthesia providers have transformed their practice to benefit patients and the health systems include participation in the Perioperative Surgical Home (PSH)[13] and leadership roles in the implementation of Enhanced Recovery After Surgery (ERAS) protocols designed to optimize perioperative care, reduce complications, costs, and lengths of stay.[14] As a result of these efforts, the role for anesthesiologists expanded and provided opportunities to work collaboratively with a more diverse group of providers and health system leaders to improve care for patients beyond the specific needs of the surgical patient population.[3]

Many anesthesia groups are adapting their practices to these new models of care and payment; however, the transition is challenging. The emphasis on value represents an opportunity for anesthesiologists to redefine their role and the scope of anesthesia practice. To do so will require that they develop new skills related to quality, safety, and management beyond what was a part of the core curriculum of anesthesia training.

Table 1.3 Drivers of Value-Based Health Care

Program	Description	Cost Savings	Advantages	Disadvantages
Centers of Excellence	Multidisciplinary, comprehensive program for patient care in a highly focused area (e.g., orthopedics, bariatric surgery).	Standardized approach to equipment; reduction in complications, readmissions, and discharge to facility.	Potentially improved patient outcomes and financial performance.	May lead to decreased access to care. Some studies indicate no improvement in care.
Accountable Care Organizations	Group of physicians, hospitals, and other health care providers joining together to coordinate care among Medicare patients.	Health care teams meet specific quality benchmarks, increasing efficiency of care and reducing costs.	Streamlined communication, reduced medical errors, and reduced duplication of services and cost of care.	May not demonstrate mortality reduction in surgical patients.
Insurance specialty programs (e.g., bundled payments, shared cost savings, population-based payments, merit-based incentive payment)	Engages physicians and health care systems to coordinate care and reduce cost. Fosters competition among providers to create value. Hospital administration negotiates with department chairs or practice managers for reimbursement, including anesthesiology/perioperative medicine.	Hospital retains more money from bundle if there is a reduction in complications, readmissions, or discharge to facility.	Total allowable expenditures for an episode of care are predetermined. Merit-based incentive payments tie payment to quality, cost, and use of health care information.	May penalize physicians caring for the sickest patients. May not really improve quality or cost.

Adapted from Table 1 in Mahajan A, Esper SA, Cole DJ, et al. Anesthesiologists' role in value-based perioperative care and healthcare transformation. Anesthesiology. 2021;134(4):526–540.

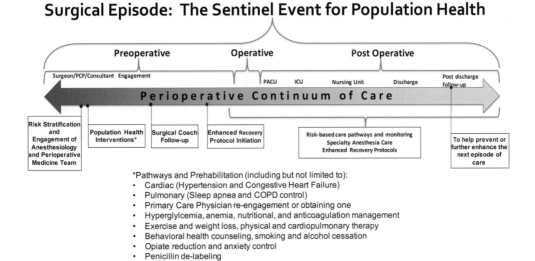

Fig. 1.1 An approach to coordinated perioperative patient care with targeted population health interventions and risk-based care pathways designed to improve patient outcomes.
(From Mahajan A, Esper SA, Cole DJ, et al. Anesthesiologists' role in value-based perioperative care and healthcare transformation. *Anesthesiology*. 2021;134[4]:526–540, Fig. 4.)

Residency programs are refining the curriculum to meet these new needs. Practicing anesthesiologists are also acquiring these additional skills needed to succeed in this new model of care and payment. Fig. 1.1 describes an approach to proactively improving population health in the perioperative setting.[12]

FUTURE OF ANESTHESIA CARE

Anesthesiology is a vibrant and exciting specialty that has undergone dramatic changes over the past few decades. Advances in clinical management and new drugs and technologies have transformed clinical practice and significantly improved patient outcomes. New models of care, including the PSH, and an expanded scope of practice represent major advances for the specialty. At the same time, anesthesia practices must continue to evolve, to reassess traditional approaches to clinical care and identify opportunities to improve quality and safety across the entire continuum of care. Many have taken a broader role in the health care system in order to continue to improve value for the populations served, implement patient-centered care, and manage the financial burdens confronting the health care system.

Anesthesiologists, along with their colleagues, must also contribute to efforts to improve access and address health disparities faced by those of low socioeconomic status and for racial and ethnic minorities. Although health care is undergoing significant change and new models of care will continue to evolve, for learners just entering the field of anesthesiology, the opportunities are exciting and diverse and provide the foundation for a rewarding career.

ACKNOWLEDGMENT

The editors and publisher would like to thank Dr Ronald D. Miller for contributing to this chapter in the previous edition of this work. It has served as a foundation for the current chapter.

REFERENCES

1. Carli F, Awasthi R, Gillis C, et al. Integrating prehabilitation in the Ppreoperative clinic: A paradigm shift in perioperative care. *Anesth Analg.* 2021 May 1;132(5):1494–1500. doi:10.1213/ANE.0000000000005471 PMID: 33724962.

2. Prielipp RC, Cohen NH. The future of anesthesiology: Implications of the changing healthcare environment. *Curr Opin Anaesthesiol.* 2016 Apr;29(2):198–205. doi:10.1097/ACO.0000000000000301 PMID: 26705129.

3. Mathis MR, Schonberger RB, Whitlock EL, et al. Opportunities beyond the anesthesiology department: Broader impact through broader thinking. *Anesth Analg.* 2021 Mar 8:10.1213/ANE.0000000000005428. doi:10.1213/ANE.0000000000005428 Epub ahead of print PMID: 33684091; PMCID: PMC8423864.

4. Kempthorne P, Morriss WW, Mellin-Olsen J, Gore-Booth J. The WFSA Global Anesthesia Workforce Survey. *Anesth Analg.* 2017 Sep;125(3):981–990. doi:10.1213/ANE.0000000000002258 PMID: 28753173.

5. IHS Markit Ltd. *The Complexities of Physician Supply and Demand: Projections From 2019 to 2034.* Washington, DC: AAMC; 2021.

6. Council on Accreditation of Nurse Anesthesia Educational Programs. Accreditation Standards, Policies and Procedures, and Guidelines. https://www.coacrna.org/accreditation/accreditation-standards-policies-and-procedures-and-guidelines/ Accessed January 6, 2022.

7. Institute of Medicine (US) Committee on Quality of Health Care in America. To Err is Human: Building a Safer Health System. Kohn LT, Corrigan JM, Donaldson MS, editors. Washington (DC): National Academies Press (US); 2000. PMID: 25077248.

8. American Society of Anesthesiologists Guidelines, Statements, Clinical Resources. https://www.asahq.org/standards-and-guidelines Accessed January 8, 2022.

9. APSF Newsletter. https://www.apsf.org/apsf-newsletter/ Accessed January 8, 2022.

10. Centers for Medicare and Medicaid Services. National Health Expenditure Data. https://www.cms.gov/Research-Statistics-Data-and-Systems/Statistics-Trends-and-Reports/NationalHealthExpendData/NationalHealthAccountsHistorical Accessed January 9, 2022.

11. Institute of Medicine (US) Committee on Quality of Health Care in America. *Crossing the Quality Chasm: A New Health System for the 21st Century.* Washington (DC): National Academies Press (US); 2001 PMID: 25057539.

12. Mahajan A, Esper SA, Cole DJ, Fleisher LA. Anesthesiologists' Role in Value-based Perioperative Care and Healthcare Transformation. *Anesthesiology.* 2021 Apr 1;134(4):526–540. doi:10.1097/ALN.0000000000003717 PMID: 33630039.

13. Vetter TR. Perioperative Surgical Home Models. *Anesthesiol Clin.* 2018 Dec;36(4):677–687. doi:10.1016/j.anclin.2018.07.015 Epub 2018 Oct 12. PMID: 30390787.

14. Ljungqvist O, Scott M, Fearon KC. Enhanced Recovery After Surgery: A Review. *JAMA Surg.* 2017 Mar 1;152(3):292–298. doi:10.1001/jamasurg.2016.4952 PMID: 28097305.

2 LEARNING ANESTHESIA

Kristina R. Sullivan, Manuel C. Pardo, Jr.

The challenges of learning perioperative anesthesia care have grown considerably as the specialty has evolved. The beginning anesthesia trainee is faced with an ever-increasing quantity of literature and the need for increased knowledge and adequate patient care experiences. Healthcare systems increasingly focus on improving the patient experience of care (including quality and satisfaction), improving population health, reducing the cost of healthcare,[1] and improving environmental sustainability.[2]

Most training programs begin with close clinical supervision by an attending anesthesiologist. More experienced trainees may also offer their perspectives, coaching, and practical advice to junior trainees. Programs use a variety of teaching modalities to facilitate learning, including problem-based learning, various forms of e-learning, hands-on task training, mannequin-based patient simulation, and standardized patient sessions.[3] The practice of anesthesia involves the development of flexible patient care routines, factual and theoretical knowledge, manual and procedural skills, and the mental abilities to adapt to changing situations.[4]

COMPETENCIES, MILESTONES, AND ENTRUSTABLE PROFESSIONAL ACTIVITIES

Physician anesthesiologists must attain a broad fund of knowledge and skills. Over the past few decades, the Accreditation Council for Graduate Medical Education (ACGME) has carefully considered how to ensure physician competence. In the late 1990s it launched the Outcome Project, which includes a focus on six core competencies: patient care, medical knowledge, professionalism, interpersonal and communication skills, systems-based practice, and practice-based learning and improvement. The ACGME then advanced the core competencies approach by adopting the Dreyfus model of skill acquisition to create a framework of "milestones." Milestones specific to anesthesiology, published in 2014, defined the development

Table 2.1 Example of Anesthesia Resident Milestones: Patient Care Competency, Perioperative Care, and Management

Level 1	Level 2	Level 3	Level 4	Level 5
Identifies the components of an anesthetic plan	Develops an anesthetic plan for a healthy patient undergoing uncomplicated procedures	Develops an anesthetic plan for patients with well-controlled comorbidities or undergoing complicated procedures	Develops an anesthetic plan for patients with multiple, uncontrolled comorbidities and undergoing complicated procedures	
Identifies the components of a pain management plan	Implements simple perioperative pain management plan	Identifies patients with a history of chronic pain who require a modified perioperative pain management plan	Implements the anesthetic plan for patients with complex pain history and polypharmacy	In collaboration with other specialists, develops protocols for multimodal analgesia plan for patients with a complex pain history and substance use disorder
Identifies potential impact of anesthesia beyond intraoperative period	Identifies patient-specific risks factors for long-term anesthetic effects	Develops the anesthetic plan based on risk factors to mitigate the long-term impact of anesthesia	Implements the anesthetic plan to mitigate the long-term impact of anesthesia	Develops departmental or institutional protocols for reduction of the long-term impact of anesthesia

Milestones are arranged into levels from 1 to 5. These levels do not correspond with postgraduate year of education. Level 4 is designed as a graduation goal (but not a graduation requirement).
From Anesthesiology Milestones 2.0. Accreditation Council for Graduate Medical Education (ACGME), 2020. Available at https://www.acgme.org/globalassets/PDFs/Milestones/AnesthesiologyMilestones2.0.pdf. Accessed December 17, 2021.

of anesthesia residents during 4 years of training.[5] These milestones were updated in 2020 to account for advancements in the field of anesthesiology.[6] For example, an entire milestone devoted to point-of-care ultrasound was added in the 2020 revisions. Table 2.1 shows an example of a milestone in the patient care competency. The milestones incorporate several aspects of residency training, including a description of expected behavior, the complexity of the patient and the surgical procedure, and the level of supervision needed by the resident.

Over the last decade, Entrustable Professional Activities (EPAs) have gained traction as a tool to advance competency-based assessment.[7,8] EPAs are defined as tasks or responsibilities that trainees are entrusted to perform without supervision once relevant competencies are attained.[7,9] An EPA, or task, can be mapped to multiple milestones and competencies and thus provide a framework for assessment. Entrustment decisions by supervisors are documented along a continuum (Box 2.1). Feedback related to these decisions can help trainees form individualized learning plans that will help inform future goals.

> **Box 2.1** Example of Entrustable Professional Activity (EPA) in Anesthesiology
>
> *Task:* Induction of anesthesia for a fasted ASA 1/2 patient without a known difficult airway
> *Competencies involved:* medical knowledge, patient care, interpersonal and communication skills
> *Milestones addressed:* perioperative care and management, application and interpretation of monitors, intraoperative care, airway management
> *Entrustment decisions by supervisors:* observed, performed under supervision, performed independently

ASA, American Society of Anesthesiologists.

(Box 2.2). Important patient care decisions involve assessing the preoperative evaluation; creating the anesthesia plan; preparing the operating room; and managing the intraoperative anesthetic, postoperative care, and outcome. An understanding of this framework will facilitate the learning process.

STRUCTURED APPROACH TO ANESTHESIA CARE

Anesthesia providers care for the surgical patient in the preoperative, intraoperative, and postoperative periods

Preoperative Evaluation

The goals of preoperative evaluation include assessing the risk of coexisting diseases, modifying risks, addressing patients' concerns, and discussing options for anesthesia care (see Chapters 13 and 14). The beginning

Table 2.2 Questions to Consider in Preoperative Evaluation

Question	Anesthetic Considerations
What is the indication for the proposed surgery?	The indication for surgery may have anesthetic implications. For example, a patient requiring esophageal fundoplication will likely have severe gastroesophageal reflux disease, which may require modification of the anesthesia plan (e.g., preoperative nonparticulate antacid, intraoperative rapid-sequence induction of anesthesia).
What is the proposed surgery?	A given procedure may have implications for anesthetic choice. Anesthesia for hand surgery, for example, can be accomplished with local anesthesia, peripheral nerve blockade, general anesthesia, or sometimes a combination of techniques.
Is the procedure elective, urgent, or an emergency?	The urgency of a given procedure (e.g., acute appendicitis) may preclude lengthy delay of the surgery for additional testing, without increasing the risk of complications (e.g., appendiceal rupture, peritonitis). Surgical procedures related to a cancer diagnosis may also present a degree of urgency depending on the risk of metastasis.
What are the inherent risks of this surgery?	Surgical procedures have different inherent risks. For example, a patient undergoing coronary artery bypass graft has a significant risk of problems such as death, stroke, or myocardial infarction. A patient undergoing cataract extraction is unlikely to sustain perioperative morbidity.
Does the patient have coexisting medical conditions? Does the surgery or anesthesia care plan need to be modified because of them?	The anesthesia provider must understand the physiologic effects of the surgery and anesthetic and the potential interaction with the medical condition. For example, a patient with poorly controlled systemic hypertension is more likely to have an exaggerated hypertensive response to direct laryngoscopy. The anesthetic plan may be modified to increase the induction dose of intravenously administered anesthetic (e.g., propofol) and administer a short-acting beta-adrenergic blocker (e.g., esmolol) before instrumentation of the airway.
Has the patient had anesthesia before? Were there complications such as difficult airway management? Does the patient have risk factors for difficult airway management?	Anesthesia records from previous surgery can yield much useful information. The most important fact is the ease of airway management techniques such as direct laryngoscopy. If physical examination reveals some risk factors for difficult tracheal intubation but the patient had a clearly documented uncomplicated direct laryngoscopy for recent surgery, the anesthesia provider may choose to proceed with routine laryngoscopy. Other useful historical information includes intraoperative hemodynamic and respiratory instability and occurrence of postoperative nausea.

trainee should learn the types of questions that are the most important to understanding the patient and the proposed surgery (Table 2.2).

Box 2.2 Phases of Anesthesia Care

Preoperative Phase
Preoperative evaluation
Choice of anesthesia
Premedication

Intraoperative Phase
Physiologic monitoring and vascular access
General anesthesia (i.e., plan for induction, maintenance, and emergence)
Regional anesthesia (i.e., plan for type of block, needle, local anesthetic)

Postoperative Phase
Postoperative pain control method
Special monitoring or treatment based on surgery or anesthetic course
Disposition (e.g., home, postanesthesia care unit, ward, monitored ward, step-down unit, intensive care unit)
Follow-up (anesthesia complications, patient outcome)

Creating the Anesthesia Plan

After the preoperative evaluation, the anesthesia plan can be completed. The plan should list drug choices and doses in detail, in addition to anticipated problems (Boxes 2.3 and 2.4). Many alternatives to a given plan may be acceptable, but the trainee and the supervising anesthesia provider should agree in advance on the details.

Preparing the Operating Room

After determining the anesthesia plan, the trainee must prepare the operating room. Routine operating room preparation includes tasks such as checking the anesthesia workstation (see Chapter 15). The specific anesthesia plan may have implications for preparing additional equipment. For example, fiber-optic tracheal intubation requires special equipment that may be kept in a cart dedicated to difficult airway management.

Managing the Intraoperative Anesthetic

Intraoperative anesthesia management generally follows the anesthesia plan but should be adjusted based

---

Box 2.3   Sample General Anesthesia Plan

Case
A 47-year-old, 75-kg female with biliary colic and well-controlled asthma requires anesthesia for laparoscopic cholecystectomy.

Preoperative Phase
Premedication:
Midazolam 1–2 mg intravenous (IV) to reduce anxiety
Albuterol, two puffs, to prevent bronchospasm

Intraoperative Phase
Vascular Access and Monitoring
Vascular access: one peripheral IV catheter
Monitors: pulse oximetry, capnography, electrocardiogram, noninvasive blood pressure with standard adult cuff size, temperature

Induction
Propofol 2 mg/kg (150 mg) IV (preceded by lidocaine 60 mg IV to reduce propofol injection pain)
Neuromuscular blocking drug to facilitate tracheal intubation: rocuronium 0.6 mg/kg (50 mg) IV
Airway management
Facemask: adult medium size
Direct laryngoscopy: Macintosh 3 blade, 7.0-mm internal diameter (ID) endotracheal tube

Maintenance
Inhaled anesthetic: sevoflurane

Opioid: fentanyl, anticipate 2–4 µg/kg IV total during procedure
Neuromuscular blocking drug titrated to train-of-four monitor (peripheral nerve stimulator) at the ulnar nerve

Emergence
Antagonize effects of nondepolarizing neuromuscular blocking drug: sugammadex 2–4 mg/kg based on train-of-four monitoring
Antiemetic: dexamethasone 4 mg IV at start of procedure; ondansetron 4 mg IV at end of procedure
Tracheal extubation: when patient is awake, breathing, and following commands
Possible intraoperative problem and approach: bronchospasm: increase inspired oxygen and inhaled anesthetic concentrations, decrease surgical stimulation if possible, administer albuterol through endotracheal tube (5–10 puffs), adjust ventilator to maximize expiratory flow

Postoperative Phase
Postanesthesia care unit (PACU) orders to include fentanyl IV prn for postoperative analgesia, in addition to oxycodone 5 mg PO before PACU discharge; prn antiemetics include prochlorperazine, because antiemetics of two different drug classes were administered intraoperatively
Disposition: PACU, then hospital ward once PACU discharge criteria are met

---

Box 2.4   Sample Regional Anesthesia Plan

Case
A 27-year-old, 80-kg male requires diagnostic right shoulder arthroscopy for chronic pain. He has no known medical problems.

Preoperative Phase
Premedication: midazolam 1–2 mg intravenous (IV) to reduce anxiety
Nerve block placed in preoperative area with electrocardiogram (ECG), blood pressure, and pulse oximetry monitoring
Type of block: interscalene
Needle: 22-gauge short-bevel, 5 cm long, echogenic
Local anesthetic: 0.5% ropivacaine, 20 mL
Ancillary equipment: ultrasound machine with linear transducer, sterile sheath, ultrasound gel
Technique: chlorhexidine skin preparation, localize nerve in

posterior triangle of neck, use ultrasound to guide in-plane needle insertion, inject local anesthetic
Precautions: because of the risk of local anesthetic systemic toxicity (LAST), the location of 20% intralipid is confirmed before block placement

Intraoperative Phase
Intraoperative sedation and analgesia:
Midazolam 0.5–1 mg IV given every 5–10 minutes as indicated
Fentanyl 25–50 µg IV given every 5–10 minutes as indicated

Postoperative Phase
Postanesthesia care unit (PACU) orders will include prn IV fentanyl for analgesia, but will most likely not be required because of the long-acting local anesthetic used for the nerve block
Disposition: PACU, then home once PACU discharge criteria are met

---

on the patient's responses to anesthesia and surgery. The anesthesia provider must evaluate several different information pathways from which a decision on whether to change the patient's management can be made. The trainee must learn to process these different information sources and attend to multiple tasks simultaneously. The general cycle of mental activity involves observation, decision making, action, and repeat evaluation[10]

(Fig. 2.1). Vigilance, being watchful and alert, is necessary for safe patient care, but vigilance alone is not enough. The anesthesia provider must weigh the significance of each observation and can become overwhelmed by the amount of information or by rapidly changing information. Intraoperative clinical events can stimulate thinking and promote an interactive discussion between the trainee and supervisor (Table 2.3).

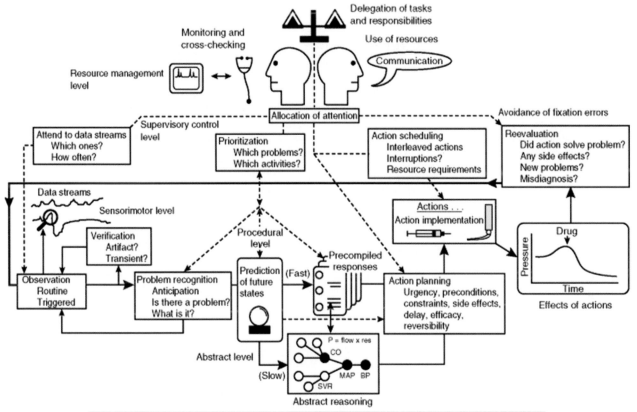

Fig. 2.1 Model of the anesthesia professional's complex process of intraoperative decision making. There is a primary loop (*heavy black arrows*) of observation, decision, action, and reevaluation. This loop is controlled by higher levels of supervisory control (allocation of attention) and resource management. *BP*, Blood pressure; *CO*, cardiac output; *MAP*, mean arterial pressure; *P*, pressure; *res*, resistance; *SVR*, systemic vascular resistance. (From Gaba DM, Fish KJ, Howard SK, et al. Crisis Management in Anesthesiology, 2nd ed. Philadelphia: Saunders; 2014, Figure 1.4.)

Patient Follow-up

The patient should be reassessed after recovery from anesthesia. This follow-up includes assessing general satisfaction with the anesthetic; postoperative pain; and a review for complications such as dental injury, nausea, nerve injury, and intraoperative recall.

LEARNING STRATEGIES

Learning during supervised direct patient care is the foundation of clinical training. Because the scope of anesthesia practice is so broad (see Chapter 1) and the competencies trainees are required to master are diverse, direct patient care cannot be the only component of the teaching program. Other modalities include independent reading, in-person or synchronous virtual lectures or small-group discussions, simulations, and various forms of e-learning.[3] Independent reading should include basic textbooks and selected portions of comprehensive textbooks in addition to anesthesia specialty journals and general medical journals. In-person or synchronous virtual lectures can be efficient methods for transmitting large amounts of information. However, the large group lecture format is not conducive to audience interaction. In-person or synchronous virtual group discussions are most effective when they are small (fewer than 12 participants) and interactive. Journal clubs, quality assurance conferences, and problem-based case discussions lend themselves to this format.

A teaching method termed *the flipped classroom* can combine aspects of asynchronous e-learning and in-person or synchronous group discussions.[11] One popular approach to the flipped classroom involves the use of an asynchronous video lecture that must be viewed before the class session. Interactive class time involves discussions or other active learning modalities that are only effective if the trainee has viewed the material beforehand.

Table 2.3 Examples of Intraoperative Events to Discuss

Event	Questions to Consider	Possible Discussion Topics
Tachycardia after increase in surgical stimulation	Is the depth of anesthesia adequate? Could there be another cause for the tachycardia? Is the patient in sinus rhythm, or could this be a primary arrhythmia?	Assessment of anesthetic depth Approaches to increasing depth of anesthesia Diagnosis of tachycardia
End-tidal CO_2 increases after laparoscopic insufflation	Is the patient having a potentially life-threatening complication of laparoscopy such as CO_2 embolism? What is the expected rise in end-tidal CO_2 with laparoscopic procedures? How should the mechanical ventilator settings be adjusted?	Complications of laparoscopy Mechanical ventilation modes Causes of intraoperative hypercarbia
Peripheral nerve stimulator indicates train-of-four 0/4 15 minutes before the end of surgery	Is the nerve stimulator functioning properly? Is there a reason for prolonged neuromuscular blockade? Can the blockade be reversed safely?	Neuromuscular stimulation patterns Clinical implications of residual neuromuscular blockade Pharmacology of neuromuscular blockade reversal

Simulations can take several forms: task-based simulators to practice discrete procedures such as laryngoscopy or intravenous catheter placement, mannequin-based simulators to recreate an intraoperative crisis such as malignant hyperthermia or cardiac arrest, and computer-based simulators designed to repetitively manage advanced cardiac life support algorithms. The wide variety of web-based material that is readily accessible to trainees includes podcasts and videocasts, ultrasound learning modules, and other procedure-based instructional videos.[3]

The beginning trainee is typically focused on learning to care for one patient at a time, that is, case-based learning. When developing an individual anesthesia plan, the trainee should also set learning goals for a case (Box 2.5). Trainees should regularly reflect on their practice and on how they can improve their individual patient care and their institution's systems of patient care.

Learning Orientation

The trainee's approach to a learning challenge can be described as a "performance orientation" or a "learning orientation."[12] Trainees with a performance orientation have a goal of validating their abilities, whereas trainees with a learning orientation have the goal of increasing their mastery of the situation. Feedback is more likely to be viewed as beneficial for trainees with a learning orientation, whereas a trainee with a performance orientation is likely to view feedback as merely a mechanism to highlight an area of weakness. If the training setting is challenging and demanding, an individual with a strong learning orientation is more likely to thrive.

Box 2.5 Sample Learning Goals for Operating Room Case

A 47-year-old, 75-kg female with biliary colic and well-controlled asthma requires anesthesia for laparoscopic cholecystectomy. Possible learning goals to be addressed by directed reading before the case or discussion during the case include the following:

What complications of laparoscopic surgery can present intraoperatively?

What are the manifestations?

How should these complications be treated?

How will the severity of the patient's asthma be assessed?

What if the patient had wheezing and dyspnea in the preoperative area?

The growth mindset theory suggests that performance versus learning orientation is influenced by an individual's beliefs about their intelligence and abilities. People with a growth mindset believe that intelligence and abilities are not fixed and can be developed. Other features of a growth mindset include embracing challenges, viewing effort as necessary for success, and considering feedback as important for ongoing learning.[13] Individuals with a growth mindset focus on mastery of learning goals rather than performance (either performing more poorly than others or trying to outperform others). Although growth mindset theory has been studied in primary and secondary schools for decades, the theory as it relates to health professions education is in its early phase of exploration. Although more research is warranted, potential benefits of the growth mindset include helping health professions learners be more receptive to feedback, which can support the relationship between learners and educators.[13]

Cognitive Load

Providing anesthesia in the operating room is a complex process that requires processing and using enormous amounts of information. Anesthesia trainees, especially those in the beginning of their training, encounter an enormous cognitive load as they learn new information. In brief, cognitive load theory suggests that new information must be processed by the working memory, which has a limited capacity.[14] The working memory faces three types of cognitive load: intrinsic load, extraneous load, and germane load.[15] Intrinsic load is related to the degree of difficulty of the material and the expertise of the person processing the information (i.e., load associated with the task). Extraneous load is the load imposed that is not necessary to learning the information (i.e., load *not* essential to the task). Germane load is the load imposed by the learner's use of strategies to organize and process information and may be viewed as a learner's level of concentration devoted to learning. Optimizing germane load allows learners to organize knowledge into schemas or scripts. These act as a single element in working memory and therefore reduce intrinsic load. Extensive practice allows for schemas and scripts to become automated and performed with ease and without effort. This opens space in the working memory to process and learn more information.

Using cognitive load theory, instructors can facilitate learning in one of three ways: (1) teach at the level and expertise of the learner (decrease intrinsic load); (2) remove content or other interruptions not pertinent to the task or subject (decrease extraneous load); and (3) encourage strategies that allow for processing of information (optimize germane load).[14,16] If intrinsic and extraneous load are too high, a learner will not have enough working memory to allow for the germane load needed to develop schemas and scripts. Trainees who understand these processes, including the importance of practice, are more likely to excel in their learning and grow as clinicians.

REFERENCES

1. Whittington JW, Nolan K, Lewis N, Torres T. Pursuing the triple aim: The first 7 years. Milbank Q. 2015;93(2):263–300. doi: 10.1111/1468-0009.12122. PMID: 26044630; PMCID: PMC4462878.
2. MacNeill AJ, McGain F, Sherman JD. Planetary health care: A framework for sustainable health systems. *Lancet Planet Health*. 2021;5(2):e66–e68. doi:10.1016/S2542-5196(21)00005-X PMID: 33581064.
3. Martinelli SM, Isaak RS, Schell RM, Mitchell JD, McEvoy MD, Chen F. Learners and Luddites in the twenty-first century: Bringing evidence-based education to anesthesiology. *Anesthesiology*. 2019;131(4):908–928. doi:10.1097/ALN.0000000000002827 PMID: 31365369.
4. St Pierre M, Nyce JM. How novice and expert anaesthetists understand expertise in anaesthesia: A qualitative study. *BMC Med Educ.* 2020 12;20(1):262. doi:10.1186/s12909-020-02180-8 PMID: 32787964; PMCID: PMC7425048.
5. The anesthesiology milestone project. *J Grad Med Educ.* 2014;6(1 Suppl 1):15–28. doi:10.4300/JGME-06-01s1-30 PMID: 24701262; PMCID: PMC3966579.
6. Anesthesiology Milestones 2.0. Accreditation Council for Graduate Medical Education (ACGME), 2020. https://www.acgme.org/globalassets/PDFs/Milestones/AnesthesiologyMilestones2.0.pdf Accessed December 17, 2021.
7. Ten Cate O, Schwartz A, Chen HC. Assessing trainees and making entrustment decisions: On the nature and use of entrustment-supervision scales. *Acad Med.* 2020;95(11):1662–1669. doi:10.1097/ACM.0000000000003427 PMID: 32324633.
8. Marty AP, Schmelzer S, Thomasin RA, Braun J, Zalunardo MP, Spahn DR, Breckwoldt J. Agreement between trainees and supervisors on first-year entrustable professional activities for anaesthesia training. *Br J Anaesth.* 2020;125(1):98–103. doi:10.1016/j.bja.2020.04.009 Epub 2020 May 16. PMID: 32423610.
9. Woodworth GE, Marty AP, Tanaka PP, Ambardekar AP, Chen F, Duncan MJ, Fromer IR, Hallman MR, Klesius LL, Ladlie BL, Mitchell SA, AK Miller Juve, McGrath BJ, Shepler JA, 3rd Sims C, Spofford CM, Van Cleve W, Maniker RB. Development and Pilot Testing of Entrustable Professional Activities for US Anesthesiology Residency Training. *Anesth Analg.* 2021 1;132(6):1579–1591. doi:10.1213/ANE.0000000000005434 PMID: 33661789.
10. Gaba DM, Fish KJ, Howard SK, Burden A. *Crisis Management in Anesthesiology.* 2nd ed Philadephia: Sauders; 2014.
11. Tainter CR, Wong NL, Cudemus-Deseda GA, Bittner EA. "Flipped Classroom" model for teaching in the intensive care unit. *J Intensive Care Med.* 2017;32(3):187–196. doi:10.1177/0885066616632156 Epub 2016 Jul 7. PMID: 26912409.
12. Weidman J, Baker K. The cognitive science of learning: Concepts and strategies for the educator and learner. *Anesth Analg.* 2015;121(6):1586–1599.
13. Wolcott MD, McLaughlin JE, Hann A, Miklavec A, Beck Dallaghan GL, Rhoney DH, Zomorodi M. A review to characterise and map the growth mindset theory in health professions education. *Med Educ.* 2021;55(4):430–440. doi:10.1111/medu.14381 Epub 2020 Oct 9. PMID: 32955728.
14. van Merriënboer JJ, Sweller J. Cognitive load theory in health professional education: Design principles and strategies. *Med Educ.* 2010;44(1):85–93. doi:10.1111/j.1365-2923.2009.03498.x PMID: 20078759.
15. Rana J, Burgin S. Teaching & learning tips 2: Cognitive load theory. *Int J Dermatol.* 2017;56(12):1438–1441. doi:10.1111/ijd.13707 PMID: 29130491.
16. Castro-Alonso JC, de Koning BB, Fiorella L, Paas F. Five Strategies for Optimizing Instructional Materials: Instructor- and Learner-Managed Cognitive Load. *Educ Psychol Rev.* 2021 9:1–29. doi:10.1007/s10648-021-09606-9 Epub ahead of print. PMID: 33716467; PMCID: PMC7940870.

3 CLINICIAN WELL-BEING

Laura Berenstain, Jina Sinskey

Clinician well-being has emerged as a critical issue because of widespread clinician burnout. There is growing recognition that a combination of individual strategies and systems-level solutions is required to successfully promote clinician well-being. Interventions to prevent burnout are more effective than those that address burnout after it has occurred.

DEFINING TERMS

Burnout

In its 11 revision of the International Classification of Diseases (ICD-11) the World Health Organization (WHO) defines burnout as an occupational phenomenon rather than an individual mental health diagnosis (e.g., depression).[1] The term burnout was initially coined by Freudenberger in the 1970s, who described 12 progressive stages of burnout experienced by individuals in the helping professions in response to severe stress: (1) compulsion to prove oneself, (2) working harder, (3) neglecting of needs, (4) displacement of conflicts, (5) revision of values, (6) denial of emerging problems, (7) withdrawal, (8) obvious behavioral changes, (9) depersonalization, (10) inner emptiness, (11) depression, and (12) burnout.[2] Three key dimensions of burnout are commonly evaluated: emotional exhaustion, depersonalization, and a diminished sense of personal accomplishment.[3] Burnout rates in U.S. anesthesiologists and anesthesiology trainees range from 14% to 51%.[4,5] Clinician burnout is associated with negative consequences for (1) patient care, (2) the clinician workforce and health care system costs, and (3) clinicians' own health and safety.[1] Both work environment and individual factors can influence the risk of burnout in anesthesiology (Table 3.1).

Table 3.1	Work Environment and Individual Factors as Risk Factors for Burnout in Anesthesiology

Anesthesia Work Environment Factors	Individual Factors
• Front-line providers of acute care • Work associated with time pressure • Rapid pace of work • Need for sustained vigilance • Chaotic setting • Limited control over schedule • Lack of respect as a consulting clinician	• Perceived lack of support at work • Perceived lack of support at home • Working more than 40 hours per week • Lesbian, gay, transgender/transsexual, queer/questioning, intersex, asexual status • Perceived staffing shortages

From Pinyavat T, Mulaikal TA. Fostering physician well-being in anesthesiology. *Int Anesthesiol Clin.* 2020;58(4):36–40 and Afonso AM, Cadwell JB, Staffa SJ, et al. Burnout rate and risk factors among anesthesiologists in the United States. *Anesthesiology.* 2021;134(5):683–696.

Resilience

Resilience refers to the ability of both individuals and social groups to withstand, adapt, recover, or even grow from adversity, stress, or trauma; in other words, the ability to bounce back from challenging life experiences. Traditionally, resilience in the context of clinician well-being has focused on individual personality traits, behaviors, and attitudes. Resilience is a continuous, dynamic state that can be nurtured and trained.[1]

Moral Injury

Moral injury was first described in war veterans. It refers to the lasting negative effects on an individual's conscience or moral compass when that person perpetrates, fails to prevent, or witnesses acts that transgress one's own deeply held moral beliefs and expectations.[6] Emotions of guilt, shame, and remorse are frequently associated with moral injury. In medicine moral injury describes the distress that clinicians experience when they are unable to provide high-quality patient care because of factors beyond their control. During the coronavirus disease 2019 (COVID-19) pandemic, concerns about adequate personal protective equipment (PPE), witnessing patients dying alone in isolation, and the need to make allocation decisions to ration scarce medical resources were among numerous factors that contributed to clinician moral injury.

Well-Being

Well-being is not simply the absence of burnout. It also includes the presence of positive emotions (e.g.,

contentment and happiness), the absence of negative emotions, satisfaction with life, fulfillment, engagement, and positive functioning. Professional well-being allows clinicians to thrive and achieve their full potential through the experience of positive perceptions and an environment that supports a high quality of life at work.[1] The terms *wellness* and *well-being* are often used interchangeably. Efforts to promote wellness have traditionally focused on physical and emotional health and maintaining a healthy lifestyle. Although physical and emotional health are critical to overall well-being, they are only part of the equation. In addition to these two domains, well-being encompasses several distinctive, interdependent dimensions that can be internal or external to the individual (Fig. 3.1). Drivers of clinician well-being can be organized into a hierarchy of needs, starting with basic needs at the lowest level and leading to self-actualization at the highest level (Fig. 3.2).

WHY WELL-BEING IS IMPORTANT

Physicians with high levels of well-being generally have enthusiasm for life and work, along with a sense of accomplishment and belonging. However, personal characteristics such as perfectionism, self-doubt, inability to delegate, and high levels of commitment despite adversity can contribute to emotional exhaustion. Maslach and colleagues suggested that the best workers are more predisposed to burnout because they will continue to expend significant energy to meet their goals even in the face of barriers.[7] Not surprisingly, the prevalence of burnout observed among physicians compared with other U.S. workers is significantly higher even after adjustment for work hours, age, and gender.[1]

Chronic occupational stress is linked to neurobiologic findings. High levels of norepinephrine and dopamine are released in the brain during episodes of uncontrollable stress, weakening the abilities of the prefrontal cortex and impairing higher-order functions, including reasoning, social cognition, attention regulation, and complex decision making. In contrast, controllable stressors (such as a meaningful challenge) do not result in the same chemical changes.[8] Structural magnetic resonance imaging (MRI) findings obtained longitudinally in both a control population and a group with occupational exhaustion syndrome strongly suggested links between chronic occupational stress and thinning of the prefrontal cortex, enlargement of the amygdala, and caudate reduction. These findings were gender-specific, with women affected to a greater degree than men.

Professionalism, teamwork, and patient safety can all suffer as a result of burnout. Multiple studies have suggested a relationship between physician burnout and an increased incidence of both self-perceived medical errors and suboptimal care. Anesthesia residents at greater

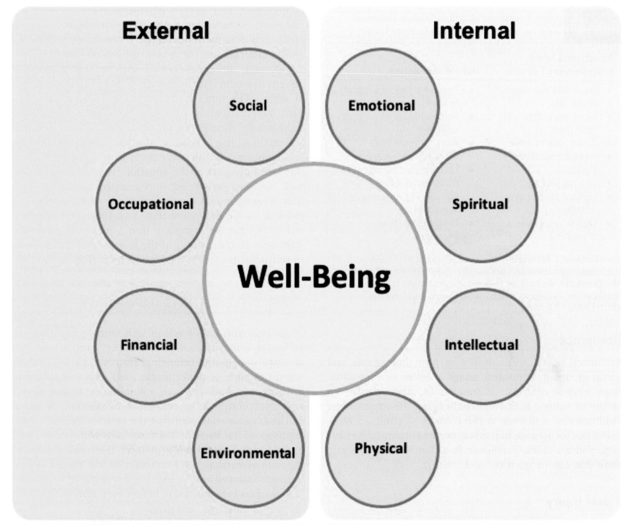

Fig. 3.1 The eight dimensions of well-being. (Adapted from Substance Abuse and Mental Health Services Administration [SAMHSA]. *Creating a Healthier Life: A Step-by-Step Guide to Wellness.* Washington, DC: SAMSHA; 2016.)

risk for burnout and depression reported more medication errors and mistakes with negative consequences for patients than residents with lesser risk.[9] Perhaps most concerning is the finding that emotional distress demonstrated during residency can have implications for future burnout as a practicing physician. In a longitudinal study of internal medicine physicians with early signs of emotional distress the persistence of emotional distress along with an association with depersonalization was identified 10 years after residency.[10]

The negative financial impact of burnout on health care systems is considerable. Studies have found that physicians with self-reported burnout were approximately twice as likely to leave the institution; the societal cost of turnover and reduced productivity caused by physician burnout in the United States is estimated to be greater than $4 billion annually.[1] Clinicians may also elect to reduce their work hours or retire early, resulting in decreased system productivity and reduced access to care for patients. Physician turnover also adversely affects colleagues and increases the risk of burnout for other health care team members.

The provision of optimal health care is the end product of a successful relationship between those providing care and those seeking care. Recognizing the negative impact of clinician burnout on health care organizations, the American Medical Association (AMA) has outlined five critical arguments for supporting well-being: (1) moral and ethical, (2) business, (3) recognition, (4) regulatory, and (5) tragedy.[11] The moral and ethical case may be the most important, as clinician burnout may contribute to excessive alcohol use and suicide.[1]

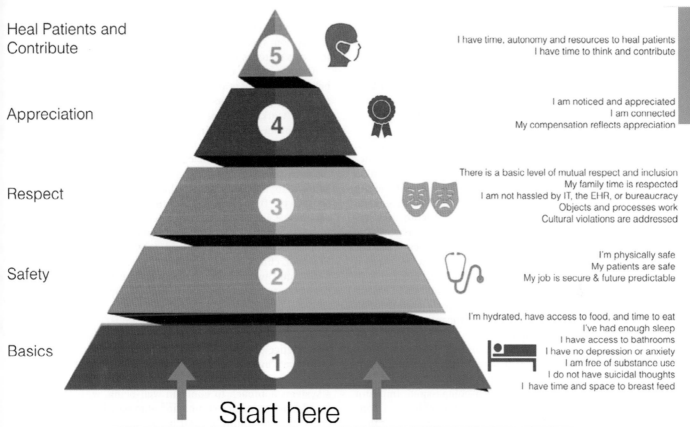

Fig. 3.2 Health professional wellness hierarchy. (*From Shapiro DE, Duquette C, Abbott LM, et al. Beyond burnout: A physician wellness hierarchy designed to prioritize interventions at the systems level. Am J Med. 2019;132[5]:556–563.*)

FACTORS AFFECTING CLINICIAN WELL-BEING

Autonomy, competence, and relatedness (or belonging) are basic psychological needs recognized as critical for achieving life satisfaction and supporting well-being.[12] Motivation also plays a critical role in well-being. Intrinsic motivators such as honoring one's values and finding meaning in one's work and life are associated with increased satisfaction.[12] The Charter on Physician Well-Being acknowledges the need for commitment on the individual, organizational, and societal levels to improve clinician well-being.[13]

Individual Factors

The incidence of burnout symptoms varies across medical specialties and practice settings. Professional characteristics correlated with a higher risk of burnout or dissatisfaction with work–life integration include medical specialty,[14] hours worked per week, and the number of call nights per week.[15] Factors unique to the practice of anesthesiology have been shown to result in a higher practitioner risk for burnout than seen in other specialties. Within the specialty itself, anesthesiology residents show the highest risk of developing burnout.[16] A National Aeronautics and Space Administration (NASA) Task Load Index assessing mental, physical, and time demands and perceived effort by the physician was used to determine physician task load. Higher task load scores were strongly correlated with burnout independent of other variables, with anesthesiology demonstrating one of the highest task load scores.[14]

Overall, physicians have a lower rate of satisfaction with work–life integration than the general U.S. working population, even after adjusting for age, sex, relationship status, and hours worked per week.[1] A 2021 survey of over 4000 American Society of Anesthesiologists (ASA) members evaluated the presence of burnout with the Maslach Burnout Inventory Human Services Survey.[4] Of the respondents, 59% were at high risk of burnout and 14% met criteria for burnout syndrome. The risk factors independently associated with a high risk of burnout included perceived lack of support at work; working more than 40 hours per week; lesbian, gay, bisexual, transgender/transsexual, queer/questioning, intersex, or asexual status; and perceived staffing shortages.

In a 2021 cross-sectional study of over 4000 U.S. physicians lower work–life integration scores were independently associated with female gender; age between 35 and 44 years; working more hours per week; and certain medical specialties, including anesthesiology, general surgery, and emergency medicine. The relationship status of "single" was also associated with lower work–life integration. Among females, the most significant adverse effect on work–life integration was seen in women identifying as Black/African American.[15] Compared with other physician mothers, physician mothers carrying additional caregiving responsibilities (e.g., caring for ill parents or other relatives) had significantly higher rates of mood or anxiety disorders.[17]

An overdeveloped sense of responsibility to others coupled with a culture that deprioritizes personal needs can consistently lead to difficulty finding adequate time for self-care and a lack of self-compassion. Impostor syndrome, or feelings of not being "enough," can contribute as well. A multicenter study suggested a strong association and dose–response relationship between physician self-valuation and both sleep deprivation and burnout, with self-valuation accounting for nearly 27% of the variability in physician burnout. Differences in self-valuation also accounted for most of the observed differences between male and female physicians in burnout rates.[18]

Organizational Level

Although individual factors influence clinician well-being, most clinicians already tend to exhibit high levels of resilience, underscoring the importance of organizational factors in promoting well-being.[1] A supportive work environment can profoundly affect clinician engagement. A 2021 study found that perceived lack of support at work is strongly associated with a high risk for burnout in practicing anesthesiologists.[4] A survey of anesthesiology trainees found that factors associated with a lower risk of burnout include perceived workplace resource availability, perceived ability to maintain work–life balance, and having a strong social support system.[5]

Numerous factors at the organizational level influence clinician well-being. The areas of the work–life model proposed by Maslach and Leiter provide an organizational context of burnout by looking at six areas: workload, control, reward, community, fairness, and values.[19] The degree of mismatch existing in these six areas is predictive of burnout, representing opportunities to develop specific strategies targeted to each area to improve matches between people and their work.

Culture refers to the collective norms, values, and beliefs of members of a particular group or society. By encouraging behaviors such as the compulsion to prove oneself, working harder, and neglecting one's needs, the culture of medical training often drives clinicians toward the initial stages of burnout described previously in this chapter.[20] Historically, the culture of medicine has upheld the idea that the responsibility for clinician well-being belongs to the individual rather than the organization or society. Organizational culture permeates the work experience and can affect and intensify factors perceived to be individual in nature. For example, work–life integration is typically considered to vary by individual. However, clinicians feel comfortable tending to nonwork needs only when cultural norms in the workplace also demonstrate a commitment to work–life integration.[21]

Societal Level

The practice of medicine happens within, and is strongly influenced by, the broader context of society. In 2019 the National Academy of Medicine (NAM) advocated for a systems approach to clinician well-being, with recommendations to reduce stigma and eliminate barriers associated with obtaining mental health support (Table 3.2).[1] Clinicians are often reluctant to seek help for mental health conditions because mental health–related stigma and structural issues such as medical licensure can have serious repercussions for clinicians' ability to practice medicine. This is especially concerning because failure to seek professional mental help is thought to contribute to a higher risk of suicide among physicians versus the general population. Although the Federation of State Medical Boards (FSMB) published recommendations for physician well-being in 2018, a review of initial medical license applications from 54 states and territories and Washington, DC in 2021 found that only 1 state was consistent with all recommendations and 5 states were consistent with none.[22]

The rapidly changing and stressful environment created by the COVID-19 pandemic exacerbated existing clinician burnout. Health care professionals' experiences during COVID-19 compromised the foundation of clinician well-being by threatening not only their basic needs but also their safety (physical safety and job security). Anesthesia care team members and other individuals participating in endotracheal intubation procedures experienced an even greater threat to their physical safety and mental health because of the heightened risk of exposure to, and transmission of, severe acute respiratory syndrome coronavirus 2 (SARS-CoV-2). The surge of physical and mental health issues in clinicians has

Table 3.2 National Academy of Medicine Goals for Eliminating Clinician Burnout and Enhancing Professional Well-Being

Goal	Description
Create positive work environments	Transform health care work systems by creating positive work environments that prevent and reduce burnout, foster professional well-being, and support quality care
Create positive learning environments	Transform health professions education and training to optimize learning environments that prevent and reduce burnout and foster professional well-being
Reduce administrative burden	Prevent and reduce the negative consequences on clinicians' professional well-being that result from laws, regulations, policies, and standards promulgated by health care policy, regulatory, and standards-setting entities, including government agencies (federal, state, and local), professional organizations, and accreditors
Enable technology solutions	Optimize the use of health information technologies to support clinicians in providing high-quality patient care
Provide support to clinicians and learners	Reduce the stigma and eliminate the barriers associated with obtaining the support and services needed to prevent and alleviate burnout symptoms, facilitate recovery from burnout, and foster professional well-being among learners and practicing clinicians
Invest in research	Provide dedicated funding for research on clinician professional well-being

From National Academies of Sciences, Engineering, and Medicine. National Academy of Medicine: Taking Action Against Clinician Burnout: A Systems Approach to Professional Well - Being. 2019.

accentuated the need for a national strategy to protect their well-being.

The NAM recommends creating positive work and learning environments to foster professional well-being in medicine,[1] underscoring the importance of inclusive environments that allow all clinicians to thrive. The recognition that structural racism and health inequities exist in medicine and the medical community must be acknowledged and addressed. Bias and discrimination occur regularly in medicine and can create a harsh work environment that can lead to burnout and suicidality.[23] Microaggressions refer to everyday slights, insults, putdowns, invalidations, and offensive behaviors experienced by members of a marginalized group. Microaggressions may be intentional or unintentional.[24] In medicine microaggressions often take the form of verbal and nonverbal reminders of how an individual, such as a member of an underrepresented minority or a woman, differs from the traditional image of someone in their field. This can lead to attrition, continuing and perpetuating inequities that ultimately hurt the entire medical community. In contrast, *microinterventions* can be a powerful tool to nurture an environment of diversity, equity, and inclusion by providing support and affirmation to individuals targeted by microaggressions.

MENTAL HEALTH

Fatigue Mitigation

Fatigue is defined as mental and physical exhaustion and tiredness. Practicing anesthesiologists and anesthesiology residents often work 24-hour or overnight shifts, which can lead to sleep deprivation and disruption of their circadian rhythm. Sleep-related impairment is associated with decreased professional fulfillment, increased burnout, and increased self-reported medical errors.[25] The Accreditation Council for Graduate Medical Education (ACGME) includes guidelines for fatigue mitigation as part of its common program requirements for anesthesiology residents.[26] Potential strategies for fatigue mitigation include scheduling interventions (e.g., 16-hour vs. 24-hour shifts), strategic naps, and the use of bright lights in clinical settings if feasible.

Substance Use Disorders

Substance use disorders are a serious issue in the anesthesia workplace with potentially devastating consequences for the involved clinician and their patients. Ease of access to venous cannulation equipment and potent drugs with abuse potential, and proficiency with both, create a unique risk for substance use disorders. The incidence of substance use disorders in practicing anesthesiologists and anesthesiology residents ranges between 1% and 2%,[27] with a high risk of relapse in both groups.[28,29] The risk of substance use disorder in certified registered nurse anesthetists (CRNAs) appears similar.[30] Substance use disorders can prove fatal, and one study of practicing anesthesiologists demonstrated that nearly 20% of physicians with a substance use disorder died of a substance use disorder–related cause.[28]

Behavioral changes described in affected anesthesiologists include withdrawal from family and friends; mood swings; increased episodes of anger, irritability, and hostility; spending more time at the hospital (even when off duty); volunteering for extra calls; refusing relief for lunch or coffee breaks; requesting frequent bathroom breaks; and signing out increasing amounts of opioids or quantities inappropriate for the given case.[31] Treatment generally involves referral to an inpatient facility that specializes in the treatment of health care professionals and includes detoxification, monitored abstinence, intensive education, exposure to self-help groups, and psychotherapy.[31] Substance use disorder prevention programs composed of education, strict substance control practices, structured interventions, and testing have been proposed as a potential strategy to reduce substance use disorders.[27] Reentry into clinical practice must be carefully planned with appropriate staging and monitoring to mitigate the risk of relapse.

Depression

Physicians with a high level of distress, whether because of burnout, depression, or both, can potentially enter a downward cycle that can result in tragic consequences. Burnout can be conceptualized as a process that proceeds through stages beginning with exhaustion and potentially culminating in physical symptoms and despair. As a clinician progresses through the various stages, patient care is often maintained at the expense of the clinician's own well-being and mental health. This perspective also aids in determining the most appropriate and helpful interventions for the clinician who is suffering.

Burnout and major depressive disorder (MDD) can share many of the same symptoms, including anhedonia, fatigue, impaired concentration and cognition, and changes in appetite and sleep. Burnout is described as a workplace phenomenon, whereas MDD is a clinical disorder with well-defined diagnostic criteria published by the American Psychiatric Association. Consideration for the distinction is essential in order not to prevent or delay treatment for clinicians with MDD.

The proportion of physicians screening positive for MDD showed a modest but steady increase between 2011 and 2017, reaching 42%.[32] Burnout, depression, and suicidal ideation are frequent among anesthesiology residents. A 22% incidence of depression risk has been described in anesthesiology residents, with a rate of suicidal ideation more than twice the age-adjusted rate observed in developed countries.[9] In a repeated cross-sectional study approximately half of residents were at high risk for burnout, and one in eight screened positive for depression.[5] These estimates may be low because of underreporting and undertreatment of depression as a result of the stigmatization in medical culture.

Depression is linked to patient safety. Physicians with depression are more likely to experience suboptimal functioning and report medical errors. In a study of anesthesiology residents those at high risk for burnout and depression reported more medical errors and less vigilant patient monitoring than their fellow residents.[9]

Suicide

Physicians have the highest suicide rate of any profession, twice that of the general population, with female physicians at greater risk than males.[33] Although female physicians attempt suicide less often than women in the general population, their completion rate equals male physicians and is estimated to be 2.5 to 4 times that of the general population. A 2020 meta analysis evaluated physician suicide rates since 1980.[34] Although the age-standardized suicide mortality ratio (SMR) for male physicians was significantly lower than the SMR of the general male population, female physicians' SMR remained substantially greater than the SMR for the general female population. Career-associated factors were the most prominent risk factor, and physician specialties associated with a greater risk of suicide included psychiatry and anesthesiology.[34] Although overall rates of suicide were lower than the rates for the age- and gender-matched general population, suicide is the leading cause of death among male residents and the second leading cause among female residents.

Physicians are more likely to commit suicide because of a job-related problem than the general population.[35] Risk factors for suicide in the medical profession include fatigue, social or professional isolation, stress resulting from complaints of bullying, the effects of aging, a perfectionist personality type, and reluctance to seek medical help.[33] Depression, substance abuse, impaired relationships, and self-destructive tendency have also been associated with physician suicide.[34] Early recognition of warning signs, continued efforts to enhance access to mental health resources, and the availability of a national suicide hotline (National Suicide Prevention Lifeline: 1-800-273-8255) will hopefully decrease the risk and promote emotional wellness for all.

INTERVENTIONS TO IMPROVE WELL-BEING

Personal Strategies

Anesthesiology poses more complex challenges to well-being than most medical specialties, ranging from constant scheduling changes to the frequency of exposure to stressful patient care situations. In concert with fatigue and duty to others practice-related challenges can complicate developing reliable personal strategies to enhance well-being and resiliency. Individual factors related to resilience include self-monitoring, setting limits, promotion of social engagement, and the capacity for mindfulness. Choosing the best personal strategies to promote well-being and how and when to implement them is an individual process, with success related to the sustainability of one's choices. One size does not fit all.

Adequate nutrition, hydration, exercise, and sleep are the cornerstones of self-care and fit into the "basics" level of the health professional wellness hierarchy (see Fig 3.2). Yet even these can prove difficult to achieve consistently, as most clinicians become conditioned to ignore or defer their own needs in response to work demands. Although meeting basic needs can be considered personal strategies, they should also remain departmental and institutional priorities. The individual's ability to consistently fill these human needs is greatly facilitated by providing adequate breaks, accessibility to nutritional food, and conveniently located exercise facilities. Seeking social support and having trusted confidants are also crucial for regenerating energy.

Clinicians with burnout often experience an inability to be "present" and are obsessed with thoughts of the past or anxiety about the future. The practice of mindfulness provides a path to allow the mind respite by fully engaging in the present moment. By creating intentional and nonjudgmental awareness of the moment, mindfulness can be practiced during hand hygiene and while washing the dishes, eating, walking, or sitting. Meditation is a way of cultivating and facilitating mindfulness through the self-regulation of attention and awareness. In mindfulness meditation an anchor, usually the breath, is used as a focus to return to when the mind wanders. Recognizing it as a "practice" helps one remember that perfection is not the goal. Instead, the aim is to return to the present moment as many times as necessary, with nonjudgment and acceptance. A greater level of mindfulness has been shown to facilitate self-reflection, decrease anxiety, and promote emotional self-regulation, with less reactivity to stressful situations and emotional triggers.[36]

As humans, we constantly judge our thoughts, feelings, and experiences, many times harshly. Self-compassion is defined as being open and sensitive to one's own suffering, experiencing feelings of care and kindness to oneself, and not judging one's own inadequacies and failures. Self-compassion allows us to recognize and accept our common humanity and is also associated with compassion towards others.[37] Loving-kindness ("metta") or compassion meditations use the self as the object of practice, cultivating compassion for oneself and spreading it to others. Multiple studies have suggested a complementary effect between mindfulness and compassion practices, with mindfulness practices reducing negative affect system activity (amygdala) and compassion increasing positive emotion brain systems.[38]

Clinicians often find it hard to permit themselves to spend time on self-care. We must shift our mindset and learn to choose ourselves, understanding that self-care is not selfish and that if we do not care for ourselves, we will not be able to care for others effectively. The sustained effort necessary to implement and continue self-care strategies is not easy, and recognizing this may necessitate self-compassion.

Systemic Approaches

The NAM has put forth recommendations for health care organizations to address clinician well-being using a systems approach (see Table 3.2).[1] To address trainee well-being, the ACGME includes well-being requirements for all accredited residency and fellowship programs.[26] Professional societies, including the ASA, are supporting clinician well-being by providing open, accessible, and practical resources and websites for clinician well-being.

Most anesthesia providers will be involved in a medical error or adverse event during their career. A survey of anesthesiologists showed that 84% of respondents were involved in an unanticipated death or serious injury of a perioperative patient, and most were emotionally affected by the event with feelings of guilt, anxiety, and reliving of the episode.[39] Sixty-seven percent stated that their ability to provide patient care was compromised immediately after the event, and 19% acknowledged that they had never fully recovered. The term "second victim" refers to health care professionals who are injured by the same errors as their patients who are harmed. Second victims tend to migrate toward one of three paths: dropping out, surviving, or thriving.[40] Many institutions have formal peer support programs in place to provide social support after critical events. Peer support can and should also be made available outside of specific critical events.

There is a growing emphasis on well-being education for trainees and practicing clinicians, with an increasing number of anesthesiology programs developing formal well-being curricula. Published well-being curricula for anesthesiology residency programs incorporate a combination of education modalities beyond the traditional lecture format, including facilitated small-group discussions and simulation.[41] A study comparing facilitated small-group discussions with providing the same amount of free time found that a facilitated small-group curriculum aimed at promoting collegiality and community reduced depersonalization and increased meaning and engagement in work, with sustained results at 12 months.[42]

Coaching can be defined as "partnering with a client in a thought-provoking and creative process that inspires the client to maximize their personal and professional well-being."[43] Coaching is distinct from other workplace interventions, as it addresses the whole person and can explore both professional and personal issues to facilitate well-being. Through an ongoing trusting and confidential relationship, coaching encourages the development of self-awareness and recognition of individual strengths, enabling the coachee to question self-defeating beliefs and assumptions and focus on future possibilities. Unlike a traditional mentoring relationship, coach and client work as equals, with the client presumed to have the resources and wisdom to tackle life's challenges. Mindfulness and self-reflection are encouraged. Coaching can also be used for leadership or career development and to enhance team performance. In a randomized study of physicians a 6-month coaching intervention decreased overall burnout by 17.1% in the intervention group, whereas burnout in the control group during the same period increased by 4.9%. Improvements in emotional exhaustion, resiliency, and quality of life were also noted.[44] Coaching is not psychological treatment, however, and clinicians suffering from depression or substance abuse should be referred to appropriate sources for help.

Extensive evidence supports the fact that organizational culture and work environment are crucial elements in whether clinicians remain engaged or enter the burnout cascade. When individual strategies to combat burnout are placed at the center of leadership's efforts, there may be skepticism regarding leadership's commitment to the problem. The NAM has advocated for a systemic approach to promoting engagement and reducing burnout.[1] An organizational infrastructure to support well-being can potentially include a chief well-being officer, well-being committees, and associate/vice chair positions for well-being.

A 2021 report proposed a new integrative model for wellness-centered leadership (WCL) that has three key elements. The first and foremost element requires that leaders *care about people always,* seeking to understand the complex needs and contributions of both individuals and teams.[45] The importance of practicing self-care should also be emphasized for leaders, as a leader's personal level of burnout and self-valuation has been shown to predict their leadership behavior scores.[46] Flexibility and work–life integration should be encouraged. The second element of WCL requires the *cultivation of individual and team relationships.* This involves articulating a vision, creating a shared sense of alignment, and nurturing individualized professional development for team members. Building community at work leads to increased engagement and decreases in burnout. The final component for WCL is transformational: *to inspire change* by empowering teams and encouraging innovative thinking.

Intrinsic motivators, including meaning, purpose, alignment in values, and professional development, are emphasized. Leadership is transformational rather than transactional, and the psychological needs of autonomy, competence, and belonging are honored.

Policies to Support Well-Being

The NAM Action Collaborative on Clinician Well-Being and Resilience was created in 2017 in response to the rising rates of clinician burnout and its consequences. Its mission is to improve the understanding of clinician well-being challenges and seek and elevate evidence-based, multidisciplinary solutions. Sponsors of the Action Collaborative on Clinician Well-Being and Resilience include the ACGME, the AMA, the ASA, and multiple academic medical centers.

Several national policies are currently in progress to advocate for clinician well-being. The Dr. Lorna Breen Health Care Provider Protection Act (HR1667) was passed by both the U.S. House of Representatives and the U.S. Senate in 2021 after the death by suicide of Dr. Lorna Breen.[47] The bill specifies that the secretary of Health and Human Services will establish evidence-based education and awareness campaigns encouraging health care professionals to seek support and treatment for mental health concerns. It will further establish grants to health professions schools and academic health centers for training in evidence-informed strategies to reduce and prevent suicide, burnout, and behavioral health conditions among health care professionals and provide funding for evidence-informed strategies to improve clinician well-being and job satisfaction. Currently, in early 2022, HR1667 is awaiting resolution of technical differences between the two bills before being signed into law by President Biden.

Challenges related to well-being exist in a spectrum across all stages of a health care professional's career. The results of burnout are detrimental to clinicians, patients, colleagues, and the health care system. Efforts to enhance clinician well-being must occur at all levels: individual, organizational, and societal.

REFERENCES

1. National Academies of Sciences, Engineering, and Medicine; National Academy of Medicine. Taking Action Against Clinician Burnout: A Systems Approach to Professional Well-Being. 2019.
2. Freudenberger HJ. Staff burn-out. *Journal of Social Issues.* 1974;30:159–165.
3. Maslach C, Zimbardo PG. *Burnout: The Cost of Caring.* Englewood Cliffs: Prentice Hall; 1982.
4. Afonso AM, Cadwell JB, Staffa SJ, et al. Burnout rate and risk factors among anesthesiologists in the United States. *Anesthesiology.* 2021;134(5):683–696.
5. Sun H, Warner DO, Macario A, et al. Repeated cross-sectional surveys of burnout, distress, and depression among anesthesiology residents and first-year graduates. *Anesthesiology.* 2019;131(3):668–677.
6. Litz BT, Stein N, Delaney E, et al. Moral injury and moral repair in war veterans: a preliminary model and intervention strategy. *Clin Psychol Rev.* 2009;29(8):695–706.
7. Maslach C, Schaufeli WB, Leiter MP. Job burnout. *Annu Rev Psychol.* 2001;52:397–422.
8. Arnsten AFT, Shanafelt T. Physician distress and burnout: the neurobiological perspective. *Mayo Clin Proc.* 2021;96(3):763–769.
9. de Oliveira Jr GS, Chang R, Fitzgerald PC, et al. The prevalence of burnout and depression and their association with adherence to safety and practice standards: a survey of United States anesthesiology trainees. *Anesth Analg.* 2013;117(1):182–193.
10. Raimo J, LaVine S, Spielmann K, et al. The correlation of stress in residency with future stress and burnout: a

10-year prospective cohort study. *J Grad Med Educ.* 2018;10(5):524–531.

11. AMA STEPS Forward. Establishing a Chief Wellness Officer Position. https://edhub.ama-assn.org/steps-forward/module/2767739. Accessed November 20, 2021.

12. Ryan RM, Deci EL. Self-determination theory and the facilitation of intrinsic motivation, social development, and well-being. *Am Psychol.* 2000;55(1):68–78.

13. Thomas LR, Ripp JA, West CP. Charter on physician well-being. *JAMA.* 2018;319(15):1541–1542.

14. Harry E, Sinsky C, Dyrbye LN, et al. Physician task load and the risk of burnout among US physicians in a national survey. *Jt Comm J Qual Patient Saf.* 2021;47(2):76–85.

15. Tawfik DS, Shanafelt TD, Dyrbye LN, et al. Personal and professional factors associated with work-life integration among US physicians. *JAMA Netw Open.* 2021;4(5):e2111575.

16. Pinyavat T, Mulaikal TA. Fostering physician well-being in anesthesiology. *Int Anesthesiol Clin.* 2020;58(4):36–40.

17. Yank V, Rennels C, Linos E, et al. Behavioral health and burnout among physician mothers who care for a person with a serious health problem, long-term illness, or disability. *JAMA Intern Med.* 2019;179(4):571–574.

18. Trockel MT, Hamidi MS, Menon NK, et al. Self-valuation: Attending to the Most Important Instrument in the Practice of Medicine. *Mayo Clin Proc.* 2019;94(10):2022–2031.

19. Maslach C, Leiter MP. New insights into burnout and health care: strategies for improving civility and alleviating burnout. *Med Teach.* 2017;39(2):160–163.

20. Vinson AE, Bachiller PR. It's the Culture!—How systemic and societal constructs impact well-being. *Paediatr Anaesth.* 2021;31(1):16–23.

21. Schwartz SP, Adair KC, Bae J, et al. Consistency between state medical license applications and recommendations regarding physician mental health. *BMJ Qual Saf.* 2019;28(2):142–150.

22. Saddawi-Konefka D, Brown A, Eisenhart I, et al. Consistency between state medical license applications and recommendations regarding physician mental health. *JAMA.* 2021;325(19):2017–2018.

23. Ehie O, Muse I, Hill L, et al. Professionalism: microaggression in the healthcare setting. *Curr Opin Anaesthesiol.* 2021;34(2):131–136.

24. Sue DW, Alsaidi S, Awad MN, et al. Disarming racial microaggressions: microintervention strategies for targets, White allies, and bystanders. *Am Psychol.* 2019;74(1):128–142.

25. Trockel MT, Menon NK, Rowe SG, et al. Assessment of physician sleep and wellness, burnout, and clinically significant medical errors. *JAMA Netw Open.* 2020;3(12):e2028111.

26. Accreditation Council for Graduate Medical Education (ACGME). Common Program Requirements for Graduate Medical Education in Anesthesiology. https://www.acgme.org/Portals/0/PFAssets/ProgramRequirements/040_Anesthesiology_2020.pdf?ver2020-06-18-132902-423. Accessed November 20,2021.

27. Fitzsimons MG, Baker K, Malhotra R, et al. Reducing the Incidence of Substance Use Disorders in Anesthesiology Residents: 13 Years of Comprehensive Urine Drug Screening. *Anesthesiology.* 2018;129(4):821–828.

28. Warner DO, Berge K, Sun H, et al. Substance use disorder in physicians after completion of training in anesthesiology in the United States from 1977 to 2013.. *Anesthesiology.* 2020;133(2):342–349.

29. Warner DO, Berge K, Sun H, et al. Substance Use Disorder Among Anesthesiology Residents, 1975–2009. *JAMA.* 2013;310(21):2289–2296.

30. Taylor L. Substance abuse and misuse identification and prevention: an evidence-based protocol for CRNAs in the workplace. *AANA J.* 2020;88(3):213–221 PMID: 32442099.

31. Bryson EO, Silverstein JH. Addiction and substance abuse in anesthesiology. *Anesthesiology.* 2008;109(5):905–917.

32. Shanafelt TD, West CP, Sinsky C, et al. Changes in burnout and satisfaction with work-life integration in physicians and the general US working population between 2011 and 2017. *Mayo Clin Proc.* 2019;94(9):1681–1694.

33. Schernhammer ES, Colditz GA. Suicide rates among physicians: a quantitative and gender assessment (meta-analysis). *Am J Psychiatry.* 2004;161(12):2295–2302.

34. Duarte D, El-Hagrassy MM, Couto TCE, et al. Male and female physician suicidality: a systematic review and meta-analysis. *JAMA Psychiatry.* 2020;77(6):587–597.

35. Gold KJ, Sen A, Schwenk TL. Details on suicide among US physicians: data from the National Violent Death Reporting System. *Gen Hosp Psychiatry.* 2013;35(1):45–49.

36. Lomas T, Medina JC, Ivtzan I, et al. A systematic review of the impact of mindfulness on the well-being of healthcare professionals. *J Clin Psychol.* 2018;74(3):319–355.

37. Neff KD. The development and validation of a scale to measure self-compassion. *Self and Identity.* 2003;2(3):223–250.

38. Conversano C, Ciacchini R, Orrù G, et al. Mindfulness, compassion, and self-compassion among health care professionals: what's new? A systematic review. *Front Psychol.* 2020;11:1683.

39. Gazoni FM, Amato PE, Malik ZM, et al. The impact of perioperative catastrophes on anesthesiologists: results of a national survey. *Anesth Analg.* 2012;114(3):596–603.

40. Scott SD, Hirschinger LE, Cox KR, et al. The natural history of recovery for the healthcare provider "second victim" after adverse patient events. *Qual Saf Health Care.* 2009;18(5):325–330.

41. Thornton KC, Sinskey JL, Boscardin CK, et al. Design and implementation of an innovative, longitudinal wellness curriculum in an anesthesiology residency program. *A A Pract.* 2021;15(2):e01387.

42. West CP, Dyrbye LN, Rabatin JT, et al. Intervention to promote physician well-being, job satisfaction, and professionalism: a randomized clinical trial. *JAMA Intern Med.* 2014;174(4):527–533.

43. International Coaching Federation (ICF). About ICF. https://coachfederation.org/about. Accessed June 17, 2021.

44. Dyrbye LN, Shanafelt TD, Gill PR, et al. Effect of a professional coaching intervention on the well-being and distress of physicians: a pilot randomized clinical trial. *JAMA Intern Med.* 2019;179(10):1406–1414.

45. Shanafelt T, Trockel M, Rodriguez A, et al. Wellness-centered leadership: equipping health care leaders to cultivate physician well-being and professional fulfillment. *Acad Med.* 2021;96(5):641–651.

46. Shanafelt TD, Makowski MS, Wang H, et al. Association of burnout, professional fulfillment, and self-care practices of physician leaders with their independently rated leadership effectiveness. *JAMA Netw Open.* 2020;3(6):e207961.

47. U.S. Congress. Dr. Lorna Breen Health Care Provider Protection Act. https://www.congress.gov/bill/117th-congress/house-bill/1667 Accessed February 20, 2022 Accessed November 20, 2021.

PHARMACOLOGY AND PHYSIOLOGY

4 BASIC PHARMACOLOGIC PRINCIPLES

Tae Kyun Kim, Shinju Obara, Ken B. Johnson

The basic principles of pharmacology are a fundamental element of an anesthesia provider's knowledge base. This chapter provides an overview of key principles in clinical pharmacology used to describe anesthetic drug behavior. Box 4.1 lists definitions of some basic pharmacologic terms. Pharmacokinetic concepts include volumes of distribution, drug clearance, transfer of drugs between plasma and tissues, and binding of drugs to circulating plasma proteins. The section on pharmacokinetics introduces both the physiologic processes that determine pharmacokinetics and the mathematical models used to relate dose to concentration. Pharmacodynamic concepts include the concentration–drug effect relationship and drug–drug interactions for selected anesthetic interactions for selected anesthetic effects. Anesthesia providers rarely administer just one drug. Most anesthetics are a combination of several drugs with specific goals in analgesia, sedation, and muscle relaxation. Thus pharmacodynamic interactions can profoundly influence anesthetic effect. Formulating the *right dose* of an anesthetic requires consideration of many patient factors: age; body habitus; sex; chronic exposure to opioids, benzodiazepines, or alcohol; presence of heart, lung, kidney, or liver disease; and the extent of blood loss or dehydration, among others. Two of these factors, body habitus and age, will be discussed as examples of patient factors influencing anesthetic drug pharmacology.

PHARMACOKINETIC PRINCIPLES

Pharmacokinetics describes the relationship between drug dose and drug concentration in plasma or at the site of drug effect over time. The processes of absorption, distribution, and elimination (metabolism and excretion) govern this relationship. Absorption is not relevant to intravenously administered drugs but is relevant to all other routes of drug delivery. The time course of intravenously administered drugs is a function of distribution

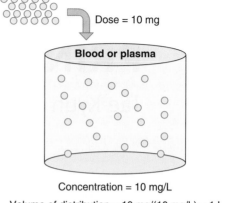

Concentration = 10 mg/L

Volume of distribution = 10 mg/(10 mg/L) = 1 L

Fig. 4.1 Schematic of a single-tank model of distribution volume. The group of red dots at the top left represent a bolus dose that, when administered to the tank of water, evenly distributes within the tank. (Modified from Miller RD, Cohen NH, Eriksson LI, et al., eds. *Miller's Anesthesia*. 8th ed. Philadelphia: Saunders Elsevier; 2014:Fig. 24.1.)

volume and clearance. Estimates of distribution volumes and clearances are described by pharmacokinetic parameters. Pharmacokinetic parameters are derived from mathematical formulas fit to measured blood or plasma concentrations over time after a known drug dose.

Fundamental Pharmacokinetic Concepts

Volume of Distribution

An oversimplified model of drug distribution throughout plasma and tissues is the dilution of a drug dose into a tank of water. The volume of distribution (Vd) is the apparent size of the tank required to explain a measured drug concentration from the tank water once the drug has had enough time to thoroughly mix within the tank (Fig. 4.1). The distribution volume is estimated using the simple relationship between dose (e.g., mg) and measured concentration (e.g., mg/L) as presented in Eq. 4.1.

$$\text{Volume of distribution} = \frac{\text{Amount of dose (mg)}}{\text{Concentration (mg/L)}}$$

With an estimate of tank volume, drug concentration after any bolus dose can be calculated. Just as the tank has a volume regardless of whether there is drug in it, distribution volumes in people are an intrinsic property regardless of whether any drug has been given.

Human bodies are not water tanks. As soon as a drug is injected, it begins to be cleared from the body. To account for this in the schematic presented in Fig. 4.1, a faucet is added to the tank to mimic drug elimination

from the body (Fig. 4.2). Using Eq. 4.1, estimating the volume of distribution without accounting for elimination leads to volume of distribution estimates that become larger than the initial volume. To refine the definition of distribution volume, the amount of drug that is present at a given time t is divided by the concentration at the same time.

$$Vd = \frac{\text{Amount } (t)}{\text{Concentration } (t)}$$

If elimination occurs as a first-order process (i.e., elimination is proportional to the concentration at that time), the volume of distribution calculated by Eq. 4.2 will be constant (Figs. 4.2 and 4.3).

When a drug is administered intravenously, some drug stays in the vascular volume, but most of the drug distributes to peripheral tissues. This distribution is often represented as additional volumes of distribution (tanks) connected to a central tank (blood or plasma volume). Peripheral distribution volumes increase the total volume of distribution (Fig. 4.4).

The schematic in Fig. 4.4 presents a plasma volume and tissue volume. The peripheral tank represents distribution of drug in peripheral tissues. There may be more than one peripheral tank (volume) to best describe the entire drug disposition in the body. The size of the peripheral volumes represents a drug's solubility in tissue relative to blood or plasma. The more soluble a drug is in peripheral tissue relative to blood or plasma, the larger the peripheral volumes of distribution.

An important point illustrated in Fig. 4.4 is that drug not only distributes to the peripheral tank and thus

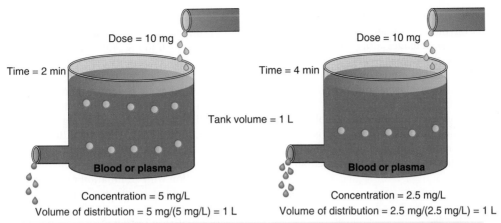

Fig. 4.2 Schematic of a single-tank model of elimination as a first-order process. At 2 minutes (*left panel*) and 4 minutes (*right panel*) after a 10-mg drug bolus, tank concentrations are decreasing from 5 to 2.5 mg/mL. Accounting for elimination, estimates of the distribution volume at each time point are both 1 L. (From Miller RD, Cohen NH, Eriksson LI, et al., eds. *Miller's Anesthesia.* 8th ed. Philadelphia: Saunders Elsevier; 2014:Fig. 24.2.)

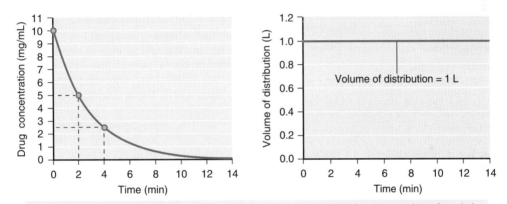

Fig. 4.3 Simulation of concentration (*left*) and distribution volume (*right*) changes over time after a bolus dose for a single-tank (one-compartment) model. The distribution volume remains constant throughout. (From Miller RD, Cohen NH, Eriksson LI, et al., eds. *Miller's Anesthesia.* 8th ed. Philadelphia: Saunders Elsevier; 2014:Fig. 24.3.)

increases the volume of distribution, but it also binds to tissue in that tank. This process further lowers the measurable concentration in the central tank. Thus the total volume of distribution may even be larger than the two tanks added together. In fact, some anesthetics have huge distribution volumes (e.g., fentanyl has an apparent distribution volume of 4 L/kg) that are substantially larger than an individual's vascular volume (0.07 L/kg) or extracellular volume (0.2 L/kg).

With an additional tank, the volume of distribution no longer remains constant over time. As illustrated in Fig. 4.5, at time = 0, the volume of distribution is estimated as 4.3 L, the same as that of the model presented in Fig. 4.3, which has only one tank. The volume of distribution then increases to 48 L over the next 10 minutes. The increase is due to the distribution of drug to the peripheral volume. This illustrates how the volume of distribution changes over time. To model distribution of volume changes over time, pharmacokinetic model structures consist of one or more tanks connected with pipes. The tanks have a fixed volume, and the rate of drug movement from one tank to another is modeled with rate constants. This allows modeling of changes in distribution volumes over time.

The amount of drug that moves to the peripheral tissue commonly surpasses the amount that is eliminated during the first few minutes after drug administration. As an example, consider a simulation of a propofol bolus that plots the accumulation of propofol in peripheral tissues and the amount eliminated over time (Fig. 4.6). During the first 4 minutes, the amount distributed to the peripheral tissue is larger than the amount eliminated from the body. After 4 minutes, the amounts reverse.

Clearance

Clearance describes the rate of drug removal from the plasma or blood. Two processes contribute to drug clearance: systemic (out of the tank) and intercompartmental (between the tanks) clearance (Fig. 4.7). Systemic clearance permanently removes drug from the body, either by eliminating the parent molecule or by transforming it into metabolites. Intercompartmental clearance moves drug between plasma and peripheral tissue tanks. By way of clarification, in this chapter the words *compartment* and *tank* are used interchangeably.

Clearance is defined in units of flow, that is, the volume completely cleared of drug per unit of time (e.g., L/min). Clearance is not to be confused with elimination

rate (e.g., mg/min). To explain why elimination rates do not accurately characterize clearance, consider the simulation presented in Fig. 4.8. Using the volume of distribution, the total amount of drug can be calculated at every measured drug concentration. The concentration change in time window *A* is larger than that in time window *B* even though they are both 1 minute in duration. The elimination rates are 28 and 10 mg/min for time windows *A* and *B*, respectively. They are different, and neither can be used as a parameter to predict drug concentrations when another dose of drug is administered. Because of this limitation with elimination rate, clearance was developed to provide a single number to describe the decay in drug concentration presented in Fig. 4.8.

For discussion purposes, assume that concentration is the power necessary to push drug out of the water tank. The higher the concentration, the larger the amount of drug eliminated. To standardize the elimination rate, the eliminated amount of drug is scaled to concentration. For example, the elimination rate in time window *A* (28.4 mg/min) scaled to the mean concentration during that time window (14 μg/mL) is 2 L/min. Normalizing the elimination rate in time window *B* (10.4 mg/min) to concentration (5 μg/mL) gives the same result as *A*. If the time interval is narrowed so that the time window approaches zero, the definition of clearance becomes:

$$\text{Clearance} = \frac{dA/dt}{C\,(t)}$$

where dA/dt is the rate of drug elimination at given time t and $C\,(t)$ is the corresponding concentration at time t. The elimination rate (dA/dt) can be expressed

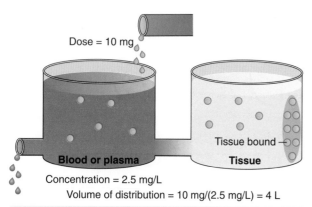

Dose = 10 mg

Tissue bound

Blood or plasma

Tissue

Concentration = 2.5 mg/L

Volume of distribution = 10 mg/(2.5 mg/L) = 4 L

Fig. 4.4 Schematic of a two-tank model. The total volume of distribution consists of the sum of the two tanks. The blue dots in the ellipse in the peripheral volume represent tissue-bound drug. The measured concentration in the blood or plasma is 2.5 mg/mL just after a bolus dose of 10 mg. Using Fig. 4.1, this leads to a distribution volume of 4 L. (From Miller RD, Cohen NH, Eriksson LI, et al., eds. *Miller's Anesthesia.* 8th ed. Philadelphia: Saunders Elsevier; 2015:Fig. 24.4.)

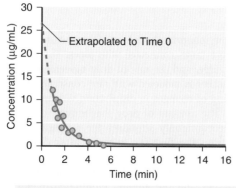

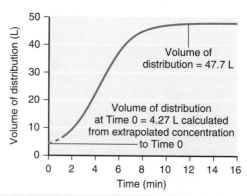

Fig. 4.5 Simulation of concentration and apparent distribution volume changes over time after a bolus dose for a two-tank (two-compartment) model. On the left, the *dots* represent measured drug concentrations. The *solid line* represents a mathematical equation fit to the measured concentrations. The *dotted line* represents an extrapolation of the mathematical equation (i.e., pharmacokinetic model) to time 0. On the right, the apparent distribution volume is time dependent, with the initial volume of distribution much smaller than the distribution volume at near steady state. The apparent distribution volume of time 0 is not a true reflection of the actual volume of distribution. (From Miller RD, Cohen NH, Eriksson LI, et al., eds. *Miller's Anesthesia.* 8th ed. Philadelphia: Saunders Elsevier; 2015:Fig. 24.5.)

as $Q(C_{in} - C_{out})$. Rearranging Eq. 4.3, clearance can be expressed as follows:

$$\text{Clearance} = \frac{Q(C_{in} - C_{out})}{C_{in}}$$

where Q is the blood flow to metabolic organs, C_{in} is the concentration of drug delivered to metabolic organs, and C_{out} is the concentration of drug leaving metabolic organs. The fraction of inflowing drug extracted by the organ is $(C_{in} - C_{out})/C_{in}$ and is called the *extraction ratio*

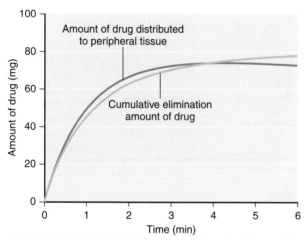

Fig. 4.6 Simulation of propofol accumulation in the peripheral tissues *(blue line)* and the cumulative amount of propofol eliminated *(yellow line)* after a 2-mg/kg propofol bolus to a 77-kg (170-lb), 177-cm (5 ft 10 in) tall 53-year-old man, using published pharmacokinetic model parameters.[31] Drug indicates propofol. (From Miller RD, Cohen NH, Eriksson LI, et al., eds. *Miller's Anesthesia*. 8th ed. Philadelphia: Saunders Elsevier; 2015:Fig. 24.6.)

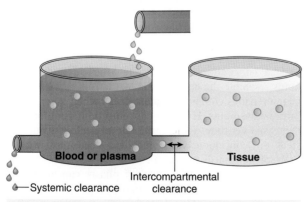

Fig. 4.7 Schematic of a two-tank model illustrating two sources of drug removal from the central tank (blood or plasma): systemic and intercompartmental clearance. (From Miller RD, Cohen NH, Eriksson LI, et al., eds. *Miller's Anesthesia*. 8th ed. Philadelphia: Saunders Elsevier; 2015:Fig. 24.8.)

(ER). Clearance can be estimated as organ blood flow multiplied by the ER. Eq. 4.4 can be simplified as shown here (Eq. 4.5):

$$\text{Clearance} = Q \times ER$$

The total clearance is the sum of each clearance by metabolic organs such as the liver, kidney, and other tissues (Fig. 4.9).

Hepatic clearance has been well characterized. For example, the relationship between clearance, liver blood flow, and the ER is presented in Fig. 4.10.[1] For drugs with an ER of nearly 1 (e.g., propofol), a change in liver blood flow produces a nearly proportional change in clearance. For drugs with a low ER (e.g., alfentanil), clearance is nearly independent of the rate of liver blood flow. If nearly 100% of the drug is extracted by the liver, this implies that the liver has tremendous metabolic capacity for the drug. In this case the rate-limiting step in metabolism is flow of drug to the liver, and such drugs are said to be "flow limited." Any reduction in liver blood flow, such as usually accompanies anesthesia, can be expected to reduce clearance. However, moderate changes in hepatic metabolic function per se will have little impact on clearance because hepatic metabolic capacity is overwhelmingly in excess of demand.

For many drugs (e.g., alfentanil), the ER is considerably less than 1. For these drugs, clearance is limited by the capacity of the liver to take up and metabolize drug. These drugs are said to be "capacity limited." Clearance will change in response to any change in the capacity of the liver to metabolize such drugs, as might be caused by liver disease or enzymatic induction. However, changes in liver blood flow, as might be caused by the anesthetic state itself, usually have little influence on clearance because the liver handles only a fraction of the drug that it sees anyway.

Front-End Kinetics

Front-end kinetics refers to the description of intravenous drug behavior immediately after administration. How rapidly a drug moves from the blood into peripheral tissues directly influences the peak plasma drug concentration. With compartmental models, an important assumption is that an intravenous bolus instantly mixes in the central volume, with the peak concentration occurring at the moment of injection without elimination or distribution to peripheral tissues. For simulation purposes, the initial concentration and volume of distribution at time = 0 are extrapolated as if the circulation had been infinitely fast. This, of course, is not real. If a drug is injected into an arm vein and that initial concentration is measured in a radial artery, the drug appears in the arterial circulation 30 to 40 seconds after injection. The delay likely represents the time required for the drug to pass through the venous volume of the upper part of the arm, heart, great vessels, and peripheral arterial circulation.

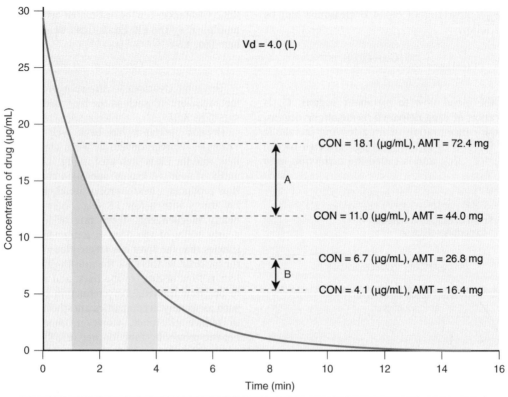

Fig. 4.8 Simulation of drug concentration changes when a drug is administered to a single-tank model with linear elimination (see Fig. 4.2). The concentration changes for two time windows are labeled with dashed lines from 1 to 2 minutes (time window *A*) and from 3 to 4 minutes (time window *B*), respectively. The concentrations *(CON)* at the beginning and end of each time window are used to calculate the amount *(AMT)* of drug that is eliminated (see text). *Vd*, Volume of distribution. (Modified from Miller RD, Cohen NH, Eriksson LI, et al., eds. *Miller's Anesthesia.* 8th ed. Philadelphia: Saunders Elsevier; 2015:Fig. 24.9.)

More sophisticated models (e.g., a recirculatory model)[2] account for this delay and are useful when characterizing the behavior of a drug immediately after bolus administration, such as with induction agents, when the speed of onset and duration of action are of interest.

Compartmental Pharmacokinetic Models
Compartmental models have no physiologic correlate. They are built by using mathematical expressions fit to concentration over time data and then reparameterized in terms of *volumes and clearances*. The *one-compartment model* presented in Fig. 4.11 contains a single volume and a single clearance. Although used for several drugs, this model is perhaps oversimplified for anesthetic drugs. To better model anesthetic drugs, clinical pharmacologists have developed two- or three-compartment models that contain several tanks connected by pipes. As illustrated in Fig. 4.11, the volume to the right in the two-compartment model—and in the center of the three-compartment model—is the central volume. The other volumes are peripheral volumes. The sum of all volumes is the volume of distribution at steady state, Vdss. Clearance in which the drug leaves the central compartment to the outside is the *central* or *metabolic* clearance. Clearances between the central compartment and the peripheral compartments are the intercompartmental clearances.

Multicompartment Models
Plasma concentrations over time after an intravenous bolus resemble the curve in Fig. 4.12. This curve has the characteristics common to most drugs when given as an intravenous bolus. First, the concentrations continuously decrease over time. Second, the rate of decline is initially steep but continuously becomes less steep, until we get to a portion that is *log-linear.*

For many drugs, three distinct phases can be distinguished, as illustrated for fentanyl in Fig. 4.12. A *rapid-distribution* phase (*blue line*) begins immediately after injection of the bolus. Very rapid movement of the drug from plasma to the rapidly equilibrating tissues characterizes this phase. Next, a second *slow-distribution* phase (*red line*) is characterized by movement of the drug into

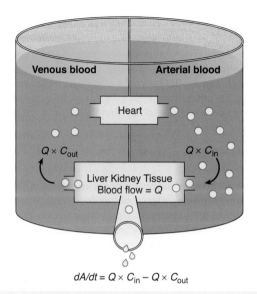

$$dA/dt = Q \times C_{in} - Q \times C_{out}$$

Fig. 4.9 Schematic of drug extraction. *A*, Amount of drug; C_{in} and C_{out}, drug concentrations presented to and leaving metabolic organs; *dA/dt*, drug elimination rate; *Q*, blood flow. (From Miller RD, Cohen NH, Eriksson LI, et al., eds. *Miller's Anesthesia*. 8th ed. Philadelphia: Saunders Elsevier; 2015:Fig. 24.10.)

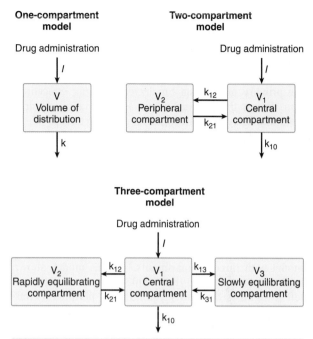

Fig. 4.11 One-, two-, and three-compartment mammillary models. (From Miller RD, Cohen NH, Eriksson LI, et al., eds. *Miller's Anesthesia*. 8th ed. Philadelphia: Saunders Elsevier; 2015:Fig. 24.12.)

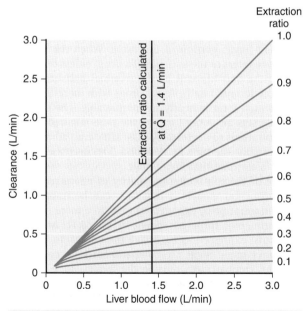

Fig. 4.10 Relationship among liver blood flow (*Q*), clearance, and extraction ratio. For drugs with a high extraction ratio, clearance is nearly identical to liver blood flow. For drugs with a low extraction ratio, changes in liver blood flow have almost no effect on clearance.[1] (From Miller RD, Cohen NH, Eriksson LI, et al., eds. *Miller's Anesthesia*. 8th ed. Philadelphia: Saunders Elsevier; 2015:Fig. 24.11.)

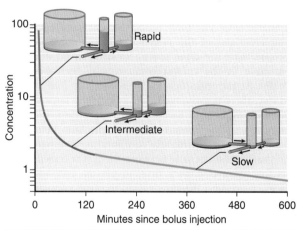

Fig. 4.12 Hydraulic model of fentanyl pharmacokinetics. Drug is administered into the central tank, from which it can distribute into two peripheral tanks, or it may be eliminated. The volume of the tanks is proportional to the volumes of distribution. The cross-sectional area of the pipes is proportional to clearance.[3] (From Miller RD, Cohen NH, Eriksson LI, et al., eds. *Miller's Anesthesia*. 8th ed. Philadelphia: Saunders Elsevier; 2015:Fig. 24.13.)

more slowly equilibrating tissues and return of the drug to plasma from the most rapidly equilibrating tissues. Third, the terminal phase (*green line*) is nearly a straight line when plotted on a semilogarithmic graph. The terminal phase is often called the "elimination phase" because the primary mechanism for decreasing drug concentration during the terminal phase is elimination of drug from the body. The distinguishing characteristic of the terminal elimination phase is that the plasma concentration is lower than tissue concentrations and the relative proportion of drug in plasma and peripheral volumes of distribution remains constant. During this terminal phase, drug returns from the rapid- and slow-distribution volumes to plasma and is permanently removed from plasma by metabolism or excretion.

The presence of three distinct phases after bolus injection is a defining characteristic of a mammillary model with three compartments.[3] In this model, shown in Fig. 4.12, there are three tanks corresponding (from left to right) to the slowly equilibrating peripheral compartment, the central compartment (the plasma into which drug is injected), and the rapidly equilibrating peripheral compartment. The horizontal pipes represent intercompartmental clearance or (for the pipe draining onto the page) metabolic clearance. The volumes of each tank correspond to the volumes of the compartments for fentanyl. The cross-sectional areas of the pipes correlate with fentanyl's systemic and intercompartmental clearance. The height of water in each tank corresponds to drug concentration. By using this hydraulic model, we can follow the processes that decrease drug concentration over time after bolus injection. Initially, drug flows from the central compartment to both peripheral compartments via intercompartmental clearance and completely out of the model via metabolic clearance. Because there are three places for drug to go, the concentration in the central compartment decreases very rapidly. At the transition between the *blue line* and the *red line*, there is a change in the role of the most rapidly equilibrating compartment. At this transition, the concentration in the central compartment falls below the concentration in the rapidly equilibrating compartment, and the direction of flow between them is reversed. After this transition (*red line*), drug in plasma has only two places to go: into the slowly equilibrating compartment or out the drain pipe. These processes are partly offset by the return of drug to plasma from the rapidly equilibrating compartment. The net effect is that once the rapidly equilibrating compartment has come to equilibration, the concentration in the central compartment falls far more slowly than before.

Once the concentration in the central compartment decreases below both the rapidly and slowly equilibrating compartments (*green line*), the only method of decreasing the plasma concentration is metabolic clearance, the drain pipe. Return of the drug from both peripheral compartments to the central compartment greatly slows the rate of decrease in plasma drug concentration.

Curves that continuously decrease over time, with a continuously increasing slope (i.e., like the curve in Fig. 4.12), can be described by a sum of negative exponentials. In pharmacokinetics, one way of denoting this sum of exponentials is to say that the plasma concentration over time is as follows:

$$C(t) = Ae^{-\alpha t} + Be^{-\beta t} + Ce^{-\gamma t}$$

where t is the time since the bolus injection; $C(t)$ is the drug concentration after a bolus dose; and A, α, B, β, C, and γ are parameters of a pharmacokinetic model. A, B, and C are coefficients, whereas α, β, and γ are exponents. After a bolus injection, all six of the parameters in Eq. 4.6 will be greater than 0. Polyexponential equations are used mainly because they describe the plasma concentrations observed after bolus injection, except for the misspecification in the first few minutes, mentioned previously. Compartmental pharmacokinetic models are strictly empiric. These models have no anatomic correlate. They are based solely on fitting equations to measured plasma concentrations after a known dose. Kinetic models are transformed into models that characterize concentration changes over time in terms of volumes and clearances. Although more intuitive, they have no physiologic correlate.

Special significance is often ascribed to the smallest exponent. This exponent determines the slope of the final log-linear portion of the curve. When the medical literature refers to the half-life of a drug, unless otherwise stated, the half-life will be the terminal half-life. However, the terminal half-life for drugs with more than one exponential term is nearly uninterpretable. The terminal half-life sets an upper limit on the time required for the concentrations to decrease by 50% after drug administration. Usually, the time needed for a 50% decrease will be much faster than that upper limit.

Part of the continuing popularity of pharmacokinetic compartmental models is that they can be transformed from an unintuitive exponential form to a more intuitive compartmental form, as shown in Fig. 4.11. Microrate constants, expressed as k_{ij}, define the rate of drug transfer from compartment i to compartment j. Compartment 0 is the compartment outside the model, so k_{10} is the microrate constant for processes acting through metabolism or elimination that irreversibly remove the drug from the central compartment (analogous to k for a one-compartment model). The intercompartmental microrate constants (k_{12}, k_{21}, etc.) describe movement of the drug between the central and peripheral compartments. Each peripheral compartment has at least two microrate constants, one for drug entry and one for drug exit. The microrate constants for the two- and three-compartment models can be seen in Fig. 4.11.

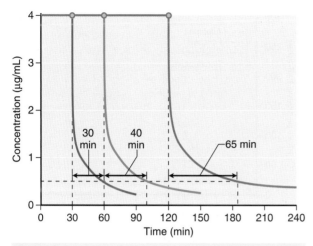

Fig. 4.13 Simulation of decrement times for a target-controlled infusion set to maintain a target propofol concentration of 4 µg/mL for 30, 60, and 120 minutes. Once terminated, the time required to reach 0.5 µg/mL was 30, 40, and 65 minutes for each infusion, respectively. Simulations of the decrement times used a published pharmacokinetic model.[31] (From Miller RD, Cohen NH, Eriksson LI, et al., eds. *Miller's Anesthesia*. 8th ed. Philadelphia: Saunders Elsevier; 2015:Fig. 24.14.)

Back-End Kinetics

Using estimates of distribution volume and clearance, back-end kinetics is a useful tool that describes the behavior of intravenous drugs when administered as continuous infusions. Back-end kinetics provide descriptors of how plasma drug concentrations decrease once a continuous infusion is terminated. An example is decrement time. This predicts the time required to reach a certain plasma concentration once an infusion is terminated. Decrement times are a function of infusion duration. Consider the example of decrement times for a set of continuous target-controlled infusions (TCIs) (Fig. 4.13). In this simulation TCI of propofol is set to maintain a concentration of 4 µg/mL for 30, 60, and 120 minutes. Once the infusion is stopped, the time to reach 0.5 µg/mL is estimated. As illustrated, the longer the infusion, the longer the time required to reach 0.5 µg/mL. This example demonstrates how drugs accumulate in peripheral tissues with prolonged infusions. This accumulation prolongs the decrement time.

Another use of decrement times is as a tool to compare drugs within a drug class (e.g., opioids). As a comparator, plots of decrement times are presented as a function of infusion duration. When used this way, decrement times are determined as the time required to reach a target percentage of the concentration immediately after termination of a continuous infusion. Examples of 50% and 80% decrement times for selected opioids and sedatives are presented in Fig. 4.14. Of note, for shorter infusions, the decrement times are similar for both classes of anesthetic drugs. Once infusion duration exceeds 2 hours, the decrement times vary substantially. A popular decrement time is the 50% decrement time, also known as the *context-sensitive half-time.*[4] The term *context-sensitive* refers to infusion duration. The term *half-time* refers to the 50% decrement time.

Biophase

Biophase refers to the time delay between changes in plasma concentration and drug effect. Biophase accounts for the time required for a drug to diffuse from the plasma to the site of action plus the time required, once drug is at the site of action, to elicit a drug effect. A simulation of various propofol bolus doses and their predicted effect on the electroencephalogram (EEG) bispectral index scale (BIS) is presented in Fig. 4.15. The time to peak effect for each dose is identical (approximately 1.5 minutes after the peak plasma concentration). The difference between each dose is the magnitude and duration of effect. A key principle is that when drug concentrations are in flux (i.e., during induction of anesthesia and emergence from anesthesia), changes in drug effect will lag behind changes in drug concentration. This lag between the plasma concentration and effect usually results in the phenomenon called *hysteresis,* in which two different plasma concentrations correspond to one drug effect or one plasma concentration corresponds to two drug effects. For example, Fig. 4.15 shows that the different concentrations at *C* and *c* correspond to the same BIS score.

To collapse the hysteresis between plasma concentration and effect and to match one plasma concentration to one drug effect, this lag is often modeled with an "effect-site" compartment added to the central compartment. Kinetic microrate constants used to describe biophase include k_{1e} and k_{e0}. The k_{1e} describes drug movement from the central compartment to the effect site, and k_{e0} describes the elimination of drug from the effect-site compartment. There are two important assumptions with the effect-site compartment: (1) The amount of drug that moves from the central compartment to the effect-site compartment is negligible and vice versa, and (2) there is no *volume* estimate to the effect-site compartment.

Typically, the relationship between plasma and the site of drug effect is modeled with an *effect-site* model, as shown in Fig. 4.16. The site of drug effect is connected to plasma by a first-order process. Eq. 4.7 relates effect-site concentration to plasma concentration:

$$dCe = \frac{k_{e0} \times (Cp - Ce)}{dt}$$

where *Ce* is the effect-site concentration, *Cp* is the plasma drug concentration, and k_{e0} is the rate constant for elimination of the drug. The constant k_{e0} describes the rate of rise and offset of drug effect (Fig. 4.17).

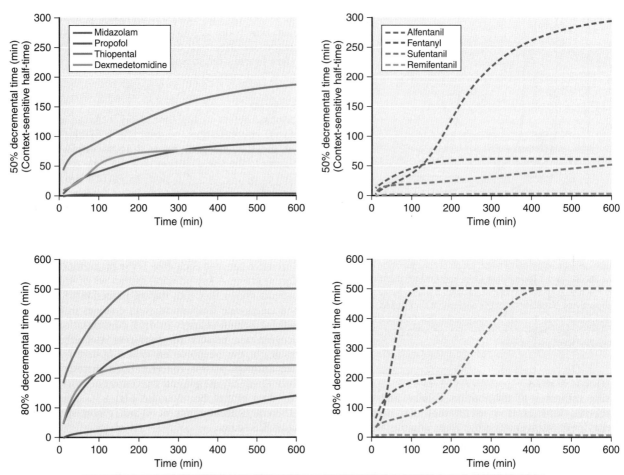

Fig. 4.14 These graphs show 50% and 80% decrement times for selected sedatives *(left side)* and opioids *(right side)*. The vertical axis refers to the time required to reach the desired decrement time. The horizontal axis refers to infusion duration. Simulations of the decrement times used published pharmacokinetic models for each sedative and analgesic.[5,31,32,41–43] (From Miller RD, Cohen NH, Eriksson LI, et al., eds. *Miller's Anesthesia*. 8th ed. Philadelphia: Saunders Elsevier; 2015:Fig. 24.15.)

In summary the conventional pharmacokinetic term *half-life* has little meaning to anesthesia providers, who work with drugs whose clinical behavior is not well described by half-life. The pharmacokinetic principles discussed in this section (such as volume of distribution, clearance, elimination, front-end kinetics, back-end kinetics, context-sensitive half-time, and biophase) better illustrate how an anesthetic will behave.

PHARMACODYNAMIC PRINCIPLES

Simply stated, pharmacokinetics describes what the body does to the drug, whereas pharmacodynamics describes what the drug does to the body. In particular, pharmacodynamics describes the relationship between drug concentration and pharmacologic effect.

Models used to describe the concentration–effect relationships are created in much the same way as pharmacokinetic models; they are based on observations and used to create a mathematical model. To create a pharmacodynamic model, plasma drug levels and a selected drug effect are measured simultaneously. For example, consider the measured plasma concentrations of an intravenous anesthetic drug after a bolus dose and the associated changes on the EEG spectral edge frequency (a measure of anesthetic depth) from one individual, presented in Fig. 4.18. Shortly after the plasma concentration peaks, the spectral edge starts to decrease, reaches a nadir, and then returns to baseline as the plasma concentrations drop to near 0.

Combining data from several individuals and plotting the measured concentrations versus the observed effect (modified to be a percentage of the maximal effect across

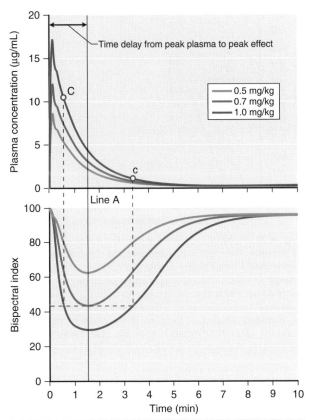

Fig. 4.15 Demonstration of biophase. The *top plot* presents a simulation of three propofol doses and the resultant plasma concentrations. The *bottom plot* presents a simulation of the predicted effect on the bispectral index scale (BIS). These simulations assume linear kinetics: regardless of the dose, effects peak at the same time *(Line A)*, as do the plasma concentration. The time to peak effect is 1.5 minutes. Even the plasma concentrations of points *C* and *c* are different; however, the BIS scores of those two points are the same. This finding demonstrates the hysteresis between plasma concentration and BIS score. Simulations used published pharmacokinetic and pharmacodynamic models.[30,32] (From Miller RD, Cohen NH, Eriksson LI, et al., eds. *Miller's Anesthesia.* 8th ed. Philadelphia: Saunders Elsevier; 2015:Fig. 24.16.)

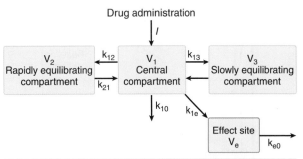

Fig. 4.16 A three-compartment model with an added effect site to account for the delay in equilibration between the rise and fall in arterial drug concentrations and the onset and offset of drug effect. The effect site is assumed to have a negligible volume. (From Miller RD, Cohen NH, Eriksson LI, et al., eds. *Miller's Anesthesia.* 8th ed. Philadelphia: Saunders Elsevier; 2015:Fig. 24.17.)

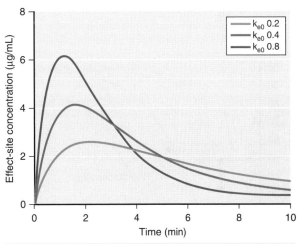

Fig. 4.17 Simulations of predicted plasma and effect-site concentrations for three different k_{e0} values. As the k_{e0} increases, the time to peak effect increases and the peak predicted effect-site concentration decreases.[30,32,44] (From Miller RD, Cohen NH, Eriksson LI, et al., eds. *Miller's Anesthesia.* 8th ed. Philadelphia: Saunders Elsevier; 2015:Fig. 24.18.)

all individuals) creates a hysteresis loop (Fig. 4.19). The ascending portion of the loop represents rising drug concentrations (see *arrow*). While rising, the increase in drug effect lags behind the increase in drug concentration. For the descending loop, the decrease in drug effect lags behind the decrease in drug concentration.

To create a pharmacodynamic model, the hysteresis loop is collapsed using modeling techniques that account for the lag time between plasma concentrations and the observed effect. These modeling techniques provide an estimate of the lag time, known as the $t_{1/2}k_{e0}$, and an estimate of the effect-site concentration (Ce) associated with a 50% probability of drug effect (C_{50}).

Most concentration–effect relationships in anesthesia are described with a sigmoid curve. The standard equation for this relationship is the Hill equation, also known as the *sigmoid Emax relationship* (Eq. 4.8):

$$\text{Effect} = E_0 + \left(E_{max} - E_0 \right)\left(C^\gamma / \left(C_{50}^\gamma + C^\gamma \right) \right)$$

where E_0 is the baseline effect, E_{max} is the maximal effect, C is the drug concentration, and γ represents the slope of the concentration–effect relationship; γ is also known as the Hill coefficient. For values of γ less than 1, the curve is hyperbolic, and for values greater than

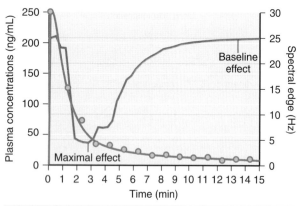

Fig. 4.18 Schematic representation of drug plasma concentrations *(blue circles)* after a bolus and the associated changes in the electroencephalogram's spectral edge *(red line)* measured in one individual. Note that changes in the spectral edge lag behind changes in plasma concentrations. (From Miller RD, Cohen NH, Eriksson LI, et al., eds. *Miller's Anesthesia.* 8th ed. Philadelphia: Saunders Elsevier; 2015:Fig. 24.19.)

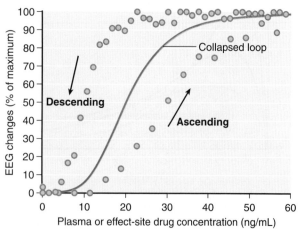

Fig. 4.19 Schematic representation of plasma concentrations versus normalized spectral edge measurements (presented as a percentage of maximal effect) from several individuals *(blue circles).* The *black arrows* indicate the ascending and descending arms of a hysteresis loop that coincide with increasing and decreasing drug concentrations. *The red* line represents the pharmacodynamic model developed from collapsing the hysteresis loop. *EEG,* electroencephalogram. (From Miller RD, Cohen NH, Eriksson LI, et al., eds. *Miller's Anesthesia.* 8th ed. Philadelphia: Saunders Elsevier; 2015:Fig. 24.20.)

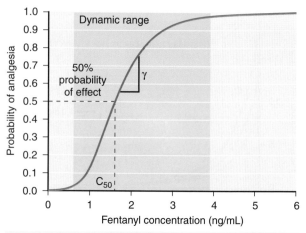

Fig. 4.20 A pharmacodynamic model for the analgesic effect of fentanyl. The *green area* represents the dynamic range, the concentration range where changes in concentration lead to a change in effect. Concentrations above or below the dynamic range do not lead to changes in drug effect. The C_{50} represents the concentration associated with 50% probability of analgesia. Gamma (γ) represents the slope of the curve in the dynamic range. (From Miller RD, Cohen NH, Eriksson LI, et al., eds. *Miller's Anesthesia.* 8th ed. Philadelphia: Saunders Elsevier; 2015:Fig. 24.21.)

Potency and Efficacy

Two important concepts are relevant to this relationship: potency and efficacy. Potency describes the amount of drug required to elicit an effect. The C_{50} is a common parameter used to describe potency. For drugs that have a concentration-versus-effect relationship that is shifted to the left (small C_{50}), the drug is considered to be more potent, and the reverse is true for drugs that have a concentration-versus-effect relationship shifted to the right. For example, as illustrated in Fig. 4.21, the analgesia C_{50} for some of the fentanyl congeners ranges from small for sufentanil (0.04 ng/mL) to large for alfentanil (75 ng/mL). Thus sufentanil is more potent than alfentanil.

Efficacy is a measure of drug effectiveness once it occupies a receptor. Similar drugs that work through the same receptor may have varying degrees of effectiveness despite having the same receptor occupancy. For example, with G protein–coupled receptors, some drugs may bind the receptor in such a way as to produce a more pronounced activation of second messengers, causing more of an effect than others. Drugs that achieve maximal effect are known as *full agonists* and those that have a less-than-maximal effect are known as *partial agonists.*

Anesthetic Drug Interactions

An average clinical anesthetic rarely consists of one drug, but rather a combination of drugs to achieve desired levels of hypnosis, analgesia, and muscle relaxation. Hypnotics, analgesics (also see Chapters 8 and 9),

1, the curve is sigmoid. Fig. 4.20 presents an example of this relationship: a fentanyl effect-site concentration–effect curve for analgesia. This example illustrates how C_{50} and γ characterize the concentration–effect relationship.

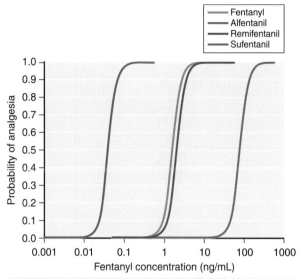

Fig. 4.21 Pharmacodynamic models for fentanyl congeners. The C_{50} for each drug is different, but the slope and maximal effect are similar.[45] (From Miller RD, Cohen NH, Eriksson LI, et al., eds. *Miller's Anesthesia*. 8th ed. Philadelphia: Saunders Elsevier; 2015:Fig. 24.22.)

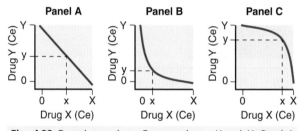

Fig. 4.22 Drug interactions. For two drugs, *X* and *Y*, *Panel A* represents additive, *Panel B* represents synergistic, and *Panel C* represents antagonistic interactions. Ce, Effect-site concentration. (From Miller RD, Cohen NH, Eriksson LI, et al., eds. *Miller's Anesthesia*. 8th ed. Philadelphia: Saunders Elsevier; 2015:Fig. 24.26.)

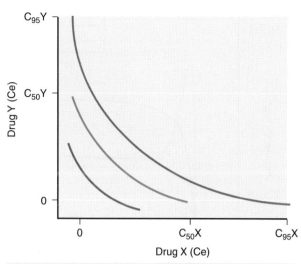

Fig. 4.23 Schematic illustration of isoeffect (isobole) lines. The *red, green,* and *blue lines* represent the 50% and 95% isoboles for a synergistic interaction between drugs *X* and *Y*. Isoboles represent concentration pairs with an equivalent effect. A set of 5%, 50%, and 95% isoboles can be used to describe the dynamic range of the concentrations for drugs *X* and *Y* for a given effect. As with single concentration effect curves, the ideal dosing leads to concentration pairs that are near the 95% isobole. Ce, Effect-site concentration. (From Miller RD, Cohen NH, Eriksson LI, et al., eds. *Miller's Anesthesia*. 8th ed. Philadelphia: Saunders Elsevier; 2015:Fig. 24.27.)

and muscle relaxants (also see Chapter 11) all interact with one another such that each drug, when administered in the presence of other drugs, rarely behaves as if it were administered alone. For example, when an analgesic is administered in the presence of a hypnotic, analgesia is more profound with the hypnotic than by itself, and hypnosis is more profound with the analgesic than by itself. Thus anesthesia is the practice of applied drug interactions. This phenomenon is likely a function of each class of drug exerting an effect on different receptors.

Substantial studies have been performed exploring how anesthetic drugs interact with one another. As illustrated in Fig. 4.22, interactions have been characterized as antagonistic, additive, and synergistic. When drugs that have an additive interaction are coadministered, their overall effect is the sum of the two individual effects. With antagonistic interactions, the overall effect is less than if the drug combination was additive; with synergistic interactions, the overall effect is greater than if the drug combination was additive.

A term used to characterize the continuum of drug concentrations across various combinations of drug pairs (X in combination with Y) is the isobole. The isobole is an isoeffect line for a selected probability of effect. A common isobole is the 50% isobole line. It represents all possible combinations of two-drug effect-site concentrations that would lead to a 50% probability of a given effect. Other isoboles are of more clinical interest. For example, the 95% isobole for loss of responsiveness represents the concentration pairs necessary to ensure a 95% probability of unresponsiveness. Similarly, the 5% isobole represents the concentration pairs having a low likelihood of that effect (i.e., most patients would be responsive). When formulating an anesthetic dosing regimen, dosing an anesthetic to achieve a probability of effect just above but not far beyond the 95% isobole is ideal (Fig. 4.23).

Several researchers have developed mathematical models that characterize anesthetic drug interactions in three dimensions. These models are known as *response surface models* and include effect-site concentrations for each drug in addition to a probability estimate of the overall effect. Fig. 4.24 presents the propofol–remifentanil interaction for loss of responsiveness as published by Bouillon and associates.[5] The response surface presents the full range of remifentanil–propofol isoboles (0%–100%) for loss of

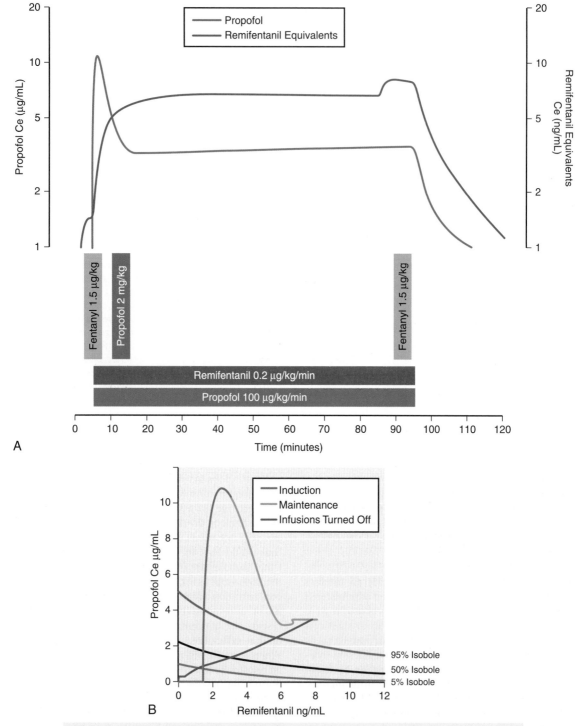

Fig. 4.24 Simulation of a 90-minute total intravenous anesthetic consisting of propofol bolus (2 mg/kg) and infusion (100 μg/kg/min), remifentanil infusion (0.2 μg/kg/min), and intermittent fentanyl boluses (1.5 μg/kg). (A) Resultant effect-site concentrations *(Ce)* are presented. (B) Predictions of loss of responsiveness are presented on a topographic (top-down) view.

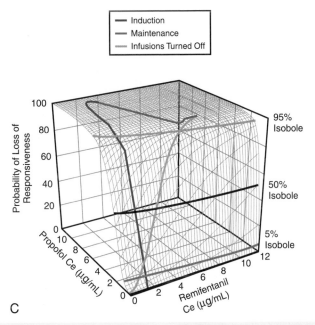

Fig. 4.24 cont'd (C) On a three-dimensional response surface plot, the *green, black,* and *yellow lines* represent the 5%, 50%, and 95% isoboles, respectively. Each isobole presents the propofol-remifentanil pairs that yield the same effect. The inward bow of the isoboles indicates that the interaction is synergistic. The isoboles are in close proximity to one another, indicating a steep transition from responsive to unresponsive. (From Miller RD, Cohen NH, Eriksson LI, et al., eds. *Miller's Anesthesia.* 8th ed. Philadelphia: Saunders Elsevier; 2015:Fig. 24.29. Author's representation based on data from Bouillon TW, Bruhn J, Radulescu L, et al. Pharmacodynamic interaction between propofol and remifentanil regarding hypnosis, tolerance of laryngoscopy, bispectral index, and electroencephalographic approximate entropy. *Anesthesiology.* 2004;100[6]:1353-1372.)

responsiveness. There are two common representations of the response surface model: the three-dimensional plot and the topographic plot. The topographic plot represents a top-down view of the response surface with drug concentrations on the vertical and horizontal axes. Drug effect is represented with selected isobole lines (i.e., 5%, 50%, and 95%).

Response surface models have been developed for a variety of anesthetic effects to include responses to verbal and tactile stimuli, painful stimuli, hemodynamic or respiratory effects, and changes in electrical brain activity. For example, with airway instrumentation, response surface models have been developed for loss of response to placing a laryngeal mask airway,[6] laryngoscopy,[7,8] tracheal intubation,[9] and esophageal instrumentation[10] for selected combinations of anesthetic drugs. Although many response surface models exist, there are several gaps in available models covering all common combinations of anesthetic drugs and various forms of stimuli encountered in the perioperative environment.

SPECIAL POPULATIONS

When formulating an anesthetic, many aspects of patient demographics and medical history need to be considered to determine the correct dose. Such factors include age; body habitus; gender; chronic exposure to opioids, benzodiazepines, or alcohol; presence of heart, lung, kidney, or liver disease; and the extent of blood loss or dehydration. Each of them can dramatically affect anesthetic drug kinetics and dynamics. How some patient characteristics (e.g., obesity) influence anesthetic drug behavior has been studied, whereas other patient characteristics remain difficult to assess (e.g., chronic opioid exposure). The findings are briefly summarized to characterize the pharmacokinetics and pharmacodynamics in a few unique special populations.

Influence of Obesity on Anesthetic Drugs

Obesity is a worldwide epidemic, and overweight patients frequently undergo anesthesia and surgery. Therefore anesthesia providers should be familiar with the pharmacologic alterations of anesthetics in obese individuals. In general, manufacturer dosing recommendations are scaled to kilograms of actual total body weight (TBW). However, anesthesia providers rarely use mg/kg dosing in obese patients for fear of administering an excessive dose (e.g., a 136-kg patient does not require twice as much drug as a patient of the same height who weighs 68 kg). Accordingly, researchers have developed several

Table 4.1 Common Weight Scalars

Scalar[a]	Equations
Ideal body weight	Male: 50 kg + 2.3 kg for each 2.54 cm (1 inch) over 152 cm (5 feet) Female: 45.5 kg + 2.3 kg for each 2.54 cm (1 inch) over 152 cm (5 feet)
Lean body mass	Male: $1.1 \times TBW - 128 \times (TBW/Ht)^2$ Female: $1.07 \times TBW - 148 \times (TBW/Ht)^2$
Fat-free mass[46]	Male: $(9.27 \times 10^3 \times TBW)/(6.68 \times 10^3 + 216 \times BMI)$ Female: $(9.27 \times 10^3 \times TBW)/(8.78 \times 10^3 + 244 \times BMI)$
Pharmacokinetic mass[24,25]	$52/(1 + [196.4 \times e^{-0.025\ TBW} - 53.66]/100)$ (fentanyl only)
Modified fat-free mass[13,47]	$FFM + 0.4^b (TBW - FFM)$

[a]Superscript numbers in this column indicate references at the end of the chapter.
[b]The dose/kg using IBW, TBW, or FFM in an obese person are all less than the dose/kg using TBW in a nonobese patient.
BMI, Body mass index; *FFM*, fat-free mass; *Ht*, height in centimeters; *IBW*, ideal body weight; *LBM*, lean body mass; *MFFM*, modified fat-free mass; *TBW*, total body weight in kg.

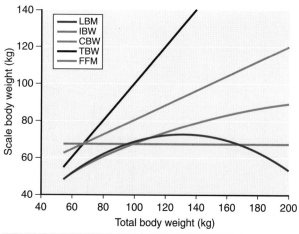

Fig. 4.25 Scaled weights as a function of total body weight *(TBW)*. Key points in this plot: IBW remains the same regardless of the TBW, and LBM starts to decline for weight increases above 127 kg. *CBW*, Corrected body weight; *FFM*, fat-free mass; *IBW*, ideal body weight; *LBM*, lean body mass (for a 40-year-old man, 176 cm tall). (From Miller RD, Cohen NH, Eriksson LI, et al., eds. *Miller's Anesthesia.* 8th ed. Philadelphia: Saunders Elsevier; 2015:Fig. 24.31.)

weight scalars in an attempt to avoid excessive dosing or underdosing in this patient population. Some of these scalars include lean body mass (LBM), ideal body weight (IBW), and fat-free mass (FFM). Table 4.1 presents the formulas used to estimate these weight scalars. Table 4.2 presents samples of the resultant scaled weight for a lean individual and an obese individual. In general, the aim of weight scalars is to match dosing regimens for obese patients with what is required for normal-size patients. These scaled weights are usually smaller than TBW in obese patients and thus help prevent excessive drug administration (Fig. 4.25). Scaled weights have been used in place of TBW for both bolus (mg/kg) and infusion (mg/kg/hr) dosing and for TCIs.

This section will discuss the pharmacologic alterations of select intravenous anesthetic drugs (propofol, remifentanil, and fentanyl) in obese patients, including shortcomings of weight scalars when used in bolus and continuous infusion dosing.

Propofol

The influence of obesity on propofol pharmacokinetics is becoming clearer (also see Chapter 8). Generally, in obese patients the blood distributes more to nonadipose than to adipose tissues, resulting in higher plasma drug concentrations in obese patients with mg/kg dosing than in normal patients with less adipose mass. Furthermore, propofol clearance increases because of the increased liver volume and liver blood flow associated with obesity (and increased cardiac output). Changes to volumes of distribution likely influence concentration peaks with bolus dosing, whereas changes in clearance likely influence concentrations during and after infusions. Various weight scalars in propofol bolus and continuous infusion dosing have been studied.

Table 4.2 Dosing Weights Based on Various Dosing Scalars

Dosing Scalar	Dosing Weight, 176-cm (6-foot)-Tall Male	
	68 kg BMI = 22	185 kg BMI = 60
Total body weight (TBW)	68	185
Ideal body weight (IBW)	72	72
Lean body mass (LBM)	56	62
Fat-free mass (FFM)	55	88
Modified fat-free mass (MFFM)	60	127

BMI, Body mass index (kg/m²).

Dosing Scalars for Propofol

Simulations of an infusion using various weight scalars are presented in Fig. 4.26. The simulations predict propofol effect-site concentrations from a 60-minute infusion

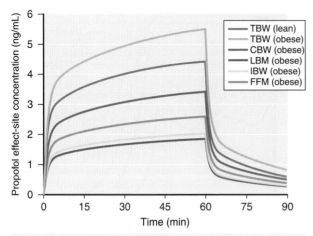

Fig. 4.26 Simulations of propofol plasma concentrations that result from a 60-minute infusion (10 mg/kg/hr [167 µg/kg/min]) to a 40-year-old man who is 176 cm tall. Simulations include the following dosing weights: total body weights (TBWs) of 68 kg and 185 kg (body mass indices of 22 and 60, respectively) and scaled weights for the 185-kg weight to include Servin's corrected body weight (CBW), lean body mass (LBM), ideal body weight (IBW), and fat-free mass (FFM). Key points: At the 185-kg weight, when dosed to TBW, the infusion leads to high propofol concentrations, whereas when dosed to IBW or LBM, the infusion leads to low propofol concentrations. When the 185-kg individual is dosed using CBW, it best approximates the propofol concentrations that result from TBW in a lean individual. (From Miller RD, Cohen NH, Eriksson LI, et al., eds. *Miller's Anesthesia.* 8th ed. Philadelphia: Saunders Elsevier; 2014:Fig. 24.32.)

(167 µg/kg/min) in a 176-cm (6-foot)-tall obese (185 kg) and lean (68 kg) male patient. If dosed according to TBW, peak plasma concentrations in the lean and obese individuals are different. The other weight scalars lead to much smaller concentrations with the infusion.

Of the many available dosing scalars, authors recommend LBM[11] for bolus dosing (i.e., during induction) and TBW or corrected body weight (CBW) for infusions.[9,12] For continuous infusions, other weight scalars are likely to result in inadequate dosing (most worrisome for LBM).

One concern with using TBW to dose continuous infusions (i.e., µg/kg/min) is drug accumulation. Prior investigations, however, do not support this assumption. Servin and colleagues[13] performed pharmacokinetic analyses of propofol administration to normal and obese patients using TBW and CBW. The CBW was defined as the IBW + 0.4 × (TBW – IBW).[11] They found similar concentrations at eye opening in both groups and absence of propofol accumulation in obese patients. However, some reports suggest that dosing infusions according to CBW may underdose morbidly obese patients.[12]

Other Sedatives

Only limited information is available on the behavior of other sedatives (i.e., midazolam, ketamine, etomidate, and barbiturates) in obese patients. Although not clinically validated in obese patients, bolus doses probably should be based on TBW, and use of other dosing scalars will lead to inadequate effect. For dexmedetomidine, dosing according to TBW can lead to excessive sedation and lower oxygen hemoglobin saturations in obese patients.[14] Clinical pharmacology research in obese patients suggests that the FFM scalar may be a better choice for bolus dosing.[15]

In contrast, continuous infusion rates should be dosed to IBW.[16] Remimazolam, an ultra-short-acting benzodiazepine, has recently become available. At this time, an appropriate selection of weight scalars in obese patients is unknown, which warrants future investigation.

Opioids
Remifentanil

The distribution volume and clearance of remifentanil are similar in lean and obese patients, largely because of its rapid metabolism by nonspecific esterases.[17] As with propofol, researchers have explored several scaled weights in an effort to optimize bolus dosing, continuous infusions, and TCIs.

Dosing Scalars

As described earlier, simulation is used to predict remifentanil effect-site concentrations and analgesic effect for a variety of scaled weights in a 174-cm-tall obese (185 kg, body mass index [BMI] of 60) individual and lean (68 kg, BMI of 22) individual (Fig. 4.27). Pharmacokinetic model parameters are estimated from an obese population, and pharmacodynamic model parameters are used to predict the probability of analgesia.[18,19] Several key points are illustrated in these simulations:

1. For an obese patient, dosing scaled to FFM or IBW resulted in almost identical remifentanil effect-site concentrations as in the lean patient dosed according to TBW. Unlike propofol, dosing remifentanil to CBW (red line, see Fig. 4.27A) leads to higher plasma concentrations compared with levels achieved when dosing to TBW in a lean individual.
2. Dosing scaled to LBM in the obese individual resulted in lower effect-site concentrations than those in a lean individual dosed according to TBW.
3. Dosing the obese individual to TBW was excessive.
4. All dosing scalars, except LBM, provided effect-site concentrations associated with a high probability of analgesia.

As can be appreciated in Fig. 4.27, LBM has substantial shortcomings in morbidly obese patients.[20] First, dosing remifentanil to LBM leads to plasma concentrations with a low probability of effect compared with the other dosing scalars. Second, with excessive weight (BMI over

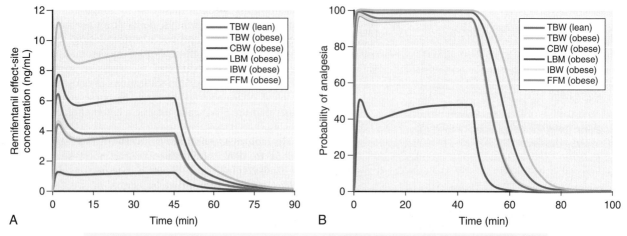

Fig. 4.27 Simulations of remifentanil effect-site concentrations (A) and analgesic effect (B) that result from a 1-μg/kg bolus and a 60-minute infusion at a rate of 0.15 μg/kg/min to a 40-year-old man who is 176 cm tall. Simulations include the following dosing weights: total body weights *(TBWs)* of 68 kg and 185 kg (body mass indices of 22 and 60, respectively) and scaled weights for the 185-kg weight to include Servin's corrected body weight *(CBW)*, lean body mass *(LBM)*, ideal body weight *(IBW)*, and fat-free mass *(FFM)*. Remifentanil effect-site concentrations and estimates of analgesic effect were estimated using published pharmacokinetic models (Kim et al., *Anesthesiology.* 2017;126:1019–1032 and Ref. 28). Analgesia was defined as loss of response to 30 psi of pressure on the anterior tibia.

40), LBM actually becomes smaller with increasing TBW, making it impractical to use (see Fig. 4.25). A modified LBM,[11] FFM eliminates the extremely low dosing weight problem.[21] In this simulation IBW also provides suitable effect-site concentrations, but this may not always be the case when using a weight scalar that is based only on patient height.

Fentanyl

Despite widespread use in the clinical arena, relatively little work has explored how obesity affects fentanyl pharmacokinetics (also see Chapter 9). Published fentanyl pharmacokinetic models[22,23] tend to overestimate fentanyl concentrations as TBW increases.[13] Investigators have[24,25] explored ways to improve predictions using published models by modifying demographic data (e.g., either height or weight). Recommendations include use of a modified weight, called the *pharmacokinetic mass,* to improve the predictive performance of one of the many available fentanyl kinetic models.

Other Opioids

Even less information regarding the impact of obesity on drug behavior is available for opioids other than remifentanil and fentanyl. Researchers have studied sufentanil in obese patients and found that its volume of distribution increases linearly with TBW,[26] and clearance was similar between lean and obese individuals. They recommend bolus dosing using TBW and "prudently reduced" dosing for continuous infusions. Although

no pharmacokinetic data are available for morphine in obese patients, one group of investigators measured morphine metabolites in morbidly obese patients.[27] They found that rate of morphine metabolism is not altered in morbidly obese patients, but the elimination of its metabolites is reduced. Specifically, there were increased levels of both morphine-3-glucuronide and morphine-6-glucuronide. Of note, the latter metabolite can cause sedation.

Inhaled Anesthetics

A widely held perception of volatile anesthetics (also see Chapter 7) is that they accumulate more in obese than in lean patients and that this leads to prolonged emergence. This concept, however, has not been confirmed.[28] Two phenomena contribute to this observation: first, blood flow to adipose tissue *decreases* with increasing obesity,[29] and second, the time required to fill adipose tissue with volatile anesthetics is long.

Influence of Increasing Age on Anesthetic Drug Pharmacology

Age is one of the most valuable covariates to consider when developing an anesthetic plan (also see Chapter 35). As with obesity, both remifentanil and propofol can serve as prototypes to understand how age influences anesthetic drug behavior. The influence of age on remifentanil and propofol is characterized in quantitative terms.[30–33]

With remifentanil, elderly patients require less drug to produce an opioid effect. The effectiveness of reduced doses in older patients is primarily a function of changes in pharmacodynamics, but may involve pharmacokinetic changes as well.[31] Based on previously published pharmacokinetic and pharmacodynamic models built from measurements over a wide age range,[30-33] simulations can be performed to explore how age may influence dosing. For example, to achieve equipotent doses in 20- and 80-year-olds, the dose for the 80-year-old should be reduced by 55%. A similar analysis for propofol recommends that the dose for an 80-year-old be reduced by 65% compared with that of a 20-year-old.

The mechanisms for these changes are not clear, especially for pharmacodynamic changes. One possible source of change in pharmacokinetic behavior may be the result of decreased cardiac output. Decreased cardiac output in the elderly[15] results in slower circulation and drug mixing. This may lead to high peak concentrations[15,34] and decreased drug delivery to metabolic organs and reduced clearance. Many intravenous anesthetics (propofol, thiopental, and etomidate) have slower clearance and a smaller volume of distribution.[30,35-37] in the elderly. Beyond age-related changes in cardiac output, other comorbid conditions may reduce cardiovascular function as well.[38] Taking this into account, anesthesia providers often consider a patient's "physiologic" age instead of solely relying on chronologic age.[39,40] For some older patients, such as those with no significant coexisting disease, normal body habitus, and good exercise tolerance, a substantial reduction in dose may not be warranted.

SUMMARY

This chapter reviewed basic principles of clinical pharmacology used to describe anesthetic drug behavior: pharmacokinetics, pharmacodynamics, and anesthetic drug interactions. These principles provide anesthesia practitioners with the information needed to make rational decisions about the selection and administration of anesthetics. From a practical aspect, these principles characterize the magnitude and time course of drug effect, but because of complex mathematics, they have limited clinical utility in everyday practice. Advances in computer simulation, however, have brought this capability to the point of real-time patient care. One of the most important advances in our understanding of clinical pharmacology is the development of interaction models that describe how different classes of anesthetic drugs influence one another. This knowledge is especially relevant to anesthesia providers, given that they rarely use just one drug when providing an anesthetic.

REFERENCES

1. Wilkinson GR, Shand DG. Commentary: a physiological approach to hepatic drug clearance. *Clin Pharmacol Ther.* 1975;18:377–390.
2. Krejcie TC, Avram MJ, Gentry WB, et al. A recirculatory model of the pulmonary uptake and pharmacokinetics of lidocaine based on analysis or arterial and mixed venous data from dogs. *J Pharmacokinet Biopharm.* 1997;25:169–190.
3. Youngs EJ, Shafer SL. Basic pharmacokinetic and pharmacodynamic principles. In: White PF, ed. *Textbook of Intravenous Anesthesia*: Baltimore: Williams & Wilkins; 1997.
4. Hughes MA, Glass PS, Jacobs JR. Context-sensitive half-time in multicompartment pharmacokinetic models for intravenous anesthetic drugs. *Anesthesiology.* 1992;76(3):334–341.
5. Bouillon TW, Bruhn J, Radulescu L, et al. Pharmacodynamic interaction between propofol and remifentanil regarding hypnosis, tolerance of laryngoscopy, bispectral index, and electroencephalographic approximate entropy. *Anesthesiology.* 2004;100(6):1353–1372.
6. Heyse B, Proost JH, Schumacher PM, et al. Sevoflurane remifentanil interaction: comparison of different response surface models. *Anesthesiology.* 2012;116(2):311–323.
7. Kern SE, Xie G, White JL, Egan TD. A response surface analysis of propofol-remifentanil pharmacodynamic interaction in volunteers. *Anesthesiology.* 2004;100(6):1373–1381.
8. Manyam SC, Gupta DK, Johnson KB, et al. Opioid-volatile anesthetic synergy: a response surface model with remifentanil and sevoflurane as prototypes. *Anesthesiology.* 2006;105(2):267–278.
9. Mertens MJ, Engbers FH, Burm AG, Vuyk J. Predictive performance of computer-controlled infusion of remifentanil during propofol/remifentanil anaesthesia. *Br J Anaesth.* 2003;90(2):132–141.
10. LaPierre CD, Johnson KB, Randall BR, et al. An exploration of remifentanil-propofol combinations that lead to a loss of response to esophageal instrumentation, a loss of responsiveness, and/or onset of intolerable ventilatory depression. *Anesth Analg.* 2011;113(3):490–499.
11. Albertin A, Poli D. La Colla L, et al. Predictive performance of "Servin's formula" during BIS-guided propofol-remifentanil target-controlled infusion in morbidly obese patients. *Br J Anaesth.* 2007;98(1):66–75.
12. Igarashi T, Nagata O, Iwakiri H, et al. Two cases of intraoperative awareness during intravenous anesthesia with propofol in morbidly obese patients. *Masui.* 2002;51(11):1243–1247.
13. Servin F, Farinotti R, Haberer JP, Desmonts JM. Propofol infusion for maintenance of anesthesia in morbidly obese patients receiving nitrous oxide. A clinical and pharmacokinetic study. *Anesthesiology.* 1993;78(4):657–665.
14. Xu B, Zhou D, Re L, et al. Pharmacokinetic and pharmacodynamics of intravenous dexmedetomidine in morbidly obese patients undergoing laparoscopic surgery. *J Anesth.* 2017;31(6):813.
15. Cortinez LI, Anderson BJ, Holford NHG, et al. Dexmedetomidine pharmacokinetics in the obese. *Eur J Clin Pharmacol.* 2015;71(12):1501–1508.
16. Greenblatt DJ, Abernethy DR, Locniskar A, et al. Effect of age, gender, and obesity on midazolam kinetics. *Anesthesiology.* 1984;61(1):27–35.
17. Upton RN, Ludbrook GL, Grant C, Martinez AM. Cardiac output is a determinant of the initial concentrations of propofol after

short-infusion administration. *Anesth Analg.* 1999;89(3):545–552.

18. Kim TK, Obara S, Egan TD, et al. Disposition of remifentanil in obesity: a new pharmacokinetic model incorporating the influence of body mass. *Anesthesiology.* 2017;126(6):1019–1032.

19. Johnson KB, Syroid ND, Gupta DK, et al. An evaluation of remifentanil propofol response surfaces for loss of responsiveness, loss of response to surrogates of painful stimuli and laryngoscopy in patients undergoing elective surgery. *Anesth Analg.* 2008;106(2):471–479.

20. La Colla L, Albertin A, La Colla G, et al. No adjustment vs. adjustment formula as input weight for propofol target-controlled infusion in morbidly obese patients. *Eur J Anaesthesiol.* 2009;26(5):362–369.

21. La Colla L, Albertin A, La Colla G, et al. Predictive performance of the "Minto" remifentanil pharmacokinetic parameter set in morbidly obese patients ensuing from a new method for calculating lean body mass. *Clin Pharmacokinet.* 2010;49(2):131–139.

22. Anderson BJ, Holford NH. Mechanistic basis of using body size and maturation to predict clearance in humans. *Drug Metab Pharmacokinet.* 2009;24(1):25–36.

23. Duffull SB, Dooley MJ, Green B, et al. A standard weight descriptor for dose adjustment in the obese patient. *Clin Pharmacokinet.* 2004;43(16):1167–1178.

24. Shibutani K, Inchiosa Jr. MA, Sawada K, Bairamian M. Accuracy of pharmacokinetic models for predicting plasma fentanyl concentrations in lean and obese surgical patients: derivation of dosing weight ("pharmacokinetic mass"). *Anesthesiology.* 2004;101(3):603–613.

25. Shibutani K, Inchiosa Jr. MA, Sawada K, Bairamian M. Pharmacokinetic mass of fentanyl for postoperative analgesia in lean and obese patients. *Br J Anaesth.* 2005;95(3):377–383.

26. Schwartz AE, Matteo RS, Ornstein E, et al. Pharmacokinetics of sufentanil in obese patients. *Anesth Analg.* 1991;73(6):790–793.

27. Hoogd S, Välitalo PAJ, Dahan A, et al. Influence of Morbid Obesity on the Pharmacokinetics of Morphine, Morphine-3-Glucuronide, and Morphine-6-Glucuronide. *Clin Pharmacokinet.* 2017;56(12):1577–1587.

28. Cortinez LI, Gambús P, Trocóniz IF, et al. Obesity does not influence the onset and offset of sevoflurane effect as measured by the hysteresis between sevoflurane concentration and bispectral index. *Anesth Analg.* 2011;113(1):70–76.

29. Lesser GT, Deutsch S. Measurement of adipose tissue blood flow and perfusion in man by uptake of ^{85}Kr. *J Appl Physiol.* 1967;23(5):621–630.

30. Schnider TW, Minto CF, Gambus PL, et al. The influence of method of administration and covariates on the pharmacokinetics of propofol in adult volunteers. *Anesthesiology.* 1998;88(5):1170–1182.

31. Minto CF, Schnider TW, Egan TD, et al. Influence of age and gender on the pharmacokinetics and pharmacodynamics of remifentanil. I. Model development. *Anesthesiology.* 1997;86(1):10–23.

32. Schnider TW, Minto CF, Shafer SL, et al. The influence of age on propofol pharmacodynamics. *Anesthesiology.* 1999;90(6):1502–1516.

33. Minto CF, Schnider TW, Shafer SL. Pharmacokinetics and pharmacodynamics of remifentanil. II. Model application.. *Anesthesiology.* 1997;86(1):24–33.

34. Krejcie TC, Avram MJ. What determines anesthetic induction dose? It's the front-end kinetics, doctor!. *Anesth Analg.* 1999;89(3):541–544.

35. Arden JR, Holley FO, Stanski DR. Increased sensitivity to etomidate in the elderly: initial distribution versus altered brain response. *Anesthesiology.* 1986;65(1):19–27.

36. Homer TD, Stanski DR. The effect of increasing age on thiopental disposition and anesthetic requirement. *Anesthesiology.* 1985;62:714–724.

37. Stanski DR, Maitre PO. Population pharmacokinetics and pharmacodynamics of thiopental: the effect of age revisited. *Anesthesiology.* 1990;72(3):412–422.

38. Rodeheffer RJ, Gerstenblith G, Becker LC, et al. Exercise cardiac output is maintained with advancing age in healthy human subjects: cardiac dilatation and increased stroke volume compensate for a diminished heart rate. *Circulation.* 1984;69(2):203–213.

39. Avram MJ, Krejcie TC, Henthorn TK. The relationship of age to the pharmacokinetics of early drug distribution: the concurrent disposition of thiopental and indocyanine green. *Anesthesiology.* 1990;72(3):403–411.

40. Williams TF. Aging or disease?. *Clin Pharmacol Ther.* 1987;42(6):663–665.

41. Lee S, Kim BH, Lim K, et al. Pharmacokinetics and pharmacodynamics of intravenous dexmedetomidine in healthy Korean subjects. *J Clin Pharm Ther.* 2012;37:698–703.

42. Hudson RJ, Bergstrom RG, Thomson IR, et al. Pharmacokinetics of sufentanil in patients undergoing abdominal aortic surgery. *Anesthesiology.* 1989;70:426–431.

43. Scott JC, Stanski DR. Decreased fentanyl and alfentanil dose requirements with age. A simultaneous pharmacokinetic and pharmacodynamic evaluation. *J Pharmacol Exp Ther.* 1987;240(1):159–166.

44. Doufas AG, Bakhshandeh M, Bjorksten AR, et al. Induction speed is not a determinant of propofol pharmacodynamics. *Anesthesiology.* 2004;101:1112–1121.

45. Egan TD, Muir KT, Hermann DJ, et al. The electroencephalogram (EEG) and clinical measures of opioid potency: defining the EEG-clinical potency relationship ("fingerprint") with application to remifentanil. *Int J Pharm Med.* 2001;15(1):11–19.

46. Janmahasatian S, Duffull SB, Ash S, et al. Quantification of lean bodyweight. *Clin Pharmacokinet.* 2005;44(10):1051–1065.

47. Cortinez LI, Anderson BJ, Penna A, et al. Influence of obesity on propofol pharmacokinetics: derivation of a pharmacokinetic model. *Br J Anaesth.* 2010;105(4):448–456.

5

CLINICAL CARDIAC AND PULMONARY PHYSIOLOGY

John Feiner, Wendy Smith

When it comes to direct, integrated, daily management of cardiac and pulmonary physiology, no specialty compares with anesthesiology.[1-3] A sound understanding of the separate and integrated fundamentals of cardiorespiratory physiology is essential for an anesthesia provider to rapidly manage both critical and common situations such as hypotension, arterial hypoxemia, hypercapnia, and high peak airway pressures. The knowledge and skills required to excel as anesthesia providers provide invaluable insight when facing novel physiologic and logistic conundrums, as evidenced by anesthesiologists during the COVID-19 pandemic.[4] This chapter reviews the basic tools and approaches every anesthesia provider must have in their armamentarium in order to provide safe, physiologically sound patient care. Although concepts are explained in discrete parts, the skilled anesthesia provider must also consider the integration and interdependence of multiple physiologic systems.

HEMODYNAMICS

Arterial Blood Pressure

Systemic arterial blood pressure and mean arterial pressure (MAP) are commonly monitored by anesthesia providers via a blood pressure cuff or an indwelling arterial cannula. Although treatment of chronic systemic hypertension is sometimes necessary, acute hypotension is more often encountered during anesthesia care. Hypotension varies from mild, clinically insignificant reductions in MAP from general anesthesia or regional anesthesia to life-threatening emergencies. Hypotension can be of sufficient magnitude to jeopardize organ perfusion, causing injury and an adverse outcome. Organs of most immediate concern are the heart and brain, followed by the kidneys, liver, and lungs. All have typical injury patterns associated with prolonged shock. Understanding the physiology behind hypotension is critical for diagnosis and treatment.

Intraoperative hemodynamic instability has long been thought to result in worse outcomes after surgery. In large retrospective studies intraoperative hypotension of even 5 minutes' duration (systolic blood pressure [SBP] <70 mm Hg, MAP <50 mm Hg, diastolic blood pressure [DBP] <30 mm Hg) is associated with increased postoperative morbidity and mortality risks.[5,6] In a large 2020 observational study of patients undergoing noncardiac surgery intraoperative hypotension was associated with acute kidney injury in those patients in higher-risk groups (based on American Society of Anesthesiologists [ASA] physical status and type of surgery).[7] Postoperative hypotension is also a risk factor for myocardial injury after noncardiac surgery.[8]

Physiologic Approach to Hypotension

This chapter will focus mainly on the physiology of the left ventricle (LV) in the discussion of hypotension. However, the contribution of the right ventricle (RV) and venous system is also important.[9] To assess and treat acute hypotension, it is logical to start with the MAP and to consider it as the product of its physiologic components:

$$MAP = SVR \times CO$$

where SVR is the systemic vascular resistance and CO is cardiac output. When faced with an inadequate MAP, one should consider which component is the primary culprit. Additionally, although the clinician's focus tends to be on MAP alone, the contributing pressures (e.g., SBP, DBP, and pulse pressure [PP = SBP – DBP]) also require attention and can provide invaluable information when formulating a differential diagnosis and treatment plan. The pulse pressure is created by the addition of stroke volume (SV) on top of the DBP within the compliant vascular tree. The aorta is responsible for most of this compliance. Increased pulse pressure can occur with an increased SV, but most often occurs because of the poor aortic compliance that accompanies aging (also see Chapter 35). Decreasing DBP can have more dramatic effects on SBP when vascular compliance is poor.

Systemic Vascular Resistance

Most drugs administered during general anesthesia and neuraxial regional anesthesia (also see Chapter 17) decrease SVR. Several pathologic conditions can produce profound reductions in SVR, including sepsis, anaphylaxis, spinal shock, and reperfusion of ischemic organs. The calculation for SVR is as follows:

$$SVR = 80 \times (MAP - CVP)/CO$$

where CVP is the central venous pressure, and the factor 80 converts units into dyne/s/cm^5 from pressure in millimeters of mercury (mm Hg) and CO given in liters per minute (L/min).

Pulmonary artery (PA) catheterization can be used to obtain the measurements necessary for calculating SVR, but this monitor is not usually immediately available. Signs of adequate perfusion (e.g., warm extremities, good pulse oximeter plethysmograph waveform and perfusion index) may sometimes be present when hypotension is caused by low SVR. On the other hand, hypertension nearly always involves excessive vasoconstriction.[1]

According to Poiseuille's law, resistance is inversely proportional to the fourth power of the radius of a vessel. Individually, small vessels offer a very high resistance to flow. However, total SVR is decreased when there are many vessels arranged in parallel. Capillaries, despite being the smallest blood vessels, are not responsible for most of the SVR because there are so many in parallel. Most of the resistance to blood flow on the arterial side of the circulation is in the arterioles.

Cardiac Output

As a cause of hypotension, decreased CO may be more difficult to treat than decreased SVR. Increased CO is not usually associated with systemic hypertension, and most hyperdynamic states, such as sepsis and liver failure, are associated with decreased systemic blood pressure, which may lead to falsely believing the issue is low SVR alone.

CO is defined as the amount of blood (in liters) pumped by the heart in 1 minute. Although the amount of blood pumped by the right side and left side of the heart can differ in the presence of certain congenital heart malformations, these amounts are usually the same. CO is the product of heart rate (HR) and SV, the net amount of blood ejected by the heart in one cycle:

$$CO = HR \times SV$$

HR is an obvious determinant, as are the components of SV: preload, afterload, and contractility, which must all be considered when determining the cause of hypotension. CO can be measured clinically by thermodilution via a PA catheter and by transesophageal echocardiography (TEE). Less invasive devices to measure CO have been developed, including esophageal Doppler and pulse contour analysis (also see Chapter 20). Because the normal CO changes according to body size, cardiac index (CO divided by body surface area) is often used.

Heart Rate

Tachycardia and bradycardia can cause hypotension if CO is decreased. The electrocardiogram (ECG), pulse oximetry, or physical examination can identify the presence

---

[1]Perfusion index is a measure of the pulsatile signal relative to the background absorption and is an important measure of signal strength.

of bradycardia or tachycardia. A determination of rhythm and an understanding of how rhythm affects filling pressures are essential for analyzing HR and its potential effects on hypotension. Loss of sinus rhythm and atrial contraction results in decreased ventricular filling. Atrial contraction constitutes a significant percentage of preload, even more so in patients with a poorly compliant ventricle. A slow HR may result in enhanced ventricular filling and an increased SV, but an excessively slow HR results in an inadequate CO in the setting of a stiff ventricle, making CO more HR dependent. Tachycardia may result in insufficient time for the LV to fill and result in low CO and hypotension.

Ejection Fraction and Stroke Volume

Ejection fraction (EF) is the percentage of ventricular blood volume that is pumped by the heart in a single contraction (SV/end-diastolic volume [EDV]). Unlike SV, the EF does not differ based on body size, and an EF of 60% to 70% is considered normal. Hyperdynamic states such as sepsis and cirrhosis are reflected by an increased EF. Poor cardiac function is indicated by a reduced EF. Because CO can be maintained by increasing HR, the SV should be calculated to better assess cardiac function. However, with chronic dilated cardiomyopathy, the SV can improve despite the smaller EF.

Preload

Preload refers to the amount the cardiac muscle is "stretched" before contraction. Preload is best defined clinically as the EDV of the heart, which can be measured directly with TEE. Filling pressures (e.g., left atrial [LA] pressure, pulmonary capillary wedge pressure [PCWP], pulmonary artery diastolic [PAD] pressure) can also assess preload. CVP measures filling pressures on the right side of the heart, which correlates with filling pressures on the left side of the heart in the absence of pulmonary disease and when cardiac function is normal. By using a balloon to stop flow in a PA, pressure equilibrates within the system so that PCWP is nearly equivalent to LA pressure and reflects the filling pressure of the left side of the heart. The relationship between pressure and volume of the heart in diastole is depicted by ventricular compliance curves (Fig. 5.1). With a poorly compliant heart, normal filling pressures may not produce an adequate EDV. Likewise, trying to fill a "stiff" LV to a normal volume may increase intracardiac and pulmonary capillary pressures excessively.

Frank–Starling Mechanism

The Frank–Starling mechanism, a physiologic description of the increased pumping action of the heart with increased filling to an ideal volume, highlights the importance of preload. For a given ventricle, achievement of the ideal preload results in increased contraction necessary to eject added ventricular volume, resulting in a larger SV and similar EF. Reduced ventricular filling, as

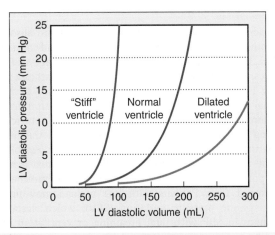

Fig. 5.1 The pressure–volume relationship of the heart in diastole is shown in the compliance curves plotting left ventricular (LV) diastolic volume versus pressure. The "stiff" heart shows a steeper rise of pressure with increased volume than the normal heart. The dilated ventricle shows a much more compliant curve.

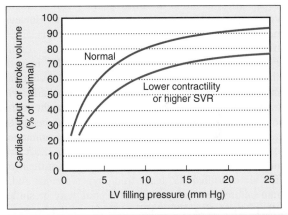

Fig. 5.2 The cardiac function curve shows the typical relationship between preload, represented by left ventricular (LV) filling pressure, and cardiac function, reflected in cardiac output or stroke volume. Filling pressure can be measured as left atrial pressure or pulmonary capillary wedge pressure. At low preload, augmentation of filling results in significantly increased cardiac output. This is the steeper portion of the curve. At higher LV filling pressures, little improvement in function occurs with increased preload, and with overfilling, a decrement in function can occur because of impaired perfusion (not shown). Lower contractility or higher systemic vascular resistance (SVR) shifts the normal curve to the right and downward.

in hypovolemia, results in reduced SV. Small increases in preload may have dramatic effects ("volume responsiveness") on SV and CO (Fig. 5.2). At higher points on the curve, little additional benefit is derived from increases in preload; for patients with heart failure, the increase in preload can be detrimental.

Causes of Low Preload

Causes of low preload can be broken down into absolute (hypovolemia) and relative (venodilation and obstruction). Hypovolemia may result from hemorrhage or fluid losses. Venodilation occurs with general anesthesia and may be even more prominent in the presence of neuraxial anesthesia (also see Chapter 17). Tension pneumothorax and pericardial tamponade prevent ventricular filling because of increased pressure around the heart, obstructing blood flow and preventing the establishment of appropriate filling pressures.[10] Thus cardiac tamponade may exist even in the setting of normal or increased CVP. Patients with low preload may manifest systolic pressure variation (SPV), which describes changes in SBP with tidal breathing or ventilation that can be observed on an arterial blood pressure tracing[11] (also see Chapter 20). The extreme form of this is pulsus paradoxus, a marked decrease in SBP during the inspiratory phase of tidal breathing. Pulse pressure variation (PPV) [$(PP_{peak} - PP_{nadir})/PP_{average}$] is analogous to SPV but requires computer calculation. Both SPV and PPV are also useful in identifying hypovolemia and are more sensitive and specific indicators of intravascular volume responsiveness than filling pressures such as CVP. However, when using low tidal volume ventilation, especially in patients with poor lung compliance (e.g., acute respiratory distress syndrome [ARDS]), SPV and PPV may not reliably predict fluid responsiveness unless tidal volume is temporarily increased (so-called *tidal volume challenge*).[12]

Additionally, pathologic problems on the right side of the heart may prevent filling of the LV. Right heart failure, pulmonary embolism, and other causes of pulmonary hypertension may prevent the right side of the heart from pumping a sufficient volume to fill the left side of the heart. With an overfilled RV (e.g., from hypervolemia and/or pump failure), the interventricular septum may be shifted, further constricting filling of the left side of the heart.

Contractility

Contractility, or the inotropic state of the heart, is a measure of the force of contraction independent of loading conditions (preload or afterload). It can be measured for research purposes by the rate at which pressure develops in the cardiac ventricles (dP/dT) or by systolic pressure–volume relationships (Fig. 5.3). Decreased myocardial contractility, alone or in conjunction with other causes discussed in this section, should be considered in the differential diagnosis of hypotension (Box 5.1).[13]

Afterload

Afterload is the resistance to ejection of blood from the LV with each contraction. For our purposes, afterload is largely determined by SVR and myocardial wall stress. When SVR is increased beyond normal values (900 to 1440 dyn/s/cm^{-5}), the heart does not empty as completely, resulting in a lower SV, EF, and CO (see Fig. 5.2).

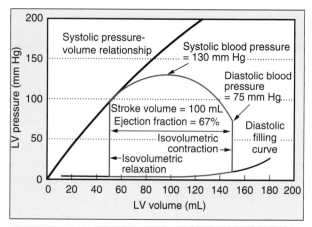

Fig. 5.3 The closed loop (*red line*) shows a typical cardiac cycle. Diastolic filling occurs along the typical diastolic curve from a volume of 50 mL to an end-diastolic volume (EDV) of 150 mL. Isovolumetric contraction increases the pressure in the left ventricle (LV) until it reaches the pressure in the aorta (at diastolic blood pressure) and the aortic valve opens. The LV then ejects blood, and volume decreases. Pressure in the LV and aorta reaches a peak at some point during ejection (systolic blood pressure), and the pressure then drops until the point at which the aortic valve closes (roughly the dicrotic notch). The LV relaxes without changing volume (isovolumetric relaxation). When the pressure decreases below left atrial pressure, the mitral valve opens, and diastolic filling begins. The plot shows a normal cycle, and the stroke volume (SV) is 100 mL, ejection fraction (EF) is SV/EDV = 67%, and blood pressure is 130/75 mm Hg. The systolic pressure–volume relationship (*black line*) can be constructed from a family of curves under different loading conditions (i.e., different preload) and reflects the inotropic state of the heart.

Box 5.1 Conditions Associated With Decreased Myocardial Contractility as a Cause of Hypotension

Myocardial ischemia
Anesthetic drugs
Cardiomyopathy
Previous myocardial infarction
Valvular heart disease (decreased stroke volume independent of preload)

High SVR also increases cardiac filling pressures, which may contribute to increased cardiac ischemia (described later) and increased wall stress. Wall stress is described using the law of Laplace: wall stress = P × r/T. In this equation P = ventricular transmural pressure, r = ventricular radius, and T = ventricular wall thickness. Low SVR improves SV and increases CO such that a low SVR is often associated with a higher CO (Fig. 5.4).

However, low SVR may also decrease cardiac filling pressures. This finding may suggest that preload rather than afterload is the cause of hypotension. Low SVR allows more extensive emptying and a lower end-systolic

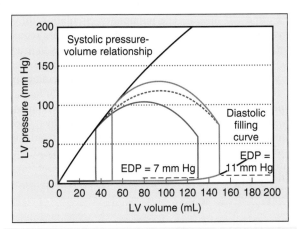

Fig. 5.4 Changes in the cardiac cycle that can occur with vasodilatation are depicted. The cycle in *green* is the same cycle shown in Fig. 5.3. The *red dashed line* suggests the transition to the new cardiac cycle shown in blue. The systolic blood pressure has decreased to 105 mm Hg. The end-systolic volume has decreased, as has the end-diastolic volume. End-diastolic pressure (EDP) has decreased from 11 to 7 mm Hg in this example. The ejection fraction is slightly increased; however, the stroke volume may decrease, but with restoration of left ventricular (LV) filling pressures to the same level as before, the stroke volume will be higher.

volume (ESV), one of the hallmarks of low SVR on TEE. With the same venous return, the heart does not fill to the same EDV, resulting in lower left ventricular filling pressures (see Fig. 5.4). A similar process occurs when the SVR is increased. Such stress-induced increases in cardiac filling pressures are more pronounced in patients with poor cardiac function. For any given patient, the goal is to find the SVR at which filling pressures allow the ventricle to operate on the most efficient portion of the Starling curve while not providing excessive afterload.

CARDIAC REFLEXES

The cardiovascular regulatory system consists of peripheral and central receptor systems that can detect various physiologic states, a central "integratory" system in the brainstem, and neurohumoral output to the heart and vascular system. A clinical understanding of cardiac reflexes is based on the concept that the cardiovascular system in the brainstem integrates the signal and provides a response through the autonomic nervous system.

Autonomic Nervous System (Also See Chapter 6)

The heart and vascular systems are controlled by the autonomic nervous system. Sympathetic and parasympathetic efferents innervate the sinoatrial and atrioventricular nodes. Sympathetic nervous system stimulation increases HR through activation of β_1-adrenergic receptors.

Parasympathetic nervous system stimulation can profoundly slow HR through stimulation of muscarinic acetylcholine receptors in the sinoatrial and atrioventricular nodes, whereas parasympathetic nervous system suppression contributes to increased HR. Conduction through the atrioventricular node is increased and decreased by sympathetic and parasympathetic nervous system innervation, respectively. Sympathetic nervous system stimulation increases myocardial contractility. Parasympathetic nervous system stimulation may decrease myocardial contractility slightly, but it has its major effect through decreasing HR.

Baroreceptors

Baroreceptors in the carotid sinus and aortic arch are activated by increased systemic blood pressure that stimulates stretch receptors to send signals through the vagus and glossopharyngeal nerves to the central nervous system. The sensitivity of baroreceptors to systemic blood pressure changes varies and is significantly altered by long-standing essential hypertension. A typical response to acute hypertension is increased parasympathetic nervous system stimulation that decreases HR. Vagal stimulation and decreases in sympathetic nervous system activity also decrease myocardial contractility and cause reflex vasodilatation. This carotid sinus reflex can be used therapeutically to produce vagal stimulation that may be an effective treatment for supraventricular tachycardia.

The atria and ventricles are innervated by a variety of sympathetic and parasympathetic receptor systems. Atrial stretch (i.e., Bainbridge reflex) can increase HR, which may help match CO to venous return.

Stimulation of the chemoreceptors in the carotid sinus has respiratory and cardiovascular effects. Arterial hypoxemia results in sympathetic nervous system stimulation. The sympathetic response is a major factor in tolerance of mild to moderate hypoxemia.[14] However, it is notable that more profound and prolonged arterial hypoxemia can result in bradycardia, possibly through central mechanisms. A variety of other reflexes causing bradycardia include increased ocular pressure (i.e., oculocardiac reflex), bradycardia with stretch of abdominal viscera, and the Cushing reflex (bradycardia in response to increased intracranial pressure).

Many anesthetics blunt cardiac reflexes in a dose-dependent fashion, with the result that sympathetic nervous system responses to hypotension are reduced. The blunting of such reflexes represents an additional mechanism by which anesthetic drugs contribute to hypotension.

CORONARY BLOOD FLOW

The coronary circulation is unique in that a larger percentage of oxygen is extracted by the heart than in any other vascular bed, up to 60% to 70%, compared with the 25% extraction for the body as a whole. The consequence of this physiology is that the heart cannot increase oxygen extraction as a reserve mechanism. In cases of threatened oxygen supply vasodilatation to increase blood flow is the primary compensatory mechanism of the heart.

Coronary reserve is the ability of the coronary circulation to increase flow more than the baseline state. Endogenous regulators of coronary blood flow include adenosine, nitric oxide, and adrenergic stimulation. With coronary artery stenosis, compensatory vasodilatation downstream can maintain coronary blood flow until about 90% stenosis, when coronary reserve begins to become exhausted.

The perfusion pressure of a vascular bed is usually calculated as the difference between MAP and venous pressure, based on the Hagen–Poiseuille law:

$$Q = (P_1 - P_2)/R$$

where Q is flow, P_1 is upstream pressure, P_2 is downstream pressure, and R is resistance. Instantaneous flow through the coronary arteries varies throughout the cardiac cycle, peaking during systole. The heart is fundamentally different from other organs because the myocardial wall tension developed during systole can completely stop blood flow in the subendocardium. The LV is therefore perfused predominantly during diastole. The end-diastolic pressure in the left ventricle (LVEDP) may exceed CVP and represents the effective downstream pressure. Perfusion pressure to most of the LV is therefore DBP minus LVEDP. Thus elevated LVEDP, as is seen in decompensated heart failure or extreme volume overload, may be associated with coronary ischemic events. The RV, with its lower intramural pressure, is perfused during diastole and systole.

PULMONARY CIRCULATION

The pulmonary circulation includes the RV, PAs, pulmonary capillary bed, and pulmonary veins, ending in the left atrium. The bronchial circulation supplies nutrients to lung tissue and empties into the pulmonary veins and left atrium. The pulmonary circulation differs substantially from the systemic circulation in its regulation, normal pressures (Table 5.1), and responses to drugs. Use of a PA catheter to measure pressures in the pulmonary circulation requires a fundamental understanding of their normal values and their meaning. Pulmonary hypertension has idiopathic causes and may accompany several common diseases (e.g., cirrhosis of the liver, sleep apnea). It is associated with significant anesthetic-related morbidity and mortality rates and, like many disease states, requires a sound understanding of cardiopulmonary physiology to mitigate complications (also see Chapter 26).

Pulmonary Artery Pressure

Pulmonary artery pressure (PAP) is much lower than systemic pressure because of low pulmonary vascular resistance (PVR). Like the systemic circulation, the pulmonary circulation accepts the entire CO and must adapt its resistance to meet different conditions.

Pulmonary Vascular Resistance

Determinants of PVR are different from SVR in the systemic circulation. During blood flow through the pulmonary circulation, resistance is thought to occur in the larger vessels, small arteries, and capillary bed. Vessels within the alveoli and the extraalveolar vessels respond differently to forces within the lung.

The most useful physiologic model for describing changes in the pulmonary circulation is the *distention* of capillaries and the *recruitment* of new capillaries. The distention and recruitment of capillaries explain the changes in PVR in a variety of circumstances. Increased PAP causes distention and recruitment of capillaries, increasing the cross-sectional area and decreasing PVR. Increased CO also decreases PVR through distention and recruitment. The reciprocal changes between CO and PVR maintain fairly constant pulmonary pressures over a wide range of CO values in nonpathologic states.

Just as cardiac contraction can affect coronary blood flow, alveolar distension can affect pulmonary blood flow.

Table 5.1	Normal Values for Pressures in the Venous and Pulmonary Arterial Systems				
Value	CVP (mm Hg)	PAS (mm Hg)	PAD (mm Hg)	PAM (mm Hg)	PCWP (mm Hg)
Normal	2–8	15–30	4–12	9–16	4–12
High	>12	>30	>12	>25	>12
Pathologic	>18	>40	>20	>35	>20

CVP, Central venous pressure; *PAD*, pulmonary artery diastolic pressure; *PAM*, pulmonary artery mean pressure; *PAS*, pulmonary artery systolic pressure; *PCWP*, pulmonary capillary wedge pressure.

Lung volumes have different effects on intraalveolar and extraalveolar vessels. With large lung volumes, intraalveolar vessels can be compressed, whereas extraalveolar vessels have lower resistance. The opposite is true at very small lung volumes. Therefore higher PVR can occur at both large and small lung volumes. Increased PVR at small lung volumes helps to divert blood flow from collapsed alveoli, such as during one-lung ventilation.

Sympathetic nervous system stimulation can cause pulmonary vasoconstriction, but the effect is not large, in contrast to the systemic circulation, in which neurohumoral influence is the primary regulator of vascular tone. The pulmonary circulation has therefore been very difficult to treat with drugs. Previously, the mainstay of treatment included nitric oxide, an important regulator of vascular tone delivered by inhalation, in addition to prostaglandins and phosphodiesterase inhibitors (e.g., sildenafil), which are both pulmonary vasodilators. Although advances in pharmacologic treatments have been made and new receptors can be targeted (e.g., endothelin receptor antagonists, guanylate cyclase stimulators, and prostacyclins), effective pulmonary hypertension treatment remains challenging.[15]

Hypoxic Pulmonary Vasoconstriction

Hypoxic pulmonary vasoconstriction (HPV) is the pulmonary vascular response to a low alveolar oxygen partial pressure (P_{AO_2}). In many patients HPV is an important adaptive response that improves gas exchange by diverting blood away from poorly ventilated areas, decreasing shunt fraction. Normal regions of the lung can easily accommodate the additional blood flow without increasing PAP. Global alveolar hypoxia, such as occurs with apnea or at high altitude, can cause significant HPV and increased PAP.

Anesthetic drugs such as the potent inhaled anesthetics can impair HPV, whereas commonly used intravenous drugs, such as propofol and opioids, demonstrate no inhibition of HPV. Calcium channel blockers may blunt HPV in the setting of preexisting V/Q mismatch.[16] During surgical procedures requiring one-lung ventilation, HPV may play a role in the resolution of hypoxemia, although many other factors are also important, including acid–base status, CO, development of atelectasis, and concomitant drug administration[17] (also see Chapter 27).

Pulmonary Emboli

Pulmonary emboli obstruct blood vessels, increasing the overall resistance to blood through the pulmonary vascular system. Common forms of emboli are blood clots and air, but they also include amniotic fluid, carbon dioxide, and fat emboli.

Arteriolar Thickening

Arteriolar thickening occurs in several clinical circumstances. It is associated with certain types of long-standing congenital heart disease. Primary pulmonary hypertension is an idiopathic disease associated with arteriolar hyperplasia. Similar changes are associated with cirrhosis of the liver (i.e., portopulmonary hypertension).

Zones of the Lung

A useful concept in pulmonary hemodynamics is West's zones of the lung. Gravity determines the way pressures change in the vascular system relative to the measurement at the level of the heart. These differences are small compared with arterial pressures, but for venous pressure and PAP, these differences are clinically significant. Every 20 cm of change in height produces a 15-mm Hg pressure difference. This can create significant positional differences in PAP that affect blood flow in the lung in various positions, such as upright and lateral positions.

In zone 1 airway pressures exceed PAP and pulmonary venous pressures. Zone 1 therefore has no blood flow despite ventilation. Normally, zone 1 does not exist, but with positive-pressure ventilation or low PAP, as may occur under anesthesia or with blood loss, zone 1 may develop. In zone 2 airway pressure is more than pulmonary venous pressure, but it is not more than PAP. In zone 2 flow is proportional to the difference between PAP and airway pressure. In zone 3 PAP and venous pressure exceed airway pressure, and a normal blood flow pattern results (i.e., flow is proportional to the difference between PAP and venous pressure). Position can also be used therapeutically to decrease blood flow to abnormal areas of the lung, such as unilateral pneumonia, and thereby improve gas exchange. Blood flow through the collapsed lung during one-lung ventilation is also reduced by this physiologic effect.

Pulmonary Edema

Intravascular fluid balance in the lung depends on hydrostatic driving forces. Excessive pulmonary capillary pressures cause fluid to leak into the interstitium and then into alveoli. Although the pulmonary lymphatic system is very effective in clearing fluid, it can be overwhelmed. Hydrostatic pulmonary edema is expected with high left ventricular filling pressures. Pulmonary edema occurs as PCWP exceeds 20 mm Hg, although patients may tolerate even higher pressures if these pressures persist chronically. Pulmonary edema can also occur with "capillary leak" from lung injury, such as acid aspiration of gastric contents, sepsis, or blood transfusion.

PULMONARY GAS EXCHANGE

Oxygen

Oxygen must pass from the environment to the tissues, where it is consumed during aerobic metabolism. Arterial hypoxemia is defined as a low partial pressure of oxygen

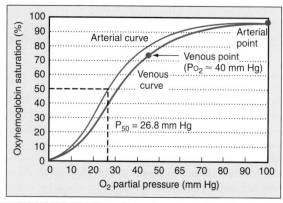

Fig. 5.5 The oxyhemoglobin dissociation curve is S-shaped and relates oxygen partial pressure to the oxyhemoglobin saturation. A typical arterial curve is shown in *red*. The higher Pco_2 and the lower pH of venous blood cause a rightward shift of the curve and facilitate unloading of oxygen in the tissues (*blue*). Normal adult P_{50}, the Po_2 at which hemoglobin is 50% saturated, is shown (26.8 mm Hg). Normal Pao_2 of about 100 mm Hg results in an Sao_2 of about 98%. Normal Pvo_2 is about 40 mm Hg, resulting in a saturation of about 75%.

Table 5.2	Events That Shift the Oxyhemoglobin Dissociation Curve	
Left Shift		**Right Shift**
(P_{50} <26.8 mm Hg)		(P_{50} >26.8 mm Hg)
Alkalosis		Acidosis
Hypothermia		Hyperthermia
Decreased 2,3-diphosphoglycerate (stored blood)		Increased 2,3-diphosphoglycerate (chronic arterial hypoxemia or anemia)

P_{50}, Po_2 value at which hemoglobin is 50% saturated with oxygen.

in arterial blood (Pao_2). An arbitrary definition of arterial hypoxemia (Pao_2 < 60 mm Hg) is commonly used but not necessary. Occasionally, arterial hypoxemia is used to describe a Pao_2 that is low relative to what might be expected based on the inspired oxygen concentration (Fio_2). Arterial hypoxemia (which reflects pulmonary gas exchange and denotes low oxygen in the blood) is distinguished from hypoxia—low oxygen content in tissues—which reflects circulatory factors.

Mild and even moderate arterial hypoxemia (e.g., at high altitude) can be well tolerated and is not usually associated with substantial injury or adverse outcomes. Anoxia, a nearly complete lack of oxygen, is potentially fatal and is often associated with permanent neurologic injury, depending on its duration. Arterial hypoxemia is most significant when anoxia is threatened, such as with apnea, and the difference between the two may be less than 1 minute.

Measurements of Oxygenation
Measurements of arterial blood oxygen levels include Pao_2, oxyhemoglobin saturation (Sao_2), and arterial oxygen content (Cao_2). Pao_2 and Sao_2 are related through the oxyhemoglobin dissociation curve (Fig. 5.5). Understanding the oxyhemoglobin dissociation curve is facilitated by the ability to measure continuous oxyhemoglobin saturation with pulse oximetry (Spo_2) and measurement of Pao_2 with arterial blood gas analysis.

Oxyhemoglobin Dissociation Curve
Rightward and leftward shifts of the oxyhemoglobin dissociation curve provide significant homeostatic adaptations

to changing oxygen availability. P_{50}, the Po_2 at which hemoglobin is 50% saturated with oxygen, is a measurement of the position of the oxyhemoglobin dissociation curve (see Fig. 5.5 and Table 5.2). The normal P_{50} value of adult hemoglobin is 26.8 mm Hg. Other points on the curve, such as the normal venous point and points for 80% and 90% oxygen saturations, may also be clinically useful.

As Fig. 5.5 shows, clinical implications of rightward and leftward shifts are more significant as Sao_2 values decrease below 100 mm Hg. Therefore a rightward shift causes little change in conditions for loading oxygen (essentially the same Sao_2 at Po_2 of 100 mm Hg), but it allows larger amounts of oxygen to dissociate from hemoglobin in the tissues where the Sao_2 is lower. This improves tissue oxygenation. Carbon dioxide and metabolic acid shift the oxyhemoglobin dissociation curve rightward, whereas alkalosis shifts it leftward. It should be noted that fetal hemoglobin is intrinsically left shifted, an adaptation uniquely suited to placental physiology (also see Chapter 33).

Oxygen in arterial blood is carried in two ways: bound to hemoglobin and dissolved in the plasma. The blood oxygen content is the sum of the two forms. Although amounts of dissolved oxygen are trivial at normal Po_2 levels, at high Fio_2 dissolved oxygen can be physiologically and clinically important. Although under normal conditions only a fraction (25%) of the oxygen on hemoglobin is used, all the dissolved oxygen, added while giving supplemental oxygen, can be used.

Arterial Oxygen Content
Cao_2 is calculated based on Sao_2 and partial pressure plus the hemoglobin concentration (Fig. 5.6):

$$Cao_2 = Sao_2 (Hb \times 1.39) + 0.003 (Pao_2)$$

In the equation Hb is the hemoglobin level, 1.39 is the capacity of hemoglobin for oxygen (1.39 mL of O_2/g of Hb fully saturated), and 0.003 mL O_2/dL/mm Hg is the solubility of oxygen. For example, if Hb = 15 g/dL and

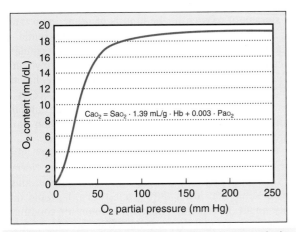

Fig. 5.6 The relationship between Pao_2 and oxygen content is also sigmoidal because most of the oxygen is bound to hemoglobin. Oxygen content at the plateau of the curve ($Po_2 > 100$ mm Hg) continues to rise because dissolved oxygen still contributes a small, but not negligible, quantity. *Hb*, Hemoglobin.

$Pao_2 = 100$ mm Hg, resulting in nearly 100% saturation, the value of Cao_2 is calculated as follows:

$$CaO_2 = 1.00\,(15 \times 1.39) + 0.003\,(100)$$
$$= 20.85 + 0.3$$
$$= 21.15\,\text{mL/dL}$$

Dissolved oxygen can continue to provide additional Cao_2, which can be clinically significant, with Fio_2 of 1.0 and with hyperbaric oxygen. The oxygen cascade depicts the passage of oxygen from the atmosphere to the tissues (Fig. 5.7).

Multiwavelength Pulse Oximetry

Complete measurement of oxygen parameters is derived not just from analysis of arterial blood gases (Pao_2) but also from multiwavelength pulse oximetry. Oximetry provides measurement of methemoglobin (MetHb) and carboxyhemoglobin (COHb). Most blood gas machines are now combined with oximeters so that the Sao_2 provided is a true measured value, not calculated. This is called the *functional saturation*, which is the percentage of oxyhemoglobin saturation relative to hemoglobin available to bind oxygen. The *fractional saturation* is relative to all hemoglobin. Therefore fractional saturation is the functional saturation minus MetHb and COHb. Newer pulse oximeters can now also measure MetHb and COHb.

Determinants of Alveolar Oxygen Partial Pressure

The alveolar gas equation describes transfer of oxygen from the environment into the alveoli:

$$PAO_2 = FIO_2 \times (PB - PH_2O) - PCO_2/RQ$$

where PB is the barometric pressure, PH_2O is the vapor pressure of water (47 mm Hg at normal body temperature

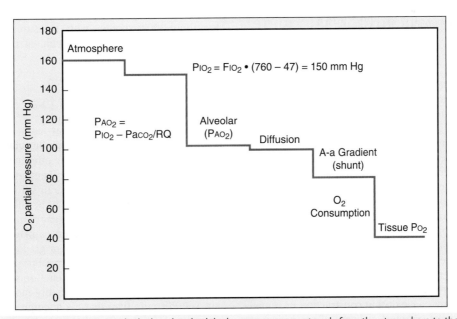

Fig. 5.7 The oxygen cascade depicts the physiologic steps as oxygen travels from the atmosphere to the tissues. Oxygen starts at 21% in the atmosphere and is initially diluted with water vapor to about 150 mm Hg, PIO_2. Alveolar PO_2 (PAO_2) is determined by the alveolar gas equation. Diffusion equilibrates PO_2 between the alveolus and the capillary. The A-a (alveolar-to-arterial) gradient occurs with intrapulmonary shunt and ventilation-to-perfusion ($\dot{V}/\dot{Q}$) mismatch. Oxygen consumption then reduces PO_2 to tissue levels (about 40 mm Hg).

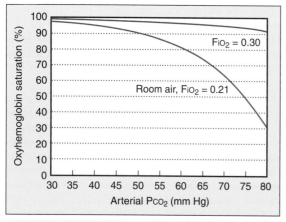

Fig. 5.8 Hypoventilation decreases oxygenation, as determined by the alveolar gas equation. The *blue curve* shows what is expected for room air (FiO$_2$ = 0.21). High PaCO$_2$ further shifts the oxyhemoglobin dissociation curve to the right. However, as little as 30% oxygen can completely negate the effects of hypoventilation (*red curve*).

of 37°C), and RQ is the respiratory quotient (the ratio of carbon dioxide production to oxygen consumption). For example, while breathing 100% oxygen (FiO$_2$ = 1.0) at sea level (PB = 760 mm Hg) and the PH$_2$O = 47 mm Hg with PaCO$_2$ = 40 mm Hg, the alveolar PO$_2$ (PaO$_2$) is calculated as follows. RQ is usually assumed to be approximately 0.8 on a normal diet.

$$PaO_2 = 1.0\,(760 - 47) - 40/0.8$$
$$= 713 - 50$$
$$= 663\ mm\,Hg$$

The alveolar gas equation describes the way in which inspired oxygen and ventilation determine PaO$_2$. It also describes the way in which supplemental oxygen improves oxygenation. One clinical consequence of this relationship is that supplemental oxygen can easily compensate for and mask the adverse effects of hypoventilation (Fig. 5.8).

A sound understanding of the differential diagnosis of arterial hypoxemia is vital for anesthesia providers because of the common and life-threatening nature of this condition. From an oxygen supply perspective, low barometric pressure is a culprit at high altitude. Though modern anesthesia workstations have multiple safety mechanisms to prevent delivery of hypoxic gas mixtures, death from delivery of gases other than oxygen is still occasionally reported. This may be because of errors in pipeline connections made during construction or remodeling. During patient transport, delivery of an inadequate FiO$_2$ may occur when oxygen tanks run out or with failure to recognize accidental disconnection of a self-inflating bag (Ambu) from its oxygen source (also see Chapter 15).

From both an oxygen supply and demand perspective, apnea is an important cause of arterial hypoxemia,

as storage of oxygen in the lung is of prime importance in delaying the appearance of arterial hypoxemia in humans. Storage of oxygen on hemoglobin is secondary, because use of this oxygen requires significant oxyhemoglobin desaturation. In contrast to voluntary breath-holding, apnea during anesthesia or sedation occurs at functional residual capacity (FRC). This substantially reduces the time to oxyhemoglobin desaturation compared with a breath-hold at total lung capacity.

The time can be estimated for SaO$_2$ to reach 90% when the FRC is 2.5 L and the PaO$_2$ is 100 mm Hg. Normal oxygen consumption is about 300 mL/min, although this is somewhat lower during anesthesia. It would take only about 30 seconds under these room air conditions to develop arterial hypoxemia. After breathing 100% oxygen, it might take 7 minutes to reach an SaO$_2$ of 90%. The time it takes to develop arterial hypoxemia after breathing 100% oxygen varies. Desaturation begins when enough alveoli have collapsed and intrapulmonary shunt develops, not simply when oxygen stores have become exhausted. Obese patients develop arterial hypoxemia with apnea substantially faster than lean patients (also see Chapter 29).

Venous Admixture

Venous admixture describes physiologic causes of arterial hypoxemia for which PaO$_2$ is normal. The alveolar-to-arterial oxygen (A-a) gradient reflects venous admixture. Normal A-a gradients are 5 to 10 mm Hg, but they increase with age. For example, if the arterial PO$_2$ while breathing 100% oxygen were measured as 310 mm Hg, the A-a gradient could be calculated from the previous example.

$$A\text{-}a\ gradient = PaO_2 - PaO_2$$
$$= 663\ mm\,Hg - 310\ mm\,Hg$$
$$= 353\ mm\,Hg$$

A picture of gas exchange can be accomplished mathematically by integrating all the effects of shunting, supplemental oxygen, and the oxyhemoglobin dissociation curve to create "isoshunt" diagrams (Fig. 5.9). Although calculating a shunt fraction may be the most exact way to quantitate problems in oxygenation, it requires information only available from a PA catheter and therefore is not always clinically useful. A-a gradients are clinically simpler and more useful to derive but do not represent a constant measurement of oxygenation with different FiO$_2$ levels. The A-a gradient is probably most useful in room air. The P/F ratio (PaO$_2$/FiO$_2$) is a simple and useful measurement of oxygenation that remains more consistent at high FiO$_2$ (Fig. 5.10).[18]

Intrapulmonary Shunt

An intrapulmonary shunt is one of the most important causes of an increased A-a gradient and the development

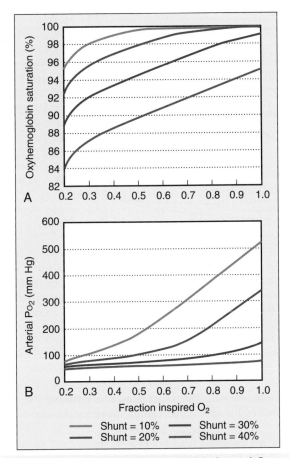

Fig. 5.9 The effect of intrapulmonary shunting and FIO_2 on PaO_2 (A) and SaO_2 (B) is shown graphically at shunt fractions from 10% (mild) to 40% (severe). Assumed values for these calculations are hemoglobin, 14 g/dL; $PaCO_2$, 40 mm Hg; arterial-to-venous oxygen content difference, 4 mL O_2/dL; and sea-level atmospheric pressure, 760 mm Hg. Increased FIO_2 still substantially improves oxygenation at high shunt fractions but is unable to fully correct it.

of arterial hypoxemia. In the presence of an intrapulmonary shunt mixed venous blood is not exposed to alveolar gas, and it continues through the lungs to mix with oxygenated blood from normal areas of the lung. This mixing lowers the PaO_2. Clinically, shunting occurs when alveoli are not ventilated, as with atelectasis, or when alveoli are filled with fluid, as with pneumonia or pulmonary edema. The quantitative effect of an intrapulmonary shunt is described by the shunt equation:

$$\dot{Q}s/\dot{Q}t = (Cc'o_2 - Cao_2)/(Cc'o_2 - C\bar{v}o_2)$$

In the equation $\dot{Q}s/\dot{Q}t$ is the shunt flow relative to total flow (i.e., shunt fraction), C is the oxygen content, c′ is end-capillary blood (for a theoretical normal alveolus), a is arterial blood, and v̄ is mixed venous blood.

Ventilation–Perfusion Mismatch

Ventilation–perfusion (V̇/Q̇) mismatch is similar to intrapulmonary shunt (V̇/Q̇ = 0), with some important distinctions. In V̇/Q̇ mismatch disparity between the amount of ventilation and perfusion in various alveoli leads to areas of high V̇/Q̇ (i.e., well-ventilated alveoli) and areas of low V̇/Q̇ (i.e., poorly ventilated alveoli). Because of the shape of the oxyhemoglobin dissociation curve, the improved oxygenation in well-ventilated areas cannot compensate for the low PO_2 in the poorly ventilated areas, resulting in lower PaO_2 or arterial hypoxemia.

Clinically, in V̇/Q̇ mismatch administering 100% oxygen can achieve a PO_2 on the plateau of the oxyhemoglobin dissociation curve even in poorly ventilated alveoli. Conversely, administering 100% oxygen in the presence of an intrapulmonary shunt only adds more dissolved oxygen in the normally perfused alveoli, although as seen in Fig. 5.9, this may result in more improvement in oxygenation than is often appreciated. Arterial hypoxemia remaining despite administration of 100% oxygen is always caused by the presence of an intrapulmonary shunt.

Diffusion Impairment

Diffusion impairment is not equivalent to low diffusing capacity. For diffusion impairment to cause an A-a gradient, equilibrium has not occurred between the PO_2 in the alveolus and the PO_2 in pulmonary capillary blood. This rarely occurs, even in patients with limited diffusing capacity. The small A-a gradient that can result from diffusion impairment is easily eliminated with supplemental oxygen, making this a clinically unimportant problem. Clinically significant diffusion impairment can occur with exercise at extreme altitude, owing both to the smaller driving oxygen partial pressure and the limited time for equilibrium because of the rapid transit of blood through the pulmonary capillaries.

Venous Oxygen Saturation

Low $S\bar{v}o_2$ causes a subtle but important effect when intrapulmonary shunt is already present.[19] Shunt is a mixture of venous blood and blood from normal regions of the lungs. If the $S\bar{v}o_2$ is lower, the resulting mixture must have a lower PaO_2. Low CO may lower $S\bar{v}o_2$ significantly. This changes the way in which we interpret intrapulmonary shunt in different clinical conditions. For example, in sepsis when the $S\bar{v}o_2$ may be quite high, the shunt fraction may be higher than expected; high $S\bar{v}o_2$ may be described as covering up a high shunt fraction.

Carbon Dioxide

Carbon dioxide is produced in the tissues and removed from the lungs by ventilation. Carbon dioxide is carried in the blood as dissolved gas, as bicarbonate, and as a small amount bound to hemoglobin as carbaminohemoglobin.

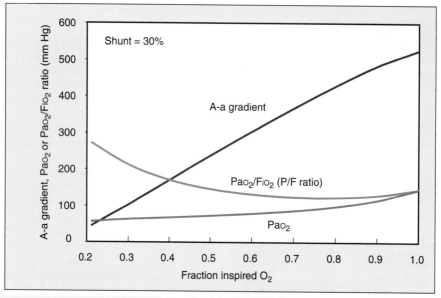

Fig. 5.10 Despite a constant shunt fraction of 0.3 (30%), the A-a gradient is much higher at high F_{IO_2}, indicating problems in its usefulness as a measurement of oxygenation with different F_{IO_2} values. The ratio of Pa_{O_2} to F_{IO_2} (the P/F ratio) is remarkably constant at high F_{IO_2}, making it a useful measurement of oxygenation when the gold standard, shunt fraction, is not available.

Unlike the oxyhemoglobin dissociation curve, the dissociation curve for carbon dioxide is essentially linear.

Hypercapnia

New-onset hypercapnia (i.e., high Pa_{CO_2}) may be a sign of respiratory difficulty or oversedation with opioids. Although hypercapnia itself may not be dangerous, Pa_{CO_2} values greater than 80 mm Hg that are uncompensated may cause CO_2 narcosis, possibly contributing to delayed awakening in the postanesthesia care unit. The greatest concern of hypercapnia is that it may indicate a risk of impending respiratory failure and apnea, in which arterial hypoxemia and anoxia can rapidly ensue. Although the presence of hypercapnia may be obvious if capnography is used, this monitor is not always available, and substantial hypercapnia may go unnoticed. Supplemental oxygen can prevent arterial hypoxemia despite severe hypercapnia, and an analysis of arterial blood gases would not necessarily be performed if hypercapnia were not suspected (see Fig. 5.8).

The organ systems affected by hypercapnia include the lungs (pulmonary vasoconstriction, right shift of hemoglobin–oxygen dissociation curve), kidneys (renal bicarbonate resorption), central nervous system (somnolence, cerebral vasodilation), and heart (coronary artery vasodilation, decreased cardiac contractility).[20,21]

Determinants of Arterial Carbon Dioxide Partial Pressure

Pa_{CO_2} is a balance of production and removal. If removal exceeds production, Pa_{CO_2} decreases. If production exceeds removal, Pa_{CO_2} increases. The resulting Pa_{CO_2} is expressed by an alveolar carbon dioxide equation:

$$Pa_{CO_2} = k \times \dot{V}_{CO_2}/\dot{V}_A$$

In the equation k is a constant (0.863) that corrects units, $\dot{V}_{CO_2}$ is carbon dioxide production, and $\dot{V}_A$ is alveolar ventilation.

Rebreathing

Because breathing circuits with rebreathing properties are frequently used in anesthesia, increased inspired P_{CO_2} concentrations are a potential cause of hypercapnia. Exhausted carbon dioxide absorbents and malfunctioning expiratory valves on the anesthesia delivery circuit are possible causes of rebreathing in the operating room that are easily detected with capnography. Use of certain transport breathing circuits may be the most common cause of clinically significant rebreathing, which may be unrecognized because capnography is not routinely used during patient transport from the operating room.

Increased Carbon Dioxide Production

Several important physiologic causes of increased carbon dioxide production may cause hypercapnia under anesthesia (Box 5.2). The anesthesia provider should not view CO_2 production in terms of cellular production, but rather as the pulmonary excretion of CO_2. This is how it would be measured clinically and how it would be detected by the homeostatic mechanisms of the body. Other brief increases in CO_2 production may occur when

Box 5.2 Causes of Increased Carbon Dioxide Production

Fever
Malignant hyperthermia
Systemic absorption during laparoscopy procedures
 (physiologically similar to increased production)
Thyroid storm
Tourniquet release
Administration of sodium bicarbonate

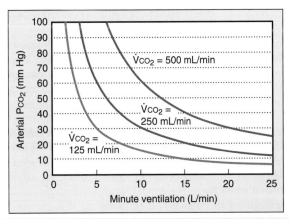

Fig. 5.11 Carbon dioxide has a hyperbolic relationship with ventilation. The depicted curves are simulated with a normal resting carbon dioxide production (250 mL/min), low carbon dioxide production (125 mL/min, as during anesthesia), and increased carbon dioxide production (500 mL/min, as during moderate exercise). The value of physiologic dead space is assumed to be 30% in these calculations.

administering sodium bicarbonate, which is converted into CO_2, or when releasing a tourniquet, where carbon dioxide has accumulated in the tissues of the leg and then returns to the circulation.

Increased Dead Space

Dead space, or "wasted ventilation," refers to areas receiving ventilation that do not participate in gas exchange. Dead space is further categorized as anatomic, alveolar, and physiologic (total) dead space. Anatomic dead space represents areas of the tracheobronchial tree that are not involved in gas exchange. This includes equipment dead space, such as the endotracheal tube and tubing distal to the Y-connector of the anesthesia delivery circuit. Alveolar dead space represents alveoli that do not participate in gas exchange owing to lack of blood flow. Physiologic or total dead space represents the sum of anatomic and alveolar dead space. Most pathologically significant changes in dead space represent increases in alveolar dead space.

Dead space is increased in many clinical conditions. Emphysema and other end-stage lung diseases, such as cystic fibrosis, are often characterized by substantial dead space. Pulmonary embolism is a potential cause of significant increases in dead space. Physiologic processes that decrease PAP, such as hemorrhagic shock, can be expected to increase dead space (increased zone 1 through decreased arterial pressure). Increased airway pressure and positive end-expiratory pressure (PEEP) can also increase dead space (increased zone 1 through increased airway pressure). Dead space has been shown to be an important prognostic indicator in patients with ARDS and can help guide PEEP management[22] (also see Chapter 41).

Quantitative estimates of dead space are described by the Bohr equation, which expresses the ratio of dead space ventilation ($\dot{V}_D$) relative to tidal ventilation ($\dot{V}_T$):

$$\dot{V}_D/\dot{V}_T = (Pa_{CO_2} - P\bar{E}_{CO_2})/Pa_{CO_2}$$

where $P\bar{E}_{CO_2}$ is the mixed-expired carbon dioxide.

For example, if the $Pa_{CO_2} = 40$ mm Hg and the $P\bar{E}_{CO_2} = 20$ mm Hg during controlled ventilation of the lungs, the $\dot{V}_D/\dot{V}_T$ can be calculated as follows:

$$\dot{V}_D/\dot{V}_T = (40 - 20)/40$$
$$= 20/40$$
$$= 0.5$$

Some physiologic dead space (25%–30%) is considered normal because some anatomic dead space is always present. The Pa_{CO_2}–Pet_{CO_2} gradient is a useful indication of the presence of alveolar dead space. However, this gradient will change as Pa_{CO_2} changes with hyperventilation or hypoventilation even when dead space is constant.

Hypoventilation

Decreased minute ventilation is the most important and common cause of hypercapnia (Fig. 5.11). This may be because of decreased tidal volume, breathing frequency, or both. Alveolar ventilation ($\dot{V}_A$) combines minute ventilation and dead space ($\dot{V}_A = \dot{V}_T - \dot{V}_D$); however, it is more clinically useful to separate these processes. Ventilatory depressant effects of anesthetic drugs are a common cause of hypoventilation. Although increased minute ventilation can often completely compensate for elevated carbon dioxide production, rebreathing, or dead space, there is no physiologically useful compensation for inadequate minute ventilation.

If alveolar ventilation decreases by one half, Pa_{CO_2} should double (see Fig. 5.11). This change occurs over several minutes as a new steady state develops. CO_2 changes during apnea are more complicated. During the first minute of apnea, Pa_{CO_2} increases from a normal of 40 mm Hg to 46 mm Hg (the normal $P\bar{V}_{CO_2}$). This increase may be higher and more rapid in patients with smaller lung volumes or high arterial-to-venous carbon dioxide differences. After the first minute, Pa_{CO_2} increases more slowly as carbon dioxide production adds carbon dioxide to the blood, at about 3 mm Hg per minute.

Differential Diagnosis of Increased Arterial Carbon Dioxide Partial Pressure

Increased $Paco_2$ values can be analyzed by assessing minute ventilation, performing capnography, and measuring an arterial blood gas value. Capnography can easily detect rebreathing. A clinical assessment of minute ventilation by physical examination and as measured by most mechanical ventilators should be adequate. Comparison of end-tidal Pco_2 with $Paco_2$ can identify abnormal alveolar dead space. Abnormal carbon dioxide production can be inferred. However, significant abnormalities of carbon dioxide physiology often are unrecognized when $Paco_2$ is normal, because increased minute ventilation can compensate for substantial increases in dead space and carbon dioxide production. Noticing the presence of increased dead space when minute ventilation is increased in volume and $Paco_2$ is 40 mm Hg is just as important as noticing abnormal dead space when the $Paco_2$ is 80 mm Hg and minute ventilation is normal.

PULMONARY MECHANICS

Pulmonary mechanics concern pressure, volume, and flow relationships in the lung and bronchial tree (Fig. 5.12). An understanding of pulmonary mechanics is essential for managing the ventilated patient. Pressures in the airway are routinely measured or sensed by the anesthesia provider delivering positive-pressure ventilation. Differentiation between static and dynamic properties can lead to important changes in patient management.

Static Properties

The lung is made of elastic tissue that stretches under pressure (Fig. 5.13). Surface tension has a significant role in the compliance of the lung because of the air–fluid interface in the alveoli. Surfactant decreases surface tension and stabilizes small alveoli, which would otherwise tend to collapse.

The chest wall has its own compliance curve. At FRC, the chest wall tends to expand, but negative (subatmospheric) intrapleural pressure keeps the chest wall collapsed. The lungs tend to collapse, but they are held expanded because of the pressure difference from the airways to the intrapleural pressure. FRC is the natural balance point between the lungs tending to collapse and chest wall tending to expand.

Dynamic Properties and Airway Resistance

Airway resistance is mainly determined by the radius of the airway, but turbulent gas flow may make resistance worse. A number of clinical processes can affect airway resistance (Box 5.3). Resistance in small airways is physiologically different, because they have no cartilaginous

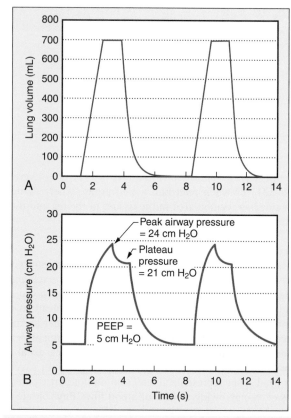

Fig. 5.12 Lung volume is shown as a function of time (A) in a typical volume-controlled ventilator with constant flow rates. Lung volume increases at a constant rate during inspiration because of constant flow. Exhalation occurs with a passive relaxation curve. The lower panel (B) shows the development of pressure over time. Pressure is produced from a static compliance component (see Fig. 5.13) and a resistance component. If flow is held during an inspiratory pause, a plateau pressure is reached, where there is no resistive pressure component. In this example peak airway pressure (PAP) is 24 cm H_2O, and positive end-expiratory pressure (PEEP) is 5 cm H_2O. Dynamic compliance is tidal volume (VT): (VT)/(PAP − PEEP) = 37 mL/cm H_2O. Plateau pressure (Pplat) is 21 cm H_2O, and static compliance is VT/(Pplat − PEEP) = 44 mL/cm H_2O.

structure or smooth muscle. Unlike capillaries, which have positive pressure inside to keep them open, small airways have zero (atmospheric) pressure during spontaneous

Box 5.3 Factors Influencing Airway Resistance
Radius of the airways
Smooth muscle tone
Bronchospasm
Inflammation of the airways (asthma, chronic bronchitis)
Foreign bodies
Compression of airways
Turbulent gas flow (helium, a temporizing measure)
Anesthesia equipment

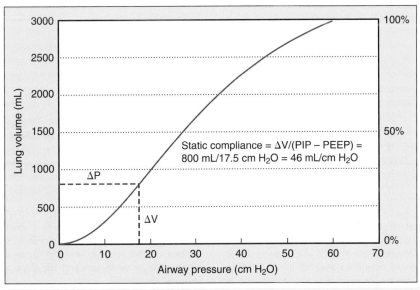

Fig. 5.13 A static compliance curve of a normal lung has a slight S shape. A slightly higher pressure can be required to open alveoli at low lung volumes (i.e., beginning of the curve), whereas higher distending pressures are needed as the lung is overdistended. Static compliance is measured as the change (Δ) in volume divided by the change in pressure (inspiratory pressure [PIP] – positive end-expiratory pressure [PEEP]), which is 46 mL/cm H_2O in this example.

ventilation. However, these airways are kept open by the same forces (i.e., pressure inside is greater than the pressure outside) that keep capillaries open. Negative pressure is transmitted from the intrapleural pressure through the structure of lung, and this pressure difference keeps small airways open. When a disease process, such as emphysema, makes pleural pressure less negative, resistance in the small airways is increased, and dynamic compression occurs during exhalation.

During positive-pressure ventilation, resistance in anesthesia breathing equipment or airways manifests as elevated airway pressures, because flow through resistance causes a pressure change. Distinguishing airway resistance effects from static compliance components is a useful first step in the differential diagnosis of high peak airway pressures. This is facilitated by anesthesia machines that are equipped to provide an inspiratory pause. During ventilation, airway pressure reaches a peak inspiratory pressure, but when ventilation is paused, the pressure component from gas flow and resistance disappears, and the airway pressure decreases toward a plateau pressure (see Fig. 5.12).

CONTROL OF BREATHING

Anesthesia providers are in a unique position to observe ventilatory control mechanisms because most drugs administered for sedation and anesthesia depress breathing.

Central Integration and Rhythm Generation

Specific areas of the brainstem are involved in generating the respiratory rhythm, processing afferent signal information, and changing the efferent output to the inspiratory and expiratory muscles.

Central Chemoreceptors

Superficial areas on the ventrolateral medullary surface respond to pH and P_{CO_2}. Carbon dioxide is in rapid equilibrium with carbonic acid and therefore immediately affects the local pH surrounding the central chemoreceptors. Although the signal is transduced by protons, not carbon dioxide directly, these chemoreceptors are described clinically as carbon dioxide responsive. The central chemoreceptors are protected from rapid changes in metabolic pH by the blood–brain barrier.

Peripheral Chemoreceptors

Carotid bodies are the primary peripheral chemoreceptors in humans; aortic bodies have no significant role. Low P_{O_2}, high P_{CO_2}, and low pH stimulate the carotid bodies.[23] Unlike the central chemoreceptors, metabolic acids immediately affect peripheral chemoreceptors. Because of high blood flow, peripheral chemoreceptors are effectively at arterial, not venous, blood values.

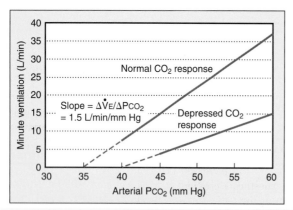

Fig. 5.14 The hypercapnic ventilatory response (HCVR) is measured as the slope of the plot of P_{CO_2} versus minute ventilation ($\dot{V}_E$). End-tidal P_{CO_2} is usually substituted for Pa_{CO_2} for clinical studies. The apneic threshold is the P_{CO_2} at which ventilation is zero. It can be extrapolated from the curve, but it is difficult to measure in awake volunteers, although it is easy to observe in patients under general anesthesia. A depressed carbon dioxide response results from opioids, which lower the slope and raise the apneic threshold.

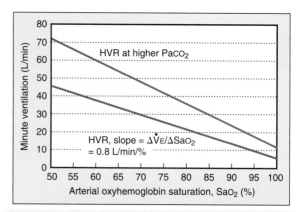

Fig. 5.15 Hypoxic ventilatory response (HVR) expressed relative to Sa_{O_2} is approximately linear, which is simpler than the curvilinear response expressed as a function of Pa_{O_2}. HVR is the slope of the linear plot. HVR is higher at higher carbon dioxide concentrations. Both absolute ventilation and the slope are shifted. Low Pa_{CO_2} likewise lowers HVR.

Hypercapnic Ventilatory Response

Ventilation increases dramatically as Pa_{CO_2} is increased. In the presence of high P_{O_2} values most of this ventilatory response results from the central chemoreceptors, whereas in the presence of room air about one-third of the response results from peripheral chemoreceptor stimulation. The ventilatory response to carbon dioxide is moderately linear, although at Pa_{CO_2} levels below resting values, minute ventilation does not tend to go to zero because of an "awake" drive to breathe (Fig. 5.14). At a high Pa_{CO_2} value, minute ventilation is eventually limited by maximal minute ventilation.

Decreasing Pa_{CO_2} during anesthesia, as produced by assisted ventilation, results in a point at which ventilation ceases, called the *apneic threshold*. As CO_2 rises, ventilation returns at the apneic threshold and then stabilizes at a Pa_{CO_2} setpoint that is about 5 mm Hg higher.

The brainstem response to carbon dioxide is slow, requiring about 5 minutes to reach 90% of steady-state ventilation. When allowing the Pa_{CO_2} to rise in an apneic patient, it may take a noticeably long time to stabilize minute ventilation, which is a direct consequence of the dynamics of the central ventilatory drive.

Hypoxic Ventilatory Response

Ventilation increases as Pa_{O_2} and Sa_{O_2} decrease, reflecting stimulation of the peripheral chemoreceptors. The central response to hypoxemia paradoxically results in decreased minute ventilation, called *hypoxic ventilatory decline* (HVD). The timing and combination of these effects mean that in prolonged arterial hypoxemia, ventilation rises to an initial peak, reflecting the rapid response of the peripheral chemoreceptors, and then decreases to an intermediate plateau in 15 to 20 minutes, reflecting the slower addition of HVD.

Although it is P_{O_2} that affects the carotid body, it is easier to consider the hypoxic ventilatory response in terms of oxyhemoglobin desaturation because minute ventilation changes linearly with Sa_{O_2} (Fig. 5.15). The effects of hypoxia and hypercapnia on the carotid body are synergistic. At high Pa_{CO_2} levels, the response to hypoxia is much larger, whereas low Pa_{CO_2} levels can dramatically decrease responsiveness. Unlike the hypercapnic ventilatory response, the response to hypoxia is rapid and takes only seconds to appear.

Effects of Anesthesia

Opioids, sedative-hypnotics, and volatile anesthetics have dose-dependent depressant effects on ventilation and ventilatory control (also see Chapters 7–9). Opioid receptors are present on neurons considered responsible for respiratory rhythm generation. Sedative-hypnotics work primarily on γ-aminobutyric acid A receptors ($GABA_A$), which provide inhibitory input in multiple neurons of the respiratory system. Volatile anesthetics decrease excitatory neurotransmission. All these drugs exert most of their depressant effects in the central integratory area and therefore clinically appear to decrease the hypoxic and hypercapnic ventilatory responses similarly. Specific effects of drugs on peripheral chemoreceptors include the inhibitory effects of dopamine and the slight excitatory effects of dopaminergic blockers such as haloperidol.

Disorders of Ventilatory Control

Neonates with a history of prematurity and of post-conceptual age <60 weeks may have episodes of apnea after anesthesia. Likewise, sudden infant death syndrome may be a result of immature ventilatory control systems. Ondine's curse, originally described after surgery near the upper cervical spinal cord, results in profound hypoventilation during sleep and anesthesia caused by abnormalities in the central integratory system that seem to blunt the hypoxic and hypercapnic ventilatory responses. Idiopathic varieties of Ondine's curse have occurred in children and are referred to as *primary central alveolar hypoventilation syndromes*. Morbidly obese patients and those with sleep apnea may exhibit abnormalities of ventilatory control (also see Chapter 48).

Periodic breathing, a pattern in which groups of sequential breaths are separated by apneic episodes, is commonly observed during drug-induced sedation. Mechanistically, this is most likely when peripheral chemoreceptors are activated by mild arterial hypoxemia. Continual overcorrection and undercorrection of the Pao_2 leads to oscillations of $Paco_2$ and Sao_2. Periodic breathing is also common during sleep at higher altitudes.

Identifying the Cause of Respiratory Failure

With a solid foundation of respiratory physiology, the anesthesia provider is particularly well suited to rapid, accurate diagnosis and correction of acute respiratory failure. The first step is differentiating between hypoxemic, hypercarbic, and mixed etiologies. Once the primary insult is identified, the differential diagnosis can focus on whether the issue is external or intrinsic to the patient, the result of dead space or shunt, or any combination of the factors discussed earlier. Additionally, understanding the signal pathways that detect and compensate for hypoxemia and/or hypercarbia allow for a deeper understanding of confusing physiologic states, such as the "silent hypoxia" that was described in the early days of the COVID-19 pandemic.[14]

INTEGRATION OF THE HEART AND LUNGS

Supply and Delivery

The interrelationship between the heart and lungs is suggested by the Fick equation, which relates oxygen consumption and oxygen needs at the tissue level:

$$\dot{V}o_2 = Co \times (Cao_2 - C\bar{v}o_2)$$

where $\dot{V}o_2$ is oxygen consumption, Cao_2 is the arterial oxygen content, $C\bar{v}o_2$ is the mixed venous oxygen content, and CO is cardiac output.

Oxygen Delivery

Oxygen delivery (Do_2) is the total amount of oxygen supplied to tissues and is a function of CO and Cao_2:

$$Do_2 = CO \times Cao_2$$

Do_2 can be limited by decreases in CO or Cao_2. Cao_2 can be limited by anemia or hypoxemia. It is important to think of supply and delivery as being inextricably linked. Under ideal circumstances, hypoxemia can be compensated for by increased CO. This is an important concept for anesthesia providers to recognize and use when caring for the patient with hypoxemia.[14]

Oxygen Extraction

Different indices can be used to assess how much oxygen is removed from blood by tissues to meet their metabolic demand. Mixed venous oxygen saturation ($S\bar{v}o_2$) is normally about 75%. If tissues extract more oxygen, $S\bar{v}o_2$ decreases. However, with high Fio_2, $S\bar{v}o_2$ may increase because of the added amount of dissolved oxygen, even though true extraction has not changed. The arteriovenous oxygen content difference ($Cao_2 - C\bar{v}o_2$) is independent of changes in Fio_2 and is therefore a useful measurement of the balance of oxygen supply and demand. On the other hand, the arteriovenous oxygen content difference decreases in anemia because extracting the same percentage of oxygen means extracting less total oxygen because of the lower hemoglobin concentration. The most reliable figure is the calculated oxygen extraction ratio:

$$O_2 \text{ extraction} = (Cao_2 - C\bar{v}o_2)/Cao_2$$

Anemia

An example of threatened oxygen supply is anemia. To adapt to anemia, the body can increase CO or extract more oxygen. The normal physiologic response is to increase CO and maintain Do_2. Increased HR and SV are responsible for this compensation. However, during anesthesia with a near-absent HR response, increased oxygen extraction is a more important mechanism of compensation.[24]

Metabolic Demand

Increased oxygen consumption is usually met with a combination of increased CO and increased oxygen extraction. Whereas oxygen consumption is usually constant and relatively low under anesthesia, recovery from anesthesia may be associated with significant increases in metabolic demands. Shivering and early ambulation after outpatient surgery are stresses that may affect patients still recovering from anesthesia or after significant blood loss. Increased minute ventilation is required to meet increased oxygen needs and to eliminate the extra carbon dioxide produced.

Mechanical Relationships

The relationship between the heart and lungs is further highlighted during periods of extreme physiologic stress such as refractory hypoxemia. Whereas most treatment approaches for refractory hypoxemia have little effect on the heart (e.g., lung-protective ventilation, neuromuscular blockade), lung recruitment maneuvers and prone positioning can lead to hemodynamic compromise.[25-27] Given their colocation in the thoracic cavity, it is not surprising that the cardiac and respiratory systems have a mechanical relationship. In an underfilled state a recruitment maneuver (e.g., a sustained inspiration of 30 seconds) or a switch to prone positioning, although helpful for improving V/Q matching, may impede venous return to the right heart, leading to clinically significant hypotension. More commonly, a switch to positive-pressure ventilation will increase RV afterload while decreasing LV afterload through a reduction in LV wall stress.

REFERENCES

1. Berne RM, Levy MN. *Cardiovascular Physiology.* 8th ed. Mosby; 2001.
2. Lumb AB, Thomas CR. *Nunn and Lumb's Applied Respiratory Physiology.* 9th ed: Elsevier; 2021.
3. West JB. *Respiratory Physiology: The Essentials.* 9th ed. Wolters Kluwer Health/Lippincott Williams & Wilkins; 2012.
4. van Klei WA, Hollmann MW, Sneyd JR. The value of anaesthesiologists in the COVID-19 pandemic: A model for our future practice? *Br J Anaesth.* 2020;125(5):652–655. doi:10.1016/j.bja.2020.08.014.
5. Walsh M, Devereaux PJ, Garg AX, et al. Relationship between intraoperative mean arterial pressure and clinical outcomes after noncardiac surgery: Toward an empirical definition of hypotension. *Anesthesiology.* 2013;119(3):507–515. doi:10.1097/ALN.0b013e3182a10e26.
6. Wesselink EM, Kappen TH, Torn HM, Slooter AJC, van Klei WA. Intraoperative hypotension and the risk of postoperative adverse outcomes: A systematic review. *Br J Anaesth.* 2018;121(4):706–721. doi:10.1016/j.bja.2018.04.036.
7. Mathis MR, Naik BI, Freundlich R, et al. Preoperative risk and the association between hypotension and postoperative acute kidney injury. *Anesthesiology.* 2020;132:461–475.
8. Liem VG, Hoeks SE, Mol KH, et al. Postoperative hypotension after noncardiac surgery and the association with myocardial injury. *Anesthesiology.* 2020;133:519–522.
9. Funk DJ, Jacobsohn E, Kumar A. The role of venous return in critical illness and shock-part I: Physiology. *Crit Care Med.* 2013;41(1):255–262. doi:10.1097/CCM.0b013e3182772ab6.
10. Gelman S, Warner DS, Warner MA. Venous function and central venous pressure: A physiologic story. *Anesthesiology.* 2008;108(4):735–748. doi:10.1097/ALN.0b013e3181672607.
11. Michard F. Changes in arterial pressure during mechanical ventilation. *Anesthesiology.* 2005;103(2):419–428. doi:10.1097/00000542-200508000-00026.
12. Myatra SN, Prabu NR, Divatia JV, Monnet X, Kulkarni AP, Teboul JL. The changes in pulse pressure variation or stroke volume variation after a "tidal volume challenge" reliably predict fluid responsiveness during low tidal volume ventilation. *Crit Care Med.* 2017 Mar;45(3):415–421. doi:10.1097/CCM.0000000000002183. PMID: 27922879.
13. Topalian S, Ginsberg F, Parrillo JE. Cardiogenic shock. *Crit Care Med.* 2008;36(1):S66. doi:10.1097/01.CCM.0000296268.57993.90.
14. Bickler PE, Feiner JR, Lipnick MS, McKleroy W. "Silent" presentation of hypoxemia and cardiorespiratory compensation in COVID-19. *Anesthesiology.* 2021;134(2):262–269. doi:10.1097/ALN.0000000000003578.
15. Ruopp NF. Cockrill BA. Diagnosis and treatment of pulmonary arterial hypertension: A review. *JAMA.* 2022 Apr 12;327(14):1379–1391. doi:10.1001/jama.2022.4402. PMID: 35412560.
16. Mishra A, Reed RM, Eberlein M. Severe, rapidly reversible hypoxemia in the early period after bilateral lung transplantation. *Ann Am Thorac Soc.* 2016;13(6):979–985. doi:10.1513/AnnalsATS.201602-107CC.
17. Lumb AB, Slinger P. Hypoxic pulmonary vasoconstriction: Physiology and anesthetic implications. *Anesthesiology.* 2015;122(4):932–946. doi:10.1097/ALN.0000000000000569.
18. Feiner JR, Weiskopf RB. Evaluating pulmonary function: An assessment of Pao_2/Fio_2. *Crit Care Med.* 2017;45(1):e40. doi:10.1097/CCM.0000000000002017.
19. Shepherd SJ, Pearse RM. Role of central and mixed venous oxygen saturation measurement in perioperative care. *Anesthesiology.* 2009;111(3):649–656. doi:10.1097/ALN.0b013e3181af59aa.
20. Weinberger SE, Schwartzstein RM, Weiss JW. Hypercapnia. *N Engl J Med.* 1989;321(18):1223–1231. doi:10.1056/NEJM198911023211804.
21. Crystal GJ. Carbon dioxide and the heart: Physiology and clinical implications. *Anesth Analg.* 2015;121(3):610–623. doi:10.1213/ANE.0000000000000820.
22. Kallet RH, Zhuo H, Liu KD, Calfee CS, Matthay MA. The association between physiologic dead-space fraction and mortality in subjects with ARDS enrolled in a prospective multi-center clinical trial. *Respir Care.* 2014;59(11):1611–1618. doi:10.4187/respcare.02593.
23. Weir EK, López-Barneo J, Buckler KJ, Archer SL Acute oxygen-sensing. mechanisms. doi: 10.1056/NEJMra050002.
24. Weiskopf RB, Viele MK, Feiner J, et al. Human cardiovascular and metabolic response to acute, severe isovolemic anemia. *JAMA.* 1998;279(3):217–221. doi:10.1001/jama.279.3.217.
25. Guérin C, Reignier J, Richard JC, et al. Prone positioning in severe acute respiratory distress syndrome. doi:10.1056/NEJMoa1214103.
26. Moss M, Huang DT, Brower RG, et al., National Heart, Lung, and Blood Institute PETAL Clinical Trials Network. Early neuromuscular blockade in the acute respiratory distress syndrome. *N Engl J Med.* 2019 May 23;380(21):1997–2008. Epub 2019 May 19. PMID: 31112383; PMCID: PMC6741345.
27. Fan E, Del Sorbo L, Goligher EC, et al. An official American Thoracic Society/European Society of Intensive Care Medicine/Society of Critical Care Medicine Clinical Practice Guideline: Mechanical ventilation in adult patients with acute respiratory distress syndrome. *Am J Respir Crit Care Med.* 2017;195(9):1253–1263. doi:10.1164/rccm.201703-0548ST.

6 AUTONOMIC NERVOUS SYSTEM

Erica J. Stein, David B. Glick

The autonomic nervous system (ANS) controls involuntary activities of the body outside consciousness. It is at once the most primitive and among the most essential of control systems—primitive in that its characteristics are largely preserved across all mammalian species and essential in that it oversees responses to immediate life-threatening challenges and the body's vital maintenance needs. The ANS is divided into two major branches. The sympathetic nervous system (SNS) controls the "fight or flight" response, including redistribution of blood flow from the viscera to skeletal muscle and increased cardiac output. The parasympathetic nervous system (PNS), on the other hand, oversees the body's maintenance needs, such as digestion and genitourinary function. The primary goal of anesthetic management is to modulate the body's autonomic responses. As a result, safe administration of anesthetic care requires knowledge of ANS pharmacology, disease states that may impair ANS function, and expected responses to surgery and anesthesia.

ANATOMY OF THE AUTONOMIC NERVOUS SYSTEM

The Sympathetic Nervous System

The preganglionic fibers of the SNS originate from the thoracolumbar region (T1–L2 or L3) of the spinal cord (Fig. 6.1). The cell bodies of these neurons lie in the spinal gray matter. The nerve fibers extend to paired ganglia, creating the sympathetic chains that lie immediately lateral to the vertebral column or extend to unpaired distal plexuses (e.g., the celiac and mesenteric plexuses). Preganglionic sympathetic fibers not only synapse at the ganglion of the level of their origin in the spinal cord but can also course up and down the paired ganglia. A sympathetic response therefore is not confined to the segment from which the stimulus originates, as discharge can be amplified and diffuse. The postganglionic neurons of the SNS then travel to the target organ. The sympathetic

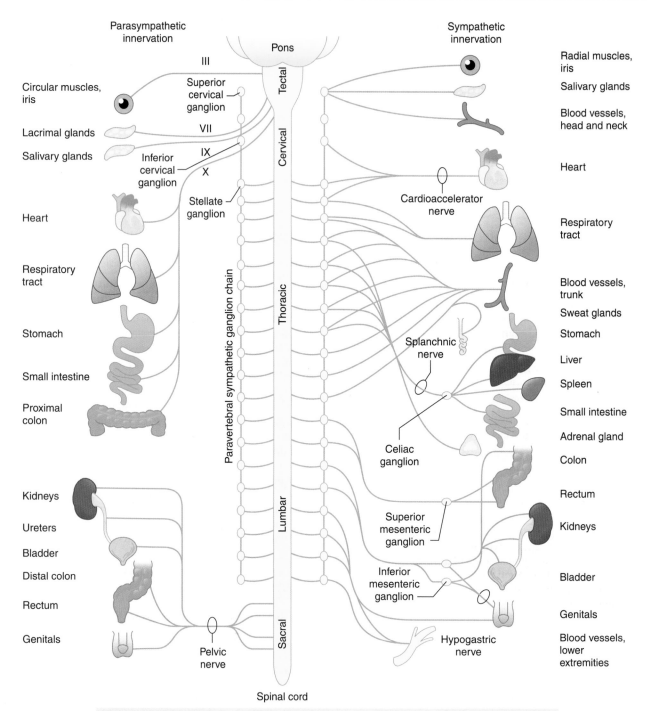

Fig. 6.1 Schematic representation of the autonomic nervous system depicting the functional innervation of peripheral effector organs and the anatomic origin of peripheral autonomic nerves from the spinal cord. Although both paravertebral sympathetic ganglia chains are presented, the sympathetic innervation to the peripheral effector organs is shown only on the right side of the figure, whereas the parasympathetic innervation of peripheral effector organs is depicted on the left. The roman numerals on nerves originating in the tectal region of the brainstem refer to the cranial nerves that provide parasympathetic outflow to the effector organs of the head, neck, and trunk. (From Ruffolo R. Physiology and biochemistry of the peripheral autonomic nervous system. In Wingard L, Brody T, Larner J, et al., eds. Human Pharmacology: Molecular to Clinical. St. Louis: Mosby-Year Book; 1991:77.)

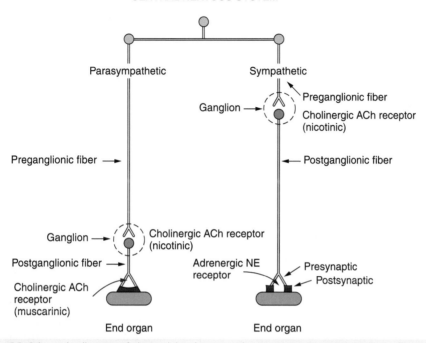

CENTRAL NERVOUS SYSTEM

Fig. 6.2 Schematic diagram of the peripheral autonomic nervous system. Preganglionic fibers and postganglionic fibers of the parasympathetic nervous system release acetylcholine (*ACh*) as the neurotransmitter. Postganglionic fibers of the sympathetic nervous system release norepinephrine (*NE*) as the neurotransmitter (exceptions are fibers to sweat glands, which release ACh). (From Lawson NW, Wallfisch HK. Cardiovascular pharmacology: A new look at the pressors. In Stoelting RK, Barash J, eds. Advances in Anesthesia. Chicago: Year Book Medical Publishers; 1986:195–270.)

preganglionic fibers are relatively short because sympathetic ganglia are generally close to the central nervous system (CNS). In contrast, the postganglionic fibers run a long course before innervating effector organs (Fig. 6.2).

The neurotransmitter released at the terminal end of the preganglionic sympathetic neuron is acetylcholine (ACh), and the cholinergic receptor on the postganglionic neuron is a nicotinic receptor. Norepinephrine is the primary neurotransmitter released at the terminal end of the postganglionic neuron at the synapse with the target organ (Fig. 6.3). Other classic neurotransmitters of the SNS include epinephrine and dopamine. Additionally, co-transmitters, such as adenosine triphosphate (ATP) and neuropeptide Y, modulate sympathetic activity. Norepinephrine and epinephrine bind postsynaptically to adrenergic receptors, which include the α_1-, β_1-, β_2-, and β-receptors. When norepinephrine binds to the α_2-receptors, located presynaptically on the postganglionic sympathetic nerve terminal, subsequent norepinephrine release is decreased (negative feedback). Dopamine (D) binds to D_1 receptors postsynaptically or D_2 receptors presynaptically.

Sympathetic neurotransmitters are synthesized from tyrosine in the postganglionic sympathetic nerve ending (Fig. 6.4). The rate-limiting step is the transformation of tyrosine to dihydroxyphenylalanine (DOPA), which is catalyzed by the enzyme tyrosine hydroxylase. DOPA is then converted to dopamine and, once inside the storage vesicle at the nerve terminal, is β-hydroxylated to norepinephrine. In the adrenal medulla norepinephrine is methylated to epinephrine. The neurotransmitters are stored in vesicles until the postganglionic nerve is stimulated. Then the vesicles merge with the cell membrane and release their contents into the synapse (Fig. 6.5). In general, only 1% of the total stored norepinephrine is released with each depolarization; thus there is a tremendous functional reserve. The released norepinephrine binds to the presynaptic and postsynaptic adrenergic receptors. The postsynaptic receptors then activate secondary messenger systems in the postsynaptic cell via G protein–linked activity. Norepinephrine is then released from these receptors and mostly taken up at the presynaptic nerve terminal and transported to storage vesicles for reuse. Norepinephrine that escapes this reuptake process and makes its way into the circulation is metabolized by either the monoamine oxidase (MAO) or catechol-*O*-methyltransferase (COMT) enzyme in the blood, liver, or kidney.

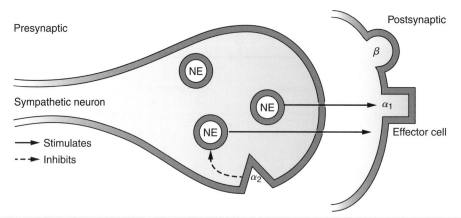

Fig. 6.3 Schematic depiction of the postganglionic sympathetic nerve ending. Release of the neurotransmitter norepinephrine (*NE*) from the nerve ending results in stimulation of postsynaptic receptors, which are classified as α_1, β_1, and β_2. Stimulation of presynaptic α_2-receptors results in inhibition of NE release from the nerve ending. (Adapted from Ram CVS, Kaplan NM. Alpha- and beta-receptor blocking drugs in the treatment of hypertension. In Harvey WP, ed. Current Problems in Cardiology. Chicago: Year Book Medical Publishers; 1970.)

The Parasympathetic Nervous System

The PNS arises from cranial nerves III, VII, IX, and X and from sacral segments S1–S4 (see Fig. 6.1). Unlike the ganglia of the SNS, the ganglia of the PNS are in close proximity to (or even within) their target organs (see Fig. 6.2). Like the SNS, the preganglionic nerve terminals release ACh into the synapse, and the postganglionic cell binds the ACh via nicotinic receptors. The postganglionic nerve terminal then releases ACh into the synapse it shares with the target organ cell. The ACh receptors of the target organ are muscarinic receptors. Like the adrenergic receptors, muscarinic receptors are coupled to G proteins and secondary messenger systems. ACh is rapidly inactivated within the synapse by the cholinesterase enzyme. The effects of stimulating adrenergic and cholinergic receptors throughout the body are listed in Table 6.1.

ADRENERGIC PHARMACOLOGY

Endogenous Catecholamines

Table 6.2 summarizes the pharmacologic effects and therapeutic doses of catecholamines.

Norepinephrine
Norepinephrine, the primary adrenergic neurotransmitter, binds to α- and β-receptors. It is used primarily for its α_1-adrenergic effects that increase systemic vascular resistance. Like all the endogenous catecholamines, the half-life of norepinephrine is short (2.5 minutes), so it is usually given as a continuous infusion at rates of 3 µg/min or more and titrated to the desired effect. The increase in systemic resistance can lead to reflex bradycardia.

Additionally, because norepinephrine vasoconstricts the pulmonary, renal, and mesenteric circulations, infusions must be carefully monitored to prevent injury to vital organs. Prolonged infusion of norepinephrine can also cause ischemia in the fingers and toes because of the marked peripheral vasoconstriction.

Epinephrine
Like norepinephrine, epinephrine binds to α- and β-adrenergic receptors. Exogenous epinephrine is used intravenously in life-threatening circumstances to treat cardiac arrest, circulatory collapse, and anaphylaxis. It is also commonly used locally to decrease the systemic absorption of local anesthetics and to reduce surgical blood loss. Among the therapeutic effects of epinephrine are positive inotropy, chronotropy, and enhanced conduction in the heart (β_1); smooth muscle relaxation in the vasculature and bronchial tree (β_2); and vasoconstriction (α_1). The effects that predominate depend on the dose of epinephrine administered. Epinephrine also has endocrine and metabolic effects that include increasing the levels of blood glucose, lactate, and free fatty acids.

An intravenous dose of 1 mg can be given for cardiovascular collapse, asystole, ventricular fibrillation, pulseless electrical activity, or anaphylactic shock to constrict the peripheral vasculature and maintain myocardial and cerebral perfusion. In less acute circumstances epinephrine can be given as a continuous infusion. The response of individual patients to epinephrine varies, so the infusion must be titrated to effect while the patient is monitored for signs of compromised renal, cerebral, or myocardial perfusion. In general, an infusion rate of 1 to 2 µg/min should primarily stimulate β_2-receptors and decrease airway resistance and vascular tone. A rate

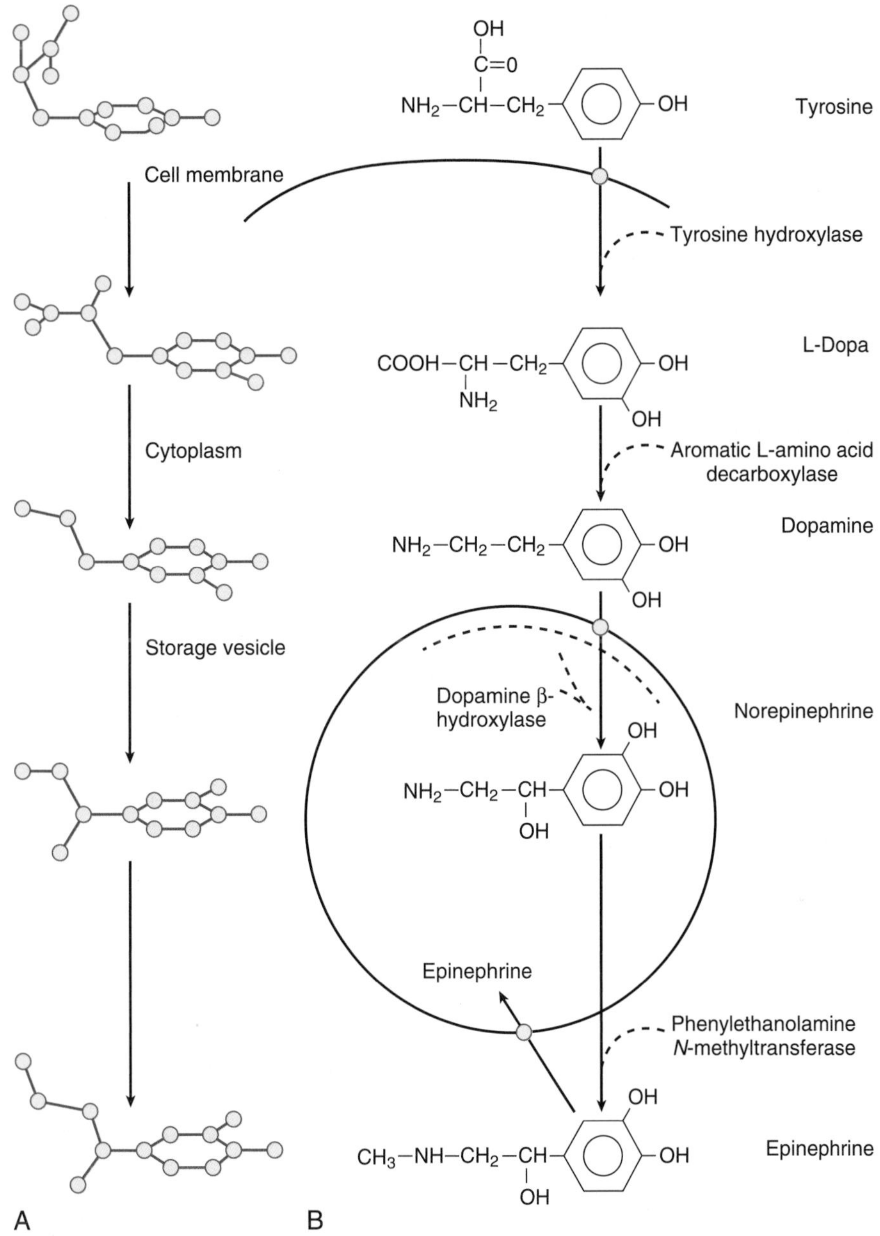

Fig. 6.4 Biosynthesis of norepinephrine and epinephrine in sympathetic nerve terminal (and adrenal medulla). (A) Perspective view of molecules. (B) Enzymatic processes. (From Tollenaeré JP. Atlas of the Three-Dimensional Structure of Drugs. Amsterdam: Elsevier North-Holland; 1979, as modified by Vanhoutte PM. Adrenergic neuroeffector interaction in the blood vessel wall. Fed Proc. 1978;37:181.)

of 2 to 10 μg/min increases heart rate, contractility, and conduction through the atrioventricular node. When doses larger than 10 μg/min are given, the α_1-adrenergic effects predominate, resulting in generalized vasoconstriction, which can lead to reflex bradycardia.

Epinephrine also can be administered as an aerosol to treat severe croup or airway edema. Bronchospasm is treated with epinephrine administered subcutaneously in doses of 300 μg every 20 minutes with a maximum of three doses. Epinephrine treats bronchospasm both via its direct effect as a bronchodilator and because it decreases antigen-induced release of bronchospastic substances (as may occur during anaphylaxis) by stabilizing the mast cells that release these substances.

Because epinephrine decreases the refractory period of the myocardium, the risk of arrhythmias during

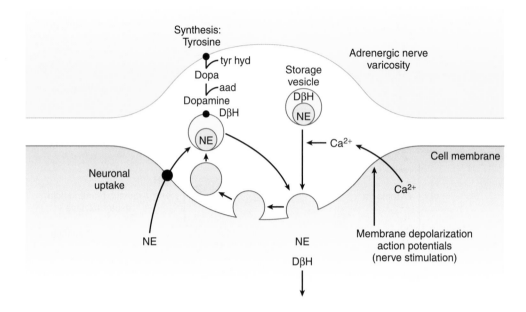

Fig. 6.5 Release and reuptake of norepinephrine at sympathetic nerve terminals. *Solid circle,* Active carrier; *aad,* aromatic L-amino acid decarboxylase; *DβH,* dopamine β-hydroxylase; *Dopa,* L-dihydroxyphenylalanine; *NE,* norepinephrine; *tyr hyd,* tyrosine hydroxylase. (From Vanhoutte PM. Adrenergic neuroeffector interaction in the blood vessel wall. Fed Proc. 1978;37:181, as modified by Shepherd J, Vanhoutte P. Neurohumoral regulation. In Shepherd S, Vanhoutte P, eds. The Human Cardiovascular System: Facts and Concepts. New York: Raven Press; 1979:107.)

halothane anesthesia is increased when epinephrine is given. The risk of arrhythmias seems to be less in children but increases with hypocapnia.

Dopamine

In addition to binding to α- and β-receptors, dopamine binds to dopaminergic receptors. Besides its direct effects, dopamine acts indirectly by stimulating the release of norepinephrine from storage vesicles. Dopamine is unique in its ability to improve blood flow through the renal and mesenteric beds in shock-like states by binding to postjunctional D_1 receptors. Dopamine is rapidly metabolized by MAO and COMT and has a half-life of 1 minute, so it must be given as a continuous infusion. At doses between 0.5 and 2.0 µg/kg/min, D_1 receptors are stimulated and renal and mesenteric beds are dilated. When the infusion is increased to 2 to 10 µg/kg/min, the $β_1$-receptors are stimulated and cardiac contractility and output are increased. At doses of 10 µg/kg/min and higher, $α_1$-receptor binding predominates and causes marked generalized constriction of the vasculature, negating any benefit to renal perfusion.

In the past dopamine was frequently used to treat patients in shock. The belief was that infusions of dopamine, by improving renal blood flow, could protect the kidney and aid in diuresis. Subsequently, dopamine was not found to have a beneficial effect on renal function in shock states. Its routine use for patients in shock is questionable because it may increase mortality risk and the incidence of arrhythmic events.[1,2]

Synthetic Catecholamines

Isoproterenol

Isoproterenol (Isuprel) provides relatively pure and nonselective β-adrenergic stimulation. Its $β_1$-adrenergic stimulation is greater than its $β_2$-adrenergic effects. Its popularity has declined because of adverse effects such as tachycardia and arrhythmias. It is no longer part of the advanced cardiac life support (ACLS) protocols (also see Chapter 45), and its principal uses now are as a chronotropic drug after cardiac transplantation and to initiate atrial fibrillation or other arrhythmias during cardiac electrophysiology ablation procedures. With larger doses, isoproterenol may cause vasodilation caused by $β_2$-adrenergic stimulation. Because isoproterenol is not taken up into the adrenergic nerve endings, its half-life is longer than that of the endogenous catecholamines, ranging from 2.5 to 5 minutes.

Table 6.1 Responses Elicited in Effector Organs by Stimulation of Sympathetic and Parasympathetic Nerves

Effector Organ	Adrenergic Response	Receptor Involved	Cholinergic Response	Receptor Involved	Dominant Response (A or C)
Heart	Increase	β_1	Decrease	M_2	C
Rate of contraction	Increase	β_1	Decrease	M_2	C
Force of contraction					
Blood vessels	Vasoconstriction	α_1			A
Arteries (most)	Vasodilation	β_2			A
Skeletal muscle	Vasoconstriction	α_2			A
Veins					
Bronchial tree	Bronchodilation	β_2	Bronchoconstriction	M_3	C
Splenic capsule	Contraction	α_1			A
Uterus	Contraction	α_1	Variable		A
Vas deferens	Contraction	α_1			A
Gastrointestinal tract	Relaxation	α_2	Contraction	M_3	C
Eye	Contraction	α_1	Contraction (miosis)	M_3	A
Radial muscle, iris	(mydriasis)	β_2	Contraction	M_3	C
Circular muscle, iris	Relaxation		(accommodation)		C
Ciliary muscle					
Kidney	Renin secretion	β_1			A
Urinary bladder	Relaxation	β_2	Contraction	M_3	C
Detrusor	Contraction	α_1	Relaxation	M_3	A, C
Trigone and sphincter					
Ureter	Contraction	α_1	Relaxation		A
Insulin release from pancreas	Decrease	α_2			A
Fat cells	Lipolysis	β_1 (β_3)			A
Liver glycogenolysis	Increase	α_1 (β_3)			A
Hair follicles, smooth muscle	Contraction (piloerection)	α_1			A
Nasal secretion	Decrease	α_1	Increase		C
Salivary glands	Increase secretion	α_1	Increase secretion		C
Sweat glands	Increase secretion	α_1	Increase secretion		C

A, Adrenergic; *C*, cholinergic; *M*, muscarinic.
From Bylund DB. Introduction to the autonomic nervous system. In Wecker L, Crespo L, Dunaway G, et al., eds. Brody's Human Pharmacology: Molecular to Clinical. 5th ed. Philadelphia: Mosby; 2010:102.

Dobutamine

Dobutamine, a synthetic analog of dopamine, has predominantly β_1-adrenergic effects. When compared with isoproterenol, inotropy is more affected than chronotropy. It exerts less of a β_2-type effect than isoproterenol does and less of an α_1-type effect than does norepinephrine. Unlike dopamine, endogenous norepinephrine is not released, and dobutamine does not act at dopaminergic receptors.

Dobutamine is potentially useful in patients with congestive heart failure (CHF) or myocardial infarction complicated by low cardiac output. Doses smaller than 20 µg/kg/min usually do not produce tachycardia. Because dobutamine directly stimulates β_1-receptors, it does not rely on endogenous norepinephrine stores for its effects and may still be useful in catecholamine-depleted states such as chronic CHF. However, prolonged treatment with dobutamine causes downregulation of β-adrenergic receptors. If given for more than 3 days, tolerance and even tachyphylaxis may occur and can be avoided by intermittent infusions of dobutamine.

Table 6.2 Pharmacologic Effects and Therapeutic Doses of Catecholamines

Catecholamine	Mean Arterial Pressure	Heart Rate	Cardiac Output	Systemic Vascular Resistance	Renal Blood Flow	Arrhythmogenicity	Preparation (mg/250 mL)	Intravenous Dose (mcg / kg/min)
Dopamine	+	+	+++	+	+++	+	200 (800 µg/mL)	2-20
Norepinephrine	+++	−	−	+++	−−−	+	4 (16 µg/mL)	0.01-0.1
Epinephrine	+	++	++	++	−−	+++	1 (4 µg/mL)	0.01-0.15
Isoproterenol	−	+++	+++	−−	−	+++	1 (4 µg/mL)	0.03-0.15
Dobutamine	+	+	+++	−	++	±	250 (1000 µg/mL)	2-20

+, Mild increase; + +, moderate increase; +++, marked increase; −, mild decrease; −−, moderate decrease; −−−, marked decrease.

However, there are no controlled trials demonstrating improved survival.[3]

Fenoldopam

Fenoldopam is a selective D_1 agonist and potent vasodilator that enhances renal blood flow and diuresis; its peak effect takes 15 minutes. Because of mixed results in clinical trials, fenoldopam is no longer used for treatment of chronic hypertension or CHF. Instead, intravenous fenoldopam, at infusion rates of 0.1 to 0.8 µg/kg/min, has been approved for treatment of severe hypertension. Fenoldopam is an alternative to sodium nitroprusside with fewer side effects (e.g., no thiocyanate toxicity, rebound effect, or coronary steal) and improved renal function. However, clinical studies on the use of fenoldopam as a nephroprotective agent have provided mixed results.[4,5]

Noncatecholamine Sympathomimetic Amines

Most noncatecholamine sympathomimetic amines act at α- and β-receptors through both direct (binding of the drug by adrenergic receptors) and indirect (release of endogenous norepinephrine stores) activity. Mephentermine and metaraminol are rarely used currently, so the only widely used noncatecholamine sympathomimetic amine at this time is ephedrine.

Ephedrine

Ephedrine increases arterial blood pressure and has a positive inotropic effect. Because it does not have detrimental effects on uterine blood flow in animal models, ephedrine became widely used as a pressor in hypotensive pregnant patients. However, phenylephrine is now the preferred treatment for hypotension in the parturient because of a decreased risk of fetal acidosis (also see Chapter 33). As a result of its $β_1$-adrenergic stimulating effects, ephedrine is helpful in treating moderate hypotension, particularly if accompanied by bradycardia. The usual dose is 2.5 to 10 mg given intravenously or 25 to 50 mg administered intramuscularly.

Tachyphylaxis caused by the indirect effects of ephedrine may develop as norepinephrine stores are depleted. In addition, although drugs with indirect activity are widely used as a first-line therapy for intraoperative hypotension, repeat doses of ephedrine administration in life-threatening events (instead of switching to epinephrine) may contribute to morbidity.[6]

SELECTIVE α-ADRENERGIC RECEPTOR AGONISTS

$α_1$-Adrenergic Agonists

Phenylephrine

Phenylephrine (Neo-Synephrine), a selective $α_1$-agonist, is frequently used for peripheral vasoconstriction when cardiac output is adequate (e.g., in the hypotension that may accompany spinal anesthesia). It is also used to maintain afterload in patients with aortic stenosis whose coronary perfusion is compromised by a decline in systemic vascular resistance. Given intravenously, phenylephrine has a rapid onset and relatively short duration of action (5-10 minutes). It may be given as a bolus of 40 to 100 µg or as an infusion starting at a rate of 10 to 20 µg/min. Larger doses of phenylephrine, up to 1 mg, may lead to conversion of supraventricular tachycardia to sinus rhythm through reflex action, but this treatment option is not part of current ACLS algorithms (also see Chapter 45). Phenylephrine is also a mydriatic and nasal decongestant. Applied topically, alone or in combination with local anesthetics, phenylephrine is used to prepare the nares for nasotracheal intubation.

$α_2$-Adrenergic Agonists

$α_2$-Agonists are assuming greater importance as anesthetic adjuvants and analgesics. Their primary effect is sympatholytic. They reduce peripheral norepinephrine release by stimulating prejunctional inhibitory $α_2$-receptors. Traditionally, they have been used as antihypertensive drugs, but applications based on their sedative, anxiolytic, and analgesic properties are becoming increasingly common.

Clonidine

Clonidine, the prototypical drug of this class, is a selective agonist for α_2-adrenoreceptors. Its antihypertensive effects result from central and peripheral attenuation of sympathetic outflow. Clonidine withdrawal may precipitate a hypertensive crisis, so it should be continued throughout the perioperative period. A transdermal patch is available if a patient cannot take clonidine orally. If it is not continued perioperatively, arterial blood pressure should be monitored closely with ready ability to treat hypertension. Labetalol is used to treat clonidine withdrawal syndrome.

Although experience with α_2-agonists as a sole anesthetic is limited (also see Chapter 8), these drugs can reduce the requirements for other intravenous or inhaled anesthetics as part of a general or regional anesthetic technique.[7] The results of a 2003 meta-analysis imply that perioperative use of clonidine and the other α_2-agonists dexmedetomidine and mivazerol also decreased myocardial infarction and perioperative mortality rates in patients who had vascular surgery.[8] However, a more recent (2014) large randomized trial of perioperative clonidine did not show a reduction in death or nonfatal myocardial infarction within 30 days of noncardiac surgery.[9]

In addition to their use in the operative setting, α_2-agonists provide effective analgesia for acute and chronic pain, particularly as adjuncts to local anesthetics and opioids. Epidural clonidine is indicated for the treatment of intractable pain, which is the basis for approval of parenteral clonidine in the United States as an orphan drug. Clonidine also is used to treat patients with reflex sympathetic dystrophy and other neuropathic pain syndromes (also see Chapter 44).

Dexmedetomidine

Like clonidine, dexmedetomidine is highly selective for the α_2-receptors. Its half-life of 2.3 hours and distribution half-life of less than 5 minutes make its clinical effect quite short. Unlike clonidine, dexmedetomidine is available as an intravenous solution in the United States. The usual dosing is an infusion of 0.3 to 0.7 µg/kg/h either with or without a 1 µg/kg initial dose given over 10 minutes.

In healthy volunteers dexmedetomidine increases sedation, analgesia, and amnesia; it decreases heart rate, cardiac output, and circulating catecholamines in a dose-dependent fashion. The inhaled anesthetic-sparing, sedative, and analgesic effects demonstrated in preclinical and volunteer studies have been borne out in clinical practice. The relatively minor impact of α_2-induced sedation on respiratory function combined with the short duration of action of dexmedetomidine has led to its use for awake fiber optic endotracheal intubation.[10] Dexmedetomidine infusions for the perioperative management of obese patients with obstructive sleep apnea minimized the need for narcotics while providing adequate analgesia.[11]

β_2-ADRENERGIC RECEPTOR AGONISTS

β_2-Agonists are used to treat asthma (also see Chapter 27). With large doses, the β_2-receptor selectivity can be lost, and severe side effects related to β_1-adrenergic stimulation are possible. Commonly used agonists include metaproterenol (Alupent, Metaprel), terbutaline (Brethine, Bricanyl), and albuterol (Proventil, Ventolin).

β_2-Agonists are also used to arrest premature labor (also see Chapter 33). Ritodrine (Yutopar) has been marketed for this purpose. Unfortunately, β_1-adrenergic adverse effects are common, particularly when the drug is given intravenously.

α-ADRENERGIC RECEPTOR ANTAGONISTS

α_1-Antagonists have long been used as antihypertensive drugs, but their side effects, which include marked orthostatic hypotension and fluid retention, have made them less popular as other medications for controlling arterial blood pressure with more attractive side effect profiles have become available.

Phenoxybenzamine

Phenoxybenzamine (Dibenzyline) is the prototypical α_1-adrenergic antagonist (though it also has α_2-antagonist effects). Because it irreversibly binds α_1-receptors, new receptors must be synthesized before complete recovery. Phenoxybenzamine decreases peripheral resistance and increases cardiac output. Its primary adverse effect is orthostatic hypotension that can lead to syncope with rapid patient movement from the supine to standing position. Nasal stuffiness is another effect. Phenoxybenzamine is most commonly used in the treatment of pheochromocytomas. It establishes a "chemical sympathectomy" preoperatively that makes arterial blood pressure less labile during surgical resection of these catecholamine-secreting tumors. When exogenous sympathomimetics are given after α_1-blockade, their vasoconstrictive effects are inhibited. Despite its irreversible binding to the receptor, the recommended treatment for a phenoxybenzamine overdose is an infusion of norepinephrine because some receptors remain free of the drug; vasopressin may also be effective in this setting.

Prazosin

Prazosin (Minipress) is a potent selective α_1-blocker that antagonizes the vasoconstrictor effects of norepinephrine and epinephrine. Orthostatic hypotension is a major problem with prazosin. Unlike other antihypertensive drugs, prazosin improves lipid profiles by lowering low-density lipoprotein levels and raising the level of high-density lipoproteins. The usual starting dose of prazosin is 0.5 to 1 mg given at bedtime because of the risk of orthostatic hypotension. Doxazosin (Cardura) and terazosin (Hytrin) have pharmacologic effects similar to those of prazosin but have longer pharmacokinetic half-lives. Because of the high cost of phenoxybenzamine, these agents are being used with greater frequency for the preoperative preparation of patients with pheochromocytomas. However, because these agents provide competitive antagonism instead of permanent binding to the α-receptors, modest intraoperative hypertensive episodes seem to be more common in these patients than in those who received phenoxybenzamine.[12] Agents such as tamsulosin (Flomax) show selectivity for the α_{1A}-receptor subtype and are effective in the treatment of benign prostatic hyperplasia without the hypotensive effects seen when the nonselective α_1-blockers are used to treat this condition.

Yohimbine

α_2-Antagonists such as yohimbine increase the release of norepinephrine, but they have found little clinical utility in anesthesia.

β-ADRENERGIC ANTAGONISTS

β-Adrenergic antagonists (i.e., β-blockers) are frequently taken by patients about to undergo surgery. Clinical indications for β-adrenergic blockade include ischemic heart disease, postinfarction management, arrhythmias, hypertrophic cardiomyopathy, hypertension, heart failure, migraine prophylaxis, thyrotoxicosis, and glaucoma. In patients with heart failure and reduced ejection fraction β-blocker therapy has been shown to reverse ventricular remodeling and reduce mortality rate.[13] In the 1990s a study by the Perioperative Ischemia Research Group demonstrated the value of initiating β-blockade perioperatively in patients at risk for coronary artery disease.[14] Study subjects given perioperative β-blockers had a markedly reduced all-cause 2-year mortality rate (68% survival rate in placebo group vs. 83% in atenolol-treated group). The presumed mechanism for this improved survival rate was a diminution of the surgical stress response by the β-blockers. These and other confirmatory findings led to tremendous political and administrative pressure to increase the use of β-blockers perioperatively. Subsequent studies, however, have questioned the value of perioperative β-blockade, including a large study of oral metoprolol started on the day of surgery and continuing for 30 days (POISE trial), which demonstrated increased mortality rate in the β-blocker group.[15] A systematic

review on perioperative β-blockade from the American College of Cardiology/American Heart Association (ACC/AHA) states that although perioperative continuation of β-blockade started 1 day or less before noncardiac surgery in high-risk patients prevents nonfatal myocardial infarctions, it increases the rate of death, hypotension, bradycardia, and stroke. In addition, there is insufficient data regarding continuation of β-blockade started 2 days or more before noncardiac surgery.[16] The 2014 ACC/AHA guideline on perioperative cardiovascular evaluation and management of patients undergoing noncardiac surgery recommends that patients on chronic β-blocker therapy continue this therapy in the perioperative period, but β-blocker therapy should not be started on the day of surgery[17] (also see Chapter 13). Additionally, other literature reviews have shown that the evidence for all-cause mortality with perioperative β-blockade is uncertain, with no evidence of a difference in ventricular arrythmias or cerebrovascular events and low-certainty evidence that β-blockers reduced atrial fibrillation and myocardial infarctions; however, β-blockers may increase bradycardia and increase hypotension.[18]

The most widely used β-adrenergic blockers in anesthetic practice are propranolol, metoprolol, labetalol, and esmolol because they are available as intravenous formulations and have well-characterized effects. The most important differences among these blockers are tied to cardioselectivity and duration of action. Nonselective β-blockers act at the β_1- and β_2-receptors. Cardioselective β-blockers have stronger affinity for β_1-adrenergic receptors than for β_2-adrenergic receptors. With β_1-receptor selective blockade, velocity of atrioventricular conduction, heart rate, and cardiac contractility decrease. The release of renin by the juxtaglomerular apparatus and lipolysis at adipocytes also decrease. With larger doses, the relative selectivity for β_1-receptors is lost and β_2-receptors are also blocked, with the potential for bronchoconstriction, peripheral vasoconstriction, and decreased glycogenolysis.

Adverse Effects of β-Adrenergic Blockade

Life-threatening bradycardia, even asystole, may occur with β-adrenergic blockade, and decreased contractility may precipitate heart failure in patients with compromised cardiac function. In patients with bronchospastic lung disease β_2-blockade may be fatal. Diabetes mellitus is a relative contraindication to the long-term use of β-adrenergic antagonists because warning signs of hypoglycemia (tachycardia and tremor) can be masked and because compensatory glycogenolysis is blunted. To avoid worsening of hypertension, use of β-blockers in patients with pheochromocytomas should be avoided unless α-receptors have already been blocked. Overdose of β-blocking drugs may be treated with atropine, but isoproterenol, dobutamine, or glucagon also may be required along with cardiac pacing to maintain an adequate rate of contraction.

Undesirable drug interactions are possible with β-blockers. The rate and contractility effects of verapamil are additive to those of β-blockers, so care must be taken when combining these drugs. Similarly, the combination of digoxin and β-blockers can have powerful effects on heart rate and conduction and should be used with special care.

Specific β-Adrenergic Blockers

Propranolol

Propranolol (Inderal, Ipran), the prototypical β-blocker, is a nonselective β-blocking drug. Because of its high lipid solubility, it is extensively metabolized in the liver, but metabolism varies greatly from patient to patient. Clearance of the drug can be affected by liver disease or altered hepatic blood flow. Propranolol is available in an intravenous form and was initially given as either a bolus or an infusion. Infusions of propranolol have largely been supplanted by the shorter-acting esmolol. For bolus administration, doses of 0.1 mg/kg may be given, but most practitioners initiate therapy with much smaller doses, typically 0.25 to 0.5 mg, and titrate to effect. Propranolol shifts the oxyhemoglobin dissociation curve to the right, which might account for its efficacy in vasospastic disorders.[19] Additionally, propranolol is commonly used in the treatment of hyperthyroidism to mitigate tachycardia that may result and because propranolol inhibits the peripheral conversion of T_4 thyroid hormone to the more active T_3 hormone.

Metoprolol

Metoprolol (Lopressor), a cardioselective β-adrenergic blocker, is approved for the treatment of angina pectoris and acute myocardial infarction. No dosing adjustments are necessary in patients with liver failure. The usual oral dose is 100 to 200 mg/day taken once or twice daily for hypertension and twice daily for angina pectoris. Intravenous doses of 2.5 to 5 mg may be administered every 2 to 5 minutes up to a total dose of 15 mg, with titration to heart rate and blood pressure.

Labetalol

Labetalol (Trandate, Normodyne) acts as a competitive antagonist at the α_1- and β-adrenergic receptors. Metabolized by the liver, its clearance is affected by hepatic perfusion. Labetalol may be given intravenously every 5 minutes in 5- to 10-mg doses or as an infusion of up to 2 mg/min. It can be effective in the treatment of patients with aortic dissection[20] and in hypertensive emergencies. Because vasodilation is not accompanied by tachycardia, labetalol has been given to patients with coronary artery disease postoperatively. It may be used to treat hypertension in pregnancy both on a long-term basis and in more acute situations.[21] Uterine blood flow is not affected,

even with significant reductions in blood pressure[22] (also see Chapter 33).

Esmolol

Because it is hydrolyzed by bloodborne esterases, esmolol (Brevibloc) has a uniquely short half-life of 9 to 10 minutes, which makes it particularly useful in anesthetic practice. It can be used when β-blockade of short duration is desired or in critically ill patients in whom the adverse effects of bradycardia, heart failure, or hypotension may require rapid withdrawal of the drug. Esmolol is cardioselective, and the peak effects of a loading dose are seen within 5 to 10 minutes and diminish within 20 to 30 minutes. It may be given as a bolus of 0.5 mg/kg or as an infusion. When used to treat supraventricular tachycardia, a bolus of 500 µg/kg is given over 1 minute, followed by an infusion of 50 µg/kg/min for 4 minutes. If the heart rate is not controlled, a repeat loading dose followed by a 4-minute infusion of 100 µg/kg/min is given. If needed, this sequence is repeated with the infusion increased in 50-µg/kg/min increments up to 300 µg/kg/min. Esmolol is safe and effective for the treatment of intraoperative and postoperative hypertension and tachycardia. If continuous use is required, it may be replaced by a longer-lasting cardioselective β-blocker such as metoprolol.

CHOLINERGIC PHARMACOLOGY

In contrast to the rich selection of drugs to manipulate adrenergic responses, there is a relative paucity of drugs that affect cholinergic transmission. A small number of direct cholinergic agents are used topically for the treatment of glaucoma or to restore gastrointestinal or urinary function. The classes of drugs with relevance to the anesthesia provider are the anticholinergic agents (muscarinic antagonists) and the anticholinesterases.

Muscarinic Antagonists

The muscarinic antagonists compete with neurally released ACh for access to muscarinic cholinoceptors and block ACh's effects. The results are faster heart rate, sedation, and dry mouth. With the exception of the quaternary ammonium compounds that do not readily cross the blood–brain barrier and have few actions on the CNS, there is no significant specificity of action among these drugs; they block all muscarinic effects with equal efficacy, although there are some quantitative differences in effect (Table 6.3).

In the era of ether anesthetics a muscarinic antagonist was added to anesthetic premedication to decrease secretions and to prevent harmful vagal reflexes. This addition is less important with modern inhaled anesthetics. Preoperative use of these drugs continues in some pediatric and otorhinolaryngologic cases or when fiber-optic intubation is planned.

Table 6.3 Comparative Effects of Anticholinergics Administered Intramuscularly as Pharmacologic Premedication

Effect	Atropine	Scopolamine	Glycopyrrolate
Antisialagogue effect	+	+++	++
Sedative and amnesic effect	+	+++	0
Increased gastric fluid pH	0	0	0/+
Central nervous system toxicity	+	++	0
Lower esophageal sphincter relaxation	++	++	++
Mydriasis and cycloplegia	+	+++	0
Heart rate	++	0/+	+

0, None; +, mild; ++, moderate; +++, marked.

Because of its tertiary structure, atropine can cross the blood–brain barrier. Thus large doses (1–2 mg) can affect the CNS. In contrast, because of its quaternary structure, the synthetic antimuscarinic drug glycopyrrolate (Robinul) does not cross the blood–brain barrier. Glycopyrrolate has a longer duration of action than atropine and has largely replaced atropine for blocking the adverse muscarinic effects (bradycardia) of the anticholinesterase drugs that reverse neuromuscular blockade (also see Chapter 11). Scopolamine also crosses the blood–brain barrier and can have profound CNS effects. The patch preparation of scopolamine is used prophylactically for postoperative nausea and vomiting, but it may be associated with adverse eye, bladder, skin, and psychological effects. The CNS side effects (e.g., delusions or delirium) that can follow treatment with atropine or scopolamine are treated with physostigmine, an anticholinesterase that is able to cross the blood–brain barrier.

Cholinesterase Inhibitors

Anticholinesterase drugs impair the inactivation of ACh by the cholinesterase enzyme and sustain cholinergic agonism at nicotinic and muscarinic receptors. These drugs are used to reverse neuromuscular blockade (see Chapter 11) and to treat myasthenia gravis. The most prominent side effect of these drugs is bradycardia. The commonly used cholinesterase inhibitors are physostigmine, neostigmine, pyridostigmine, and edrophonium. In addition to reversing the effects of neuromuscular-blocking drugs by increasing the concentration of ACh at the neuromuscular junction, cholinesterase inhibitors stimulate intestinal function or are applied topically to the eye as a miotic. One topical drug (echothiophate iodide) irreversibly binds cholinesterase and can interfere with the metabolism of succinylcholine (as the anticholinesterases impair the function of the pseudocholinesterase enzyme as well).

REFERENCES

1. Holmes CL, Walley KR. Bad medicine: Low-dose dopamine in the ICU. *Chest.* 2003;123:1266–1275.
2. DeBacker D, Aldecoa C, Nijimi H, et al. Dopamine versus norepinephrine in the treatment of septic shock: A meta-analysis. *Crit Care Med.* 2012;40(3):725–730.
3. Krell MJ, Kline EM, Bates ER, et al. Intermittent, ambulatory dobutamine infusions in patients with severe congestive heart failure. *Am Heart J.* 1986;112:787–791.
4. Sun H, Xie Q, Peng Z. Does fenoldopam protect kidney in cardiac surgery? A systemic review and meta-analysis with trail sequential analysis. *Shock.* 2019;52(3):326–333.
5. Ranucci M, Soro G, Barzaghi N, et al. Fenoldopam prophylaxis of postoperative acute renal failure in high-risk cardiac surgery patients. *Ann Thorac Surg.* 2004;78:1332–1338.
6. Caplan RA, Ward RJ, Posner K, et al. Unexpected cardiac arrest during spinal anesthesia: A closed claims analysis of predisposing factors. *Anesthesiology.* 1988;68:5–11.
7. Maze M, Tranquilli W. Alpha-2 adrenergic agonists: Defining the role in clinical anesthesia. *Anesthesiology.* 1991;74:581–605.
8. Wijeysundera DN, Naik JS, Beattie WS. Alpha-2 adrenergic agonists to prevent perioperative cardiovascular complications—A meta-analysis. *Am J Med.* 2003;114:742–752.
9. Devereaux PJ, Sessler DI, Leslie K, et al. Clonidine in patients undergoing noncardiac surgery. *N Engl J Med.* 2014;16:1504–1513.
10. Bergese SD, Khabiri B, Roberts WD, et al. Dexmedetomidine for conscious sedation in difficult awake fiberoptic intubation cases. *J Clin Anesth.* 2007;19:141–144.
11. Ramsay MA, Saha D, Hebeler RF. Tracheal resection in the morbidly obese patient: The role of dexmedetomidine. *J Clin Anesth.* 2006;18:452–454.
12. Kong H, Li N, Yang X. et al. Nonselective compared with selective α-blockade is associated with less intraoperative hypertension in patients with pheochromocytomas and paragangliomas: A retrospective cohort study with propensity score matching. *Anesth Analg.* 2021;132:140–149.
13. Florea VG, Cohn JN. The autonomic nervous system and heart failure. *Circ Res.* 2014;114:1815–1826.

14. Mangano DT, Layug EL, Wallace A, et al. Effect of atenolol on mortality and cardiovascular morbidity after noncardiac surgery. Multicenter Study of Perioperative Ischemia Research Group. *N Engl J Med.* 1996;335:1713–1720.

15. POISE Study Group. Effects of extended-release metoprolol succinate in patients undergoing non-cardiac surgery (POISE trial): A randomised controlled trial. *Lancet.* 2008;371:1839–1847.

16. Wijeysundera DN, Duncan D, Nkonde-Price C, et al. Perioperative beta blockade in noncardiac surgery: A systematic review for the 2014 ACC/AHA guideline on perioperative cardiovascular evaluation and management of patients undergoing noncardiac surgery. *J Am Coll Cardiol.* 2014;64:2406–2425.

17. Fleisher LA, Fleischmann KE, Auerbach AD, et al. ACC/AHA guideline on perioperative cardiovascular evaluation and management of patients undergoing noncardiac surgery: A report of the American College of Cardiology/American Heart Association Task Force on Practice Guidelines. *J Am Coll Cardiol.* 2014;64:e77–e137.

18. Blessberger H, Lewis SR, Pritchard MW, et al. Perioperative beta-blockers for preventing surgery-related mortality and morbidity in adults undergoing non-cardiac surgery (review). *Cochrane Database Syst Rev.* 2019;(9):CD013438.

19. Pendleton RG, Newman DJ, Sherman SS, et al. Effect of propranolol upon the hemoglobin-oxygen dissociation curve. *J Pharmacol Exp Ther.* 1972;180:647–656.

20. DeSanctis RW, Doroghazi RM, Austen WG, et al. Aortic dissection. *N Engl J Med.* 1987;317:1060–1067.

21. Lavies NG, Meiklejohn BH, May AE, et al. Hypertensive and catecholamine response to tracheal intubations in patients with pregnancy-induced hypertension. *Br J Anaesth.* 1989;63:429–434.

22. Jouppila P, Kirkinen P, Koivula A, et al. Labetalol does not alter the placental and fetal blood flow or maternal prostanoids in pre-eclampsia. *Br J Obstet Gynaecol.* 1986;93:543–547.

Chapter

7 INHALED ANESTHETICS

Daniel Charles Cook, Hugh C. Hemmings, Jr.

HISTORY

Before the introduction of anesthesia, surgery was usually excruciating and harrowing for patients, limited in duration and technique by what the patient could tolerate.[1] On October 16, 1846, the dentist William T. G. Morton administered diethyl ether for a surgery at the Massachusetts General Hospital to remove a tumor from Ebenezer Hopkins Frost's neck.[2] The patient's ability to tolerate the surgery, recalling afterwards a dulled sensation,[2] led the surgeon, John C. Warren, to famously exclaim, "Gentlemen, this is no humbug."[3] This case is generally credited as the first successful public demonstration of an inhaled anesthetic used for surgery.[3] Within a month, this and other experiences using ether for procedures were published in the *Boston Medical and Surgical Journal* (now the *New England Journal of Medicine*),[2] and within months surgeries were being performed routinely with ether anesthesia in the United States and Europe.[4]

The public demonstration of ether anesthesia by Morton was preceded by other successful applications of ether anesthesia, notably by Crawford Long in Georgia, and by consideration of the utility of nitrous oxide for surgery, such as by Sir Humphy Davy of England, and an unsuccessful public attempt of a tooth extraction under nitrous oxide anesthesia by the dentist Horace Wells.[3] Nevertheless, the immediate, far-reaching, and profound impact of the demonstration of ether anesthesia for surgery[4] underlies why this date continues to be celebrated as "Ether Day."[1] After October 16, 1846, Morton and his associates spent years quarreling for credit over the discovery and seeking to patent ether, unfortunately leading to underwhelming and tragic ends.[1] Nevertheless, the advent of inhaled anesthesia ushered in a new era of surgery and medicine, and the article describing the first surgeries performed under ether anesthesia was voted as the most important in 200 years of publications from the *New England Journal of Medicine*.[5] This recognition is well deserved for one of the most important advances in medicine.

CHEMICAL AND PHYSICAL PROPERTIES

Molecular Structures

The most commonly used inhaled anesthetics available in 2020 are isoflurane (1-chloro-2,2,2-trifluoroethyl difluoromethyl ether), sevoflurane (1,1,1,3,3,3-hexafluoro-2-(fluoromethoxy) propane), and desflurane (2-(difluoromethoxy)-1,1,1,2-tetrafluoroethane). They are halogenated ethers containing fluorine and/or chlorine (Fig. 7.1). Halothane (2-bromo-2-chloro-1,1,1-trifluoroethane), which is rarely used today, is a polyhalogenated alkane. Both sevoflurane and desflurane have fluorine exclusively as the halogen substitution, which is credited for their minimal metabolism and improved pharmacokinetic profile.[6-8] Other halogenated ethers, including isoflurane, contain both chlorine and fluorine, and halothane also contains bromine. These four drugs, and several others that preceded them, are known as *volatile anesthetics*. Volatility refers to their tendency, as liquids at standard temperature and pressure, to evaporate. The other routinely used inhaled anesthetic, nitrous oxide, is an oxide of nitrogen, with the chemical formula N_2O. Xenon, an element classified as a noble gas, is also an inhaled anesthetic, but given its limited availability, difficult delivery and expense, it is rarely used, though research suggests it may have specific applications as a neuroprotectant.

Physical Properties

Several physicochemical properties of inhaled anesthetics are critical to understanding their delivery and pharmacokinetics. To understand the pharmacology and chemistry of inhaled anesthetics, it is useful to consider the ideal gas law:

$$PV = nRT$$

where P is pressure, V is volume, n is the number of gas particles (in moles), R is the universal gas constant, and T is temperature. Other relationships, such as Charles' law ($V_1/T_1 = V_2/T_2$) and Boyle's law ($P_1 V_1 = P_2 V_2$), can be derived simply from the ideal gas law by considering the other variables as constants.

The partial pressure of a gas is the pressure exerted by one individual gas within a gaseous mixture. The total pressure of a gas mixture is the sum of the partial pressures of each of its components:

$$P_T = P_1 + P_2 + \ldots + P_n$$

where P_T is the total pressure of the gas mixture composed of n gases denoted by the subscripts. The contribution of any one gas within the gas mixture to the total

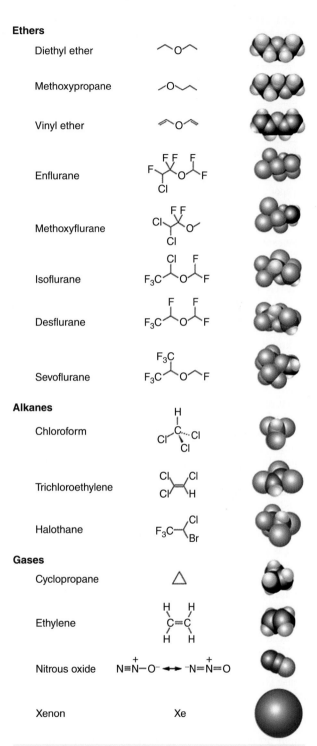

Fig. 7.1 Molecular structures and space-filling model of historical and currently used inhaled anesthetics. (From Hudson AE, Hemmings HC Jr. Pharmacokinetics of inhaled anesthetics, Ch. 3. In: Hemmings HC Jr, Egan TD, eds. *Pharmacology and Physiology for Anesthesia: Foundations and Clinical Application*, 2nd ed. Philadelphia: Elsevier; 2019:45.)

Table 7.1 Comparative Properties of Inhaled Anesthetics

Characteristic	Halothane	Methoxyflurane	Isoflurane	Sevoflurane	Desflurane	Nitrous oxide	Xenon
Partition coefficients							
Blood–gas	2.54	11	1.46	0.65	0.45	0.46	0.14
Brain–blood	1.9		1.6	1.7	1.3	1.1	
Muscle–blood	3.4		2.9	3.1	2.0	1.2	
Fat–blood	51		45	48	27	2.3	
MAC (age 40)	0.75	0.16	1.28	2.05	6.0	104	0.71
Vapor pressure at 20°C (mm Hg)	244	22.5	240	160	669		
Molecular weight	197.4	165	184.5	200.1	168.0	44.0	131.3
Percent metabolized	15–40	70	0.2	5	0.02		

Adapted from McKay RE. Inhaled anesthetics, Chapter 8 In: *Basics of Anesthesia*, 7th ed. Philadelphia: Elsevier; 2018: 81. Based on Steward A, Allott PR, Cowles AL, et al. Solubility coefficients for inhaled anaesthetics for water, oil, and biological media. *Br J Anaesth*. 1973;45:282-293. Yasuda N, Targ AG, Eger EI. Solubility of I-653, sevoflurane, isoflurane, and halothane in human tissues. *Anesth Analg*. 1989;69:370-373.

pressure is proportional to its molar fraction within the mixture:

$$P_i = XP_t$$

where X is the molar fraction (the percentage of the gas mixture for the individual gas) and Pi is the partial pressure of that gas. It is the partial pressure of a volatile anesthetic within the body that determines its pharmacologic effect. Conceptually, partial pressure is the gas equivalent of plasma concentration for an intravenous anesthetic. A striking example of this concept is the lowering of analgesia, sedation, and nausea because of a fixed concentration of nitrous oxide when ambient pressure is lowered within a pressurized chamber.[9] Because it is the absolute partial pressure of an inhaled anesthetic that is pharmacodynamically relevant, lowering ambient pressure at a constant concentration decreases its partial pressure and, thereby, its anesthetic effect. Although not well-studied, this concept likely applies to the provision of anesthesia at elevated altitudes, a setting in which the potency of an anesthetic at a given concentration will be reduced by the reduction in atmospheric pressure.[10]

Vapor pressure is the partial pressure exerted by the gaseous phase of a chemical in equilibrium with its liquid phase (Table 7.1). It can be conceptualized as the pressure exerted on a liquid to prevent molecules from escaping into the gaseous phase. Thus liquids that are more likely to evaporate (i.e., are more volatile) have higher vapor pressures. This chemical property depends on temperature; as temperature is increased, vapor pressure also increases. Boiling occurs when the temperature of a liquid is increased such that its vapor pressure exceeds ambient pressure. Thus a more volatile liquid, with a higher vapor pressure, will also boil at lower temperatures (it has a lower boiling point). Desflurane has the highest vapor pressure among the modern volatile agents. Its boiling point is 24°C (75°F), highlighting its propensity to evaporate or boil under temperature and pressure conditions that may occur in the operating room. This distinction necessitates a unique bottle design and pressurized vaporizer mechanism.[11] Although other volatile anesthetics can be poured into a vaporizer, desflurane would quickly evaporate, polluting the operating room environment, thus necessitating a closed system (see later).

The most important physicochemical property to explain the pharmacokinetics of inhaled anesthetics is their solubility, which is the amount of a gas that can be homogeneously dissolved into a liquid. At low concentrations, the solubility of a gas can be defined by Henry's law,

$$C = kP_{gas}$$

where C is the concentration, P is the partial pressure, and k is the solubility constant that depends on the gas, solvent, and temperature (as temperature increases, solubility decreases). In anesthetic pharmacology the partition coefficient is the metric generally used to convey and compare solubility. The partition coefficient is the ratio of concentrations at equilibrium of a solute dissolved in two different solvents (Fig. 7.2). Applied to inhaled anesthesia, the partition coefficient is the concentrations of the anesthetic in two different body compartments when the partial pressure of the drug has equilibrated.[7] Anesthetic uptake from lung alveoli into the blood is described by the blood:gas partition coefficient. Anesthetics with lower blood:gas partition coefficients are less soluble, and therefore a lower amount (mass) of anesthetic is required to reach a given partial pressure in the blood. Partition coefficients between the blood and other organs approximate the relative accumulation of the anesthetic

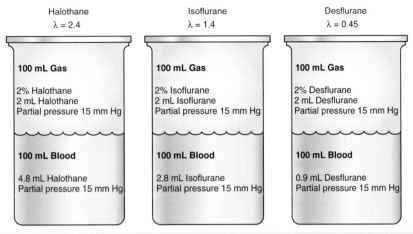

Fig. 7.2 Blood-gas partition coefficients reflect the solubility of inhaled anesthetics in blood. The partition coefficient is the ratio of concentrations of the anesthetic in blood to that in alveoli at steady state when partial pressures are equal in each compartment. (From Hudson AE, Hemmings HC Jr. Pharmacokinetics of inhaled anesthetics, Ch. 3. In: Hemmings HC Jr, Egan TD, eds. *Pharmacology and Physiology for Anesthesia: Foundations and Clinical Application,* 2nd ed. Philadelphia: Elsevier; 2019:47.)

throughout the body and, importantly, between the blood and brain (i.e., the brain:blood partition coefficient).

UPTAKE AND DISTRIBUTION IN THE BODY

Vaporizers

Maintaining general anesthesia with inhaled anesthetics requires precise delivery. For the potent, volatile anesthetics, vaporizers are used to deliver specific gas concentrations (dose) to a patient. Most modern vaporizers use a variable bypass design (Fig. 7.3). Gas from the anesthesia machine that enters into the vaporizer is split between two paths in a specific ratio: one path proceeds without accumulating anesthetic (bypasses), while the other path is through a chamber saturated with vaporized anesthetic agent. The two pathways are recombined such that the bypassing gas dilutes the gas saturated with anesthetic to achieve the desired output as volume percent (vol%)[12] (also see Chapter 44).

The vaporizer for desflurane is an exception to the variable bypass design. The high vapor pressure of desflurane would require substantial fresh gas flows to dilute the anesthetic to clinical concentrations. Moreover, because of its low boiling point, it can boil under ambient conditions, which would preclude a precise output of anesthetic with a variable bypass vaporizer design. Thus desflurane vaporizers heat the anesthetic above its boiling point to achieve a constant vapor pressure, which can then be injected in controlled volumes into the gas flow pathway (see Fig. 7.3).[12]

Nitrous oxide and xenon exist as gases at standard temperature and pressure, and are known as *gaseous anesthetics.* Nitrous oxide is supplied from a central supply wall outlet or from a tank connected to the anesthesia workstation. The concentration of nitrous oxide (vol%) is controlled by adjusting the flows of oxygen, air, and nitrous oxide through a mixer. Older machines used manual adjustments of flowmeters, but newer machines use electronic controls to set overall fresh gas flow and the percentage of nitrous oxide.

Anesthetic Circuit

The anesthesia work station delivers a gas mixture determined by the settings of the vaporizers and fresh gas flows. However, it is important to account for the nontrivial volume of the breathing circuit. Adjusting the vaporizer will not immediately change the mixture received by the patient because the gases must first reach steady state within the circuit. This process is described by

$$F_C = F_{FGF}(1 - e^{-t/t})$$

where F_C is the concentration of anesthetic in the circuit, F_{FGF} is the concentration of anesthetic in the fresh gas delivered to the circuit, and τ is the time constant of the circuit, defined as

$$\tau = V_C / FGF$$

where V_C is the volume of the circuit and *FGF* is the fresh gas flow.[13]

Partition Coefficients

Aqueous solubility is the chemical property of inhaled anesthetics that determines the kinetics of uptake and distribution, and induction of anesthesia. The solubility of inhaled anesthetics is conveyed in their blood:gas partition

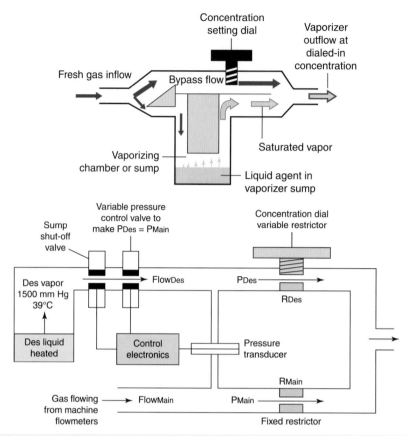

Fig. 7.3 Schematic of vaporizers for volatile anesthetic delivery. (A) Inhaled anesthetics require specialized equipment to deliver them to patients in accurate concentrations. The most common design is the variable-bypass vaporizer, which works by diluting gas saturated with anesthetic with fresh gas to achieve the desired concentration. (B) The boiling point of desflurane is near room temperature, thus preventing reliable administration of desflurane by a variable-bypass vaporizer. The Tec 6, designed specifically to administer desflurane, heats and pressurizes the anesthetic chamber to achieve a steady vapor pressure. Injection of desflurane vapor into the fresh gas dilutes the anesthetic to the desired concentration. *Des,* Desflurane. (From Eisenkraft JB. Anesthesia vaporizers, Ch. 2. In: Ehrenwerth J, Eienkraft JB, Berry JB, eds. *Anesthesia Equipment: Principles and Applications,* 2nd ed. Philadelphia, PA: Elsevier; 2013:68, 86.)

coefficients. Anesthetics with lower solubility (lower blood:gas partition coefficients) have quicker onset and recovery profiles.[14] The partial pressure of an anesthetic determines the magnitude of its effect; in other words, partial pressure is the effective concentration of an inhaled anesthetic in the blood, brain, and other organ systems. Once a therapeutic steady state has been achieved, the partial pressure of the anesthetic will be the same in the alveoli, blood, and brain, while concentrations in each of these compartments will differ according to the relevant partition coefficients. Anesthetics with lower solubility require lower concentrations in the blood to achieve a given partial pressure, thus speeding the rate of induction. An analogy can be made with the administration of intravenous drugs and their volume of distribution (V_D), which is defined as the bolus dose of a drug divided by the plasma concentration achieved. Drugs that are more lipophilic redistribute more widely from the plasma into other tissues; thus the plasma concentration reached will be relatively low, leading to a greater V_D. In effect, the drug distributes to a plasma volume that is larger than its actual volume. Solubility of inhaled anesthetics is similar conceptually to the V_D for intravenous drugs. Inhaled anesthetics that are more soluble, and therefore have higher blood:gas partition coefficients, distribute to a virtual plasma volume that is relatively large and have higher plasma molar concentrations (Fig. 7.4). Thus higher concentrations are required to reach a given partial pressure. In other words, more drug uptake is required to achieve the target partial pressure to reach the desired anesthetic effect.

The brain:blood partition coefficient is an important consideration for the induction of and recovery from

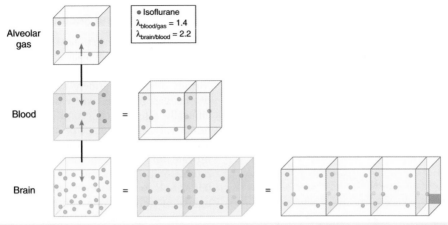

Alveolar gas

Blood

Brain

● Isoflurane
$\lambda_{blood/gas} = 1.4$
$\lambda_{brain/blood} = 2.2$

Fig. 7.4 Blood and tissue solubilities of inhaled anesthetics determine their pharmacokinetic distribution and relative concentrations in each compartment. At steady state, partial pressure equalizes across body compartments (represented by cubic volumes) but concentrations of anesthetics within compartments will differ based on the relevant partition coefficients. In the example of isoflurane the concentration increases relative to alveolar gas in blood and in the brain. (From Forman SA, Ishizawa Y. Inhaled anesthetic pharmacokinetics: Uptake, distribution, metabolism, and toxicity, Ch. 20. In: Gropper MA, ed. *Miller's Anesthesia*, 9th ed. Philadelphia: Elsevier; 2020:512.)

general anesthesia because the nervous system is the major target organ. Lower tissue solubility will lead to more rapid equilibration from the blood and, by extension, from alveoli to that tissue.[15] However, the brain:blood partition coefficients of inhaled anesthetics have a smaller range (from 1.1 to 1.9 for nitrous oxide and halothane, respectively) than the blood:gas partition coefficients (from 0.45 to 2.54 for desflurane and halothane, respectively).[16] Thus the parameter that differs more between agents is the blood:gas coefficient, which has a greater impact on how anesthetic selection determines pharmacokinetics for a given patient. Moreover, various diseases affect the uptake of inhaled anesthetics from the alveolus, and these effects are influenced by the blood:gas partition coefficient, as described further later in the chapter. Conversely, there is relatively little the anesthesiologist can do to change the equilibration of an anesthetic from the blood into the brain. For these reasons, the blood:gas partition coefficient is the critical parameter determining onset, and practitioners need to understand how the solubility of an agent affects the conduct of the anesthetic procedure.

Gas Exchange

The driving force of gas diffusion is the gradient in partial pressure. Gas exchange continues until partial pressures across the diffusion barrier are equalized. To induce general anesthesia, a target partial pressure of an inhaled anesthetic must be reached in the brain and spinal cord. At steady state, the partial pressure in the brain and alveoli are equal. According to Dalton's law of partial pressure, partial pressure is determined by the fractional concentration of the drug relative to that of total alveolar gas, so achieving a specific volume fraction of inhaled anesthetic in the alveolus, F_A, is necessary to induce general anesthesia, with the rate of induction depending on how rapidly the target F_A is reached. The anesthetist controls the fraction of inspired gas made up by the inhaled anesthetic delivered to the patient in the inspired gas (F_I). As the lungs are ventilated, F_A approaches and eventually equals F_I, with the rate of induction depending on how quickly the F_A/F_I ratio approaches 1.[7]

The rate of the rise of F_A/F_I is determined by anesthetic solubility, expressed as the blood:gas partition coefficient (Fig. 7.5).[7] Drugs with lower blood:gas partition coefficients are less soluble in blood, and thus F_A increases more quickly and target anesthetic partial pressure is reached faster. As anesthetic diffuses across the alveolar membrane, its partial pressure in blood increases, thereby decreasing the partial pressure gradient, such that more anesthetic remains in the alveolus to contribute to F_A.

A variety of other factors, determined by either the anesthetist or physiologic states, affect the rate of rise of F_A/F_I.[7] Increasing anesthetic delivery to the alveoli, either through higher fresh gas flow, anesthetic concentration, or alveolar ventilation, speeds the rise in F_A/F_I. Processes that decrease anesthetic uptake from the alveoli also increase the rate of rise of F_A/F_I. An example is a decrease in cardiac output, which allows the partial pressure in the alveolus to equilibrate with the blood in the pulmonary capillaries more quickly, this reduces the partial pressure difference and retains more anesthetic in the alveoli to increase F_A. Ventilation-perfusion mismatching reduces

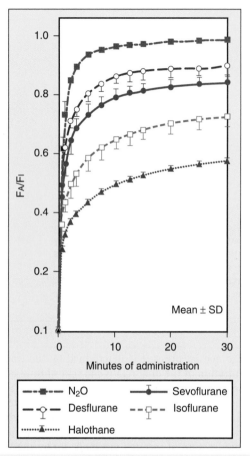

Fig. 7.5 Solubility in blood is the primary property of inhaled anesthetics governing equilibration between alveoli and blood and, thereby, the rate of induction of anesthesia. F_A, Fraction of alveolar gas; F_I, fraction of inhaled gas. (From McKay RE. Inhaled anesthetics, Ch. 7. In Pardo M, ed. *Basics of Anesthesia*, 7th ed. Philadelphia: Elsevier; 2018:91.)

anesthetic uptake. In the case of dead space ventilation alveolar ventilation is diverted, so anesthesia uptake is decreased. For a right-to-left shunt, the shunt fraction reduces the mixed venous content of anesthetic, thereby increasing the partial pressure gradient from alveolus to pulmonary capillary blood, slowing the rise in F_A. In contrast, a left-to-right shunt does not significantly alter F_A/F_I.

Inhaled anesthetic solubility remains an important consideration, even in patient-specific situations. For instance, a decrease in cardiac output speeds the rise in F_A/F_I, more so for anesthetics that are relatively insoluble. For soluble anesthetics, equilibration of partial pressures between the alveolus and blood takes longer and is affected less by lower cardiac output. Conversely, a right-to-left shunt will have a greater impact in slowing the rate of the rise of F_A/F_I with insoluble anesthetics.

Concentration and Second Gas Effects

The effective concentration of nitrous oxide as a percentage of gas volume (vol%) is substantially higher than for the volatile anesthetics because of its lower potency. Nitrous oxide is routinely administered at 60% to 70% of the gas mixture, whereas volatile anesthetics have clinically relevant concentrations in the range of 1.5% to 6.5 vol%. Thus uptake of nitrous oxide into the blood affects alveolar volume, whereas these changes are insignificant for volatile anesthetics. This unique property of nitrous oxide affects the rate of induction of anesthesia (Fig. 7.6).[17] As nitrous oxide diffuses out of the alveoli, the uptake of nitrous oxide into blood and the reduction in alveolar volume concentrates the coadministered volatile anesthetic. For a volatile anesthetic, if 50% of the agent diffuses into the blood, its F_A will decrease by 50% because the corresponding decrease in alveolar volume is negligible. However, if nitrous oxide is administered at 80 vol% of a gas mixture and half of it (40% of alveolar volume) is taken up into the blood, the remaining alveolar volume is 60%, so the F_A has changed from 0.8 (80/100) to 0.67 (40/60). The concurrent change in alveolar volume with uptake of nitrous oxide serves to increase nitrous oxide delivery as fresh gas replaces the absorbed anesthetic. This phenomenon, known as the *concentration effect*, increases the rate of rise of F_A/F_I for nitrous oxide relative to volatile anesthetics with similar blood-gas coefficients, explaining, in part, its rapid induction profile.[17]

A similar principle applies to the effect that high concentrations of nitrous oxide have on other inhaled anesthetics. The substantial decrease in alveolar volume as nitrous oxide diffuses into the blood partly offsets the uptake of a coadministered volatile anesthetic and concentrates the remaining anesthetic within the alveoli (see Fig. 7.6). Thus the rate of rise of F_A/F_I for a volatile anesthetic is greater in the presence of nitrous oxide than without it, a phenomenon known as the *second gas effect*.[17]

MINIMUM ALVEOLAR CONCENTRATION

Volatile anesthetic potencies are measured and compared as minimum alveolar concentration (MAC), the concentration necessary to prevent movement in response to a painful surgical stimulus in 50% of subjects in a population (Fig. 7.7). This concept was pioneered by Edmond Eger II and his colleagues in the early 1960s.[18] A MAC of 1.0 indicates that the end-tidal concentration of the inhaled anesthetic is such that half of patients would be immobile in response to surgical incision. Though achieving a desirable outcome in only 50% of patients is not a clinically useful endpoint, MAC has a variety of properties that make it useful in comparing between anesthetic properties and, in practice, for dosing them.[19]

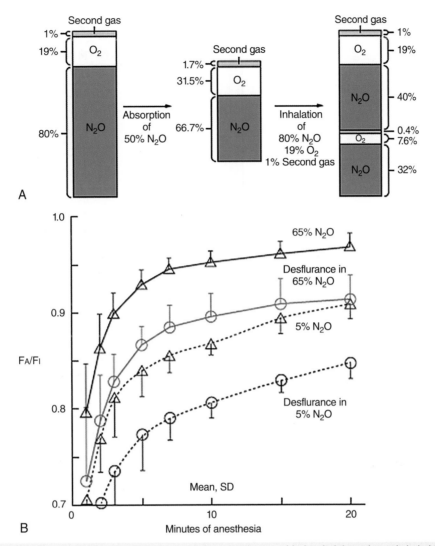

Fig. 7.6 Uptake of nitrous oxide during induction. (A) Nitrous oxide is administered at relatively high concentrations. The resultant decrease in alveolar volume concentrates the remaining alveolar nitrous oxide and other anesthetic gases, which is termed the *concentration effect* and *second gas effect*, respectively. These effects offset gas uptake during induction to maintain a high alveolar partial pressure, thereby increasing the rate of induction. (B) Increasing the concentration of nitrous oxide results in a more rapid rise of F_A/F_I for nitrous oxide alone (concentration effect) and desflurane in nitrous oxide (second gas effect). F_A, Fraction of alveolar gas; F_I, fraction of inhaled gas. (A, Modified from Stoelting RK, Eger EI 2nd. An additional explanation for the second gas effect: A concentrating effect. *Anesthesiology*. 1969;30:273–277.
B, Modified from Taheri S, Eger EI 2nd. A demonstration of the concentration and second gas effects in humans anesthetized with nitrous oxide and desflurane. *Anesth Analg*. 1999;89:774–780. From Hudson AE, Hemmings HC Jr. Pharmacokinetics of inhaled anesthetics, Ch. 3. In: Hemmings HC Jr, Egan TD, eds. *Pharmacology and Physiology for Anesthesia: Foundations and Clinical Application*, 2nd ed. Philadelphia: Elsevier; 2019:54.)

Once a steady anesthetic concentration is reached (equilibrium or steady state), end-tidal anesthetic concentration is proportional to the alveolar partial pressure, which is in equilibrium with all organ systems, including the central nervous system. Thus MAC is a surrogate measure for the partial pressure of anesthetic in the brain and spinal cord (Table 7.2). Inhaled anesthetics with lower MAC values are more potent, as lower anesthetic concentrations are required to achieve the clinical endpoint. The dose at which movement is prevented is

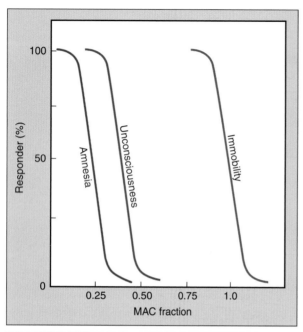

Fig. 7.7 Definition of minimum alveolar concentration *(MAC)*. MAC is defined as the concentration of an inhaled anesthetic required to produce immobility in response to a noxious stimulus in 50% of the population. This definition has been applied to other clinical endpoints, such as amnesia and unconsciousness, in addition to immobility. The slope reflects the small population variability in sensitivity to inhaled anesthesia. (From Hudson AE, Herold KF, Hemmings HC Jr. Pharmacology of inhaled anesthetics, Ch. 11. In: Hemmings HC Jr, Egan TD, eds. *Pharmacology and Physiology for Anesthesia: Foundations and Clinical Application,* 2nd ed. Philadelphia: Elsevier; 2019:222.)

Table 7.2	Expression of MAC as Partial Pressure	
Agent	**MAC (vol%)**	**P$_{MAC}$ (mm Hg)**
Halothane	0.75	5.7
Enflurane	1.68	12.8
Isoflurane	1.15	8.7
Methoxyflurane	0.16	1.2
Sevoflurane	2.10	16
Desflurane	7.25	55
Nitrous oxide	104	790
Xenon	71	540

From Eisenkraft JB. Anesthesia vaporizers, Ch. 3. In: Ehrenwerth J, Eienkraft JB, Berry JB, eds. *Anesthesia Equipment: Principles and Applications,* 3rd ed. Philadelphia: Elsevier: 2021:66–99.

reproducible within subjects, and the range of concentrations across a population is narrow, thus allowing precise determinations of MAC for each anesthetic.[19]

The standard deviation for MAC across anesthetics is about 0.1 (i.e., 10% of the concentration defining MAC). Therefore 1.2 times MAC, an increase in the dose of 20% over MAC, or two standard deviations, will produce immobility to a surgical stimulus in 95% of patients.[19] MAC values are additive. Two inhaled anesthetics delivered in a gas mixture will have a combined MAC that is the sum of the individual MAC values for the concentrations employed. Thus administering nitrous oxide and sevoflurane each at half their MAC (0.5 MAC) will yield a gas mixture with a combined MAC of 1.0.[7]

Other clinical endpoints to compare potencies of inhaled anesthetics have been defined. For isoflurane, sevoflurane, and desflurane, these other definitions are generally related to the MAC for immobility by a multiplicative factor. MAC-awake is the end-tidal anesthetic concentration that allows a patient to respond meaningfully (in the absence of noxious stimuli). MAC-awake is about one-third of MAC. For halothane and nitrous oxide, it is higher relative to MAC immobility (0.55 and 0.64 MAC, respectively).[19] Similarly, MAC-amnesia is the concentration to prevent recall in 50% of a population. This value is not as well defined, but it is likely less than MAC-awake, and it is assumed that conscious recall is abolished at anesthetic concentrations preventing a meaningful response (again, when measured in the absence of noxious stimuli). Another endpoint is MAC-BAR, or blunted autonomic response, at which 50% of a population will not mount an adrenergic response, evidenced by tachycardia, hypertension, and other signs, in response to a surgical stimulus. The MAC-BAR is approximately 1.5 to 1.6 times MAC.[19]

MAC is a measurement of a response to an anesthetic across a population. However, individual patients can have different anesthetic requirements depending on physiology, pathology, and other medications (Box 7.1). Age is an important and well-validated factor influencing anesthetic potency. MAC values are generally referenced to a specific age, usually 40 years. Increasing age reduces MAC by 6% to 7% for each decade. This trend is broken for infants less than 1 year of age, where MAC increases from neonates to older children. Other nonmodifiable patient factors that increase MAC are red hair and chronic ethanol use, whereas pregnancy and chronic amphetamine use decrease MAC. Certain pathophysiologic conditions affect MAC. Hyperthermia and hypernatremia increase MAC, whereas hypothermia, hyponatremia, hypercarbia, hypoxia, and anemia decrease MAC. A variety of drugs can affect MAC, including many that are used regularly for surgery under general anesthesia. Acute alcohol intoxication decreases, whereas amphetamine use increases MAC. Benzodiazepines, ketamine, barbiturates, propofol, etomidate, dexmedetomidine, opioids, and local anesthetics decrease MAC. Other nonanesthetic medications, such as lithium and verapamil, can also lower MAC.[19]

Box 7.1 Factors That Increase or Decrease Anesthetic Requirements

Factors Increasing MAC

Drugs
- Amphetamine (acute use)
- Cocaine
- Ephedrine
- Ethanol (chronic use)

Age
- Highest at age 6 months

Electrolytes
- Hypernatremia
- Hyperthermia

Red hair

Factors Decreasing MAC

Drugs
- Propofol
- Etomidate
- Barbiturates
- Benzodiazepines
- Ketamine
- α_2 -Agonists (clonidine, dexmedetomidine)
- Ethanol (acute use)
- Local anesthetics
- Opioids
- Amphetamines (chronic use)
- Lithium
- Verapamil

Age
- Elderly patients

Electrolyte disturbance
- Hyponatremia

Other factors
- Anemia (hemoglobin <5 g/dL)
- Hypercarbia
- Hypothermia
- Hypoxia
- Pregnancy

From McKay RE. Inhaled anesthetics. Ch. 7. In Pardo M, ed. *Basics of Anesthesia*, 7th ed. Philadelphia, PA: Elsevier; 2018:86.

MECHANISMS

Molecular Mechanisms

Despite 175 years of using inhaled anesthetics, the molecular mechanisms leading to amnesia, unconsciousness, and immobility remain elusive. Although the molecular targets of intravenous anesthetics are better defined, an equivalent reductionist understanding for inhaled anesthetics has not been achieved. An emerging consensus holds that multiple targets that can vary between agents are responsible for the characteristic endpoints of general anesthesia. After the widespread use of inhaled anesthetics began, much of the scientific exploration sought to discover a common target of their effects, an approach that was influenced by the work of the French physiologist Claude Bernard.[20] The lipophilicity of inhaled anesthetics led to theories that attributed anesthetic action to disruption of lipid membranes. Early experimental support for this concept at the turn of the 20th century correlated anesthetic potencies with their oil–water partition coefficients, which was known as the *Meyer–Overton correlation* for the two pharmacologists involved (Fig. 7.8).[20] Since the late 1970s, rigorous biophysical studies, led by Nicholas Franks and William Lieb, demonstrated inhibition of the purified firefly protein luciferase in the absence of lipids. The degree of inhibition of luciferase, as determined by its light-generating chemical reaction, correlated with anesthetic potency, signifying that the clinical characteristics of inhaled anesthetics could be attributed to effects on proteins as opposed to lipids (see Fig. 7.8).[21] These findings ushered in an era of defining target proteins in the central nervous system. Lipophilicity of inhaled anesthetics is likely important to determining their ability to access specific sites in target protein complexes, including ion channels. However, inhaled anesthetics do not affect lipid membrane properties at clinically relevant concentrations, so direct membrane-mediated effects are unlikely to explain the clinical effects of anesthetics.[22]

A variety of voltage- and ligand-gated ion channels are modulated by inhaled anesthetics and are thought to represent their critical neuronal targets for their neurophysiologic effects (Fig. 7.9). These effects can be divided into presynaptic and postsynaptic targets. Postsynaptically, volatile anesthetics potentiate inhibitory GABA$_A$ and glycine receptors, causing hyperpolarization and thus inhibiting action potential generation; however, these channels are not modulated by the inhaled anesthetics nitrous oxide or xenon.[23] All the inhaled anesthetics inhibit acetylcholine, α-amino-3-hydroxy-5-methyl-4-isoxazole propionic acid (AMPA), and *N*-methyl-D-aspartate (NMDA) receptors.[24] Voltage-gated ion channels are also modulated by volatile anesthetics. Two-pore potassium channels are potentiated, causing hyperpolarization of neurons, thus inhibiting depolarization and action potential generation and propagation. Voltage-gated sodium and calcium channels are also targets of volatile anesthetics.[24] Studies have yielded conflicting results for anesthetic effects on synaptic vesicle exocytotic SNARE proteins. Volatile anesthetics also inhibit mitochondrial function, in particular by inhibiting complex I of the electron transport chain. Notably, patients with mutations in complex I exhibit a substantial increase in sensitivity to volatile anesthesia, confirming involvement of this target in potentiating anesthetic potency.[25] Nevertheless, the degree to which each of these various targets contribute to produce general anesthesia remains unclear.

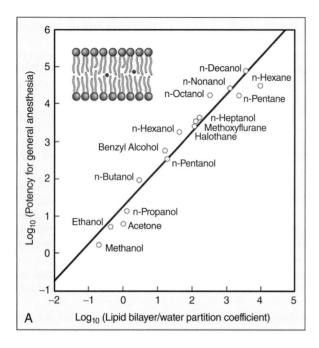

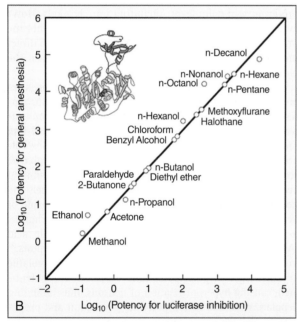

Fig. 7.8 The potency of inhaled anesthetics correlates with their lipophilicity. This relationship was originally described as the Meyer–Overton correlation. More recently, inhibition of purified luciferase was also shown to correlate with anesthetic potency. This seminal experiment focused further research on anesthetic interactions with proteins, which indicates that inhaled anesthesia acts through modulation of various proteins involved in neuronal function, not via bulk effects on lipid bilayers. (From Hudson AE, Herold KF, Hemmings HC Jr. Pharmacology of inhaled anesthetics, Ch. 11. In Hemmings HC Jr., Egan TD, eds. *Pharmacology and Physiology for Anesthesia: Foundations and Clinical Application*, 2nd ed. Philadelphia: Elsevier; 2019:219.)

Neuronal Network Mechanisms

At the neural network level, volatile anesthetics reduce functional connectivity between brain regions, with the most consistent effects observed on frontoparietal cortical interactions.[26] Studies employing electroencephalography (EEG) to monitor patterns of activity under anesthesia show discrete brain states that transition nonrandomly and independently of surgical stimuli. Thus anesthesia-induced unconsciousness caused by inhaled anesthetics may be the result of alterations in connections and patterns of brain activity, preventing integration of multiple systems that underlie consciousness (Fig. 7.10).[26] Additional studies are required to understand how modulation of molecular targets gives rise to alterations in brain connectivity and how these processes relate to the clinical endpoints of sedation, amnesia, and unconsciousness, although effects on ion channels to reduce neuronal excitability are likely important.

Volatile anesthetics produce immobility primarily by actions on the spinal cord, not the brain.[27] Delivery of volatile anesthetics into the vasculature of the spinal cord of animal models reduced the dose required to prevent movement in response to noxious stimuli compared with selective delivery to brain.[28] Moreover, transection of the spinal cord in rats did not alter sensitivity to isoflurane of reflex movement in response to noxious stimuli.[29] These studies strongly implicate the spinal cord as primarily responsible for mediating the immobility caused by volatile anesthesia.

ORGAN SYSTEM EFFECTS

Inhaled anesthetics alter normal physiologic mechanisms and can have pronounced, organ-specific effects. The clinical pharmacology of inhaled anesthesia can be exploited to achieve intraoperative goals, but, conversely, anesthetics can have undesirable detrimental effects on patients. Understanding organ-specific effects and toxicity is thus critical to the safe use of inhaled anesthetics.

Central Nervous System

With increasing doses of volatile anesthetics, neuronal activity is progressively inhibited. These effects can be readily observed by EEG, which shows a transition to higher-amplitude and lower-frequency electrical patterns, primarily in the alpha (8 to 13 Hz) and slow delta (1 Hz) frequencies, with theta oscillations (5 to 8 Hz) appearing at MAC doses of anesthetics.[30] Further increases beyond typical surgical levels of anesthesia produce burst suppression and, ultimately, an isolectric EEG. Once an isolectric EEG is induced, detectable neuronal electrophysiologic activity is mostly absent, and cerebral metabolism, reflected in the cerebral metabolic

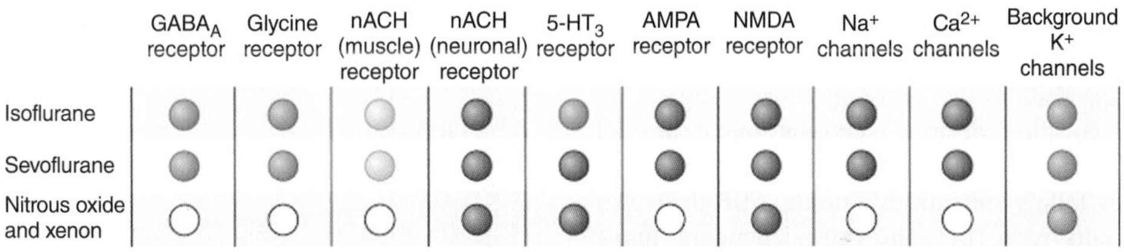

	GABA$_A$ receptor	Glycine receptor	nACH (muscle) receptor	nACH (neuronal) receptor	5-HT$_3$ receptor	AMPA receptor	NMDA receptor	Na$^+$ channels	Ca^{2+} channels	Background K$^+$ channels
Isoflurane	●	●	○	●	●	●	●	●	●	●
Sevoflurane	●	●	○	●	●	●	●	●	●	●
Nitrous oxide and xenon	○	○	○	●	●	○	●	○	○	●

Fig. 7.9 Inhaled anesthetics inhibit or potentiate various ion channels and neurotransmitter receptors involved in neurotransmission within the central nervous system, with agent-specific differences. (From Hudson AE, Herold KF, Hemmings HC Jr. Pharmacology of inhaled anesthetics, Ch. 11. In: Hemmings HC Jr., Egan TD, eds. *Pharmacology and Physiology for Anesthesia: Foundations and Clinical Application*, 2nd ed. Philadelphia: Elsevier; 2019:220.)

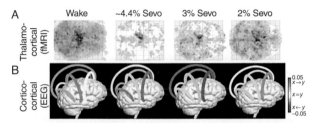

Fig. 7.10 Inhaled anesthetics at clinically relevant concentrations disrupt normal functional connectivity in the brain, which may contribute to unconsciousness. (From Hemmings HC, Riegelhaupt PM, Kelz MB, et al. Towards a comprehensive understanding of anesthetic mechanisms of action: A decade of discovery. *Trends Pharmacol Sci.* 2019;40[7]:464–481.)

rate for oxygen (CMRO$_2$), is reduced to 40% to 50% of normal, with the remaining metabolic demand needed to maintain baseline ion gradients and cellular integrity.[31] For most agents, further decreases can be achieved only by hypothermia. Halothane can produce dose-dependent reductions even after cessation of cortical activity, which has been interpreted as evidence of neurotoxicity.[31] An isoelectric EEG under anesthesia is considered excessive for the purposes of surgery. Burst suppression has been targeted to prevent ischemic neuronal injury, but no advantage in neurologic outcomes has been shown.[32] Isoelectricity is also targeted in patients with status epilepticus unresponsive to other treatments.

Stereotypic, dose-dependent changes in the EEG pattern occur with volatile anesthesia. At sub-MAC concentrations, beta frequencies (13 to 24 Hz) are reduced and alpha and delta (8 to 13 and 1 to 4 Hz, respectively) frequencies predominate. Increasing anesthetic concentration further causes theta frequencies (4 to 7 Hz) to emerge (Fig. 7.11).[30] At doses of 1.3 times MAC and above, burst suppression can be observed.[33] These dose-dependent effects on the EEG have led to the development of devices to monitor the "brain state" under anesthesia, with the BIS monitor being the most widely used and studied. However, large trials investigating BIS have not shown reduced rates of intraoperative awareness when compared with maintaining end-tidal anesthetic above 0.7 times MAC,[34] nor has there been a mortality benefit associated with targeting BIS values to a lighter depth of anesthesia[35] (also see Chapter 20).

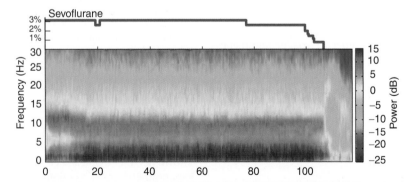

Fig. 7.11 Stereotypic changes in the electroencephalogram occur with volatile anesthetics. Increases in delta and alpha frequencies with sevoflurane are shown in the spectrogram by intense bands centered around frequencies of ~1 Hz and ~10 Hz. (From Purdon PL, Sampson A, Pavone KJ, et al. Clinical electroencephalography for anesthesiologists part I: Background and basic signatures. *Anesthesiology.* 2015;123[4]:937–960.)

Cerebral autoregulation describes the relationship between cerebral blood flow (CBF) and cerebral or systemic arterial pressures. Within the autoregulatory range, CBF remains nearly constant despite changing mean arterial blood pressure. With excessively low or excessively high arterial pressures falling outside this range, CBF decreases or increases, respectively, in a pressure-dependent manner.[36] Cerebral autoregulation is inhibited by relatively high doses (above 1.5 times MAC) of halothane, isoflurane, and desflurane, while sevoflurane affects autoregulation less.[37,38]

CBF is coupled to metabolic demands, a process called *flow–metabolism coupling*. This process is altered by volatile anesthesia. Volatile anesthetics are direct vasodilators, and at higher concentrations, this can lead to an increase in CBF. However, as noted earlier, volatile anesthetics also reduce $CMRO_2$. Whether CBF is increased depends on the relative effects on vasodilation and suppression of $CMRO_2$.[37,38] Volatile anesthetic concentrations below MAC generally do not cause an increase in CBF or intracranial pressure (ICP) because vasodilation is offset by the decreased $CMRO_2$. However, above MAC, the vasodilatory effects predominate and ICP increases.

Cardiovascular System

All volatile anesthetics produce hypotension, mediated primarily by systemic vasodilation.[39,40] The reduction in systemic vascular resistance (SVR) caused by arterial vasodilation is accompanied by inhibition of the baroreceptor reflex, particularly with halothane, thereby augmenting the hypotension from vasodilation (Fig. 7.12).[41,42] Volatile anesthetics also depress myocardial contractility; at MAC or greater, isoflurane, sevoflurane, and desflurane can decrease cardiac index.[39,40] The depressed cardiac function may be partially offset by reduced SVR; for instance, at 2.0 times MAC of sevoflurane, cardiac index normalizes despite reduced contractility because afterload is also decreased (Fig. 7.13).[40]

Volatile anesthetics at higher concentrations, or with a sudden change in concentration, can cause tachycardia, an effect most prominent with desflurane; this phenomenon is likely the result of a vagolytic effect.[43] Volatile anesthetics can prolong the QT interval, which can predispose patients with prolonged QT interval to torsades de pointes. Halothane, in particular, predisposes to ventricular tachycardia resulting from epinephrine. However, volatile anesthetics can have either proarrhythmic or antiarrhythmic effects depending on the underlying predisposing pathology and the part of the conduction system at risk.[44]

Pulmonary System

Volatile anesthetics alter many aspects of pulmonary physiology. Although they increase respiratory rate, they concurrently decrease tidal volume such that minute ventilation is reduced in a dose-dependent fashion.[45]

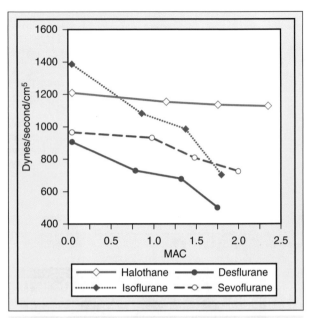

Fig. 7.12 Volatile anesthetics reduce vascular resistance. The reduction in systemic vascular resistance is dose-dependent and agent-specific (isoflurane > desflurane > sevoflurane > halothane).

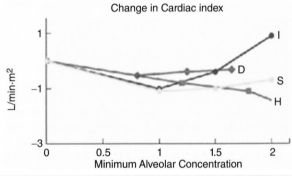

Fig. 7.13 Volatile anesthetics variably affect cardiac index. Halothane > sevoflurane > isoflurane produce dose-dependent reductions in cardiac index, whereas desflurane has comparatively little effect. Cardiac index increases with 2 MAC isoflurane. (From Ebert TJ, Naze SA. Inhaled anesthetics, Ch. 18. In: Barash PG, Cahalan MK, Cullen BF, et al., eds. *Clinical Anesthesia*, 8th ed. Philadelphia: Lippincott Williams & Wilkins; 2017:474.)

They also affect respiratory drive in response to oxygen and carbon dioxide. In unanesthetized subjects decreasing oxygenation increases minute ventilation, an effect known as the *hypoxic ventilatory response (HVR)*. At subanesthetic doses, as might occur during postanesthetic recovery, volatile anesthetics potently suppress HVR, and at surgical concentrations, HVR can be completely abolished.[46] Volatile anesthetics also profoundly inhibit the peripheral chemoreceptor response to hypercarbia.[47] However, the central chemoreceptor response remains,

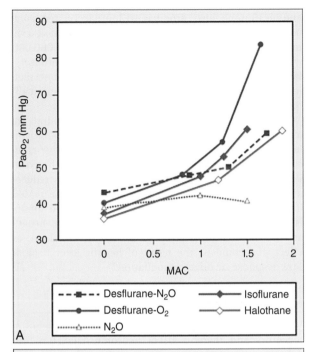

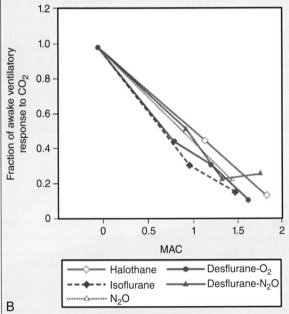

Fig. 7.14 Volatile anesthetics suppress the ventilatory response to carbon dioxide. (A) Progressive hypercarbia occurs in a dose-dependent and agent-specific manner. (B) All agents similarly depress the ventilatory response to inhaled carbon dioxide. $Paco_2$, Arterial partial pressure of CO_2. (From McKay RE. Inhaled anesthetics, Ch. 7. In: Pardo M, ed. *Basics of Anesthesia*, 7th ed. Philadelphia: Elsevier; 2018:99.)

Volatile anesthetics are all bronchodilators because of their smooth muscle–relaxing effects; however, there are agent-specific differences, such that sevoflurane and halothane exert greater effects than isoflurane or desflurane.[48] Mucociliary clearance is decreased by volatile anesthetics and nitrous oxide in a dose-dependent fashion,[49] with sevoflurane causing the least impairment in vitro.[50] Volatile anesthetics may also decrease surfactant production.[51] These effects may contribute to postoperative pulmonary complications, including atelectasis, hypoxemia, and pneumonia.

As vasodilators, volatile anesthetics diminish hypoxic pulmonary vasoconstriction in a dose-dependent fashion. Halothane is most potent, but isoflurane, sevoflurane, and desflurane have similar effects.[52] The net impact on pulmonary shunt during one-lung ventilation is minimal, so it is unlikely to have a clinically relevant impact in worsening gas exchange.[53]

Renal System

Historically, kidney injury caused by volatile anesthesia was a concern. Methoxyflurane is capable of causing high-output renal failure as a result of elevated plasma levels of fluoride from its metabolism (Fig. 7.15).[54] This toxicity led to discontinuation of its use in anesthetic practice, although it continues to be used outside the United States in nonanesthetic doses via inhaler as an analgesic for trauma and procedural pain.[55] Production of compound A from sevoflurane breakdown by alkaline carbon dioxide absorbents can cause nephrotoxicity in animal models; however, compound A has not been shown to lead to kidney injury in humans.[56]

Ischemic preconditioning by volatile anesthetics may be protective in ischemia-reperfusion injury that can lead to acute kidney injury (AKI).[57] However, in animal models, volatile anesthesia is also capable of reducing renal blood flow and oxygen delivery when compared with propofol anesthesia.[58] There are few randomized controlled trials (RCTs) to assess whether volatile anesthesia may be nephrotoxic or protective. In the small VAPOR-1 trial the sevoflurane group had a lower incidence of kidney transplant graft failure compared with the propofol group despite higher kidney injury biomarkers after surgery.[58] Further studies are needed to assess if volatile anesthetics can be used to mitigate ischemic kidney injury and improve kidney function postoperatively.

Hepatic System

Certain volatile anesthetics can cause hepatotoxicity. Most notably, halothane can lead to fulminant hepatitis in 1/15,000 cases, attributed to trifluoroacetylated compounds generated by CYP2E1 oxidative metabolism, triggering adduct and neoantigen formation and resulting in autoimmune liver injury (Fig. 7.16).[59] Isoflurane

but is depressed up to 70% at surgical levels of volatile anesthesia (Fig. 7.14). Thus volatile anesthesia makes a patient reliant on $Paco_2$ to stimulate ventilation.

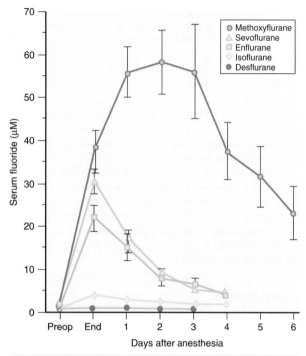

Fig. 7.15 Metabolism of certain volatile anesthetics can increase serum fluoride concentration. Volatile anesthetics exhibit agent-specific metabolism and release of fluoride. This effect is greatest with anesthetic doses of methoxyflurane and can precipitate nephrotoxicity. (From Forman SA, Ishizawa Y. Inhaled anesthetic pharmacokinetics: Uptake, distribution, metabolism, and toxicity, Ch. 20. In: Gropper MA, ed. *Miller's Anesthesia*, 9th ed. Philadelphia: Elsevier; 2020:530.)

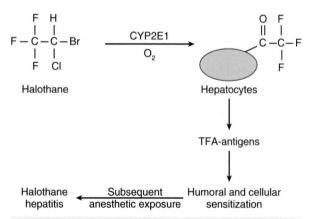

Fig. 7.16 Hepatic metabolism of halothane produces trifluoroacetylated adducts. Adducted liver proteins can form neoantigens that trigger an autoimmune reaction, causing fulminant hepatotoxicity. *TFA*, Trifluroacetyl. (From Forman SA, Ishizawa Y. Inhaled anesthetic pharmacokinetics: Uptake, distribution, metabolism, and toxicity, Ch. 20. In: Gropper MA, ed. *Miller's Anesthesia*, 9th ed. Philadelphia: Elsevier; 2020:529.)

and desflurane also produce trifluoroacetylated compounds, but substantially less, and therefore have estimated rates of hepatic failure less than 1/1,000,000, whereas sevoflurane does not produce trifluoroacetylated by-products. Thus the modern volatile anesthetics have a substantially reduced incidence of clinically relevant hepatotoxicity.[59]

The phenomenon of ischemic preconditioning has led to interest in using volatile anesthetics to mitigate hepatic injury in liver transplant,[60] but supportive clinical evidence is lacking. Hepatic blood flow is altered by volatile anesthetics. Total hepatic blood flow is reduced at doses above MAC. Portal blood flow is decreased, likely secondary to reduced cardiac output and diminished blood flow to preportal organs. However, hepatic arterial blood flow is either preserved or increased, an effect that could be the result of hepatic arterial blood flow response or direct vasodilation.[61]

Neuromuscular Function

Volatile anesthetics inhibit nicotinic acetylcholine receptors and thereby affect neuromuscular function. All volatile anesthetics potentiate the effects of nondepolarizing neuromuscular blocking drugs in a dose-dependent, agent-specific fashion.[62] This effect appears to result from direct, noncompetitive antagonism of nicotinic acetylcholine receptors. However, decreased acetylcholine release from presynaptic nerve terminals at the neuromuscular junction may also contribute.[63] The primary effect appears to be potentiation of neuromuscular blockade. Studies on the duration or recovery of neuromuscular function have yielded inconsistent results.[62,64]

UNIQUE ISSUES WITH NITROUS OXIDE

Nitrous oxide has unique properties that distinguish it pharmacologically from other inhaled anesthetics. The MAC of nitrous oxide is 104 vol%, and the MAC-awake is higher than for volatile anesthetics (~0.6 MAC).[65] Thus nitrous oxide must be used with other anesthetic agents to achieve general anesthesia and minimize the risk of awareness. The relatively high concentrations required for surgical anesthesia give rise to the concentration and second gas effects (see earlier). A similar pharmacologic principle applies on emergence from nitrous oxide. Once nitrous oxide is discontinued, the partial pressure of nitrous oxide in blood exceeds the partial pressure of nitrous oxide in the alveoli; the resulting diffusion of nitrous oxide from blood to alveoli causes dilution of other alveolar gases. Dilution of oxygen, known as *diffusion hypoxia*, can predispose patients to hypoxemia on emergence from nitrous oxide anesthesia.[65] However, this process also contributes to the rapid emergence profile of nitrous oxide.

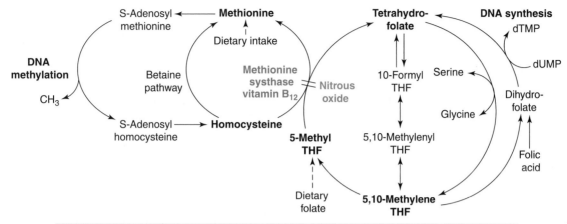

Fig. 7.17 Nitrous oxide inhibits methionine synthetase. Prolonged use of nitrous oxide can cause homocystinemia and reduce tetrahydrofolate formation, which promotes megaloblastic anemia. (From Forman SA, Ishizawa Y. Inhaled anesthetic pharmacokinetics: Uptake, distribution, metabolism, and toxicity, Ch. 20. In: Gropper MA, ed. *Miller's Anesthesia*, 9th ed. Philadelphia: Elsevier; 2020:534.)

Because it is used clinically at high partial pressures and its solubility exceeds nitrogen, nitrous oxide diffuses into enclosed gas-filled compartments and can generate pressures that may be harmful. For this reason, nitrous oxide is contraindicated in conditions or surgeries generating enclosed compartments of gas, for example, closed-loop bowel obstruction, pneumocephalus, pneumothorax, middle ear surgery, and ophthalmic surgeries using injections of insoluble gases such as sulfur hexafluoride.[65]

Nitrous oxide inhibits methionine synthetase. Prolonged use in patients with vitamin B_{12} deficiency can promote neuropathy and megaloblastic anemia.[65] Homocysteine levels may also be increased by nitrous oxide, which has raised concern for increased cardiovascular morbidity because of the deleterious effects of elevated homocysteine (Fig. 7.17). In the large ENIGMA RCT comparing volatile anesthesia with nitrous oxide in 30% oxygen with volatile anesthesia in 80% oxygen patients in the nitrous group had a higher rate of myocardial infarction (MI), though stroke and death were the same in both groups.[66] A follow-up study, ENIGMA II, examined cardiovascular morbidity and death in high-risk patients, maintaining the same fraction of inspired oxygen (FiO_2) between groups. This trial, which was better powered and designed to evaluate cardiovascular morbidity resulting from nitrous oxide, failed to detect differences in MI, stroke, or death. Thus nitrous oxide is likely safe to use with regard to cardiovascular outcomes, even in high-risk patients.[67]

TOXICITY AND ADVERSE EVENTS

Postoperative Nausea and Vomiting

Postoperative nausea and vomiting (PONV) are common complications of general anesthesia with inhaled anesthesia, occurring in 30% of patients, that have profound effects on patient satisfaction.[68] A variety of risk factors have been shown to increase the likelihood of PONV (Fig. 7.18).[68] The Apfel score enables risk stratification for PONV, with 1 point each assigned for postoperative opioid use, being a nonsmoker, having a history of PONV or motion sickness, and female sex; a score of 4 predicts an 80% risk of PONV.[68] Other factors also contribute to the development of PONV, including type and duration of surgery, age, and the use of volatile

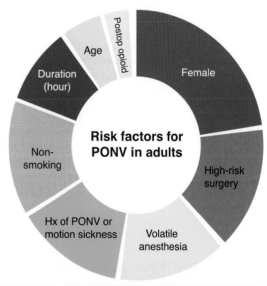

Fig. 7.18 Use of volatile anesthetics is a major risk factor for postoperative nausea and vomiting (PONV). (From Gan TJ, Belani KG, Bergese S, et al. Fourth consensus guidelines for the management of postoperative nausea and vomiting. *Anesth Analg.* 2020;131[2]:411–448.)

anesthesia. The pathogenesis of PONV is likely the result of anesthetic and surgical effects affecting serotoninergic, dopaminergic, and μ opioid receptors of the area postrema of the brainstem, with vagal and vestibular afferents contributing.[69] It is unclear how volatile anesthetics specifically affect these pathways. Nitrous oxide used for more than an hour further increases risk, but prophylactic antiemetics can ameliorate the impact of nitrous oxide.[68]

Malignant Hyperthermia

Malignant hyperthermia (MH) is a pharmacogenetic reaction that can lead to a lethal response to volatile anesthesia or succinylcholine. MH is caused most commonly by mutations in the ryanodine receptor 1 (RyR1) isoform, but about 25% of patients have mutations in other genes, such as the *CACNA1* gene that encodes the L-type voltage-gated calcium channel responsible for triggering the opening of RyR1 in skeletal muscle.[69] These mutations result in excessive calcium efflux from the sarcoplasmic reticulum, which is the major intracellular store of calcium (Fig. 7.19). This overwhelming rise in cytosolic calcium in skeletal muscle leads to uncontrolled, sustained muscle contraction, muscle rigidity,

myonecrosis, hypermetabolism, and severe hyperthermia. The presenting symptoms are often an unexplained increase in temperature or end-tidal CO_2, tachycardia, lactic acidosis, hyperkalemia, and rhabdomylosis.[70]

Without treatment, mortality is 60% to 80%. However, prompt recognition and aggressive treatment can reduce mortality to <2%.[70,71] The specific therapy for MH is dantrolene, which is an inhibitor of RyR1 that prevents excessive release of calcium from the sarcoplasmic reticulum. Supportive care with cooling, hyperventilation with 100% oxygen, intravenous bicarbonate and fluids, electrolyte management, and hemodynamic support are also critical (Table 7.3).[70] The severity of the disease requires that, in patients who have MH or may be MH susceptible, precautions must be taken to avoid any exposure to volatile anesthetic or succinylcholine triggers.[70] The disease phenotype can be tested at limited centers by the caffeine halothane contracture test and confirmed with genetic testing that shows a pathogenic mutation.[70] The Malignant Hyperthermia Association of the United States (MHAUS; https://www.mhaus.org/) is an excellent resource for information and offers a 24-hour hotline that can be called during an emergency possibly caused by MH.

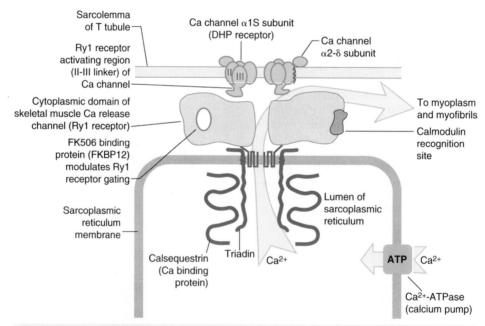

Fig. 7.19 Pathophysiology of malignant hyperthermia (MH). MH is a pharmacogenetic syndrome, often inherited in an autosomal dominant fashion, that is caused primarily by mutations in the ryanodine receptor isoform 1 (RyR1), which is expressed in skeletal muscle. In patients with MH, exposure to volatile anesthetics and succinylcholine triggers excessive release of calcium from the sarcoplasmic reticulum, leading to multisystem toxicity from hypermetabolism, hyperthermia, and myonecrosis. *DHP*, Dihydropyridine. (From Zhou J, Nozri A, Bateman B, et al. Malignant hyperthermia and muscle-related disorders, Ch. 35. In: Gropper MA, ed. *Miller's Anesthesia*, 9th ed. Philadelphia: Elsevier; 2020:1118.)

Table 7.3 Managing a Malignant Hyperthermia Crisis

Action	Notes
Stop potent inhalation agents	Turn vaporizers "OFF" and/or insert activated charcoal filters into the circuit
Do not repeat succinylcholine if it has been previously administered	
Increase minute ventilation to lower ETCO$_2$	Eliminate the inhalational agent
Get help	Duty anesthetist
	Consultant anesthetist
Prepare and administer dantrolene	2.5 mg/kg initial dose
	Every 10–15 min until acidosis, pyrexia, muscle rigidity are resolving
Begin cooling measures if hyperthermic	Tissue destruction will occur at 41.5°C (106.7°F)
	Use intravenous normal saline at 4°C (39.2°F)
	Ice packs to all exposed areas
	More aggressive measures as needed
Stop cooling measures at 38.5°C (101.3°F)	
Treat arrhythmias as needed	Amiodarone is the first choice
	Lignocaine
	Do not use calcium channel blockers
Secure blood gases, electrolytes, creatine kinase, blood, and urine for myoglobin	Coagulation profile; check values regularly
	Treat hyperkalemia with hyperventilation, glucose and insulin as needed
	Once crisis is under control, an MH hotline should be contacted for further guidance
Continue dantrolene	1 mg/kg every 4–8 h for 24–48 h
	Alternatively and only if recrudescence occurs, dantrolene at 2.5 mg/kg bolus
Ensure urine output of 2 mL/kg/h with	Mannitol
	Furosemide
	Fluids as needed
Evaluate need for invasive monitoring and continued mechanical ventilation	
Observe patient in intensive care unit	At least 24 h
Refer patient and family for MH testing	Contracture or DNA testing

From Rosenberg H, Pollock N, Schiemann A, et al. Malignant hyperthermia: A review. *Orphanet J Rare Dis.* 2015;10:93.

Developmental Neurotoxicity (also see Chapter 12)

Whether commonly used inhaled anesthetics can cause neurotoxicity and long-lasting cognitive dysfunction has been studied intensively since the early 2000s. Initial studies identified that gamma-aminobutyric acid type A receptor (GABA$_A$R) agonists, such as volatile anesthetics, and NMDA receptor antagonists, such as nitrous oxide and ketamine, caused widespread apoptosis of neurons and oligodendrocytes in fetal and neonatal rodents.[72] These effects were accompanied by evidence of persistent

cognitive deficits in adult animals. Studies in nonhuman primates confirmed increased neuroapoptosis and behavioral changes, such as increased social anxiety responses, in young animals exposed to volatile anesthetics.[72] These preclinical studies suggest that exposure to many commonly used anesthetics in mammals during early life, during the phase of rapid synaptogenesis, can cause acute toxicity leading to persistent neurodevelopmental deficits.

Large, retrospective cohort studies in young children requiring general anesthesia have yielded inconsistent findings regarding neurocognitive impairment, though developmental deficits may be more likely with multiple exposures and underlying risk factors.[73] The accumulated evidence prompted the US Food and Drug Administration (FDA) to release a statement in 2016 that lengthy or repeated exposure to general anesthesia may affect the cognitive development of children, with a recommendation to postpone procedures requiring anesthesia when reasonable.[74] International and US anesthesia experts have developed advocacy and research initiatives, SafeTots and SmartTots, respectively.[73] The publication of two large, prospective cohort studies with rigorous neurocognitive evaluations found no difference in outcomes in children exposed once to general anesthesia compared with nonexposed children,[75,76] though deficits were found in secondary outcomes of learning and behavior in multiply exposed children.[76] To date, only one study, the general anesthesia or awake-regional anesthesia in infancy (GAS) trial, has randomized young children to either general anesthesia or regional anesthesia without sedation to assess neurodevelopmental impairment. In prespecified analyses at 2 and 5 years of age, no differences in neurocognitive assessments were found for children receiving a mean of 1 hour of sevoflurane compared with spinal anesthesia.[77,78] Thus inhaled anesthesia for a single surgery lasting an hour or less is likely safe. Whether longer or multiple exposures to general anesthesia or preexisting neurologic disease predispose to developmental deficits in young children remains unresolved.

Postoperative Cognitive Dysfunction

The risk of postoperative neurocognitive disorder (PND), also known as *postoperative cognitive dysfunction (POCD)*, after surgery has been studied for nearly 70 years.[79] Nevertheless, controversy continues as to whether anesthesia, surgery, or both lead to lasting cognitive impairments. Possible mechanisms that have been explored in preclinical models include inflammation and increased proinflammatory cytokines, increased tau protein phosphorylation, increased Aβ peptide, mitochondrial dysfunction, calcium dysregulation, decreased neuronal dendritic spines, and alterations in neurotransmitter receptor expression.[80] In clinical studies higher rates of cognitive dysfunction occur 1 week after surgery and anesthesia compared with nonoperative control subjects, but there are mixed results as to whether cognitive impairment persists at 3 months. In a study with assessments at 1 to 2 years postoperatively there was no difference in cognitive impairments between operative and control subjects, and only 1% of subjects had cognitive impairment at all three assessment intervals (1 week, 3 months, and 1 to 2 years).[81]

It is possible that neurocognitive dysfunction does not result from general anesthesia, as randomized

---

Box 7.2 Intraoperative Recommendations to Promote Perioperative Brain Health

Avoid (or use with caution) centrally acting anticholinergics, benzodiazepines, meperidine, first- and second-generation antipsychotics, corticosteroids, and H$_2$ receptor antagonists

Avoid relative hypotension

Maintain normothermia

Monitor age-adjusted end-tidal MAC fraction

Use EEG-based intraoperative brain monitoring to titrate anesthetic administration

Adapted from Berger M, Schenning KJ, Brown CH, et al. Best practices for postoperative brain health: Recommendations from the fifth international perioperative neurotoxicity working group. *Anesth Analg.* 2018;127:1406–1413.*EEG,* Electroencephalogram; *MAC,* minimum alveolar concentration.

---

studies comparing neuraxial anesthesia with volatile anesthesia report similar rates of cognitive dysfunction at 3 months.[82–84] However, studies comparing volatile anesthesia with intravenous anesthesia have found worse cognitive function with volatile anesthesia within 1 week. Overall, it remains difficult to draw firm conclusions as to whether cognitive impairment can be attributed to general anesthesia, surgery, or both as a result of significant heterogeneity in research methods.[85] Nevertheless, in 2018 the Perioperative Neurotoxicity Working Group, convened as part of the American Society of Anesthesiologists Brain Health Initiative, provided recommendations for screening, counseling, and management goals in patients at risk of POCD (Box 7.2).[86]

Cancer Recurrence and Morbidity

Volatile anesthetics can inhibit the immune response, raising concern for worsened outcomes after resections for cancer. A recent meta analysis of nine retrospective analyses and a single RCT reported greater recurrence-free and overall survival using total intravenous anesthesia (TIVA) as opposed to volatile anesthesia.[87] However, the authors noted that substantial heterogeneity of study design and outcomes weakened the conclusion. In the single RCT included in the meta analysis there was no difference at 2 years in women randomized to receive propofol and remifentanil or sevoflurane for breast cancer resection; however, the relatively short follow-up and small trial size (80 patients) may have limited the ability of the trial to detect survival differences.[88] Large RCTs are underway to better assess whether volatile anesthesia worsens cancer outcomes compared with TIVA.

Table 7.4 Composition of Base Chemicals and Water Content of Carbon Dioxide Absorbents*

CO_2 Absorbent	$Ca(OH)_2$ (%)	$Ba(OH)_2$ (%)	KOH (%)	NaOH (%)	LiOH (%)	H_2O (%)
Baralyme[†]	70	10	4.6	–	–	14
Soda lime I	80	–	2.6	1.3	–	15
Sodasorb	90	–	0.0005	3.8	–	16
Drägersorb 800 plus	82	–	0.003	2	–	16
Soda lime II/Medisorb	81	–	0.003	2.6	–	16
Spherasorb	84.5	–	0.003	1.5	–	14
Amsorb	83.2	–	–	–	–	14.4
LofloSorb	84	–	–	–	–	16
Superia	79.5	–	–	–	–	17.5
Lithium hydroxide	–	–	–	–	99	1

From Forman SA, Ishizawa Y. Inhaled anesthetic pharmacokinetics: Uptake, distribution, metabolism, and toxicity, Ch. 20. In: Gropper MA, ed. *Miller's Anesthesia*, 9th ed. Philadelphia: Elsevier; 2020:509–539. Data from Keijzer C, Perez RSGM, De Lange JJ. Compound A and carbon monoxide production from sevoflurane and seven different types of carbon dioxide absorbent in a patient model. *Acta Anaesthesiol Scand.* 2007;51:31–37 and Kharasch ED, Powers KM, Artru AA. Comparison of Amsorb, sodalime, and Baralyme degradation of volatile anesthetics and formation of carbon monoxide and compound A in swine in vivo. *Anesthesiology.* 2002;96:173–182.
*Various absorbents also contain other components, such as polyvinylpyrrolidone, calcium chloride, calcium sulfate, magnesium chloride, and aluminosilicate.
[†]Baralyme was withdrawn from the market in 2004.

Reactions With Carbon Dioxide Absorbents (also see Chapter 15)

Modern anesthesia workstations are designed to work with circle circuits that allow rebreathing of expired gas; this design conserves inhaled anesthetics, reduces the release of anesthetics to the atmosphere, and helps to maintain physiologic airway temperature and humidity. To prevent excessive buildup and rebreathing of CO_2, circuits include CO_2 absorbent in the expiratory limb that consists of a mixture of sodium, potassium, calcium, or barium hydroxides to catalyze a chemical reaction converting CO_2 and water into carbonates (Table 7.4). However, with desiccated absorbent, toxic by-products can be formed. Carbon monoxide (CO) can be generated, potentially causing CO poisoning. The propensity to generate CO is dependent on the makeup of the absorbent (KOH > NaOH >> $Ba(OH)_2$ > $Ca(OH)_2$) and the volatile anesthetic used (primarily desflurane and isoflurane).[89] Additionally, the reactions are exothermic, and prolonged use of desiccated absorbent, particularly with sevoflurane, can generate substantial heat and, rarely, cause a fire or explosion.[89,90] Although newer CO_2 absorbents are less hazardous, it is important to replace the absorbent regularly, particularly once the pH indicator shows it is exhausted.

Compound A is a breakdown product formed by the reaction of sevoflurane with strong alkali absorbents (Fig. 7.20). It can cause nephrotoxicity in rodent models, but has not been shown to cause toxicity in human subjects.[91] The theoretical risk of injury has led to the recommendation to maintain a fresh gas flow of at least 1 L min^{-1} if used for over 2 MAC-hours.[54]

METABOLISM, ELIMINATION, AND RECOVERY

The modern volatile anesthetics isoflurane, sevoflurane, and desflurane are minimally metabolized (0.2%, 5%, and 0.02%, respectively). Halothane, however, undergoes substantial hepatic metabolism (46%).[92,93] Metabolism occurs primarily by the cytochrome P450 system in the liver, specifically by CYP2E1, although other enzymes contribute to other volatile anesthetics. The breakdown of volatile anesthetics liberates fluoride.[93] Only methoxyflurane has been shown to release sufficient fluoride to generate clinical renal injury.

Similar to intravenous anesthetics, the duration of inhaled anesthesia affects their elimination, a concept referred to as *context-sensitive decrement time* (Fig. 7.21) (also see Chapter 4). For procedures of short duration, there are minimal differences in the time to eliminate volatile anesthetics. However, longer durations of administration increase the decrement time. This phenomenon is explained by a multicompartment pharmacokinetic model in which the anesthetic accumulates in slowly equilibrating, lipophilic tissues

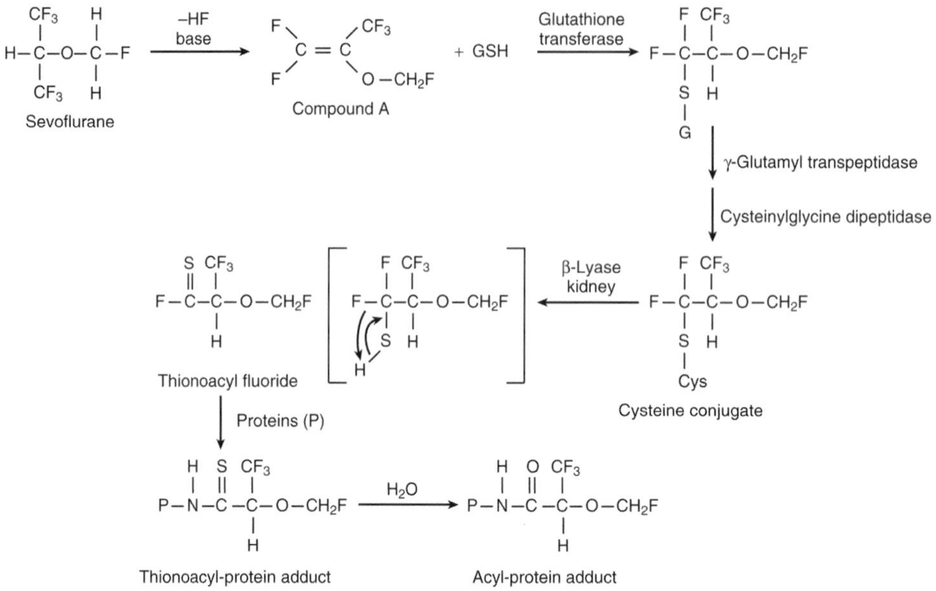

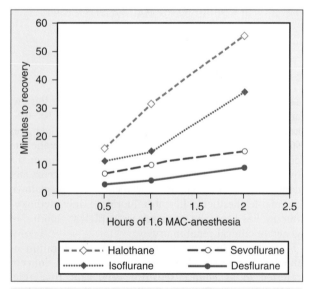

Fig. 7.20 Degradation of sevoflurane. Compound A is formed by the breakdown of sevoflurane catalyzed by strong bases in carbon dioxide absorbents. Compound A can be inhaled and undergo metabolism in the body. Although compound A mediates nephrotoxicity in animal models, it has not been shown to cause clinically relevant kidney injury in human patients. (Adapted from Martin JL, Kandel L, Laster MJ, et al. Studies of the mechanism of nephrotoxicity of compound A in rats. *J Anesth.* 1997;11:32–37. From Forman SA, Ishizawa Y. Inhaled anesthetic pharmacokinetics: Uptake, distribution, metabolism, and toxicity, Ch. 20. In: Gropper MA, ed. *Miller's Anesthesia,* 9th ed. Philadelphia: Elsevier; 2020:531.)

Fig. 7.21 Context-sensitive elimination of volatile anesthetics. Similar to intravenous anesthetics, inhaled anesthetics exhibit context-sensitive decrement times, whereby longer durations of administration prolong the time from cessation of delivery to elimination and recovery. Anesthetics with greater blood and tissue solubility have longer recovery times. (From Eger EI II. *Desflurane (Suprane): A Compendium and Reference.* Nutley: Anaquest; 1993:111.)

such as fat.[94] Thus the critical pharmacologic parameters dictating the context-sensitive decrement time of inhaled anesthetics are their blood–gas and blood–tissue partition coefficients, particularly blood–fat, and relative perfusion of the various compartments. The blood–gas partition coefficient largely determines elimination and recovery for shorter procedures, whereas the blood–fat partition coefficient affects elimination for longer procedures.

Beyond these pharmacokinetic considerations, emergence from general anesthesia shows hysteresis with respect to the partial pressure of inhaled anesthetic, meaning less anesthetic is required to maintain anesthesia than to induce it. This phenomenon, also referred to as *neural inertia,* may be best explained if emergence is considered as a series of transitions through discrete brain states under anesthesia with resistance to state transitions.[95] Thus patients can remain anesthetized despite minimal inhaled anesthetic concentrations. Moreover, greater population variability is observed for doses of anesthetics required for emergence as opposed to induction. Thus emergence is more complex than pharmacokinetic elimination of inhaled anesthetics and is not linearly related to partial pressure (Fig. 7.22).

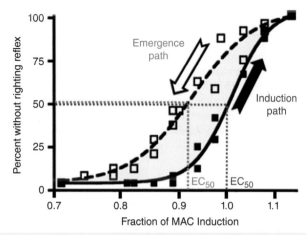

Fig. 7.22 Hysteresis in induction of and emergence from general anesthesia. Induction of anesthesia requires higher concentrations than are required for maintenance of anesthesia. Loss of righting reflex is a surrogate measure for loss of consciousness/immobility in rodents. (From Aranake A, Mashour GA, Avidan MS. Minimum alveolar concentration: Ongoing relevance and clinical utility. *Anaesthesia*. 2013;68:512–522.)

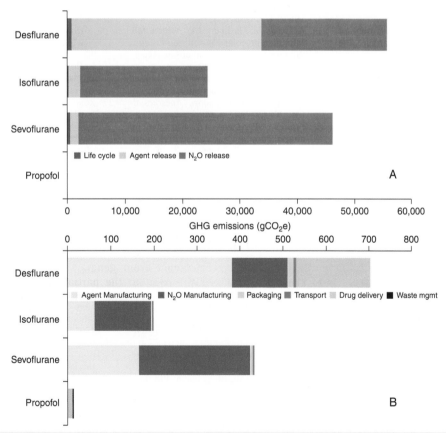

Fig. 7.23 The production and clinical use of inhaled anesthetics have agent-specific adverse environmental effects. Environmental impact is determined largely by atmospheric release of wasted gases. (From Sherman J, Le C, Lamers V, et al. Life cycle greenhouse gas emissions of anesthetic drugs. *Anesth Analg*. 2012;114[5]:1086–1090.)

ENVIRONMENTAL CONSIDERATIONS (ALSO SEE CHAPTER 49)

Evidence of ozone depletion by halogenated chemicals in the atmosphere elicited concern for the environmental impact of inhaled anesthesia as early as 1975.[96] Wasted inhaled anesthetics are scavenged, and the exhaust is released from health care facility ventilation systems into the environment. Inhaled anesthetics can cause deleterious effects in two major ways: a greenhouse gas effect and ozone depletion.[97] Nitrous oxide can deplete ozone, and it is also a potent greenhouse gas, with a global warming potential 300 times higher than carbon dioxide.[98] The medical and dental industries account for 86% of nitrous oxide generated for use as a product, comprising nearly 1% of nitrous oxide released into the atmosphere.[98] The modern halogenated agents exert environmental effects as greenhouse gases, with atmospheric lifetimes and global warming potentials in the order of desflurane > isoflurane > sevoflurane (Fig. 7.23).[99,100]

REFERENCES

1. Fenster JM. *Ether Day: The Strange Tale of America's Greatest Medical Discovery and the Haunted Men Who Made It.* New York: HaperCollins Publishers Inc.; 2002.
2. Bigelow HJ. Insensibility during surgical operations by inhalation. *Bost Med Surg J.* 1847;35:518–519.
3. Eger EI, Saidman LJ, Westhorpe RN. *The Wondrous Story of Anesthesia.* New York: Springer; 2014.
4. Warren JC. *Etherization, With Surgical Remarks*: Ticknor & Fields; 1848.
5. Kliff S. The New England Journal of Medicine's most important article. *The Washington Post.* 2012.
6. Targ AG, Nobuhiko Y, Eger EI, et al. Halogenation and anesthetic potency. *Anesth Analg.* 1989;68:599–602.
7. Eger EI. Current and future perspectives on inhaled anesthetics. *Pharmacotherapy.* 1998;18:895–910.
8. Fiserova-Bergerova V, Holaday DA. Uptake and clearance of inhalation anesthetics in man. *Drug Metab Rev.* 1979;9:43–60.
9. James MF, Manson ED, Dennett JE. Nitrous oxide analgesia and altitude. *Anaesthesia.* 1982;37:285–288.
10. Safar P, Tenicela R. High altitude physiology in relation to anesthesia and inhalation therapy. *Anesthesiology.* 1964;25:515–531.
11. Graham SG. The desflurane Tec 6 vaporizer. *Br J Anaesth.* 1994;72:470–473.
12. Boumphrey S, Marshall N. Understanding vaporizers. *Contin Educ Anaesthesia Crit Care Pain.* 2011;11:199–203.
13. Kern D, Larcher C, Basset B, et al. Inside anesthesia breathing circuits: time to reach a set sevoflurane concentration in toddlers and newborns: simulation using a test lung. *Anesth Analg.* 2012;115:310–314.
14. Yasuda N, Lockhart SH, Eger EI, et al. Kinetics of desflurane, isoflurane, and halothane in humans. *Anesthesiology.* 1991;74:489–498.
15. Yasuda N, Targ AG, Eger EI, et al. Pharmacokinetics of desflurane, sevoflurane, isoflurane, and halothane in pigs. *Anesth Analg.* 1990;71:340–348.
16. Eger EI. Physicochemical properties and pharmacodynamics of desflurane. *Anaesthesia.* 1995;50:3–8.
17. Taheri S, Eger EI. A demonstration of the concentration and second gas effects in humans anesthetized with nitrous oxide and desflurane. *Anesth Analg.* 1999;89:774–780.
18. Merkel G, Eger EI. A comparative study of halothane and halopropane anesthesia including method for determining equipotency. *Anesthesiology.* 1963;24:346–357.
19. Aranake A, Mashour GA, Avidan MS. Minimum alveolar concentration: ongoing relevance and clinical utility. *Anaesthesia.* 2013;68:512–522.
20. Perouansky M. The quest for a unified model of anesthetic action: a century in Claude Bernard's shadow. *Anesthesiology.* 2012;117:465–474.
21. Franks NP, Lieb WR. Do general anaesthetics act by competitive binding to specific receptors?. *Nature.* 1984;310:599–601.
22. Herold KF, Sanford RL, Lee W, et al. Clinical concentrations of chemically diverse general anesthetics minimally affect lipid bilayer properties. *Proc Natl Acad Sci USA.* 2017;114:3109–3114.
23. Forman SA, Chin VA. General anesthetics and molecular mechanisms of unconsciousness. *Int Anesth Clin.* 2008;46:43–53.
24. Campagna JA, Miller KW, Forman SA. Mechanisms of actions of inhaled anesthetics. *N Engl J Med.* 2003;348:2110–2124.
25. Morgan PG, Hoppel CL, Sedensky MM. Mitochondrial defects and anesthetic sensitivity. *Anesthesiology.* 2002;96:1268–1270.
26. Hemmings Jr HC, Riegelhaupt PM, Kelz MB, et al. Towards a comprehensive understanding of anesthetic mechanisms of action: a decade of discovery. *Trends Pharmacol Sci.* 2019;40:464–481.
27. Sonner JM, Antognini JF, Dutton RC, et al. Inhaled anesthetics and immobility: mechanisms, mysteries, and minimum alveolar anesthetic concentration. *Anesth Analg.* 2003;97:718–740.
28. Yang J, Chai Y, Gong C, et al. Further proof that the spinal cord, and not the brain, mediates the immobility produced by inhaled anesthetics. *Anesthesiology.* 2009;110:591–595.
29. Rampil IJ. Anesthetic potency is not altered after hypothermic spinal cord transfection in rats. *Anesthesiology.* 1994;80:606–610.
30. Purdon PL, Sampson A, Pavone KJ, et al. Clinical electroencephalography for anesthesiologists, Part 1: Background and basic signatures. *Anesthesiology.* 2015;123:937–960.
31. Newberg LA, Milde JH, Michenfelder JD. The cerebral metabolic effects of isoflurane at and above concentrations that suppress corticla electrical activity. *Anesthesiology.* 1983;59:23–28.
32. Roach GW, Newman MF, Murkin JM, et al. Ineffectiveness of burst suppression therapy in mitigating perioperative cerebrovascular dysfunction. *Anesthesiology.* 1999;90:1255–1264.
33. Pilge S, Jordan D, Kreuzer M, et al. Burst suppression-MAC and burst suppression-CP50 as measures of cerebral effects of anaesthetics. *Br J Anaesth.* 2014;112:1067–1074.
34. Avidan MS, Mashour GA. Prevention of intraoperative awareness with explicit recall: making sense of the evidence. *Anesthesiology.* 2013;118:449–456.
35. Short TG, Campbell D, Framptom C, et al: Anaesthetic depth and complications after major surgery: an international, randomised controlled trial. Lancet 394: 1907–1914, 2019.
36. Dagal A, Lam AM. Cerebral autoregulation and anesthesia. *Curr Opin Anaesthesiol.* 2009;22:547–552.
37. Matta BF, Mayberg TS, Lam AM. Direct cerebrovasodilatory effects of halothane, isoflurane, and desflurane during propofol-induced isoelectric electroencephalogram in humans. *Anesthesiology.* 1995;83:980–985.
38. Matta BF, Heath KJ, Tipping K, et al. Direct cerebral vasodilatory effects of sevoflurane and isoflurane. *Anesthesiology.* 1999;91:677–680.

39. McKinney MS, Fee JP, Clarke RS. Cardiovascular effects of isoflurane and halothane in young and elderly adult patients. *Br J Anaesth*. 1993;71:696–701.

40. Jr. Malan TP, DiNardo JA, Isner RJ, et al. Cardiovascular effects of sevoflurane compared with those of isoflurane in volunteers. *Anesthesiology*. 1995;83:918–928.

41. Muzi M, Ebert TJ. A comparison of baroreflex sensitivity during isoflurane and desflurane anesthesia in humans. *Anesthesiology*. 1995;82:919–925.

42. Duke PC, Fownes D, Wade JG. Halothane depress baroreflex control of heart rate in man. *Anesthesiology*. 1977;46:184–187.

43. Picker O, Scheeren TW, Arndt JO. Inhalation anaesthetics increase heart rate by decreasing cardiac vagal activity in dogs. *Br J Anaesth*. 2001;87:748–754.

44. Gallagher JD, McClernan CA. The effects of halothane on ventricular tachycardia in intact dogs. *Anesthesiology*. 1991;75:866–875.

45. Canet J, Sanchis J, Segri A, Llorente C, et al. Effects of halothane and isoflurane on ventilation and occlusion pressure. *Anesthesiology*. 1994;81:563–571.

46. Knill RL, Gelb AW. Ventilatory responses to hypoxia and hypercapnia during halothane sedation and anesthesia in man. *Anesthesiology*. 1978;49:244–251.

47. Sollevi A, Lindahl SG. Hypoxic and hypercapnic ventilatory responses during isoflurane sedation and anaesthesia in women. *Acta Anaesthesiol Scand*. 1995;39:931–938.

48. Dikmen Y, Eminoglu E, Salihoglu Z, et al. Pulmonary mechanics during isoflurane, sevoflurane and desflurane anaesthesia. *Anaesthesia*. 2003;58:745–748.

49. Forbes AR, Horrigan RW. Mucociliary flow in the trachea during anesthesia with enflurane, ether, nitrous oxide, and morphine. *Anesthesiology*. 1977;46:319–321.

50. Matsuura S, Shirakami G, Iida H, et al. The effect of sevoflurane on ciliary motility in rat cultured tracheal epithelial cells: a comparison with isoflurane and halothane. *Anesth Analg*. 2006;102:1703–1708.

51. Araújo MN, Santos CL, Samary CS, et al. Sevoflurane, compared with isoflurane, minimizes lung damage in pulmonary but not in extrapulmonary acute respiratory distress syndrome in rats. *Anesth Analg*. 2017;125:491–498.

52. Lumb AB, Slinger P. Hypoxic pulmonary vasoconstriction. *Anesthesiology*. 2015;122:932–946.

53. Benumof JL. Isoflurane anesthesia and arterial oxygenation during one-lung ventilation. *Anesthesiology*. 1986;64:419–422.

54. Fukazawa K, Lee HT. Volatile anesthetics and AKI: risks, mechanisms, and a potential therapeutic window. *J Am Soc Nephrol*. 2014;25:884–892.

55. Jephcott C, Grummet J, Nguyen N, et al. A review of the safety and efficacy of inhaled methoxyflurane as an analgesic for outpatient procedures. *Br J Anaesth*. 2018;120:1040–1048.

56. Eger EI. Compound A: does it matter?. *Can J Anesth*. 2001;48:427–430.

57. Iguchi N, Kosaka J, Booth LC, et al. Renal perfusion, oxygenation, and sympathetic nerve activity during volatile or intravenous general anaesthesia in sheep. *Br J Anaesth*. 2019;122:342–349.

58. Nieuwenhuijs-Moeke GJ, Nieuwenhuijs VB, Seelen MAJ, et al. Propofol-based anaesthesia versus sevoflurane-based anaesthesia for living donor kidney transplantation: results of the VAPOR-1 randomized controlled trial. *Br J Anaesth*. 2017;118:720–732.

59. Safari S, Motavaf M, Siamdoust SAS, et al. Hepatotoxicity of halogenated inhalational anesthetics. *Iran Red Crescent Med J*. 2014;16:e20153.

60. Rao Z, Xiongxiong P, Zhang H, et al. Isoflurane preconditioning alleviated murine liver ischemia and reperfusion injury by restoring AMPK/mTOR-mediated autophagy. *Anesth Analg*. 2017;125:1355–1363.

61. Gelman S: Hepatic oxygen supply during surgery and anesthesia, Clinical Aspects of O2 Transport and Tissue Oxygenation, 384–396, 1989.

62. Wulf H, Ledowski T, Linstedt U, et al. Neuromuscular blocking effects of rocuronium during desflurane, isoflurane, and sevoflurane anaesthesia. *Can J Anesth*. 1998;45:526–532.

63. De Castro Fonseca M, Da Silva JH, Perpetua Ferraz V, et al. Comparative presynaptic effects of the volatile anesthetics sevoflurane and isoflurane at the mouse neuromuscular junction. *Muscle Nerve*. 2015;52:876–884.

64. Taivainen T, Meretoja OA. The neuromuscular blocking effects of vecuronium during sevoflurane, halothane and balanced anaesthesia in children. *Anaesthesia*. 1995;50:1046–1049.

65. Buhre W, Disma N, Hendrickx J, et al. European Society of Anaesthesiology Task Force on Nitrous Oxide: a narrative review of its role in clinical practice. *Br J Anaesth*. 2019;122:587–604.

66. Leslie K, Myles PS, Chan MT, et al. Nitrous oxide and long-term morbidity and mortality in the ENIGMA trial. *Anesth Analg*. 2011;112:387–393.

67. Leslie K, Myles PS, Kasza J, et al. Nitrous oxide and serious long-term morbidity and mortality in the evaluation of nitrous oxide in the gas mixture for anaesthesia (ENIGMA)-II trial. *Anesthesiology*. 2015;123:1267–1280.

68. Gan TJ, Belani KG, Bergese S, et al. Fourth Consensus Guidelines for the Management of Postoperative Nausea and Vomiting. *Anesth and Analg*. 2020;131:411–448.

69. Horn CC, Wallisch WJ, Homanics GE, et al. Pathophysiological and neurochemical mechanisms of postoperative nausea and vomiting. *Eur J Pharmacol*. 2014;722:55–66.

70. Rosenberg H, Pollock N, Schiemann A, et al. Malignant hyperthermia: a review. *Orphanet J Rare Dis*. 2015;10:1–19.

71. Larach MG, Brandom BW, Allen GC, et al. Cardiac arrests and deaths associated with malignant hyperthermia in North America from 1987 to 2006: a report from the North American Malignant Hyperthermia Registry of the Malignant Hyperthermia Association of the United States. *Anesthesiology*. 2008;108:603–611.

72. Jevtovic-Todorovic V. Exposure of developing brain to general anesthesia: what is the animal evidence?. *Anesthesiology*. 2018;128:832–839.

73. McCann ME, Soriano SG. Does general anesthesia affect neurodevelopment in infants and children?. *BMJ*. 2019;367: 1–12.

74. FDA Drug Safety Communication: FDA approves label changes for use of general anesthetic and sedation drugs in young children, https://www.fda.gov/drugs/drug-safety-and-availability/fda-drug-safety-communication-fda-approves-label-changes-use-general-anesthetic-and-sedation-drugs.

75. Sun LS, Li G, Miller TLK, et al. Association between a single general anesthesia exposure before age 36 months and neurocognitive outcomes in later childhood. *JAMA*. 2016;315:2312–2320.

76. Warner DO, Zaccariello MJ, Katusic SK, et al. Neuropsychological and behavioral outcomes after exposure of young children to procedures requiring general anesthesia: the Mayo anesthesia safety in kids (MASK) study. *Anesthesiology*. 2018;129:89–105.

77. Davidson AJ, Disma N, de Graaf JC, et al. Neurodevelopmental outcome at 2 years of age after general anaesthesia and awake-regional anaesthesia in infancy (GAS): an international multicentre, randomised controlled trial. *Lancet*. 2016;387:239–250.

78. McCann ME, de Graaff JC, Dorris L, et al. Neurodevelopmental outcome at 5 years of age after general anaesthesia or awake-regional anaesthesia in infancy (GAS): an international, multicentre, randomised, controlled equivalence trial. *Lancet*. 2019;393:664–677.

79. Bedford PD. Adverse cerebral effects of anaesthesia on old people. *Lancet*. 1953;269:259–263.

80. Belrose JC, Noppens RR. Anesthesiology and cognitive impairment: a narrative review of current clinical literature. *BMC Anesthesiol.* 2019;19:1–12.

81. Abildstrom H, Rasmussen LS, Rentowl P, et al. Cognitive dysfunction 1–2 years after non-cardiac surgery in the elderly. *Acta Anaesthesiol Scand.* 2000;44:1246–1251.

82. Rasmussen LS, Johnson T, Kuipers HM, et al. Does anaesthesia cause postoperative cognitive dysfunction? A randomised study of regional versus general anaesthesia in 438 elderly patients. *Acta Anaesthesiol Scand.* 2003;47:260–266.

83. Silbert BS, Evered LA, Scott DA. Incidence of postoperative cognitive dysfunction after general or spinal anaesthesia for extracorporeal shock wave lithotripsy. *Br J Anaesth.* 2014;113:784–791.

84. Evered LA, Scott DA, Silbert B, et al. Postoperative cognitive dysfunction is independent of type of surgery and anesthetic. *Anesth Analg.* 2011;112:1179–1185.

85. Evered LA, Silbert BS. Postoperative cognitive dysfunction and noncardiac surgery. *Anesth Analg.* 2018;127:496–505.

86. Berger M, Schenning KJ, Brown CH, et al. Best practices for postoperative brain health: recommendations from the fifth international perioperative neurotoxicity working group. *Anesth Analg.* 2018;127:1406–1413.

87. Yap A, Lopez-Olivo MA, Dubowitz J, et al. Anesthetic technique and cancer outcomes: a meta analysis of total intravenous versus volatile anesthesia. *Can J Anesth.* 2019;66:546–561.

88. Yan T, Zhang GH, Wang BN, et al. Effects of propofol/remifentanil-based total intravenous anesthesia versus sevoflurane-based inhalational anesthesia on the release of VEGF-C and TGF-β and prognosis after breast cancer surgery: a prospective, randomized and controlled study. *BMC Anesthesiol.* 2018;18:1–9.

89. Coppens MJ, Versichelen LFM, Rolly G, et al. The mechanisms of carbon monoxide production by inhalational agents. *Anaesthesia.* 2006;61:462–468.

90. Olympio MA. Carbon dioxide absorbent dessication safety conference convened by APSF. *APSF Newsletter.* 2005;20:25–44.

91. Sondekoppam RV, Narsingani KH, Schimmel TA, et al. The impact of sevoflurane anesthesia on postoperative renal function: a systematic review and meta-analysis of randomized-controlled trials. *Can J Anesth.* 2020;67:1595–1623.

92. Eger EI. Characteristics of anesthetic agents used for induction and maintenance of general anesthesia. *Am J Heal Pharm.* 2004;61:3–10.

93. Karasch ED, Thummel KE. Identification of cytochrome P450 2E1 as the predominant enzyme catalyzing human liver microsomal defluorination of sevoflurane, isoflurane, and methoxyflurane. *Anesthesiology.* 1993;79:795–807.

94. Carpenter RL, Eger EI, Johnson BH, et al. Does the duration of anesthetic administration affect the pharmacokinetics or metabolism of inhaled anesthetics in humans?. *Anesth Analg.* 1987;66:1–8.

95. McKinstry-Wu AR, Proekt A, Kelz MB. Neural inertia: a sticky situation for anesthesia. *J Neurosurg Anesthesiol.* 2020;32:190–192.

96. Fox JW, Fox EJ, Villaneuva R. Stratospheric ozone destruction and halogenated anaesthetics. *Lancet.* 1975;305:864.

97. Ishizawa Y. General anesthetic gases and the global environment. *Anesth Analg.* 2011;112:213–217.

98. Inventory of U.S. greenhouse gas emissions and sinks: 1990–2018. United States Environmental Protection Agency. https://www.epa.gov/ghgemissions/inventory-us-greenhouse-gas-emissions-and-sinks-1990-2018

99. Sulbaek Andersen MP, Sander SP, Nielsen OJ, Wagner DS, et al. Inhalation anaesthetics and climate change. *Br J Anaesth.* 2010;105:760–766.

100. Ryan SM, Nielsen CJ. Global warming potential of inhaled anesthetics: application to clinical use. *Anesth Analg.* 2010;111:92–98.

8 INTRAVENOUS ANESTHETICS

Michael P. Bokoch, Po-Yi Paul Su

WHY INTRAVENOUS ANESTHETICS?

Intravenous (IV) anesthetics are fundamental tools in the daily practice of modern anesthesia (Box 8.1). One or more IV anesthetics will be administered in essentially any clinical encounter where a provider delivers anesthesia or sedation, regardless of the setting (operating room, non–operating room, or intensive care unit [ICU]). When used appropriately, IV anesthetics have many advantages and only a few drawbacks (Table 8.1). A *chief advantage* is the rapid onset of hypnosis (within seconds when given as a bolus) with sufficient depth of anesthesia for laryngoscopy. A *relative disadvantage* is the current inability to quantify effect site (i.e., brain) concentrations of IV anesthetics in real time, analogous to the end-tidal inhaled anesthetic measurements on modern anesthesia machines. Therefore anesthesia providers rely on knowledge of pharmacokinetics, careful and repeated observation of clinical endpoints (such as respiratory

Box 8.1	Classification of Intravenous Anesthetic Drugs

Isopropylphenol
  Propofol
Barbiturates
  Thiopental
  Methohexital
Benzodiazepines
  Diazepam
  Midazolam
  Lorazepam
  Remimazolam
Arylcyclohexylamine
  Ketamine
Carboxylated imidazole
  Etomidate
α_2-adrenergic agonists
  Dexmedetomidine

| Table 8.1 | Pros and Cons of Intravenous Anesthetics (as Compared With Volatile Anesthetics) |

Advantages	Disadvantages
Rapid onset of induction with deep anesthesia for airway instrumentation	Hard to measure effect-site concentration during clinical use, depth of anesthesia less predictable (i.e., no end-tidal concentration, no minimum alveolar concentration)
Rapid recovery after bolus dose	
Organ system effects and side effects vary by agent	Elimination depends on hepatic and/or renal function
Portable (no vaporizer/ special delivery equipment/ scavenger required)	Slow recovery after prolonged infusion (context-sensitive half-time)
No environmental hazard (no direct greenhouse gas generation)	May impair spontaneous ventilation
Beneficial ancillary properties (e.g., antiemetic)	Hard to ensure immobility if used alone

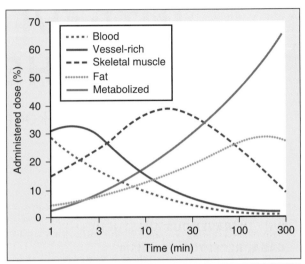

Fig. 8.1 After rapid intravenous injection of thiopental, the percentage of the administered dose remaining in blood (*brown line*) rapidly decreases as the drug moves from the blood to highly perfused vessel-rich tissues (*blue line*), especially the brain. Subsequently, thiopental is redistributed to skeletal muscles (*red line*) and, to a lesser extent, to fat (*pink line*). Ultimately, most of the administered dose of thiopental undergoes metabolism (*green line*). (From Saidman LJ. Uptake, distribution, and elimination of barbiturates. In: Eger EI, ed. Anesthetic Uptake and Action. Baltimore, MA: Williams & Wilkins; 1974:264–284, used with permission.)

rate), surrogate monitors (such as the processed electroencephalogram), and clinical experience to optimally and safely use IV anesthetics—topics that we aim to introduce in this chapter.

IV anesthetics used for induction of general anesthesia are lipophilic and preferentially partition into highly perfused, lipid-rich tissues (brain and spinal cord). This pharmacokinetic property accounts for the rapid onset of action. Redistribution of the drug into less perfused and inactive tissues such as skeletal muscles and fat leads to rapid termination of effect after a single IV bolus (Fig. 8.1). Thus many different IV anesthetics share a similar time to recovery (~5 to 10 minutes) after a single dose despite significant differences in their metabolism and elimination (Fig. 8.2 and Table 8.2).

Similar to inhaled anesthetics, IV anesthetics can provide the key components of anesthesia (hypnosis, amnesia, analgesia, and immobility) and are extremely useful as part of "balanced anesthesia" techniques—the practice of using smaller doses of multiple drugs in synergy rather than a large dose of a single drug in order to limit associated side effects. Other drug classes used as part of balanced anesthesia include inhaled anesthetics, opioids, and neuromuscular blockers (see Chapters 7, 9, and 11). Together, IV anesthetics represent an indispensable toolkit for tailoring an anesthetic plan to any given patient and clinical scenario.

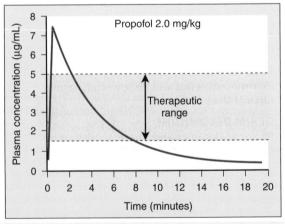

Fig. 8.2 Time course of the propofol plasma concentration after a simulated single bolus injection of 2.0 mg/kg. The shape of this curve is similar for other induction drugs, although the slope and the absolute concentrations are different. (From Vuyk J, Sitsen E, Reekers M. Intravenous anesthetics. In: Miller RD, ed. Miller's Anesthesia. 8th ed. Philadelphia, PA: Elsevier; 2015: 821–863. [Original chapter: Reves JG, Glass PSA. Chapter 9, Nonbarbiturate intravenous anesthetics. In: Miller RD, ed. Miller's Anesthesia. 3rd ed. New York, NY: Churchill Livingstone; 1990: 243–279.])

GABA_A RECEPTOR AGONISM

γ-aminobutyric acid type-A receptors (GABA_ARs) are ligand-gated ion channels that are the common target of most IV anesthetics. GABA is the main inhibitory neurotransmitter in the central nervous system (CNS). Upon activation, GABA_ARs conduct inhibitory (hyperpolarizing) chloride currents across the plasma membrane of neurons. Four types of IV anesthetic discussed in this chapter (propofol, barbiturates, benzodiazepines, and etomidate) behave as *agonists,* or activators, of GABA_ARs. Only two IV anesthetics act by different mechanisms: ketamine is primarily an *antagonist* of N-methyl-D-aspartate (NMDA) glutamate receptors, and dexmedetomidine is an agonist of α_2-adrenergic receptors.

The IV anesthetics targeting GABA_ARs exhibit distinct clinical differences. Such differences may seem surprising given the shared common target. However, the biology of these receptors is complex. First, GABA_ARs are a diverse family of pentameric receptors, not a single gene product. Nineteen possible subunits exist in the human genome. The most common type of GABA_AR in the brain is composed of two α, two β, and one γ subunit (Fig. 8.3).[1] Second, GABA_ARs may be located either within or outside of synapses. This diversity may explain why several different types of GABA-mediated currents are found in the CNS (*fast* versus *slow, phasic* versus *tonic*). Different IV anesthetics likely have some selectivity for certain types of GABA_ARs. Third, multiple drug binding sites exist on each receptor (see Fig. 8.3). Benzodiazepines bind at a site in the extracellular portion of the receptor that is different from the endogenous neurotransmitter GABA. Propofol, barbiturates, and etomidate most likely bind to distinct sites within the transmembrane region of GABA_ARs.[2]

The properties of IV anesthetics on the GABA_AR almost certainly depend on the binding site. For example, benzodiazepines are unlikely to open the channel independent of endogenous GABA. Instead, benzodiazepines assist GABA in triggering a rotational motion that opens the ion channel. Propofol and barbiturates, on the other hand, may act independently (directly open the channel) or synergistically with GABA. Although the complex pharmacology of GABA_ARs remains incompletely understood, the aforementioned factors explain in part the diverse effects of IV anesthetics.

PROPOFOL

Propofol, a GABA_AR agonist, is the most frequently administered IV anesthetic because of its many favorable properties. When administered as a bolus for the induction of general anesthesia, propofol provides rapid hypnosis, excellent suppression of airway reflexes, short duration of action, and largely predictable hemodynamic side effects. Before the introduction of propofol in the late 1980s, the prevailing induction techniques (barbiturate injection or inhalational) could not produce this constellation of effects. Since that time, propofol has also

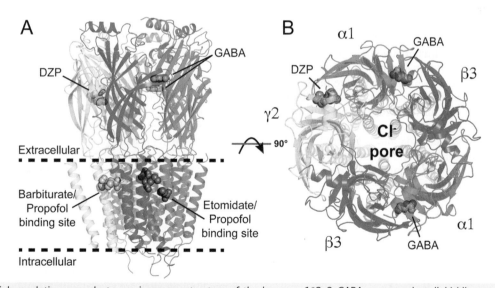

Fig. 8.3 High-resolution cryo-electron microscopy structure of the human α1β3γ2 GABA_A receptor in a lipid bilayer as viewed (A) from within the plane of the membrane and (B) from the extracellular face looking down the chloride (Cl-) pore. The position of bound GABA (*green*) and diazepam (DZP, *orange*) molecules are shown, as are the approximate binding sites for etomidate/propofol (*purple*) and barbiturates/propofol (*light blue*). Receptor subunits are shown as transparent ribbons and color-coded (*red* = α1, *blue* = β3, and *yellow* = γ2). (PDB ID: 6HUP, structure originally published in Masiulis S, Desai R, Uchanski T, et al. GABA_A receptor signalling mechanisms revealed by structural pharmacology. *Nature.* 2019;565[7740]:454–459. Images prepared using PyMOL v1.7.0.3, Schrödinger LLC.)

risen to become the leading drug for sedation by airway-trained providers during endoscopy, radiology, and other non-operating room procedures (also see Chapter 38). Propofol is also a mainstay of ICU sedation for patients requiring mechanical ventilation. Propofol infusion is often combined with volatile anesthetics to maintain general anesthesia, and it may be used as the sole hypnotic agent during total intravenous anesthesia (TIVA) techniques. TIVA with propofol may be the anesthetic technique of choice for select surgical procedures and/or patient populations (Box 8.2).[3] Given the fundamental role of propofol in modern anesthetic practice and the transformative effect it has had on global health care, it is fitting that the veterinarian John (Iain) Glen was awarded a 2018 Lasker Prize for developing this indispensable drug.[4]

Box 8.2 Examples of Scenarios Where Total Intravenous Anesthesia (Typically Propofol-Based) Is Preferred

Severe postoperative nausea and vomiting
Neuromonitoring (evoked potential monitoring)
Malignant hyperthermia (known or suspected)
Airway surgery

Physical Properties and Pharmacokinetics

Propofol (2,6-diisopropylphenol) is insoluble in aqueous solution (Fig. 8.4). It is formulated at 1% (10 mg/mL) in an emulsion containing 10% soybean oil (to dissolve the propofol), 2.25% glycerol (to yield isotonicity), and 1.2% egg lecithin (to stabilize the soybean oil–propofol droplets).[4] The emulsion is milky white and slightly viscous, with a pH of 7 to 8.5. In some countries a 2% formulation is available. Because bacteria can grow within the emulsion, it is imperative to use aseptic technique when drawing up propofol. Unused vials and syringes should be discarded within 12 hours after opening. To slow microbial growth, most manufacturers include a preservative such as ethylenediaminetetraacetic acid (0.05 mg/mL), metabisulfite (0.25 mg/mL), or benzyl alcohol (1 mg/mL). Allergic reactions to propofol are rare, and there is no evidence for cross-reactivity in patients with immunoglobulin E-mediated allergy to egg, soy, or peanut.[5] Formulations containing metabisulfite may be of concern for patients with asthma or sulfite allergy.

Propofol is rapidly metabolized in the liver through phase I (oxidation by cytochrome P450 enzymes) and phase II (mainly glucuronidation) reactions.[6] The inactive water-soluble metabolites are excreted through the kidneys. Certain propofol metabolites occasionally color the urine green. Plasma clearance is rapid and exceeds hepatic blood flow (Table 8.2). This finding, confirmed during the anhepatic phase of liver transplantation, proves that propofol metabolism occurs at extrahepatic tissue sites. The kidney, small intestine, and lungs are major contributors and together account for 40% of plasma propofol clearance. The rapid clearance explains the more complete recovery from propofol, with less "hangover" than observed with thiopental. As with other IV drugs, the effects of propofol are well described by a three-compartment model (also see Chapter 4). The hypnotic effect is terminated by redistribution from the plasma and highly perfused compartments (such as the brain) to poorly perfused compartments (such as skeletal muscle; see Fig. 8.1). A patient usually awakens within 8 to 10 minutes after an induction dose of propofol, which tracks the period of decline in plasma concentration after a single bolus dose (see Fig. 8.2).[6]

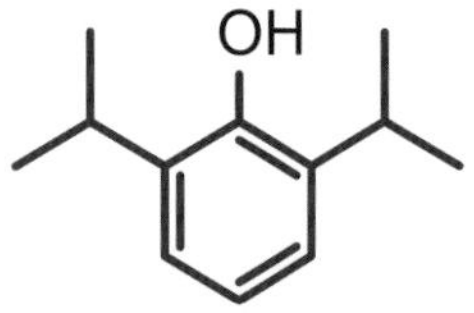

Fig. 8.4 Chemical structure of propofol. Marvin software was used for drawing all chemical structures in this chapter, MarvinSketch 6.2.2, 2014, ChemAxon (http://www.chemaxon.com).

Continuous Intravenous Infusion

Propofol has three pharmacokinetic properties that make it ideal for use as a continuous IV infusion: (1) efficient plasma clearance, (2) rapid metabolism, and (3) slow redistribution from poorly perfused compartments back into the central compartment. As a result, patients awaken relatively quickly after prolonged infusion of propofol as compared with other IV anesthetics. One way to characterize the kinetics of an anesthetic infusion is the "context-sensitive half-time," a parameter that describes the time needed for the plasma levels of a drug to drop by 50% (the "half-time") after stopping the infusion (Fig. 8.5).[7] This time depends on the duration for which an infusion has been run (the "context") (also see Chapter 4). The context-sensitive half-time of propofol remains short even after a prolonged infusion.

Pharmacodynamics

The major mechanism of action of propofol is through increasing the flow of inhibitory chloride current through $GABA_AR$s. Propofol binds nonselectively to multiple sites within the transmembrane domain of the receptor. Some binding sites are shared with etomidate and others with barbiturates (see Fig. 8.3A).[2] These sites are distinct from the GABA and benzodiazepine binding sites on the $GABA_AR$ extracellular domains. Propofol both directly activates the $GABA_AR$ and potentiates activation of the channel by endogenous GABA.

Table 8.2 Pharmacokinetic Data[a] for Intravenous Anesthetics

Drug	Induction Dose (mg/kg IV)	Duration of Action (min)	$V_{d,ss}$ (L/kg)	$t_{1/2\alpha}$ (min)	Protein Binding (%)	Clearance (mL/kg/min)	$t_{1/2\beta}$ (h)
Propofol	1–2.5	3–8	2–10	2–4	97	20–30	4–23
Thiopental	3–5	5–10	2.5	2–4	83	3.4	11
Methohexital	1–1.5	4–7	2.2	5–6	73	11	4
Midazolam	0.1–0.3	15–20	1.1–1.7	7–15	94	6.4–11	1.7–2.6
Diazepam	0.3–0.6	15–30	0.7–1.7	10–15	98	0.2–0.5	20–50
Lorazepam	0.03–0.1	60–120	0.8–1.3	3–10	98	0.8–1.8	11–22
Ketamine	1–2	5–10	3.1	11–16	12	12–17	2–4
Etomidate	0.2–0.3	3–8	2.5–4.5	2–4	77	18–25	2.9–5.3
Dexmedetomidine	N/A	N/A	2–3	6	94	10–30	2–3

[a]Data are for average adult patients. The duration of action reflects the duration after an average single IV dose.

IV, Intravenous; N/A, not applicable; $t_{1/2\alpha}$, distribution half-time; $t_{1/2\beta}$, elimination half-time; $V_{d,ss}$, volume of distribution at steady state.

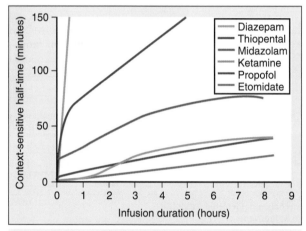

Fig. 8.5 Context-sensitive half-time for the most commonly used intravenous anesthetics. Propofol, etomidate, and ketamine have the smallest increase in context-sensitive half-times, with prolonged infusions making these drugs more suitable for use as continuous infusions. (From Vuyk J, Sitsen E, Reekers M. Intravenous anesthetics. In: Miller RD, ed. Miller's Anesthesia. 8th ed. Philadelphia, PA: Elsevier; 2015:821–863.)

Central Nervous System

In the CNS propofol primarily acts as a hypnotic without analgesia. It reduces the cerebral metabolic rate for oxygen ($CMRO_2$), which leads to decreased cerebral blood flow (CBF) through preserved flow-metabolism coupling (Table 8.3). This results in decreases in cerebral blood volume, intracranial pressure (ICP), and intraocular pressure. Propofol preserves cerebral autoregulation (the relationship between CBF and cerebral perfusion pressure) better than higher doses of volatile anesthetics (>0.5 minimum alveolar concentration). Although propofol can reduce ICP, it must be used with caution in brain-injured patients, as the combination of systemic hypotension and reduced CBF may compromise cerebral perfusion.

The direct effect of propofol on neuron viability, whether neuroprotective or neurotoxic, likely depends on the exact dose and context. At high doses, propofol induces burst suppression on the electroencephalogram (EEG), an endpoint that has been used for the titration of IV anesthetics for neuroprotection during neurosurgical procedures. Although propofol may be toxic to developing neurons in animals and cell culture, no human study has demonstrated long-term cognitive or memory problems in children who have received propofol anesthesia (see also Chapter 12). Occasionally, excitatory effects such as twitching or spontaneous movement occur during propofol induction. Although these motor effects may resemble seizure activity, propofol is actually an anticonvulsant and may be safely administered to patients with seizure disorders or to emergently treat seizures.

Cardiovascular System

Propofol produces a larger decrease in systemic arterial blood pressure than any other drug used for induction of anesthesia.[8] It causes profound vasodilation but does not affect myocardial contractility at clinical doses.[6] Vasodilation occurs in both the arterial and venous circulation and leads to reductions in preload and afterload. The effect is worse with rapid injection and is more pronounced in elderly patients, especially those with reduced intravascular fluid volume (also see Chapter 35). The degree of vasodilation may also be altered in patients with diabetes, hypertension, or obesity. Propofol inhibits the normal baroreflex response, often blunting a compensatory increase in heart rate and exacerbating hypotension during IV induction. Extreme decreases

Table 8.3 Summary of the Pharmacodynamic Effects of Commonly Used Intravenous Anesthetics

Dose/Effect	Propofol	Thiopental	Midazolam	Ketamine	Etomidate	Dexmedetomidine
Dose for induction of anesthesia (mg/kg IV)	1.5–2.5	3–5	0.1–0.3	1–2	0.2–0.3	
Systemic blood pressure	Decreased	Decreased	Unchanged to decreased	Increased[a]	Unchanged to decreased	Decreased[b]
Heart rate	Unchanged to decreased	Increased	Unchanged	Increased	Unchanged to increased	Decreased
Systemic vascular resistance	Decreased	Decreased	Unchanged to decreased	Increased	Unchanged to decreased	Decreased[b]
Ventilation	Decreased	Decreased	Unchanged	Unchanged	Unchanged to decreased	Unchanged to decreased
Respiratory rate	Decreased	Decreased	Unchanged to decreased	Unchanged	Unchanged to decreased	Unchanged
Response to carbon dioxide	Decreased	Decreased	Decreased	Unchanged	Decreased	Unchanged
Cerebral blood flow	Decreased	Decreased	Decreased	Increased to unchanged	Decreased	Decreased
Cerebral metabolic requirements for oxygen	Decreased	Decreased	Decreased	Increased to unchanged	Decreased	Unchanged
Intracranial pressure	Decreased	Decreased	Unchanged	Increased to unchanged	Decreased	Unchanged
Anticonvulsant	Yes	Yes	Yes	Yes?	No	No
Anxiolysis	Yes	No	Yes	No	No	Yes
Analgesia	No	No	No	Yes	No	Yes
Emergence delirium	No	No	No	Yes	No	May reduce
Nausea and vomiting	Decreased	Unchanged	Decreased	Unchanged	Increased	Unchanged
Pain on injection	Yes	No	No	No	Yes	No

[a]May cause direct myocardial depression and hypotension in critically ill or catecholamine-depleted patients.
[b]Bolus injection may increase systemic vascular resistance and blood pressure. *IV,* Intravenous.

in blood pressure may occur in patients with cardiac tamponade, cardiomyopathy, coronary artery disease, or valvular heart disease, as these groups are less able to compensate for the peripheral vasodilation. Severe bradycardia and, rarely, asystole may occur with propofol administration.

Respiratory System

Propofol is a respiratory depressant and often produces apnea after an IV induction dose. Propofol infusion decreases minute ventilation by reducing tidal volume and respiratory rate, with a more pronounced effect on tidal volume. The ventilatory response to hypoxia and hypercapnia is also blunted. Propofol increases upper airway collapsibility by inhibiting oropharyngeal muscles, including the genioglossus (the major tongue muscle).[9] Consequently, upper airway obstruction frequently occurs with sedative doses or during emergence from propofol anesthesia.

Propofol suppresses upper airway reflexes to a greater extent than other IV anesthetics, making it well suited for supraglottic airway placement or upper endoscopy procedures. Propofol also inhibits lower airway irritability and reduces the incidence of bronchoconstriction after tracheal intubation as compared with thiopental or etomidate.[10] Given these properties, propofol often provides excellent intubating conditions even without neuromuscular blocking drugs if sufficient doses are given.

Other Effects

Two other properties of propofol increase its utility as a first-line anesthetic: (1) it is an antiemetic and (2) it does not prolong the action of neuromuscular blocking drugs as much as volatile anesthetics. A rare but potentially fatal side effect is *propofol infusion syndrome*, which is usually characterized by unexpected arrhythmias or electrocardiogram changes after prolonged high-dose administration (>20 hours). These findings should prompt discontinuation of propofol and laboratory investigation for possible metabolic acidosis, rhabdomyolysis, elevated triglycerides, and hyperkalemia.[11]

Clinical Uses

Pain from injection of propofol is a common complaint that can lead to patient distress or dissatisfaction. The most effective means to reduce injection pain is to inject into an antecubital vein (larger, faster venous flow rate). Alternatively, if a hand vein is chosen, (1) premedication with a small dose of opioid and (2) IV lidocaine injection (up to 1.5 mg/kg) through the same IV, with or without proximal venous occlusion, are effective to reduce pain. Lidocaine may be administered alone or as an admixture with propofol.[12]

Induction and Maintenance of General Anesthesia
Propofol (1 to 2.5 mg/kg IV) is the most common drug for induction of general anesthesia. The dose should be decreased in the elderly, especially those who have a reduced cardiovascular reserve, or after premedication with benzodiazepines or opioids. Children generally require larger doses (2.5 to 3.5 mg/kg IV). Obese patients require a larger total dose compared with nonobese patients of similar height and age. Propofol boluses for morbidly obese patients should be calculated per kilogram of lean body weight rather than total body weight to avoid excess hypotension.[13] Generally, titration of the induction dose of propofol (rather than a single bolus) helps prevent severe hemodynamic changes. Propofol, like its predecessor thiopental, is an excellent choice for rapid-sequence intubation when combined with a fast-acting neuromuscular blocking drug such as succinylcholine or rocuronium.

Propofol is also often used to maintain general anesthesia as part of a balanced regimen along with volatile anesthetics, opioids, nitrous oxide, and/or other IV anesthetics. When combined with nitrous oxide or opioids, the therapeutic plasma propofol concentration for maintenance of anesthesia normally ranges between 2 and 8 µg/mL. This typically requires a continuous infusion rate between 100 and 200 µg/kg/min. Propofol may also serve as the sole sedative-hypnotic agent in TIVA techniques, where it is usually combined with opioids. Some clinical trials suggest a reduction in postoperative pain scores and opioid consumption for patients receiving propofol-based TIVA as compared with volatile anesthesia, but it is difficult to draw firm conclusions because of the small trial sizes and significant heterogeneity.[3] Propofol itself is not thought to provide significant analgesia. A current area of investigation is the role of propofol in cancer surgery. Preclinical propofol studies have demonstrated beneficial immune, antiinflammatory, and antitumor properties as compared with volatile anesthetics.[3] Some retrospective studies suggest that propofol TIVA may be associated with better long-term outcomes after cancer surgery. However, this exciting possibility is not yet supported by prospective clinical trials.

Sedation
Propofol is a popular choice for sedation of mechanically ventilated patients in the ICU (also see Chapter 41) and for sedation during procedures in or outside the operating room. The typical continuous infusion rate is between 25 and 75 µg/kg/min. Because of its pronounced respiratory depressant effect and its narrow therapeutic range, propofol should be administered only by individuals trained in airway management. Spontaneous ventilation is usually preserved in children at quite rapid propofol infusion rates (200 to 250 µg/kg/min), making it a good choice for pediatric procedures such as magnetic resonance imaging scans (also see Chapter 34).[14] Small boluses of propofol (10 to 20 mg IV) may provide useful anxiolysis.

Antiemetic
Subanesthetic bolus doses of propofol or a subanesthetic infusion can be used to treat postoperative nausea and vomiting (PONV) (10 to 20 mg IV or 10 to 20 µg/kg/min as an infusion).[15] Propofol TIVA, as compared with volatile anesthetics, reduces PONV but may not reduce unplanned admissions, postdischarge nausea and vomiting, or the cost of anesthesia in the ambulatory setting.[16,17]

Alternative Formulations

Because of the widespread use of propofol for sedation during non–operating room procedures such as endoscopy, great interest and intense research have focused on finding an alternative drug with more favorable properties (namely, less respiratory depression). *Fospropofol*, a water-soluble prodrug of propofol, was one such compound that was approved by the Food and Drug Administration (FDA) in 2008. Similar to propofol, respiratory depression and airway compromise were major concerns. The FDA concluded that fospropofol should be administered only by anesthesia providers trained in airway management. Fospropofol has since been discontinued, and some of the pharmacokinetic data leading to its approval were eventually retracted.

BARBITURATES

Barbiturates (e.g., *thiopental*) were the most common IV anesthetic induction agents before the introduction of propofol. These GABA$_A$R agonists are hypnotics with similar speed of onset to propofol, but have fallen out of use because of inferior kinetics (prolonged context-sensitive half-time), suboptimal suppression of airway reflexes, and problems with the alkaline chemical formulation.[18] *Methohexital,* the shortest-acting barbiturate, still plays a niche role in contemporary anesthesia practice as a common induction agent for electroconvulsive therapy (ECT) procedures.

Pharmacokinetics and Pharmacodynamics

Barbiturates activate $GABA_ARs$ by binding within the transmembrane domain of the pentameric ion channel. There is evidence for at least partial overlap between the propofol and barbiturate binding sites (see Fig. 8.3A).[2] Similar to propofol, and unlike benzodiazepines, high barbiturate concentrations are able to directly open the chloride channel even in the absence of endogenous GABA molecules.

Thiopental and methohexital (Fig. 8.6) are formulated as sodium salts mixed with anhydrous sodium carbonate. After reconstitution with water or normal saline, the solutions (2.5% thiopental and 1% methohexital) are alkaline, with a pH higher than 10. Although this property prevents bacterial growth and helps increase the shelf life of the solution after reconstitution, it will lead to precipitation when mixed with acidic drug preparations such as neuromuscular blockers. These precipitates can irreversibly block IV delivery lines if mixing occurs during administration. Furthermore, accidental injection into an artery or infiltration into subcutaneous tissue will cause extreme pain and may lead to severe tissue injury.

Most barbiturates undergo hepatic metabolism. The most important phase I reaction is oxidation; the resulting metabolites are inactive and excreted in the urine (directly) or in the bile (after conjugation). Chronic administration of barbiturates or other drugs that induce oxidative microsomal enzymes enhances barbiturate metabolism. Through stimulation of *aminolevulinic acid synthetase,* the production of porphyrins is increased. Therefore barbiturates should not be administered to patients with acute intermittent porphyria.

Methohexital is cleared more rapidly by the liver than thiopental and thus has a shorter elimination half-time. This allows for faster and more complete recovery. Although thiopental is metabolized slowly and has a long elimination half-time, clinical recovery after a single bolus is comparable to methohexital and propofol because it depends on redistribution to inactive tissue sites rather than metabolism (see Fig. 8.1). However, even single induction doses of thiopental may lead to psychomotor impairment lasting several hours. If administered as repeated boluses or as a continuous infusion, especially when using larger doses to produce burst suppression on the EEG, thiopental recovery is markedly prolonged because of the long context-sensitive half-time (see Fig. 8.5).

Central Nervous System

Barbiturates produce dose-dependent CNS depression ranging from sedation to general anesthesia. They do not have analgesic properties and may even reduce the pain threshold. Barbiturates are potent cerebral vasoconstrictors and produce predictable decreases in CBF, cerebral blood volume, and ICP (see Table 8.3). As a result, they decrease $CMRO_2$ in a dose-dependent manner up to the point where the EEG becomes isoelectric. Because of this property, IV infusions may be useful in the critical care setting to treat refractory status epilepticus. An exception to this rule is methohexital, which activates epileptic foci, thus facilitating seizure-mapping surgeries. For the same reason, methohexital is also a popular choice for anesthesia to facilitate ECT (also see Chapter 38).

Cardiovascular System

Induction doses of barbiturates produce modest decreases in systemic arterial blood pressure that are smaller than those produced by propofol. This effect is principally the result of peripheral vasodilation and reflects barbiturate-induced depression of the medullary vasomotor center and decreased sympathetic nervous system outflow from the CNS. Although barbiturates blunt the baroreceptor reflex, compensatory increases in heart rate limit the magnitude and duration of hypotension. Negative inotropic effects of barbiturates, which can be demonstrated in isolated heart preparations, are usually masked in vivo by baroreceptor reflex–mediated responses.

Respiratory System

Barbiturates cause respiratory depression similar to propofol: decreased minute ventilation via reduced tidal

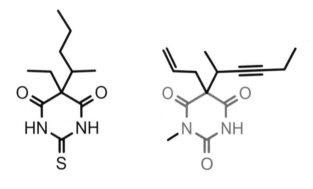

Fig. 8.6 Chemical structure of the barbiturate drugs thiopental (*left*) and methohexital (*right*), The common barbituric acid skeleton is shown in *red*.

volume and respiratory rate. Suppression of laryngeal and cough reflexes is not as profound as with propofol administration, making barbiturates an inferior choice for airway instrumentation in the absence of neuromuscular blocking drugs. Furthermore, stimulation of the upper airway or trachea (e.g., from secretions, supraglottic airway placement, direct laryngoscopy, tracheal intubation) during inadequate depression of airway reflexes may result in laryngospasm or bronchospasm. This phenomenon is not unique to barbiturates but is true in general when anesthetic depth is insufficient.

Side Effects

Accidental intraarterial injection of barbiturates results in excruciating pain and intense vasoconstriction, often leading to severe tissue injury involving gangrene. Aggressive therapy is directed at reversing the vasoconstriction to maintain perfusion and reduce the drug concentration by dilution. One approach is to block the sympathetic nervous system in the involved extremity (stellate ganglion block) to facilitate vasodilation. Barbiturate crystal formation probably results in the occlusion of distal, small-diameter arterioles. Crystal formation in veins is less hazardous because of the greater capacity of venodilation. Accidental subcutaneous injection (extravasation) of barbiturates results in local tissue irritation, thus emphasizing the importance of using dilute concentrations (2.5% thiopental, 1% methohexital). If extravasation occurs, some recommend local injection of the tissues with 0.5% lidocaine (5 to 10 mL) in an attempt to dilute the barbiturate concentration.

Life-threatening allergic reactions to barbiturates are rare. However, barbiturate-induced histamine release is occasionally seen.

Clinical Uses

The principal clinical use of barbiturates is rapid IV induction of anesthesia. A continuous IV infusion of a barbiturate such as thiopental is rarely used to maintain anesthesia because of its long context-sensitive half-time and prolonged recovery period (see Fig. 8.5).[7]

Induction of Anesthesia
Administration of thiopental (3 to 5 mg/kg IV) or methohexital (1 to 1.5 mg/kg IV) produces unconsciousness in less than 30 seconds. Patients may experience a garlic or onion taste during induction of anesthesia. When used as an anesthetic for ECT, methohexital may allow for longer seizure duration when compared with propofol.[19]

Neuroprotection
When used for neuroprotection, barbiturates have traditionally been titrated to achieve an isoelectric EEG, an endpoint that indicates maximal reduction of $CMRO_2$. The ability of barbiturates to decrease ICP makes these drugs an option for managing patients with space-occupying intracranial lesions (also see Chapter 30).[20] Furthermore, they may provide neuroprotection from focal cerebral ischemia (stroke, surgical retraction, temporary clips during aneurysm surgery) but probably not from global cerebral ischemia (cardiac arrest). Barbiturates are unlikely to provide cerebral protection during cardiac surgery. A clear risk of high-dose barbiturate therapy to decrease ICP is the associated hypotension, which can critically reduce cerebral perfusion pressure. Although barbiturates can lower ICP after traumatic brain injury, their use commonly causes hypotension and reduced cerebral perfusion pressure; there is no evidence for improved outcomes in this setting.[21] Prolonged infusions to achieve "barbiturate coma" for neuroprotection may cause immune suppression, electrolyte disturbances, and hypothermia.

BENZODIAZEPINES

Benzodiazepines commonly used in the perioperative period include diazepam, midazolam, and lorazepam. These drugs generally lack the hypnotic efficacy and rapid recovery kinetics required to be useful as sole agents for IV induction of general anesthesia. Nevertheless, they remain extremely useful in the perioperative period. Benzodiazepines are most often used as premedication or part of sedation regimens for the desirable effects of anxiolysis and anterograde amnesia. They have a favorable side effect profile and cause minimal cardiovascular or respiratory depression when used alone and in moderate doses. Benzodiazepines are unique among IV anesthetics in that their action is readily reversed by administration of flumazenil, a selective antagonist.

Pharmacokinetics and Pharmacodynamics

The shared chemical structure of benzodiazepines consists of a benzene ring fused to a seven-member diazepine ring (Fig. 8.7). Similar to propofol and barbiturates, benzodiazepines bind to $GABA_ARs$ and enhance the conduction of chloride currents, thereby leading to hyperpolarization of neurons and reduced excitability. Unlike other IV anesthetics that bind in the $GABA_AR$ transmembrane domain, benzodiazepines bind in the extracellular domain (see Fig. 8.3). Benzodiazepine binding alone is insufficient to activate the $GABA_AR$. Rather, these drugs enhance the ability of endogenous GABA to open the channel by inducing a rotational conformational change in the receptor. Consistent with its greater potency, midazolam has an affinity for $GABA_ARs$ that is approximately twice that of diazepam. $GABA_ARs$ that respond to benzodiazepines occur almost exclusively on

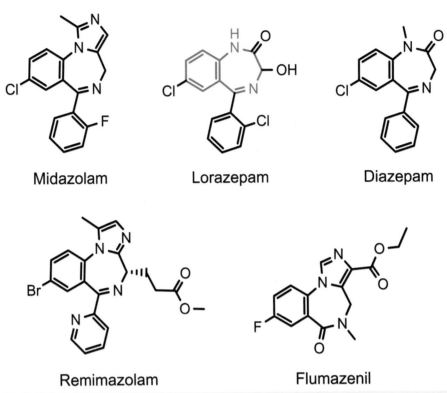

Fig. 8.7 Chemical structure of the most commonly used benzodiazepine drugs (midazolam, lorazepam, and diazepam), the new short-acting drug remimazolam, and the antagonist flumazenil. The common benzodiazepine ring structure is shown in *red*.

postsynaptic nerve endings in the CNS, with the greatest density found in the cerebral cortex. This anatomic distribution explains the minimal effects of benzodiazepines outside the CNS (see Table 8.3).

Midazolam is the most lipophilic of the three benzodiazepines most commonly used in the perioperative setting. However, it is packaged in an acidic formulation that solubilizes the drug in an open-ring structure. Once absorbed into the blood at physiologic pH, the diazepine structure rapidly forms through spontaneous ring closure. Midazolam, lorazepam, and diazepam are all highly protein bound, mainly to serum albumin. Although they are discussed here as IV formulations, they may be absorbed orally. Other possible routes of administration include intramuscular (IM), intranasal, and sublingual. Midazolam rapidly crosses into the CNS, but is considered to have a slower effect-site equilibration time than propofol and thiopental. In this regard, IV doses of midazolam should be sufficiently spaced to permit the peak clinical effect to be recognized before a repeat dose is considered. Midazolam has the shortest context-sensitive half-time of the group, making it the most suitable for continuous infusion (see Fig. 8.5).[7]

Similar to other IV anesthetics, termination of bolus action occurs by rapid redistribution to inactive tissue sites (see Table 8.2). The primary metabolic pathway for midazolam and diazepam is oxidation by hepatic cytochrome P450 3A4, a process susceptible to factors such as age, liver disease, and interaction with drugs that modulate the efficiency of the enzyme systems. Midazolam is selectively metabolized to a single dominant metabolite, 1-hydroxymidazolam, which has some sedative effects but undergoes rapid glucuronidation and clearance. This metabolite does not cause significant sedation in patients with normal hepatic and renal function unless midazolam is given as a prolonged infusion. The long elimination half-time of diazepam explains the prolonged CNS effects, especially in elderly patients. In contrast, lorazepam is one of the few benzodiazepines that does not undergo oxidative metabolism and is excreted after a single-step conjugation to glucuronic acid.

Central Nervous System
All benzodiazepines share a wide spectrum of CNS effects, although predilections for individual effects vary between drugs. The most important effects are the sedative-hypnotic and amnestic properties (anterograde, but not retrograde).[22] In addition, benzodiazepines are anticonvulsants used to treat seizures. Muscle relaxation is mediated through the spinal cord and may require larger doses.

Like propofol and barbiturates, benzodiazepines decrease $CMRO_2$ and CBF, but to a lesser extent. However, midazolam is unable to produce an isoelectric EEG even at high doses, thus emphasizing that there is a *ceiling effect* on $CMRO_2$ reduction. Patients with decreased intracranial compliance demonstrate little or no change in ICP after the administration of midazolam. Benzodiazepines have not been shown to possess neuroprotective properties. They are potent anticonvulsants for the treatment of status epilepticus, alcohol withdrawal, and local anesthetic–induced seizures.

Cardiovascular System

When administered alone and in small doses, benzodiazepines cause minimal changes in heart rate or blood pressure. If given in sufficient doses to induce general anesthesia, midazolam produces a larger decrease in arterial blood pressure than diazepam. This change is most likely the result of peripheral vasodilation. Hypotension is more likely in hypovolemic patients.

Respiratory System

Benzodiazepines produce minimal depression of ventilation. Transient apnea may occur with rapid IV administration of midazolam for induction of anesthesia. Benzodiazepines decrease the ventilatory response to carbon dioxide, but this effect is not usually significant if they are administered alone. More severe respiratory depression can occur when benzodiazepines are coadministered with opioids.

Side Effects

Allergic reactions to benzodiazepines are extremely rare to nonexistent. Pain during IV injection and subsequent thrombophlebitis are most pronounced with diazepam. Propylene glycol, the organic solvent required to dissolve diazepam and lorazepam, is most likely responsible for pain during IM or IV administration and for the unpredictable absorption after IM injection. Midazolam is water soluble in the low pH formulation, which obviates the need for an organic solvent and decreases the likelihood of pain during injection or erratic absorption.

Clinical Uses

Benzodiazepines are used for (1) preoperative medication, (2) sedation, (3) IV induction of anesthesia, and (4) suppression of seizure activity. The slow onset and prolonged duration of action of lorazepam limit its usefulness in the perioperative setting, especially when rapid and sustained awakening at the end of surgery is desirable. Flumazenil (8 to 15 µg/kg IV) may be useful for treating patients experiencing delayed awakening, but its duration of action is brief (about 20 minutes) and resedation may

occur. Administration of flumazenil in patients receiving chronic benzodiazepine therapy may induce seizures.

Preoperative Medication and Sedation

The amnestic, anxiolytic, and sedative effects of benzodiazepines are the basis for their use as preoperative medication. Midazolam (1 to 2 mg IV) is effective for premedication, sedation during regional anesthesia, and brief procedures. The addition of midazolam to propofol sedation for colonoscopy may improve operating conditions without slowing recovery time or worsening cognitive impairment at discharge.[23] When compared with diazepam, midazolam produces a more rapid onset, with more intense amnesia and less postoperative sedation. Many patients who receive preoperative midazolam do not recall the operating room, and some have no memory of the preoperative holding area.[24] Both anesthesia providers and surgeons should be aware of this fact when providing information to patients and families before surgery. Although awareness during anesthesia is rare, benzodiazepines seem to be superior to ketamine and barbiturates for prevention of recall. Midazolam is commonly used for oral premedication of children. For example, 0.5 mg/kg administered orally 30 minutes before induction of anesthesia provides reliable sedation and anxiolysis in children without delayed awakening (also see Chapter 34). Midazolam also lowers the incidence of PONV.[25] Despite these possible benefits, the routine use of premedication with benzodiazepines for elective surgery may not improve patient experience.[26]

The synergistic effects between benzodiazepines and other drugs, especially opioids and propofol, facilitate better sedation and analgesia. However, the combination of these drugs also exacerbates respiratory depression and may lead to airway obstruction or apnea. These drugs may also increase the risk for aspiration of gastric contents by impairing pharyngeal function and the coordination between breathing and swallowing.[27] Benzodiazepine effects, in addition to synergy with other respiratory depressants, are more pronounced in the elderly (also see Chapter 35), so smaller doses and careful titration may be necessary. Caution is advised when using benzodiazepines for sedation of critically ill, mechanically ventilated patients, as this drug class has been linked to longer duration of ICU stay and increased delirium compared with alternative regimens (propofol or dexmedetomidine)[28] (also see Chapter 41).

Induction of Anesthesia

Although rarely used for this purpose, general anesthesia can be induced by the administration of midazolam (0.1 to 0.3 mg/kg IV). The onset of unconsciousness, however, is slower than induction with thiopental, propofol, or etomidate. Unconsciousness is facilitated when a small dose of opioid (fentanyl, 50 to 100 µg IV) is injected 1 to 3 minutes before midazolam. Despite the possible reduction of cardiovascular side effects, it is unlikely that the use of a benzodiazepine for induction of anesthesia offers any advantage over propofol, and delayed awakening may occur.

Suppression of Seizure Activity

The efficacy of benzodiazepines as anticonvulsants is the result of their ability to enhance the inhibitory effects of GABA, particularly in the limbic system. Indeed, diazepam (0.1 mg/kg IV) is often effective in abolishing seizure activity produced by local anesthetics or alcohol withdrawal. Lorazepam (0.1 mg/kg IV) is the IV benzodiazepine of choice for status epilepticus. Diazepam (0.2 mg/kg IV) may also be used. For prehospital treatment of status epilepticus, IM administration of midazolam (10 mg IM for patients >40 kg; 5 mg IM for patients 13 to 40 kg) is effective and can be performed more rapidly than IV therapy.

Remimazolam

In 2020 the FDA approved a new ultrashort-acting benzodiazepine named *remimazolam* based on the results of several clinical trials demonstrating its utility and safety in procedural sedation (mostly endoscopy). Remimazolam contains a carboxylic ester group that is rapidly hydrolyzed by tissue esterases, analogous to remifentanil (also see Chapter 9). Compared with midazolam, remimazolam has a smaller volume of distribution, faster clearance, clearance independent of body weight, and a markedly shorter context-sensitive half time.[29] The kinetic properties of remimazolam make it a promising IV anesthetic drug that may yield less prolonged sedation compared with midazolam, particularly in patients with liver disease or those taking cytochrome P450–inhibiting drugs. However, at least one study suggests moderate hemodynamic effects (elevated heart rate and decreased blood pressure) during remimazolam infusion.[29]

KETAMINE

Ketamine is an arylcyclohexylamine and relative of phencyclidine (PCP) that works uniquely through antagonism of NMDA receptors to facilitate a characteristic hypnotic state known as *dissociative anesthesia,* wherein the patient's eyes remain open with a slow nystagmic gaze (see Table 8.3). Additionally, ketamine is different from most other IV anesthetics in that it produces significant analgesia. In anesthetic doses ketamine produces full anesthesia with an increase in blood pressure and without significant respiratory depression or upper airway collapse. However, when ketamine is administered as the sole anesthetic, amnesia is not as complete as with the administration of a benzodiazepine.

After its approval by the FDA in 1970, ketamine was established as a safe anesthetic and was widely used during the Vietnam War. However, with the unpleasant psychomimetic side effects, the abuse potential of ketamine, and the introduction of propofol, the popularity of ketamine as the primary or sole IV anesthetic has since declined. Still, the unique features of ketamine (potent analgesia with minimal respiratory depression and relative cardiovascular stability) and its versatile routes of administration (IV, IM, oral, intranasal, rectal, epidural) make it a very valuable alternative in certain settings (Box 8.3). In pain medicine subanesthetic doses of ketamine are administered to limit or reverse opioid tolerance and opioid-induced hyperalgesia and to treat refractory chronic pain (also see Chapter 44). More recently, ketamine is recognized for its benefits in the treatment of refractory major depression.

Pharmacokinetics and Pharmacodynamics

The mechanism of action of ketamine is complex, but the major anesthetic effect is produced through noncompetitive inhibition of the NMDA receptor complex. Ketamine conventionally exists as a racemic mixture, with the S(+) form being more potent than the R(−) enantiomer (Fig. 8.8). More recently, the S(+) enantiomer–only formulation, appropriately named *esketamine,* was approved by the FDA for major depression treatment. The high lipid solubility of ketamine ensures a rapid onset of effect. Like other IV induction drugs, the effect of a single bolus injection is terminated by redistribution to inactive tissue sites. Metabolism occurs primarily in the liver and involves *N*-demethylation by the cytochrome P450 system. Norketamine, the primary active metabolite, is less potent (one-third to one-fifth the potency of ketamine) and is subsequently further

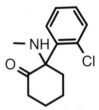

Fig. 8.8 Chemical structure of racemic ketamine.

Box 8.3 Clinical Scenarios for Potential Ketamine Use
• Sedation for painful procedures
• Infusion for analgesia, especially with opioid-tolerant patients or those with anticipated difficult pain management
• Intramuscular induction for uncooperative patients
• IV induction while maintaining spontaneous respiration and hemodynamics
• IV rapid-sequence induction to maintain hemodynamics

IV, Intravenous.

metabolized and excreted in urine. Ketamine has many possible routes of administration with good bioavailability, except enterically where it undergoes extensive first-pass metabolism. Ketamine is the only IV anesthetic that has low protein binding (12%) (see Table 8.2).[30]

Central Nervous System

In contrast to other IV anesthetics, ketamine is a cerebral vasodilator that increases both CBF and $CMRO_2$ (also see Chapter 30). The historical literature emphasizes concerns of elevated ICP with ketamine administration because of the increased CBF and thus it has been avoided in patients with intracranial disease. More recent studies argue against this notion in both traumatic and nontraumatic neurologic illnesses, and in fact, ketamine may lower ICP in some cases.[31,32] At low doses, ketamine may facilitate seizures; however, at anesthetic doses, it is considered an anticonvulsant and may be considered for treatment of status epilepticus when more conventional drugs are ineffective.

Transient, self-resolving psychotomimetic and schizophrenia-like symptoms can occur after ketamine administration in healthy patients.[33] Such reactions may include vivid colorful dreams; hallucinations; out-of-body experiences; and increased and distorted visual, tactile, and auditory sensitivity. These reactions can be distressing, particularly to those with underlying psychiatric history. A euphoric state may also be induced, which explains the abuse potential of the drug. Administration of a benzodiazepine in combination with ketamine may help limit the unpleasant experiences and provide amnesia. Although ketamine has been largely avoided in patients with psychosis and schizophrenia, this is not an absolute contraindication and may be considered by evaluating the risks, benefits, and alternatives in a particular clinical context.

Cardiovascular System

Ketamine can produce significant, but transient, increases in systemic arterial blood pressure, heart rate, and cardiac output via centrally mediated sympathetic stimulation, adrenocortical stimulation, and inhibition of norepinephrine reuptake. These effects, which are associated with increased cardiac work and myocardial oxygen demand, are not always desirable and can be blunted by coadministration of benzodiazepines, opioids, or inhaled anesthetics. Ketamine is a direct myocardial depressant, but this property is usually masked by its stimulation of the sympathetic nervous system. However, hypotension can develop in critically ill patients with limited ability to increase their sympathetic nervous system activity or patients with limited cardiovascular reserve.

Respiratory System

Ketamine does not produce significant respiratory depression. When used as a single drug, the respiratory response to hypercapnia is preserved and arterial blood gases remain stable. Transient hypoventilation and, in rare cases, a short period of apnea can follow rapid administration of large IV doses for induction of anesthesia. The ability to protect the upper airway in the presence of ketamine cannot be assumed despite the presence of active airway reflexes and maintenance of pharyngeal muscle tone. Frequently, lacrimation and salivation are increased, and premedication with an anticholinergic drug may be required to limit this effect. Especially in children the risk for laryngospasm may be increased because of excess salivation. Ketamine relaxes bronchial smooth muscles and may be helpful in the management of patients experiencing bronchospasm.

Clinical Uses

Induction and Maintenance of Anesthesia

Induction of anesthesia can be achieved with ketamine, 1 to 2 mg/kg IV or 4 to 6 mg/kg IM. Ketamine can be used for rapid-sequence intubation. Though not commonly used for maintenance of anesthesia, the short context-sensitive half-time makes ketamine an option for this purpose (see Fig. 8.3).[7] For example, general anesthesia can be achieved with the infusion of ketamine, 15 to 45 µg/kg/min, plus 50% to 70% nitrous oxide or by ketamine alone, 30 to 90 µg/kg/min. Ketamine can also be mixed in the same syringe as propofol ("ketofol") for procedural sedation to provide significant analgesia and to minimize the need for supplemental opioids. For example, a final ketamine concentration of 1 to 2 mg/mL in propofol can be given as a sedative infusion at a rate based on propofol dosing and titrated by the anesthesia provider to effect.

Analgesia

Small bolus doses of ketamine (0.2 to 0.8 mg/kg IV) can provide effective analgesia without compromise of the airway (e.g., cesarean section under neuraxial anesthesia when the regional block becomes insufficient). An infusion of a subanesthetic dose of ketamine (3 to 5 µg/kg/min) during general anesthesia and in the early postoperative period may be useful to produce analgesia or reduce opioid tolerance and opioid-induced hyperalgesia, although not all studies examining the use of ketamine as an adjunct show the desired improvement in pain scores and recovery.[34] Moderate-quality evidence supports the use of moderate-dose ketamine infusions (80 mg infused over 2 hours) to improve pain from complex regional pain syndrome. Analgesic outcomes for other refractory pain conditions such as fibromyalgia, headaches, and phantom limb pain remain controversial. Nevertheless, ketamine infusions continue to be safely administered for these difficult-to-treat conditions (also see Chapter 44).[35]

Treatment of Major Depression

Ketamine is receiving attention as a rapid-onset therapeutic option for treatment-resistant major depression. Intranasal and IV ketamine can improve depressive symptoms, and the antidepressant efficacy is sustained with repeated administration.[36,37] ECT is the alternative treatment modality for refractory depression. Whether using ketamine as part of the anesthesia for ECT can provide additive or synergistic antidepressant effect is controversial. With optimization of dose, timing, and frequency of treatments, ketamine may prove useful for maintenance of antidepressant effects in treatment-resistant patients.

ETOMIDATE

Etomidate is an IV anesthetic with hypnotic (but not analgesic) properties and a favorable hemodynamic effect profile (Fig. 8.9). However, it uniquely causes reversible, dose-dependent adrenocortical suppression, which has sparked debates about the risks and benefits of its use in specific settings.

Pharmacokinetics and Pharmacodynamics

Etomidate has GABA-like effects and seems to primarily act through potentiation of $GABA_AR$-mediated chloride currents, like most other IV anesthetics. An induction dose of etomidate produces rapid onset of anesthesia, and recovery depends on redistribution to inactive tissue sites (comparable to thiopental and propofol). Metabolism is primarily hepatic by ester hydrolysis to inactive metabolites, which are then excreted in urine and bile. The duration of action is linearly related to the dose, with each 0.1 mg/kg providing about 100 seconds of unconsciousness. Because of its minimal effects on hemodynamics and short context-sensitive half-time, larger doses, repeated boluses, or continuous infusions can safely be administered (see Fig. 8.5).[7] Etomidate, like most other IV anesthetics, is highly protein bound (77%), primarily to albumin.

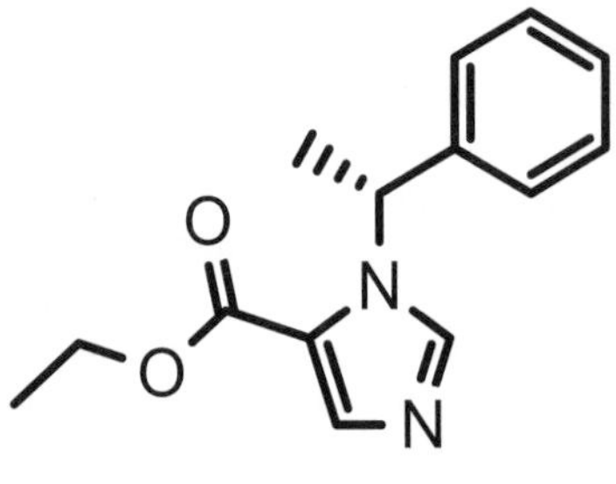

Fig. 8.9 Chemical structure of R(+)-etomidate.

Central Nervous System

Etomidate reduces $CMRO_2$ and is, in parallel, also a potent direct cerebral vasoconstrictor resulting in decreased CBF and ICP (also see Chapter 30). Despite its reduction of $CMRO_2$, etomidate showed mixed neuroprotection results in animal studies, and human studies are lacking. Excitatory spikes on the EEG are more frequent after etomidate than from thiopental. Similar to methohexital, etomidate may activate seizure foci, manifested as fast activity on the EEG. Etomidate can be used in ECT to facilitate longer motor seizure activity (also see Chapter 38).

Cardiovascular System

A characteristic and desired feature of etomidate bolus injection for induction of anesthesia is cardiovascular stability. Arterial blood pressure remains unchanged or minimally decreased and principally reflects small decreases in systemic vascular resistance. Any hypotensive effects of etomidate can be exaggerated in the presence of hypovolemia. Etomidate produces minimal changes in heart rate and cardiac output. The depressive effects on myocardial contractility are minimal at clinically used concentrations.

Respiratory System

The depressant effects of etomidate on ventilation are less pronounced than those of barbiturates, although apnea may occasionally follow rapid IV injection. Etomidate may decrease tidal volume but is compensated for by an increase in respiratory rate. Depression of ventilation may be exaggerated when etomidate is combined with inhaled anesthetics or opioids.

Endocrine System

Etomidate causes adrenocortical suppression by producing a dose-dependent inhibition of 11β-hydroxylase, an enzyme necessary for the conversion of cholesterol to cortisol (Fig. 8.10). This suppression lasts at least 4 to 8 hours after a single induction dose of etomidate, and relative adrenal insufficiency may last up to 24 to 48 hours. Infusion of etomidate for sedation in patients with sepsis (or critically ill patients in general) is no longer used because of low-level evidence and inferences from cortisol testing, but whether etomidate contributes causally to mortality has not been definitely established. The safety of single-dose etomidate for intubation of critically ill patients and as an induction drug for general anesthesia continues to generate controversy. Some high-quality randomized trials show no mortality risk related to single administration of etomidate; other metaanalyses find significant associations between single-dose etomidate, with an increased risk of adrenal insufficiency and mortality in patients with or at risk of sepsis.[38-40] Development of novel short-acting etomidate derivatives (e.g., ABP-700) is underway with promising results (including no adrenocortical side effects) in healthy human volunteers.[41]

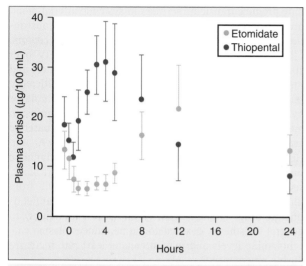

Fig. 8.10 Etomidate, but not thiopental, is associated with decreases in the plasma concentrations of cortisol. $P < 0.005$ versus thiopental, mean ± SD (standard deviation). (From Fragen RT, Shanks CA, Molteni A, et al. Effects of etomidate on hormonal responses to surgical stress. *Anesthesiology.* 1984;61:652–656, used with permission.)

Clinical Uses

Etomidate is an alternative to propofol and barbiturates for the rapid IV induction of anesthesia, especially in patients with compromised myocardial contractility, coronary artery disease, or severe aortic stenosis. After a standard induction dose (0.2 to 0.3 mg/kg IV), the onset of unconsciousness is comparable to that achieved by thiopental and propofol but is superior in avoidance of postinduction hypotension (Box 8.4). Etomidate is superior to propofol and thiopental in achieving ideal intubating conditions by preserving the hemodynamics, and hence distribution pharmacokinetics, of neuromuscular blocking agents.

There is a frequent incidence of pain followed by venous irritation during IV injection of propylene glycol–formulated etomidate; newer lipid emulsion formulations without the organic solvent are much better tolerated. Involuntary myoclonic movements are common from the transient imbalance of excitatory and inhibitory signaling in the thalamocortical tract and are not reflective of seizures. Myoclonus may be masked by the concomitant administration of neuromuscular blocking agents, benzodiazepines, and/or opioids. Awakening after a single IV dose of etomidate is rapid, with little evidence of any residual depressant effects. Etomidate does not produce analgesia, and PONV may be more common than after the administration of thiopental or propofol. The principal limiting factor in the clinical use of etomidate for induction of anesthesia is its undesired ability to transiently depress adrenocortical function. The clinical significance of transient etomidate-induced adrenal suppression is

---

Box 8.4 Clinical Scenarios for Potential Etomidate Use

- IV rapid-sequence induction to maintain hemodynamics
- IV induction for patients with cardiovascular risk factors where hemodynamic stability is critically important
- IV induction for ECT to help facilitate seizures

ECT, Electroconvulsive therapy; *IV,* intravenous.

unclear in nonseptic perioperative patients. Theoretically, this suppression may be either desirable if it reduces neurohormonal stresses during surgery and anesthesia, or undesirable if it prevents useful protective responses against perioperative stresses. Although controversy remains regarding the risk of mortality with single-dose etomidate in septic patients, one should be prompted to perform an assessment of risks and benefits of etomidate use (e.g., patients with cardiovascular risk factors or risk of postinduction hypotension) and alternative induction agents (for example, ketamine).

DEXMEDETOMIDINE

Dexmedetomidine is a highly selective and potent α_2-adrenergic agonist used most prevalently as a sedative agent in the procedure suites and ICUs. It has the ability to induce a unique cooperative-sedative response with minimal respiratory depression, which allows for a smooth transition between wakefulness and sleeplike state upon gentle stimulation (Box 8.5). Additionally, it has anxiolytic, sympatholytic, and analgesic properties and can be used as an anesthetic adjunct to decrease the dose of other inhaled or IV anesthetics.

Pharmacokinetics and Pharmacodynamics

Dexmedetomidine produces its effects through activation of CNS α_2-receptors; these effects can be reversed with α_2-antagonists. Dexmedetomidine is the active S-enantiomer of medetomidine, a highly selective α_2-adrenergic agonist and imidazole derivative that is used in veterinary medicine (Fig. 8.11). Dexmedetomidine is water soluble and undergoes rapid hepatic metabolism involving *N*-methylation, hydroxylation, and conjugation.

Box 8.5 Clinical Scenarios for Potential Dexmedetomidine Use

- Continuous infusion for sedation in the intensive care unit
- Sedation for procedures such as colonoscopies, endoscopies, awake fiber-optics, and awake seizure mapping
- Continuous infusion as part of balanced anesthesia for neuromonitoring, multimodal analgesia
- Prevention of postoperative delirium/emergence agitation

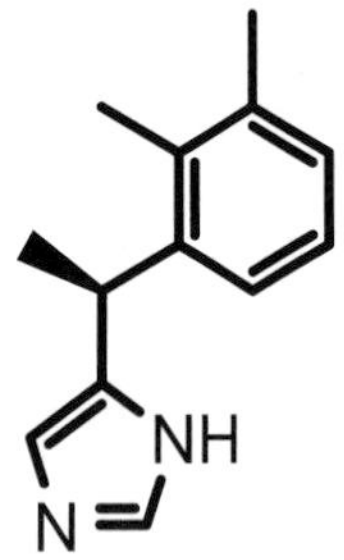

Fig. 8.11 Chemical structure of S-dexmedetomidine.

Inactive metabolites are excreted through urine and bile. Clearance is high, and the elimination half-time is short (see Table 8.2). However, there is a significant increase in the context-sensitive half-time from 4 minutes after a 10-minute infusion to 250 minutes after an 8-hour infusion.

Central Nervous System

Recognition of the usefulness of α_2-agonists was based on the observation that patients receiving chronic clonidine therapy have decreased anesthetic requirements. Hypnosis presumably results from stimulation of α_2-receptors in the locus ceruleus, and the analgesic effect originates at the level of the spinal cord. The sedative effect produced by dexmedetomidine has a different quality than that of other IV anesthetics: it more resembles a physiologic sleep state through activation of endogenous sleep pathways. Dexmedetomidine has a synergistic sedative effect when combined with other sedative-hypnotics. Dexmedetomidine decreases CBF without significant changes in ICP and $CMRO_2$ (see Table 8.3). Tolerance and dependence can develop, and patients can exhibit withdrawal symptoms upon cessation of a prolonged infusion of dexmedetomidine. Although changes in the EEG do occur, spikes from seizure foci are not suppressed, making dexmedetomidine a useful drug for epilepsy surgery.[42] Evoked potentials monitored during spine surgery are not suppressed at usual infusion doses (<0.6 µg/kg/hr).[43]

Dexmedetomidine has been associated with a decreased risk of postoperative cognitive dysfunction (including delirium) in the ICU and after various types of surgeries in the immediate perioperative period.[44–46] However, whether dexmedetomidine influences long-term postoperative cognitive outcomes remains an active area of research (also see Chapter 35).

Cardiovascular System

Dexmedetomidine infusion produces moderate decreases in heart rate and systemic vascular resistance and, consequently, decreases systemic arterial blood pressure through its effect on central α_2 receptos. A bolus or loading dose may produce transient *increases* in systemic arterial blood pressure and reflex bradycardia because of vasoconstriction mediated by peripheral α_2-adrenergic receptors. Clinically useful loading doses (0.5 to 1 µg/kg IV over 10 minutes) increase systemic vascular resistance and mean arterial pressure, but probably do not significantly increase pulmonary vascular resistance.[47] Bradycardia or hypotension associated with dexmedetomidine infusion may require treatment. Increasing age, decreased baseline arterial blood pressure (mean arterial pressure <70 mm Hg), and hypovolemia are risk factors for hemodynamic instability during dexmedetomidine infusion. Heart block, severe bradycardia, or even asystole may result from unopposed vagal stimulation; the response to anticholinergic drugs is unchanged. When used as an adjunct to general anesthesia, dexmedetomidine reduces plasma catecholamine levels and may attenuate heart rate increases during emergence.[48]

Respiratory System

One favorable property of dexmedetomidine is its minimal depression on the respiratory system—in fact, dexmedetomidine can be safely used through tracheal extubation. A small to moderate decrease in tidal volume and minimal change in the respiratory rate can be seen with dexmedetomidine infusion. The ventilatory response to carbon dioxide is largely unchanged, but the response to hypoxia seems reduced to a similar degree as propofol. Importantly, although the respiratory effects are mild, upper airway obstruction as a result of sedation is possible and comparable to propofol.[49]

Immune System

Surgery induces a stress endocrine, metabolic, and immune response. This response can be a risk factor for poor outcomes in patients with cardiovascular, endocrine, metabolic, immune, or infectious disorders. Dexmedetomidine is capable of blunting the surgical stress response comparable to epidural anesthesia.[48] Dexmedetomidine infusion inhibits the release of epinephrine, norepinephrine, cortisol, and other proinflammatory factors in the blood. These antiinflammatory effects may play a part in the possible renal, myocardial, and cognitive protective effects of dexmedetomidine.[50]

Clinical Uses

Dexmedetomidine was approved by the FDA in 1999 for sedation of intubated and mechanically ventilated patients during treatment in an intensive care setting and for sedation of nonintubated patients before and/or during surgical and other procedures. Although there is no evidence of mortality benefit, some clinical studies suggest that dexmedetomidine may reduce the duration of mechanical ventilation, shorten the length of ICU stay, and improve sleep quality. In the operating room dexmedetomidine may be used as an adjunct to general anesthesia or to provide sedation during regional anesthesia or awake fiber-optic tracheal intubation. When administered during general anesthesia, dexmedetomidine (0.5 to 1 µg/kg IV initial dose over a period of 10 to 15 minutes, followed by an infusion of 0.2 to 0.7 µg/kg/hr) decreases the dose requirements for inhaled and IV anesthetics. Awakening and the transition to the postoperative setting may benefit from dexmedetomidine-produced sedative and analgesic effects without respiratory depression. Dexmedetomidine decreases perioperative opioid consumption and may improve pain scores, but analgesic benefit has not been shown in all settings. Perineural dexmedetomidine is also used as a potent adjunct to local anesthetics in neuraxial and peripheral regional anesthesia. It has been shown to facilitate better postoperative analgesia and prolong the duration of the block.

Dexmedetomidine has been used extensively in children and has demonstrated efficacy in this population. Specifically, it may be beneficial for prevention of emergence delirium after pediatric anesthesia without affecting time to extubation or discharge (also see Chapter 34).[51]

ACKNOWLEDGMENTS

The editors and publisher would like to thank Dr. Helge Eilers for his contributions to prior editions of this chapter. The authors thank Hamed Darbanian for suggesting helpful corrections to Table 8.3.

REFERENCES

1. Scott S, Aricescu AR. A structural perspective on GABAA receptor pharmacology. *Curr Opin Struct Biol.* 2019;54:189–197. http://doi.org/10.1016/j.sbi.2019.03.023.
2. Kent DE, Savechenkov PY, Bruzik KS, Miller KW. Binding site location on GABAA receptors determines whether mixtures of intravenous general anaesthetics interact synergistically or additively in vivo. *Br J Pharmacol.* 2019;176(24):4760–4772. http://doi.org/10.1111/bph.14843.
3. Irwin MG, Chung CKE, Ip KY, Wiles MD. Influence of propofol-based total intravenous anaesthesia on peri-operative outcome measures: A narrative review. *Anaesthesia.* 2020;75(Suppl 1):e90–e100. http://doi.org/10.1111/anae.14905.
4. Walsh CT. Propofol: Milk of amnesia. *Cell.* 2018;175(1):10–13. http://doi.org/10.1016/j.cell.2018.08.031.
5. Asserhøj LL, Mosbech H, Krøigaard M, Garvey LH. No evidence for contraindications to the use of propofol in adults allergic to egg, soy or peanut. *Br J Anaesth.* 2016;116(1):77–82. http://doi.org/10.1093/bja/aev360.
6. Sahinovic MM, Struys MMRF, Absalom AR. Clinical pharmacokinetics and pharmacodynamics of propofol. *Clin Pharmacokinet.* 2018;57(12):1539–1558. http://doi.org/10.1007/s40262-018-0672-3.
7. Hughes MA, Glass PS, Jacobs JR. Context-sensitive half-time in multicompartment pharmacokinetic models for intravenous anesthetic drugs. *Anesthesiology.* 1992;76(3):334–341. http://doi.org/10.1097/00000542-199203000-00003.
8. Hannam JA, Mitchell SJ, Cumin D, et al. Haemodynamic profiles of etomidate vs propofol for induction of anaesthesia: A randomised controlled trial in patients undergoing cardiac surgery. *Br J Anaesth.* 2019;122(2):198–205. http://doi.org/10.1016/j.bja.2018.09.027.
9. Simons JCP, Pierce E, Diaz-Gil D, et al. Effects of depth of propofol and sevoflurane anesthesia on upper airway collapsibility, respiratory genioglossus activation, and breathing in healthy volunteers. *Anesthesiology.* 2016;125(3):525–534. http://doi.org/10.1097/ALN.0000000000001225.
10. Eames WO, Rooke GA, Wu RS, Bishop MJ. Comparison of the effects of etomidate, propofol, and thiopental on respiratory resistance after tracheal intubation. *Anesthesiology.* 1996;84(6):1307–1311. http://doi.org/10.1097/00000542-199606000-00005.
11. Krajčová A, Waldauf P, Anděl M, et al. Propofol infusion syndrome: A structured review of experimental studies and 153 published case reports. *Crit Care.* 2015;19(398):1–9. http://doi.org/10.1186/s13054-015-1112-5
12. Euasobhon P, Dej-arkom S, Siriussawakul A, et al. Lidocaine for reducing propofol-induced pain on induction of anaesthesia in adults. *Cochrane Database Syst Rev Online.* 2016;2:CD007874. http://doi.org/10.1002/14651858.CD007874.pub2.
13. Ingrande J, Brodsky JB, Lemmens HJ Lean body weight scalar for the anesthetic induction dose of propofol in morbidly obese subjects. *Anesth Analg.* 2011;113(1):57–62. doi: 10.1213/ANE.0b013e3181f6d9c0
14. Heard C, Harutunians M, Houck J, Joshi P, Johnson K, Lerman J Propofol anesthesia for children undergoing magnetic resonance imaging. *Anesth Analg.* 2015;120(1):157–164. http://doi.org/10.1213/ANE.0000000000000504
15. Borgeat A, Wilder-Smith OH, Saiah M, Rifat K. Subhypnotic doses of propofol possess direct antiemetic properties. *Anesth Analg.* 1992;74(4):539–541. doi: 10.1213/00000539-199204000-00013.
16. Apfel CC, Korttila K, Abdalla M, et al. A factorial trial of six interventions for the prevention of postoperative nausea and vomiting. *N Engl J Med.* 2004;350(24):2441–2451. http://doi.org/10.1056/NEJMoa032196.
17. Kumar G, Stendall C, Mistry R, Gurusamy K, Walker D. A comparison of total intravenous anaesthesia using propofol with sevoflurane or desflurane in ambulatory surgery: Systematic review and meta-analysis. *Anaesthesia.* 2014;69(10):1138–1150. http://doi.org/10.1111/anae.12713.
18. Sneyd JR. Thiopental to desflurane–An anaesthetic journey. Where are we going next?. *Br J Anaesth.* 2017;119(suppl_1):i44–i52. http://doi.org/10.1093/bja/aex328.
19. Lihua P, Su M, Ke W, Ziemann-Gimmel P. Different regimens of intravenous sedatives or hypnotics for electroconvulsive therapy (ECT) in adult patients with depression. *Cochrane Database Syst Rev Online.* 2014;4:CD009763. http://doi.org/10.1002/14651858.CD009763.pub2.
20. Roberts I, Sydenham E. Barbiturates for acute traumatic brain injury. *Cochrane Database Syst Rev Online.* 2012;12:CD000033. http://doi.org/10.1002/14651858.CD000033.pub2.
21. Ellens N, Figueroa B, Clark J. The use of barbiturate-induced coma during cerebrovascular neurosurgery procedures: A review of the literature. *Brain Circ.* 2015;1(2):140–146. http://doi.org/10.4103/2394-8108.172887.
22. Bulach R, Myles PS, Russnak M. Double-blind randomized controlled trial to determine extent of amnesia with midazolam given immediately before general anaesthesia. *Br J Anaesth.* 2005;94(3):300–305. http://doi.org/10.1093/bja/aei040.
23. Padmanabhan U, Leslie K, Eer AS, Maruff P, Silbert BS. Early cognitive impairment after sedation for colonoscopy: The effect of adding midazolam

and/or fentanyl to propofol. *Anesth Analg.* 2009;109(5):1448–1455. http://doi.org/10.1213/ane.0b013e3181a6ad31.

24. Chen Y, Cai A, Fritz BA, et al. Amnesia of the operating room in the B-unaware and BAG-RECALL clinical trials. *Anesth Analg.* 2016;122(4):1158–1168. http://doi.org/10.1213/ANE.0000000000001175.

25. Grant MC, Kim J, Page AJ, Hobson D, Wick E, Wu CL The effect of intravenous midazolam on postoperative nausea and vomiting. *Anesth Analg.* 2016;122(3):656–663 http://doi.org/10.1213/ANE.0000000000000941.

26. Maurice-Szamburski A, Auquier P, Viarre-Oreal V, et al. Effect of sedative premedication on patient experience after general anesthesia: A randomized clinical trial. *JAMA.* 2015;313(9):916–925. doi: http://doi.org/10.1001/jama.2015.1108.

27. Cedborg AIH, Sundman E, Boden K, et al. Effects of morphine and midazolam on pharyngeal function, airway protection, and coordination of breathing and swallowing in healthy adults. *Anesthesiology.* 2015;122(6):1253–1267. http://doi.org/10.1097/ALN.0000000000000657.

28. Kok L, Slooter AJ, Hillegers MH, van Dijk D, Veldhuijzen DS. Benzodiazepine use and neuropsychiatric outcomes in the ICU: A systematic review. *Crit Care Med.* 2018;46(10):1673–1680. http://doi.org/10.1097/CCM.0000000000003300.

29. Schüttler J, Eisenried A, Lerch M, Fechner J, Jeleazcov C, Ihmsen H. Pharmacokinetics and pharmacodynamics of remimazolam (CNS 7056) after continuous infusion in healthy male volunteers: Part I. Pharmacokinetics and clinical pharmacodynamics. *Anesthesiology.* 2020;132(4):636–651. http://doi.org/10.1097/ALN.0000000000003103.

30. Peltoniemi MA, Hagelberg NM, Olkkola KT, Saari TI. Ketamine: A review of clinical pharmacokinetics and pharmacodynamics in anesthesia and pain therapy. *Clin Pharmacokinet.* 2016;55(9):1059–1077. http://doi.org/10.1007/s40262-016-0383-6.

31. Zeiler FA, Teitelbaum J, West M, Gillman LM. The ketamine effect on intracranial pressure in nontraumatic neurological illness. *J Crit Care.* 2014;29(6):1096–1106. http://doi.org/10.1016/j.jcrc.2014.05.024.

32. Zeiler FA, Teitelbaum J, West M, Gillman LM. The ketamine effect on ICP in traumatic brain injury. *Neurocrit Care.* 2014;21(1):163–173. http://doi.org/10.1007/s12028-013-9950-y.

33. Beck K, Hindley G, Borgan F, et al. Association of ketamine with psychiatric symptoms and implications for its therapeutic use and for understanding schizophrenia: A systematic review and meta-analysis. *JAMA Netw Open.* 2020;3(5):e204693. doi: 10.1001/jamanetworkopen.2020.4693.

34. Gorlin AW, Rosenfeld DM, Ramakrishna H. Intravenous sub-anesthetic ketamine for perioperative analgesia. *J Anaesthesiol Clin Pharmacol.* 2016;32(2):160–167. http://doi.org/10.4103/0970-9185.182085.

35. Pickering G, Pereira B, Morel V, et al. Ketamine and magnesium for refractory neuropathic pain: A randomized, double-blind, crossover trial. *Anesthesiology.* 2020;133(1):154–164. http://doi.org/10.1097/ALN.0000000000003345.

36. Daly EJ, Singh JB, Fedgchin M, et al. Efficacy and safety of intranasal esketamine adjunctive to oral antidepressant therapy in treatment-resistant depression: A randomized clinical trial. *JAMA Psychiatry.* 2018;75(2):139–148. http://doi.org/10.1001/jamapsychiatry.2017.3739.

37. Singh JB, Fedgchin M, Daly EJ, et al. A double-blind, randomized, placebo-controlled, dose-frequency study of intravenous ketamine in patients with treatment-resistant depression. *Am J Psychiatry.* 2016;173(8):816–826. http://doi.org/10.1176/appi.ajp.2016.16010037.

38. Bruder EA, Ball IM, Ridi S, Pickett W, Hohl C. Single induction dose of etomidate versus other induction agents for endotracheal intubation in critically ill patients. *Cochrane Database Syst Rev Online.* 2015;1:CD010225. http://doi.org/10.1002/14651858.CD010225.pub2.

39. Gu W-J, Wang F, Tang L, Liu J-C. Single-dose etomidate does not increase mortality in patients with sepsis: A systematic review and meta-analysis of randomized controlled trials and observational studies. *Chest.* 2015;147(2):335–346. http://doi.org/10.1378/chest.14-1012.

40. Erdoes G, Basciani RM, Eberle B. Etomidate—A review of robust evidence for its use in various clinical scenarios. *Acta Anaesthesiol Scand.* 2014;58(4):380–389. https://doi.org/10.1111/aas.12289.

41. Valk BI, Absalom AR, Meyer P, et al. Safety and clinical effect of i.v. infusion of cyclopropyl-methoxycarbonyl etomidate (ABP-700), a soft analogue of etomidate, in healthy subjects. *Br J Anaesth.* 2018;120(6):1401–1411. http://doi.org/10.1016/j.bja.2018.01.038.

42. Oda Y, Toriyama S, Tanaka K, et al. The effect of dexmedetomidine on electrocorticography in patients with temporal lobe epilepsy under sevoflurane anesthesia. *Anesth Analg.* 2007;105(5):1272-1277. http://doi.org/10.1213/01.ane.0000281075.77316.98

43. Rozet I, Metzner J, Brown M, et al. Dexmedetomidine does not affect evoked potentials during spine surgery. *Anesth Analg.* 2015;121(2):492–501. http://doi.org/10.1213/ANE.0000000000000840.

44. Su X, Meng Z-T, Wu X-H, et al. Dexmedetomidine for prevention of delirium in elderly patients after non-cardiac surgery: A randomised, double-blind, placebo-controlled trial. *Lancet.* 2016;388(10054):1893–1902. http://doi.org/10.1016/S0140-6736(16)30580-3.

45. Djaiani G, Silverton N, Fedorko L, et al. Dexmedetomidine versus propofol sedation reduces delirium after cardiac surgery: A randomized controlled trial. *Anesthesiology.* 2016;124(2):362–368. http://doi.org/10.1097/ALN.0000000000000951.

46. Duan X, Coburn M, Rossaint R, Sanders RD, Waesberghe JV, Kowark A. Efficacy of perioperative dexmedetomidine on postoperative delirium: Systematic review and meta-analysis with trial sequential analysis of randomised controlled trials. *Br J Anaesth.* 2018;121(2):384–397. http://doi.org/10.1016/j.bja.2018.04.046.

47. Friesen RH, Nichols CS, Twite MD, et al. The hemodynamic response to dexmedetomidine loading dose in children with and without pulmonary hypertension. *Anesth Analg.* 2013;117(4):953–959. http://doi.org/10.1213/ANE.0b013e3182a15aa6.

48. Li Y, Wang B, Zhang L, et al. Dexmedetomidine combined with general anesthesia provides similar intraoperative stress response reduction when compared with a combined general and epidural anesthetic technique. *Anesth Analg.* 2016;122(4):1202–1210. http://doi.org/10.1213/ANE.0000000000001165.

49. Lodenius Å, Maddison KJ, Lawther BK, et al. Upper airway collapsibility during dexmedetomidine and propofol sedation in healthy volunteers: A nonblinded randomized crossover study. *Anesthesiology.* 2019;131(5):962–973. http://doi.org/10.1097/ALN.0000000000002883.

50. Wang K, Wu M, Xu J, et al. Effects of dexmedetomidine on perioperative stress, inflammation, and immune function: Systematic review and meta-analysis. *Br J Anaesth.* 2019;123(6):777–794. http://doi.org/10.1016/j.bja.2019.07.027.

51. Dahmani S, Delivet H, Hilly J. Emergence delirium in children: An update. *Curr Opin Anaesthesiol.* 2014;27(3):309–315. http://doi.org/10.1097/ACO.0000000000000076.

OPIOIDS

Talmage D. Egan

Opioids play an indispensable role in the practice of anesthesiology, critical care, and pain management. A sound understanding of opioid pharmacology, including both basic science and clinical aspects, is critical for the safe and effective use of these important drugs. This chapter will focus almost exclusively on the intravenous opioid receptor agonists used perioperatively.

BASIC PHARMACOLOGY

Structure and Activity

The opioids of clinical interest in anesthesiology share many structural features. Morphine is a benzylisoquinoline alkaloid (Fig. 9.1). Many commonly used semisynthetic opioids are created by simple modification of the morphine molecule. Codeine, for example, is the 3-methyl derivative of morphine. Similarly, hydromorphone, hydrocodone, and oxycodone are also synthesized by relatively simple modifications of morphine. More complex alteration of the morphine molecular skeleton results in mixed agonist-antagonists like nalbuphine and even complete antagonists like naloxone.

The fentanyl series of opioids are chemically related to meperidine. Meperidine is the first completely synthetic opioid and can be regarded as the prototype clinical phenylpiperidine (see Fig. 9.1). Fentanyl is a simple modification of the basic phenylpiperidine structure. Other commonly used fentanyl congeners like alfentanil and sufentanil are somewhat more complex versions of the same phenylpiperidine skeleton.

Opioids share many physicochemical features in common, although some individual drugs have unique features (Table 9.1). In general, opioids are highly soluble weak bases that are highly protein bound and largely ionized at physiologic pH. Opioid physicochemical properties influence their clinical behavior. For example, relatively unbound, unionized molecules such as alfentanil

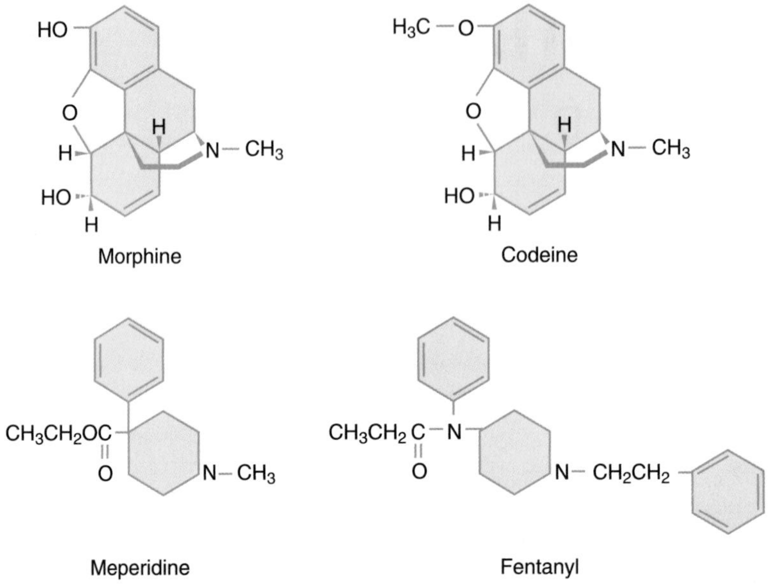

Fig. 9.1 The molecular structures of morphine, codeine, meperidine, and fentanyl. Note that codeine is a simple modification of morphine (as are many other opiates); fentanyl and its congeners are more complex modifications of meperidine, a phenylpiperidine derivative.

Table 9.1 Selected Opioid Physicochemical and Pharmacokinetic Parameters

	Morphine	Fentanyl	Sufentanil	Alfentanil	Remifentanil
pKa	8.0	8.4	8.0	6.5	7.1
% Un ionized at pH 7.4	23	<10	20	90	67?
Octanol–H_2O partition coefficient	1.4	813	1778	145	17.9
% Bound to plasma protein	20–40	84	93	92	80
Diffusible fraction (%)	16.8	1.5	1.6	8.0	13.3
Vdc (L/kg)	0.1–0.4	0.4–1.0	0.2	1.1–0.3	0.06–0.08
Vdss (L/kg)	3–5	3–5	2.5–3.0	0.4–1.0	0.2–0.3
Clearance (mL/min/kg)	15–30	10.20	10–15	4–9	30–40
Hepatic extraction ratio	0.6–0.8	0.8–1.0	0.7–0.9	0.3–0.5	NA

From Bailey, P.L., Egan, T.D., Stanley, T. H. Intravenous opioid anesthetics. In: Miller, R.D., ed. *Anesthesia*, 5th ed. New York, Churchill Livingstone; 2000:312.
NA, Not applicable; *Vdc,* volume of distribution of central compartment; *Vdss,* volume of distribution at steady state; ? indicates greater uncertainty about the value.

and remifentanil have a shorter latency to peak effect after bolus injection.

Mechanism

Opioids produce their main pharmacologic effects by interacting with opioid receptors, which are typical of the G protein–coupled family of receptors widely found in biology (e.g., beta-adrenergic and dopaminergic, among others). Expression of cloned opioid receptors in cultured cells has facilitated analysis of the intracellular signal transduction mechanisms activated by the opioid receptors.[1] Binding of opioid agonists with the receptors leads to activation of the G protein, producing effects that are primarily inhibitory (Fig. 9.2); these effects ultimately culminate in hyperpolarization of the cell and reduction of neuronal excitability.

Three classical opioid receptors have been identified using molecular biology techniques: mu, kappa, and delta. More recently, a fourth opioid receptor, ORL1 (also known as *NOP*), has also been identified, although its function is quite different from that of the classical opioid

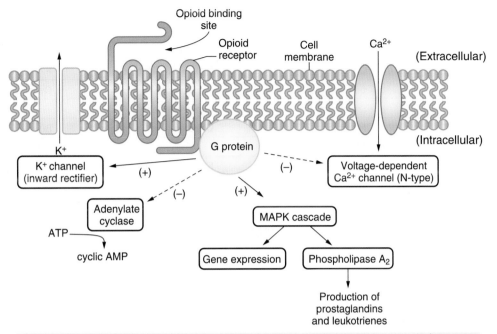

Fig. 9.2 Opioid mechanisms of action. The endogenous ligand or drug binds to the opioid receptor and activates the G protein, resulting in multiple effects that are primarily inhibitory. The activities of adenylate cyclase and the voltage-dependent Ca2+ channels are depressed. The inwardly rectifying K+ channels and mitogen activated protein kinase *(MAPK)* cascade are activated. *AMP,* Adenosine monophosphate; *ATP,* adenosine triphosphate.

receptors. Each of these opioid receptors has a commonly employed experimental bioassay, associated endogenous ligand(s), a set of agonists and antagonists, and a spectrum of physiologic effects when the receptor is agonized (Table 9.2). Although the existence of opioid receptor subtypes (e.g., mu-1, mu-2) has been proposed, it is not clear from molecular biology techniques that distinct genes code for them. Posttranslational modification of opioid receptors certainly occurs and may be responsible for conflicting data regarding opioid receptor subtypes.[2]

Opioids exert their therapeutic effects at multiple sites. They inhibit the release of substance P from primary sensory neurons in the dorsal horn of the spinal cord, mitigating the transfer of painful sensations to the brain. Opioid actions in the brainstem modulate nociceptive transmission in the dorsal horn of the spinal cord through descending inhibitory pathways. Opioids are thought to change the affective response to pain through actions in the forebrain; decerebration prevents opioid analgesic efficacy in rats.[3] Furthermore, morphine induces signal changes in "reward structures" in the human brain.[4]

Studies in genetically altered mice have yielded important information about opioid receptor function. In mu opioid receptor knockout mice morphine-induced analgesia, reward effect and withdrawal effect are absent.[5,6] Importantly, mu receptor knockout mice also fail to exhibit respiratory depression in response to morphine.[7]

Metabolism

The intravenous opioids in common perioperative clinical use are transformed and excreted by a wide variety of metabolic pathways. In general, opioids are metabolized by the hepatic microsomal system, although hepatic conjugation and subsequent excretion by the kidney are important for some drugs. For certain opioids, the specific metabolic pathway involved has important clinical implications in terms of active metabolites (e.g., morphine, meperidine) or an ultrashort duration of action (e.g., remifentanil). For other opioids, genetic variation in the metabolic pathway can drastically alter the clinical effects (e.g., codeine). These nuances are addressed in a subsequent section focused on individual drugs.

CLINICAL PHARMACOLOGY

Pharmacokinetics (also see Chapter 4)

Pharmacokinetic differences are the primary basis for the rational selection and administration of opioids in perioperative anesthesia practice. Key pharmacokinetic behaviors are (1) the latency to peak effect-site concentration after bolus injection (i.e., bolus front-end kinetics), (2) the time to clinically relevant decay of concentration after bolus injection (i.e., bolus back-end kinetics), (3) the time

Table 9.2 A Summary of Selected Features of Opioid Receptors

	Mu (μ)	Delta (δ)	Kappa (κ)
Tissue bioassay*	Guinea pig ileum	Mouse vas deferens	Rabbit vas deferens
Endogenous ligand	β-Endorphin	Leu-enkephalin	Dynorphin
	Endomorphin	Met-enkephalin	
Agonist prototype	Morphine	Deltorphin	Buprenorphine
	Fentanyl		Pentazocine
Antagonist prototype	Naloxone	Naloxone	Naloxone
Supraspinal analgesia	Yes	Yes	Yes
Spinal analgesia	Yes	Yes	Yes
Ventilatory depression	Yes	No	No
Gastrointestinal effects	Yes	No	Yes
Sedation	Yes	No	Yes

From Bailey, P.L., Egan, T.D., Stanley, T.H. Intravenous opioid anesthetics. In: Miller, R.D., ed. *Anesthesia,* 5th ed. New York, Churchill Livingstone; 2000:312.
*Traditional experimental method to assess opioid receptor activity in vivo.

to steady-state concentration after starting a continuous infusion (i.e., infusion front-end kinetics), and (4) the time to clinically relevant decay in concentration after stopping a continuous infusion (i.e., infusion back-end kinetics).

Applying opioid pharmacokinetic concepts to clinical anesthesiology requires recognition of several fundamental principles. First, a table of pharmacokinetic parameters has limited clinical value (see Table 9.1). Understanding pharmacokinetic behavior is best achieved through computer simulation. Second, opioids administered by bolus injection or continuous infusion must be considered separately.[8] Third, pharmacokinetic information must be integrated with knowledge about the concentration–effect relationship and drug interactions (i.e., pharmacodynamics) in order to be clinically useful.

The latency to peak effect and the offset of effect after bolus injection (i.e., bolus front-end kinetics and bolus back-end kinetics) of various intravenous opioids can be explored by predicting the time course of effect-site concentrations after a bolus is administered. Because the opioids differ in terms of potency (and thus the required dosages), for comparison purposes, the effect-site concentrations must be normalized to the percentage of peak concentration for each drug. Considering morphine, fentanyl, sufentanil, alfentanil, and remifentanil as among the most commonly used opioids intraoperatively, pharmacokinetic simulation illustrates how opioids differ in terms of latency to peak effect after a bolus is administered (Fig. 9.3, *top panel*).

The simulation of a bolus injection (see Fig. 9.3, *top panel*) has obvious clinical implications. For example, when a rapid onset of opioid effect is desirable, morphine may not be a good choice. Similarly, when the clinical goal is a brief duration of opioid effect followed by rapid dissipation, remifentanil or alfentanil might be preferred. Note how remifentanil's concentration has declined very substantially before fentanyl's peak concentration has even been achieved. The simulation illustrates why the front-end kinetics of fentanyl make it a drug well suited for patient-controlled analgesia (PCA) (also see Chapter 40). In contrast to morphine, the peak effect of a fentanyl bolus is manifest before a typical PCA lockout period has elapsed, thus mitigating a "dose stacking" problem.

The latency to peak effect is governed by the speed with which the plasma and effect site come to equilibrium (i.e., the k_{e0} parameter; also see Chapter 4). Drugs with a more rapid equilibration typically have a higher "diffusible" fraction (i.e., the proportion of drug that is unionized and unbound) and high lipid solubility (see Table 9.1). However, a very large dose of a typically slow-onset opioid can produce a rapid onset because a supratherapeutic drug level in the effect site is reached even though the peak concentration comes later.

The time to steady state after beginning a continuous infusion is also best examined by pharmacokinetic simulation. Using the same prototypes as with bolus administration, pharmacokinetic simulation (see Fig. 9.3, *middle panel*) shows the time required to achieve steady-state effect-site concentrations (i.e., infusion front-end kinetics).

This simulation of simple, constant-rate infusions has obvious clinical implications. First, the time required to reach a substantial fraction of the ultimate steady-state concentration is very long in the context of intraoperative

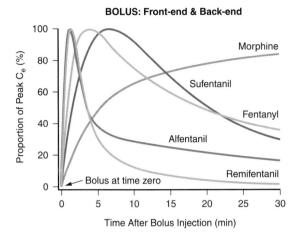

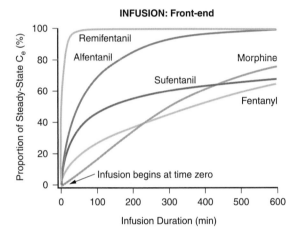

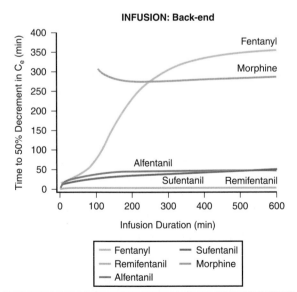

Fig. 9.3 Opioid pharmacokinetics. Simulations illustrating front-end and back-end pharmacokinetic behavior after administration by bolus injection or continuous infusions for morphine, fentanyl, alfentanil, sufentanil, and remifentanil using pharmacokinetic parameters from the literature (see text for details).[49,87-90]

use. To reach a near steady state more quickly requires a bolus to be administered before the infusion is commenced (or increased). Remifentanil perhaps represents a partial exception to this general rule. Also, for many drugs, opioid concentrations will increase for many hours after an infusion is commenced; in other words, concentrations are typically increasing even though the infusion rate may have been the same for hours! That remifentanil achieves a near steady state relatively quickly is certainly part of why it has emerged as a popular drug for total intravenous anesthesia (TIVA).

The time to offset of effect after stopping a steady-state infusion is best expressed by the context-sensitive half-time (CSHT) simulation.[9] Defined as the time required to achieve a 50% decrease in concentration after stopping a continuous, steady-state infusion, the CSHT is a means of normalizing the pharmacokinetic behavior of drugs so that rational comparisons can be made regarding the predicted offset of drug effect. The CSHT is thus focused on "infusion back-end" kinetics (also see Chapter 4).

The bottom panel of Fig. 9.3 is a CSHT simulation for commonly used opioids. For most drugs, the CSHT changes with time. Thus for brief infusions, the predicted back-end kinetics for the various drugs do not differ much (remifentanil is a notable exception to this general rule). As the infusion time lengthens, the CSHTs begin to differentiate, providing a rational basis for drug selection. Second, depending on the desired duration of opioid effect, either the shorter-acting or longer-acting drugs can be chosen. Finally, the shapes of these curves differ depending on the degree of concentration decline required. In other words, the curves representing the time required to achieve a 20% or an 80% decrease in concentration (e.g., the 20% or 80% decrement time simulations) are quite different.[8] Thus depending on the anesthesia technique applied, the CSHT simulations are not necessarily the clinically relevant simulations (i.e., a 50% decrease may not be the clinical goal). Also, CSHT simulation for morphine does not account for active metabolites (see the section on individual drugs).

Pharmacodynamics

In most respects the mu agonist opioids can be considered pharmacodynamic equals with important pharmacokinetic differences; that is, both the therapeutic and adverse effects are essentially the same. Their efficacy as analgesics and their propensity to produce ventilatory depression are indistinguishable from each other. Pharmacodynamic differences do exist in part as a function of non–opioid receptor mechanisms such as histamine release.

Because the nervous system profoundly influences the function of the entire body, mu opioid agonist pharmacodynamic effects are observed in many organ systems. Fig. 9.4 summarizes the major pharmacodynamic effects of the fentanyl congeners. Depending on the clinical

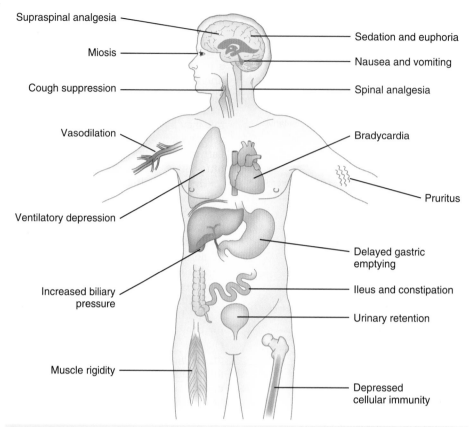

Supraspinal analgesia

Miosis

Cough suppression

Vasodilation

Ventilatory depression

Increased biliary pressure

Muscle rigidity

Sedation and euphoria

Nausea and vomiting

Spinal analgesia

Bradycardia

Pruritus

Delayed gastric emptying

Ileus and constipation

Urinary retention

Depressed cellular immunity

Fig. 9.4 Opioid pharmacodynamics. A summary chart of selected effects of the fentanyl congeners (see text for details).

circumstances and clinical goals of treatment, some of these widespread effects can be viewed as therapeutic or adverse. For example, in some clinical settings the sedation produced by mu agonists might be viewed as a goal of therapy. In others drowsiness would clearly be thought of as an adverse effect.

Therapeutic Effects

The relief of pain is the primary therapeutic effect of opioid analgesics. Acting at spinal and brain mu receptors, opioids provide analgesia both by attenuating the nociceptive traffic from the periphery and by altering the affective response to painful stimulation centrally. Mu agonists are most effective in treating "second pain" sensations carried by slowly conducting, unmyelinated C fibers; they are less effective in treating "first pain" sensations (carried by small, myelinated A-delta fibers) and neuropathic pain. A unique aspect of opioid-induced analgesia (in contrast to drugs like local anesthetics) is that other sensory modalities are not affected (e.g., touch and temperature, among others).

Perioperatively (certainly intraoperatively), the drowsiness produced by mu agonists is also one of the targeted

effects. The brain is the anatomic substrate for the sedative action of mu agonists. With increasing doses, mu agonists eventually produce drowsiness and sleep (the relief of pain no doubt contributes to the promotion of sleep in uncomfortable patients both preoperatively and postoperatively). With sufficient doses, the mu agonists produce pronounced delta wave activity on the electroencephalogram, which resembles the pattern observed during natural sleep.

Mu agonists can of course produce significant pain relief at doses that do not produce sleep. This is the basis of their clinical utility in the treatment of pain in ambulatory patients. On the other hand, the fact that increasing doses eventually produce drowsiness (and therefore the inability to request additional doses) is the essential scientific foundation for the safety of PCA devices. However, even large doses of opioids do not reliably produce unresponsiveness and amnesia, and thus opioids cannot be viewed as complete anesthetics when used alone.

Opioids also suppress the cough reflex via the cough centers in the medulla. Attenuation of the cough reflex presumably makes coughing and "bucking" against the indwelling endotracheal tube less likely.

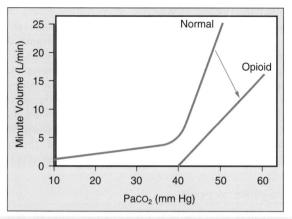

Fig. 9.5 Opioid-induced ventilatory depression study methodology. The method characterizes the relationship between Pa_{CO_2} and minute volume. The curve labeled "Normal" represents the expected response of minute volume to rising Pa_{CO_2} levels in an awake human. Note the dramatic increase in minute volume as CO_2 tension rises. The curve labeled "Opioid" represents the blunted response of minute volume to rising CO_2 levels after administration of an opioid. Note that the slope of the curve decreases and the curve no longer has a "hockey stick" shape; this means that at physiologic Pa_{CO_2} levels, the patient receiving sufficient opioid may be apneic or severely hypoventilatory. (Adapted with permission from Gross.[11])

Adverse Effects

Depression of ventilation is the primary adverse effect associated with mu agonist drugs. When the airway is secured and ventilation is controlled intraoperatively, opioid-induced depression of ventilation is of little consequence. However, opioid-induced respiratory depression in the postoperative period can lead to hypoxemic brain injury and death.

Mu agonists alter the ventilatory response to arterial carbon dioxide at the ventilatory control center in the medulla. The depression of ventilation is mediated by the mu receptor; mu receptor knockout mice do not exhibit respiratory depression from morphine.[10]

In unmedicated humans increases in arterial carbon dioxide partial pressure markedly increase minute volume (Fig. 9.5). Under the influence of opioid analgesics, the curve is flattened and shifted to the right; for a given carbon dioxide partial pressure, the minute volume is lower.[11] More importantly, the "hockey stick" shape of the normal curve is lost; there may be a partial pressure of carbon dioxide below which the patient will not breathe (i.e., the "apneic threshold") in the presence of opioids.

The clinical signs of depressed ventilation are quite subtle with moderate opioid doses. Postoperative patients receiving opioid analgesic therapy can be awake and alert and yet have a significantly decreased minute volume. Respiratory rate decreases, whereas initially tidal volume may increase slightly. As the opioid concentration is increased, both respiratory rate and tidal volume progressively decrease, eventually culminating in an irregular ventilatory rhythm and then complete apnea.

A variety of factors can increase the risk of opioid-induced ventilatory depression. Clear risk factors include large opioid dose, advanced age, concomitant use of other central nervous system (CNS) depressants, and renal insufficiency (for morphine). Natural sleep also increases the ventilatory depressant effect of opioids.[12]

Opioids can alter cardiovascular physiology by a variety of different mechanisms. Compared with many other anesthetic drugs (e.g., propofol, volatile anesthetics), however, the cardiovascular effects of opioids, particularly the fentanyl congeners, are relatively minimal (morphine and meperidine are exceptions, see later).

The fentanyl congeners cause bradycardia by directly increasing vagal nerve tone in the brainstem, which experimentally can be blocked by microinjection of naloxone into the vagal nerve nucleus or by peripheral vagotomy.[13,14]

Opioids also produce vasodilation by depressing vasomotor centers in the brainstem and, to a lesser extent, by a direct effect on vessels. This action decreases both preload and afterload. Decreases in arterial blood pressure are more pronounced in patients with increased sympathetic tone, such as patients with congestive heart failure or hypertension. Clinical doses of opioids do not appreciably alter myocardial contractility.

Opioids can induce muscle rigidity, usually from the rapid administration of large bolus doses of the fentanyl congeners. This rigidity can even make bag and mask ventilation during induction of anesthesia nearly impossible as a result of vocal cord rigidity and closure.[15] The rigidity tends to coincide with the onset of unresponsiveness.[16] Although the mechanism of opioid-induced muscle rigidity is unknown, it is not a direct action on muscle because it can be eliminated by neuromuscular blocking drugs.

Opioids also cause nausea and vomiting. They stimulate the chemoreceptor trigger zone in the area postrema on the floor of the fourth ventricle in the brain. This can lead to nausea and vomiting, which are exacerbated by movement. This perhaps explains why ambulatory surgery patients are more likely to be troubled by postoperative nausea and vomiting, PONV (also see Chapter 39).

Pupillary constriction induced by mu agonists can be a useful diagnostic sign indicating some ongoing opioid effect. Opioids stimulate the Edinger–Westphal nucleus of the oculomotor nerve to produce miosis. Even small doses of opioids elicit this response, and very little tolerance to the effect develops. Thus miosis is a useful, albeit nonspecific, indicator of opioid exposure even in opioid-tolerant patients. Opioid-induced pupillary constriction is reversible with naloxone.

Opioids have important effects on gastrointestinal physiology. Opioid receptors are found throughout the enteric plexus of the bowel. Stimulation of these receptors by opioids causes tonic contraction of gastrointestinal smooth muscle, thereby decreasing coordinated, peristaltic contractions. Clinically, this results in delayed gastric emptying and presumably larger gastric volumes in patients receiving opioid therapy preoperatively. Postoperatively, patients can develop opioid-induced ileus that can potentially delay the resumption of proper nutrition and discharge from the hospital. An extension of this acute problem is the chronic constipation associated with long-term opioid therapy. Methylnaltrexone, alvimopan, and several other more recently approved drugs are mu receptor antagonists whose physicochemical properties prevent them from crossing the blood–brain barrier in appreciable amounts, thus rendering their mu receptor antagonism active in the gut but not in the CNS. These drugs have been shown to be effective in the treatment of postoperative ileus and the constipation associated with chronic opioid use,[17] but the conventional wisdom about the clinical use of these agents is still evolving.[18]

Similar effects are observed in the biliary system, which also has an abundance of mu receptors. Mu agonists can produce contraction of the gallbladder smooth muscle and spasm of the sphincter of Oddi, potentially causing a falsely positive cholangiogram during gallbladder and bile duct surgery. These effects are completely reversible with naloxone and can be partially reversed by glucagon treatment.

Although the urologic effects are minimal, opioids can sometimes cause urinary retention by decreasing bladder detrusor tone and by increasing the tone of the urinary sphincter. These effects are in part centrally mediated, although peripheral effects are also likely, given the widespread presence of opioid receptors in the genitourinary tract.[19,20] Although the urinary retention associated with opioid therapy is not typically pronounced, it can be troublesome in males, particularly when the opioid is administered intrathecally or epidurally.

Although not an acute effect relevant to intraoperative management, opioids depress cellular immunity. Morphine and the endogenous opioid beta-endorphin, for example, inhibit the transcription of interleukin-2 in activated T cells, among other immunologic effects.[21] Individual opioids (and perhaps classes of opioids) may differ in terms of the exact nature and extent of their immunomodulatory effects. Although opioid-induced impairment of cellular immunity is not well understood, impaired wound healing, perioperative infections, and cancer recurrence are possible adverse outcomes.

Opioid therapy produces adaptations in the CNS that result in tolerance and opioid-induced hyperalgesia (OIH). These phenomena are pharmacologically distinct, but both can result in poorly controlled pain and the need for an escalation in dosage. Opioid tolerance is a decrease in the analgesic response over time secondary to continued opioid administration. OIH, in contrast, is an increased pain response to a noxious stimulus while undergoing opioid treatment.[22,23] Whether acute tolerance and OIH play important roles in the management of perioperative patients is somewhat controversial, in part because the data from animal and human studies are inconsistent.[23,24] Current thinking suggests that both phenomena may coexist to some degree in certain perioperative settings. Key risk factors for the occurrence of both tolerance and OIH include prolonged therapy and higher opioid dosages. There is some evidence that N-methyl-D-aspartic acid (NMDA) receptor antagonism mediated through drugs like ketamine may mitigate the severity of OIH.[25]

Drug Interactions

Drug interactions can be based on two mechanisms: pharmacokinetic (i.e., where one drug influences the concentration of the other) or pharmacodynamic (i.e., where one drug influences the effect of the other). In anesthesia practice although unintended pharmacokinetic interactions sometimes occur, pharmacodynamic interactions occur with virtually every anesthetic and are produced by design.

The most common pharmacokinetic interaction in opioid clinical pharmacology is observed when intravenous opioids are combined with propofol. Perhaps because of the hemodynamic changes induced by propofol and their impact on pharmacokinetic processes, opioid concentrations may be higher when given in combination with a continuous propofol infusion.[26]

The most important pharmacodynamic drug interaction involving opioids is the synergistic interaction that occurs when opioids are combined with sedatives.[27] When combined with volatile anesthetics, opioids dramatically reduce the minimum alveolar concentration (MAC) of a volatile anesthetic (Fig. 9.6) Careful examination of "opioid-MAC reduction" data reveals several clinically critical concepts (see Fig. 9.6). First, opioids synergistically reduce MAC. Second, the MAC reduction is substantial (as much as 75% or more). Third, most of the MAC reduction occurs at moderate opioid levels (i.e., even modest opioid doses substantially reduce MAC). Fourth, the MAC reduction is not complete; that is, opioids are not complete anesthetics. The addition of the opioid cannot completely eliminate the need for the other anesthetic. And fifth, an infinite number of hypnotic-opioid combinations will achieve MAC (this implies that clinicians must choose the optimal combination based on the goals of the anesthetic and operation). All of these concepts also apply when opioids are used in combination with propofol for TIVA.[28]

Special Populations

Hepatic Failure

Even though the liver is the metabolic organ primarily responsible for the biotransformation of most opioids, liver failure is usually not severe enough to have a major impact on opioid pharmacokinetics. Of course, the anhepatic

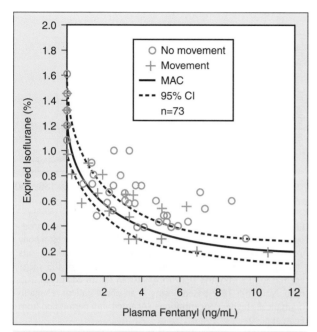

Fig. 9.6 Volatile anesthetic minimum alveolar concentration *(MAC)* reduction by opioids: the prototype example of isoflurane and fentanyl. The solid curve is MAC; the dotted curves are the 95% confidence intervals (see text for details). (Adapted with permission from McEwan et al.[27])

phase of orthotopic liver transplantation is a notable exception to this general rule (also see Chapter 36). With ongoing drug administration, concentrations of opioids that rely on hepatic metabolism increase when the patient has no liver. Even after partial liver resection, an increase in the ratio of morphine glucuronides to morphine occurs, indicating a decrease in the rate of morphine metabolism.[29] Because remifentanil's metabolism is completely unrelated to hepatic clearance mechanisms, its disposition is not affected during liver transplantation.[30]

Pharmacodynamic considerations can be important for opioid therapy in patients with severe liver disease. Patients with ongoing hepatic encephalopathy are especially vulnerable to the sedative effects of opioids. As a consequence, this drug class must be used with caution in this patient population.

Kidney Failure

Renal failure has implications of major clinical importance with respect to morphine and meperidine (see the section on individual drugs later). For the fentanyl congeners, the clinical importance of kidney failure is much less marked. Remifentanil's metabolism is not affected by kidney disease.[31]

Morphine is principally metabolized by conjugation in the liver; the resulting water-soluble glucuronides (i.e., morphine 3-glucuronide and morphine 6-glucuronide,

M3G and M6G) are excreted via the kidney. The kidney also plays a role in the conjugation of morphine and may account for as much as half of its conversion to M3G and M6G.

M3G is inactive, but M6G is an analgesic with a potency rivaling morphine. Very high levels of M6G and life-threatening respiratory depression can develop in patients with renal failure (Fig. 9.7).[32] Consequently, morphine may not be a good choice in patients with severely altered renal clearance mechanisms.

The clinical pharmacology of meperidine is also significantly altered by renal failure. Normeperidine, the main metabolite, has analgesic and excitatory CNS effects that range from anxiety and tremulousness to myoclonus and

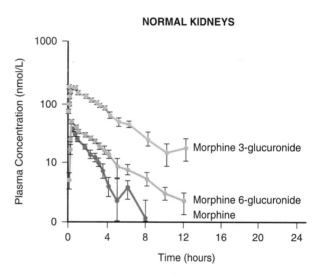

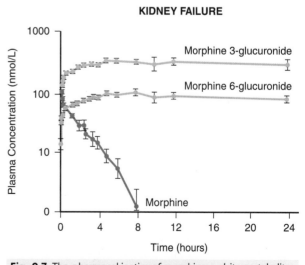

Fig. 9.7 The pharmacokinetics of morphine and its metabolites in normal volunteers versus kidney failure patients. Note the significant accumulation of the metabolites in renal failure. (Adapted with permission from Osborne et al.[32])

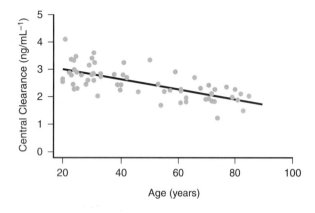

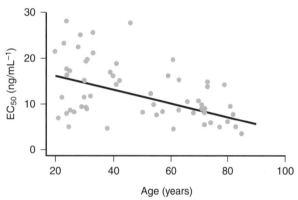

Fig. 9.8 The influence of age on the clinical pharmacology of remifentanil. Although there is considerable variability, in general, older subjects have a lower central clearance and a higher potency (i.e., lower EC$_{50}$).[34]

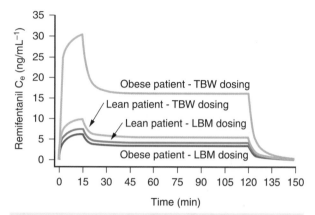

Fig. 9.9 A pharmacokinetic simulation illustrating the consequences of calculating the remifentanil dosage based on total body weight *(TBW)* or lean body mass *(LBM)* in obese and lean patients (1 mcg/kg bolus injection followed by an infusion of 0.5 mcg/kg/min for 15 min and 0.25 mcg/kg/min for an additional 105 min). Note that TBW-based dosing in an obese patient results in dramatically higher concentrations. (Adapted with permission from Egan et al.[37])

frank seizures. Because the active metabolites are subject to renal excretion, CNS toxicity secondary to accumulation of normeperidine is especially a concern in patients with renal failure. This shortcoming of meperidine has caused many hospital formularies to restrict its use or to remove it from the formulary altogether.

Gender
Gender may have an important influence on opioid pharmacology. Morphine is more potent in women than in men and has a slower onset of action in women.[33] Some of these differences may be related to cyclic gonadal hormones and psychosocial factors.

Age (also see Chapter 35)
Advancing age is clearly an important factor influencing the clinical pharmacology of opioids. For example, fentanyl congeners are more potent in the older patient (Fig. 9.8).[34,35] Decreases in clearance and central distribution volume also occur in older patients.

With advanced age, although pharmacokinetic changes also play a role, pharmacodynamic differences are primarily responsible for the decreased dose requirement in older patients (>65 years of age). Remifentanil doses should be decreased by at least 50% or more in elderly patients. Similar dosage reductions are prudent for the other opioids as well.

Obesity
Although detailed information is unavailable for many of the commonly used opioids, evidence from the study of drugs introduced more recently suggests that body weight is an important factor influencing the clinical pharmacology of opioids. Opioid pharmacokinetic parameters, especially clearance, appear to be more closely related to lean body mass (LBM) rather than to total body weight. In practical terms this means that morbidly obese patients do indeed require a higher dosage than lean patients in order to achieve the same target concentration, but the very obese patients do not need nearly as much as would be suggested by their total body weight.[36]

For example, as illustrated through pharmacokinetic simulation (Fig. 9.9), a total body weight (TBW)–based dosing scheme results in much higher remifentanil effect-site concentrations than a dosing calculation based on LBM.[37] In contrast, TBW and LBM dosing schemes result in similar concentrations for lean patients. More recent information from two larger studies has confirmed these concepts,[38,39] which likely apply to other opioids as well.

Unique Features of Individual Opioids

Codeine
Codeine, although not commonly used intraoperatively, has special importance among opioids because of the well-characterized pharmacogenomic nuance associated with it.

Codeine is actually a prodrug; morphine is the active compound. Codeine is metabolized (in part) by O-demethylation into morphine, a metabolic process mediated by the liver microsomal isoform CYP2D6.[40] Patients who lack CYP2D6 because of deletions, frameshift, or splice mutations (i.e., approximately 10% of the Caucasian population) or whose CYP2D6 is inhibited (e.g., patients taking quinidine) would not be expected to benefit from codeine even though they exhibit a normal response to morphine.[41,42] Conversely, patients with *CYP2D6* gene duplications are expected to exhibit excessive effect with codeine administration (this genotype can be especially troublesome for a mother with a nursing infant; the child may exhibit morphine toxicity).

Morphine

Morphine is the prototype opioid against which all newcomers are compared. There is no evidence that any synthetic opioid is more effective in controlling pain than nature's morphine, derived from the opium poppy plant. Were it not for the histamine release and the resulting hypotension associated with morphine, fentanyl may not have replaced morphine as the most commonly used opioid intraoperatively

Morphine has a slow onset time. Morphine's pKa renders it almost completely ionized at physiologic pH. This property and its low lipid solubility account for morphine's prolonged latency to peak effect; morphine penetrates the CNS slowly. This feature has both advantages and disadvantages associated with it. The prolonged latency to peak effect means that morphine is perhaps less likely to cause acute respiratory depression after bolus injection of typical analgesic doses compared with the more rapid-acting opioids. On the other hand, the slow onset time means that clinicians are perhaps more likely to inappropriately "stack" multiple morphine doses in a patient experiencing severe pain, thus creating the potential for a toxic "overshoot."[43]

Morphine's active metabolite, M6G, has important clinical implications. Although conversion to M6G accounts for only 10% of morphine's metabolism, M6G may contribute to morphine's analgesic effects even in patients with normal renal function, particularly with longer-term use. Because of morphine's high hepatic extraction ratio, the bioavailability of orally administered morphine is significantly lower than after parenteral injection. The hepatic first-pass effect on orally administered morphine results in high M6G levels. In fact, M6G may be the primary active compound when morphine is administered orally.[44] As noted in the section on kidney failure, M6G's accumulation to potentially toxic levels in dialysis patients is another important implication of this active metabolite.

Fentanyl

Fentanyl may be the most important opioid used in modern anesthesia practice. As the original fentanyl congener, its clinical application is well entrenched and highly diverse. Fentanyl can be delivered in numerous ways. In addition to the intravenous route, fentanyl can be delivered by transdermal, transmucosal, transnasal, and transpulmonary routes.

Oral transmucosal delivery of fentanyl citrate (OTFC) results in the faster achievement of higher peak levels than when the same dose is swallowed.[45] Avoidance of the first-pass effect results in substantially greater bioavailability. Because OTFC is noninvasive and rapid in onset, it is a successful therapy for breakthrough pain in opioid-tolerant cancer patients, often in combination with a transdermal fentanyl patch.

Alfentanil

Alfentanil was the first opioid to be administered almost exclusively by continuous infusion. Because of its relatively short terminal half-life, alfentanil was originally predicted to have a rapid offset of effect after termination of a continuous infusion.[46] Subsequent advances in pharmacokinetic theory (i.e., the CSHT) proved this assertion to be false.[8] However, alfentanil is in fact a short-acting drug after a single bolus injection because of its high "diffusible fraction"; it reaches peak effect-site concentrations quickly and then begins to decline (see the relevant "Pharmacokinetics" section earlier). Alfentanil illustrates how a drug can exhibit different pharmacokinetic profiles depending on the method of administration (i.e., bolus versus continuous infusion). More so than fentanyl and sufentanil, alfentanil's metabolism by the liver may be more unpredictable because of the significant interindividual variability of hepatic CYP3A4, the primary enzyme responsible for alfentanil biotransformation.

Sufentanil

Sufentanil's distinguishing feature is that it is the most potent opioid commonly used in anesthesia practice. Because it is more intrinsically efficacious at the opioid receptor, the absolute doses used are much smaller compared with the other less potent drugs (e.g., a 1000-fold less than morphine doses).

Remifentanil

Remifentanil is a prototype example of how specific clinical goals can be achieved by designing molecules with specialized structure–activity (or structure–metabolism) relationships. By losing its mu receptor agonist activity upon ester hydrolysis, a very short-acting opioid results (Fig. 9.10).[47] The perceived unmet need driving remifentanil's development was having an opioid with a rapid onset and offset so that the drug could be titrated up and down as necessary to meet the dynamic needs of the patient during the rapidly changing conditions of anesthesia and surgery.

Compared with the currently marketed fentanyl congeners, remifentanil's CSHT is short, on the order of about 5 minutes.[48] Pharmacodynamically, remifentanil

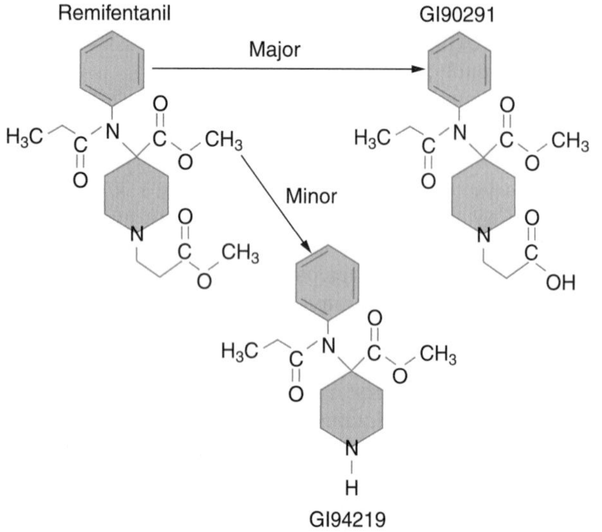

Fig. 9.10 Remifentanil's metabolic pathway. De esterification (i.e., ester hydrolysis) by nonspecific plasma and tissue esterases to an inactive acid metabolite (GI-90291) accounts for the vast majority of remifentanil's metabolism. (Adapted with permission from Egan et al.[48])

exhibits a short latency to peak effect similar to alfentanil and a potency slightly less than fentanyl.[49]

Remifentanil's role in modern anesthesia practice is now well established. Remifentanil is perhaps best suited for cases where its responsive pharmacokinetic profile can be exploited to advantage. These cases include the following: (1) when rapid recovery is desirable, (2) when the anesthetic requirement rapidly fluctuates, (3) when opioid titration is unpredictable or difficult, (4) when there is a substantial danger to opioid overdose, or (5) when a "high dose" opioid technique is advantageous but the patient is not going to be mechanically ventilated postoperatively.[50] Remifentanil's most common clinical application is the provision of TIVA in combination with propofol. Perhaps remifentanil's principal advantage in the context of TIVA is that it quickly reaches a steady state after dosage adjustment. Remifentanil is also commonly given by bolus when only a very brief pulse of opioid effect followed by rapid recovery is desired (e.g., in preparation for local anesthetic injection during Monitored Anesthesia Care).[51]

Opioid Agonist-Antagonists and Pure Antagonists

Opioid agonist-antagonists act as partial agonists at the mu receptor, while having competitive antagonist properties at the same receptors. These drugs serve as analgesics with more limited ventilatory depression and a lower potential for dependence, as they demonstrate a "ceiling effect," producing less analgesia compared with pure agonists. The lower abuse potential was the primary perceived unmet need underlying the development of these drugs. Drugs in this category are used for the treatment of chronic pain and for the treatment of opioid addiction. These drugs cause some degree of competitive antagonism when administered in the presence of ongoing full agonist activity (e.g., when administered after morphine and other pure agonists).

Pure opioid antagonists, of which naloxone is the prototype, are complete competitive antagonists of the opioid receptor that are devoid of any agonist activity. These pure antagonists are used in the management of acute opioid overdose and chronic abuse.

Tramadol
Tramadol is a centrally acting analgesic with moderate mu receptor affinity and weak kappa and delta receptor affinity. Notably, tramadol also has antagonist activity at the 5HT and nicotinic acetylcholine (NA) receptors. Although providing analgesia both through opioid and serotonin receptor pathways, tramadol carries less risk of respiratory depression. However, when combined with serotonin reuptake inhibitors or other serotonergic medications, it does carry the risk of serotonin syndrome and of CNS excitability and seizures.[52]

Buprenorphine
Buprenorphine is an opioid agonist-antagonist with increasing clinical implications in the perioperative patient. (Also see Chapter 40.) It is 25 times more potent than morphine with a 50 times greater affinity for the mu receptor. It can be administered sublingually, transdermally, or parenterally, but undergoes extensive first-pass hepatic metabolism with oral administration. Although moderate doses can be used to treat chronic pain, higher doses used in the treatment of chronic pain can antagonize the effects of other opioids, making the treatment of acute-on-chronic pain difficult. Because it binds opioid receptors so tightly and its elimination half-life is in the range of 20 to 72 hours, high-dose opioid full agonists are required to overcome its effects.[53] Buprenorphine, including long acting injectable formulations, is playing an increasing role in the treatment of opioid use disorder.[92]

Nalbuphine
Also an opioid agonist-antagonist, nalbuphine has a potency and duration of action similar to morphine. It can be used as a sole agent for sedation with more limited ventilatory depression and as an agent to reverse ventilatory depression in opioid overdose while maintaining some analgesia, such as at the end of an anesthetic when a patient is exhibiting excessive opioid effect (usually in very small doses).[54]

Naloxone/Naltrexone
Naloxone is an injectable mu antagonist that reverses both the therapeutic and adverse effects of mu agonists.[55] Naloxone's most common indication is the emergency reversal of opioid-induced ventilatory depression after acute overdose. Its important role in this regard has merited

naloxone's inclusion on the World Health Organization's "List of Essential Medicines." Naloxone is sometimes used in much smaller doses during emergence from anesthesia to restore adequate ventilatory effort and thereby expedite extubation of the trachea. The treatment of opioid-induced pruritus is another common therapeutic application.

Although the drug is very effective in reversing the ventilatory depression associated with opioids, it can cause numerous untoward effects, including acute withdrawal syndrome, nausea, vomiting, tachycardia, hypertension, seizures, and pulmonary edema, among others.[56] Recognizing that naloxone's duration of action is shorter than most of the mu agonists is a key point in determining the dosing schedule; repeated doses may be necessary to sustain its effects.

In response to the opioid abuse epidemic in the United States, new delivery systems have been developed that are intended for emergency use by lay persons in the event of opioid overdose; these include nasal spray and autoinjector preparations.[57,58]

Naltrexone, a longer-acting mu opioid antagonist available in oral, injectable, and implantable forms, is used in the long-term management of opioid addiction in combination with other nonpharmacologic therapies.[59]

CLINICAL APPLICATION

Opioids play a vital role in virtually every area of anesthesia practice. In the treatment of postoperative pain (also see Chapter 40) opioids are of prime importance, whereas in most other settings in perioperative medicine, opioids are therapeutic adjuncts used in combination with other drugs.

Common Clinical Indications

Postoperative analgesia is the longest-standing indication for opioid therapy in anesthesia practice. In the modern era, opioid administration via PCA devices is perhaps the most common mode of delivery (also see Chapter 40). In recent years opioids are increasingly combined postoperatively with various other analgesics, such as nonsteroidal anti-inflammatory drugs (NSAIDs), to increase efficacy and safety.

Internationally, the most common clinical indication for opioids in anesthesia practice is their use for what has come to be known as "balanced anesthesia." This perhaps misguided term connotes the use of multiple drugs (e.g., volatile anesthetics, neuromuscular blockers, sedative-hypnotics, and opioids) in smaller doses to produce the state of anesthesia. With this technique, the opioids are primarily used for their ability to decrease MAC. A basic assumption underlying this balanced anesthesia approach is that the drugs used in combination mitigate the disadvantages of the individual drugs (i.e., the volatile anesthetics) used in larger doses as single-drug therapy.

"High-dose opioid anesthesia," a technique originally described for morphine in the early days of open heart surgery[60] and later associated with the fentanyl congeners,[61] is another common application of opioids in clinical anesthesia. The original scientific underpinning of this approach was that high doses of opioids enabled the clinician to reduce the concentration of volatile anesthetic to a minimum, thereby avoiding the direct myocardial depression and other untoward hemodynamic effects in patients whose cardiovascular systems were already compromised. In addition, fentanyl often produces a relative bradycardia that could be helpful in patients vulnerable to myocardial ischemia. Currently, although the general concept is still applied, the opioid doses used are smaller. Opioids are also sometimes administered for their possible beneficial effects in terms of cardioprotection (i.e., preconditioning).

TIVA is a more recently developed and increasingly popular indication for opioids in anesthesia practice. As the name implies, this technique relies entirely upon intravenous agents for the provision of general anesthesia. Most commonly, continuous infusions of remifentanil or alfentanil are combined with a propofol infusion. Both the opioid and the sedative can be delivered by target controlled infusion (TCI)–enabled pumps. A clear advantage of this technique, perhaps among others, is the enhanced patient well-being in the early postoperative period, including less nausea and vomiting and often a feeling of euphoria.[62]

Rational Drug Selection and Administration

In articulating a scientific foundation for rational opioid selection, pharmacokinetic considerations are extremely important. Indeed, the mu agonists (opioids) can be considered pharmacodynamic equals (in most respects) with important pharmacokinetic differences.[63] Thus rational selection of one mu opioid agonist over another requires the clinician to identify the desired temporal profile of drug effect and then choose an opioid that best enables the clinician to achieve it (within obvious constraints such as pharmacoeconomic concerns).

In selecting the appropriate opioid, among the key questions to address are: How quickly must the desired opioid effect be achieved? How long must the opioid effect be maintained? How critical is it that opioid-induced ventilatory depression or sedation dissipate quickly (e.g., will the patient be mechanically ventilated postoperatively)? Is the capability to raise and lower the level of opioid effect quickly during the anesthetic critical? Will there be significant pain postoperatively that will require opioid treatment? All of these questions relate to the optimal temporal profile of opioid effect. The answers to these questions are addressed through the application of pharmacokinetic concepts.

For example, when a brief pulse of opioid effect followed by rapid recovery is desired (e.g., to provide analgesia for a retrobulbar block), a bolus of remifentanil or alfentanil might be preferred. When long-lasting opioid effect is desired, such as when there will be significant postoperative pain or when the trachea will remain intubated, a fentanyl infusion is a prudent choice. If the patient should be awake and alert shortly after the procedure is finished (e.g., a craniotomy in which the surgeons hope to perform a neurologic examination in the operating room immediately postoperatively), a remifentanil infusion might be advantageous.

The formulation of a rational administration strategy also requires the proper application of pharmacokinetic principles. An important goal of any dosing scheme is to reach and maintain a steady-state level of opioid effect. To achieve a steady-state concentration in the site of action, opioids are frequently administered by continuous infusion. This is increasingly accomplished through the use of TCI technology, which requires that the clinician be familiar with the appropriate pharmacokinetic model for the opioid of interest. When these systems are not available, the clinician must remember that infusions must be preceded by a bolus in order to reach steady state in a timely fashion.

EMERGING DEVELOPMENTS

Opioid Abuse Epidemic

Deaths related to the abuse and diversion of prescription opioids have skyrocketed in the United States and elsewhere.[64] In addition to fatalities, this pervasive pattern of prescription and illicit opioid abuse has resulted in a huge surge in admissions to facilities specializing in the treatment of opioid use disorder (OUD), although this is controversial[65] The trend is partly the result of opioid prescribing practices for chronic pain conditions that may predispose some patients to addiction.[66,67] Perioperative opioid prescribing practices also likely influence the incidence of OUD, although this is controversial.[68] Tragically, viewing pain as the "fifth vital sign," as promulgated by The Joint Commission on accreditation of health care organizations beginning in the late 1990s, is thought to have contributed to the development of the opioid abuse epidemic.[69]

The epidemic has reached such a crisis level that federal and state government authorities in the United States have enacted legislation and set aside funding to support research, prevention, and treatment of the problem.[70,71] State-approved pharmacy-based naloxone dispensing (without a physician's prescription) for patients filling opioid prescriptions is a notable example of the efforts supported by such legislation.[72] In addition, professional societies and the Centers for Disease Control and Prevention (CDC) have produced new guidelines for opioid prescribing.[73] Properly viewed as a "disease of despair,"[74] OUD is currently an area of intense public discussion and medical investigation.[75]

In the perioperative arena efforts to prevent the development of persistent opioid use after surgery and OUD have focused on improved opioid stewardship (e.g., multimodal analgesia regimens to reduce opioid exposure and limited prescribing of opioids for use after hospital discharge, among others).[76] A particular question of contemporary interest is whether intraoperative opioid usage patterns influence the incidence of persistent opioid use after surgery.[77] This question has given rise to increased interest in "multimodal general anesthesia."

Multimodal General Anesthesia (and Opioid-Free Anesthesia)

In recent years the concept of "multimodal general anesthesia" has extended the concept of balanced anesthesia to include more drugs that target different neuroanatomic circuits and multiple neurophysiologic mechanisms.[78] The opioid epidemic has provided much of the motivation to move away from opioids toward other adjunct drugs. Multimodal general anesthesia does not call for the total abandonment of intraoperative opioids, but rather a more eclectic pharmacologic assortment that decreases the total opioid exposure.

The suggested pharmacopeia includes a host of anesthetic adjuncts, including opioids (e.g., remifentanil), alpha-2 agonists (e.g., dexmedetomidine), local anesthetics (e.g., lidocaine), cations (e.g., magnesium), and NMDA antagonists (e.g., ketamine, N_2O). The pharmacologic foundation of the concept is grounded in the firmly established observation that when anesthetic drugs of different mechanisms are administered together, they typically interact with synergism. This approach will almost certainly reduce dose-related opioid adverse effects perioperatively and may have some impact on postoperative opioid abuse, although this is still speculative.[79]

Opioid-free anesthesia (OFA) can be viewed as a subset of this multimodal general anesthesia concept; the overriding goal is to further decrease (or eliminate) perioperative opioid exposure. Although the OFA anesthesia technique has gained some momentum in contemporary anesthesia practice, whether the technique is broadly and practically feasible and whether the desired goals can be fully achieved remain controversial.[80,81]

Biased mu-Receptor Agonists

The most serious adverse effects of conventional opioids, both clinically and in a social context, are their ventilatory depressive and addictive properties, both of which are manifest prominently by the opioid epidemic. An ideal opioid would have the analgesic potential of the traditional opioids while avoiding their respiratory depressive effects and addictive potential. Recent advances in the understanding of the mu opioid receptor mechanisms have made some improvement in opioids a possibility, at least in terms of ventilatory depressant effects.

Two distinct transduction pathways have been described in connection with mu opioid receptor

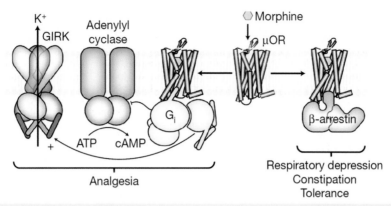

Fig. 9.11 The role of the beta-arrestin pathway in mu agonist adverse effects. Opiate-induced MOR signaling through Gi activates G protein–gated inwardly rectifying potassium channels (GIRKs) and inhibits adenylyl cyclase, leading to analgesia. Conversely, recruitment of beta-arrestin is implicated in tolerance, respiratory depression, and constipation. (Adapted with permission from Manglik et al.[91])

activation, as shown in Fig. 9.11. The G protein–coupled signaling pathway is responsible for the analgesic, reward, and pleasure effects. The beta-arrestin pathway mediates the respiratory depression and gastrointestinal effects.[82,83] Findings in experiments using beta-arrestin knockout mice provide support for these observations.[84]

Improved understanding of these signaling pathways has led to the development of a novel class of opioids: the biased agonists. The biased agonists are full agonists of the G protein–mediated pathway, but produce less recruitment of the beta-arrestin pathway. Biased agonists, therefore, have the full analgesic effects of conventional opioids with less risk of constipation and respiratory depression. The nomenclature connotes a bias toward the G protein–signaling pathway.

The biased agonist oliceridine was recently approved by the U.S. Food and Drug Administration. Oliceridine has been shown to be equianalgesic to morphine with similar potency, but with significantly less respiratory depression.[85] Other candidate molecules are being developed for their potential as biased agonists.[86]

Although biased agonists show promise in the treatment of pain and the curbing of opioid epidemic deaths, they do not eliminate all of the adverse effects of the previously marketed opioids. Notably, they exert the same sedative effects as classic opioids. And because the G protein pathway mediates the reward signals that lead to opioid addiction, there is a possibility that the biased agonists may decrease deaths associated with opioid abuse but increase the overall prevalence, although this is entirely speculative. Nonopiate strategies for analgesia continue to be a prominent part of the strategy to stem the tide against the opioid epidemic.

ACKNOWLEDGMENT

Dr. Ezekiel D. Egan contributed to the Emerging Developments section in a substantive way through literature review, discussion of key points, the creation of text, and editing of the final manuscript. His contributions to the chapter are gratefully acknowledged.

REFERENCES

1. Minami M, Satoh M. Molecular biology of the opioid receptors: structures, functions and distributions. *Neurosci Res.* 1995;23:121–145.
2. Pan L, Xu J, Yu R, Xu MM, Pan YX, Pasternak GW. Identification and characterization of six new alternatively spliced variants of the human mu opioid receptor gene. *Oprm Neuroscience.* 2005;133:209–220.
3. Matthies BK, Franklin KB. Formalin pain is expressed in decerebrate rats but not attenuated by morphine. *Pain.* 1992;51:199–206.
4. Becerra L, Harter K, Gonzalez RG, Borsook D. Functional magnetic resonance imaging measures of the effects of morphine on central nervous system circuitry in opioid-naive healthy volunteers. *Anesth Analg.* 2006;103:208–216 Table of contents.
5. Matthes HW, Maldonado R, Simonin F, Valverde O, Slowe S, Kitchen I, Befort K, Dierich A, Le Meur M, Dolle P, Tzavara E, Hanoune J, Roques BP, Kieffer BL. Loss of morphine-induced analgesia, reward effect and withdrawal symptoms in mice lacking the mu-opioid-receptor gene. *Nature.* 1996;383:819–823.
6. Sora I, Takahashi N, Funada M, Ujike H, Revay RS, Donovan DM, Miner LL, Uhl GR, Matthies BK, Franklin KB, Minami M, Satoh M. Opiate receptor knockout mice define mu receptor roles in endogenous nociceptive responses and morphine-induced analgesia. *Proc Natl Acad Sci U S A.* 1997;94:1544–1549.
7. Dahan A, Sarton E, Teppema L, Olievier C, Nieuwenhuijs D, Matthes HW, Kieffer BL. Anesthetic potency and influence of morphine and sevoflurane on respiration in mu-opioid receptor knockout mice. *Anesthesiology.* 2001;94:824–832.
8. Shafer SL, Varvel JR. Pharmacokinetics, pharmacodynamics, and rational opioid selection. *Anesthesiology.* 1991;74:53–63.
9. Hughes MA, Glass PS, Jacobs JR. Context-sensitive half-time in multicompartment pharmacokinetic models for intravenous anesthetic drugs [see

comments]. *Anesthesiology*. 1992;76:334–341.

10. Romberg R, Sarton E, Teppema L, Matthes HW, Kieffer BL, Dahan A. Comparison of morphine-6-glucuronide and morphine on respiratory depressant and antinociceptive responses in wild type and mu-opioid receptor deficient mice. *Br J Anaesth*. 2003;91:862–870.

11. Gross JB. When you breathe IN you inspire, when you DON'T breathe, you ... expire: new insights regarding opioid-induced ventilatory depression. *Anesthesiology*. 2003;99:767–770.

12. Jr. Forrest WH, Bellville JW. The effect of sleep plus morphine on the respiratory response to carbon dioxide. *Anesthesiology*. 1964;25:137–141.

13. Laubie M, Schmitt H, Vincent M. Vagal bradycardia produced by microinjections of morphine-like drugs into the nucleus ambiguus in anaesthetized dogs. *Eur J Pharmacol*. 1979;59:287–291.

14. Reitan JA, Stengert KB, Wymore ML, Martucci RW. Central vagal control of fentanyl-induced bradycardia during halothane anesthesia. *Anesth Analg*. 1978;57:31–36.

15. Bennett JA, Abrams JT, Van Riper DF, Horrow JC. Difficult or impossible ventilation after sufentanil-induced anesthesia is caused primarily by vocal cord closure. *Anesthesiology*. 1997;87:1070–1074.

16. Streisand JB, Bailey PL, LeMaire L, Ashburn MA, Tarver SD, Varvel J, Stanley TH. Fentanyl-induced rigidity and unconsciousness in human volunteers. Incidence, duration, and plasma concentrations. *Anesthesiology*. 1993;78:629–634.

17. Nee J, Zakari M, Sugarman MA, Whelan J, Hirsch W, Sultan S, Ballou S, Iturrino J, Lembo A. Efficacy of treatments for opioid-induced constipation: systematic review and meta-analysis. *Clin Gastroenterol Hepatol*. 2018;16:1569–1584 e2.

18. Chamie K, Golla V, Lenis AT, Lec PM, Rahman S, Viscusi ER. Peripherally acting µ-opioid receptor antagonists in the management of postoperative ileus: a clinical review. *J Gastrointest Surg*. 2020.

19. Dray A, Metsch R. Inhibition of urinary bladder contractions by a spinal action of morphine and other opioids. *J Pharmacol Exp Ther*. 1984;231:254–260.

20. Dray A, Metsch R. Spinal opioid receptors and inhibition of urinary bladder motility in vivo. *Neurosci Lett*. 1984;47:81–84.

21. Borner C, Warnick B, Smida M, Hartig R, Lindquist JA, Schraven B, Hollt V, Kraus J. Mechanisms of opioid-mediated inhibition of human T cell receptor signaling. *J Immunol*. 2009;183:882–889.

22. Konopka KH, van Wijhe M. Opioid-induced hyperalgesia: pain hurts?. *Br J Anaesth*. 2010;105:555–557.

23. Angst MS. Intraoperative use of remifentanil for TIVA: postoperative pain, acute tolerance, and opioid-induced hyperalgesia. *J Cardiothorac Vasc Anesth*. 2015;29(Suppl 1):S16–S22.

24. Colvin LA, Bull F, Hales TG. Perioperative opioid analgesia-when is enough too much? A review of opioid-induced tolerance and hyperalgesia. *Lancet*. 2019;393:1558–1568.

25. Joly V, Richebe P, Guignard B, Fletcher D, Maurette P, Sessler DI, Chauvin M. Remifentanil-induced postoperative hyperalgesia and its prevention with small-dose ketamine. *Anesthesiology*. 2005;103:147–155.

26. Bouillon T, Bruhn J, Radu-Radulescu L, Bertaccini E, Park S, Shafer S. Non-steady state analysis of the pharmacokinetic interaction between propofol and remifentanil. *Anesthesiology*. 2002;97:1350–1362.

27. McEwan AI, Smith C, Dyar O, Goodman D, Smith LR, Glass PS. Isoflurane minimum alveolar concentration reduction by fentanyl. *Anesthesiology*. 1993;78:864–869.

28. Vuyk J, Lim T, Engbers FH, Burm AG, Vletter AA, Bovill JG. The pharmacodynamic interaction of propofol and alfentanil during lower abdominal surgery in women. *Anesthesiology*. 1995;83:8–22.

29. Rudin A, Lundberg JF, Hammarlund-Udenaes M, Flisberg P, Werner MU. Morphine metabolism after major liver surgery. *Anesth Analg*. 2007;104:1409–1414 table of contents.

30. Dershwitz M, Hoke JF, Rosow CE, Michalowski P, Connors PM, Muir KT, Dienstag JL. Pharmacokinetics and pharmacodynamics of remifentanil in volunteer subjects with severe liver disease. *Anesthesiology*. 1996;84:812–820.

31. Hoke JF, Shlugman D, Dershwitz M, Michalowski P, Malthouse-Dufore S, Connors PM, Martel D, Rosow CE, Muir KT, Rubin N, Glass PS. Pharmacokinetics and pharmacodynamics of remifentanil in persons with renal failure compared with healthy volunteers. *Anesthesiology*. 1997;87:533–541.

32. Osborne R, Joel S, Grebenik K, Trew D, Slevin M. The pharmacokinetics of morphine and morphine glucuronides in kidney failure. *Clin Pharmacol Ther*. 1993;54:158–167.

33. Sarton E, Olofsen E, Romberg R, den Hartigh J, Kest B, Nieuwenhuijs D, Burm A, Teppema L, Dahan A. Sex differences in morphine analgesia: an experimental study in healthy volunteers. *Anesthesiology*. 2000;93:1245–1254 discussion 6A.

34. Minto CF, Schnider TW, Egan TD, Youngs E, Lemmens HJ, Gambus PL, Billard V, Hoke JF, Moore KH, Hermann DJ, Muir KT, Mandema JW, Shafer SL. Influence of age and gender on the pharmacokinetics and pharmacodynamics of remifentanil. I. Model development. *Anesthesiology*. 1997;86:10–23.

35. Scott JC, Stanski DR. Decreased fentanyl and alfentanil dose requirements with age. A simultaneous pharmacokinetic and pharmacodynamic evaluation. *J Pharmacol Exp Ther*. 1987;240:159–166.

36. Bouillon T, Shafer SL. Does size matter?. *Anesthesiology*. 1998;89:557–560.

37. Egan TD, Huizinga B, Gupta SK, Jaarsma RL, Sperry RJ, Yee JB, Muir KT. Remifentanil pharmacokinetics in obese versus lean patients. *Anesthesiology*. 1998;89:562–573.

38. Eleveld DJ, Proost JH, Vereecke H, Absalom AR, Olofsen E, Vuyk J, Struys M. An allometric model of remifentanil pharmacokinetics and pharmacodynamics. *Anesthesiology*. 2017;126:1005–1018.

39. Kim TK, Obara S, Egan TD, Minto CF, La Colla L, Drover DR, Vuyk J, Mertens M. Disposition of remifentanil in obesity: a new pharmacokinetic model incorporating the influence of body mass. *Anesthesiology*. 2017;126:1019–1032.

40. Poulsen L, Brosen K, Arendt-Nielsen L, Gram LF, Elbaek K, Sindrup SH. Codeine and morphine in extensive and poor metabolizers of sparteine: pharmacokinetics, analgesic effect and side effects. *Eur J Clin Pharmacol*. 1996;51:289–295.

41. Caraco Y, Sheller J, Wood AJ. Pharmacogenetic determination of the effects of codeine and prediction of drug interactions. *J Pharmacol Exp Ther*. 1996;278:1165–1174.

42. Eckhardt K, Li S, Ammon S, Schanzle G, Mikus G, Eichelbaum M. Same incidence of adverse drug events after codeine administration irrespective of the genetically determined differences in morphine formation. *Pain*. 1998;76:27–33.

43. Lotsch J, Dudziak R, Freynhagen R, Marschner J, Geisslinger G. Fatal respiratory depression after multiple intravenous morphine injections. *Clin Pharmacokinet*. 2006;45:1051–1060.

44. Osborne R, Joel S, Trew D, Slevin M. Morphine and metabolite behavior after different routes of morphine administration: demonstration of the importance of the active metabolite morphine-6-glucuronide. *Clin Pharmacol Ther*. 1990;47:12–19.

45. Streisand JB, Varvel JR, Stanski DR, Le Maire L, Ashburn MA, Hague BI, Tarver SD, Stanley TH. Absorption and bioavailability of oral transmucosal fentanyl citrate. *Anesthesiology*. 1991;75:223–229.

46. Stanski DR, Jr. Hug CC. Alfentanil-a kinetically predictable narcotic analgesic. *Anesthesiology*. 1982;57:435–438.

47. Egan TD. Remifentanil pharmacokinetics and pharmacodynamics. A

preliminary appraisal. *Clin Pharmacokinet.* 1995;29:80–94.

48. Egan TD, Lemmens HJ, Fiset P, Hermann DJ, Muir KT, Stanski DR, Shafer SL. The pharmacokinetics of the new short-acting opioid remifentanil (GI87084B) in healthy adult male volunteers. *Anesthesiology.* 1993;79:881–892.

49. Egan TD, Minto CF, Hermann DJ, Barr J, Muir KT, Shafer SL. Remifentanil versus alfentanil: comparative pharmacokinetics and pharmacodynamics in healthy adult male volunteers [published erratum appears in Anesthesiology. 1996 Sep;85(3):695]. *Anesthesiology.* 1996;84:821–833.

50. Egan TD. The clinical pharmacology of remifentanil: a brief review. *J Anesth.* 1998;12:195–204.

51. Egan TD, Kern SE, Muir KT, White J. Remifentanil by bolus injection: a safety, pharmacokinetic, pharmacodynamic, and age effect investigation in human volunteers. *Br J Anaesth.* 2004;92:335–343.

52. Grond S, Sablotzki A. Clinical pharmacology of tramadol. *Clin Pharmacokinet.* 2004;43:879–923.

53. Chen KY, Chen L, Mao J. Buprenorphine-naloxone therapy in pain management. *Anesthesiology.* 2014;120:1262–1274.

54. Errick JK, Heel RC. Nalbuphine. A preliminary review of its pharmacological properties and therapeutic efficacy. *Drugs.* 1983;26:191–211.

55. Jasinski DR, Martin WR, Haertzen CA. The human pharmacology and abuse potential of N-allylnoroxymorphone (naloxone). *J Pharmacol Exp Ther.* 1967;157:420–426.

56. Jasinski DR, Martin WR, Sapira JD. Antagonism of the subjective, behavioral, pupillary, and respiratory depressant effects of cyclazocine by naloxone. *Clin Pharmacol Ther.* 1968;9:215–222.

57. Edwards ET, Edwards ES, Davis E, Mulcare M, Wiklund M, Kelley G. Comparative usability study of a novel auto-injector and an intranasal system for naloxone delivery. *Pain Ther.* 2015;4:89–105.

58. Krieter P, Chiang N, Gyaw S, Skolnick P, Crystal R, Keegan F, Aker J, Beck M, Harris J. Pharmacokinetic properties and human use characteristics of an FDA approved intranasal naloxone product for the treatment of opioid overdose. *J Clin Pharmacol.* 2016;56:1243–1253.

59. Kunoe N, Lobmaier P, Ngo H, Hulse G. Injectable and implantable sustained release naltrexone in the treatment of opioid addiction. *Br J Clin Pharmacol.* 2014;77:264–271.

60. Lowenstein E, Hallowell P, Levine FH, Daggett WM, Austen WG, Laver MB. Cardiovascular response to large doses of intravenous morphine in man. *N Engl J Med.* 1969;281:1389–1393.

61. Lunn JK, Stanley TH, Eisele J, Webster L, Woodward A. High dose fentanyl anesthesia for coronary artery surgery: plasma fentanyl concentrations and influence of nitrous oxide on cardiovascular responses. *Anesth Analg.* 1979;58:390–395.

62. Hofer CK, Zollinger A, Buchi S, Klaghofer R, Serafino D, Buhlmann S, Buddeberg C, Pasch T, Spahn DR. Patient well-being after general anaesthesia: a prospective, randomized, controlled multi-centre trial comparing intravenous and inhalation anaesthesia. *Br J Anaesth.* 2003;91:631–637.

63. Mather LE. Pharmacokinetic and pharmacodynamic profiles of opioid analgesics: a sameness amongst equals?. *Pain.* 1990;43:3–6.

64. Rudd RA, Aleshire N, Zibbell JE, Gladden RM. Increases in drug and opioid overdose deaths–United States, 2000–2014. *MMWR Morb Mortal Wkly Rep.* 2016;64:1378–1382.

65. Brady KT, McCauley JL, Back SE. Prescription opioid misuse, abuse, and treatment in the United States: an update. *Am J Psychiatry.* 2016;173:18–26.

66. Johnson SR. The opioid abuse epidemic: How healthcare helped create a crisis. *Mod Healthc.* 2016;46:8–9.

67. Weisberg DF, Becker WC, Fiellin DA, Stannard C. Prescription opioid misuse in the United States and the United Kingdom: cautionary lessons. *Int J Drug Policy.* 2014;25:1124–1130.

68. Yaster M, Benzon HT, Anderson TA. "Houston, We Have a Problem!": The role of the anesthesiologist in the current opioid epidemic. *Anesth Analg.* 2017;125:1429–1431.

69. Chidgey BA, McGinigle KL, McNaull PP. When a vital sign leads a country astray-The opioid epidemic. *JAMA Surg.* 2019;154:987–988.

70. Kharasch ED, Brunt LM. Perioperative opioids and public health. *Anesthesiology.* 2016;124:960–965.

71. Office of the Press Secretary the White House President Obama proposes $1.1 billion in new funding to address the prescription opioid abuse and heroin use epidemic. *J Pain Palliat Care Pharmacother.* 2016;30:134–137.

72. Bachyrycz A, Shrestha S, Bleske BE, Tinker D, Bakhireva LN. Opioid overdose prevention through pharmacy-based naloxone prescription program: innovations in healthcare delivery. *Subst Abus.* 2017;38:55–60.

73. Frieden TR, Houry D. Reducing the risks of relief–The CDC opioid-prescribing guideline. *N Engl J Med.* 2016;374:1501–1504.

74. Feinberg J. Tackle the epidemic, not the opioids. *Nature.* 2019;573:165.

75. Strang J, Volkow ND, Degenhardt L, Hickman M, Johnson K, Koob GF, Marshall BDL, Tyndall M, Walsh SL. Opioid use disorder. *Nat Rev Dis Primers.* 2020;6:3.

76. Ashburn MA, Fleisher LA. Perioperative opioid management-An opportunity to put the genie back into the bottle. *JAMA Surg.* 2018;153:938.

77. Egan TD. Are opioids indispensable for general anaesthesia?. *Br J Anaesth.* 2019;122:e127–e135.

78. Brown EN, Pavone KJ, Naranjo M. Multimodal general anesthesia: theory and practice. *Anesth Analg.* 2018;127:1246–1258.

79. Egan TD, Svensen CH. Multimodal general anesthesia: a principled approach to producing the drug-induced, reversible coma of anesthesia. *Anesth Analg.* 2018;127:1104–1106.

80. Edwards DA, Hedrick TL, Jayaram J, Argoff C, Gulur P, Holubar SD, Gan TJ, Mythen MG, Miller TE, Shaw AD, Thacker JKM, McEvoy MD. American Society for Enhanced Recovery and Perioperative Quality Initiative joint consensus statement on perioperative management of patients on preoperative opioid therapy. *Anesth Analg.* 2019;129:567–577.

81. Shanthanna H, Ladha KS, Kehlet H, Joshi GP. Perioperative opioid administration: a critical review of opioid-free versus opioid-sparing approaches. *Anesthesiology.* 2021;134:645–659.

82. Violin JD, Lefkowitz RJ. Beta-arrestin-biased ligands at seven-transmembrane receptors. *Trends Pharmacol Sci.* 2007;28:416–422.

83. Siuda ER, 3rd Carr R, Rominger DH, Violin JD. Biased mu-opioid receptor ligands: a promising new generation of pain therapeutics. *Curr Opin Pharmacol.* 2017;32:77–84.

84. Raehal KM, Walker JK, Bohn LM. Morphine side effects in beta-arrestin 2 knockout mice. *J Pharmacol Exp Ther.* 2005;314:1195–1201.

85. Dahan A, van Dam CJ, Niesters M, van Velzen M, Fossler MJ, Demitrack MA, Olofsen E. Benefit and risk evaluation of biased μ-receptor agonist oliceridine versus morphine. *Anesthesiology.* 2020;133:559–568.

86. Kudla L, Bugno R, Skupio U, Wiktorowska L, Solecki W, Wojtas A, Golembiowska K, Zádor F, Benyhe S, Buda S, Makuch W, Przewlocka B, Bojarski AJ, Przewlocki R. Functional characterization of a novel opioid, PZM21, and its effects on the behavioural responses to morphine. *Br J Pharmacol.* 2019;176:4434–4445.

87. Lotsch J, Skarke C, Schmidt H, Liefhold J, Geisslinger G. Pharmacokinetic modeling to predict morphine and morphine-6-glucuronide plasma concentrations in healthy young volunteers. *Clin Pharmacol Ther.* 2002;72:151–162.

88. Lotsch J, Skarke C, Schmidt H, Grosch S, Geisslinger G. The transfer half-life

of morphine-6-glucuronide from plasma to effect site assessed by pupil size measurement in healthy volunteers. *Anesthesiology*. 2001;95:1329–1338.

89. Gepts E, Shafer SL, Camu F, Stanski DR, Woestenborghs R, Van Peer A, Heykants JJ. Linearity of pharmacokinetics and model estimation of sufentanil. *Anesthesiology*. 1995;83:1194–1204.

90. Scott JC, Cooke JE, Stanski DR. Electroencephalographic quantitation of opioid effect: comparative pharmacodynamics of fentanyl and sufentanil. *Anesthesiology*. 1991;74:34–42.

91. Manglik A, Lin H, Aryal DK, McCorvy JD, Dengler D, Corder G, Levit A, Kling RC, Bernat V, Hubner H, Huang XP, Sassano MF, Giguere PM, Lober S, Da D, Scherrer G, Kobilka BK, Gmeiner P, Roth BL, Shoichet BK. Structure-based discovery of opioid analgesics with reduced side effects. *Nature*. 2016;537:185–190.

92. Shulman M, Wai JM, Nunes EV. Buprenorphine treatment for opioid use disorder: an overview. *CNS Drugs*. 2019;33(6):567–580.

10 LOCAL ANESTHETICS

Charles B. Berde, Anjali Koka

Local anesthesia can be defined as loss of sensation in a discrete region of the body caused by disruption of nerve impulse generation or propagation. Local anesthesia can be produced by various chemical and physical means. However, in routine clinical practice local anesthesia is produced by several compounds whose mechanism of action is similar. Although they have different durations of action, recovery is normally spontaneous, predictable, and complete. The clinical duration of local anesthesia can be extended in various ways, including continuous infusion via indwelling catheters or pumps, additives, and other formulations that prolong the duration of local anesthetics.

HISTORY

Clinical use of local anesthetics began with cocaine in the 1880s.[1] The topically applied local anesthetic benzocaine and the injectable drugs procaine, tetracaine, and chloroprocaine were subsequently developed as adaptations of cocaine's structure as an amino ester (Figs. 10.1 and 10.2).

In 1948 lidocaine was introduced as the first member of a new class of local anesthetics, the amino amides. Advantages of the amino amides over the earlier amino esters included more stability and a reduced frequency of allergic reactions. Because of these favorable properties, lidocaine became the template for the development of a series of amino-amide anesthetics (see Fig. 10.2).

Along with lidocaine, most amino-amide local anesthetics are derived from the aromatic amine xylidine, including mepivacaine, bupivacaine, ropivacaine, and levobupivacaine. Ropivacaine and levobupivacaine share an additional distinctive characteristic: they are single enantiomers rather than racemic mixtures. They are products of a developmental strategy that takes advantage of the differential stereoselectivity of

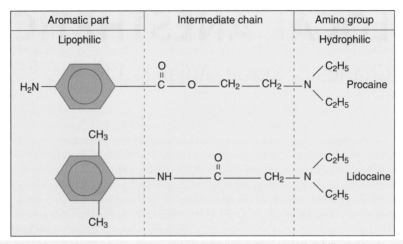

Fig. 10.1 Local anesthetics have three portions: (1) lipophilic, (2) hydrophilic, and a connecting (3) hydrocarbon chain. This figure illustrates creative ways of altering this basic structure for desired pharmacologic characteristics (duration of action, cardiovascular).

neuronal and cardiac sodium ion channels in an effort to reduce the potential for cardiac toxicity (see "Adverse Effects" later). Almost all of the amides undergo biotransformation in the liver, whereas the esters undergo hydrolysis in plasma.

NERVE CONDUCTION

Under normal or resting circumstances, the neural membrane is characterized by a negative potential of roughly –90 mV (the potential inside the nerve fiber is negative relative to the extracellular fluid). This negative potential is created by energy-dependent outward transport of sodium and inward transport of potassium ions, combined with greater membrane permeability to potassium ions relative to sodium ions. With excitation of the nerve, there is an increase in the membrane permeability to sodium ions, causing a decrease in the transmembrane potential. If a critical potential is reached (i.e., threshold potential), there is a rapid and self-sustaining influx of sodium ions resulting in a propagating wave of depolarization,—the action potential, after which the resting membrane potential is reestablished.

Nerve fibers can be classified according to fiber diameter, presence (type A and B) or absence (type C) of myelin, and function (Table 10.1). The nerve fiber diameter influences conduction velocity; a larger diameter correlates with more rapid nerve conduction. The presence of myelin also increases conduction velocity. This effect results from insulation of the axolemma from the surrounding media, forcing current to flow through periodic interruptions in the myelin sheath (i.e., nodes of Ranvier) (Fig. 10.3).

LOCAL ANESTHETIC ACTIONS ON SODIUM CHANNELS

Local anesthetics act on a wide range of molecular targets, but they exert their predominant desired clinical effects by blocking sodium ion flux through voltage-gated sodium channels. Voltage-gated sodium channels are complex transmembrane proteins comprising large α-subunits and much smaller β-subunits[2] (Fig. 10.4).

The α-subunits have four homologous domains arranged in a square, each composed of six transmembrane helices, and the pore lies in the center of these four domains. β-Subunits modulate electrophysiologic properties of the channel, and they also have prominent roles in channel localization, binding to adhesion molecules, and connection to intracellular cytoskeletons. There are nine major subtypes of sodium channel α-subunits in mammalian tissues and four major subtypes of β-subunits.

Different sodium channel subtypes are expressed in different tissues, at diverse developmental stages, and in a range of disease states. Sodium channel subtypes are an active area of investigation around human diseases with spontaneous pain and pain insensitivity, as targets of new analgesics, and in other areas of medicine, including cardiology and neurology.[2,3] Sodium channel subtypes will be discussed again later in this chapter (see "When Local Anesthesia Fails" and "Future Local Anesthetics").

From an electrophysiologic standpoint, local anesthetics block conduction of impulses by decreasing the rate of depolarization in response to excitation, preventing achievement of the threshold potential. They do not alter the resting transmembrane potential, and they have little effect on the threshold potential.

Sodium channels cycle between resting, open, and inactive conformations. During excitation, the sodium

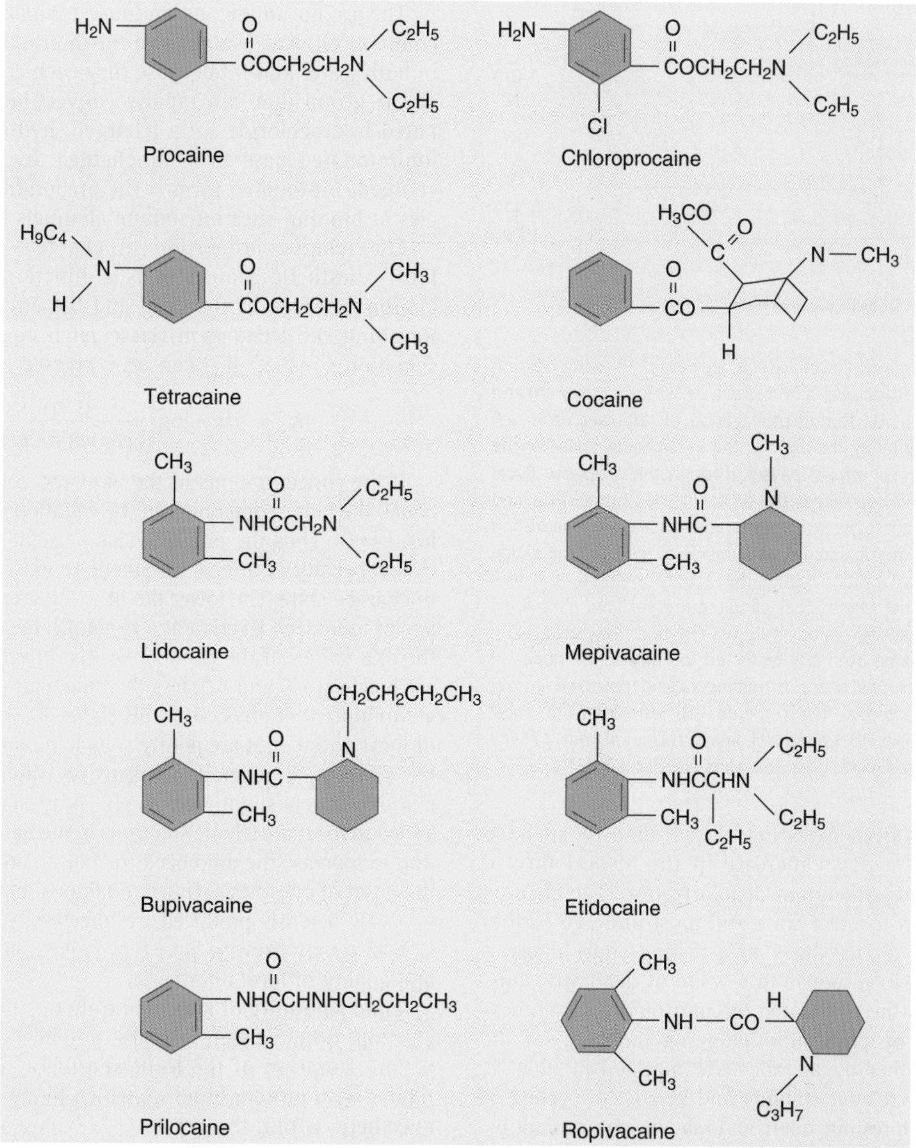

Fig. 10.2 Chemical structures of ester (i.e., procaine, chloroprocaine, tetracaine, and cocaine) and amide (i.e., lidocaine, mepivacaine, bupivacaine, etidocaine, prilocaine, and ropivacaine) local anesthetics.

Table 10.1 Classification of Nerve Fibers

Type	Fiber Subtype	Diameter (μm)	Conduction Velocity (m/s)	Function
A (myelinated)	Alpha	12–20	80–120	Proprioception, large motor
	Beta	5–15	35–80	Small motor, touch, pressure
	Gamma	3–8	10–35	Muscle tone
	Delta	2–5	5–25	Pain, temperature, touch
B (myelinated)		3	5–15	Preganglionic autonomic
C (unmyelinated)		0.3–1.5	0.5–2.5	Dull pain, temperature, touch

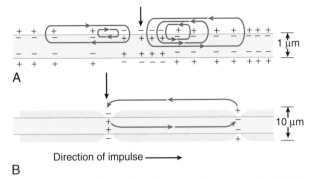

A

B

Direction of impulse ⟶

Fig. 10.3 Pattern of "local circuit currents" flowing during propagation of an impulse in a nonmyelinated C fiber's axon (A) and a myelinated axon (B). During propagation of impulses, from *left* to *right*, current entering the axon at the initial rising phase of the impulse (*large vertical arrows*) passes through the axoplasm (local circuit current) and depolarizes the adjacent membrane. Plus and minus signs adjacent to the axon membrane indicate the polarization state of the axon membrane: negative inside at rest, positive inside during active depolarization under the action potential, and less negative in regions where local circuit currents flow. This ionic current passes relatively uniformly across the nonmyelinated axon, but in the myelinated axon it is restricted to entry at the nodes of Ranvier, several of which are simultaneously depolarized during a single action potential. (From Berde CB, Strichartz GR. Local anesthetics. In: Miller RD, Cohen NH, Eriksson LI, et al., eds. Miller's Anesthesia. 8th ed. Philadelphia: Saunders Elsevier; 2015.)

channel moves from a resting closed state to an open activated state, with an increase in the inward flux of sodium ions and consequent depolarization. The channel transitions to an inactive state and must undergo further conformational change back to a resting state before it can again open in response to a wave of depolarization.

According to the modulated receptor model, local anesthetics act not by physically "plugging the pore" of the channel, but rather by an allosteric mechanism; that is, by changing the relative stability and kinetics of cycling of channels through resting, open, and inactive conformations. In so doing, the fraction of channels accessible to opening and conducting inward sodium currents in response to a wave of depolarization is reduced.[4] This mechanism provides nerve blocks that are either a "use-dependent" or "frequency-dependent" type of block; that is, the block intensifies with more frequent rates of nerve firing.

pH, Net Charge, and Lipid Solubility

The predominant binding site for local anesthetics on sodium channels is near the cytoplasmic side of the plasma membrane. A major structural requirement for a molecule to be an effective local anesthetic is sufficient solubility and rapid diffusion in both hydrophilic environments (extracellular fluid, cytosol, and the headgroup region of membrane phospholipids) and in the hydrophobic environment of the lipid bilayers in plasma membranes.

The amino-amide and amino-ester local anesthetics in common clinical use achieve this aim of good solubility in both water and fat because they each contain a tertiary amine group that can rapidly convert between a protonated hydrochloride form (charged, hydrophilic) and an unprotonated base form (uncharged, hydrophobic). The charged, protonated form is the predominant active species at binding sites on sodium channels (Fig. 10.5).[5]

The relative proportion of charged and uncharged local anesthetic molecules is a function of the dissociation constant of the drug and the environmental pH. Recalling the Henderson-Hasselbalch equation, the dissociation constant (K_a) can be expressed as follows:

$$pK_a = pH - \log\left(\frac{[base]}{[conjugate\ acid]}\right)$$

If the concentrations of the base and conjugate acid are equal, the latter component of the equation cancels (because log 1 = 0). Thus the pKa provides a useful way to describe the propensity of a local anesthetic to exist in a charged or uncharged state. The lower the pKa, the greater the percentage of unionized fraction at a given pH. In contrast, because the pKa values of the commonly used injectable anesthetics are between 7.6 and 8.9, less than one half of the molecules are unionized at physiologic pH (Table 10.2). The base forms of local anesthetics are poorly soluble in water and less stable, so they are generally marketed as water-soluble hydrochloride salts at slightly acidic pH. Bicarbonate is sometimes added to local anesthetic solutions immediately before injection to increase the unionized fraction in an effort to hasten the onset of anesthesia. Other conditions that lower pH, such as tissue acidosis produced by infection, inflammation, or ischemia, may likewise have a negative impact on the onset and quality of local anesthesia.

Lipid solubility of a local anesthetic affects tissue penetration, time course of uptake, potency, and duration of action. Duration of the local anesthetic action also correlates with protein binding, which likely serves to retain anesthetic within the nerve.

Degrees of anesthetic potency may be altered by the in vitro or in vivo system in which these effects are determined. For example, tetracaine is approximately 20 times more potent than bupivacaine when assessed in isolated nerves, but these drugs are nearly equipotent when assessed in vivo. Even when assessed in vivo, comparisons among local anesthetics may vary based on the specific site of application (spinal vs. peripheral block) because of secondary effects such as the inherent vasoactive properties of the anesthetic.

DIFFERENTIAL LOCAL ANESTHETIC BLOCKADE

From a clinical viewpoint and from electrophysiologic measurements, local anesthesia is not an all-or-none

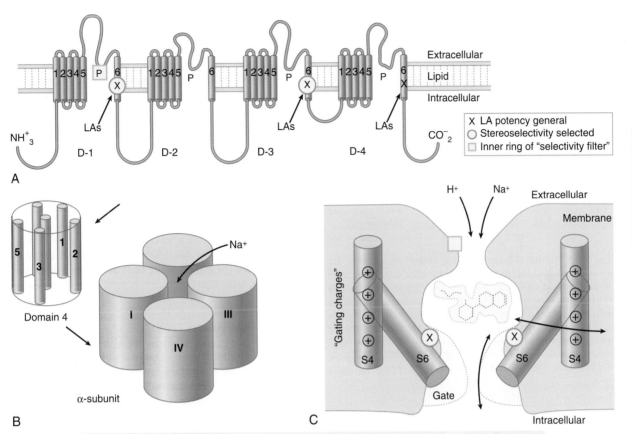

Fig. 10.4 Structural features of the Na+ channel that determine local anesthetic (LA) interactions. (A) Consensus arrangement of the single peptide of the Na+ channel α-subunit in a plasma membrane. Four domains with homologous sequences (D-1 through D-4) each contain six α-helical segments that span the membrane (S1 to S6). Each domain folds within itself to form one cylindrical bundle of segments, and these bundles converge to form the functional channel's quaternary structure (B). Activation gating leading to channel opening results from primary movement of the positively charged S4 segments in response to membrane depolarization (see panel C). Fast inactivation of the channel follows binding to the cytoplasmic end of the channel of part of the small loop that connects D-3 to D-4. Ions travel through an open channel along a pore defined at its narrowest dimension by the P region formed by partial membrane penetration of the four extracellular loops of protein connecting S5 and S6 in each domain. Intentional, directed mutations of different amino acids on the channel indicate residues that are involved in LA binding in the inner vestibule of the channel (X on S6 segments), at the interior regions of the ion-discriminating "selectivity filter (*square* on the P region), and also are known to influence stereoselectivity for phasic inhibition (*circle*, also on S6 segments). (C) Schematic cross section of the channel speculating on the manner in which S6 segments, forming a "gate," may realign during activation to open the channel and allow entry and departure of a bupivacaine molecule by the "hydrophilic" pathway. The closed (inactivated) channel has a more intimate association with the LA molecule, whose favored pathway for dissociation is no longer between S6 segments (the former pore) but now, much more slowly, laterally between segments and then through the membrane, the "hydrophobic" pathway. Na+ ions entering the pore will compete with the LA for a site in the channel, and H+ ions, which pass very slowly through the pore, can enter and leave from the extracellular opening, thereby protonating and deprotonating a bound LA molecule and thus regulating its rate of dissociation from the channel. (From Berde CB, Strichartz GR. Local anesthetics. In: Miller RD, Cohen NH, Eriksson LI, et al., eds. Miller's Anesthesia. 8th ed. Philadelphia: Saunders Elsevier; 2015.)

phenomenon: patients experience gradations in the intensity of sensory and motor blockade that vary over time after local anesthetic injections. Clinically apparent "numbness" generally correlates with intraneural concentrations of local anesthetics but also reflects complex integration and processing of inputs in the spinal dorsal horn and at supraspinal sites in the somatosensory pathway. When compound action potentials are recorded in peripheral

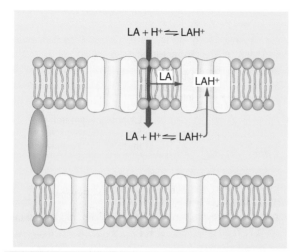

Fig. 10.5 During diffusion of local anesthetic across the nerve sheath and membrane to receptor sites within the inner vestibule of the sodium channel, only the uncharged base (LA) can penetrate the lipid membrane. After reaching the axoplasm, ionization occurs, and the charged cationic form (LAH+) attaches to the receptor. Anesthetic may also reach the channel laterally (i.e., hydrophobic pathway). (From Covino BG, Scott DB, Lambert DH. Handbook of Spinal Anesthesia and Analgesia. Philadelphia: WB Saunders; 1994:7, used with permission.)

nerves exposed to local anesthetics in varying concentrations and lengths of nerve exposed, conduction blockade is facilitated either by increasing the concentration of local anesthetic or by increasing the length of nerve exposed to more dilute concentrations. At the limit of short lengths of nerve exposed to local anesthetic, conduction blockade requires exposure of at least three successive nodes of Ranvier to prevent the action potential from "skipping over" the region of local anesthetic exposure.

Historically, the term *differential blockade* in clinical textbooks referred to the observation that infusions of dilute concentrations of local anesthetic could produce analgesia and signs of autonomic blockade with relative sparing of motor strength. This clinical trend is not readily explained by the electrophysiologic observations of action potential blockade in large and small fibers perfused to steady state.[6] The mechanisms underlying this divergence between clinical experience and experimental data are poorly understood, but they may be related to the anatomic and geographic arrangement of nerve fibers, variability in the longitudinal spread required for neural blockade, effects on other ion channels, and inherent impulse activity.

SPREAD OF LOCAL ANESTHESIA AFTER INJECTION

When local anesthetics are deposited around a peripheral nerve, they must cross a series of diffusion barriers

to access sodium channels in nerve axons (Fig. 10.6). With large nerve trunks, they diffuse from the outer surface (mantle) toward the center (core) of the nerve along a concentration gradient (Fig. 10.7).[7] As a result, nerve fibers located in the mantle of the mixed nerve are blocked first. These mantle fibers are generally distributed to more proximal anatomic structures, whereas distal structures are innervated by fibers near the core. This anatomic arrangement accounts for the initial development of proximal anesthesia with subsequent distal involvement as local anesthetic diffuses to reach more central core nerve fibers. Skeletal muscle weakness may precede sensory blockade if the motor nerve fibers are more superficial. The sequence of onset and recovery from conduction blockade of sympathetic, sensory, and motor nerve fibers in a mixed peripheral nerve depends as much or more on the anatomic location of the nerve fibers within the mixed nerve than on their intrinsic sensitivity to local anesthetics.

PHARMACOKINETICS

For most oral and intravenous drugs, systemic uptake carries the drug from the administration site to the effect site. Local anesthetics are different: when drug is deposited near the target site, systemic absorption competes with drug entry into effect sites in nerves. Thus rapid and efficient systemic uptake from an injection site diminishes, rather than increases, efficacy in nerve blockade. This principle is illustrated in Fig. 10.8. High plasma concentrations of local anesthetics after absorption from injection sites (or unintended intravascular injection) are undesirable and are the origin of their potential toxicity. Peak plasma concentrations achieved are determined by the rate of systemic uptake and, to a lesser extent, the rate of clearance of the local anesthetic. Uptake is affected by several factors related to the physiochemical properties of the local anesthetic and local tissue blood flow. Uptake tends to be delayed for local anesthetics with high lipophilicity and protein binding.

Local Anesthetic Vasoactivity

Anesthetics differ in their tendencies to cause either vasoconstriction or vasodilation of blood vessels. These effects vary with site of injection, concentration, and balance of local direct actions on vascular smooth muscle versus indirect actions via blockade of sympathetic efferent fibers. Such differences may be clinically important. For example, the less frequent incidence of systemic toxicity of S (–) ropivacaine compared with the R (+) enantiomer in part may result from its vasoconstrictive activity (see "Adverse Effects"). The variable effect of vasoconstrictors added to local anesthetic solutions used for spinal anesthesia is another example. In contrast to

Table 10.2 Comparative Pharmacology and Common Current Use of Local Anesthetics

Classification and Compounds	pKa	% Nonionized at pH 7.4	Potency[a]	Max. Dose (mg) for Infiltration[b]	Duration After Infiltration (min)	Topical	Local	IV	Periph	Epi	Spinal
Esters											
Procaine	8.9	3	1	500	45–60	No	Yes	No	Yes	No	Yes
Chloroprocaine	8.7	5	2	600	30–60	No	Yes	Yes	Yes	Yes	Yes[c]
Tetracaine	8.5	7	8	N/A	N/A	Yes[d]	No	No	No	No	Yes
Amides											
Lidocaine	7.9	24	2	300	60–120	Yes	Yes	Yes	Yes	Yes	Yes[c]
Mepivacaine	7.6	39	2	300	90–180	No	Yes	No	Yes	Yes	Yes[c]
Prilocaine	7.9	24	2	400	60–120	Yes[e]	Yes	Yes	Yes	Yes	Yes[c]
Bupivacaine, levobupivacaine	8.1	17	8	150	240–480	No	Yes	No	Yes	Yes	Yes
Ropivacaine	8.1	17	6	200	240–480	No	Yes	No	Yes	Yes	Yes

[a]Relative potencies vary based on experimental model or route of administration.
[b]Dosage should take into account the site of injection, use of a vasoconstrictor, and patient-related factors.
[c]Use of procaine, lidocaine, mepivacaine, prilocaine, and chloroprocaine for spinal anesthesia is somewhat controversial; indications are evolving (see text).
[d]Used in combination with another local anesthetic to increase duration.
[e]Formulated with lidocaine as a eutectic mixture.
Epi, Epidural; *IV,* intravenous; *Periph,* peripheral.

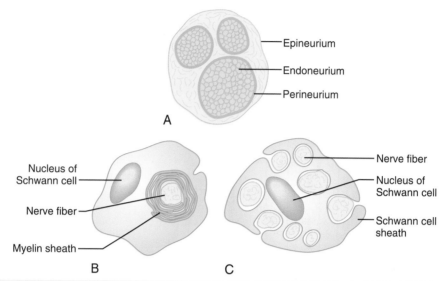

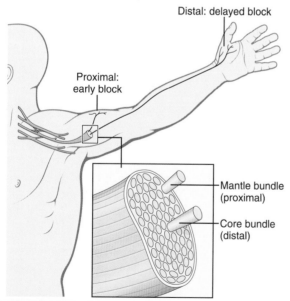

Fig. 10.6 Transverse sections of a peripheral nerve (A) showing the outermost epineurium; the inner perineurium, which collects nerve axons in fascicles; and the endoneurium, which surrounds each myelinated fiber. Each myelinated axon (B) is encased in the multiple membranous wrappings of myelin formed by one Schwann cell, each of which stretches longitudinally more than approximately 100 times the diameter of the axon. The narrow span of axon between these myelinated segments, the node of Ranvier, contains the ion channels that support action potentials. Nonmyelinated fibers (C) are enclosed in bundles of 5 to 10 axons by a chain of Schwann cells that tightly embrace each axon with but one layer of membrane. (From Berde CB, Strichartz GR. Local anesthetics. In: Miller RD, Cohen NH, Eriksson LI, et al., eds. Miller's Anesthesia. 8th ed. Philadelphia: Saunders Elsevier; 2015.)

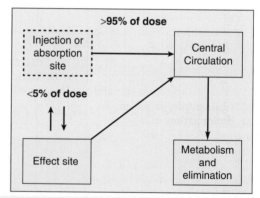

Fig. 10.8 Heuristic model of local anesthetic uptake and distribution. Systemic uptake of local anesthetics from the perineural injection compartment competes with drug entry into nerves. Vasoconstrictors delay systemic uptake from the perineural injection compartment, reducing peak blood concentrations of local anesthetics and maintaining a higher concentration gradient favoring drug entry into nerves over the first 30 minutes after injection.

Fig. 10.7 Local anesthetics deposited around a peripheral nerve diffuse along a concentration gradient to block nerve fibers on the outer surface (mantle) before more centrally located (core) fibers. This accounts for early manifestations of anesthesia in more proximal areas of the extremity.

lidocaine or bupivacaine, there is some evidence that tetracaine produces a significant increase in spinal cord blood flow. Consequently, prolongation of spinal anesthesia by epinephrine or other vasoconstrictors is more pronounced with tetracaine than with other commonly used spinal anesthetics.

Metabolism

The amino-ester local anesthetics undergo hydrolysis by plasma esterases, whereas the amino-amide local anesthetics undergo metabolism by hepatic microsomal enzymes. The lungs are also capable of extracting local anesthetics such as lidocaine, bupivacaine, and prilocaine from the circulation. The rate of this metabolism and first-pass pulmonary extraction may influence toxicity (see "Systemic Toxicity"). In this regard, the relatively rapid hydrolysis of the ester local anesthetic chloroprocaine makes it less likely to produce sustained plasma concentrations than other local anesthetics, particularly the amino amides. However, patients with atypical plasma cholinesterase levels may be at increased risk of developing excessive plasma concentrations of chloroprocaine or other ester local anesthetics because of absent or limited plasma hydrolysis. Hepatic metabolism of lidocaine is extensive, and clearance of this local anesthetic from plasma parallels hepatic blood flow. Liver disease or decreases in hepatic blood flow, as occur with congestive heart failure or general anesthesia, can decrease the rate of metabolism of lidocaine. Less than 5% of injected local anesthetics are excreted unchanged in the urine.

Additives

Epinephrine is the most common additive in local anesthetic solutions. In a typical concentration of 5 µg/mL (1:200,000), epinephrine produces local vasoconstriction, which slows the rate of tissue absorption and therefore reduces peak systemic concentrations, decreasing the odds of systemic toxicity (see "Systemic Toxicity"). Depending on the injection site and the local anesthetic to which epinephrine is added, epinephrine may result in some prolongation of sensory or motor block. Epinephrine can also be used as a marker for detection of intravascular injection based on effects on heart rate, arterial blood pressure, or symptoms. However, systemic absorption of epinephrine may contribute to cardiac dysrhythmias or accentuate systemic hypertension in vulnerable patients. Epinephrine should be avoided when performing peripheral nerve blocks in areas that may lack collateral flow (e.g., digital blocks). In contrast, epinephrine-induced vasoconstriction decreases local bleeding and may provide added benefit when combined with local anesthetics used for infiltration anesthesia.

In addition to the vasoconstrictive agent epinephrine, other additives are used clinically to prolong analgesia from peripheral nerve blocks, including α_2 agonists, opioids, and antiinflammatories. Of the perineural additives studied, the off-label use of buprenorphine, clonidine, dexamethasone, dexmedetomidine, and magnesium most consistently prolong clinical analgesia from peripheral nerve blocks. Additive doses vary clinically and may correlate with side effects, which can include bradycardia, hypotension, and nausea.[8] Traditionally, anesthesia providers have exercised considerable freedom in mixing their own additives and combinations. There is a growing recognition that this practice sometimes produces drug administration errors. In addition, although some additives have undergone proper preclinical testing to ensure the absence of local tissue toxicities on nerve and muscle, others have not (see "Local Tissue Toxicity"). Caution should be exercised when using additives that lack sufficient preclinical safety data and a regulatory evaluation process.

ADVERSE EFFECTS

Important adverse effects of local anesthetics, although rare, may occur from systemic absorption, local tissue toxicity, allergic reactions, and drug-specific effects.

Systemic Toxicity

Systemic toxicity of local anesthetics results from excessive plasma concentrations of these drugs, most often from accidental intravascular injection during performance of epidural and caudal blocks. Less often, excessive plasma concentrations result from absorption of local anesthetics from tissue injection sites. The magnitude of local anesthetic systemic absorption depends on the dose injected, the specific site of injection, and the inclusion of a vasoconstrictor in the local anesthetic solution. Systemic absorption of local anesthetic is greatest after injection for intercostal nerve blocks and caudal anesthesia, intermediate after epidural anesthesia, and least after brachial plexus and lower extremity blocks (Fig. 10.9).[9]

Clinically significant systemic toxicity results from effects on the central nervous system and cardiovascular system. Establishment of maximal acceptable local anesthetic doses for performance of regional anesthesia is an attempt to limit plasma concentrations that can result from systemic absorption of these drugs (see Table 10.2). However, standard dosage recommendations are not entirely evidence based and are inconsistent, and they fail to consider the specific injection-site and patient-related factors.[10] Nonetheless, dosage recommendations represent a starting point for dose adjustments based on clinical circumstances and evolving evidence.

Central Nervous System Toxicity

Increasing plasma concentrations of local anesthetics classically produce circumoral numbness, facial tingling, restlessness, vertigo, tinnitus, and slurred speech, culminating in tonic-clonic seizures, though marked variation from this pattern is quite common.[11] Local anesthetics are neuronal depressants, and onset of seizures likely

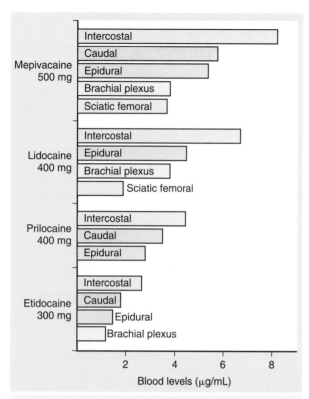

Fig. 10.9 Peak plasma concentrations of local anesthetics resulting during performance of various types of regional anesthetic procedures. (From Covino BD, Vassals HG. Local Anesthetics: Mechanism of Action in Clinical Use. Orlando: Grune & Stratton; 1976:97, used with permission.)

reflects selective depression of cortical inhibitory neurons, leaving excitatory pathways unopposed. However, larger doses may affect inhibitory and excitatory pathways, resulting in central nervous system depression and even coma. These effects generally parallel anesthetic potency. Arterial hypoxemia and metabolic acidosis can occur rapidly during seizure activity, and hypoxemia and acidosis both can enhance the central nervous system toxicity of the local anesthetics.

Treatment of central nervous system toxic reactions begins with prompt intervention, with administration of supplemental oxygen and assisting ventilation as indicated to prevent hypoxemia and hypercarbia. Benzodiazepines (i.e., midazolam, lorazepam, diazepam) are generally the drugs of first choice to terminate seizures because of their efficacy and relative hemodynamic stability. Propofol, although more immediately accessible, should be used with caution for seizure suppression, as it can compromise cardiac function.

Cardiovascular System Toxicity

High plasma concentrations of local anesthetics can produce profound hypotension caused by relaxation of arteriolar vascular smooth muscle and direct myocardial depression. The cardiac toxicity, in part, reflects the ability of local anesthetics to block cardiac sodium ion channels in addition to other ion channels, including calcium channels. As a result, cardiac automaticity and conduction of cardiac impulses are impaired, manifesting on the electrocardiogram as prolongation of the PR interval and widening of the QRS complex. Local anesthetics may profoundly depress myocardial contractility to varying degrees. For example, the ratio of the dose required to produce cardiovascular collapse compared with that producing seizures for lidocaine is about twice that for bupivacaine.[12] Such findings support the concept that bupivacaine is more likely to cause cardiac toxicity, which has been the driving force for the development of single-enantiomer anesthetics, such as ropivacaine and levobupivacaine.

Lipid Resuscitation

Intravenous infusions of lipid emulsions have become a standard treatment of local anesthetic systemic toxicity (LAST) (also see Chapters 18 and 45). The mechanism by which lipid is effective is not clear but is likely related to its ability to extract bupivacaine (or other lipophilic drugs) from aqueous plasma or tissue targets, thus reducing their effective free concentration ("lipid sink").[13] Accordingly, solutions of lipid emulsion should be stocked and readily accessible in any area where major conduction blockade is performed, and in locations where overdoses from any lipophilic drug might be treated. A more detailed discussion of this topic and guidelines for administration of lipid emulsions (20%), checklists, and treatment protocols can be found in a publication by the American Society of Regional Anesthesia and Pain Medicine (ASRA) Task Force on Local Anesthetic Systemic Toxicity.[10,14]

According to the ASRA guidelines, an intravenous bolus dose of 20% lipid emulsion starts with a bolus of 1.5 mL/kg over 2 to 3 minutes (100 mL if greater than 70 kg) followed by a continuous infusion at 0.25 mL/kg/min. Although lipid rescue is important and should be used, it is not 100% effective and not a substitute for following dosing guidelines and safe practice regarding patient monitoring, fractionated dosing, and observation for early warning signs of systemic toxicity.

ASRA guidelines recommend additional modifications of standard advanced cardiac life support (ACLS) protocols, including avoidance of vasopressin, calcium channel blockers, β-blockers, and other local anesthetics (lidocaine, amiodarone). Incremental dosing of epinephrine should be decreased to less than 1 mcg/kg[14].

Local Tissue Toxicity

Local anesthetics are in general well tolerated in terms of their local tissue effects. Nevertheless, all currently available local anesthetics have intrinsic toxicities to nerve and muscle that occasionally become clinically apparent. These incidences of toxicities increase with local tissue concentration[15] and duration of exposure, and these risks may be exacerbated by factors that increase nerve vulnerability and predispose to nerve ischemia, including preexisting nerve dysfunction, metabolic and inflammatory conditions, increased tissue pressure, and systemic hypotension. Intraneural concentrations can rise steadily during prolonged perineural infusions. For these reasons, for prolonged perineural infusions, we recommend use of relatively dilute local anesthetic concentrations, generally no more than 0.2% for bupivacaine or ropivacaine.

Allergic Reactions

Allergic reactions to local anesthetics are rare, despite the frequent use of these drugs. Less than 1% of all adverse reactions to local anesthetics are caused by allergic mechanisms. Most adverse responses attributed to allergic reactions are instead caused by additives or are manifestations of systemic toxicity from excessive plasma concentrations of the local anesthetic. Hypotension associated with syncope may be vagally mediated, whereas tachycardia and palpitations may occur from systemic absorption of epinephrine.

Cross-Sensitivity

The amino-ester local anesthetics, which produce metabolites related to para-aminobenzoic acid, are more likely to evoke hypersensitivity reactions than the amino amides. Allergic reactions may also be caused by methylparaben or similar compounds that resemble para-aminobenzoic acid, which are used as preservatives in commercial formulations of ester and amide local anesthetics. Although patients known to be allergic to amino-ester local anesthetics can receive amino-amide local anesthetics, this recommendation should be cautiously accepted because it assumes that the local anesthetic was responsible for evoking the initial allergic reaction, rather than a common preservative.

Documentation

Documentation of an allergy to local anesthetics is based principally on clinical history (e.g., rash, laryngeal edema, hypotension, bronchospasm). However, increases in serum tryptase, a marker of mast cell degranulation, may have some value with respect to confirmation, and intradermal testing may help establish the local anesthetic as the offending antigen if other drugs (e.g., sedative-hypnotics, opioids) have been administered concurrently.

SPECIFIC LOCAL ANESTHETICS

Amino Esters

Procaine

The earliest injectable local anesthetic, procaine, enjoyed extensive use during the first half of the past century, primarily as a spinal anesthetic. Its instability and the considerable potential for hypersensitivity reactions resulted in limited use after the introduction of lidocaine. Transient neurologic symptoms (TNS) is a rare condition characterized by severe pain of the buttocks and lower extremities after spinal anesthesia. Concerns regarding TNS associated with spinal lidocaine (see "Lidocaine") have renewed interest in procaine as a spinal anesthetic. Limited data suggest that procaine offers a small advantage with respect to TNS; however, spinal procaine is associated with a significantly greater incidence of nausea.[16]

Tetracaine

Tetracaine is still commonly used for spinal anesthesia. As such, it has a long duration of action, particularly if used with a vasoconstrictor, although this combination results in a surprisingly high risk of TNS.[17] Tetracaine is available as a 1% solution or as Niphanoid crystals; the crystal form is preferable because of the relative instability of the anesthetic in solution. Tetracaine is rarely used for epidural anesthesia or peripheral nerve blocks because of its slow onset, profound motor blockade, and potential toxicity when administered at high doses. Although it is an ester, its rate of metabolism is one-fourth that of procaine and one-tenth that of chloroprocaine.

Chloroprocaine

Chloroprocaine initially gained popularity as an epidural anesthetic, particularly in obstetrics, because its rapid hydrolysis virtually eliminated concern about systemic toxicity and fetal exposure to the local anesthetic. Unfortunately, neurotoxic injury, presumed to occur from accidental intrathecal injection of large doses intended for the epidural space, tempered enthusiasm for neuraxial administration of chloroprocaine. This toxicity was thought to be caused by the preservative sodium bisulfite contained in the commercial formulation. However, subsequent studies do not demonstrate neurotoxicity from intrathecal bisulfite; instead, it was found not to be neurotoxic and may even have neuroprotective effects.[18] In any event a formulation of chloroprocaine devoid of preservatives and antioxidants is available.

Chloroprocaine produces epidural anesthesia of a relatively short duration. Epidural administration of chloroprocaine is sometimes avoided because it impairs the anesthetic or analgesic action of epidural bupivacaine and of opioids used concurrently or sequentially.[19] Chloroprocaine has been reevaluated as a spinal anesthetic, and the risk of TNS appears low.[20] Chloroprocaine solutions used for spinal anesthesia should be bisulfite-free. Commonly used intrathecal doses in adults range from 30 to 60 mg.

Because of its rapid plasma clearance, chloroprocaine has two unique roles in pediatric regional anesthesia: (1) as a continuous epidural infusion in neonates and very young infants and (2) for repeat loading doses in patients receiving postoperative epidural or peripheral perineural infusions in the setting where a repeat loading dose with the more commonly used amino-amide local anesthetics would result in stepwise increase of blood concentrations into a toxic range.

Amino Amides

Lidocaine

Lidocaine is the most commonly used local anesthetic. It is used for local, topical, and regional intravenous block; peripheral nerve block; and spinal and epidural anesthesia. Although recent issues have led to restricted use of lidocaine for spinal anesthesia, this local anesthetic remains popular for all other applications, including epidural anesthesia.

Potential neurotoxicity (i.e., cauda equina syndrome) when lidocaine is administered for spinal anesthesia has emerged as a concern, especially when used with a continuous spinal technique.[21] Most of the initial injuries resulted from neurotoxic concentrations of anesthetic in the caudal region of the subarachnoid space achieved by the combination of maldistribution and relatively large doses of anesthetic administered through small-gauge spinal catheters.[22] However, even doses of lidocaine routinely used for single-injection spinal anesthesia (75–100 mg) have been associated with neurotoxicity.

As described earlier, TNS is pain of the lower extremities after spinal anesthesia. Symptoms of TNS generally manifest within the first 12 to 24 hours after surgery, most often resolve within 3 days, and rarely persist beyond a week. Nonsteroidal antiinflammatory drugs are often effective and should be used as first-line treatment. TNS is not associated with sensory loss, motor weakness, or bowel and bladder dysfunction. Additionally, magnetic resonance imaging (MRI) and electrophysiologic examinations are normal. The cause and significance of TNS symptoms remain to be established, but discrepancies between factors affecting TNS and experimental animal toxicity cast doubt that TNS and persistent neurologic deficits (e.g., cauda equina syndrome) are mediated by the same mechanism.

All local anesthetics can cause TNS; however, the risk is 5-to 10-fold higher when patients receive intrathecal doses of lidocaine or mepivacaine compared with bupivacaine, levobupivacaine, prilocaine, procaine, and ropivacaine. There is a suggestion that the risk of TNS with intrathecal chloroprocaine may be lower, though authors of a recent systematic review regarded this conclusion as preliminary.[23] In addition to the use of intrathecal lidocaine, factors that may contribute to the occurrence of TNS include the lithotomy position and outpatient status. In contrast, local anesthetic concentration, the presence of glucose, concomitant administration of epinephrine, and technique-related factors such as the size or type of needle do not alter the incidence of TNS with lidocaine.[17]

Mepivacaine

Mepivacaine was the first in the series of pipecholyl xylidines, combining the piperidine ring of cocaine with the xylidine ring of lidocaine (see Fig. 10.2). This resulted in an anesthetic with characteristics similar to lidocaine, although with less vasodilation, and a slightly longer duration of action. The clinical use of mepivacaine parallels lidocaine, with the exception that it is relatively ineffective as a topical local anesthetic. Mepivacaine is often used for short-duration spinal anesthesia, although its use still carries a risk for developing TNS.

Prilocaine

Prilocaine was introduced into clinical practice with the anticipation that its rapid metabolism and infrequent acute toxicity (central nervous system toxicity about 40% less than lidocaine) would make it a useful drug. Unfortunately, administration of large doses (>600 mg) may result in clinically significant accumulation of the metabolite ortho-toluidine, an oxidizing compound capable of converting hemoglobin to methemoglobin. Prilocaine-induced methemoglobinemia spontaneously subsides and can be reversed by the administration of methylene blue (1 to 2 mg/kg given intravenously over a 5-minute period). Nevertheless, the capacity to induce dose-related methemoglobinemia has limited the clinical acceptance of prilocaine.

Bupivacaine

Bupivacaine is a congener of mepivacaine, with a butyl rather than a methyl group on the piperidine ring, a modification that imparts a longer duration of action. This characteristic, combined with its high-quality sensory anesthesia relative to motor blockade, has established bupivacaine as one of the most commonly used local anesthetics for epidural anesthesia during labor and for postoperative pain management. Bupivacaine is also commonly used for peripheral nerve block, and it has a relatively unblemished record as a spinal anesthetic.

Refractory cardiac arrest has been associated with the use of 0.75% bupivacaine when accidentally injected intravenously during attempted epidural anesthesia,[24] and this concentration is no longer recommended for epidural anesthesia. The most likely mechanism for bupivacaine's cardiotoxicity relates to the nature of its interaction with cardiac sodium ion channels.[25] When electrophysiologic differences between anesthetics are compared, lidocaine enters the sodium ion channel quickly and leaves quickly. In contrast, recovery from bupivacaine blockade during diastole is relatively prolonged, making it far more potent with respect to depressing the maximum upstroke velocity of the cardiac action potential (Vmax) in ventricular cardiac muscle. As a result, bupivacaine has been labeled a "fast-in, slow-out" local anesthetic. This characteristic likely creates conditions favorable for unidirectional block and reentry. Other mechanisms may contribute to bupivacaine's cardiotoxicity, including disruption of atrioventricular nodal conduction, depression of myocardial contractility, and indirect effects mediated by the central nervous system.[26] This potential for cardiotoxicity places important limitations on the total dose of bupivacaine, and it underscores the vital role of fractional dosing and methods to detect inadvertent intravascular injection when large doses of local anesthetic (especially bupivacaine) are given for regional block. The recent identification of lipid emulsion as a therapeutic intervention for bupivacaine cardiotoxicity does not diminish the critical importance of these preventive measures. Cardiotoxicity is of no concern when small doses are administered for spinal anesthesia.

Single Enantiomers

Concerns for bupivacaine cardiotoxicity have focused attention on the stereoisomers of bupivacaine and on its homolog, ropivacaine.

Stereochemistry

Isomers are different compounds that have the same molecular formula. Subsets of isomers that have atoms connected by the same sequence of bonds but that have different spatial orientations are called *stereoisomers*. Enantiomers are a particular class of stereoisomers that exist as mirror images. The term *chiral* is derived from the Greek *cheir*, meaning "hand," because the forms can be considered nonsuperimposable mirror images. Enantiomers have identical physical properties except for the direction of the rotation of the plane of polarized light. This property is used to classify the enantiomer as dextrorotatory (+) if the rotation is to the right, or clockwise, and as levorotatory (–) if it is to the left, or counterclockwise. A racemic mixture is a mixture of equal parts of enantiomers and is optically inactive because the rotation caused by the molecules of one isomer is canceled by the opposite rotation of its enantiomer. Chiral compounds can also be classified on the basis of absolute configuration, generally designated as R (rectus) or S (sinister). Enantiomers may differ with respect to specific biologic activity. For example, the S (–) enantiomer of bupivacaine has inherently less cardiotoxicity than its R (+) mirror image.

Ropivacaine

Ropivacaine (levopropivacaine) is the S (–) enantiomer of the homolog of mepivacaine and bupivacaine with a propyl tail on the piperidine ring. In addition to a more favorable interaction with cardiac sodium ion channels, it is more likely to produce vasoconstriction. Motor blockade is less pronounced, and electrophysiologic studies raise the possibility that C fibers are preferentially blocked, together suggesting that ropivacaine may more easily produce a differential block. However, as expected from its lower lipid solubility, ropivacaine is less potent than bupivacaine. The question of potency is critical to any comparison of these anesthetics; if more drug needs to be administered to achieve a desired effect, the apparent benefits with respect to cardiotoxicity (or differential block) may not exist when more appropriate equipotent dose comparisons are made. Ropivacaine likely offers some advantage with respect to cardiotoxicity, but any benefit over bupivacaine with respect to differential block is marginal, at best.

Levobupivacaine

Levobupivacaine is the single S (–) enantiomer of bupivacaine. Similar to ropivacaine, cardiotoxicity is reduced, but there is no advantage over bupivacaine with respect to differential blockade. As with ropivacaine, the clinically significant advantage of this compound over the racemic mixture is restricted to situations in which relatively high doses of anesthetic are administered.

Topical Local Anesthetics

Local anesthetics are commonly administered on mucosal surfaces,[27] on cut skin to facilitate laceration repair,[28] and on intact skin, especially for needle procedures in children. Systemic absorption through mucosal surfaces is relatively rapid and efficient. Systemic toxicity is a recognized problem with excessive dosing of local anesthetic sprays and gels from the oral, nasal, or tracheobronchial mucosa, particularly in infants and children.

The keratinized layer of the skin provides an effective barrier to diffusion of topical anesthetics, making it relatively more difficult to achieve anesthesia of intact skin by topical application. This limitation can be overcome by using relatively high concentrations of local anesthetic (e.g., 4% lidocaine as in LMX or tetracaine 4% gel as in Ametop). A combination of 2.5% lidocaine and 2.5% prilocaine cream (i.e., eutectic mixture of local anesthetics [EMLA]) is widely used on intact skin. This mixture has a lower melting point than either component, and it exists as an oil at room temperature that is capable of overcoming the barrier of the skin. EMLA cream is particularly useful in children (also see Chapter 34) for the prevention or attenuation of pain associated with venipuncture or placement of an intravenous catheter, although it may take up to an hour before adequate topical anesthesia is produced.[29] Another product, Synera, uses a heating element to accelerate the onset of skin analgesia from a lidocaine–tetracaine patch.

Tumescent Local Anesthesia

A variety of plastic and cosmetic surgical procedures are commonly performed by a technique known as *tumescent local anesthesia,* which involves subcutaneous infusion of large volumes of very dilute local anesthetic. The total lidocaine doses used in this approach are very large, such as eightfold larger than recommended doses for infiltration or peripheral nerve blockade. Nevertheless, there is a pharmacokinetic basis for this approach. When recommended dose guidelines and techniques are followed, plasma lidocaine concentrations remain in a safe range, though plasma concentrations commonly peak more than 12 hours after injection.[30] Several case series support the general safety of this approach when recommended guidelines are followed. Conversely, adverse events have occurred when guidelines were not followed. In particular, additional dosing of other local anesthetics over the next day has resulted in toxic reactions. Any health facility using this technique should have resources and protocols for treatment of LAST.

Systemic Local Anesthetics for Acute and Chronic Pain

Local anesthetics and related sodium channel blockers such as mexiletine can be administered as systemic analgesics and for local anesthesia. There is evidence for effectiveness as adjuvant analgesics for postoperative pain[31] and for several types of neuropathic pain.[32] For some patients with neuropathic pain, brief intravenous lidocaine infusions may produce a remarkable, though poorly understood, extended duration of pain relief (e.g., for days or weeks) that far outlasts any apparent pharmacologic duration of lidocaine.[15,33]

WHEN LOCAL ANESTHESIA FAILS

Anesthesia providers and all clinicians should strive to improve the reliability of clinical use of local anesthetics. Historically, a common cause of failed local anesthesia has been technical failure; that is, needle placement and injection of the solution not sufficiently close to the intended site of action. The widespread use of ultrasound guidance has clearly improved the technical success of many forms of regional anesthesia, especially involving peripheral nerve and plexus blocks (also see Chapter 18). Although multiple studies indicate that ultrasound facilitates more successful rates of regional anesthesia with much smaller volumes of local anesthetics, the median effective dose or volume (i.e., effectiveness for 50% of subjects) is not a relevant variable for clinical practice; what is more relevant is an ED95 (an effective dose in 95% of subjects).[34] Long-established techniques, such as thoracic epidural anesthesia, have significant technical failure rates when inserted using solely "blind" techniques such as loss of resistance. There is a growing appreciation for more objective approaches to confirmation of needle and catheter placement for many forms

of regional anesthesia in addition to ultrasound, such as Tsui and colleagues' nerve stimulation approach for epidural catheter placement,[35] transduction of epidural space pressure waves, and selective use of fluoroscopy[36] (also see Chapters 17 and 18).

Aside from technical failure in needle location, local anesthesia can fail for a range of other reasons. Clinicians can make erroneous assumptions about the relevant neuroanatomy of pain arising from a surgical procedure, leading to coverage of an inadequate subset of the nerves innervating a surgical site. In addition, there is an under-appreciation of biologic sources of variation in local anesthetic responsiveness. For example, some patients with Ehlers–Danlos syndrome type III show relative resistance to local anesthetics.[37]

Local anesthetics commonly have diminished effectiveness in sites of infection or inflammation. Inflammation-induced local anesthetic resistance probably results from both pharmacokinetic factors (local acidosis, edema, hyperemia) that reduce drug entry into nerves and pharmacodynamic factors, including peripheral and central sensitization.[38]

Rapidly developing tolerance (tachyphylaxis) can occur in some patients with repeated dosing or prolonged infusion. Animal studies[39] and clinical observations[40] associate tachyphylaxis with the development of hyperalgesia. Tachyphylaxis can be diminished or prevented by coadministration of antihyperalgesic drugs or other analgesics with central actions.[41]

Patients with long-standing chronic pain and hyperalgesia often appear to require larger volumes or concentrations, or both, of local anesthetics to achieve adequate analgesia in addition to coadministration of other analgesic or antihyperalgesic drugs. Although psychological factors may influence a patient's ability to tolerate surgery with regional anesthesia, clinicians should avoid "blaming the patient" for insufficient degrees of sensory block or analgesia caused by a variety of technical or biologic factors that influence block effectiveness.

There are other possible effects of chronic pain and its treatment on peripheral nerves and sodium channels. Nerve injury and inflammation change the expression of different sodium channel subtypes. Although the α-subunit of the sodium channel composes the "pore," β-subunits are also differentially expressed after nerve injury or inflammation, and these β-subunits modulate channel electrophysiology and thereby may alter local anesthetic responsiveness. In a rat model chronic, but not acute, opioid exposure caused impaired local anesthetic responsiveness in the sciatic nerve.[42]

FUTURE LOCAL ANESTHETICS

Local anesthetics play a central role in modern anesthetic practice. However, despite major advances in pharmacology and techniques for administration over the past century, this class of compounds has a relatively narrow therapeutic index with respect to their potential for neurotoxicity and for adverse cardiovascular and central nervous system effects. Another class of molecules that block sodium channels by a different site and mechanism are called the *site 1 sodium channel blockers*. They appear to be devoid of neurotoxicity and myotoxicity in some preliminary studies.[43] These observations suggest that sodium channel blockade and local tissue toxicity to nerve and muscle may not be mediated by a common mechanism. Site 1 blockers also appear to have minimal cardiotoxicity,[44] probably because of their much weaker affinity for the predominant sodium channel subtype in the myocardium, Nav1.5.

Regional anesthesia has grown in safety and importance in intraoperative and postoperative analgesia (also see Chapters 17, 18, and 40). Opioid sparing per se is recognized as a beneficial consequence of using regional anesthesia and analgesia. Available local anesthetics typically provide less than 12 hours of analgesia after a single injection. Although analgesia can be prolonged using additives or continuous catheters, these approaches carry risks. Continuous catheter infusions involve potential for dislodgement and additional postoperative care and expense. Therefore there have been several approaches to producing prolonged local anesthesia for wound infiltration or peripheral nerve blockade via a single injection. Controlled release or on-demand release[45] of local anesthetics has been achieved from microparticles, liposomes, hydrogels, and other vehicles. One liposomal bupivacaine product, Exparel, was approved in 2011 in the United States with approval for surgical site infiltration. Clinical trial outcomes have been mixed, but recent reviews and metaanalysis show no advantage to using liposomal bupivacaine compared with nonliposomal bupivacaine.[46–48]

Our group[*] is actively investigating the site 1 sodium channel blockers in animals[49] and in early clinical trials.[50] Site 1 blockers show profound synergism with existing local anesthetics and marked prolongation by epinephrine.

Another limitation of existing local anesthetics is the absence of modality selectivity. For example, in epidural analgesia for labor it would be very desirable to have intense analgesia, avoidance of weakness and hypotension, and preservation of sufficient sensation to feel an urge to push (also see Chapter 33). Recent research has approached sensory-selective blockade by two predominant strategies: (1) targeting local anesthetic entry preferentially into small sensory nerve fibers[51] and (2) developing drugs that bind preferentially to subtypes of sodium channels located predominantly in small sensory fibers.

CONCLUSIONS

Local anesthetics are used widely in anesthesiology and many areas of medicine. They have some risks and side effects, but they can be used with very good safety and clinical effectiveness by attention to safe dosing guidelines, early recognition of intravascular injection, and optimal technique. Local anesthetics are not a "solved problem," and current research may lead to improvements in regional anesthesia and postoperative care in the future.

ACKNOWLEDGMENTS

The authors, editor, and publisher would like to thank Dr. Kenneth Drasner for contributing to this chapter in previous editions of this work. It has served as the foundation for the current chapter.

*Disclosure: Charles B. Berde, his collaborator Dr. Daniel Kohane, and Boston Children's Hospital have licensed the site 1 blocker neosaxitoxin for commercial development and have received milestone payments, with a potential for future milestone payments and royalties.

REFERENCES

1. Drasner K. Local anesthetic systemic toxicity: A historical perspective. *Reg Anesth Pain Med.* 2010;35:162–166.
2. Catterall WA. Voltage-gated sodium channels at 60: Structure, function and pathophysiology. *J Physiol.* 2012;590:2577–2589.
3. Dib-Hajj SD, Cummins TR, Black JA, Waxman SG. Sodium channels in normal and pathological pain. *Annu Rev Neurosci.* 2010;33:325–347.
4. Wang GK, Strichartz GR. State-dependent inhibition of sodium channels by local anesthetics: A 40-year evolution. *Biochem (Mosc) Suppl Ser A Membr Cell Biol.* 2012;6:120–127.
5. Covino BG, Scott DB, Lambert DH. *Handbook of Spinal Anaesthesia and Analgesia.* Philadelphia: WB Saunders; 1994:7.
6. Gissen AJ, Covino BG, Gregus J. Differential sensitivities of mammalian nerve fibers to local anesthetic agents. *Anesthesiology.* 1980;53:467–474.
7. Winnie AP, Tay CH, Patel KP, et al. Pharmacokinetics of local anesthetics during plexus blocks. *Anesth Analg.* 1977;56:852–861.
8. Kirksey MA, Haskins SC, Cheng J, Liu SS. Local anesthetic peripheral nerve block adjuvants for prolongation of analgesia: A systematic qualitative review. *PLoS One.* 2015;10:e0137312.
9. Covino BG, Vassallo HG. *Local Anesthetics: Mechanisms of Action and Clinical Use.* Philadelphia: Grune & Stratton; 1976.
10. Rosenberg PH, Veering BT, Urmey WF. Maximum recommended doses of local anesthetics: A multifactorial concept. *Reg Anesth Pain Med.* 2004;29:564–575 discussion 524.
11. Neal JM, Bernards CM, Butterworth JF, et al. ASRA practice advisory on local anesthetic systemic toxicity. *Reg Anesth Pain Med.* 2010;35:152–161.
12. de Jong RH, Ronfeld RA, DeRosa RA. Cardiovascular effects of convulsant and supraconvulsant doses of amide local anesthetics. *Anesth Analg.* 1982;61:3–9.
13. Weinberg G, Ripper R, Feinstein DL, Hoffman W. Lipid emulsion infusion rescues dogs from bupivacaine-induced cardiac toxicity. *Reg Anesth Pain Med.* 2003;28:198–202.
14. Neal JM, Neal EJ, Weinberg GL. American Society of Regional Anesthesia and Pain Medicine Local Anesthetic Systemic Toxicity checklist: 2020 version. *Reg Anesth Pain Med.* 2021 Jan;46(1):81–82. www.asra.com/content/documents/asra_last_checklist.
15. Lambert LA, Lambert DH, Strichartz GR. Irreversible conduction block in isolated nerve by high concentrations of local anesthetics. *Anesthesiology.* 1994;80:1082–1093.
16. Hodgson PS, Liu SS, Batra MS, et al. Procaine compared with lidocaine for incidence of transient neurologic symptoms. *Reg Anesth Pain Med.* 2000;25:218–222.
17. Freedman JM, Li DK, Drasner K, et al. Transient neurologic symptoms after spinal anesthesia: An epidemiologic study of 1,863 patients. *Anesthesiology.* 1998;89:633–641.
18. Taniguchi M, Bollen AW, Drasner K. Sodium bisulfite: Scapegoat for chloroprocaine neurotoxicity *Anesthesiology.* 2004;100:85–91.
19. Eisenach JC, Schlairet TJ, Dobson 2nd CE, Hood DH. Effect of prior anesthetic solution on epidural morphine analgesia. *Anesth Analg.* 1991;73:119–123.
20. Casati A, Fanelli G, Danelli G, et al. Spinal anesthesia with lidocaine or preservative-free 2-chloroprocaine for outpatient knee arthroscopy: A prospective, randomized, double-blind comparison. *Anesth Analg.* 2007;104:959–964.
21. Drasner K. Local anesthetic neurotoxicity: Clinical injury and strategies that may minimize risk. *Reg Anesth Pain Med.* 2002;27:576–580.
22. Rigler ML, Drasner K. Distribution of catheter-injected local anesthetic in a model of the subarachnoid space. *Anesthesiology.* 1991;75:684–692.
23. Forget P, Borovac JA, Thackeray EM, Pace NL. Transient neurological symptoms (TNS) following spinal anaesthesia with lidocaine versus other local anaesthetics in adult surgical patients: A network meta-analysis. *Cochrane Database Syst Rev.* 2019 Dec 1;12(12):CD003006.
24. Albright GA. Cardiac arrest following regional anesthesia with etidocaine or bupivacaine. *Anesthesiology.* 1979;51:285–287.
25. Clarkson CW, Hondeghem LM. Mechanism for bupivacaine depression of cardiac conduction: Fast block of sodium channels during the action potential with slow recovery from block during diastole. *Anesthesiology.* 1985;62:396–405.
26. Bernards CM, Artu AA. Hexamethonium and midazolam terminate dysrhythmias and hypertension caused by intracerebroventricular bupivacaine in rabbits. *Anesthesiology.* 1991;74:89–96.
27. Qi X, Lai Z, Li S, Liu X, Wang Z, Tan W. The efficacy of lidocaine in laryngospasm prevention in pediatric surgery: A network meta-analysis. *Sci Rep.* 2016;6:32308 Sep 2.
28. Tayeb BO, Eidelman A, Eidelman CL, McNicol ED, Carr DB. Topical anaesthetics for pain control during repair of dermal laceration. *Cochrane Database Syst Rev.* 2017;2(2):CD005364 Feb 22.
29. Shahid S, Florez ID, Mbuagbaw L. Efficacy and safety of EMLA cream for pain control due to venipuncture in infants: A meta-analysis. *Pediatrics.* 2019 Jan;1 43(1):e20181173.
30. Klein JA, Jeske DR. Estimated maximal safe dosages of tumescent lidocaine. *Anesth Analg.* 2016 May;122(5):1350–1359.
31. Weibel S, Jelting Y, Pace NL, et al. Continuous intravenous perioperative lidocaine infusion for postoperative pain and recovery in adults. *Cochrane Database Syst Rev.* 2018 Jun 4;6(6):CD009642.
32. Challapalli V, Tremont-Lukats IW, McNicol ED, Lau J, Carr DB. Systemic administration of local anesthetic agents to relieve neuropathic pain. Cochrane Database Syst Rev. 2019 Oct 7;2019(10).
33. Araujo MC, Sinnott CJ, Strichartz GR. Multiple phases of relief from experimental mechanical allodynia by systemic lidocaine: Responses to early and late infusions. *Pain.* 2003;103:21–29.
34. Fisher D. What if half of your patients moved (or remembered or did something else bad) at incision? *Anesthesiology.* 2007;107:1–2.
35. Tsui BC, Wagner A, Cave D, Kearney R. Thoracic and lumbar epidural analgesia via the caudal approach using electrical stimulation guidance in pediatric patients: A review of 289 patients. *Anesthesiology.* 2004;100:683–689.
36. Taenzer AH, Ct Clark, Kovarik WD. Experience with 724 epidurograms for epidural catheter placement in pediatric children. *Reg Anesth Pain Med.* 2010;35:432–435.
37. Arendt-Nielsen L, Kaalund S, Bjerring P, Hogsaa B. Insufficient effect of local analgesics in Ehlers Danlos type III patients (connective tissue disorder). *Acta Anaesthesiol Scand.* 1990;34:358–361.
38. Cairns BE, Gambarota G, Dunning PS, et al. Activation of peripheral excitatory amino acid receptors decreases the duration of local anesthesia. *Anesthesiology.* 2003;98:521–529.
39. Lee KC, Wilder RT, Smith RL, Berde CB. Thermal hyperalgesia accelerates and MK-801 prevents the development of tachyphylaxis to rat sciatic nerve blockade. *Anesthesiology.* 1994;81:1284–1293.
40. Bromage PR, Pettigrew RT, Crowell DE. Tachyphylaxis in epidural analgesia: I. Augmentation and decay of local anesthesia. *J Clin Pharmacol J New Drugs.* 1969;9:30–38.
41. Lund C, Mogensen T, Hjortso NC, Kehlet H. Systemic morphine enhances spread of sensory analgesia during postoperative epidural bupivacaine infusion. *Lancet.* 1985;2:1156–1157.

42. Liu Q, Gold MS. Opioid-induced loss of local anesthetic potency in the rat sciatic nerve. *Anesthesiology*. 2016;125(4):755–764.

43. Epstein-Barash H, Shichor I, Kwon AH, et al. Prolonged duration local anesthesia with minimal toxicity. *Proc Natl Acad Sci USA*. 2009;106:7125–7130.

44. Wylie MC, Johnson VM, Carpino E, et al. Respiratory, neuromuscular, and cardiovascular effects of neosaxitoxin in isoflurane-anesthetized sheep. *Reg Anesth Pain Med*. 2012;37:152–158.

45. Cullion K, Petishnok LC, Sun T, Santamaria CM, Pemberton GL, McDannold NJ, Kohane DS. Local anesthesia enhanced with increasing high-frequency ultrasound intensity. *Drug Deliv Transl Res*. 2020 Oct;10(5):1507–1516.

46. Hamilton TW, Athanassoglou V, Mellon S, et al. Liposomal bupivacaine infiltration at the surgical site for the management of postoperative pain. *Cochrane Database Syst Rev*. 2017 Feb 1;2(2):CD011419.

47. Ilfeld BM, Eisenach JC, Gabriel RA. Clinical effectiveness of liposomal bupivacaine administered by infiltration or peripheral nerve block to treat postoperative pain. *Anesthesiology*. 2021 Feb 1;134(2):283–344.

48. Hussain N, Brull R, Sheehy B, et al. Perineural liposomal bupivacaine is not superior to nonliposomal bupivacaine for peripheral nerve block analgesia. *Anesthesiology*. 2021 Feb 1;134(2):147–164.

49. Templin JS, Wylie MC, Kim JD, et al. Neosaxitoxin in rat sciatic block: Improved therapeutic index using combinations with bupivacaine, with and without epinephrine. *Anesthesiology*. 2015;123:886–898.

50. Lobo K, Donado C, Cornelissen L, et al. A phase 1, dose-escalation, double-blind, block-randomized, controlled trial of safety and efficacy of neosaxitoxin alone and in combination with 0.2% bupivacaine, with and without epinephrine, for cutaneous anesthesia. *Anesthesiology*. 2015;123:873–885.

51. Binshtok AM, Bean BP, Woolf CJ. Inhibition of nociceptors by TRPV1-mediated entry of impermeant sodium channel blockers. *Nature*. 2007;449:607–610.

52. Relland LM, Beltran R, Kim SS, et al. Continuous epidural chloroprocaine after abdominal surgery is associated with lower postoperative opioid exposure in NICU infants.. *J Pediatr Surg*. 2021. doi:10.1016/j.jpedsurg.2021.05.015. 34154813.

11 NEUROMUSCULAR BLOCKING AND REVERSAL AGENTS

Cynthia A. Lien

INTRODUCTION

Neuromuscular blocking agents (NMBAs) interrupt the usual transmission of nerve impulses at the neuromuscular junction (NMJ) by one of two mechanisms to interfere with neuromuscular transmission and produce paralysis of skeletal muscles. On the basis of differences in their mechanisms of action, these drugs can be classified as depolarizing NMBAs (which mimic the actions of acetylcholine [ACh] at the acetylcholine receptor [AChR]) and nondepolarizing NMBAs (which interfere with the actions of ACh by blocking binding sites on the AChR). Nondepolarizing NMBAs are further subdivided into long-, intermediate-, and short-acting drugs (Table 11.1) based on their duration of action. Succinylcholine (SCh) is the only depolarizing NMBA that is used clinically.

This chapter will describe the choice of NMBA, dosing of NMBAs, monitoring depth of neuromuscular blockade (NMB), and pharmacologic reversal of NMB.

Table 11.1	Classification of Neuromuscular Blocking Agents	
Mechanism of Action	**Neuromuscular Blocking Agent**	**Duration of Action**
Depolarizing	Succinylcholine	Ultrashort-acting
Nondepolarizing	Pancuronium	Long-acting
	Vecuronium	Intermediate-acting
	Rocuronium	Intermediate-acting
	Atracurium	Intermediate-acting
	Cisatracurium	Intermediate-acting
	Mivacurium	Short-acting

Clinical Uses

NMBAs are used of NMBAs in the operating room to facilitate endotracheal intubation and optimize surgical conditions. They may also be administered in other clinical settings to facilitate emergent intubations, and to facilitate mechanical ventilation of intubated patients. NMBAs do not have analgesic or anesthetic effects and should not be used to render an inadequately anesthetized patient immobile. Patient airways must be secured and ventilation supported once an NMBA has been administered and this support continued until muscle strength has returned to baseline (a train-of-four ratio [TOFR] ≥0.9). Intraoperative evaluation of depth of NMB is monitored by the muscular response to stimulation of a peripheral nerve, and the results of monitoring are used to determine whether additional NMB is necessary and how to dose reversal agents.

Choice of Neuromuscular Blocking Agent

The choice of NMBA is influenced by its speed of onset, duration of action, route of elimination, and associated adverse effects. The rapid onset and brief duration of skeletal muscle paralysis, characteristic of SCh-induced NMB, are useful when tracheal intubation is the only reason for administering an NMBA. Although SCh could be given intermittently for shorter procedures, doing so is associated with an increased risk of bradycardia, asystolic cardiac arrest, and prolonged duration of NMB. For intubation and maintenance of NMB, administration of short- or intermediate-acting nondepolarizing NMBAs may be appropriate. The choice of long-, intermediate-, or short-acting agent will depend on the duration of NMB that is necessary and the anticipated means of administration of the NMBA (intermittent boluses or an infusion). The choice of specific NMBA in each of these categories will also depend on availability of the NMBA, the presence of patient comorbidities, and plans for antagonism of residual NMB.

THE NEUROMUSCULAR JUNCTION

The NMJ consists of a prejunctional motor nerve ending separated from the highly folded postjunctional membrane of the skeletal muscle by a synaptic cleft (Fig. 11.1). Nicotinic acetylcholine receptors (nAChRs) are located at prejunctional and postjunctional sites.[1] Neuromuscular transmission is initiated by arrival of an impulse at the motor nerve terminal with an associated influx of calcium ions and subsequent release of the ligand ACh. ACh binds to AChRs (the ligand-gated channel) on the postjunctional muscle membrane, opening the AChR channel and causing a change in membrane permeability to ions through the cell membrane, principally potassium and sodium. This change in permeability and movement of ions causes a decrease in the transmembrane potential from about −90 mV to −45 mV (threshold potential), at which point a propagated action potential spreads over the surfaces of skeletal muscle fibers and leads to muscular contraction. ACh is rapidly hydrolyzed at the NMJ (within 15 ms) by the enzyme acetylcholinesterase (true cholinesterase) (AChE), so that it can no longer bind with the nAChR, restoring membrane permeability (repolarization) and preventing sustained depolarization.

The release of ACh in response to neural stimulation is a calcium-dependent process, resulting in the release of 50 to 100 vesicles containing ACh. The connection between the impulse and depolarization and the rise in intracellular calcium is a voltage-gated calcium channel, which allows for intracellular movement of calcium in response to an electrical current. In response to the increase in intracellular calcium, the ACh-containing synaptic vesicles move to release sites on the nerve terminal membrane. The release of ACh from the synaptic vesicles is mediated by a series of proteins. The protein synapsin anchors the ACh vesicle to the release site of the nerve terminal through the formation of a ternary complex with syntaxin during depolarization and calcium entry. Assembly of the ternary complex forces the vesicle in close apposition to the nerve membrane at the active zone of the nerve terminal with release of its contents, ACh. The fusion is disassembled once the ACh has been released, and the vesicle is recycled.

Small amounts of ACh are released from nerve terminals without a nerve impulse. These result in miniature end-plate potentials (MEPPs). Although not large enough to cause a muscle depolarization, MEPPs are diminished by the administration of nondepolarizing NMBAs and increased by the administration of anticholinesterases.

Synchronized release of ACh from the synaptic vesicles of the nerve terminal in an amount adequate to generate an action potential occurs in response to an electrical impulse. The rapid release of ACh once an impulse arrives at the motor nerve terminal indicates that only those vesicles close to the membrane of the nerve terminal can participate in the process of exocytosis. With repetitive stimulation, vesicles are moved toward the motor nerve terminal for subsequent release, accounting for the post tetanic potentiation observed during NMB.

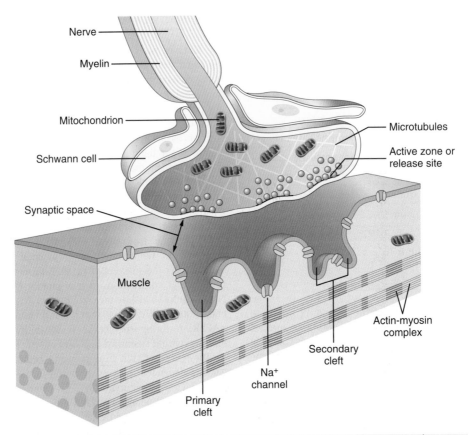

Fig. 11.1 Adult neuromuscular junction with the three cells that constitute the synapse: the motor neuron (i.e., nerve terminal), muscle fiber, and Schwann cell. The motor neuron from the ventral horn of the spinal cord innervates the muscle. Each fiber receives only one synapse. The motor nerve loses its myelin and terminates on the muscle fiber. The nerve terminal, covered by a Schwann cell, has vesicles clustered about the membrane thickenings, which are the active zones, toward its synaptic side and mitochondria and microtubules toward its other side. A synaptic gutter, made up of a primary and many secondary clefts, separates the nerve from the muscle. The muscle surface is corrugated, and dense areas on the shoulders of each fold contain acetylcholine receptors. Sodium channels are present at the clefts and throughout the muscle membrane. (From Martyn JA. Neuromuscular physiology and pharmacology. In: Miller RD, ed. Miller's Anesthesia. 8th ed. Philadelphia, PA: Elsevier Saunders; 2015.)

Not all of the released ACh binds to the AChR of the motor end plate. Most of it is hydrolyzed by AChE at the NMJ. The AChE is anchored to the basal lamina of the postjunctional membrane. Although firmly anchored to the motor end plate region, its catalytic sites have ready access to ACh in the junctional cleft. A different cholinesterase, butyrylcholinesterase, which metabolizes SCh, does not exist in the synaptic cleft of the NMJ.

Prejunctional Receptors and Release of Acetylcholine

Cholinergic receptors are found presynaptically, at the motor nerve terminal, and at the postsynaptic region of the NMJ. The prejunctional receptors are involved in the modulation of the release of ACh into the NMJ. Prejunctional nicotinic receptors are activated by ACh and are believed to function in a positive-feedback control system that serves to maintain the availability of ACh when demand for it is high. They are involved with the mobilization of ACh, but not the actual process of its release.

Presynaptic receptors, aided by calcium, facilitate replenishment of the motor nerve terminal. In addition to being stimulated by ACh, they are stimulated by SCh and neostigmine and depressed by small doses of nondepolarizing NMBAs. Inhibition of these presynaptic nAChRs explains the fade in response to high-frequency repetitive stimulation such as tetanic or even train-of-four (TOF) stimulation.[1]

Postjunctional Receptors

The postjunctional, mature AChR is an intrinsic membrane glycoprotein with five distinct subunits (Fig. 11.2): two α, one β, one δ, and one ε. The α-subunits contain the major portion of the ACh receptor binding site. Each of the subunits contains four helical domains, M1 to M4, that traverse the cell membrane. The ion channel of each subunit has permeability that is equal to that of Na^+ and K^+, allowing for the flow of ions across the cell membrane along their concentration gradients, with Na^+ entering and K^+ leaving the muscle cell. Calcium contributes ≈2.5% to the total permeability. This flow of ions is the basis of normal neuromuscular transmission. There are two distinct pockets for binding of ACh formed by the N and C termini of the protein. One occurs at the intersection of the α to ε subunits and the other at the intersection of the α to δ subunits. These binding sites have different affinities for different NMBAs. Occupation of one or both α-subunits by a nondepolarizing NMBA causes the ion channel to remain closed, in spite of the release of ACh from the prejunctional neuron so that the ion flow to produce depolarization cannot occur. SCh binds to the AChR binding sites and acts as an agonist, causing the ion channel to remain open (mimicking ACh) and resulting in prolonged depolarization. Its duration of action is longer than that of ACh because it remains in the NMJ available to bind to the AChR until it diffuses away from the NMJ, where it is metabolized by butyrylcholinesterase. SCh is not a metabolite for AChE.

Nondepolarizing NMBAs may, in addition to competitively binding to the AChR, inhibit neuromuscular transmission by occluding the AChR channel preventing the normal flow of ions required for subsequent depolarization. NMB secondary to occlusion of channels is resistant to drug-enhanced antagonism with anticholinesterase drugs. The lipid environment around cholinergic receptors can be altered by volatile anesthetics, which change the properties of the ion channels. This may account in part for the augmentation of NMB by volatile anesthetics.

Extrajunctional Receptors

Extrajunctional receptors are different in structure than the postjunctional nAChRs. They retain the two α-subunits but have γ-unit replacing the ε-subunit. Additionally, whereas postjunctional receptors are confined to the area of the end plate of skeletal muscle that is opposite the prejunctional motor neurons (as a component of the motor end plate), extrajunctional receptors are present throughout skeletal muscles. Extrajunctional receptor synthesis is normally suppressed by neural activity. Prolonged inactivity, sepsis, skeletal muscle denervation, burn injury, or trauma may be associated with a proliferation of extrajunctional receptors. When activated, extrajunctional receptors stay open longer and permit more ions to flow across the muscle cell membrane,[2] which in part explains the exaggerated hyperkalemic response when SCh is administered to patients with denervation or burn injury. Proliferation of these receptors also accounts for the resistance or tolerance to nondepolarizing NMBAs, which can be observed in patients with burns or prolonged immobilization.[2,3]

STRUCTURE-ACTIVITY RELATIONSHIPS

NMBAs are quaternary ammonium compounds with at least one positively charged nitrogen atom (Fig. 11.3) that will bind to one or both of the binding sites present on the postsynaptic cholinergic receptors. In addition, these

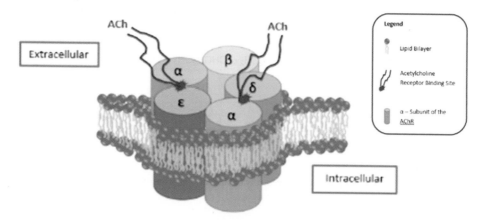

Fig. 11.2 The nicotinic acetylcholine receptor within the lipid bilayer of the postjunctional muscle membrane. The acetylcholine receptor is composed of five subunits: two α, one ε, one δ, and one β. The binding sites for acetylcholine are located at the extracellular portion of the α to ε and α to δ subunits.

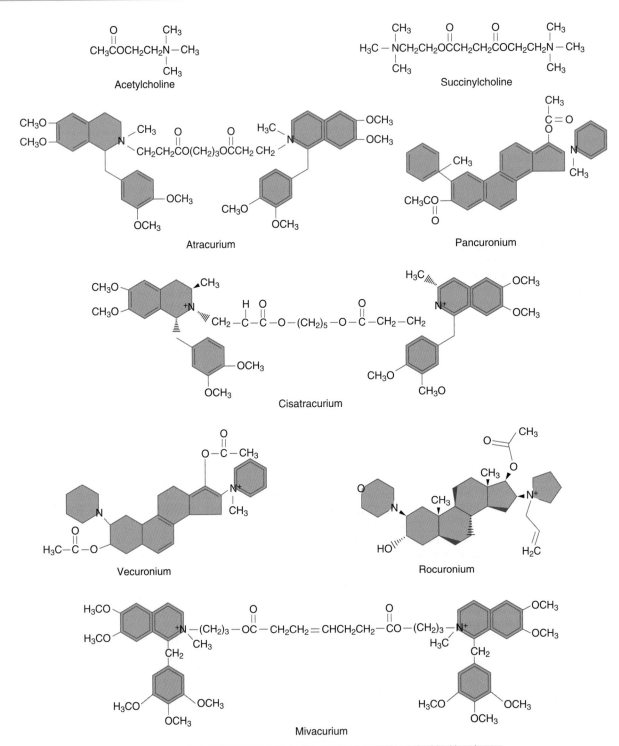

Fig. 11.3 Chemical structure of acetylcholine and neuromuscular blocking drugs.

compounds have structural similarities to the endogenous neurotransmitter ACh. For example, SCh is two molecules of ACh linked by methyl groups. The long, slender, flexible structure of ACh allows it to bind to and activate cholinergic receptors. Although the bulky rigid nondepolarizing NMBAs contain structural elements similar to ACh, they do not activate cholinergic receptors.

Nondepolarizing NMBAs are either aminosteroid compounds (pancuronium, vecuronium, rocuronium) or benzylisoquinolinium compounds (atracurium, cisatracurium, mivacurium). Pancuronium is the bisquaternary aminosteroid NMBA most closely related to ACh structurally. The ACh-like fragments of pancuronium give the steroidal molecule its high degree of neuromuscular blocking activity. Vecuronium and rocuronium are monoquaternary analogs of pancuronium. Their different structures account for the differing means of elimination of the amino steroidal NMBAs and the benzylisoquinolinium NMBAs from the body (Table 11.2).

DEPOLARIZING NEUROMUSCULAR BLOCKING AGENTS: SUCCINYLCHOLINE

Characteristics of Blockade

SCh mimics the action of ACh and produces a sustained depolarization of the postjunctional membrane. Skeletal muscle paralysis occurs because a depolarized postjunctional membrane and inactivated sodium channels cannot respond to subsequent release of ACh. Depolarizing NMB is also referred to as *phase I blockade*. Phase II blockade is present when the postjunctional membrane has become repolarized but still does not respond normally to ACh (desensitization NMB). The mechanism of phase II blockade is unknown but may reflect the development of nonexcitable areas around the end plates that become repolarized but unable to promote the spread of impulses initiated by ACh. With the initial dose of SCh, subtle signs of a phase II blockade begin to appear (fade to tetanic stimulation).[4] Phase II blockade, which resembles the blockade produced by nondepolarizing NMBAs, predominates when the intravenous dose of SCh exceeds 3 to 5 mg/kg.

Pharmacodynamics

SCh is the only depolarizing NMBA used clinically. Its mechanism of action and its relatively rapid metabolism (Fig. 11.4) are responsible for its unique pharmacodynamic properties, which include both a rapid onset and an ultrashort duration of action. Typically, doses of 0.5 to 1.5 mg/kg are administered intravenously to produce a rapid onset of skeletal muscle paralysis (30 to 60 seconds) that lasts 5 to 10 minutes. These pharmacodynamic characteristics are useful in a compound that is administered to facilitate tracheal intubation. SCh has been used clinically for more than 60 years, and despite consistent industrial efforts, no NMBA has been developed that has these pharmacodynamic properties.[5] Although an intravenous dose of 0.5 mg/kg may be adequate, larger doses are commonly administered to facilitate tracheal intubation. If a subparalyzing dose of a nondepolarizing NMBA (pretreatment with 5% to 10% ED_{95}—the dose that, on average, will cause 95% suppression of muscle response to neural stimulation) is administered 2 to 4 minutes before administration of SCh to blunt fasciculations, the dose of SCh should be increased by about 70%. It is important to remember that the administration of even small, precurarizing or defasciculating doses of NMBAs can cause symptomatic muscle weakness and put patients at risk of difficulty breathing or swallowing.

The sustained depolarization produced by the initial administration of SCh is initially manifested as transient generalized skeletal muscle contractions known as *fasciculations*. The sustained opening of sodium channels produced by SCh is associated with leakage of potassium from the interior of cells sufficient to increase plasma

Table 11.2 Elimination of Neuromuscular Blocking Agents

NMBA	Hepatic		Renal	Metabolism	
	Unchanged, Biliary Excretion	Degradation		%	Means of Elimination
Pancuronium	5-10%	10%	80%		
Vecuronium	40-75%	20-30%	15-25%		
Rocuronium	50-70%	10-20%	10-25%		
Atracurium			10-40%	60-90%	Hofmann Elimination, Nonspecific Esterases
Cisatracurium			16%	77%	Hofmann Elimination
Mivacurium			<5%	95-99%	Butyrylcholinesterase

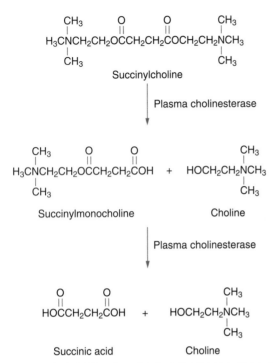

Fig. 11.4 The brief duration of action of succinylcholine is the result of its rapid hydrolysis in plasma by cholinesterase enzyme to inactive metabolites (succinylmonocholine has 1/20 to 1/80 the activity of succinylcholine at the neuromuscular junction).

concentrations of potassium by about 0.1 to 0.4 mEq/L in a healthy patient. In patients with denervation, burns, or trauma, where there is likely to be proliferation of extrajunctional nAChRs and damaged muscle membranes, many more channels will leak potassium, causing hyperkalemia.[2]

Metabolism

Hydrolysis of SCh to inactive metabolites is accomplished by plasma cholinesterase (pseudocholinesterase, butyrylcholinesterase), which is produced in the liver. Plasma cholinesterase has an enormous capacity to hydrolyze SCh at a rate rapid enough that only a small fraction of the original intravenous dose of SCh reaches the NMJ. Because plasma cholinesterase is not present at the NMJ, the NMB produced by SCh is terminated by its diffusion from the NMJ into plasma. Therefore plasma cholinesterase influences the duration of action of SCh by controlling the amount of SCh that is hydrolyzed before it reaches the NMJ. Liver disease must be severe before decreases in the synthesis of plasma cholinesterase are sufficient to prolong the effects of SCh. Anticholinesterases, as used in the treatment of myasthenia gravis, and certain chemotherapeutic drugs (nitrogen mustard, cyclophosphamide) may decrease plasma cholinesterase

activity enough that prolonged skeletal muscle paralysis follows the administration of SCh.

Atypical Plasma Cholinesterase

Atypical plasma cholinesterase lacks the ability to hydrolyze ester bonds in drugs such as SCh and mivacurium. The presence of this atypical enzyme is often recognized only after an otherwise healthy patient experiences prolonged skeletal muscle paralysis (>1 hour) after the administration of a conventional dose of SCh or mivacurium. Subsequent determination of the dibucaine number permits diagnosis of the presence of atypical plasma cholinesterase. Dibucaine is an amide local anesthetic that inhibits normal plasma cholinesterase activity by about 80%, whereas the activity of atypical enzyme is inhibited by only 20% (Table 11.3). The dibucaine number reflects the quality of plasma cholinesterase (ability to metabolize SCh and mivacurium) and not the quantity of enzyme that is circulating in plasma. For example, decreases in plasma cholinesterase activity because of liver disease, advanced age, pregnancy, or treatment with an anticholinesterase are often associated with a normal dibucaine number.

Adverse Side Effects

In spite of its utility in facilitating tracheal intubation, SCh has many adverse effects (Box 11.1). Adverse side effects after the administration of SCh are numerous and may limit or even contraindicate the use of this NMBA in certain patients. SCh should not be given to patients more than 24 hours after major burns, trauma, and extensive denervation of skeletal muscles because it may cause acute hyperkalemia and cardiac arrest.[2] When administered to boys with unrecognized muscular dystrophy, SCh has resulted in acute hyperkalemia and cardiac arrest. Because of this, the U.S. Food and Drug Administration (FDA) issued a warning against the use of SCh in children, except for emergency control of the airway. When administered with volatile anesthetics in susceptible patients it can trigger malignant hyperthermia.[6]

Cardiac Dysrhythmias

Sinus bradycardia, junctional rhythm, and sinus arrest may follow the administration of SCh. These responses are the result of the action of SCh at cardiac postganglionic muscarinic receptors, where this drug mimics the normal effects of ACh. Cardiac dysrhythmias are most likely to occur when a second intravenous dose of SCh is administered within minutes of the first dose. Whereas intravenous administration of atropine 1 to 3 minutes before SCh decreases the likelihood of these cardiac responses, atropine administered intramuscularly with the preoperative medication can cause tachycardia and does not reliably protect against SCh-induced decreases in heart rate.[7]

Table 11.3 Variants of Plasma Cholinesterase and Duration of Action of Succinylcholine (SCh)

Variants of Plasma Cholinesterase	Incidence	Dibucaine Number (% inhibition of enzyme activity)	Duration of SCh-Induced Neuromuscular Blockade (min)
Homozygous, typical	Normal	70-80	5-10
Heterozygous	1/480	50-60	20
Homozygous, atypical	1/3200	20-30	60-180

Box 11.1 Adverse Effects of Succinylcholine

Cardiac dysrhythmias
- Sinus bradycardia
- Junctional rhythm
- Sinus arrest

Fasciculations
Hyperkalemia
Myalgia
Myoglobinuria
Increased intraocular pressure
Increased intragastric pressure
Trismus
Malignant hyperthermia

Hyperkalemia

Administration of SCh can result in rapid development of hyperkalemia, serious cardiac arrythmias, and cardiac arrest.[2] In susceptible patients potassium levels can exceed 10 mEq/L. The classic conditions that lead to hyperkalemia after SCh include burns, trauma, and spinal cord or other major neurologic damage, with the risk of hyperkalemia beginning 24 hours after the injury. The delay in the hyperkalemic response to SCh is because of the time needed for development of extrajunctional, atypical receptors, as previously described.[2,3] When muscle has returned to its normal state, hyperkalemia will not occur. However, the judgment as to the "normal" state of the muscle is a clinically difficult estimation. Extrajunctional receptors and hyperkalemia will also develop in any patient who is immobile (such as critical care patients) for several days if SCh is administered. For example, cardiac arrest has occurred when SCh has been used for emergency endotracheal intubation in the intensive care unit (ICU). The duration of susceptibility to the hyperkalemic effects of SCh is unknown, but the risk is likely decreased several months after denervation injury. All factors considered, it is prudent to avoid administration of SCh to any patient more than 24 hours after a burn injury, extensive trauma, or spinal cord transection.

Even though they may have increased baseline potassium levels, patients with renal failure are not susceptible to an exaggerated release of potassium, and SCh can be administered to these patients.

Myalgia

Postoperative skeletal muscle myalgias, manifested particularly in the muscles of the neck, back, and abdomen, may follow the administration of SCh. Young adults undergoing minor surgical procedures are most likely to report postoperative myalgias. Unsynchronized contractions of skeletal muscle fibers (fasciculations) associated with generalized depolarization lead to myalgia. Prevention of fasciculations by prior administration of subparalyzing doses of a nondepolarizing NMBA (pretreatment) or lidocaine will decrease the incidence of, but will not totally prevent, myalgia.[8] Magnesium will prevent fasciculations but not myalgia. Nonsteroidal antiinflammatory medications are effective in treating the myalgias.

Increased Intraocular Pressure and Increased Intracranial Pressure

SCh causes an increase in intraocular pressure that peaks 2 to 4 minutes after its administration. This increase in intraocular pressure is transient and lasts 5 to 10 minutes.[2] The mechanism by which SCh increases intraocular pressure is unknown, although contraction of extraocular muscles with associated compression of the globe may be involved. The concern that contraction of extraocular muscles could cause extrusion of intraocular contents in the presence of an open eye injury has resulted in the common clinical practice of avoiding the administration of SCh to these patients. This theory has never been substantiated and is challenged by the report of patients with an open eye injury in whom intravenous administration of SCh did not cause extrusion of globe contents. Furthermore, there is evidence that contraction of extraocular muscles does not contribute to the increase in intraocular pressure that accompanies the administration of SCh.[9]

Similarly, increases in intracranial pressure (ICP) after the administration of SCh can occur but have not been reported to be of clinical consequence in patients with intracranial pathology.

Increased Intragastric Pressure

SCh causes unpredictable increases in intragastric pressure, and increases in pressure are not correlated with the dose of SCh administered. When intragastric pressure does increase, it appears to be related to the intensity of fasciculations. Observed increases in sustained intragastric pressure may be large enough to increase the risk of aspiration in patients with compromised lower esophageal sphincter tone.

Trismus

Incomplete jaw relaxation with masseter jaw rigidity after a halothane–SCh induction sequence is not uncommon in children and is considered a normal response. Trismus can occur in adults and has been reported to be severe.[10] In extreme cases this response may be so severe that the ability to mechanically open the patient's mouth is limited. The difficulty lies in separating the normal response to SCh from the masseter rigidity that may be associated with malignant hyperthermia. Because SCh is not recommended for use in children, the occurrence of trismus is decreased in current clinical practice.

NONDEPOLARIZING NEUROMUSCULAR BLOCKING AGENTS

Nondepolarizing NMBAs are classified as long-, intermediate-, and short-acting compounds. These agents act by competing with ACh for binding sites at the α-subunits at the postjunctional nicotinic cholinergic receptors, blocking ACh from binding with the AChRs and preventing changes in ion permeability. As a result, depolarization cannot occur, and skeletal muscle paralysis develops. Differences in onset, duration of action, rate of recovery, metabolism, and clearance influence the clinical decision to select one NMBA or another (Table 11.4).

Pharmacokinetics

Nondepolarizing NMBAs, because of their quaternary ammonium groups, are highly ionized, water-soluble compounds at physiologic pH and possess limited lipid solubility. As a result, these compounds cannot easily cross lipid membrane barriers, such as the blood–brain barrier, renal tubular epithelium, gastrointestinal epithelium, or placenta. Therefore nondepolarizing NMBAs do not produce central nervous system effects, renal tubular reabsorption is minimal, oral administration is ineffective, and maternal administration does not adversely affect the fetus. Redistribution of nondepolarizing NMBAs also exerts a role in the pharmacokinetics of these agents.

Many of the variable pharmacologic responses of patients to nondepolarizing NMBAs can be explained by differences in pharmacokinetics, which are influenced by many factors, such as hypovolemia, hypothermia, and the presence of hepatic or renal disease (or both). Renal and hepatic elimination is aided by access to a large fraction of the administered drug because of the high degree of ionization, which both maintains high plasma concentrations of nondepolarizing NMBAs and prevents renal reabsorption of excreted drug.

Renal disease markedly alters the pharmacokinetics of the long-acting nondepolarizing NMBAs, such as pancuronium. Although a small fraction of vecuronium is eliminated through the kidney, repeated administration of maintenance doses of vecuronium to patients with renal failure results in the prolongation of the duration of action (the time required for the first twitch in the TOF to recover to 25% of its baseline value) after each subsequent dose[11,12] because of redistribution to the liver and decreased elimination. The intermediate- and short-acting NMBAs are also eliminated by the liver (rocuronium), by metabolism by plasma cholinesterase (mivacurium), by Hofmann elimination (atracurium and cisatracurium), or by a combination of these mechanisms.

Pharmacodynamic Responses

NMBAs can be classified on the basis of their underlying structure, their potency as NMBAs, their onset of effect, their duration of action, and their means of elimination from the body (see Tables 11.1, 11.2, and 11.4). When compared on the basis of molar potency (the number of molecules rather than the mass of the molecules), potent

---

Table 11.4 Comparative Pharmacology of Nondepolarizing NMBAs

NMBA	ED$_{95}$ (mg/kg)	Min to Maximal Twitch Depression	Min to Return to ≥25% of Control Twitch Height	Intubating Dose (mg/kg)	Continuous Infusion (mg/kg/min)
Pancuronium	0.07	3–5	60–90	0.1	
Vecuronium	0.05	3–5	20–35	0.08–0.1	1
Rocuronium	0.3	1–2	20–35	0.6–1.2	
Atracurium	0.2	3–5	20–35	0.4–0.5	6–8
Cisatracurium	0.05	4–6	20–35	0.15	1–1.5
Mivacurium	0.08	2–3	12–20	0.25	5–6

NMBAs have a slower onset of effect (Fig. 11.5) than less potent NMBAs, in part because fewer molecules of the NMBA are being administered and there is less of a driving force to move it from the plasma to the NMJ. Other factors that are likely to influence the onset of NMB include protein binding, clearance, the rate of transport between plasma and effect compartment, and molecular mass.[13,14] Onset of potent NMBAs can be shortened by increasing the dose that is administered. This, though, comes with the potential downside of increasing the duration of action of an intermediate-acting NMBA so that it is similar to that of a long-acting NMBA (Fig. 11.6).[15]

Potentiation of NMB by volatile anesthetics results in lower plasma concentrations of nondepolarizing NMBAs being required to produce a given depth of NMB when a volatile anesthetic is being administered. In addition to volatile anesthetics, other medications, such as aminoglycoside antibiotics, local anesthetics, cardiac antiarrhythmic drugs, dantrolene, magnesium, lithium, and tamoxifen, may enhance the NMB produced by nondepolarizing NMBAs. A few medications can diminish the effects of a nondepolarizing NMBA. These medications include calcium, corticosteroids, and anticonvulsant medications. Electrolyte abnormalities can also increase or decrease resistance to NMBAs. Neuromuscular diseases, including myopathies, myasthenic syndrome, Guillain–Barré,

myasthenia gravis, and Duchenne muscular dystrophy, are associated with altered pharmacodynamic responses to NMBAs. Burn injury causes resistance to the effects of nondepolarizing NMBAs, as reflected by the need to establish a higher plasma concentration of drug to achieve the same pharmacologic effect as in patients without a burn injury. There is resistance to the effects of nondepolarizing NMBAs in skeletal muscles affected by a cerebrovascular accident, perhaps reflecting proliferation of extrajunctional receptors that respond to ACh.

Adverse Effects

Cardiovascular Effects

Clinically significant cardiovascular effects are most likely after the administration of long-acting NMBAs. At commonly used doses, they cause drug-induced release of histamine, blockade of cardiac muscarinic receptors, or blockade of nicotinic receptors at the autonomic ganglia. The intermediate- and short-acting NMBAs, atracurium and mivacurium, may cause transient hypotension after the rapid administration of relatively large doses [>0.45 mg/kg ($2.5 \times \mathrm{ED}_{95}$) and 0.2 mg/kg ($2.5 \times \mathrm{ED}_{95}$), respectively].[16,17] The relative magnitude of circulatory effects varies from patient to patient and depends on factors such as underlying autonomic nervous system

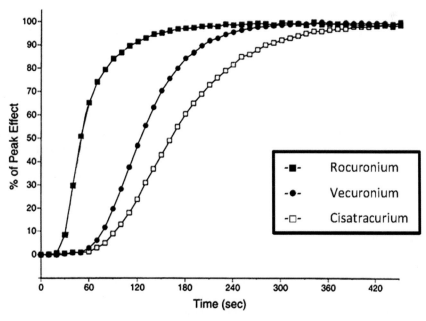

Fig. 11.5 The onset of equipotent doses of cisatracurium, vecuronium, and rocuronium. The percentage of maximal effect of a single ED_{95} dose of cisatracurium (-□-), vecuronium (-●-) or rocuronium (-■-). The percentage of maximal effect at 60 seconds is greatest after the administration of rocuronium, which is the least potent of the NMBAs tested, and least with cisatracurium, which is the most potent of the three NMBAs. (Adapted with permission from Kopman AF, Klewicka MM, Kopman DJ, et al. Molar potency is predictive of the speed of onset of neuromuscular block for agents of intermediate, short, and ultrashort duration. Anesthesiology. 1999;90(2):425–431.[14])

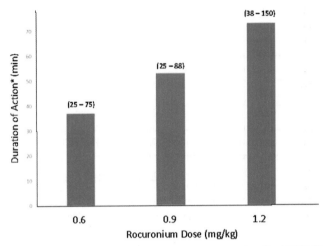

Fig. 11.6 The average duration of action of increasing doses of rocuronium ($2 \times ED_{95}$, $3 \times ED_{95}$, and $4 \times ED_{95}$). The range of values are shown in the () above each bar. As the dose of rocuronium increases, the time required to return to 25% of baseline T1 strength increases and almost doubles with increasing the dose of rocuronium.[31]
*Duration of action: The time (minutes) required to spontaneously recover to 25% of baseline muscle strength after bolus administration of a NMBA.

activity, blood volume status, preoperative medication, medications administered for induction and maintenance of anesthesia, and concurrent medication therapy.

Critical Illness Myopathy and Polyneuropathy

NMBAs are not used as often in the ICU as they had been in the past. The most common uses of NMBAs in this setting include facilitation of intubation, mechanical ventilation in patients with acute respiratory failure, and avoidance of coughing in patients with increased ICP. Patients with asthma (receiving corticosteroids) or acutely injured patients with multiple organ system failure (including sepsis) who require mechanical ventilation of the lungs for prolonged periods may develop prolonged weakness.[18] These patients exhibit moderate to severe quadriparesis with or without areflexia. The time course of the weakness is unpredictable, and in some patients the weakness may progress and persist for weeks or months. The risks and benefits of NMBAs in critically ill individuals should be considered when deciding on their use (also see Chapter 41). Use of NMBAs during mechanical ventilation may decrease barotrauma risk, but ventilator support of spontaneous ventilation improves matching of ventilation and perfusion.[19] NMBAs have also been associated with exacerbation of mechanical ventilation–induced diaphragmatic dysfunction.[20] Although myopathy can occur in critically ill patients who are not receiving NMBAs, their administration can augment the severity of this condition.

Hypersensitivity Reactions

The overall incidence of life-threatening anesthetic-related hypersensitivity reactions varies widely between countries and ranges from between 1/10,000 and 1/20,000.

Although hypersensitivity refers to the constellation of symptoms related to an immune-type response, the Sampson Criteria[21] provided a description of the distinct criteria to be used in diagnosing anaphylaxis. Since its redefinition in 2006, all immunoglobulin E (IgE)–mediated and non-IgE-mediated reactions are considered anaphylactic reactions.[22] The reported severity of anaphylactic reactions varies greatly. Patients in the operating room may not be able to describe the cutaneous symptoms, such as itching, which can affect the interpretation and grading of severity of a reaction.[23] A three-point grading system developed by Rose and colleagues[24] is useful for intraoperative diagnosis of anaphylaxis and initiating treatment (Table 11.5).

Recognition of anaphylaxis-inducing mediators is important to prevent unnecessary exposure to allergens during an anesthetic. Skin-prick testing and intradermal testing remain the gold standard for allergen testing. Testing should wait 4 to 6 weeks after an allergic reaction to avoid a false-negative response.

Perioperative hypersensitivity-related reactions and anaphylaxis are rare but serious events, and aminosteroidal NMBAs are the most common cause of intraoperative anaphylaxis in most countries. Antibiotics are the second most common cause of anaphylaxis in the United States,[25] France,[26] and Western Australia.[27] Anaphylaxis caused by aminosteroidal NMBAs is likely related to its quaternary ammonium structure.[28,29] Women are 2.5 times more likely than men to have an anaphylactic reaction to aminosteroidal NMBAs.[25] Their higher incidence of anaphylaxis may be the result of either chronic skin sensitization caused by allergenic amines in cosmetics or to hormonal changes during puberty. Overall, anaphylaxis to steroidal

NMBAs occurs in approximately 1 in 2500 individuals receiving either vecuronium or rocuronium.[30]

Effective treatment of a life-threatening hypersensitivity reaction requires early recognition and immediate therapy, including CPR and epinephrine.

Long-Acting Nondepolarizing Neuromuscular Blocking Agent: Pancuronium

Pancuronium (see Fig. 11.3) is a bisquaternary aminosteroid nondepolarizing NMBA with an ED_{95} of 70 µg/kg; it has an onset of action of 3 to 5 minutes and a duration of action of 60 to 90 minutes. An estimated 80% of a single dose of pancuronium is eliminated unchanged in urine. In the presence of renal failure, plasma clearance of pancuronium is decreased 30% to 50%, resulting in a prolonged duration of action. An estimated 10% to 40% of pancuronium undergoes hepatic deacetylation to inactive metabolites, with the exception of 3-desacetylpancuronium, which has neuromuscular blocking activity and is approximately 50% as potent as pancuronium.

Pancuronium typically produces a 10% to 15% increase in heart rate, mean arterial pressure, and cardiac output after administration of an intubating dose $(1.4 \times ED_{95})$. The increase in heart rate reflects pancuronium-induced selective blockade of cardiac muscarinic receptors, principally in the sinoatrial node.

Intermediate-Acting Nondepolarizing Neuromuscular Blocking Agents

Rocuronium, vecuronium, atracurium, and cisatracurium are classified as nondepolarizing NMBAs with an intermediate duration of action. In contrast to the long-acting pancuronium, these agents are cleared from the body more rapidly, allowing them to have a shorter duration of action.

When compared with pancuronium, these NMBAs have (1) approximately one-third the duration of action, (2) a 30% to 50% more rapid clearance, and (3) minimal to no cardiovascular effects. Neostigmine or sugammadex antagonism of residual NMB produced by intermediate-acting nondepolarizing NMBAs is facilitated by the concomitant spontaneous recovery that occurs because of the rapid clearance of the NMBAs.

Vecuronium

Vecuronium (see Fig. 11.3) is a monoquaternary aminosteroid nondepolarizing NMBA with an ED_{95} of 50 µg/kg that has an onset of action of 3 to 5 minutes and a duration of action of 20 to 35 minutes. This NMBA undergoes both hepatic and renal excretion. Metabolites are largely pharmacologically inactive, with the exception of 3-desacetylvecuronium, which is approximately 50% to 70% as potent as its parent compound, vecuronium, and has a longer duration of action than vecuronium. The increased lipid solubility of vecuronium as compared with pancuronium also facilitates its biliary excretion. The effect of renal failure on the duration of action of vecuronium is small, but repeated or large doses may result in prolonged NMB. Vecuronium does not cause adverse circulatory effects.

Rocuronium

Rocuronium (see Fig. 11.3) is a monoquaternary aminosteroid nondepolarizing NMBA with an ED_{95} of 0.3 mg/kg that has an onset of action of 1 to 2 minutes and a duration of action of 20 to 35 minutes. The lack of potency of rocuronium in comparison with vecuronium is an important factor in its rapid onset of effect. As noted previously, when a large number of molecules are administered, the result is a larger number of molecules that are available to

Table 11.5 Perioperative Anaphylaxis Grading System

Grade	Definition	Clinical Findings
A	Moderate	Measurable derangements in one of more major organ systems; non–life-threatening Cardiovascular: hypotension, tachycardia or bradycardia, arrhythmia Respiratory: cough, wheeze, difficult ventilation, oxygen desaturation, difficulty swallowing, rhinorrhea Other: change in LOC, agitation, GI upset
B	Life-threatening	Cardiovascular and/or respiratory derangement that is life-threatening Cardiovascular: systolic blood pressure <60 mm Hg, life-threatening tachyarrhythmia or bradyarrhythmia Respiratory: oxygen saturation <90%, inspiratory pressures >40 cm H_2O, severe difficulty inflating the lungs, airway angioedema
C	Cardiac arrest with or without respiratory arrest	Cardiac and/or respiratory arrest Cardiovascular: cardiac arrest Respiratory: respiratory arrest or complete failure of ventilation

GI, Gastrointestinal; *LOC*, loss of consciousness.

diffuse to the NMJ. Thus a rapid onset of action is more likely to be achieved with a less potent compound, such as rocuronium. The onset of maximum single-twitch depression after the administration of rocuronium, $4 \times ED_{95}$ (1.2 mg/kg), resembles the onset of action of SCh after the administration of 1 mg/kg (Fig. 11.7).[15] However, the large doses of rocuronium (3 to $4 \times ED_{95}$) needed to mimic the onset time of SCh produces a substantially longer duration of action, resembling that of pancuronium (see Fig. 11.6).[31]

Clearance of rocuronium is largely as an unchanged drug in bile; deacetylation does not occur. Renal excretion of the drug may account for as much as 30% of a dose, and administration of this drug to patients in renal failure could result in a longer duration of action, especially with repeated doses or prolonged intravenous infusion.

Atracurium

Atracurium (see Fig. 11.3) is a bisquaternary benzylisoquinolinium nondepolarizing NMBA that consists of a mixture of 10 stereoisomers. It has an ED_{95} of 0.2 mg/kg and an onset of action of 3 to 5 minutes. Like other intermediate-acting NMBAs, its duration of action is 20 to 35 minutes. This NMBA is cleared by Hofmann elimination, which is a chemical process of spontaneous, nonenzymatic degradation at normal body temperature and pH. It is also eliminated through hydrolysis by nonspecific plasma esterases, which are different than the plasma cholinesterase that metabolizes SCh and mivacurium, and AChE, which metabolizes ACh. Laudanosine is the major metabolite of both Hofmann degradation and ester hydrolysis. The two routes of metabolism occur simultaneously and are independent of hepatic and renal function. As such, the duration of atracurium-induced NMB is similar in healthy patients and those with absent or impaired renal or hepatic function. Ester hydrolysis accounts for an estimated two-thirds of degraded atracurium. Hofmann elimination accounts for the remaining breakdown of atracurium.

In large doses atracurium can, especially with rapid bolus administration, cause histamine release resulting in transient hypotension and tachycardia. Doses smaller than $2 \times ED_{95}$ rarely cause histamine release.

Cisatracurium

Cisatracurium is one of the 10 stereoisomers comprising atracurium and, as such, is a benzylisoquinolinium nondepolarizing NMBA. It has an ED_{95} of 50 µg/kg and an onset of action of 7 and 5 minutes after administration of either $1 \times ED_{95}$ or $2 \times ED_{95}$, respectively (reflective of its greater potency). Like atracurium, it has an intermediate duration of action. Cisatracurium is primarily degraded by a spontaneous chemical process—Hofmann elimination. In contrast to atracurium, nonspecific plasma esterases are not involved in its clearance. Because of the organ-independent clearance of cisatracurium, it can, like atracurium, be administered to patients with renal or hepatic failure or advanced age without a change in its duration of action. Cisatracurium is often used in patients undergoing renal transplantation. In contrast to atracurium, cisatracurium does not cause histamine release, so administration of large doses, as are frequently used to

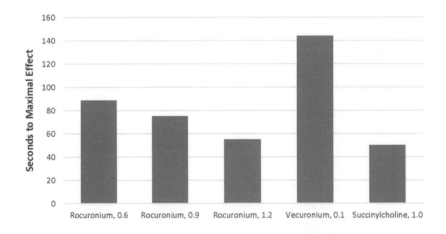

Fig. 11.7 The average onset of maximal effect of increasing doses of rocuronium compared with vecuronium 0.1 mg/kg and succinylcholine 1.0 mg/kg. $2 \times ED_{95}$ of rocuronium has a faster onset of effect than an equipotent dose of vecuronium, likely because of its lesser potency as an NMBA. Increasing the dose of rocuronium to 1.2 mg/kg, or $4 \times ED_{95}$, shortens its onset to 100% NMB to, on average, less than 60 seconds, comparable to succinylcholine 1 mg/kg.[31]

shorten its onset of effect, is free of adverse cardiovascular effects.

Short-Acting Nondepolarizing Neuromuscular Blocking Agent: Mivacurium

Mivacurium (see Fig. 11.3) is a benzylisoquinolinium nondepolarizing NMBA with an ED_{95} of 80 µg/kg that has an onset of action of 2 to 3 minutes and a duration of action of 15 minutes. The duration of action of mivacurium is approximately twice that of SCh and 30% to 40% that of the intermediate-acting nondepolarizing NMBAs. Mivacurium consists of a mixture of three stereoisomers (a *cis-trans*, a *trans-trans*, and a *cis-cis* isomer), and the two most active isomers are hydrolyzed by plasma cholinesterase at a rate equivalent to 88% that of SCh. Hydrolysis of these two isomers is responsible for the short duration of action of mivacurium. The *cis-cis* isomer comprises only a small fraction of the mixture of isomers (~5%), is a relatively impotent NMBA, and has an intermediate duration of action. Because it is metabolized by plasma cholinesterase, the clearance of mivacurium is decreased and its duration of action is increased in patients with atypical plasma cholinesterase. Mivacurium disappeared from the U.S. market in 2006 and was reintroduced in 2016.

Because of its short duration of action, mivacurium would be an appropriate NMBA for short surgical procedures. If used for longer procedures, it should be administered as an infusion.

Like atracurium, rapid administration of large doses of mivacurium can cause histamine release, resulting in transient hypotension and tachycardia.

MONITORING THE EFFECTS OF NONDEPOLARIZING NEUROMUSCULAR BLOCKING AGENTS

Routine monitoring of the depth of NMB and adequacy of recovery of neuromuscular function is both recommended by all experts in the field and supported by large multicenter trials. Monitoring provides a necessary guide for NMBA requirements intraoperatively and for the effective antagonism of residual NMB by either neostigmine or sugammadex. In spite of its import, monitoring of the depth of NMB is not routine when NMBAs are administered as part of a general anesthetic. Surveys have found that only 30% to 70% of anesthesiologists in the United States, Australia, and Europe monitor depth of paralysis when an NMBA is administered.[32,33]

Mechanically evoked responses used for monitoring the effects of NMBAs include the single-twitch response, TOF ratio, double burst stimulation, and post tetanic stimulation. The response to peripheral nerve stimulation should be used to answer the following questions: (1) Is the depth of NMB adequate for surgery? (2) Is the depth of NMB excessive? (3) Can the NMB be antagonized?

Adequate recovery of muscle strength is defined as a TOF ratio (TOFR), measured at the adductor pollicis, of 0.9 (90%). When there are four responses to TOF stimulation, the strength of the fourth response is compared with the strength of the first response to determine the TOFR (Fig. 11.8). In volunteers even a TOFR <0.9 is associated with impaired ability to swallow, increased incidence of aspiration,[34] and decreased hypoxic drive to breathe[35]; facial weakness; diplopia[36]; and in patients, decreased patient satisfaction with their postoperative experience, increased respiratory complications, and death.[37,38]

When monitoring return of muscle strength, either clinically (with tests such as a head lift or grip strength) or with qualitative monitoring of depth of neuromuscular block (through either visual or tactile assessment of the muscle response to a TOF stimulus), it is impossible to tell when a patient is strong enough for safe tracheal extubation.[39] Clinical monitoring of muscle strength is, at best, inadequate. Tidal volume is generated by the diaphragm, which is resistant to NMB, and patients can generate a tidal volume of 300 mL even when profoundly paralyzed. To paralyze the diaphragm, patients must have a profound level of NMB and a post tetanic count of 3 to 5 (Fig. 11.9).[40] At this depth of NMB, a patient would have no respone to TOF stimulation at the adductor pollicis. Similarly, the results of clinical tests of muscle strength can be misleading. A 5-second head lift, a 5-second leg lift, and a strong and sustained hand grip can each be performed over a relatively wide range of TOFRs, and unanesthetized volunteers can accomplish these tasks with a TOFR as low as 0.50.[36]

When it is monitored, depth of NMB is most commonly assessed qualitatively; that is, a nerve stimulator is used to apply a stimulus to a superficial nerve, and the response of the muscle it innervates to that stimulation is "measured" either tactilely or visually. In assessing the TOFR qualitatively the number of responses to stimulation is determined (Fig. 11.10), and when there are four responses, the strength of the fourth response relative to the first is determined (Fig. 11.8). TOF stimulation (four electrical stimulations at 2 Hz delivered every 0.5 second) is delivered through superficial electrodes placed over the course of the ulnar nerve most commonly, and the response of the adductor pollicis to stimulation is determined. The rationale for the use of TOF stimulation is based on the concept that ACh is depleted by successive stimulations. Generally, during a balanced anesthetic, two to four responses to TOF stimulation (Fig. 11.10) are maintained, with repeated boluses of NMBA; recovery of muscle strength is monitored through an increase in the strength of the fourth response to stimulation relative to the first (Figs. 11.8 and 11.11). Clinicians cannot, regardless of their level of expertise, reliably detect anything less than 60% fade in the TOFR. Even with a TOFR of

0.4,[36] the four responses to ulnar nerve stimulation may look and feel as if they are all the same (Fig. 11.8); the fourth response will more reliably appear weaker only once the TOFR is <0.4.[39] Difficulty in estimating the TOFR may be caused by the fact that the two middle twitch responses interfere with comparison of the first and last twitch response.

Although it will not provide information about whether or not recovery of muscle strength is complete, simply counting the number of responses to TOF stimulation is likely to be reproducible and will provide information about how reversal agents should be dosed. Counting the number of visible TOF responses may be helpful in predicting the ease with which NMB can be antagonized with an anticholinesterase drug, and recommendations for specific doses of reversal agents based on the response to TOF count have been made (Fig. 11.12).[41]

Double burst stimulation of the ulnar nerve may improve the clinician's ability to detect more subtle degrees of neuromuscular block. It allows detection of 40% fade between the first and the second response (the equivalent of a TOFR of 0.6). Double burst stimulation (two bursts of three electrical stimulations separated by 750 ms) is perceived by the observer as two separate twitches (Fig. 11.13), eliminating some of the challenges in interpreting the TOFR. The observer's ability to detect a TOFR less than 0.4 is improved with double burst stimulation, but the ability to conclude that the TOF ratio is greater than 0.9, or even 0.7, is still not ensured.

Profound paralysis that is too deep to be measured by TOF stimulation can be assessed by the post tetanic count. This depth of block is observed after administration of an intubating dose of NMBA, where the TOF count is zero. Applying a tetanic stimulus (50 Hz for 5 seconds) and observing the response to single twitch at 1 Hz that is begun 3 seconds after the tetanic stimulation allows for these profound depths of NMB to be quantified (Fig. 11.9). For the intermediate-acting NMBAs, once the number of post tetanic responses is 3, the first twitch in the TOF will appear in approximately 10 minutes, and once the post tetanic response is 10, the first response to TOF stimulation should reappear in 1 to 2 minutes.[42] This information is valuable when maintaining a profound level of NMB for a surgery, such as an airway procedure, when patient movement or coughing can be detrimental. In these situations it is important to gauge spontaneous recovery of neuromuscular strength in order to anticipate when to administer and how to dose the reversal agent.

Because of their lack of sensitivity, the use of qualitative monitors of NMB (those monitors to which response to TOF stimulation has to be assessed by the clinician) does not eliminate the possibility of extubating patients before adequate recovery of muscle strength.

The only way to confirm complete recovery of neuromuscular function is with a quantitative monitor. Quantitative monitors stimulate the ulnar nerve and then interpret the response to TOF stimulation and provide a display of the measured response, eliminating the

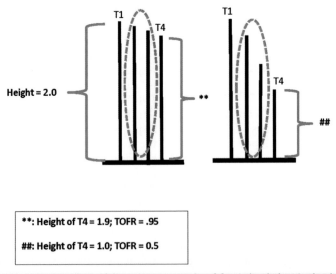

**: Height of T4 = 1.9; TOFR = .95

##: Height of T4 = 1.0; TOFR = 0.5

Fig. 11.8 Graphic representations of the response to train-of-four stimulation. In the depiction in the left-hand panel, the train-of-four ratio = 0.95 (the fourth response [T4] is 95% of the first response [T1]). In the panel on the right side of the diagram the TOFR = 0.5, T4/T1 = 0.5. In both of these situations the clinician is likely to interpret the response, either by touch or by sight, as being the same. Fade is not reliably detectable given this degree of NMB with TOF monitoring because the second and third responses (T2 and T3, respectively) confuse interpretation of the ratio.

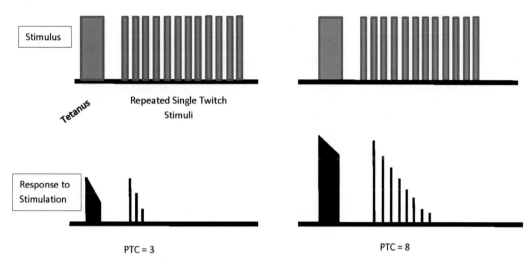

Fig. 11.9 Examples of two different responses to post tetanic stimulation. In each example as indicated in the top portion of the panel, a 50 Hz stimulus is applied for 5 seconds followed by a series of single twitches at 1 Hz beginning 3 seconds after the tetanic stimulus. Responses to the stimulation are shown in the bottom portion of the diagram. On the left-hand side of the figure, there are three responses to the post tetanic stimulus. On the right-hand side of the diagram, the depth of paralysis is less but still relatively profound; there are eight responses to post tetanic stimulation.

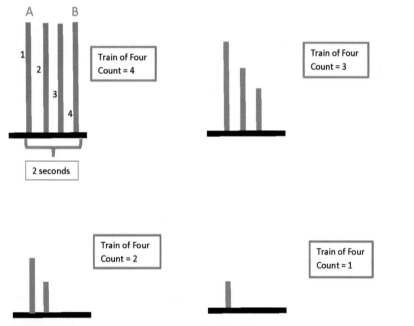

Fig. 11.10 Different responses to train-of-four stimulation, as commonly used to determine degree of neuromuscular blockade during anesthesia. A train-of-four stimulus is a series of four stimuli delivered over 2 seconds at a frequency of 2 Hz. Clinicians cannot reliably determine the degree of fade between the first and the fourth response (the train-of-four ratio). They can, though, more reliably count the number of responses to stimulation and on the basis of the response determine either the need for more NMBA or the dose of reversal agent to administer. With profound levels of neuromuscular block, there is no response to TOF stimulation. As recovery of neuromuscular function occurs after an intubating dose of NMBA, one response to TOF stimulation appears, then two, then three, and finally four. As recovery continues, the fourth response becomes as strong as the first response, T4 = T1 and the TOFR = 1.0. Typically two to three twitches in response to TOF stimulation are maintained intraoperatively through administration of small maintenance doses of NMBA. See the text for additional detail.

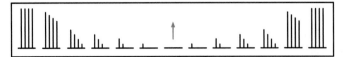

Fig. 11.11 Stylized graphic representation of the onset of neuromuscular blockade and recovery of neuromuscular function as documented with repetitive train-of-four stimuli. The train-of-four stimulus consists of four supramaximal stimuli separated by 0.5 second administered to a superficially located neural unit, such as the ulnar nerve, and the muscular response that it causes in the adductor pollicis. In the patient with no neuromuscular blockade there are four equal responses to stimulation. As neuromuscular blockade becomes more profound, the strength of those responses diminishes and the number of responses falls off to three, then two, and then one response. Recovery of neuromuscular function is indicated by the ↑ in the diagram. The train-of-four ratio (TOFR) is determined by the strength of the fourth response relative to the first response. A patient is considered to have recovered enough muscle strength when their TOFR is ≥0.9.

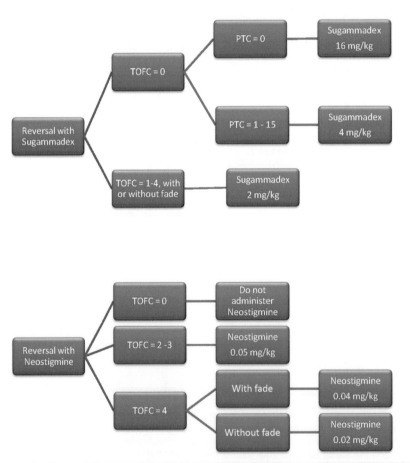

Fig. 11.12 Dosing of reversal agents based on the train-of-four count—when only a qualitative monitor is available to determine the depth of NMB or when qualitative monitoring is unreliable. (See Ref. 41 and package insert for sugammadex.)

need for the clinician to estimate the TOFR. Four types of quantitative monitors have been described: mechanomyography (MMG), kinemyography (KMG), acceleromyography (AMG), and electromyography (EMG) (Fig. 11.14). MMG had been the gold standard for monitoring and measures the strength of response to stimulation. Its setup, though, is cumbersome and the equipment required, complex. Acceleromyographs are available for use in the clinical setting. These devices monitor the acceleration of the thumb as it responds to ulnar nerve stimulation. Although the setup is less cumbersome, the results can be variable, with the AMG overinterpreting recovery of neuromuscular function (TOF response is greater than it would have been with an MMG).[43] In addition, the thumb must be able to move freely in response to stimulation of the ulnar nerve. Similarly, KMG requires movement of the thumb to gauge muscle strength. It measures the bending of a mechanosensory strip placed between the thumb and the index finger in response to stimulation of the ulnar nerve. As with AMG, the KMG will overinterpret the degree of recovery of muscle strength. EMG, the oldest of the monitoring modalities, is different than MMG, AMG, or KMG in that it does not measure movement in response to stimulation. EMG measures the action potential generated by stimulation of the nerve. The results of EMG monitoring are most consistent with those obtained with MMG monitoring and do not overestimate recovery of neuromuscular function.[43]

All recommendations for dosing of neuromuscular blocking and reversal agents are based on the response of the adductor pollicis to TOF stimulation of the ulnar nerve. Although the adductor pollicis is not always readily accessible intraoperatively, the potency of all NMBAs is determined by the response of this neuromuscular unit to stimulation. Sensitivity to the effects of NMBAs is different in different muscles.[44] The more centrally located muscles, such as the diaphragm and the orbicularis oculi, are resistant to the NMB caused by nondepolarizing NMBAs. Although onset of NMBA occurs more quickly in these muscles, the depth of NMB that results from a single dose of NMBA is not as profound as it is in the adductor pollicis (Fig. 11.15). Additionally, recovery of muscle strength occurs more slowly in the adductor pollicis than it does in the orbicularis oculi or diaphragm. Because of the different response of muscles to NMBAs, dosing based on the result of the orbicularis oculi will result in overdosing of NMBAs and overestimation of the degree of recovery and, as a result, increases the incidence of postoperative residual NMB in the postanesthesia care unit (PACU).[45]

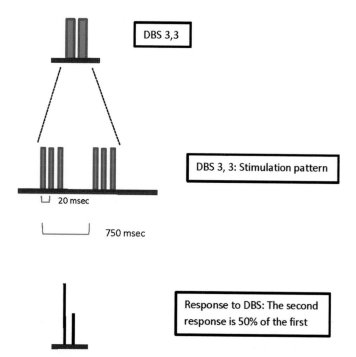

Fig. 11.13 Schematic illustration of the pattern of double burst stimulation (DBS; three electrical impulses at 50 Hz separated by 750 ms). Monitoring with DBS, when compared with TOF stimulation, allows for a small increase in sensitivity to detect residual neuromuscular blockade. Fade in the second when compared with the first response will be reliably detected once there is 40% fade (a TOFR = 0.6). In this figure the second response is 50% of the first response and would feel diminished when compared with the first.

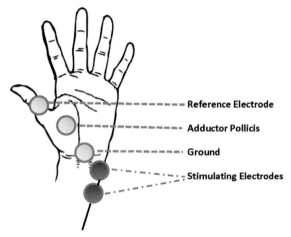

Fig. 11.14 Monitoring the EMG in response to ulnar nerve stimulation. The stimulating electrodes are placed over the course of the ulnar, with the negative one being the more distal. To monitor the EMG of the adductor pollicis, three electrodes are placed over the palm of the hand, as indicated in the figure, with the ground being close to the crease of the wrist, the reference electrode being over the thumb, and the third electrode over the belly of the adductor pollicis muscle.

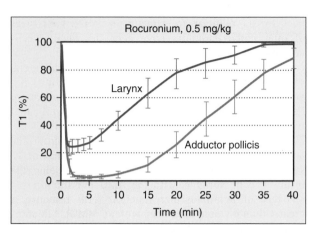

Fig. 11.15 The maximal depression of the response to neuromuscular stimulation (as determined by % suppression of T1) at the larynx and the adductor pollicis after administration of 0.5 mg/kg rocuronium. Maximal effect of NMB is observed more quickly in the larynx and is less intense than what is observed at the adductor pollicis. Recovery occurs more slowly in the adductor pollicis than it does in the larynx. All dosing recommendations for neuromuscular blocking and their reversal agents are based on the response of the adductor pollicis to ulnar nerve stimulation. (From Meistelman C, Plaud B, Donati F. Rocuronium [ORG 9426] neuromuscular blockade at the adductor muscles of the larynx and adductor pollicis in humans. Can J Anaesth. 1992;39:665–669, used with permission.)

No matter which type of peripheral nerve stimulator is used, clinical care will be improved if monitoring is employed. Despite the presence of studies designed to establish the relative efficacy of different types of monitors, the specific monitor is of secondary importance. Nevertheless, understanding of the various types of monitoring modalities used is important when NMB is part of a general anesthetic.

ANTAGONISM OF RESIDUAL NEUROMUSCULAR BLOCK

The time starting with the extubation of the trachea, transport to the PACU, and the first 30 minutes in the PACU can be among the most dangerous times in the perioperative period. Inadequately antagonized or residual NMB can impair the integrity of the airway and cause critical respiratory events in the PACU.[38] Residual NMB is usually a component of adverse outcomes and even death. Specifically, residual NMB contributes to airway obstruction, inadequate ventilation, and hypoxia and occurs with an incidence of 0.8% to 6.9%.[38] Other factors contributing to adverse effects in the PACU include obesity, opioids, emergency surgery, long duration of surgery, and abdominal surgery. It is important to assure that residual NMB does not persist into the postoperative period by careful monitoring.[46] Close observation and awareness of the likelihood of residual NMB will facilitate its diagnosis and management.

There is significant variation in antagonism of residual NMB. In contrast to most European countries, where routine antagonism is not the typical practice, the majority of anesthesiologists in the United States antagonize the residual effects of nondepolarizing NMBAs at the end of surgery.[33] Routine antagonism of neuromuscular block is recommended by some anesthesiologists to ensure complete recovery in all patients, regardless of whether depth of block was monitored objectively. This practice, however, is not without risk, as unnecessary administration of reversal agents is associated with adverse effects.

To effectively enhance recovery of neuromuscular function, the ACh concentration at the NMJ needs to be increased or the plasma concentrations of the NMBA at the NMJ need to be decreased (Fig. 11.16). For the available NMBAs, pharmacologic options for reversal include increasing ACH at the NMJ by inhibiting AChE with neostigmine or encapsulating the NMBA with sugammadex in the plasma, so that it cannot enter the NMJ.

Anticholinesterases

Neostigmine, an anticholinesterase used for reversal of NMB, inhibits AChE at the NMJ, which increases the concentration of ACh at the motor end plate. Increased amounts of ACh in the NMJ improve the chance that two ACh molecules will bind to the α-subunits of the nicotinic cholinergic receptors (Figs. 11.2 and 11.16). This action alters the balance of the competition between ACh and a nondepolarizing NMBA in favor of the neurotransmitter (ACh) and restores neuromuscular transmission. In addition, neostigmine may generate antidromic action potentials and repetitive firing of motor nerve endings (presynaptic effects).

Determinants of Speed and Adequacy of Recovery

During anticholinesterase-facilitated antagonism, recovery of neuromuscular transmission is the function of primarily two processes: ongoing spontaneous recovery of neuromuscular function as the NMBA concentration at the NMJ decreases, and increasing ACh at the NMJ after administration of the anticholinesterase. Antagonism of nondepolarizing neuromuscular block with anticholinesterases requires a variable amount of time that depends on several factors. Time from administration to peak effect varies with presynaptic ACh reserve, in addition to the degree of spontaneous rate of recovery from NMB. A number of clinical factors may render reversal of NMB more difficult (Box 11.2). Anticholinesterases should be administered only once spontaneous recovery of neuromuscular function has begun. It takes longer to antagonize profound neuromuscular block than it does moderate or shallow neuromuscular block. Anticholinesterase-facilitated recovery from an intermediate-acting NMBA occurs more quickly than that induced with a long-acting compound. Speed of recovery also depends on the anticholinesterase used for reversal. Recovery from a moderate depth of block occurs more quickly after the administration of edrophonium than neostigmine.

There is a limit to what an anticholinesterase can effectively antagonize; profound NMB cannot be reversed. Once the maximum dose of neostigmine has been administered, AChE has been maximally inhibited, and administration of additional anticholinesterase will not produce greater recovery from residual NMB.[47]

Adverse Effects

The effects of anticholinesterases are not limited to the motor end plate. Administration of these compounds also increases acetylcholine at other sites, and their effects are more widespread than just the NMJ. The muscarinic and nAChRs in the parasympathetic system can be activated by administration of an anticholinesterase, causing pronounced vagal effects such as bradycardia, prolonged QT interval, and asystole. Other muscarinic parasympathetic side effects include bronchospasm, increased bronchial and pharyngeal secretions, miosis, and increased intestinal tone. Because of these parasympathetic side effects, anticholinesterases are typically administered in combination with antimuscarinic drugs, such as glycopyrrolate or atropine. These compounds block muscarinic, but not nicotinic, receptors so that neuromuscular block can be antagonized while muscarinic effects are minimized.

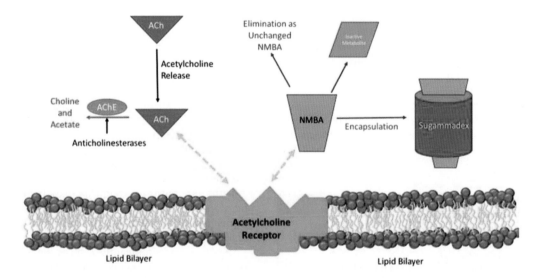

Fig. 11.16 Schematic representation of the molecular mechanisms of neuromuscular blockade and its reversal. In a very simplistic way acetylcholine competes with the NMBA for binding sites on the acetylcholine receptor. To overcome neuromuscular block, acetylcholine concentration can be increased by blocking the activity of acetylcholinesterase with an anticholinesterase (neostigmine). At the same time, the quantity of NMBA at the NMJ is decreased as the NMBA diffuses away from the NMJ and is eliminated from the body, metabolized, or encapsulated with a selective relaxant binding agent (sugammadex).

Antimuscarinic compounds increase the risk of tachyarrhythmias and other effects of antagonism of muscarinic receptors, such as urinary retention, blurred vision, photophobia, mydriasis, xerostomia, dry skin, constipation, nausea, urinary retention, insomnia, and dizziness.

Neostigmine can also block AChR, increasing the availability of ACh at the NMJ. Excessive ACh can cause both a depolarizing and an open-channel block.[48]

Dosing

The optimal dose of anticholinesterase depends on the depth of block, the duration of action of the NMBA used, the timing of the last dose of NMBA relative to administration of the anticholinesterase, and the monitoring technique used. Fig. 11.12 summarizes general recommendations for dosing of anticholinesterases; the actual range of doses varies between studies. Simply, though, smaller doses of anticholinesterases should be administered to antagonize shallower degrees of NMB, and ideally, anticholinesterases should be administered only when necessary (i.e., in the presence of residual paralysis). Without objective monitoring of neuromuscular function, it is not possible to discriminate between TOFR values of 0.4 or 0.9.[39] The administration of anticholinesterases should optimally be guided by quantitative evaluation of the TOFR. The typical dose of neostigmine for antagonism of profound neuromuscular block (a TOF count of 2-3) is 0.05 mg/kg and 0.015 to 0.025 mg/kg for antagonism of lesser degrees of neuromuscular block (a TOF count of 4 with no fade).[41,49] Profound block with a TOF count below 2 should not be antagonized with neostigmine because of the risk of inadequate recovery of neuromuscular function.[47] No anticholinesterase is required if TOFR is >0.9, as determined by monitoring with a quantitative monitor of neuromuscular function.

Pharmacokinetics and Pharmacodynamics

Bolus doses of either neostigmine or edrophonium result in peak plasma concentrations within 5 to 10 minutes that decrease rapidly, followed by a slower elimination phase. Anticholinesterases are eliminated through active secretion by the kidneys. In patients with renal failure where the duration of action of NMBAs may be increased, clearance of anticholinesterases is also reduced and their elimination half-life increased, making dose adjustment of anticholinesterases in patients with renal dysfunction unnecessary.

The anticholinesterases have markedly different onset characteristics, possibly because of the different potency of each agent. Neostigmine is more potent than edrophonium, and smaller doses are required to antagonize residual neuromuscular block. During a steady-state infusion of NMBA, the onset of action of edrophonium is 1 to 2 minutes and that of neostigmine is 7 to 11 minutes. Edrophonium has approximately one-twelfth the potency of neostigmine, and its potency increases as spontaneous recovery from neuromuscular block occurs.

Selective Relaxant Binding Agents: Sugammadex

Sugammadex is a modified γ-cyclodextrin (Fig. 11.17) designed specifically to encapsulate steroidal NMBAs so that they are unable to move into the NMJ and bind to the AChR. In developing sugammadex the depth of the cavity of the molecule was increased to 11 Å through the addition of eight side chains to encapsulate the four steroidal rings of rocuronium and leave the hydrophilic portions of the steroidal NMBA exposed to the surrounding environment. Additionally, the negatively charged carboxyl groups on the added side chains enhanced electrostatic binding to the quaternary nitrogen of rocuronium. Sugammadex forms a complex with either vecuronium or rocuronium in a 1:1 ratio, with an affinity that is greater for rocuronium than it is for vecuronium. Administration of an appropriate dose of sugammadex results in the binding of all free NMBA and rapidly eliminates free NMBA from the plasma. Sugammadex remains in the plasma and has no action at the NMJ. The rate that it reverses even a profound neuromuscular block is rapid (2 to 3 minutes) and complete.

The sugammadex:rocuronium complex (Fig. 11.18) is eliminated through the kidney. It can be removed from the circulation through dialysis in patients with end-stage renal disease, and a recent review of its use in this patient population identified no adverse outcomes.[50]

Sugammadex significantly reduces the time to recovery from rocuronium-induced NMB when compared with neostigmine reversal.[51] As a consequence of its rapid reversal of NMB, sugammadex may be used when a large dose of either rocuronium or vecuronium has been administered to patients who subsequently cannot be intubated or ventilated.[52,53]

Although sugammadex should be able to eliminate residual postoperative paralysis,[54] there is an increasing

---

Box 11.2 Factors That Increase Difficulty of NMB Reversal

- Intensity of depth of NMB at the time that the pharmacologic antagonist is administered
- Dose of the reversal agent
- Rate of spontaneous recovery from the NMBA
- Patient temperature
- Electrolyte abnormalities
- Concomitant medications
- Presence of significant concentrations of the volatile anesthetic

NMB, Neuromuscular blockade; *NMBA*, neuromuscular blocking agent.

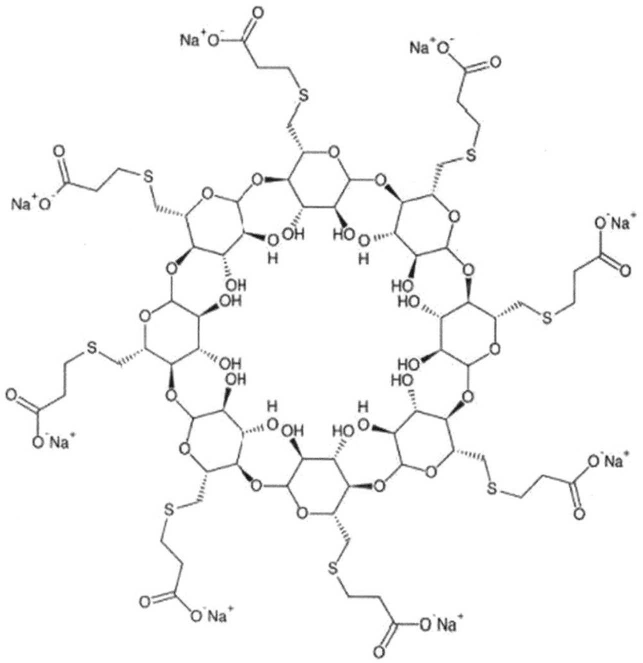

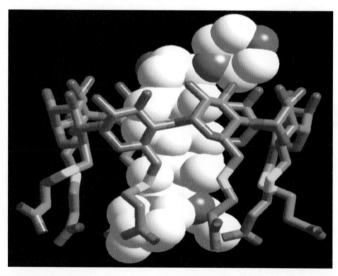

Fig. 11.17 The chemical structure of sugammadex.

Fig. 11.18 The sugammadex–rocuronium complex. The white central structure is rocuronium. The green, red, and a bit of yellow tubular structure is sugammadex. A simple explanation is that sugammadex "encircles" rocuronium so that it cannot move into the NMJ and bind to the acetylcholine receptor. The rocuronium:sugammadex complex is excreted through the kidneys. (Used with permission from Bom A, Bradley M, Cameron K, et al. A novel concept of reversing neuromuscular block: Chemical encapsulation of rocuronium bromide by a cyclodextrin-based synthetic host. Angew Chem Int Ed Engl. 2002;41:266–270.)

body of evidence indicating that when administered in an unwarranted fashion (e.g., without TOF monitoring or by using an inadequate dose), an incidence of residual NMB occurs in about 5% of patients.[55] Of note, incomplete reversal after sugammadex occurs when the number of circulating sugammadex molecules is insufficient to bind to a critical number of the rocuronium molecules present in the body. When a large dose of rocuronium is followed by an inadequate dose of sugammadex, previously redistributed rocuronium may be mobilized to produce recurrence of NMB.[56] Sugammadex dosing recommendations in adults are in Fig. 11.12.

Adverse effects of sugammadex are listed in Box 11.3, and many can be related to displacement by endogenous molecules or to nonspecific binding, such as to coagulation factor Xa. Sugammadex can cause a dose-dependent, transient prolongation of activated partial thromboplastin time (aPTT) and prothrombin time (PT; international normalized ratio [INR])[57]; however, it does not increase the risk of bleeding.[58]

Sugammadex-associated anaphylaxis occurs infrequently; the incidence is equal to, or lower than, the overall incidence of anaphylaxis caused by aminosteroidal NMBAs and antibiotics. There appears to be a geographical variation of hypersensitivity and anaphylactic reactions to sugammadex.[28] In the United States anaphylaxis to sugammadex occurs at a rate of approximately 1 in 3500 to 10,000, whereas in Japan, a country with high rates of sugammadex administration, the incidence is estimated to be as low as 1 in 35,000.[59]

Sugammadex also causes bradycardia. Bradycardia was first noted as a side effect during premarket trials. Since its approval, there have been case reports of patients having either transient or severe bradycardic episodes, occasionally resulting in asystole requiring CPR and use of a transient pacemaker.[60,61] Between 2009 and 2017, 138 cardiac events, including bradycardia and transient heart block, and nine deaths were reported after administration of sugammadex.[61,62] Most of the patients in these reports had no history of cardiopulmonary disease that would have rendered them more susceptible to developing transient heart block. The cause of sugammadex-induced bradycardia remains unknown. Because it may occur after an orthotopic heart transplant,[63] it is not likely to be parasympathetic-mediated.

Sugammadex is ineffective in reversing NMB induced with the benzylisoquinolines, which is why these agents may be preferable when NMB has to be reinstated after reversal with sugammadex.

SUMMARY

NMBAs are vital components of anesthetic care and airway management. Significant improvements to NMBAs and their reversal agents have been made since their original introduction more than 50 years ago. We now appreciate the adverse effects that can result from administration of NMBAs and have evidence that use of NMBAs can add a measure of safety if properly used, and that, without attention to the potential adverse effects of NMBAs, patient outcomes can be worsened. With use of quantitative monitors of depth of neuromuscular block to guide dosing of NMBAs and their reversal agents, NMBAs can be safely administered to facilitate airway management, ventilation and surgery.

ACKNOWLEDGMENT

The author, editors and publisher would like to thank Dr. Ronald D. Miller for contributing to this chapter in the previous edition of this work. It has served as the foundation for the current chapter.

Box 11.3 Adverse Effects of Sugammadex
Nausea and vomiting
Dry mouth
Tachycardia, bradycardia
Dizziness
Cough
Anxiety, depression
Hypotension, hypertension
Myalgias
Headache

REFERENCES

1. Fagerlund MJ, Eriksson LI. Current concepts in neuromuscular transmission. *Br J Anaesth.* 2009;103(1):108–114.
2. Martyn JAJ, Richtsfeld M. Succinylcholine-induced hyperkalemia in acquired pathologic states: Etiologic factors and molecular mechanisms. *Anesthesiology.* 2006;104(1):158–169.
3. Gronert GA. Succinylcholine-induced hyperkalemia and beyond. 1975. *Anesthesiology.* 2009;111(6):1372–1377.
4. Naguib M, Lien CA, Aker J, Eliazo R. Posttetanic potentiation and fade in the response to tetanic and train-of-four stimulation during succinylcholine-induced block. *Anesth Analg.* 2004;98(6):1686–1691 Table of contents.
5. Miller R. Will succinylcholine ever disappear? *Anesth Analg.* 2004;98(6):1674–1675.
6. Larach MG, Klumpner TT, Brandom BW, Vaughn MT, Belani KG, Herlich A, et al. Succinylcholine use and dantrolene availability for malignant hyperthermia treatment: database analyses and systematic review. *Anesthesiology.* 2019;130(1):41–54.
7. Fastle RK, Roback MG. Pediatric rapid sequence intubation: Incidence of reflex bradycardia and effects of pretreatment with atropine. *Pediatr Emerg Care.* 2004;20(10):651–655.
8. Schreiber JU, Lysakowski C, Fuchs-Buder T, Tramèr MR. Prevention of succinylcholine-induced fasciculation and myalgia: A meta-analysis of randomized trials. *Anesthesiology.* 2005;103(4):877–884.
9. Kelly RE, Dinner M, Turner LS, Haik B, Abramson DH, Daines P. Succinylcholine increases intraocular pressure in the human eye with the extraocular muscles detached. *Anesthesiology.* 1993;79(5):948–952.
10. Gill M, Graeme K, Guenterberg K. Masseter spasm after succinylcholine administration. *J Emerg Med.* 2005;29(2):167–171.
11. Bevan DR, Donati F, Gyasi H, Williams A. Vecuronium in renal failure. *Can Anaesth Soc J.* 1984;31(5):491–496.
12. Lepage JY, Malinge M, Cozian A, Pinaud M, Blanloeil Y, Souron R. Vecuronium and atracurium in patients with end-stage renal failure. A comparative study. *Br J Anaesth.* 1987;59(8):1004–1010.
13. Bartkowski RR, Witkowski TA, Azad S, Lessin J, Marr A. Rocuronium onset of action: A comparison with atracurium and vecuronium. *Anesth Analg.* 1993;77(3):574–578.
14. Kopman AF, Klewicka MM, Kopman DJ, Neuman GG. Molar potency is predictive of the speed of onset of neuromuscular block for agents of intermediate, short, and ultrashort duration. *Anesthesiology.* 1999;90(2):425–431.
15. Magorian T, Flannery KB, Miller RD. Comparison of rocuronium, succinylcholine, and vecuronium for rapid-sequence induction of anesthesia in adult patients. *Anesthesiology.* 1993;79(5):913–918.
16. Basta SJ, Ali HH, Savarese JJ, Sunder N, Gionfriddo M, Cloutier G, et al. Clinical pharmacology of atracurium besylate (BW 33A): A new non-depolarizing muscle relaxant. *Anest Analg.* 1982;61(9):723–729.
17. Savarese JJ, Ali HH, Basta SJ, Scott RP, Embree PB, Wastila WB, et al. The cardiovascular effects of mivacurium chloride (BW B1090U) in patients receiving nitrous oxide-opiate-barbiturate anesthesia. *Anesthesiology.* 1989;70(3):386–394.
18. Farhan H, Moreno-Duarte I, Latronico N, Zafonte R, Eikermann M. Acquired muscle weakness in the surgical intensive care unit: Nosology, epidemiology, diagnosis, and prevention. *Anesthesiology.* 2016;124(1):207–234.
19. Doorduin J, Nollet JL, Roesthuis LH, van Hees HW, Brochard LJ, Sinderby CA, et al. Partial neuromuscular blockade during partial ventilatory support in sedated patients with high tidal volumes. *Am J Respir Crit Care Med.* 2017;195(8):1033–1042.
20. Price DR, Mikkelsen ME, Umscheid CA, Armstrong EJ. Neuromuscular blocking agents and neuromuscular dysfunction acquired in critical illness: A systematic review and meta-analysis. *Crit Care Med.* 2016;44(11):2070–2078.
21. Sampson HA, Munoz-Furlong A, Campbell RL, Adkinson NF, Jr Bock SA, Branum A, et al. Second symposium on the definition and management of anaphylaxis: Summary report–second National Institute of Allergy and Infectious Disease/Food Allergy and Anaphylaxis Network symposium. *Ann Emerg Med.* 2006;47(4):373–380.
22. Simons FE, Ardusso LR, Bilo MB, Cardona V, Ebisawa M, El-Gamal YM, et al. International consensus on (ICON) anaphylaxis. *World Allergy Organ J.* 2014;7(1):9.
23. Matsumura T, Mitani S, Fukayama H. Sugammadex-induced anaphylaxis involving sudden onset of severe abdominal pain. *J Clin Anesth.* 2019;57:119–120.
24. Rose MA, Green SL, Crilly HM, Kolawole H. Perioperative anaphylaxis grading system: 'making the grade.' *Br J Anaesth.* 2016;117(5):551–553.
25. Mertes PM, Alla F, Trechot P, Auroy Y, Jougla E. Groupe d'Etudes des Reactions Anaphylactoides P. Anaphylaxis during anesthesia in France: an 8-year national survey. *J Allergy Clin Immunol.* 2011;128(2):366–373.
26. Tacquard C, Collange O, Gomis P, Malinovsky JM, Petitpain N, Demoly P, et al. Anaesthetic hypersensitivity reactions in France between 2011 and 2012: The 10th GERAP Epidemiologic Survey. *Acta Anaesthesiol Scand.* 2017;61(3):290–299.
27. Sadleir PH, Clarke RC, Bunning DL, Platt PR. Anaphylaxis to neuromuscular blocking drugs: Incidence and cross-reactivity in Western Australia from 2002 to 2011. *Br J Anaesth.* 2013;110(6):981–987.
28. Mertes PM, Ebo DG, Garcez T, Rose M, Sabato V, Takazawa T, et al. Comparative epidemiology of suspected perioperative hypersensitivity reactions. *Br J Anaesth.* 2019;123(1):e16–e28.
29. Harper NJN, Cook TM, Garcez T, Farmer L, Floss K, Marinho S, et al. Anaesthesia, surgery, and life-threatening allergic reactions: Epidemiology and clinical features of perioperative anaphylaxis in the 6th National Audit Project (NAP6). *Br J Anaesth.* 2018;121(1):159–171.
30. Reddy JI, Cooke PJ, van Schalkwyk JM, Hannam JA, Fitzharris P, Mitchell SJ. Anaphylaxis is more common with rocuronium and succinylcholine than with atracurium. *Anesthesiology.* 2015;122(1):39–45.
31. Magorian T, Flannery KB, Miller RD. Comparison of rocuronium, succinylcholine, and vecuronium for rapid-sequence induction of anesthesia in adult patients. *Anesthesiology.* 1993;79(5):913–918.
32. Phillips S, Stewart PA, Bilgin AB. A survey of the management of neuromuscular blockade monitoring in Australia and New Zealand. *Anaesth Intensive Care.* 2013;41(3):374–379.
33. Naguib M, Kopman AF, Lien CA, Hunter JM, Lopez A, Brull SJ. A survey of current management of neuromuscular block in the United States and Europe. *Anesth Analg.* 2010;111(1):110–119.
34. Sundman E, Witt H, Olsson R, Ekberg O, Kuylenstierna R, Eriksson LI. The incidence and mechanisms of pharyngeal and upper esophageal dysfunction in partially paralyzed humans: Pharyngeal videoradiography and simultaneous manometry after atracurium. *Anesthesiology.* 2000;92(4):977–984.
35. Jonsson M, Wyon N, Lindahl SG, Fredholm BB, Eriksson LI. Neuromuscular blocking agents block carotid body neuronal nicotinic acetylcholine receptors. *Eur J Pharmacol.* 2004;497(2):173–180.
36. Kopman AF, Yee PS, Neuman GG. Relationship of the train-of-four fade ratio to clinical signs and symptoms of residual paralysis in awake volunteers. *Anesthesiology.* 1997;86(4):765–771.
37. Kirmeier E, Eriksson LI, Lewald H, Jonsson Fagerlund M, Hoeft A, Hollmann M,

et al. Post-anaesthesia pulmonary complications after use of muscle relaxants (POPULAR): A multicentre, prospective observational study. *Lancet Respir Med.* 2019;7(2):129–140.

38. Murphy GS, Szokol JW, Marymont JH, Greenberg SB, Avram MJ, Vender JS. Residual neuromuscular blockade and critical respiratory events in the postanesthesia care unit. *Anesth Analg.* 2008;107(1):130–137.

39. Viby-Mogensen J, Jensen NH, Engbaek J. Tactile and visual evaluation of the response to train-of-four nerve stimulation. *Anesthesiology.* 1985;63:440–443.

40. Dhonneur G, Kirov K, Motamed C, Amathieu R, Kamoun W, Slavov V, et al. Post-tetanic count at adductor pollicis is a better indicator of early diaphragmatic recovery than train-of-four count at corrugator supercilii. *Br J Anaesth.* 2007;99(3):376–379.

41. Kopman AF, Eikermann M. Antagonism of non-depolarising neuromuscular block: Current practice. *Anaesthesia.* 2009;64(s1):22–30.

42. El-Orbany MI, Joseph NJ, Salem MR. The relationship of posttetanic count and train-of-four responses during recovery from intense cisatracurium-induced neuromuscular blockade. *Anesth Analg.* 2003;97(1):80–84.

43. Bowdle A, Bussey L, Michaelsen K, Jelacic S, Nair B, Togashi K, et al. A comparison of a prototype electromyograph vs. a mechanomyograph and an acceleromyograph for assessment of neuromuscular blockade. *Anaesthesia.* 2020;75(2):187–195.

44. Donati F, Meistelman C, Plaud B. Vecuronium neuromuscular blockade at the adductor muscles of the larynx and adductor pollicis. *Anesthesiology.* 1991;74(5):833–837.

45. Thilen SR, Hansen BE, Ramaiah R, Kent CD, Treggiari MM, Bhananker SM. Intraoperative neuromuscular monitoring site and residual paralysis. *Anesthesiology.* 2012;117(5):964–972.

46. Murphy GS, Szokol JW, Marymont JH, Greenberg SB, Avram MJ, Vender JS, et al. Intraoperative acceleromyographic monitoring reduces the risk of residual neuromuscular blockade and adverse respiratory events in the postanesthesia care unit. *Anesthesiology.* 2008;109(3):389–398.

47. Srivastava A, Hunter JM. Reversal of neuromuscular block. *Br J Anaesth.* 2009;103(1):115–129.

48. Legendre P, Ali DW, Drapeau P. Recovery from open channel block by acetylcholine during neuromuscular transmission in zebrafish. *J Neurosci.* 2000;20(1):140–148.

49. Fuchs-Buder T, Meistelman C, Alla F, Grandjean A, Wuthrich Y, Donati F. Antagonism of low degrees of atracurium-induced neuromuscular blockade: Dose-effect relationship for neostigmine. *Anesthesiology.* 2010;112(1):34–40.

50. Paredes S, Porter SB, Porter IE, Renew JR. Sugammadex use in patients with endstage renal disease: A historical cohort study. *Can J Anaesth.* 2020;67:1789–1797 December.

51. Sacan O, White PF, Tufanogullari B, Klein K. Sugammadex reversal of rocuronium-induced neuromuscular blockade: A comparison with neostigmine-glycopyrrolate and edrophonium-atropine. *Anesthesia and Analgesia.* 2007;104(3):569–574.

52. Lee C, Jahr JS, Candiotti KA, Warriner B, Zornow MH, Naguib M. Reversal of profound neuromuscular block by sugammadex administered three minutes after rocuronium: A comparison with spontaneous recovery from succinylcholine. *Anesthesiology.* 2009;110(5):1020–1025.

53. Curtis R, Lomax S, Patel B. Use of sugammadex in a "can't intubate, can't ventilate" situation. *Br J Anaesth.* 2012;108(4):612–614.

54. Brueckmann B, Sasaki N, Grobara P, Li MK, Woo T, de Bie J, et al. Effects of sugammadex on incidence of postoperative residual neuromuscular blockade: A randomized, controlled study. *Br J Anaesth.* 2015;115(5):743–751.

55. Kotake Y, Ochiai R, Suzuki T, Ogawa S, Takagi S, Ozaki M, et al. Reversal with sugammadex in the absence of monitoring did not preclude residual neuromuscular block. *Anesth Analg.* 2013;117(2):345–351.

56. Le Corre F, Nejmeddine S, Fatahine C, Tayar C, Marty J, Plaud B. Recurarization after sugammadex reversal in an obese patient. *Can J Anaesth.* 2011;58(10):944–947.

57. De Kam PJ, Grobara P, Prohn M, Hoppener F, Kluft C, Burggraaf J, et al. Effects of sugammadex on activated partial thromboplastin time and prothrombin time in healthy subjects. *Int J Clin Pharmacol Ther.* 2014;52(3):227–236.

58. Rahe-Meyer N, Fennema H, Schulman S, Klimscha W, Przemeck M, Blobner M, et al. Effect of reversal of neuromuscular blockade with sugammadex versus usual care on bleeding risk in a randomized study of surgical patients. *Anesthesiology.* 2014;121(5):969–977.

59. Binczak M, Fischler M, Le Guen M. Efficacy of sugammadex in preventing skin test reaction in a patient with confirmed rocuronium anaphylaxis: A case report. *A A Pract.* 2019;13(1):17–19.

60. Bhavani SS. Severe bradycardia and asystole after sugammadex. *Br J Anaesth.* 2018;121(1):95–96.

61. Saito I, Osaka Y, Shimada M. Transient third-degree AV block following sugammadex. *J Anesth.* 2015;29(4):641.

62. Hunter JM, Naguib M. Sugammadex-induced bradycardia and asystole: How great is the risk? *Br J Anaesth.* 2018;121(1):8–12.

63. King A, Naguib A, Tobias JD. Bradycardia in a pediatric heart transplant recipient: Is it the sugammadex? *J Pediatr Pharmacol Ther.* 2017;22(5):378–381.

12 ANESTHETIC NEUROTOXICITY*

Mary Ellen McCann, Sulpicio G. Soriano

ANESTHETIC DRUGS AS A CAUSE FOR NEURODEGENERATION AND LONG-TERM NEUROCOGNITIVE DEFICITS
Basic Science of Anesthetic-Induced Developmental Neurotoxicity
Age-Dependent Vulnerability of Anesthetic
Characterization of AIDN
Relevant Anesthetic Durations and Concentrations
Anesthetic and Sedative Drugs
Alleviation of AIDN

CLINICAL EVIDENCE FOR NEUROTOXICITY

INTRAOPERATIVE COURSE AND NEUROCOGNITIVE OUTCOMES
Arterial Blood Pressure
Hypocapnia and the Brain
Oxygen Management
Temperature

CONCLUSION

A major concern within the specialty of anesthesiology is the impact of general anesthesia and sedative drugs on neurodevelopment and cognition across the life span. Although definitive conclusions cannot be made, anesthesia providers should follow the progress of our knowledge regarding long-term effects of anesthesia on the developing central nervous system (CNS). Neuronal cell death and neurocognitive impairments after general anesthesia have been unequivocally demonstrated in laboratory animal models.[1] This public health concern has prompted the Food and Drug Administration to issue a Drug Safety Communication "warning that repeated or lengthy use of general anesthetic and sedation drugs during surgeries or procedures in children younger than 3 years of age or in pregnant women during their third trimester may affect the development of children's brains"[2] (also see Chapter 34). However, this is not a new concern.

In 1953 Eckenhoff warned about an abnormal incidence of postoperative personality changes in children.[3] Since then, preclinical reports on juvenile animal models unequivocally demonstrate a causal effect of general anesthesia on subsequent neurotoxic and neurocognitive dysfunction.[4] In addition, in 1955 Bedford wrote about behavioral changes in the elderly after general anesthesia.[5]

Anesthetic drugs are potent modulators of the CNS and render patients insensate to painful procedures and surgery.[6] Although the exact molecular mechanisms that produce immobility, analgesia, and amnesia are not completely known, most anesthetic and sedative drugs are either γ-aminobutyric acid (GABA) receptor agonists, N-methyl-D-aspartate (NMDA) glutamate receptor antagonists, or a combination of the two. General anesthesia and sedation can be achieved by inhaled or intravenous administration of specific drugs. Both GABA agonists

*This work was supported by the National Institutes of Health grant 1-R01 HD06 1136–01A1 (MEM) and the Boston Children's Hospital Endowed Chair in Pediatric Neuroanesthesia (SGS).

and NMDA antagonists have been implicated in causing anesthetic-induced developmental neurotoxicity (AIDN). Both the short-term and long-term neurocognitive effects of general anesthesia should be considered.

ANESTHETIC DRUGS AS A CAUSE FOR NEURODEGENERATION AND LONG-TERM NEUROCOGNITIVE DEFICITS

Basic Science of Anesthetic-Induced Developmental Neurotoxicity

Determining the root cause of the neurotoxic effect of CNS depressant drugs on the developing brain is complicated by the myriad of molecular targets and the still unknown mechanistic pathway to achieve general anesthesia. AIDN has been demonstrated in laboratory models, both in vivo and in vitro, by exposure to most anesthetic and sedative drugs commonly administered to pediatric patients (also see Chapter 34). A comparable pattern of neurodegeneration and impaired neurocognitive development has been described with the perinatal administration of inhibitory drugs.[7] AIDN was first described more than 40 years ago in fetal and postnatal rats exposed to halothane,[8] but its impact was not fully publicized to both the scientific and lay community until a 1999 report that emphasized that ketamine increased neurodegeneration in neonatal rat pups.[9] Subsequently, it was found that the combination of commonly used anesthetic drugs, isoflurane, nitrous oxide, and midazolam, not only induced neuroapoptosis but resulted in deficits in hippocampal synaptic function and learning behavior.[10]

Anesthesia removes sensory input and suppresses normal neural traffic, which in turn diminishes the trophic support required for neurogenesis and context-dependent modulation of neuroplasticity. However, several reports have described neuronal cell death mechanisms such as excitotoxicity, mitochondrial dysfunction, aberrant cell cycle reentry, trophic factor dysregulation, and disruption of cytoskeletal assembly.[11-13] Although GABA acts as an inhibitory drug in the mature brain, it is an excitatory agent during early stages of brain development because of the preponderance of the immature Na/K/2Cl transporter protein NKCC1, which produces a chloride influx leading to neuron depolarization. Therefore GABA remains excitatory until the GABA receptors are switched to the normal inhibitory mode, when the mature chloride transporter, KCC2, is expressed, which actively transports chloride out of the neural cell.[14]

Age-Dependent Vulnerability of Anesthetic

Neural development progresses through several steps that include neurogenesis, neuronal morphogenesis, and synaptogenesis. Neurogenesis starts with the creation of progenitor cells, which proliferate and differentiate into neurons or glial cells. As neurons undergo terminal differentiation into a postmitotic state, they can no longer replicate. Dendrites and axons extend from the cell body to form functional synapses with other neurons. CNS neural development (up to 70%) is regulated by early elimination during the embryonal stage and programmed cell death after birth. Redundant neural progenitor cells and neurons that do not migrate properly or make synapses are physiologically pruned by apoptosis.[15]

Critical periods of plasticity during brain development are modulated by environmental cues and have been implicated in perceptual development.[16] Likewise, the perioperative environment can influence brain development. Anesthetic drugs are powerful modulators of neuronal circuits and have an impact on the constant flux of CNS development and remodeling in both health and disease states. Because neurogenesis is ongoing throughout life, from the fetus to the elderly, these neural progenitor cells are vulnerable to the toxic effects of anesthetic drugs. Exposure to isoflurane produces neuronal cell death in brain regions where neural progenitor cells reside.[17] Therefore susceptibility to AIDN extends from the fetal period to late adulthood.

Brain growth spurt in most species is likely the time of maximal susceptibility to AIDN. This time corresponds with the time of maximal synaptogenesis. The growth spurt of the human brain occurs in the last trimester of gestation until about 3 to 4 years of age. Neuroinformatic mapping of the development of corticospinal tracts across species demonstrates that 7-day-old rat pups (the most common laboratory animal model) are neurodevelopmentally closer to 20- to 22-week-old human fetuses.[18] The timing of maximal brain growth during development is species dependent. Rodents are altricial species, and much of their neurodevelopment occurs postnatally. This time period occurs from about postnatal day 6 through postnatal day 21. Simian species, including humans, are usually considered precocial and typically have a longer gestation because offspring are born at a relatively advanced stage of development. Rhesus monkeys are susceptible to anesthetic-induced neuroapoptosis when exposed as fetuses or up to day 6 of life.[19-21] Exposure of pregnant rats to anesthetics results in increased apoptosis in the brains of the fetuses.[22] Administration of anesthetics to neonatal rodents leads to increased apoptosis and stunted axonal growth and dendritic arborization. In contrast, anesthetic exposure in juvenile rat models does not increase apoptosis but leads to enhanced dendritic formation and synaptic density.[23]

Characterization of AIDN

Pathologic Apoptosis

Accelerated apoptosis is the hallmark of AIDN (Table 12.1). Although an essential process in controlling neural development, the apoptotic pathway is also activated by cellular

Table 12.1	Key Features of Anesthetic-Induced Developmental Neurotoxicity (AIDN)
Feature	**Comment (see text for details)**
Pathologic apoptosis	The hallmark of AIDN Can be induced by extrinsic or intrinsic pathways
Impeded neurogenesis	Effect of anesthetics on neurogenesis is age-dependent
Altered dendritic development	Anesthetics affect dendritic morphogenesis in age-dependent manner
Aberrant glial development	Isoflurane can interfere with release of trophic factors by astrocytes

stress. Such stresses include glucocorticoids, heat, radiation, starvation, infection, hypoxia, pain, and anesthetics. Apoptosis is almost always executed by caspase enzymes, which are cysteine-dependent aspartate proteases that play an integral part in programmed cell death. The two main pathways are the extrinsic and intrinsic pathways. The extrinsic pathway is mediated by death receptors on the cell membrane wall, whereas the intrinsic pathway is dependent on mitochondrial activation.

Impeded Neurogenesis

Anesthetics affect neurogenesis in animals in an age-dependent manner. Isoflurane causes loss of neural stem cells and reduced neurogenesis in neonatal cohorts but a transient increase in neurogenesis in older cohorts.[24] Based on both in vivo and in vitro evidence, general anesthetics may decrease the pool of neural stem cells, especially in juveniles and adults.

Altered Dendritic Development

Dendritic spines are small protrusions of the neurons that typically receive input from a single synapse of an axon and are essential components of synaptogenesis. Exposure to ketamine and isoflurane decreases synapse and spine density in very young infant rats. As noted earlier, juvenile rats exposed to anesthetic drugs had an increase in dendritic spine formation.[23] The implications of a decrease in dendritic spine formation at a very young age and an increase in slightly older animals are unclear. Taken together, the impact of anesthetics on dendritic morphogenesis clearly differs with the age at which exposure occurs.

Aberrant Glial Development

The glial cells within the CNS form the scaffolding, which guides the migration and synaptogenesis of the neurons during development. Astrocytes are impaired during neural development by exposure to isoflurane.[25] This anesthetic interferes with the release of brain-derived neurotrophic factor (BDNF) by astrocytes, which in turn deprive the developing neurons of trophic support for axonal outgrowth. Isoflurane also induces apoptosis of oligodendrocytes in fetuses and neonate rhesus monkeys.[20]

Anesthetic Effects on Spinal Cord

General anesthetic exposure (isoflurane, nitrous oxide) in very young rat pups causes an increase in apoptosis in the spinal cord, with a preponderance of injury in the ventral horns.[26] However, no motor functional disabilities were detected in exposed rats. Postnatal day 3 rat pups that received an intrathecal injection of ketamine had increased apoptosis and microglial activation on histologic examination of their spinal cords and deranged spinal function at adulthood.[27] Intrathecal local anesthetic (bupivacaine) in the same population did not cause an increase in apoptosis.[28]

Neuroinflammation and Alzheimer-Related Neuropathology

Activation of neuroinflammatory cascades may influence the development of postoperative cognitive dysfunction (also see Chapter 35).[29] Surgical trauma clearly activates neuroinflammation. Therefore the administration of anesthetic and analgesic drugs during surgery and painful procedures should minimize this response. However, sevoflurane increases markers of neuroinflammation in young, but not adult, mice.[30] It is unclear if the impact of surgical trauma and anesthetic exposure are additive in inducing neuroinflammation. Preclinical reports demonstrate that surgery and general anesthesia increased expression of β-amyloid, a biologic precursor of Alzheimer disease.[31] Therefore neuroinflammation and Alzheimer disease neuropathology is a potent combination that could diminish neurocognitive function.

Neurocognitive Function

Decrements in neurocognitive function clearly occur after fetal and neonatal exposure to anesthetic drugs in rodents. Standard behavioral measures in rodents include the Morris water navigation test, radial arm maze, startle, prepulse inhibition of the startle reflex, and odor recognition testing. Behavioral tests were also described in rhesus monkeys exposed to ketamine or sevoflurane with operant test battery or human intruder paradigm, respectively.[19,32] The operant test battery is a measure of motivation and recognition memory, whereas the human intruder paradigm is a test for emotional reactivity. Both reports demonstrated a diminution of performance at an older age after neonatal exposure to these drugs.

Exposure to anesthetic drugs also adversely affects neurobehavioral assessments of elderly rats. Six- and 20-month-old rats anesthetized with isoflurane and nitrous oxide equally developed persistent deficits in the radial arm maze test, which confirms that exposure to anesthetic drugs can lead to neurobehavioral functional consequences at a later age.[33]

Relevant Anesthetic Durations and Concentrations

The duration of exposure may be more relevant than the concentration of exposure, although both are important. Almost all the animal studies involved an anesthetic exposure of at least 4 hours, with some trials exposing primates to 24 hours of continuous anesthesia. Exposures of less than 1 hour, regardless of the animal studied, did not cause increased neuroapoptosis. There is inconsistency about the relative neurotoxic potential of individual volatile anesthetics and whether anesthetics given in combinations are more neurotoxic than solitary anesthetics because of the higher minimum alveolar concentration (MAC) exposure in combination.

Anesthetic and Sedative Drugs

GABAergic general anesthetics act on the GABA$_A$ receptor. Although GABA is inhibitory in the mature brain, it is an excitatory agent during early stages of brain development. The immature Na/K/2Cl transporter protein NKCC1 produces a chloride influx leading to neuron depolarization. As a consequence, GABA remains excitatory until the GABA neurons switch to the normal inhibitory mode, when the mature chloride transporter, KCC2, is expressed, which actively transports chloride out of the neural cell.[14] This switch begins around the 15th postnatal week in term human infants but is not complete until about 1 year of age.

The NMDA glutamate receptor (NMDAR) is found in neurons and is activated when glutamate, glycine, or D-serine binds to it. It is critical for synaptic plasticity, which is needed for learning and memory. Structurally the NMDAR is a protein composed of four subunits, two GluN1 (formerly called NR1) and two GluN2 (formerly called NR2). Ketamine, which is a noncompetitive NMDAR antagonist, has been associated with AIDN in animals and causes an upregulation of the GluN1 subunit.[34]

In general, opioids do not increase neuroapoptosis, but under some experimental conditions, repeated morphine administration over 7 days is associated with increased apoptosis in the sensory cortex and amygdala of neonatal rats.[35] However, a single dose of morphine given to postnatal day 7 rat pups did not increase neuroapoptosis. These areas of the brain are not affected by volatile and intravenous anesthetics, which preferentially affect the learning and memory areas (hippocampus) of developing brains.

Alleviation of AIDN

Several molecular mechanisms for anesthetic-induced apoptosis have been elucidated. This finding has led to studies designed to determine whether there are clinically available neuroprotective strategies that can ameliorate the negative effects of general anesthetics on developing young children. Several nonspecific drugs that have neuroprotective properties (lithium, melatonin, estrogen, erythropoietin, estradiol, and dexmedetomidine) alleviate AIDN. Dexmedetomidine mitigates isoflurane-induced neuroapoptosis and behavioral impairment.[36] However, high doses of dexmedetomidine can induce neuroapoptosis.[37] The neuroprotective effect of dexmedetomidine probably induces cell survival signaling pathways at clinical doses. Finally, an enhanced and stimulating environment mitigates neurobehavioral deficits after neonatal exposure to sevoflurane.[30,38]

CLINICAL EVIDENCE FOR NEUROTOXICITY

Taken together, three factors appear to induce AIDN in laboratory models: (1) susceptibility during a critical period of development, (2) large dose of the anesthetic, and (3) prolonged duration of exposure. Extrapolation of these laboratory data to the human neonate is problematic. A rat brain develops over a matter of weeks, whereas a human brain develops over years. Six hours of anesthesia in a neonatal rat pup may equate to weeks in a human neonate. With the exception of sedation in intensive care patients, this extreme condition is not common in clinical practice. Therefore uncovering the effect of an equivalent exposure on the neurologic outcome in a human neonate is difficult. Prolonged and repetitive exposure and exposure at a young age to general anesthesia cause neuroapoptosis and neurodevelopmental delays in laboratory animals. Children who need frequent examinations under anesthesia or radiation treatments for cancer theoretically are at increased risk for the neurotoxic effects of general anesthesia.[39]

The implication that general anesthesia may be harmful to children is limited to retrospective epidemiologic analyses (also see Chapter 34). This evidence may be confounded by the effects of surgery and the effects of the underlying comorbid conditions. Although control for obvious confounders has been attempted, the retrospective nature of these investigations makes it impossible to control for all the known and unknown confounders. There have been several epidemiologic studies originating from the Mayo Clinic. A retrospective cohort study of over 5000 children born from 1976 through 1982 found more reading, written language, and math learning disabilities in the 593 patients who were exposed to anesthesia before the age of 4 years.[40] Risk factors included more than one anesthetic exposure and general anesthesia lasting longer than 2 hours. The Mayo Anesthesia Safety in Kids (MASK) study evaluated a more recent cohort of 997 children and demonstrated negligible deficits in singly exposed patients. However, although children who had multiple exposures to anesthesia and surgery did not have significant reductions in their IQ or operant test battery (tasks thought to represent specific brain functions), a secondary analysis did reveal a pattern of deficits in several neuropsychological tests.[41,42]

A prospective evaluation of 28 children exposed to anesthesia before 1 year of age revealed deficits in measures of long-term recognition memory, but no differences in familiarity, IQ, and Child Behavior Checklist scores.[43]

A database of over 200,000 children developed using the New York State Medicaid billing codes revealed that children undergoing inguinal hernia repair at less than 1 year of age had almost a threefold increase in diagnoses relating to developmental and behavioral issues, which was significantly higher than nonanesthetic-exposed siblings.[44] The general consensus is that there is an increased risk to children who have had two or more anesthetic exposures A subsequent report based on this cohort revealed increased utilization of attention deficit hyperactivity disorder medications in the exposed group.[45]

A prospective analysis of an obstetrical cohort from Raines, Australia, found that even a single exposure to general anesthesia was related to decreased performance on receptive and expressive language and cognitive testing performed at age 10 years.[46] The Avon Longitudinal Study of Parents and Children, a prospective cohort study of 13,433 children born in Southwest England, revealed significantly lower motor and social linguistic performance, but not neurocognitive measures, in those exposed to general anesthesia and surgery in early childhood (less than 4 years old).[47]

Large database clinical investigations from Canada and Sweden reveal that exposure to surgery and anesthesia at an age older than 2 to 4 years increased the odds ratio of cognitive deficits, though not to the extent of previously published retrospective reports from smaller populations.[48-50] Scrutiny of these large datasets reveals a lower percentage in academic achievement scores for toddlers undergoing ear, nose, and throat surgery. This finding suggests that early derangements in hearing and speech may have an impact on subsequent cognitive domains as assessed by school performance.

Other studies have cast doubt on the association between exposure to general anesthesia at a young age and later school problems. A study from the Netherlands evaluating the educational achievements of 1143 identical twin pairs found that twin pairs in which any member of the twin pair was exposed to general anesthesia had lesser educational achievements than unexposed twin pairs.[51] However, the educational achievements of discordant twin pairs (one twin exposed, one twin nonexposed) were similar to each other, meaning that the receipt of general anesthesia did not appear to be a relevant factor. Similarly, a large cohort study of 2689 children born in Denmark between 1986 and 1990 who underwent inguinal herniorrhaphy as infants were matched to control subjects who were randomly selected from an age-matched sample representing 5% of the population.[52] This study found no statistically significant differences between the exposed and nonexposed children after adjusting for known confounders.

Two published large prospective cohort studies support the contention that there is no impact of anesthetic exposure on subsequent neurocognitive domains in children. The GAS study is the only prospective randomized controlled trial to date comparing the effects of general anesthesia with regional anesthesia for inguinal hernia surgery in early infancy.[53] This study found no evidence that 1 hour of sevoflurane anesthesia in infancy increases the risk of adverse neurodevelopmental outcomes at 2 years of age compared with awake-regional anesthesia. The primary outcome, which was a full-scale IQ test done at age 5 years, confirmed no significant differences (mean difference of 0.23 [95% confidence interval (CI) −2.59 to 3.06]) on the full-scale intelligence quotient (FSIQ) of the Wechsler Preschool and Primary Scale of Intelligence.[54] The PANDA study prospectively examined the impact of inguinal hernia surgery in infants younger than 36 months of age. An extensive battery of neurocognitive tests was used to compare each anesthetized infant with a sibling who had no anesthesia exposure.[55] When compared with a sibling cohort naïve to surgery and general anesthesia, there was no significant difference in the tested neurocognitive domains. Both negative studies only examined the impact of short exposures to general anesthesia and surgery. These findings are consistent with the lack of AIDN after exposures of short duration in laboratory animals. Furthermore, the neurocognitive assessments in all the clinical reports were performed in childhood and adolescence, not at adulthood. Therefore the relationship between prolonged exposure to anesthetic drugs and neurocognitive performance in later stages of the life span needs to be addressed in future investigations.

On the other end of the age spectrum, elderly patients are at increased risk of developing postoperative cognitive dysfunction after surgery and anesthesia (also see Chapter 35).[56]

INTRAOPERATIVE COURSE AND NEUROCOGNITIVE OUTCOMES

Anesthetic drugs are not clinically administered in a vacuum. The developing CNS is an exquisitely sensitive internal milieu. Because critical periods of plasticity during brain development are modulated by the environment,[19] the perioperative environment has the potential to influence brain development. Anesthetic drugs are powerful modulators of neuronal circuits and have an impact on the constant flux of CNS development and remodeling in both health and disease states. Therefore nonphysiologic exposure to various drugs and stressors (painful stimuli, maternal deprivation, hypoglycemia, hypoxia, and ischemia) during these critical periods of development may lead to neuronal injury and altered neuroplasticity.[57] The potential contribution of surgical lesion, genetic syndromes, coexisting medical conditions, and therapeutic interventions should be considered.[58]

In anesthetized or sedated patients undergoing surgery or painful procedures, respectively, hemodynamic and metabolic changes may influence the neurocognitive outcomes of patients exposed to general anesthesia. These influences could work in concert with the neurotoxic potential of general anesthetics or independently to cause poor neurocognitive outcomes. Some of the factors that are implicated in causing poor outcomes in babies receiving neonatal intensive care may be important to infants undergoing general anesthesia. These factors include perioperative blood pressure, carbon dioxide tensions, hyperoxia or hypoxia, temperature, and serum glucose levels (Table 12.2).

Arterial Blood Pressure

Determining the optimal arterial blood pressure management for very young infants is complicated by the many definitions for hypotension in the neonate and young infant. Two commonly used definitions are a mean arterial blood pressure (MAP) below the fifth or tenth percentile for age or a MAP less than the infant's gestational age in weeks for infants who were born premature. Furthermore, normal arterial blood pressures for very young infants rapidly increase during the first 6 weeks of life and thereafter are fairly constant for the first year of life. Maintaining arterial blood pressure within the limits of cerebral autoregulation is optimal for cerebral protection, although sustaining adequate cerebral perfusion less than the limits of cerebral autoregulation is sometimes necessary. The lower limits of cerebral autoregulation in neonates are likely variable and not precisely known, and a wide range of variability likely exists. Most general anesthetics cause some degree of hypotension, which can be ameliorated by surgical stimulation. Prolonged inductions of anesthesia or surgical preparation times may lead to protracted periods of hypotension in neonates.

Hypocapnia and the Brain

The partial arterial carbon dioxide pressure (Pa_{CO_2}) is an important modulator of the cerebral blood flow (CBF), with its main effect on cerebral arteries (also see Chapter 30). Hypocapnia results in vasoconstriction of cerebral vessels, leading to decreases in CBF. Hypocapnia-induced vasoconstriction may alter neuronal nuclear membranes and increase nuclear Ca^{2+} influx through ischemia-induced tissue hypoxia and free radical generation, through alterations in the NMDAR or by changes in cerebral energy metabolism, leading to apoptotic cell death. Hypocapnia, which leads to cerebral alkalosis, not only decreases cerebral perfusion but also decreases the ability of hemoglobin to release oxygen. Premature infants may be particularly susceptible to the effects of hypocapnia. In general, it is recommended to keep the end-tidal CO_2 levels above 35 mm Hg in infants and children undergoing general anesthesia.

Oxygen Management

Excessive administered oxygen delivered during general anesthesia can lead to an increased production of reactive oxygen species (ROS), causing cell stress and apoptosis. Ordinarily, there is a balance between ROS and cell antioxidants. This balance is easily overwhelmed in young infants because their antioxidant defenses are not well developed at birth. During the last stages of fetal development, there is an increase in endogenous production of antioxidants in addition to an increase in maternal-fetal transfer of antioxidants in order to prepare the fetus for the relatively hyperoxic environment after birth compared with the relatively hypoxic fetal environment. Premature infants are at greater risk than term infants from oxygen damage because they are deficient in both of the previous factors. The antioxidant enzymes involved include superoxide dismutase, catalase, and glutathione peroxidase. These enzymes convert reactive superoxide radicals to hydrogen peroxide and then to water. Hyperoxia in young animals leads to neuroapoptosis, presumably by oxidative stress and inflammation.

Hypoxia and anoxia can cause brain ischemia. Neurons begin to lose their electrochemical gradients, and there is an influx of calcium into the cytosol as a result of glutamate release from synaptic vesicles. This leads to early necrotic cell death. This is heralded by nuclear swelling, mitochondrial collapse, and inflammation. A proportion of neurons that are stressed by ischemia will not die immediately, but will go on to die an apoptotic death sometime after the ischemic stress is eliminated.

Table 12.2	Intraoperative Factors Influencing Neurocognitive Outcomes
Factor	**Comment (see text for details)**
Arterial blood pressure	Interpatient variability in lower limits of cerebral autoregulation
Carbon dioxide tension	Hypocapnia causes cerebral vasoconstriction
Hyperoxia or hypoxia	Hyperoxia produces reactive oxygen species Hypoxia can cause cerebral ischemia
Temperature	Mild hypothermia is protective in neonate with prior ischemic injury Hyperthermia with prior ischemic injury is associated with neurocognitive disability
Serum glucose	Extremes of hypoglycemia and hyperglycemia are associated with adverse outcomes

Temperature

Temperature maintenance during anesthesia is one of the challenges of pediatric anesthesia (also see Chapter 34). Infants have a large skin surface area/body mass ratio and a high basal metabolic rate, which accelerate radiant and evaporative heat loss. In addition, reduced vasoconstriction and decreased subcutaneous fat increase their radiant and conductive heat losses during procedures. Infants who are hypothermic at the conclusion of anesthesia may not have the energy stores to both rewarm themselves and spontaneously ventilate, necessitating postoperative ventilation in these infants. However, mild hypothermia (core temperature 32 to 34°C) is neuroprotective in neonates who have suffered prior hypoxic-ischemic injury. Hyperthermia in these same neonates was associated with more neurocognitive disabilities when these children underwent testing at age 18 months.

CONCLUSION

Accumulating evidence from laboratory investigations definitively demonstrates that anesthetic and sedative drugs are potent modulators of CNS development and function throughout the life span, which in turn can lead to neuroapoptosis, altered dendritic formation, synaptogenesis, and subsequent neurocognitive deficits. Yet evidence from retrospective clinical reports in pediatric and elderly surgical populations is inconclusive.

Because anesthetic and sedative drugs are essential in the management of surgical patients, the problem of AIDN must be eventually addressed. In the meantime, anesthesia providers should be sensitive to the possibility that brain development in younger years and its decline in older patients can be an issue for perioperative care and identify contributory factors.[59]

REFERENCES

1. McCann ME, Soriano SG. Does general anesthesia affect neurodevelopment in infants and children? *BMJ.* 2019 Dec 9;367:l6459. doi:10.1136/bmj.l6459 PMID: 31818811.
2. Rappaport B, Mellon RD, Simone A, Woodcock J. Defining safe use of anesthesia in children. *N Engl J Med.* 2011;364:1387–1390.
3. Eckenhoff JE. Relationship of anesthesia to postoperative personality changes in children. *Am J Dis Child.* 1953;86:587–591.
4. Xie Z, Vutskits L. Lasting impact of general anaesthesia on the brain: Mechanisms and relevance. *Nat Rev Neurosci.* 2016;17(11):705–717.
5. Bedford PD. Adverse cerebral effects of anaesthesia on old people. *Lancet.* 1955;269:259–263.
6. Hemmings HC Jr, Riegelhaupt PM, Kelz MB, Solt K, Eckenhoff RG, Orser BA, Goldstein PA. Towards a comprehensive understanding of anesthetic mechanisms of action: A decade of discovery. *Trends Pharmacol Sci.* 2019;40(7):464–481 Jul.
7. Bittigau P, Sifringer M, Genz K, et al. Antiepileptic drugs and apoptotic neurodegeneration in the developing brain. *Proc Natl Acad Sci U S A.* 2002;99(23): 15089–15094.
8. Quimby KL, Katz J, Bowman RE. Behavioral consequences in rats from chronic exposure to 10 ppm halothane during early development. *Anesth Analg.* 1975;54:628–633.
9. Ikonomidou C, Bosch F, Miksa M, et al. Blockade of NMDA receptors and apoptotic neurodegeneration in the developing brain. *Science.* 1999;283:70–74.
10. Jevtovic-Todorovic V, Hartman RE, Izumi Y, et al. Early exposure to common anesthetic agents causes widespread neurodegeneration in the developing rat brain and persistent learning deficits. *J Neurosci.* 2003;23:876–882.
11. Sanchez V, Feinstein SD, Lunardi N, et al. General anesthesia causes long-term impairment of mitochondrial morphogenesis and synaptic transmission in developing rat brain. *Anesthesiology.* 2011;115:992–1002.
12. Soriano SG, Liu Q, Li J, et al. Ketamine activates cell cycle signaling and apoptosis in the neonatal rat brain. *Anesthesiology.* 2010;112:1155–1163.
13. Head BP, Patel HH, Niesman IR, et al. Inhibition of p75 neurotrophin receptor attenuates isoflurane-mediated neuronal apoptosis in the neonatal central nervous system. *Anesthesiology.* 2009;110:813–825.
14. Ben-Ari Y. Excitatory actions of GABA during development: The nature of the nurture. *Nat Rev Neurosci.* 2002;3:728–739.
15. Buss RR, Sun W, Oppenheim RW. Adaptive roles of programmed cell death during nervous system development. *Annu Rev Neurosci.* 2006;29:1–35.
16. Hensch TK. Critical period plasticity in local cortical circuits. *Nat Rev Neurosci.* 2005;6:877–888.
17. Hofacer RD, Deng M, Ward CG, et al. Cell-age specific vulnerability of neurons to anesthetic toxicity. *Ann Neurol.* 2013;73:695–704.
18. Clancy B, Kersh B, Hyde J, et al. Web-based method for translating neurodevelopment from laboratory species to humans. *Neuroinformatics.* 2007;5:79–94.
19. Paule MG, Li M, Allen RR, et al. Ketamine anesthesia during the first week of life can cause long-lasting cognitive deficits in rhesus monkeys. *Neurotoxicol Teratol.* 2011;33:220–230.
20. Creeley CE, Dikranian KT, Dissen GA, et al. Isoflurane-induced apoptosis of neurons and oligodendrocytes in the fetal rhesus macaque brain. *Anesthesiology.* 2014;120:626–638.
21. Raper J, Alvarado MC, Murphy KL, et al. Multiple anesthetic exposure in infant monkeys alters emotional reactivity to an acute stressor. *Anesthesiology.* 2015;123(5):1084–1092.
22. Wang S, Peretich K, Zhao Y, et al. Anesthesia-induced neurodegeneration in fetal rat brains. *Pediatr Res.* 2009;66:435–440.
23. Briner A, De Roo M, Dayer A, et al. Volatile anesthetics rapidly increase dendritic spine density in the rat medial prefrontal cortex during synaptogenesis. *Anesthesiology.* 2010;112:546–556.
24. Stratmann G, Sall JW, May LD, et al. Isoflurane differentially affects neurogenesis and long-term neurocognitive function in 60-day-old and 7-day-old rats. *Anesthesiology.* 2009;110:834–848.
25. Ryu YK, Khan S, Smith SC, Mintz CD. Isoflurane impairs the capacity of astrocytes to support neuronal development in a mouse dissociated coculture model. *J Neurosurg Anesthesiol.* 2014;26:363–368.
26. Sanders RD, Xu J, Shu Y, et al. General anesthetics induce apoptotic neurodegeneration in the neonatal rat spinal cord. *Anesth Analg.* 2008;106:1708–1711.
27. Walker SM, Westin BD, Deumens R, et al. Effects of intrathecal ketamine in the neonatal rat: Evaluation of apoptosis and long-term functional outcome. *Anesthesiology.* 2010;113:147–159.
28. Yahalom B, Athiraman U, Soriano SG, et al. Spinal anesthesia in infant rats: Development of a model and assessment of neurologic outcomes. *Anesthesiology.* 2011;114:1325–1335.
29. Vacas S, Degos V, Feng X, Maze M. The neuroinflammatory response of

postoperative cognitive decline. *Br Med Bull.* 2013;106:161–178.

30. Shen X, Dong Y, Xu Z, et al. Selective anesthesia-induced neuroinflammation in developing mouse brain and cognitive impairment. *Anesthesiology.* 2013;118:502–515.

31. Xu Z, Dong Y, Wang H, et al. Age-dependent postoperative cognitive impairment and Alzheimer-related neuropathology in mice. *Sci Rep.* 2014;4:3766.

32. Raper J, Alvarado MC, Murphy KL, Baxter MG. Multiple anesthetic exposure in infant monkeys alters emotional reactivity to an acute stressor. *Anesthesiology.* 2015;123:1084–1092.

33. Culley DJ, Baxter MG, Yukhananov R, Crosby G. Long-term impairment of acquisition of a spatial memory task following isoflurane-nitrous oxide anesthesia in rats. *Anesthesiology.* 2004;100:309–314.

34. Wang C, Sadovova N, Hotchkiss C, et al. Blockade of N-methyl-D-aspartate receptors by ketamine produces loss of postnatal day 3 monkey frontal cortical neurons in culture. *Toxicol Sci.* 2006;91:192–201.

35. Bajic D, Commons KG, Soriano SG. Morphine-enhanced apoptosis in selective brain regions of neonatal rats. *Int J Dev Neurosci.* 2013;31:258–266.

36. Sanders RD, Xu J, Shu Y, et al. Dexmedetomidine attenuates isoflurane-induced neurocognitive impairment in neonatal rats. *Anesthesiology.* 2009;110:1077–1085.

37. Liu JR, Yuki K, Baek C, et al. Dexmedetomidine-induced neuroapoptosis is dependent on its cumulative dose. *Anesth Analg.* 2016;123(4):1008–1017.

38. Shih J, May LD, Gonzalez HE, et al. Delayed environmental enrichment reverses sevoflurane-induced memory impairment in rats. *Anesthesiology.* 2012;116:586–602.

39. Banerjee P, Rossi MG, Anghelescu DL, et al. Association between anesthesia exposure and neurocognitive and neuroimaging outcomes in long-term survivors of childhood acute lymphoblastic leukemia. *JAMA Oncol.* 2019 Oct 1;5(10):1456–1463.

40. Wilder RT, Flick RP, Sprung J, et al. Early exposure to anesthesia and learning disabilities in a population-based birth cohort. *Anesthesiology.* 2009;110:796–804.

41. Warner DO, Zaccariello MJ, Katusic SK, et al. Neuropsychological and behavioral outcomes after exposure of young children to procedures requiring general anesthesia: The Mayo Anesthesia Safety in Kids (MASK) study. *Anesthesiology.* 2018;129(1):89–105.

42. Zaccariello MJ, Frank RD, Lee M, et al. Patterns of neuropsychological changes after general anaesthesia in young children: Secondary analysis of the Mayo Anesthesia Safety in Kids study. *Br J Anaesth.* 2019;122(5):671–681.

43. Stratmann G, Lee J, Sall JW, et al. Effect of general anesthesia in infancy on long-term recognition memory in humans and rats. *Neuropsychopharmacology.* 2014;39:2275–2287.

44. Dimaggio C, Sun L, Li G. Early childhood exposure to anesthesia and risk of developmental and behavioral disorders in a sibling birth cohort. *Anesth Analg.* 2011;113:1143–1151.

45. Ing C, Ma X, Sun M, et al. Exposure to surgery and anesthesia in early childhood and subsequent use of attention deficit hyperactivity disorder medications. *Anesth Analg.* 2020;131(3):723–733.

46. Ing C, DiMaggio C, Whitehouse A, et al. Long-term differences in language and cognitive function after childhood exposure to anesthesia. *Pediatrics.* 2012;130:e476–e485.

47. Walkden GJ, Gill H, Davies NM, Peters AE, Wright I, Pickering AE. Early childhood general anesthesia and neurodevelopmental outcomes in the Avon Longitudinal Study of Parents and Children Birth cohort. *Anesthesiology.* 2020;133(5):1007–1020 Nov 1.

48. O'Leary JD, Janus M, Duku E, et al. A population-based study evaluating the association between surgery in early life and child development at primary school entry. *Anesthesiology.* 2016;125:272–279.

49. Graham MR, Brownell M, Chateau DG, et al. Neurodevelopmental assessment in kindergarten in children exposed to general anesthesia before the age of 4 years: A retrospective matched cohort study. *Anesthesiology.* 2016;125(4):667–677.

50. Glatz P, Sandin RH, Pedersen NL, et al. Association of anesthesia and surgery during childhood with long-term academic performance. *JAMA Pediatr.* 2017;171(1):e163470.

51. Bartels M, Althoff RR, Boomsma DI. Anesthesia and cognitive performance in children: No evidence for a causal relationship. *Twin Res Hum Genet.* 2009;12:246–253.

52. Hansen TG, Pedersen JK, Henneberg SW, et al. Academic performance in adolescence after inguinal hernia repair in infancy: a nationwide cohort study. *Anesthesiology.* 2011;114(5):1076–1085.

53. Davidson AJ, Disma N, de Graaff JC, et al. GAS Consortium Neurodevelopmental outcome at 2 years of age after general anaesthesia and awake-regional anaesthesia in infancy (GAS): An international multicentre, randomised controlled trial. *Lancet.* 2015;387(10015):239–250.

54. McCann ME, de Graaff JC, Dorris L, et al. GAS Consortium Neurodevelopmental outcome at 5 years of age after general anaesthesia or awake-regional anaesthesia in infancy (GAS): An international, multicentre, randomised, controlled equivalence trial. *Lancet.* 2019 Feb 16;393(10172):664–677.

55. Sun LS, Li G, Miller TL, et al. Association between a single general anesthesia exposure before age 36 months and neurocognitive outcomes in later childhood. *JAMA.* 2016;315:2312–2320.

56. Berger M, Nadler JW, Browndyke J, et al. Postoperative cognitive dysfunction: Minding the gaps in our knowledge of a common postoperative complication in the elderly. *Anesthesiol Clin.* 2015;33(3):517–550.

57. McCann ME, Lee JK, Inder T. Beyond anesthesia toxicity: Anesthetic considerations to lessen the risk of neonatal neurological injury. *Anesth Analg.* 2019 Nov;129(5):1354–1364.

58. Jacola LM, Anghelescu DL, Hall L, Russell K, Zhang H, Wang F, Peters JB, Rossi M, Schreiber JE, Gajjar A. Anesthesia exposure during therapy predicts neurocognitive outcomes in survivors of childhood medulloblastoma. *J Pediatr.* 2020;223:141–147.

59. Ing C, Warner DO, Sun L. Anesthesia and developing brains: Unanswered questions and proposed paths forward. *Anesthesiology.* 2022;136(3):500–512.

Section III

PREOPERATIVE PREPARATION AND INTRAOPERATIVE MANAGEMENT

13 PREOPERATIVE EVALUATION

Manuel C. Pardo, Jr.

High-quality anesthesia care begins with the preoperative evaluation. The goals of preoperative evaluation include understanding the proposed surgery, assessing the risk of coexisting medical conditions, deciding whether additional testing is needed to prepare the patient for the procedure, discussing options for anesthesia care, and understanding and addressing patient concerns. Preoperative (or preanesthesia) evaluation can be defined as the process of clinical assessment that precedes the delivery of anesthesia care for surgery and for nonsurgical procedures.[1] The American Society of Anesthesiologists (ASA) developed standards for preanesthesia care, listed in Box 13.1.[2]

Settings for preoperative evaluation include both outpatient (e.g., in-person or virtual preoperative evaluation clinic) and inpatient (e.g., a patient preadmitted before surgery or already an inpatient in the emergency department, hospital ward, or intensive care unit). Most patients undergoing elective surgery are evaluated as outpatients at varying time intervals before the date of surgery. The timing of preoperative evaluation with respect to the proposed date of surgery has practical implications for preoperative consultation, testing, and communication between providers and patients.

This chapter will focus on the preoperative evaluation of an individual patient before a surgical or nonsurgical procedure requiring anesthesia care. This process is part of the specialty's contribution to perioperative medicine (also see Chapter 42), which includes preoperative assessment, nonsurgical patient optimization, the surgical procedure itself, and postoperative care until the patient can return to their primary care and other long-term providers after surgery.

HISTORY AND PHYSICAL EXAMINATION

The preoperative history and physical follow the same basic structure as a general medical encounter. However, each element has perioperative implications that must be explored

---

Box 13.1 American Society of Anesthesiologists Basic Standards for Preanesthesia Care

An anesthesiologist shall be responsible for determining the medical status of the patient and developing a plan of anesthesia care. The anesthesiologist, before the delivery of anesthesia care, is responsible for:

1. Reviewing the available medical record.
2. Interviewing and performing a focused examination of the patient to:
   2.1 Discuss the medical history, including previous anesthetic experiences and medical therapy.
   2.2 Assess those aspects of the patient's physical condition that might affect decisions regarding perioperative risk management.
3. Ordering and reviewing pertinent available tests and consultations as necessary for the delivery of anesthesia care.
4. Ordering appropriate preoperative medications.
5. Ensuring that consent has been obtained for the anesthesia care.
6. Documenting in the chart that the above has been performed.

These standards apply to all patients who receive anesthesia care. Under exceptional circumstances, these standards may be modified. When this is the case, the circumstances shall be documented in the patient's record.

American Society of Anesthesiologists. Basic Standards for Preanesthesia Care. Developed by Committee on Standards and Practice Parameters (CSPP). Last affirmed: December 13, 2020 (original approval: October 14, 1987).

---

further. For example, the history of present illness begins with the following: the patient is a *(age)*-year old *(sex/gender)* with *(surgical diagnosis)* who is scheduled for *(proposed procedure)* with *(surgeon/proceduralist)* on *(proposed date of surgery)* at *(health care facility)*. Some implications of these seven initial elements are described in Table 13.1.

The past medical history includes a discussion of current medical conditions and past hospitalizations. Certain medical conditions have significant perioperative implications for management and will be discussed later. The review of current medications should include prescription and nonprescription medications, topical medications, vitamins, and herbal preparations. If the patient has allergies, the date and nature of the reaction are helpful in determining their relevance. For example, even though 10% of the U.S. population has a history of penicillin allergy, few have clinically significant reactions.[3]

The past surgical and anesthetic history is of particular importance in the preoperative evaluation. Prior anesthesia records can indicate the presence of difficult airway management, intraoperative hemodynamic or respiratory issues, or postoperative nausea and vomiting. For patients undergoing the same procedure on a repeat basis (e.g., endoscopic retrograde cholangiopancreatography [ERCP] or electroconvulsive therapy [ECT]), the anesthesia medications administered should be noted as well. The patient's prior experience with regional

anesthesia can be discussed, which is relevant for procedures amenable to regional anesthesia and analgesia (also see Chapters 17 and 18).

The social history includes a discussion of risk factors for disease, such as tobacco use, alcohol use, and substance use. Social circumstances also contribute to a patient's risk of morbidity or mortality after surgical procedures. Social determinants of health are defined by the World Health Organization as the nonmedical factors that influence health outcomes, including the conditions in which people are born, grow, work, live, and age and the wider set of forces and systems shaping the conditions of daily life.[4] Specific factors include housing, transportation, education, employment, and access to care.

Family history of reactions to anesthesia often include nonspecific descriptions. Potential complications of most relevance for future anesthesia care include malignant hyperthermia or atypical plasma pseudocholinesterase (also see Chapters 7 and 11).

The review of systems is designed to elicit symptoms not already discussed in the history of present illness or past medical history. In the preoperative evaluation the review of systems should include a discussion of weight loss (relevant to nutritional status and frailty), functional status (described further later), screening for sleep apnea (e.g., STOP-BANG score, described in Chapter 48), and baseline cognitive function (for elderly patients, as described in Chapter 35).

The physical examination of a preoperative patient includes determination of vital signs, weight, and overall patient appearance. In the outpatient setting these vital signs serve as a reasonable baseline, although a single elevated blood pressure is insufficient for the diagnosis of hypertension. Table 13.2 describes the physical examination for a preoperative patient. Based on the patient's history, additional physical examination and documentation may be indicated. The American Society of Anesthesiologists (ASA) Practice Advisory for Preanesthesia Evaluation recommends that, at a minimum, a preanesthetic physical examination should include an airway examination, a pulmonary examination (including lung auscultation), and a cardiovascular examination.[1]

During the COVID-19 pandemic, the use of telehealth visits increased, leading to fewer in-person outpatient preoperative evaluations and a decrease in physical examinations until the date of surgery. The use of video and digital home monitoring devices can facilitate a virtual focused physical examination.[5]

PREOPERATIVE EVALUATION OF COMMON COEXISTING DISEASES

The patient history and review of past medical records may reveal the presence of coexisting medical conditions. The following section reviews common conditions

Table 13.1 History of Present Illness (HPI) With Anesthetic Considerations

HPI Element	Anesthetic Considerations
Age	Extremes of age are associated with changes in physiology (also see Chapters 34 and 35).
Sex/Gender	Some anesthetic complications, such as postoperative nausea and vomiting, are more likely in female patients.
Surgical Diagnosis	The surgical diagnosis may be associated with medical issues that have anesthetic implications. For example, a patient with severe back pain scheduled for spinal fusion may be receiving long-term opiate medications. A patient with small bowel obstruction may have electrolyte abnormalities and hypovolemia.
Proposed Procedure	The surgical procedure has implications for anesthesia choice. For example, extremity surgery can typically be performed with general or regional anesthesia. Certain procedures may benefit from regional anesthesia for postoperative pain management (also see Chapter 40). The risk of major adverse cardiovascular events is greater in vascular, intraperitoneal, and intrathoracic procedures, which may alter the risk/benefit ratio of further workup for coronary artery disease. Nonoperating room procedures (NORA) have different implications (also see Chapter 38).
Surgeon	At a given health care facility, different surgeons performing the same procedure may have different preferences for patient management and participation in enhanced recovery pathways.
Proposed Date of Surgery	Earlier anesthesiologist access may allow time for necessary preoperative testing and consultation, especially for a patient with severe systemic disease undergoing major surgery.
Health Care Facility	Procedures performed in a free-standing ambulatory facility likely have different resources in the event of postoperative complications (also see Chapter 37). Access to an intensive care unit and blood bank may be required depending on the proposed surgery and patient's coexisting diseases.

Table 13.2 Physical Examination in Preoperative Evaluation

Physical Examination Component	Anesthetic Considerations
Vital Signs	Markedly abnormal vital signs require a focused and rapid evaluation. In an outpatient preoperative clinic the patient may even require transfer to an emergency department for further care.
Weight	This is part of the assessment of nutrition and frailty. Patients with obesity are at greater risk for many perioperative complications (also see Chapter 29).
Overall Appearance	For inpatients scheduled for emergency procedures, the overall appearance of distress may be a clue to impending hemodynamic instability or respiratory compromise.
Airway	The basic elements include determination of mouth opening, pharyngeal space, cervical spine extension, and submandibular space/compliance. Airway examination is described in detail in Chapter 16.
Pulmonary	The lung examination is particularly important in patients with pulmonary disease or heart failure (also see Chapters 26 and 27).
Cardiovascular	The location, timing, intensity, and radiation of heart murmurs should be noted. Quiet systolic murmurs are unlikely to be associated with severe valvular disease. Peripheral pulses should be palpated, especially if arterial line placement is being considered.
Abdomen	Abdominal distension and obesity are associated with reduced lung/chest wall compliance during general anesthesia and mechanical ventilation. For patients with liver disease, the presence of ascites is a marker of disease severity (also see Chapter 28).
Musculoskeletal	In addition to evaluating for extremity edema (a potential sign of deep venous thrombosis or heart failure), consider evaluating range of motion of joints that will be affected by intraoperative patient positioning (also see Chapter 19).
Neurologic/Psychiatric	Neurologic changes such as weakness or numbness should be documented at baseline. For patients undergoing regional anesthesia, this baseline documentation is particularly important if postoperative changes are detected. Psychiatric illnesses, if severe, may affect the patient's ability to consent for surgery and anesthesia.
Skin	Skin lesions should be noted, because pressure injuries related to positioning may occur (also see Chapter 19). If regional anesthesia is planned, inspection of the skin near sites of planned needle insertion is required.

encountered in preoperative evaluation, organized by organ system. Many conditions are addressed by evidence-based clinical practice guidelines from anesthesiology and other specialties. However, substantial clinical judgment is still required to determine how guidelines apply to an individual patient. In many instances clinical practice guidelines provide advice based on expert opinion and not necessarily evidence from clinical trials. In addition, practice guidelines must be considered in conjunction with patient preferences, although it is the anesthesia provider's responsibility to emphasize appropriate evidence when presenting management options to the patient.

Additional discussion of the pathophysiology and anesthetic implications of coexisting disease may be found in other sources.[6]

Neurologic

Preoperative evaluation of patients with an intracranial mass lesion is discussed in Chapter 30. Patients with epilepsy syndromes are treated with antiepileptic drugs, which should be continued perioperatively unless the patient is undergoing epilepsy surgery, in which case the management of the antiepileptic drugs should be coordinated with the neurosurgery team. Patients with a history of acute ischemic stroke may be receiving antiplatelet or anticoagulant therapy for secondary prevention. Preoperative management of these medications is discussed later.

Parkinson Disease

Parkinson disease is the second most common neurodegenerative disorder, characterized by bradykinesia, rigidity, and tremor. Patients with Parkinson disease have a greater risk of perioperative morbidity and mortality related to the cardiovascular (e.g., orthostatic hypotension, autonomic dysfunction), pulmonary (e.g., dysphagia, impaired cough, aspiration pneumonia), neurologic (e.g., bradykinesia and fall risk, insufficient respiratory muscle strength), and infectious (e.g., increased risk of urinary tract and bacterial infections) implications of the disease.[7] Issues to address in the preoperative evaluation include the presence of comorbidities and treatment regimen, which may include both pharmacologic and deep brain stimulation. Important aspects of preoperative medication management include continuing the patient's home medication regimen as closely as possible, which is typically a strict schedule.[8] Continuing the home medication schedule will help avoid exacerbation of Parkinson disease symptoms on the day of surgery. This is particularly important for levodopa, which has a half-life of only 1 to 2 hours. Although patients must follow *nil per os* (NPO) guidelines, the Parkinson disease medications should be allowed with a sip of water. For procedures requiring general anesthesia, it is recommended that monoamine oxidase-B inhibitors (e.g., rasagiline, selegiline) be stopped 1 to 2 weeks before surgery to reduce

the risk of drug interactions with opioids and the risk of serotonin syndrome.[8]

Cardiovascular

Several specialty societies have published clinical practice guidelines on perioperative cardiovascular evaluation and management of patients undergoing noncardiac surgery, including the American College of Cardiology/American Heart Association (ACC/AHA),[9] the European Society of Cardiology and European Society of Anaesthesiology,[10] and the Canadian Cardiovascular Society.[11] The 2014 ACC/AHA practice guideline includes a stepwise approach to perioperative cardiac assessment and addresses coronary artery disease, heart failure, cardiomyopathy, valvular heart disease, arrhythmias and conduction disorders, pulmonary vascular disease, and adult congenital heart disease.

This section will review the following cardiovascular conditions commonly encountered in preoperative evaluation of the patient undergoing noncardiac surgery: coronary artery disease (also discussed in Chapter 26), hypertension, the patient receiving anticoagulant therapy (for mechanical heart valve, atrial fibrillation, or venous thromboembolism), and the patient receiving antiplatelet therapy (for coronary artery disease or stroke).

The following conditions are discussed in Chapter 26 and will not be addressed here: valvular heart disease, cardiac conduction and rhythm disturbances, cardiac implantable electronic devices, heart failure, hypertrophic cardiomyopathy, and pulmonary hypertension.

Coronary Artery Disease

Because ischemic heart disease is the leading cause of death in the world and a risk factor for perioperative mortality, preoperative assessment of coronary artery disease is an important part of the preoperative evaluation. Cardiovascular risk factors (hypertension, dyslipidemia, diabetes mellitus, obesity, chronic kidney disease) are present in 45% of patients aged 45 years or older undergoing noncardiac surgery in the United States.[12] Important concepts in the evaluation of patients with coronary artery disease include ruling out acute coronary syndrome, which includes unstable angina, ST-segment elevation myocardial infarction, and non–ST-segment-elevation myocardial infarction–these conditions require guideline-directed medical therapy by a cardiologist.

A stepwise approach for perioperative cardiac assessment from the 2014 ACC/AHA perioperative clinical practice guideline is shown in Fig. 13.1. Key concepts of this approach include use of a risk calculator to estimate the risk of major adverse cardiac events and using functional capacity to help determine the need for additional testing. An example of the metabolic equivalents for common physical activities is listed in Table 13.3. However, subjective assessment of functional status based on patient history may not be as accurate as a more formal

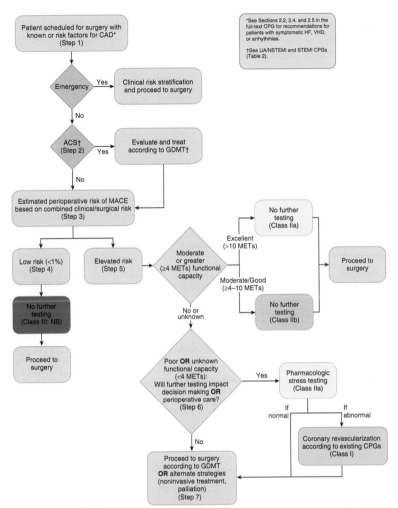

Fig. 13.1 ACC/AHA stepwise approach to perioperative cardiac assessment for CAD. **Step 1**: In patients scheduled for surgery with risk factors for or known CAD determine the urgency of surgery. If an emergency, then determine the clinical risk factors that may influence perioperative management and proceed to surgery with appropriate monitoring and management strategies based on the clinical assessment. **Step 2**: If the surgery is urgent or elective, determine if the patient has an ACS. If yes, then refer patient for cardiology evaluation and management according to GDMT. **Step 3**: If the patient has risk factors for stable CAD, then estimate the perioperative risk of MACE on the basis of the combined clinical/surgical risk. This estimate can use the American College of Surgeons NSQIP risk calculator or RCRI. **Step 4**: If the patient has a low risk of MACE (<1%), then no further testing is needed and the patient may proceed to surgery. **Step 5**: If the patient is at elevated risk of MACE, then determine functional capacity with an objective measure or scale such as the DASI. If the patient has moderate, good, or excellent functional capacity (≥4 METs), then proceed to surgery without further evaluation. **Step 6**: If the patient has poor (<4 METs) or unknown functional capacity, then the clinician should consult with the patient and perioperative team to determine whether further testing will affect patient decision making (e.g., decision to perform original surgery or willingness to undergo CABG or PCI, depending on the results of the test) or perioperative care. If yes, then pharmacologic stress testing is appropriate. In those patients with unknown functional capacity, exercise stress testing may be reasonable to perform. If the stress test is abnormal, consider coronary angiography and revascularization, depending on the extent of the abnormal test. The patient can then proceed to surgery with GDMT or consider alternative strategies, such as noninvasive treatment of the indication for surgery (e.g., radiation therapy for cancer) or palliation. If the test is normal, proceed to surgery according to GDMT. **Step 7**: If testing will not affect decision making or care, then proceed to surgery according to GDMT or consider alternative strategies, such as noninvasive treatment of the indication for surgery (e.g., radiation therapy for cancer) or palliation. *ACS,* Acute coronary syndrome; *CABG,* coronary artery bypass graft; *CAD,* coronary artery disease; *CPG,* clinical practice guideline; *DASI,* Duke Activity Status Index; *GDMT,* guideline-directed medical therapy; *HF,* heart failure; *MACE,* major adverse cardiac event; *MET,* metabolic equivalent; *NB,* no benefit; *NSQIP,* National Surgical Quality Improvement Program; *PCI,* percutaneous coronary intervention; *RCRI,* Revised Cardiac Risk Index; *STEMI,* ST-elevation myocardial infarction; *UA/NSTEMI,* unstable angina/non–ST-elevation myocardial infarction; *VHD,* valvular heart disease. (From in Fleisher LA, Fleischmann KE, Auerbach AD, et al. 2014 ACC/AHA guideline on perioperative cardiovascular evaluation and management of patients undergoing noncardiac surgery: A report of the American College of Cardiology/American Heart Association Task Force on Practice Guidelines. *J Am Coll Cardiol.* 2014;64[22]:e77–e137, Fig. 1.)

Table 13.3 Metabolic Equivalents of Common Physical Activities

Category of Activity	Description of Activity	METs
Home activities	Cooking or food preparation	2.5
	Cleaning, sweeping carpet or floors	3.3
	Sweeping garage, sidewalk, or outside of house	4.0
	Raking lawn	4.0
	Yard work, general, moderate effort	4.0
Walking	Walking within house	2.0
	Walking 2.5 mph, level surface	3.0
	Stair climbing, slow pace	4.0
	Walking 3.5 mph, level surface	4.3
	Walking, climbing hills, no load	6.3
Running	Running 4 mph (13 min/mile)	6
	Running 6.7 mph (9 min/mile)	10.5
Bicycling	Bicycling, <10 mph, leisure, to work or for pleasure	4.0
	Bicycling, 14–15.9 mph, racing or leisure, fast vigorous effort	10.0
Gym/exercise	Yoga, Hatha	2.5
	Yoga, Power	4.0
	Bicycling, stationary, 51–89 watts, light-to-moderate effort	4.8
	Elliptical trainer, moderate effort	5.0
	Aerobic dance, low impact	5.0
	Aerobic dance, high impact	7.3
	Bicycling, stationary, RPM/Spin bike class	8.5
Other sports	Golf, using power cart	3.5
	Golf, walking, carrying clubs	4.3
	Skiing, downhill, alpine or snowboarding, moderate effort, general, active time only	5.3
	Tennis, doubles	6.0
	Swimming, leisurely, not lap swimming, general	6.0
	Skiing, cross country, 2.5 mph, slow or light effort, ski walking	6.8
	Soccer, casual, general	7.0
	Rollerblading, in-line skating 9 mph, recreational pace	7.5
	Rock or mountain climbing	8.0
	Tennis, singles	8.0
	Rope jumping, slow pace (<100 skips/min)	8.8
	Swimming laps, freestyle, fast, vigorous effort	9.8

From 2011 Compendium of Physical Activities. Medicine and Science in Sports and Exercise. https://links.lww.com/MSS/A82.

activity scale such as the Duke Activity Status Index (DASI).[13] Table 13.4 lists the questions asked on the DASI scale.[14] One prospective cohort study recommended a DASI score of 34 as a threshold for identifying patients at risk for cardiac complications (i.e., patients with DASI score greater than 34 are at lower risk).[15]

Several calculators can estimate the risk of perioperative cardiovascular events. Examples include the Revised Cardiac Risk Index,[16] the American College of Surgeons National Surgical Quality Improvement Program (NSQIP) risk calculator,[17] and the Cardiovascular Risk Index (CVRI).[18] These risk calculators are compared in Table 13.5.

Table 13.4 Duke Activity Status Index (DASI)

Activity	Weight
Can you ...	
1. Take care of yourself, that is, eating, dressing, bathing, or using the toilet?	2.75
2. Walk indoors, such as around your house?	1.75
3. Walk a block or two on level ground?	2.75
4. Climb a flight of stairs or walk up a hill?	5.50
5. Run a short distance?	8.00
6. Do light work around the house like dusting or washing dishes?	2.70
7. Do moderate work around the house like vacuuming, sweeping floors, or carrying in groceries?	3.50
8. Do heavy work around the house like scrubbing floors or lifting or moving heavy furniture?	8.00
9. Do yardwork like raking leaves, weeding, or pushing a power mower?	4.50
10. Have sexual relations?	5.25
11. Participate in moderate recreational activities like golf, bowling, dancing, doubles tennis, or throwing a baseball or football?	6.00
12. Participate in strenuous sports like swimming, singles tennis, football, basketball, or skiing?	7.50

Positive responses are added to get a total score, which ranges from 0 to 58.2.
From Hlatky MA, Boineau RE, Higginbotham MB, et al. A brief self-administered questionnaire to determine functional capacity (the Duke Activity Status Index). *Am J Cardiol.* 1989;64(10):651–654.

Table 13.5 Risk Scores and Calculators to Predict Adverse Cardiac Events

Risk Score or Calculator	Criteria	Comments
Revised Cardiac Risk Index (RCRI)	High-risk type of surgery (intraperitoneal, intrathoracic, or supra-inguinal vascular), ischemic heart disease, history of congestive heart failure, history of cerebral vascular disease, insulin therapy for diabetes, preoperative serum creatinine >2.0 mg/dL	Each element is worth 1 point. Rate of major cardiac complications of 1% occurred with 1 point. From Lee TH, Marcantonio ER, Mangione CM, et al. Derivation and prospective validation of a simple index for prediction of cardiac risk of major noncardiac surgery. *Circulation.* 1999;100(10):1043–1049.
Cardiovascular Risk Index (CVRI)	Age ≥75, hemoglobin less than 12 mg/dL, any history of heart disease, symptoms of angina or dyspnea, vascular surgery, emergency surgery	Each element is worth 1 point. Outcomes assessed included risk of death, MI, or stroke. Risk of MI was 1% with CVRI score of 2. From Dakik HA, Chehab O, Eldirani M, et al. A new index for pre-operative cardiovascular evaluation. *J Am Coll Cardiol.* 2019;73(24):3067–3078.
NSQIP Surgical Risk Calculator	20 elements including procedure, age, sex, functional status, emergency case, ASA class, and presence of the following medical issues: steroid use, ascites, sepsis, ventilator dependence, disseminated cancer, diabetes, hypertension on medications, CHF, dyspnea, smoking status, COPD, dialysis, acute renal failure, and BMI.	Online risk calculator at: https://riskcalculator.facs.org/RiskCalculator/ Provides risk estimates compared with average for a variety of outcomes, including serious complications, any complications, cardiac complications, discharge to nursing or rehabilitation facility, and death. From Bilimoria KY, Liu Y, Paruch JL, et al. Development and evaluation of the universal ACS NSQIP surgical risk calculator: A decision aid and informed consent tool for patients and surgeons. *J Am Coll Surg.* 2013;217(5):833–842e1-e3.

ASA, American Society of Anesthesiologists; *BMI,* body mass index; *CHF,* congestive heart failure; *COPD,* chronic obstructive pulmonary disease; *MI,* myocardial infarction.

Hypertension

Hypertension is a major cause of death worldwide and is a risk factor for cardiovascular disease, stroke, and end-stage renal disease. As a perioperative risk factor, hypertension is most significant when end-organ damage is present. There have been no high-quality randomized trials on specific blood pressure targets before major surgery. However, general recommendations for the treatment of hypertension in patients undergoing surgical procedures are provided in the 2017 ACC Guideline for the Prevention, Detection, Evaluation, and Management of High Blood Pressure in Adults, listed in Box 13.2.[19] Perioperative management of chronic therapy with angiotensin-converting enzyme (ACE) inhibitors or angiotensin receptor blockers (ARBs) is an area of controversy. These medications have clearly been associated with intraoperative hypotension. However, a 2018 metaanalysis did not demonstrate a difference in mortality, major cardiac events, stroke, or acute kidney injury when comparing patients who withheld ACE inhibitor or ARB therapy on the morning of surgery with those who continued them.[20]

The Patient Receiving Anticoagulant Therapy

Patients with the following disorders may be receiving anticoagulation therapy: mechanical heart valve, atrial fibrillation, and venous thromboembolism. Perioperative management of anticoagulation therapy includes the following risk–benefit analysis: balancing the risk of a thrombotic event with discontinuation of anticoagulation

---

Box 13.2 Recommendations for Treatment of Hypertension in Patients Undergoing Surgical Procedures

1. In patients with hypertension undergoing major surgery who have been on β-blockers chronically β-blockers should be continued.
2. In patients with hypertension undergoing planned elective major surgery it is reasonable to continue medical therapy for hypertension until surgery.
3. In patients with hypertension undergoing major surgery discontinuation of ACE inhibitors or ARBs perioperatively may be considered.
4. In patients with planned elective major surgery and SBP of 180 mm Hg or higher or DBP of 110 mm Hg or higher deferring surgery may be considered.
5. For patients undergoing surgery, abrupt preoperative discontinuation of β-blockers or clonidine is potentially harmful.
6. β-Blockers should not be started on the day of surgery in β-blocker-naïve patients.

ACE, Angiotensin-converting enzyme; *ARB*, angiotensin receptor blocker. From Whelton PK, Carey RM, Aronow WS, et al. 2017 ACC/AHA/AAPA/ABC/ACPM/AGS/APhA/ASH/ASPC/NMA/PCNA guideline for the prevention, detection, evaluation, and management of high blood pressure in adults: Executive summary: A report of the American College of Cardiology/American Heart Association Task Force on Clinical Practice Guidelines. *Circulation*. 2018;138(17):e426–e483, Table 11.5.

---

therapy (e.g., embolic stroke, new venous thromboembolism, or pulmonary embolism) compared with the risk of bleeding with surgery or an anesthetic intervention (e.g., neuraxial block). The risk of perioperative thromboembolism can be estimated as indicated in Table 13.6.[21]

A 2012 evidence-based clinical practice guideline from the American College of Chest Physicians (ACCP) recommended situations in which patients on vitamin K antagonist (VKA) therapy should receive bridging therapy during interruption of VKA therapy.[21] Patients with mechanical heart valves, atrial fibrillation, or venous thromboembolism at *high risk* for thromboembolism (as described in Table 13.6) should receive bridging anticoagulation when VKA therapy must be interrupted before surgery. The rationale for bridging is that a VKA (e.g., warfarin) must be stopped for approximately 5 days before the anticoagulant effects abate completely. As the anticoagulant effect wanes, the patient's thromboembolism risk increases, thus potentially requiring "bridging" with a short-acting anticoagulant such as subcutaneous low-molecular-weight heparin or subcutaneous unfractionated heparin.

For patients with *low risk* for thromboembolism, the 2012 ACCP guidelines suggest no bridging, and for patients at *moderate risk* for thromboembolism, the need for bridging is based on an assessment of individual patient and surgery-related risk factors, such as the risk of surgical bleeding and the ability to obtain local hemostasis.[21] For example, endoscopic or urologic procedures that do not involve a biopsy can often be performed without interrupting anticoagulation. By contrast, procedures such as neurosurgical or cardiothoracic procedures pose a higher risk of bleeding with residual anticoagulant effects. Table 13.7 provides examples of surgical and other invasive procedures with their estimated risk of surgical bleeding.[22] In addition, although some procedures are unlikely to require blood transfusion, they may involve the risk of bleeding in an enclosed space or in an area in which local hemostasis is difficult to achieve (e.g., ophthalmologic posterior chamber procedure, intracranial or spinal procedures, neuraxial block). The surgeon or proceduralist should be consulted if there are unresolved questions about the bleeding risk of a procedure for a given patient.

Since the 1950s, the VKA warfarin was administered when oral anticoagulation was needed for the prevention of stroke in patients with atrial fibrillation. In 2010 the U.S. Food and Drug Administration (FDA) approved dabigatran (Pradaxa), a direct oral anticoagulant (DOAC) whose mechanism of action is direct thrombin inhibition, to reduce the risk of stroke and systemic embolism in patients with nonvalvular atrial fibrillation (also see Chapter 23). Advantages of DOACs over warfarin include more predictable pharmacokinetics, fewer drug interactions, and lower risk of intracranial bleeding. In addition, because the DOACs have relatively short half-lives, bridging anticoagulation is not usually

Table 13.6 Risk Stratification for Perioperative Thromboembolism

Risk Stratum	Indication for VKA Therapy		
	Mechanical Heart Valve	**Atrial Fibrillation**	**VTE**
High[a]	Any mitral valve prosthesis	CHADS$_2$ score of 5 or 6 (see score at the bottom)	Recent (within 3 mo) VTE
			Severe thrombophilia (e.g., deficiency of protein C, protein S, or antithrombin; antiphospholipid antibodies; multiple abnormalities)
	Any caged-ball or tilting disc aortic valve prosthesis	Recent (within 3 mo) stroke or TIA	Severe thrombophilia (e.g., deficiency of protein C, protein S, or antithrombin; antiphospholipid antibodies; multiple abnormalities)
	Recent (within 6 mo) stroke or TIA	Rheumatic valvular heart disease	
Moderate	Bileaflet aortic valve prosthesis and one or more of the following risk factors: atrial fibrillation, prior stroke or transient ischemic attack, hypertension, diabetes, congestive heart failure, age >75 yr	CHADS$_2$ score of 3 or 4	VTE within the past 3–12 mo
			Nonsevere thrombophilia (e.g., heterozygous factor V Leiden or prothrombin gene mutation)
			Recurrent VTE
			Active cancer (treated within 6 mo or palliative)
Low	Bileaflet aortic valve prosthesis without atrial fibrillation and no other risk factors for stroke	CHADS$_2$ score of 0–2 (assuming no prior stroke or TIA)	VTE >12 mo previous and no other risk factors

[a]High-risk patients may also include those with a prior stroke or transient ischemic attack occurring >3 mo before the planned surgery and a CHADS$_2$ score <5, those with prior thromboembolism during temporary interruption of VKAs, or those undergoing certain types of surgery associated with an increased risk for stroke or other thromboembolism (e.g., cardiac valve replacement, carotid endarterectomy, major vascular surgery).

CHADS$_2$, Congestive heart failure, hypertension, age ≥75 years, diabetes mellitus, and prior stroke or TIA. If present, each item is counted as 1 point except prior stroke or TIA, which is counted as 2 points; total score is sum of the points.

Douketis JD, Spyropoulos AC, Spencer FA, et al. Perioperative management of antithrombotic therapy: Antithrombotic Therapy and Prevention of Thrombosis, 9th ed: American College of Chest Physicians Evidence-Based Clinical Practice Guidelines. *Chest.* 2012;141(2 Suppl):e326S–e350S, Table 1.

recommended when DOACs are discontinued before surgery. Disadvantages of DOACs include the requirement for dose adjustment in patients with chronic kidney disease (CKD). A related pharmacokinetic issue is that the DOAC discontinuation date before a surgical procedure depends on the procedural bleeding risk and the patient's creatinine clearance.[23] See Table 13.8 for an example.

Although clinical practice guidelines provide recommendations for the interruption of anticoagulation, they do not replace clinician judgment for an individual patient. Each patient has a different risk profile and procedural risk; patient and provider preferences may also influence recommendations for when to hold anticoagulant therapy. Challenging situations include a patient with known venous thromboembolism (and/or pulmonary embolism) and a contraindication to anticoagulation or interruption of anticoagulation in the <3 month treatment window (e.g., a patient scheduled for urgent intracranial tumor surgery). In settings like this expert opinion suggests that inferior vena cava (IVC) filter placement be considered.[24]

After the 2012 ACCP perioperative antithrombotic guidelines were published, additional clinical trials were performed in patients with atrial fibrillation. A 2015 randomized trial evaluated over 1800 patients with chronic atrial fibrillation receiving warfarin therapy who were undergoing an elective surgery or other

Table 13.7	Risk Stratification of Surgical Bleeding Risk
High bleeding risk procedures (30-day risk of major bleed >2%)[a]	• Major surgery with extensive tissue injury • Cancer surgery, especially solid tumor resection • Major orthopedic surgery, including shoulder replacement surgery • Reconstructive plastic surgery • Urologic or gastrointestinal surgery, especially anastomosis surgery • Transurethral prostate resection, bladder resection, or tumor ablation • Nephrectomy, kidney biopsy • Colonic polyp resection • Bowel resection • Percutaneous endoscopic gastrotomy (PEG) placement, endoscopic retrograde cholangiopancreatography (ERCP) • Surgery in highly vascular organs (kidneys, liver, spleen) • Cardiac, intracranial, or spinal surgery • Any major operation (procedure duration >45 min) • Neuraxial anesthesia[b]
Low/moderate bleeding risk procedures[c] (30-day risk of major bleed 0%–2%)	• Arthroscopy • Cutaneous/lymph node biopsies • Foot/hand surgery • Coronary angiography[d] • Gastrointestinal endoscopy ± biopsy • Colonoscopy ± biopsy • Abdominal hysterectomy • Laparoscopic cholecystectomy • Abdominal hernia repair • Hemorrhoidal surgery • Bronchoscopy ± biopsy • Epidural injections
Minimal bleeding risk procedures[e] (30-day risk of major bleed ~0%)	• Minor dermatologic procedures (excision of basal and squamous cell skin cancers, actinic keratoses, and premalignant or cancerous skin nevi) • Ophthalmologic (cataract) procedures • Minor dental procedures (dental extractions, restorations, prosthetics, endodontics), dental cleanings, fillings • Pacemaker or cardioverter-defibrillator device implantation

[a]No residual anticoagulant effect at time of procedure (i.e., 4–5 drug half-life interruption preprocedure).
[b]Includes spinal and epidural anesthesia, consider not only absolute major bleed event rate but catastrophic consequences of a major bleed.
[c]Some residual anticoagulant effect allowed (i.e., 2–3 drug half-life interruption preprocedure).
[d]Radial approach may be considered minimal bleed risk compared with femoral approach.
[e]Procedure can be safely done under full-dose anticoagulation (may consider holding direct oral anticoagulant dose day of procedure to avoid peak anticoagulant effects).
From Spyropoulos AC, Brohi K, Caprini J, et al. SSC Subcommittee on Perioperative and Critical Care Thrombosis and Haemostasis of the International Society on Thrombosis and Haemostasis. Scientific and Standardization Committee Communication: Guidance document on the periprocedural management of patients on chronic oral anticoagulant therapy: Recommendations for standardized reporting of procedural/surgical bleed risk and patient-specific thromboembolic risk. *J Thromb Haemost.* 2019;17(11):1966–1972, Table 1.

invasive procedure requiring interruption of warfarin.[25] One group of patients received bridging anticoagulation with low-molecular-weight heparin, whereas the other group received no bridging. In terms of arterial thromboembolism risk, the no-bridging group was noninferior to the bridging group; the incidence of major bleeding was lower in the no-bridging group. The American College of Cardiology published the 2017 ACC Expert Consensus Decision Pathway for Periprocedural Management of Anticoagulation in Patients With Nonvalvular Atrial Fibrillation.[26] The pathway includes a suggested algorithm for the bridge versus no-bridge decision-making process in this patient population (Fig. 13.2).

The Patient Receiving Antiplatelet Therapy
Coronary artery disease and stroke represent the top two causes of mortality worldwide. These patients may receive antiplatelet therapy for pharmacologic prevention of arterial thrombotic events. As with anticoagulant therapy, perioperative management involves balancing the risks of ischemia and thrombosis with the risk of bleeding. Antiplatelet agents can be used for primary and secondary prevention of thrombosis, either as monotherapy or

Table 13.8	Example of DOAC Periprocedural Management: Rivaroxaban				
Drug	Renal Function	Low Procedural Bleeding Risk (Interval Between Last Dose and Procedure)	High Procedural Bleeding Risk (Interval Between Last Dose and Procedure)	Very High Procedural Bleeding Risk (e.g., Cardiothoracic, Intracranial, Neuraxial; Interval Between Last Dose and Procedure)	Resumption of DOAC
Rivaroxaban (Xarelto)	CrCl ≥30 mL/min $t_{1/2}$ = 8-9 hr CrCl 15-29 mL/min $t_{1/2}$ = 9-10 hr CrCl <5 mL/min or on HD $t_{1/2}$ = unknown	24 hr (last dose 2 days prior) 48 hr (last dose 3 days prior) >96 hr (last dose >5 days prior)	48 hr (last dose 3 days prior) 72 hr (last dose 4 days prior) >96 hr (last dose >5 days prior)	72 hr (last dose 4 days prior) 120 hr (last dose 6 days prior) >120 hr (last dose >6 days prior)	• Low bleed risk: consider resuming no sooner than 1 day postop • High/very high risk: consider resuming 2-3 days postop • For all patients: discuss timing with proceduralist

CrCl, Creatinine clearance; *DOAC*, direct oral anticoagulant; *ESRD*, end-stage renal disease; *HD*, hemodialysis; $t_{1/2}$, half-life.
Periprocedural management of other DOACs will vary depending on drug pharmacokinetics. For patients with ESRD on DOACs, consider consultation with institutional hematology or anticoagulation service.
From Douketis JD, Spyropoulos AC, Anderson JM, et al. The Perioperative Anticoagulant Use for Surgery Evaluation (PAUSE) study for patients on a direct oral anticoagulant who need an elective surgery or procedure: Design and rationale. *Thromb Haemost.* 2017;117(12):2415-2424. Erratum in: *Thromb Haemost.* 2018;118(9):1679-1680, and author's institutional guidelines (University of California, San Francisco).

as dual antiplatelet therapy (DAPT). Primary prevention is indicated in patients at higher risk of atherosclerotic cardiovascular disease but not at increased bleeding risk.[27] Secondary prevention with antiplatelet agents may include patients with stable coronary artery disease, acute coronary syndromes, postcoronary artery bypass graft (CABG) or percutaneous coronary intervention (PCI), post-transcatheter aortic valve replacement (TAVR), peripheral arterial disease, carotid artery disease, and stroke.

Management of antiplatelet therapy in the perioperative period involves several considerations (Box 13.3). An algorithm for the perioperative management of antiplatelet therapy in patients with coronary artery disease is shown in Fig. 13.3.[28] For patients who have received PCI and are treated with DAPT, the American College of Cardiology published 2016 guidelines that recommend delaying elective noncardiac surgery for 30 days after bare-metal stent (BMS) implantation and optimally 6 months after drug-eluting stent (DES) implantation.[29] Even after this high-risk period for stent thrombosis, the decision about duration of DAPT requires individual consideration of the risk/benefit ratio and patient preference. The duration of DAPT most commonly refers to the duration of $P2Y_{12}$ inhibitor therapy; aspirin therapy is almost always recommended indefinitely in patients with known CAD.[29]

Pulmonary

This section will focus on predicting postoperative pulmonary complications (PPCs). The following pulmonary conditions are addressed in other chapters: asthma (see Chapter 27), chronic obstructive pulmonary disease (see Chapters 27 and 42), cigarette smoking and smoking cessation (see Chapter 42), obstructive sleep apnea and use of the STOP-BANG score for screening (see Chapters 42 and 48), and pulmonary hypertension (see Chapters 26 and 27).

PPCs occur commonly and are associated with increased patient mortality. The estimated incidence of PPC after major surgery ranges from <1% to 23%, based on the definition used for PPCs.[30] Table 13.9 provides definitions for PPC from a 2015 European task force.[31]

Multiple risk prediction models can be used to provide preoperative risk stratification; however, most were developed from retrospective databases or are focused on a single adverse pulmonary outcome. There is lack of agreement between comparative studies, and many prediction models are complex and impractical for routine clinical use.[30] One prospective observational study developed a score to predict postoperative respiratory failure, listed in Table 13.10.[32] This score may be useful in counseling individual patients about their risk of PPCs, including the possibility of postoperative intensive care unit (ICU) care. Currently, there are no high-quality, evidence-based perioperative interventions to reduce the risk of PPCs. However, there is moderate-quality evidence for the potential benefit of lung-protective intraoperative ventilation and goal-directed hemodynamic/fluid therapy and low-quality evidence for enhanced recovery pathways, prophylactic mucolytics, postoperative noninvasive ventilation, prophylactic respiratory physiotherapy, and epidural analgesia.[33]

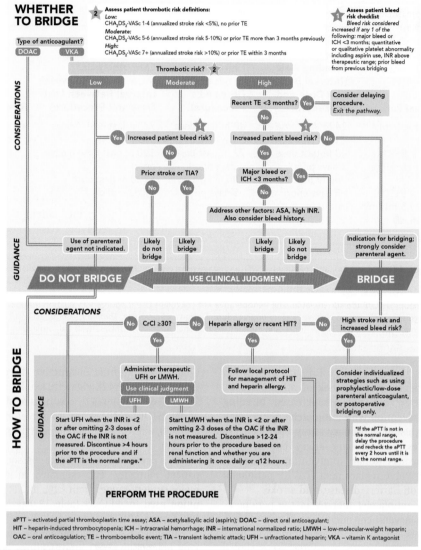

Fig. 13.2 Algorithm for Anticoagulation Bridging in Patients With Nonvalvular Atrial Fibrillation. (From Doherty JU, Gluckman TJ, Hucker WJ, et al. 2017 ACC expert consensus decision pathway for periprocedural management of anticoagulation in patients with nonvalvular atrial fibrillation: A report of the American College of Cardiology Clinical Expert Consensus Document Task Force. *J Am Coll Cardiol*. 2017;69[7]:871–898, Figure 4.)

Renal

The perioperative implications of renal disease are addressed in Chapter 28, including a discussion of preoperative risk factors for postoperative renal dysfunction, renal function tests, and pathophysiology of end-stage renal disease.

Liver

Diseases of the liver can affect nearly all organ systems. Chapter 28 describes the end-organ implications of cirrhosis,

the pathophysiology of end-stage liver disease, and complications such as ascites and hepatorenal syndrome. Preoperative evaluation of liver disease, including use of the Child–Turcotte–Pugh score and Model of End-Stage Liver Disease (MELD) score, is also addressed in Chapter 28.

Endocrine

Common endocrine disorders are discussed in Chapter 29. This section will address the preoperative medication management of patients with diabetes mellitus in more detail.

Box 13.3 Considerations for Perioperative Antiplatelet Therapy

1. What was the original indication for antiplatelet therapy (e.g., primary or secondary prevention)?
2. Did the patient complete the recommended duration of antiplatelet therapy?
3. What is the thrombotic risk of temporary stoppage of antiplatelet therapy around the time of the procedure?
4. Does the procedure require interruption of antiplatelet therapy to reduce bleeding risk?
5. What strategies can be used to decrease thrombotic risk in patients undergoing nonelective procedures?

Diabetes Mellitus

Diabetes mellitus is a risk factor for postoperative complications. Hyperglycemia is associated with cardiovascular events and with infectious complications, including wound infection, pneumonia, and sepsis. Long-term glucose control can be assessed by checking the hemoglobin A_{1C} (HbA_{1C}). Although higher levels of HbA_{1C} are associated with worse outcomes, there are no data showing that postponing surgery to improve glucose control is beneficial. However, depending on the degree of glucose imbalance and the nature of the proposed surgery, individual patients can be counseled about whether postponing surgery is warranted to achieve better glucose control.

Preoperative evaluation of a patient with diabetes includes a review of the type of diabetes; current pharmacotherapy; current glycemic control; and presence of long-term complications of diabetes such as gastroparesis, neuropathy, cardiovascular disease, and peripheral vascular disease. After evaluating the adequacy of glucose control (including frequency of both severe hypoglycemia and hyperglycemia), a plan for perioperative medication management can be developed. General recommendations are provided in Table 13.11.[34,35] Key management principles include avoiding hypoglycemia during the period when the patient is NPO beginning the night before surgery; the patient with type 1 diabetes must always be receiving basal insulin to prevent the development of diabetic ketoacidosis.

Hematologic

Preoperative anemia, including the potential role of a preoperative anemia clinic, is addressed in Chapter 42. Thrombocytopenia (defined as platelet count $<150 \times 10^9$/L) may be discovered when a patient obtains a preoperative complete blood count

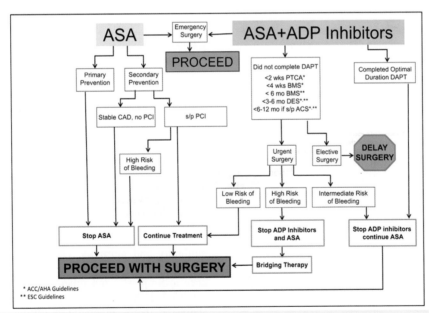

Fig. 13.3 Algorithm for perioperative management of antiplatelet therapy in patients with coronary artery disease. *ACC/AHA*, American College of Cardiology/American Heart Association; *ACS*, acute coronary syndrome; *ADP*, adenosine diphosphate; *ASA*, aspirin; *BMS*, bare-metal stents; *CAD*, coronary artery disease; *DAPT*, dual antiplatelet therapy; *DES*, drug-eluting stent; *ESC*, European Society of Cardiology; *PCI*, percutaneous coronary intervention; *PTCA*, percutaneous transluminal coronary angioplasty. (From Filipescu DC, Stefan MG, Valeanu L, et al. Perioperative management of antiplatelet therapy in noncardiac surgery. *Curr Opin Anaesthesiol.* 2020;33[3]:454–462, Figure 1. Adapted from Oprea AD, Popescu WM. Perioperative management of antiplatelet therapy. *Br J Anaesth.* 2013;111[Suppl 1]:i3–i17.)

Table 13.9	Definition of Postoperative Pulmonary Complications

Complication	Definition
Respiratory infection	Patient has received antibiotics for a suspected respiratory infection and met one or more of the following criteria: new or changed sputum, new or changed lung opacities, fever, white blood cell count $>12 \times 10^9$ /L
Respiratory failure	Postoperative PaO_2 <8 kPa (60 mm Hg) on room air, a $P_aO_2:F_IO_2$ ratio <40 kPa (300 mm Hg), or arterial oxyhemoglobin saturation measured with pulse oximetry <90% and requiring oxygen therapy
Pleural effusion	Chest radiograph changes (detailed in reference)
Atelectasis	Lung opacification with a shift of the mediastinum, hilum, or hemidiaphragm toward the affected area and compensatory overinflation in the adjacent nonatelectatic lung
Pneumothorax	Air in the pleural space with no vascular bed surrounding the visceral pleura
Bronchospasm	Newly detected expiratory wheezing treated with bronchodilators
Aspiration pneumonitis	Acute lung injury after the inhalation of regurgitated gastric contents

From Jammer I, Wickboldt N, Sander M, et al. Standards for definitions and use of outcome measures for clinical effectiveness research in perioperative medicine: European Perioperative Clinical Outcome (EPCO) definitions: A statement from the ESA-ESICM Joint Taskforce on Perioperative Outcome Measures. *Eur J Anaesthesiol.* 2015;32(2):88-105.

Table 13.10	Predictors of Postoperative Respiratory Failure (PERISCOPE-PRF) Score

Risk Factor	Risk Score Points
Patient-Related Factors	
Preoperative $S_pO_2 \geq 96\%$	0
Preoperative S_pO_2 91%–95%	7
Preoperative $S_pO_2 \leq 90\%$	10
Respiratory symptoms (at least 1)	10
History of congestive heart failure—None	0
History of congestive heart failure—NYHA I	3
History of congestive heart failure—NYHA $\geq$II	8
History of chronic liver disease	7
Procedure-Related Factors	
Emergency procedure	12
Surgical incision	
• Peripheral	0
• Closed intrathoracic/closed upper abdominal	3
• Open upper abdominal	7
• Intrathoracic open	12
Duration of surgery ≤2 hr	0
Duration of surgery >2–3 hr	5
Duration of surgery >3 hr	10

NYHA, New York Heart Association; *PRF,* postoperative respiratory failure (defined as new-onset hypoxemia appearing within the first 5 postoperative days)
The incidence (and 95% confidence interval) of PRF by sum of risk score points:
Low (<12 points): 1.1% (0.7–1.5)
Intermediate (12–22 points): 4.6% (3.4–5.6)
High (23 or more points): 18.8% (15.8–21.8)
Adapted from Canet J, Sabaté S, Mazo V, et al. PERISCOPE group. Development and validation of a score to predict postoperative respiratory failure in a multicentre European cohort: A prospective, observational study. *Eur J Anaesthesiol.* 2015;32(7):458-470, Table 3.

primarily for determination of hematocrit. The relationship between platelet count and bleeding risk is not linear and depends also on patient factors and qualitative platelet function. Based primarily on expert opinion and low-quality evidence, commonly used platelet threshold for major nonneuraxial surgery is $>50 \times 10^9$/L; for surgery on the brain or posterior eye, the recommended threshold is 100×10^9/L.[36]

Infectious Disease

Two infectious disease issues of relevance to preoperative evaluation will be discussed here: prevention of surgical site infection (SSI) and prevention of infective endocarditis (IE).

Surgical Site Infection

SSI is the most common postoperative complication in surgical patients and is associated with increased morbidity and mortality. The impact of an SSI is particularly burdensome in patients undergoing total hip or knee arthroplasty and other surgeries involving extensive medical implants. Two factors related to SSI can be addressed in the preoperative setting: glycemic control and antiseptic prophylaxis. The 2017 Centers for Disease Control and Prevention (CDC) Guideline for the Prevention of Surgical Site Infection recommends implementing perioperative glycemic control using a blood glucose target of less than 200 mg/dL in patients with and without diabetes.[37] Other organizations recommend a slightly lower maximum blood glucose target of 180 mg/dL.[34] There is no consensus recommendation for the optimal

Table 13.11	Perioperative Medication Management for Patients With Diabetes Mellitus	

Patient Type	**Medication Strategy**
Patient on oral glucose-lowering agents only	Hold oral agents on AM of surgery.
Patients on SGLT2 inhibitors	Must discontinue SGLT2 inhibitors 3–4 days before surgery to reduce the risk of "euglycemic DKA."
Patients with DM type 2 on oral agents and insulin therapy	Hold oral agents on AM of surgery; for long-acting insulin given the evening before surgery, reduce dose by 25%[a]; do not give short-acting insulin on AM of surgery.
Patients with known DM type 1 on intermittent insulin therapy	Must have basal insulin at all times to prevent DKA or other metabolic abnormalities. Reduce long-acting insulin dose by 25% on evening before surgery; on AM of surgery, may give correctional rapid-acting insulin every 2–4 hr to correct hyperglycemia.
Patients with DM type 1 on insulin pump therapy	Need to determine if insulin pump can be used perioperatively at the health care facility (based on anticipated length and stress of surgical procedure and proximity of pump to surgical field).

[a]Note: The very long-acting insulin degludec (Tresiba) has a duration of action up to 42 hours and may require dose reduction for an additional day before surgery.
From American Diabetes Association Professional Practice Committee. 16. Diabetes Care in the Hospital: Standards of Medical Care in Diabetes—2022. *Diabetes Care*. 2022;45(Suppl 1):S244-S253; Janež A, Guja C, Mitrakou A, et al. Insulin therapy in adults with type 1 diabetes mellitus: A narrative review. *Diabetes Ther*. 2020;11(2):387-409.

HbA$_{1C}$ goal for the prevention of SSI in patients with and without diabetes.

The CDC guideline also advises patients to shower or bathe with soap or an antiseptic agent on at least the night before the operative day.[37] There was no specific recommendation regarding the following factors: optimal timing of the preoperative shower, total number of soap or antiseptic agent applications, or use of chlorhexidine gluconate washcloths.

Infective Endocarditis

IE is an uncommon but potentially life-threatening infection. Since the 1950s, the AHA has made recommendations for the prevention of IE. Earlier versions of these guidelines included a list of cardiac conditions for which prophylaxis was recommended, in addition to a list of so-called bacteremia-inducing dental or surgical procedures

in which prophylaxis was recommended. The list of procedures included dental and oral surgeries, surgeries involving intestinal or respiratory mucosa, and genital-urinary tract surgeries. In 2007 the AHA made several major changes to its IE prevention guidelines including a narrower list of procedures and cardiac conditions.[38] Box 13.4 describes the key guidelines, and Box 13.5 lists the cardiac conditions with the highest risk of adverse outcomes from endocarditis.[38,39] Antimicrobial prevention regimens for a dental procedure include oral amoxicillin; or intravenous (IV) ampicillin, cefazolin, or ceftriaxone.[38]

Geriatrics

Advancing age is associated with many physiologic changes and increased likelihood of coexisting diseases. Chapter 35 describes the perioperative implications of issues that arise more frequently in this patient population, including cognitive function and decision-making capacity, functional capacity, malnutrition, and frailty.

Frailty

In older adults the syndrome of frailty is increasingly prevalent and associated with adverse health outcomes. Geriatricians defined frailty as a syndrome of decreased reserve and resistance to stressors resulting from cumulative declines across multiple physiologic systems, causing vulnerability to adverse outcomes. Multiple diagnostic tools are used to assess frailty, as described in Chapter 35. Severity of frailty syndrome is correlated with postoperative mortality and many postoperative complications.[40] However, a 2017 systematic review found that few interventions have been tested to improve the outcomes of frail patients undergoing surgery, and most available studies had substantial risk of bias.[41] For example, although postoperative exercise therapy after cardiac or orthopedic surgery was associated with improved outcomes, there have been no high-quality randomized trials of preoperative exercise in frail older patients that evaluate meaningful long-term postoperative outcomes.

PREOPERATIVE TESTING

There are two types of preoperative tests: routine and selective. A routine test is intended to discover a disease or disorder in an asymptomatic patient. Selective preoperative tests are ordered after consideration of specific information in the patient's history or medical records. The ASA Practice Advisory for Preanesthesia Evaluation states that preoperative tests should not be ordered routinely.[1] Selective tests can be used to guide or optimize perioperative decision making and management.

Historically, routine preoperative testing was common practice, even for procedures with very low risk of complications. However, despite multiple specialty society guidelines recommending against it, routine preoperative

Box 13.4 Prevention of Infective Endocarditis (IE)—Key AHA Guidelines

- Bacteremia resulting from daily activities is much more likely to cause IE than bacteremia associated with a dental procedure.
- Antibiotic prophylaxis is not recommended based solely on an increased lifetime risk of acquisition of IE.
- IE prophylaxis is only recommended for patients with the high-risk conditions (see Box 13.5).
- Antibiotic prophylaxis is reasonable for all dental procedures that involve manipulation of gingival tissues or the periapical region of teeth or perforation of oral mucosa only for patients with underlying cardiac conditions associated with the highest risk of adverse outcome from IE (see Box 13.5).
- Antibiotic prophylaxis is reasonable for procedures on the respiratory tract or infected skin, skin structures, or musculoskeletal tissue only for patients with underlying cardiac conditions associated with the highest risk of adverse outcome from IE (see Box 13.5).
- Antibiotic prophylaxis solely to prevent IE is not recommended for gastrourinary or gastrointestinal tract procedures.

Note: A 2021 scientific statement from the American Heart Association did not recommend any revisions to the 2007 IE prevention guidelines.

From Wilson W, Taubert KA, Gewitz M, et al. Prevention of infective endocarditis: Guidelines from the American Heart Association: A guideline from the American Heart Association Rheumatic Fever, Endocarditis, and Kawasaki Disease Committee, Council on Cardiovascular Disease in the Young, and the Council on Clinical Cardiology, Council on Cardiovascular Surgery and Anesthesia, and the Quality of Care and Outcomes Research Interdisciplinary Working Group. *Circulation*. 2007;116(15):1736-1754. Erratum in: *Circulation*. 20079;116(15):e376-e377; Wilson WR, Gewitz M, Lockhart PB, et al. Prevention of viridans group streptococcal infective endocarditis: A scientific statement from the American Heart Association. *Circulation*. 2021;143(20):e963-e978. Erratum in: *Circulation*. 2021;144(9):e192.

Box 13.5 Cardiac Conditions Associated With the Highest Risk of Adverse Outcome From Endocarditis for Which Prophylaxis With Dental Procedures Is Reasonable

- Prosthetic cardiac valve or prosthetic material used for cardiac valve repair
- Previous infective endocarditis (IE)
- Congenital heart disease (CHD)[a]
  - Unrepaired cyanotic CHD, including palliative shunts and conduits
  - Completely repaired congenital heart defect with prosthetic material or device, whether placed by surgery or by catheter intervention, during the first 6 months after the procedure[b]
  - Repaired CHD with residual defects at the site or adjacent to the site of a prosthetic patch or prosthetic device (which inhibits endothelialization)
- Cardiac transplantation recipients who develop cardiac valvulopathy

[a]Except for the conditions listed, antibiotic prophylaxis is no longer recommended for any other form of CHD.
[b]Prophylaxis is reasonable because endothelialization of prosthetic material occurs within 6 months after the procedure.
From Wilson W, Taubert KA, Gewitz M, et al. Prevention of infective endocarditis: Guidelines from the American Heart Association: A guideline from the American Heart Association Rheumatic Fever, Endocarditis, and Kawasaki Disease Committee, Council on Cardiovascular Disease in the Young, and the Council on Clinical Cardiology, Council on Cardiovascular Surgery and Anesthesia, and the Quality of Care and Outcomes Research Interdisciplinary Working Group. *Circulation*. 2007;116(15):1736-1754, Table 3. Erratum in: *Circulation*. 2007;116(15):e376-377.

testing frequently occurs in patients undergoing cataract extraction—one of the safest outpatient procedures performed today.[42] The increasing focus on health care value (also see Chapter 1) has led to initiatives such as the American Board of Internal Medicine (ABIM) Foundation's Choosing Wisely campaign, which aims to promote conversations between clinicians and patients to help them choose care that is supported by evidence, is not duplicative, is free from harm, and is truly necessary. The ABIM Foundation has worked with other specialty societies to identify treatments that were overused and did not provide benefit for patients.[43] Some examples of Choosing Wisely recommendations relevant to preoperative testing are provided in Table 13.12.

Rationale for Selective Testing

Although there is no evidence for explicit decision parameters for selective testing, the general principles are described in Box 13.6. Table 13.13 describes specialty society recommendations for several selected preoperative tests.[1,9,44]

Pregnancy Testing

Patients may present for surgery with early undetected pregnancy. Although some practices require all females of childbearing age to undergo a urine pregnancy test on the day of surgery, this is a controversial issue. Ethically, the patient has the right to decide whether to have pregnancy screening before receiving anesthesia. The ASA Practice Advisory for Preanesthesia Evaluation states that pregnancy testing may be offered to female patients of childbearing age for whom the result would alter the patient's management.[1] A 2016 ASA statement provided additional recommendations, stating that pregnancy testing should not be mandatory and recommending that preanesthetic educational materials should ideally be developed and given to patients to allow them to make an informed decision.[45]

Preoperative Transfusion Testing

Blood product transfusions are commonly administered during surgery (also see Chapter 25). Because the process

Table 13.12	Choosing Wisely Recommendations Relevant to Preoperative Testing

Specialty Society	Preoperative Testing Recommendation
American Society of Anesthesiologists	Do not obtain baseline laboratory studies in patients without significant systemic disease (ASA I or II) undergoing low-risk surgery—specifically complete blood count, basic or comprehensive metabolic panel, coagulation studies when blood loss (or fluid shifts) is/are expected to be minimal.
American Society of Anesthesiologists	Do not obtain baseline diagnostic cardiac testing (transthoracic/transesophageal echocardiography [TTE/TEE]) or cardiac stress testing in asymptomatic stable patients with known cardiac disease (e.g., CAD, valvular disease) undergoing low- or moderate-risk noncardiac surgery.
Society of General Internal Medicine	Do not perform routine preoperative testing before low-risk surgical procedures.
American College of Surgeons	Avoid admission or preoperative chest x-rays for ambulatory patients with unremarkable history and physical examination.
American Academy of Ophthalmology	Do not perform preoperative medical tests for eye surgery unless there are specific medical indications.
American College of Cardiology	Avoid performing stress testing, coronary calcium scoring, or advanced cardiac imaging as part of preoperative cardiovascular risk assessment in patients scheduled for low-risk noncardiac surgery.

From Clinician Lists. Choosing Wisely. An Initiative of the ABIM Foundation. https://www.choosingwisely.org/clinician-lists/.

Box 13.6 Rationale for Preoperative Testing

1. Diagnosis of a disorder that may affect perioperative anesthesia management
2. Assessment of a known medical condition that may affect perioperative care
3. Formulation of plans for perioperative anesthesia care

---

of antibody screening and crossmatching takes time, the preoperative evaluation process includes a decision whether to perform blood type and antibody screening, crossmatch for a specified quantity of red blood cells, or preparation of other blood products such as plasma or platelets. The implications of under-ordering or over-ordering transfusion tests are described in Table 13.14.

Historically, clinicians frequently overestimated the amount of blood that should be prepared for a given surgical case. The concept of the maximum surgical blood order schedule (MSBOS) was developed to compensate for this frequent overestimation; the goal was not to rigidly control clinician transfusion decisions.[46] The MSBOS was created by analyzing data on the mean number of blood units actually transfused intraoperatively and immediately postoperatively for common operations, organized by surgical service. The result is a recommendation for one of the following for a given surgical procedure: (1) no transfusion testing, (2) type and screen only, or (3) type and crossmatch for a specified number of packed red blood cell (PRBC) units. The MSBOS is institution specific; institutions use different processes to update the MSBOS as new surgical procedures are performed.[47] Table 13.15 provides an example of MSBOS recommendations for a few selected procedures. However, MSBOS recommendations do not reflect patient factors such as anemia or coagulopathy (e.g., disease or medication related) or surgical bleeding risk for a given patient. Nevertheless, the MSBOS represents a reasonable starting point for deciding whether to order a type and screen or type and crossmatch before elective surgery.

RISK ASSESSMENT

The assessment of a patient's perioperative risks is an important goal of preoperative evaluation. Tools for risk stratification can be divided into two types: risk scores and risk prediction models.[48] Examples of risk scores include ASA Physical Status (discussed later) and the Revised Cardiac Risk Index.[16] Although risk scores are simple to use and provide comparative information relative to other patients, they are not designed to provide individualized risk prediction. Risk prediction models such as the NSQIP surgical risk calculator require much more information to generate a multivariable risk assessment; the NSQIP calculator has only been validated in specific types of surgery. The practical considerations of individual risk assessment are listed in Box 13.7. Clinical judgment and the input of other specialty clinicians may be required to address the unique circumstance of a given patient.

ASA Physical Status

The ASA Physical Status classification system was developed in the 1940s to facilitate collection of statistical data in anesthesia.[49] Although the ASA Physical Status classification was not designed or developed to predict perioperative risk in an individual patient, many studies have examined the correlation between ASA Physical Status and outcomes in the aggregate. Whereas the

Table 13.13	Recommendations for Ordering Selective Preoperative Tests	
Test	**Recommendation**	**Reference**
Electrocardiogram (ECG)	Preoperative resting 12-lead electrocardiogram (ECG) is reasonable for patients with known coronary heart disease, significant arrhythmia, peripheral arterial disease, cerebrovascular disease, or other significant structural heart disease, except for those undergoing low-risk surgery.	ACC/AHA Guideline on Perioperative Cardiovascular Evaluation[9]
Electrocardiogram (ECG)	An ECG may be indicated for patients with known cardiovascular risk factors or for patients with risk factors identified in the course of a preanesthesia evaluation.	ASA Practice Advisory for Preanesthesia Evaluation[1]
Preanesthesia chest radiograph	The decision to perform a chest radiograph in the preoperative, preintervention, hospital admission, and asymptomatic outpatient settings should principally derive from a need to investigate a clinical suspicion for acute or unstable chronic cardiopulmonary disease that could influence patient care. Selective ordering is recommended, including in patients of advanced age or otherwise at increased risk.	American College of Radiology[44]
Preanesthesia hemoglobin or hematocrit	Factors to consider include type and invasiveness of procedure, patients with liver disease, extremes of age, history of anemia, bleeding, and other hematologic disorders.	ASA Practice Advisory for Preanesthesia Evaluation[1]
Preanesthesia coagulation studies	Factors to consider include bleeding disorders, renal dysfunction, liver dysfunction, and type and invasiveness of procedure.	ASA Practice Advisory for Preanesthesia Evaluation[1]
Preanesthesia serum chemistries	Clinical characteristics to consider include likely perioperative therapies, endocrine disorders, risk of renal and liver dysfunction, and use of certain medications or alternative therapies.	ASA Practice Advisory for Preanesthesia Evaluation[1]
Preanesthesia urinalysis	Urinalysis is not indicated except for specific procedures (e.g., prosthesis implantation, urologic procedures) or when urinary tract symptoms are present.	ASA Practice Advisory for Preanesthesia Evaluation[1]

initial description of the physical state system included numerous examples of each class, subsequent iterations from 1945 to 2014 omitted case examples, only providing a brief description of each class. The simplicity of the ASA Physical Status led to widespread use among many nonanesthesia clinicians and administrators. For example, the ASA Physical Status class has been used to make decisions regarding (1) inpatient versus ambulatory care locations for individual patients, (2) whether to transfer a patient to another facility, (3) assigning anesthesia providers to a given patient's case, and (4) staffing ratios when anesthesiologists cover multiple anesthetizing locations.[49] In addition, ASA Physical Status is used as a billing modifier by many insurers.

Despite these many uses of the ASA Physical Status, there have been issues with interrater reliability, including both underclassification and overclassification. In 2014 the ASA added case examples to the classification system in an effort to increase interrater reliability. However, subsequent studies have suggested that these changes were not associated with improved accuracy in classifying patients.[50] A 2020 update of the ASA Physical Status classification system included even more case descriptions, including pediatric and obstetric examples (Table 13.16).

Since 1963 the ASA Physical Status classification has included an E category denoting emergency surgery. This is now defined as a condition in which a delay in treatment will lead to a significant increase in the threat to life or body part; however, the exact duration or severity of the emergency diagnosis required to meet the E designation is not specified. According to the ASA, the final assignment of Physical Status classification is made on the day of anesthesia care by the anesthesiologist after evaluating the patient.

MEDICATION MANAGEMENT

Preoperative medication management is a critically important aspect of preoperative evaluation, especially in the outpatient setting. Because the U.S. FDA has approved over 19,000 prescription drugs for marketing—with approximately 50 new drugs approved each year—relatively few medications have been the subject of clinical trials to determine the ideal perioperative management approach. A general strategy for deciding how to manage a patient's chronic medications is listed in Box 13.8. Medications already discussed in this chapter include those for coronary artery disease, hypertension,

Table 13.14 Implications of Preoperative Transfusion Testing

Clinical Situation	Implications
Transfusion testing not ordered, patient needs urgent intraoperative PRBC transfusion	• If patient needs transfusion sooner than the time required for blood type and crossmatching (45 min or more), the patient may need emergency-release blood, which may increase likelihood of transfusion reaction. • If patient's antibody screen detects the presence of alloantibodies, the time required for crossmatching can increase significantly (by many hours), also leading to requirement for emergency-release blood, and increased risk of transfusion reaction.
Preoperative type and crossmatch for 2 units PRBC ordered for procedure with low bleeding risk	• Two units of PRBCs are crossmatched and "reserved" for that patient on the day of surgery. • Those 2 PRBC units are not available to other patients during that time.
Preoperative type and screen ordered for procedure with minimal bleeding risk	• Time and equipment for laboratory personnel to perform test represents low-value, potentially wasteful use of resources.

PRBC, Packed red blood cells.

Table 13.15 Sample MSBOS Recommendations for Given Surgical Procedures

Surgical Procedure	Blood Product and Testing Recommendation
Hand carpal tunnel release, open	None
Laparoscopic cholecystectomy	None
Laparoscopic Nissen fundoplication	Type and screen
Spine posterior laminectomy, <2 segments	Type and screen
Partial nephrectomy, laparoscopic	Type and crossmatch for 2 units PRBC
Spine posterior fusion, 7–12 segments	Type and crossmatch for 5 units PRBC
Hepatectomy, total right lobectomy	Type and crossmatch for 6 units PRBC

MSBOS, Maximum surgical blood order schedule; *PRBC,* packed red blood cells.
Examples from author's institution (University of California, San Francisco).

Box 13.7 Preoperative Risk Considerations in Individual Patients

1. Does the patient have increased perioperative risk compared with a healthy patient? If so, for what outcomes?
2. Should additional testing be pursued to evaluate risks further?
3. Can the patient's perioperative risks be reduced with additional therapy?
4. Based on the patient's perioperative risks and potential mitigating therapy, should the following aspects of the proposed surgical procedure be changed: timing of surgery, location of surgery (e.g., ambulatory surgery center versus facility with inpatient capability), assignment of subspecialty-trained anesthesia care team, intraoperative invasive monitoring, postoperative intensive care monitoring?

anticoagulant therapy (for mechanical heart valve, atrial fibrillation, venous thromboembolism), antiplatelet therapy (for coronary artery disease and stroke), and diabetes mellitus. Many institutions develop their own guidelines to ensure consistency for their perioperative clinicians, primarily based on expert opinion.[51]

NPO GUIDELINES

Fasting guidelines are commonly provided during the preoperative evaluation process. The rationale for preoperative fasting before surgery is to reduce the risk of pulmonary aspiration of gastric contents. Common practice includes withholding liquids and solids for specific periods before surgery and possibly prescribing pharmacologic agents to reduce gastric volume and pH. Patient conditions that may increase the risk of regurgitation and pulmonary aspiration include gastroesophageal reflux disease, dysphagia, and other gastrointestinal motility and metabolic disorders (e.g., diabetes mellitus with gastroparesis). Clear liquids empty from the stomach more rapidly than solid food or nonclear liquids. The ASA has published Practice Guidelines for Preoperative Fasting, listed in Table 13.17.[52] For patients with risk factors for pulmonary aspiration, there may be a role for gastrointestinal stimulants (e.g., metoclopramide), pharmacologic blockade of gastric acid secretion (proton pump inhibitors or histamine H2 blockers), or preoperative clear antacids (e.g., sodium citrate). Additional fasting instructions may be given to patients managed in an enhanced recovery pathway, such as encouraging consumption of a clear carbohydrate liquid until 2 hours before surgery (also see Chapter 14).

TABLE 13.16 ASA Physical Status Classification

ASA Physical Status Classification	Definition	Adult Examples (including but not limited to)	Pediatric Examples (including but not limited to)	Obstetric Examples (including but not limited to)
ASA I	A normal healthy patient	Healthy, nonsmoking, no or minimal alcohol use	Healthy (no acute or chronic disease), normal BMI percentile for age	
ASA II	A patient with mild systemic disease	Mild diseases only without substantive functional limitations. Current smoker, social alcohol drinker, pregnancy, obesity (30 < BMI < 40), well-controlled DM/HTN, mild lung disease	Asymptomatic congenital cardiac disease, well-controlled dysrhythmias, asthma without exacerbation, well-controlled epilepsy, non-insulin-dependent DM, abnormal BMI percentile for age, mild/moderate OSA, oncologic state in remission, autism with mild limitations	Normal pregnancy,[a] well controlled gestational HTN, controlled preeclampsia without severe features, diet-controlled gestational DM.
ASA III	A patient with severe systemic disease	Substantive functional limitations; one or more moderate to severe diseases. Poorly controlled DM or HTN, COPD, morbid obesity (BMI ≥40), active hepatitis, alcohol dependence or abuse, implanted pacemaker, moderate reduction of ejection fraction, ESRD undergoing regularly scheduled dialysis, history (>3 mo) of MI, CVA, TIA, or CAD/stents.	Uncorrected stable congenital cardiac abnormality, asthma with exacerbation, poorly controlled epilepsy, insulin-dependent DM, morbid obesity, malnutrition, severe OSA, oncologic state, renal failure, muscular dystrophy, cystic fibrosis, history of organ transplantation, brain/spinal cord malformation, symptomatic hydrocephalus, premature infant PCA <60 weeks, autism with severe limitations, metabolic disease, difficult airway, long-term parenteral nutrition, full-term infants <6 weeks of age	Preeclampsia with severe features, gestational DM with complications or high insulin requirements, a thrombophilic disease requiring anticoagulation.
ASA IV	A patient with severe systemic disease that is a constant threat to life	Recent (<3 mo) MI, CVA, TIA, or CAD/stents, ongoing cardiac ischemia or severe valve dysfunction, severe reduction of ejection fraction, shock, sepsis, DIC, ARDS, or ESRD not undergoing regularly scheduled dialysis	Symptomatic congenital cardiac abnormality, congestive heart failure, active sequelae of prematurity, acute hypoxic-ischemic encephalopathy, shock, sepsis, DIC, automatic implantable cardioverter-defibrillator, ventilator dependence, endocrinopathy, severe trauma, severe respiratory distress, advanced oncologic state.	Preeclampsia with severe features complicated by HELLP or other adverse event, peripartum cardiomyopathy with ejection fraction <40, uncorrected/decompensated heart disease, acquired or congenital.

Continued

TABLE 13.16	ASA Physical Status Classification—cont'd			
ASA Physical Status Classification	**Definition**	**Adult Examples (including but not limited to)**	**Pediatric Examples (including but not limited to)**	**Obstetric Examples (including but not limited to)**
ASA V	A moribund patient who is not expected to survive without the operation	Ruptured abdominal/ thoracic aneurysm, massive trauma, intracranial bleed with mass effect, ischemic bowel in the face of significant cardiac pathology or multiple organ/system dysfunction	Massive trauma, intracranial hemorrhage with mass effect, patient requiring ECMO, respiratory failure or arrest, malignant hypertension, decompensated congestive heart failure, hepatic encephalopathy, ischemic bowel or multiple organ/ system dysfunction.	Uterine rupture.
ASA VI	A declared brain-dead patient whose organs are being removed for donor purposes			

[a]Although pregnancy is not a disease, the parturient' s physiologic state is significantly altered from when the woman is not pregnant; hence the assignment of ASA 2 for a woman with uncomplicated pregnancy.
[b]The addition of "E" denotes emergency surgery. An emergency is defined as existing when delay in treatment of the patient would lead to a significant increase in the threat to life or body part.
ASA Physical Status Classification System. Developed by Committee on Economics. Last amended December 13, 2020 (original approval: October 15, 2014). https://www.asahq.org/standards-and-guidelines/asa-physical-status-classification-system.
ARDS, Acute respiratory distress syndrome; *BMI*, body mass index; *CAD*, coronary artery disease; *COPD*, chronic obstructive pulmonary disease; *CVA*, cerebrovascular accident; *DIC*, disseminated intravascular coagulation; *DM*, diabetes mellitus; *ECMO*, extracorporeal membrane oxygenation; *ESRD*, end-stage renal disease; *HTN*, hypertension; MI, myocardial infarction; *OSA*, obstructive sleep apnea; *PCA*, patient-controlled analgesia; *TIA*, transient ischemic attack.

INFORMED CONSENT FOR ANESTHESIA

Informed consent is the process of providing a patient with information that allows them to make an informed choice about their care. Certain aspects of anesthesia practice differ from the consent process for the surgical procedure.[53] Often, the anesthesia provider does not meet the patient until the day of surgery. For many types of surgery, there is not a real option for no treatment (i.e., no anesthesia), but there may be decisions regarding the type of anesthesia and approaches to postoperative pain management. Patient competence, or capacity for consent, includes their ability to understand the information provided, retain it, and use it to reach an informed decision. It is possible that analgesic and anxiolytic drugs administered by anesthesia providers can affect the patient's ability to retain information preoperatively and postoperatively. This reinforces the importance of documenting the informed consent discussion in the medical record at the time consent is obtained.

In terms of how much information should be disclosed to the patient during the consent process, the most commonly applied standard is the *reasonable person* standard. That is, disclosure of information should be consistent

> **Box 13.8** Perioperative Medication Management Strategy
>
> Questions to consider about a specific medication include the following:
> 1. What condition is being treated with the medication? What are the potential complications of therapy interruption and the expected time course of the complications?
> 2. Are there non-oral routes of administration for the medication that can be administered perioperatively?
> 3. Are there medication effects that can cause surgical issues such as impaired wound healing, increased risk of surgical bleeding, or increased risk of infection?
> 4. Are there medication effects that affect end-organ function, including the cardiovascular (e.g., heart rate, blood pressure, cardiac rhythm), pulmonary (e.g., hypercarbia, hypoxemia, bronchospasm), central nervous system (e.g., psychotropic, antiepileptic drugs), or renal systems?

with what a hypothetical reasonable person would want in order to make a decision. For a routine anesthetic, information discussed should include the patient's medical condition, procedures that will be performed, risks and other consequences of care, and postoperative pain

Table 13.17 ASA Preoperative Fasting Recommendations

Ingested Material	Minimum Fasting Period
Clear liquids[a]	2 hr
Breast milk	4 hr
Infant formula	6 hr
Nonhuman milk	6 hr
Light meal[b]	6 hr
Fried foods, fatty foods, or meat	Additional fasting time (e.g., 8 or more hours) may be needed

[a]Examples of clear liquids include water, fruit juices without pulp, carbonated beverages, clear tea, and black coffee.
[b]A light meal typically consists of toast and clear liquids. Meals that include fried or fatty foods or meat may prolong gastric emptying time. Both the amount and type of food ingested must be considered when determining an appropriate fasting period.
From Practice guidelines for preoperative fasting and the use of pharmacologic agents to reduce the risk of pulmonary aspiration: Application to healthy patients undergoing elective procedures: An updated report by the American Society of Anesthesiologists Task Force on Preoperative Fasting and the Use of Pharmacologic Agents to Reduce the Risk of Pulmonary Aspiration. *Anesthesiology.* 2017;126(3):376–393.
Guidelines are intended for healthy patients of all ages undergoing elective procedures. They are not intended for women in labor.

management. For procedures that do include options, such as postoperative pain management with an epidural versus IV patient-controlled analgesia (PCA), additional details and a risk–benefit discussion should be pursued. For patients with coexisting diseases associated with increased perioperative risks, those risks should be discussed as well. The level of detail in the risk discussion should be tailored to the patient circumstances, including their preferences for information, comorbidity concerns, and the planned surgical procedure. Although the U.S. Joint Commission does not require a separate written consent form for anesthesia, some institutions do require this for all anesthetics or for certain procedures such as obstetric anesthesia.

Another challenge in the informed consent process is the wide variability in patient preferences, values, and expectations of care. A systematic review of anesthesiologist-to-patient communication found that informed consent, including a discussion of risks and benefits, is highly variable and that patient comprehension of risks, benefits, and alternatives was poor when measured objectively.[54] In addition, discussions about postoperative critical care were rare, including goals of care discussions for a significant postoperative complication.

PREOPERATIVE EVALUATION CLINICS

Anesthesiologist-directed preoperative evaluation clinics are designed to facilitate early anesthesiologist access to patients, in addition to increased preoperative counseling, increased communication between providers and patients, anesthesiologist involvement in protocol development, and coordination of postoperative care. A well-designed anesthesiologist-directed preoperative evaluation clinic can reduce surgical cancellations caused by inadequate preoperative preparation, reduce costs associated with unnecessary testing, and reduce preoperative consultations with other providers.[55] A 2016 large database retrospective review also found that a visit to a preoperative evaluation clinic before elective surgery was associated with a reduction of in-hospital postoperative mortality.[56] For a learner rotating in an outpatient anesthesiology preoperative clinic, a suggested approach to evaluation of a patient is described in Box 13.9.

Enhanced Recovery Pathways

Multidisciplinary enhanced recovery pathways (also called *enhanced recovery after surgery* [ERAS]) are increasingly used for patients undergoing many types of surgery, including colorectal, orthopedic, hepatic, pancreatic, and gynecologic[57] (also see Chapter 14). ERAS pathways are developed in a multidisciplinary fashion; the local implementation almost always includes a preoperative component that may be initiated in a preoperative evaluation encounter.

Preoperative Optimization

The timing of preoperative evaluation with respect to the date of surgery influences the interventions that can be offered to patients to improve their perioperative outcomes. Most commonly, the date of surgery is a priority (especially from the perspective of the surgeon and patient), and the preoperative evaluation takes place less than 2 weeks—and often only days—before the surgical date. Thus the opportunity to manage coexisting diseases is limited. The paradigm shift to expand the focus of anesthesia and perioperative care beyond the narrow time window around the date of surgery is represented by the term *perioperative medicine,* the focus of Chapter 42. One example is the transformation of a conventional preanesthesia clinic to a *preoperative optimization clinic,* to which patients are referred 14 to 90 days before surgery. The initial multidisciplinary clinic evaluation determines whether optimization is required for certain predefined issues such as anemia, malnutrition, complex pain, smoking, frailty, or coagulation.[58] If present, optimization of these conditions is managed by an integrated, but sometimes independent, preoperative optimization clinic staffed by physicians or advanced practice providers.

A related concept is *prehabilitation,* which refers to interventions that enhance functional capacity to enable

Box 13.9 Suggested Approach to Outpatient Preoperative Evaluation

1. Receive patient assignment (at a minimum, patient name, proposed surgery and surgery date).
2. Review existing medical records, including pertinent laboratory or other diagnostic tests.
3. Review pending tests and orders from surgeon.
4. Conduct patient history and physical.
5. Decide whether further preoperative testing is indicated.[a]
6. Provide medication management instructions to patient.[a]
7. Provide NPO instructions to patient.
8. Describe perioperative course and engage in informed consent discussion with patient.
9. Communicate issues relevant to perioperative care with patient, surgeon, and patient's existing care providers (e.g., pending cardiovascular evaluation or other medical evaluation).[a]
10. Communicate with appropriate anesthesia clinical leads regarding special anesthesia concerns (e.g., anticipated difficult airway management, critical end-organ disease requiring subspecialty anesthesia care or equipment).*

[a]For a trainee, the level of supervision required for this decision should be determined at the program level.

better tolerance of a stressful event. Prehabilitation programs typically focus on several goals: (1) improved physical fitness, (2) dietary interventions to counteract the catabolic state and support anabolism with exercise, (3) antistress interventions to foster resilience and self-efficacy, and (4) cessation of adverse health habits (e.g., alcohol use disorder, smoking).[59] Several examples are described in Chapter 42.

Inpatient Preoperative Evaluation

Although much of this chapter has focused on outpatient preoperative evaluation, the principles apply to the inpatient who requires urgent or emergency surgery. However, the time course of evaluation may need to be significantly compressed. At one extreme, a patient who sustained blunt trauma in a motor vehicle collision may be brought to the operating room within minutes of arrival in the emergency department. An example of a patient group who requires surgery within 24 to 48 hours is the elderly patient with an acute hip fracture. Many patients have multiple comorbidities, including frailty; cognitive impairment; cardiovascular disease, including hypertension, heart failure, thromboembolic disease requiring anticoagulation; and anemia. The risk of death with acute hip fracture is lower for patients who undergo early surgery, defined in most studies as less than 24 to 48 hours after presentation to the emergency department.[60] In this setting the preoperative assessment must be thorough but should not generally include testing or consultation that leads to delayed surgery. Exceptions include conditions such as acute coronary syndrome or ST-segment elevation myocardial infarction. Conditions that can be addressed in a 24-hour period include occult hypovolemia, anemia, hypoxemia, electrolyte disturbances, and correction of anticoagulant effects (e.g., vitamin K for the patient on warfarin therapy).[60] ERAS pathways for the patient with hip fracture are associated with decreased time to surgery, decreased length of stay, and decreased overall complication rate.[61] Although individual studies report different preoperative ERAS elements for the patient with hip fracture, most include multimodal opiate-sparing analgesia (often with regional analgesia), short periods of fasting, and standardized nursing care.

ACKNOWLEDGMENT

The editors and publisher would like to thank Drs. Rebecca Gerlach and Bobbie Jean Sweitzer for contributing to this chapter in the previous edition of this work. It has served as the foundation for the current chapter.

REFERENCES

1. American Society of Anesthesiologists Task Force on Preanesthesia Evaluation: Practice advisory for preanesthesia evaluation: An updated report by the American Society of Anesthesiologists Task Force on Preanesthesia Evaluation. *Anesthesiology.* 2012 Mar;116(3):522–538. doi:10.1097/ALN.0b013e31823c1067. PMID: 22273990.
2. American Society of Anesthesiologists. Basic Standards for Preanesthesia Care. Developed By Committee on Standards and Practice Parameters (CSPP). Last Affirmed: December 13, 2020 (original approval: October 14, 1987). https:// www.asahq.org/standards-and-guidelines/basic-standards-for-preanesthesia-care. Accessed February 1, 2022.
3. Shenoy ES, Macy E, Rowe T, Blumenthal KG. Evaluation and management of penicillin allergy: A review. *JAMA.* 2019 Jan 15;321(2):188–199. PMID: 30644987. doi:10.1001/jama.2018.19283.
4. WHO SDH. https://www.who.int/health-topics/social-determinants-of-health#tab=tab_1. Accessed February 6, 2022.
5. Benziger CP, Huffman MD, Sweis RN, Stone NJ. The Telehealth Ten: A guide for a patient-assisted virtual physical examination. *Am J Med.* 2021 Jan;134(1):48–51. doi:10.1016/j.amjmed.2020.06.015. Epub 2020 Jul 18. PMID: 32687813; PMCID: PMC7368154.
6. Hines RL, Jones SB (eds.): *Stoelting's anesthesia and coexisting disease.* Philadelphia: Elsevier; 2021.
7. Roberts DP, Lewis SJG. Considerations for general anaesthesia in Parkinson's disease. *J Clin Neurosci.* 2018 Feb;48:34–41. doi:10.1016/j.jocn.2017.10.062. Epub 2017 Nov 10. PMID: 29133106.
8. Katus L, Shtilbans A. Perioperative management of patients with Parkinson's disease. *Am J Med.* 2014

Apr;127(4):275–280.   doi:10.1016/j.amjmed.2013.11.014. Epub 2013 Dec 11. PMID: 24333200.

9. Fleisher LA, Fleischmann KE, Auerbach AD, et al. 2014 ACC/AHA guideline on perioperative cardiovascular evaluation and management of patients undergoing noncardiac surgery: A report of the American College of Cardiology/American Heart Association Task Force on Practice Guidelines. *J Am Coll Cardiol.* 2014 Dec 9;64(22):e77–e137. doi:10.1016/j.jacc.2014.07.944. Epub 2014 Aug 1. PMID: 25091544.

10. Kristensen SD, Knuuti J, Saraste A, et al. 2014 ESC/ESA guidelines on non-cardiac surgery: Cardiovascular assessment and management: The Joint Task Force on Non-Cardiac Surgery: Cardiovascular assessment and management of the European Society of Cardiology (ESC) and the European Society of Anaesthesiology (ESA). *Eur Heart J.* 2014 Sep 14;35(35):2383–2431. doi:10.1093/eurheartj/ehu282. Epub 2014 Aug 1. PMID: 25086026.

11. Duceppe E, Parlow J, MacDonald P, et al. Canadian Cardiovascular Society Guidelines on Perioperative Cardiac Risk Assessment and Management for Patients Who Undergo Noncardiac Surgery. *Can J Cardiol.* 2017 Jan;33(1):17–32. doi:10.1016/j.cjca.2016.09.008. Epub 2016 Oct 4. Erratum in: Can J Cardiol. 2017 Dec;33(12):1735. PMID: 27865641.

12. Smilowitz NR, Gupta N, Guo Y, et al. Trends in cardiovascular risk factor and disease prevalence in patients undergoing non-cardiac surgery. *Heart.* 2018 Jul;104(14):1180–1186.   doi:10.1136/heartjnl-2017-312391. Epub 2018 Jan 5. PMID: 29305561; PMCID: PMC6102124.

13. Wijeysundera DN, Pearse RM, Shulman MA, et al. METS Study Investigators. Assessment of functional capacity before major non-cardiac surgery: An international, prospective cohort study. *Lancet.* 2018 Jun 30;391(10140):2631–2640. doi:10.1016/S0140-6736(18)31131-0. PMID: 30070222.

14. Hlatky MA, Boineau RE, Higginbotham MB, et al. A brief self-administered questionnaire to determine functional capacity (the Duke Activity Status Index). *Am J Cardiol.* 1989 Sep 15;64(10):651–654. doi:10.1016/0002-9149(89)90496-7. PMID: 2782256.

15. Wijeysundera DN, Beattie WS, Hillis GS, et al. Integration of the Duke Activity Status Index into preoperative risk evaluation: A multicentre prospective cohort study. *Br J Anaesth.* 2020 Mar;124(3):261–270.   doi:10.1016/j.bja.2019.11.025. Epub 2019 Dec 19. PMID: 31864719.

16. Lee TH, Marcantonio ER, Mangione CM, et al. Derivation and prospective validation of a simple index for prediction of cardiac risk of major noncardiac surgery. *Circulation.* 1999 Sep 7;100(10):1043–1049. PMID: 10477528. doi: 10.1161/01.cir.100.10.1043.

17. Bilimoria KY, Liu Y, Paruch JL, et al. Development and evaluation of the universal ACS NSQIP Surgical Risk Calculator: A decision aid and informed consent tool for patients and surgeons. *J Am Coll Surg.* 2013 Nov;217(5):833–842e1-3. doi:10.1016/j.jamcollsurg.2013.07.385 Epub 2013 Sep 18. PMID: 24055383; PMCID: PMC3805776.

18. Dakik HA, Chehab O, Eldirani M, et al. A new index for pre-operative cardiovascular evaluation. *J Am Coll Cardiol.* 2019 Jun 25;73(24):3067–3078. doi:10.1016/j.jacc.2019.04.023. PMID: 31221255.

19. Whelton PK, Carey RM, Aronow WS, et al. 2017 ACC/AHA/AAPA/ABC/ACPM/AGS/APhA/ASH/ASPC/NMA/PCNA guideline for the prevention, detection, evaluation, and management of high blood pressure in adults: Executive summary: A report of the American College of Cardiology/American Heart Association Task Force on Clinical Practice Guidelines. *Circulation.* 2018 Oct 23;138(17):e426–e483. doi:10.1161/CIR.0000000000000597. PMID: 30354655.

20. Hollmann C, Fernandes NL, Biccard BM. A systematic review of outcomes associated with withholding or continuing angiotensin-converting enzyme inhibitors and angiotensin receptor blockers before noncardiac surgery. *Anesth Analg.* 2018 Sep;127(3):678–687. doi:10.1213/ANE.0000000000002837. PMID: 29381513.

21. Douketis JD, Spyropoulos AC, Spencer FA, et al. Perioperative management of antithrombotic therapy: Antithrombotic Therapy and Prevention of Thrombosis, 9th ed: American College of Chest Physicians Evidence-Based Clinical Practice Guidelines. *Chest.* 2012 Feb;141(2 Suppl):e326S–e350S.   doi:10.1378/chest.11-2298. Erratum in: Chest. 2012 Apr;141(4):1129.   PMID: 22315266; PMCID: PMC3278059.

22. Spyropoulos AC, Brohi K, Caprini J, et al. SSC Subcommittee on Perioperative and Critical Care Thrombosis and Haemostasis of the International Society on Thrombosis and Haemostasis. Scientific and Standardization Committee Communication: Guidance document on the periprocedural management of patients on chronic oral anticoagulant therapy: Recommendations for standardized reporting of procedural/surgical bleed risk and patient-specific thromboembolic risk. *J Thromb Haemost.* 2019 Nov;17(11):1966–1972. doi:10.1111/jth.14598. Epub 2019 Aug 22. PMID: 31436045.

23. Douketis JD, Spyropoulos AC, Anderson JM, et al. The Perioperative Anticoagulant Use for Surgery Evaluation (PAUSE) study for patients on a direct oral anticoagulant who need an elective surgery or procedure: Design and rationale. *Thromb Haemost.* 2017 Dec;117(12):2415–2424.   doi:10.1160/TH17-08-0553. Epub 2017 Dec 6. Erratum in: Thromb Haemost. 2018 Sep;118(9):1679-1680. PMID: 29212129.

24. Kaufman JA, Barnes GD, Chaer RA, et al. Society of Interventional Radiology Clinical Practice Guideline for Inferior Vena Cava Filters in the Treatment of Patients With Venous Thromboembolic Disease: Developed in collaboration with the American College of Cardiology, American College of Chest Physicians, American College of Surgeons Committee on Trauma, American Heart Association, Society for Vascular Surgery, and Society for Vascular Medicine. *J Vasc Interv Radiol.* 2020 Oct;31(10):1529–1544.   doi:10.1016/j.jvir.2020.06.014. Epub 2020 Sep 9. PMID: 32919823.

25. Douketis JD, Spyropoulos AC, Kaatz S, et al. Perioperative bridging anticoagulation in patients with atrial fibrillation. *N Engl J Med.* 2015 Aug 27;373(9):823–833. doi:10.1056/NEJMoa1501035. Epub 2015 Jun 22. PMID: 26095867; PMCID: PMC4931686.

26. Doherty JU, Gluckman TJ, Hucker WJ, et al. 2017 ACC Expert Consensus Decision Pathway for Periprocedural Management of Anticoagulation in Patients With Nonvalvular Atrial Fibrillation: A report of the American College of Cardiology Clinical Expert Consensus Document Task Force. *J Am Coll Cardiol.* 2017 Feb 21;69(7):871–898. doi:10.1016/j.jacc.2016.11.024.   Epub 2017 Jan 9. PMID: 28081965.

27. Arnett DK, Blumenthal RS, Albert MA, et al. 2019 ACC/AHA guideline on the primary prevention of cardiovascular disease: A report of the American College of Cardiology/American Heart Association Task Force on Clinical Practice Guidelines. *Circulation.* 2019 Sep 10;140(11):e596–e646. doi:10.1161/CIR.0000000000000678. Epub 2019 Mar 17. Erratum in: Circulation. 2019 Sep 10;140(11):e649-e650. Erratum in: Circulation. 2020 Jan 28;141(4):e60. Erratum in: Circulation. 2020 Apr 21;141(16):e774.   PMID: 30879355; PMCID: PMC7734661.

28. Filipescu DC, Stefan MG, Valeanu L, Popescu WM. Perioperative management of antiplatelet therapy in noncardiac surgery. *Curr Opin Anaesthesiol.* 2020 Jun;33(3):454–462. doi:10.1097/ACO.0000000000000875.   PMID: 32371645.

29. Levine GN, Bates ER, Bittl JA, et al. 2016 ACC/AHA guideline focused update on duration of dual antiplatelet therapy in patients with coronary artery disease:

A report of the American College of Cardiology/American Heart Association Task Force on Clinical Practice Guidelines: An update of the 2011 ACCF/AHA/SCAI guideline for percutaneous coronary intervention, 2011 ACCF/AHA guideline for coronary artery bypass graft surgery, 2012 ACC/AHA/ACP/AATS/PCNA/SCAI/STS guideline for the diagnosis and management of patients with stable ischemic heart disease, 2013 ACCF/AHA guideline for the management of ST-elevation myocardial infarction, 2014 AHA/ACC guideline for the management of patients with non-ST-elevation acute coronary syndromes, and 2014 ACC/AHA guideline on perioperative cardiovascular evaluation and management of patients undergoing noncardiac surgery. *Circulation*. 2016 Sep 6;134(10):e123–e155. doi:10.1161/CIR.0000000000000404. Epub 2016 Mar 29. Erratum in: Circulation. 2016 Sep 6;134(10):e192-4. PMID: 27026020.

30. Miskovic A, Lumb AB. Postoperative pulmonary complications. *Br J Anaesth*. 2017 Mar 1;118(3):317–334. doi:10.1093/bja/aex002. PMID: 28186222.

31. Jammer I, Wickboldt N, Sander M, et al. Standards for definitions and use of outcome measures for clinical effectiveness research in perioperative medicine: European Perioperative Clinical Outcome (EPCO) definitions: A statement from the ESA-ESICM Joint Taskforce on Perioperative Outcome Measures. *Eur J Anaesthesiol*. 2015 Feb;32(2):88–105. doi:10.1097/EJA.0000000000000118. PMID: 25058504.

32. Canet J, Sabaté S, Mazo V, et al. PERISCOPE group. Development and validation of a score to predict postoperative respiratory failure in a multicentre European cohort: A prospective, observational study. *Eur J Anaesthesiol*. 2015 Jul;32(7):458–470. doi:10.1097/EJA.0000000000000223. PMID: 26020123.

33. Odor PM, Bampoe S, Gilhooly D, et al. Perioperative interventions for prevention of postoperative pulmonary complications: Systematic review and meta-analysis. *BMJ*. 2020 Mar 11;368:m540. doi:10.1136/bmj.m540. PMID: 32161042; PMCID: PMC7190038.

34. American Diabetes Association Professional Practice Committee. Diabetes care in the hospital: Standards of Medical Care in Diabetes-2022. *Diabetes Care*. 2022 Jan 1;45(Supplement_1):S244–S253. doi:10.2337/dc22-S016. PMID: 34964884.

35. Janež A, Guja C, Mitrakou A, et al. Insulin therapy in adults with type 1 diabetes mellitus: A narrative review. *Diabetes Ther*. 2020 Feb;11(2):387–409. doi:10.1007/s13300-019-00743-7. Epub 2020 Jan 4. PMID: 31902063; PMCID: PMC6995794.

36. Nagrebetsky A, Al-Samkari H, Davis NM, et al. Perioperative thrombocytopenia: Evidence, evaluation, and emerging therapies. *Br J Anaesth*. 2019 Jan;122(1):19–31. doi:10.1016/j.bja.2018.09.010. Epub 2018 Oct 25. PMID: 30579402.

37. Berríos-Torres SI, Umscheid CA, Bratzler DW, et al. Healthcare Infection Control Practices Advisory Committee. Centers for Disease Control and Prevention Guideline for the Prevention of Surgical Site Infection, 2017. *JAMA Surg*. 2017 Aug 1;152(8):784–791. doi:10.1001/jamasurg.2017.0904. Erratum in: JAMA Surg. 2017 Aug 1;152(8):803. PMID: 28467526.

38. Wilson W, Taubert KA, Gewitz M, et al. Prevention of infective endocarditis: Guidelines from the American Heart Association: A guideline from the American Heart Association Rheumatic Fever, Endocarditis, and Kawasaki Disease Committee, Council on Cardiovascular Disease in the Young, and the Council on Clinical Cardiology, Council on Cardiovascular Surgery and Anesthesia, and the Quality of Care and Outcomes Research Interdisciplinary Working Group. Circulation. 2007 Oct 9;116(15):1736–1754. doi: 10.1161/CIRCULATIONAHA.106.183095. Epub 2007 Apr 19. Erratum in: Circulation. 2007 Oct 9;116(15):e376–e377. PMID: 17446442.

39. Wilson WR, Gewitz M, Lockhart PB, et al. Prevention of viridans group streptococcal infective endocarditis: A scientific statement from the American Heart Association. *Circulation*. 2021 May 18;143(20):e963–e978. doi:10.1161/CIR.0000000000000969. Epub 2021 Apr 15. Erratum in: Circulation. 2021 Aug 31;144(9):e192. PMID: 33853363.

40. Buigues C, Juarros-Folgado P, Fernández-Garrido J, et al. Frailty syndrome and pre-operative risk evaluation: A systematic review. *Arch Gerontol Geriatr*. 2015 Nov-Dec;61(3):309–321. doi:10.1016/j.archger.2015.08.002. Epub 2015 Aug 4. PMID: 26272286.

41. McIsaac DI, Jen T, Mookerji N, et al. Interventions to improve the outcomes of frail people having surgery: A systematic review. *PLoS One*. 2017 Dec 29;12(12):e0190071. doi:10.1371/journal.pone.0190071. PMID: 29287123; PMCID: PMC5747432.

42. Chen CL, Lin GA, Bardach NS, et al. Preoperative medical testing in Medicare patients undergoing cataract surgery. *N Engl J Med*. 2015 Apr 16;372(16):1530–1538. doi:10.1056/NEJMsa1410846. PMID: 25875258; PMCID: PMC5536179.

43. Clinician Lists. Choosing Wisely. An Initiative of the ABIM Foundation. https://www.choosingwisely.org/clinician-lists/. Accessed February 16, 2022.

44. Routine Chest Radiography. American College of Radiology ACR Appropriateness Criteria. Date of origin 2000. Last review 2015. https://www.acr.org/Clinical-Resources/ACR-Appropriateness-Criteria. Accessed February 16, 2022.

45. American Society of Anesthesiologists. Pregnancy Testing Prior to Anesthesia and Surgery. Developed By: Committee on Quality Management and Departmental Administration. Last amended October 13, 2021 (original approval October 26, 2016). https://www.asahq.org/standards-and-guidelines/pregnancy-testing-prior-to-anesthesia-and-surgery. Accessed February 16, 2022.

46. Friedman BA, Oberman HA, Chadwick AR, Kingdon KI. The maximum surgical blood order schedule and surgical blood use in the United States. *Transfusion*. 1976 Jul-Aug;16(4):380–387. doi:10.1046/j.1537-2995.1976.16476247063.x. PMID: 951737.

47. White MJ, Hazard SW 3rd, Frank SM, et al. The evolution of perioperative transfusion testing and blood ordering. *Anesth Analg*. 2015 Jun;120(6):1196–1203. doi:10.1213/ANE.0000000000000619. PMID: 25988630.

48. Moonesinghe SR, Mythen MG, Das P, et al. Risk stratification tools for predicting morbidity and mortality in adult patients undergoing major surgery: Qualitative systematic review. *Anesthesiology*. 2013 Oct;119(4):959–981. doi:10.1097/ALN.0b013e3182a4e94d. PMID: 24195875.

49. Horvath B, Kloesel B, Todd MM, et al. The evolution, current value, and future of the American Society of Anesthesiologists Physical Status classification system. *Anesthesiology*. 2021 Nov 1;135(5):904–919. doi:10.1097/ALN.0000000000003947. PMID: 34491303.

50. Fielding-Singh V, Willingham MD, Grogan T, Neelankavil JP. Impact of the addition of examples to the American Society of Anesthesiologists Physical Status classification system. *Anesth Analg*. 2020 Mar;130(3):e54–e57. doi:10.1213/ANE.0000000000004482. PMID: 31651457.

51. Muluk V, Cohn SL, Whinney C. Perioperative medication management. UpToDate. https://www.uptodate.com/contents/perioperative-medication-management#H1. Accessed February 18, 2022.

52. Practice guidelines for preoperative fasting and the use of pharmacologic agents to reduce the risk of pulmonary aspiration: Application to healthy patients undergoing elective procedures: An updated report by the American Society of Anesthesiologists Task Force on Preoperative Fasting and the use of pharmacologic agents to reduce the

53. Tait AR, Teig MK, Voepel-Lewis T. Informed consent for anesthesia: A review of practice and strategies for optimizing the consent process. *Can J Anaesth.* 2014 Sep;61(9):832–842. doi:10.1007/s12630-014-0188-8. Epub 2014 Jun 5. PMID: 24898765.

54. Tylee MJ, Rubenfeld GD, Wijeysundera D, Sklar MC, Hussain S, Adhikari NKJ. Anesthesiologist to patient communication: A systematic review. *JAMA Netw Open.* 2020 Nov 2;3(11):e2023503. doi:10.1001/jamanetworkopen.2020.23503. PMID: 33180130; PMCID: PMC7662141.

55. Kash B, Cline K, Menser T, Zhang Y. The Perioperative Surgical Home (PSH) A Comprehensive Literature Review for the American Society of Anesthesiologists. https://www.asahq.org/~/media/sites/psh/files/pshlitreview.pdf. Accessed February 18, 2022.

56. Blitz JD, Kendale SM, Jain SK, Cuff GE, Kim JT, Rosenberg AD. Preoperative evaluation clinic visit is associated with decreased risk of in-hospital postoperative mortality. *Anesthesiology.* 2016 Aug;125(2):280–294. doi:10.1097/ALN.0000000000001193. PMID: 27433746.

57. Esper SA, Holder-Murray J, Subramaniam K, et al. Enhanced recovery protocols reduce mortality across eight surgical specialties at academic and university-affiliated community hospitals. *Ann Surg.* 2020 Nov 18. doi:10.1097/SLA.0000000000004642. Epub ahead of print PMID: 33214486.

58. Aronson S, Murray S, Martin G, et al. Roadmap for transforming preoperative assessment to preoperative optimization. *Anesth Analg.* 2020 Apr;130(4):811–819. doi:10.1213/ANE.0000000000004571. PMID: 31990733.

59. Carli F. Prehabilitation for the anesthesiologist. *Anesthesiology.* 2020 Sep;133(3):645–652. doi:10.1097/ALN.0000000000003331. PMID: 32358253.

60. Boddaert J, Raux M, Khiami F, Riou B. Perioperative management of elderly patients with hip fracture. *Anesthesiology.* 2014 Dec;121(6):1336–1341. doi:10.1097/ALN.0000000000000478. PMID: 25299743.

61. Liu SY, Li C, Zhang PX. Enhanced recovery after surgery for hip fractures: A systematic review and meta-analysis. *Perioper Med (Lond).* 2021 Sep 13;10(1):31. doi:10.1186/s13741-021-00201-8. PMID: 34511117; PMCID: PMC8436561.

14 CHOICE OF ANESTHETIC TECHNIQUE

Manuel C. Pardo, Jr.

The decision-making process regarding anesthetic technique begins with the proposed surgical procedure and incorporates the patient's coexisting diseases and preferences for care. The ultimate responsibility for anesthetic choice lies with the anesthesia provider. Once the anesthesia type is selected, additional management details such as choice and sequence of medications must be planned. The anesthesia provider must have the ability to implement a range of anesthetic plans and be prepared to address unexpected events that may necessitate a sudden change in plan.

TYPES OF ANESTHESIA

Choices for anesthesia include (1) general anesthesia, (2) regional anesthesia, and (3) monitored anesthesia care (MAC).

General anesthesia is a drug-induced, reversible state characterized by unconsciousness, amnesia, immobility, and control of the autonomic nervous system (ANS) responses to noxious stimulation.[1] Control of the ANS responses can be construed as "analgesia," but pain requires conscious perception. The term *nociception* refers to the propagation of impulses through the sensory system with noxious or harmful stimuli; antinociception can be considered another goal of general anesthesia.[2] Modern approaches to general anesthesia involve administration of a combination of medications, such as hypnotic drugs (see Chapters 7 and 8), neuromuscular blocking drugs (see Chapter 11), and analgesic drugs (see Chapter 9).

Regional anesthesia includes neuraxial (spinal, epidural, caudal) anesthesia (see Chapter 17) and peripheral nerve blocks (see Chapter 18). With a cooperative patient, regional anesthesia may ensure the appropriate immobility and analgesia required for surgery, without exposing the patient to the risks of general anesthesia.

Table 14.1 Continuum of Depth of Sedation: Definition of General Anesthesia and Levels of Sedation/Analgesia

	Minimal Sedation (Anxiolysis)	Moderate Sedation/Analgesia ("Conscious Sedation")	Deep Sedation/Analgesia	General Anesthesia
Responsiveness	Normal response to verbal stimulation	Purposeful[a] response to verbal or tactile stimulation	Purposeful[a] response after repeated or painful stimulation	Unarousable even with painful stimulus
Airway	Unaffected	No intervention required	Intervention may be required	Intervention often required
Spontaneous ventilation	Unaffected	Adequate	May be inadequate	Frequently inadequate
Cardiovascular function	Unaffected	Usually maintained	Usually maintained	May be impaired

[a]Reflex withdrawal from a painful stimulus is NOT considered a purposeful response.
Minimal Sedation (Anxiolysis) is a drug-induced state during which patients respond normally to verbal commands.
Moderate Sedation/Analgesia ("Conscious Sedation") is a drug-induced depression of consciousness during which patients respond purposefully to verbal commands, either alone or accompanied by light tactile stimulation.
Deep Sedation/Analgesia is a drug-induced depression of consciousness during which patients cannot be easily aroused but respond purposefully after repeated or painful stimulation.
General Anesthesia is a drug-induced loss of consciousness during which patients are not arousable, even by painful stimulation.
From American Society of Anesthesiologists. Continuum of Depth of Sedation: Definition of General Anesthesia and Levels of Sedation/Analgesia. Last amended October 23, 2019. (https://www.asahq.org/standards-and-guidelines/continuum-of-depth-of-sedation-definition-of-general-anesthesia-and-levels-of-sedationanalgesia. Accessed February 27, 2022.)

The term *monitored anesthesia care* was created by the American Society of Anesthesiologists (ASA) in the 1980s to replace the term *standby anesthesia* and to facilitate professional fee billing. The original description of MAC referred to the anesthesiologist providing anesthesia services to a patient receiving local anesthesia or no anesthesia at all.[3] The ASA currently defines MAC as "a specific anesthesia service performed by a qualified anesthesia provider, for a diagnostic or therapeutic procedure."[4] MAC may include varying levels of sedation, analgesia, and anxiolysis. The anesthesia provider of MAC must be prepared to convert to general anesthesia if necessary. The ASA has described a continuum of depth of sedation that includes progressive levels of sedation and a definition of general anesthesia (Table 14.1). The preoperative evaluation, monitoring, and other anesthesia care standards apply equally to the patient receiving MAC.

CHOOSING AN APPROPRIATE ANESTHETIC TECHNIQUE

Factors identified in the preoperative evaluation can indicate that general anesthesia may be the most appropriate anesthetic choice (Box 14.1). If general anesthesia is not chosen, other anesthetic options include regional anesthesia or MAC.

Certain patient or procedure characteristics may preclude safe regional anesthesia (Box 14.2). The planned location of the surgical incision and operative field is a major factor in determining whether regional anesthesia can provide surgical analgesia (Fig. 14.1). Depending on the level of sedation

Box 14.1 Clinical Settings Appropriate for General Anesthesia

Pain (nociception) of surgical procedure cannot be addressed with local, topical, or regional anesthesia
Surgical procedure requires secure airway (e.g., procedure compromises airway integrity, oxygenation, or ventilation)
Patient or procedure characteristics that are not suitable for regional anesthetic (see Box 14.2)
Patient or procedure characteristics that are not suitable for monitored anesthesia care (e.g., risk of airway, respiratory, or cardiovascular compromise)

Box 14.2 Situations in Which Regional Anesthesia May Not Be Appropriate

Preferences and experience of the patient, anesthesia provider, and surgeon
Need for an immediate postoperative neurologic examination in the anatomic area affected by the regional anesthetic
Coagulopathy
Preexisting neurologic disease (e.g., multiple sclerosis, neurofibromatosis)
Infected or abnormal skin at the planned cutaneous puncture site

Specific Considerations for Neuraxial Anesthesia
Hypovolemia increases the risk for significant hypotension
Coagulopathy (including anticoagulant and antiplatelet medication therapy) increases risk of epidural hematoma
Increased intracranial pressure may result in cerebral herniation with intentional or inadvertent dural puncture

required, a regional technique may allow surgical anesthesia with complete preservation of upper airway reflexes, even in the patient at risk for aspiration of gastric contents.

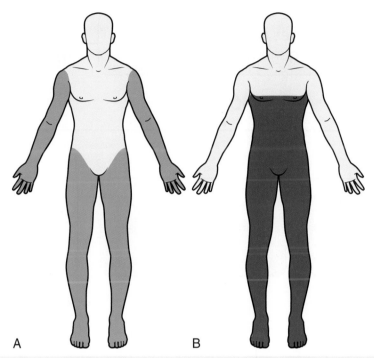

Fig. 14.1 Anatomic regions potentially amenable to peripheral nerve or neuraxial block. (A) Peripheral nerve block: *Green* areas indicate where complete surgical analgesia can typically be provided. (B) Neuraxial block: *Blue* areas indicate where complete surgical analgesia can typically be provided.

If the analgesic requirements for the planned procedure can be met with local or topical anesthesia, or if the planned procedure is not associated with pain (e.g., a diagnostic radiology procedure such as magnetic resonance imaging), MAC may be the most appropriate choice. The anesthetic risks associated with MAC are not necessarily different from general or regional anesthesia. An ASA closed claims study of patient injury documented a comparable incidence of injury severity with MAC compared with general anesthesia.[5] In patients receiving MAC respiratory depression from sedative drugs (e.g., propofol, benzodiazepines, opioids) is an important mechanism of injury.

Fig. 14.2 provides a summary of the decision-making process in choosing an appropriate anesthetic for an individual patient.

Anesthetic techniques can be combined to meet patient or surgical goals. For example, a patient with subarachnoid hemorrhage who requires diagnostic cerebral angiography may initially receive MAC. If the imaging reveals a cerebral aneurysm requiring endovascular coiling, the anesthesia provider may be asked to convert to general anesthesia to provide patient immobility and control of ventilation during the procedure.

Neuraxial and peripheral nerve blockade may be combined with general anesthesia to provide long-lasting postoperative analgesia after a surgical procedure that may not be amenable to regional anesthesia alone (also see Chapter 40). A 2018 Cochrane review evaluated randomized clinical trials comparing local anesthetics and regional anesthesia with conventional analgesia in preventing persistent postoperative pain.[6] The authors found moderate-quality evidence that regional anesthesia reduces the risk of persistent postoperative pain after thoracotomy and cesarean section and low-quality evidence for a similar benefit of regional anesthesia after breast cancer surgery.

A 2017 systematic review and metaanalysis analyzed contemporary (2010–2016) observational and randomized trials of neuraxial and combined neuraxial/general anesthesia compared with general anesthesia for major truncal and lower limb surgery.[7] Neuraxial anesthesia (alone or combined with general anesthesia) was not associated with reduced 30-day mortality compared with general anesthesia. However, there was moderate-quality evidence that pulmonary complications were reduced with neuraxial anesthesia compared with general anesthesia and moderate-quality evidence that neuraxial and neuraxial/general anesthesia were associated with reduced need for intensive care unit (ICU) admission.

The choice of anesthesia type is only one component of a patient's perioperative care plan. Increasingly, multidisciplinary enhanced recovery pathways have been used for patients undergoing a variety of surgeries, including colorectal, orthopedic, hepatic, pancreatic, and gynecologic.[8] Many studies have demonstrated improved outcomes with enhanced recovery pathways, including decreased hospital length of stay, decreased morbidity,

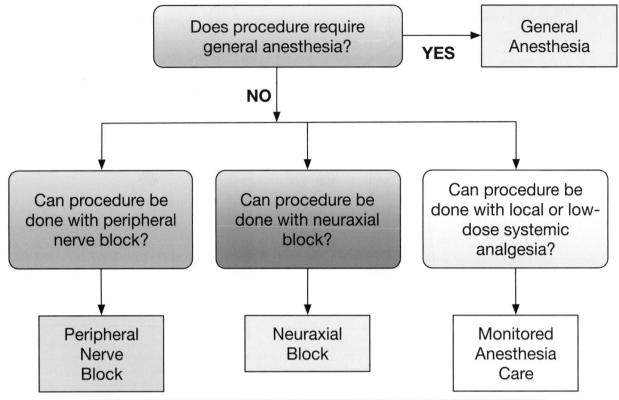

Fig. 14.2 An approach to determining the anesthetic plan based on surgical procedure, patient's coexisting diseases, and patient preferences. If general anesthesia is selected as the primary anesthetic, regional block may be performed as well for postoperative analgesia. When regional anesthesia is the primary anesthetic, additional sedation is administered along the continuum of depth of sedation (see Table 14.1).

and faster return to work. Table 14.2 provides an example of an enhanced recovery protocol used for patients scheduled for resection of colorectal cancer.[9]

PRACTICAL ASPECTS OF ANESTHESIA CHOICE

General Anesthesia

If general anesthesia is chosen, the anesthesia provider must then determine a plan for premedication, airway management, induction of anesthesia, maintenance of anesthesia, and postoperative analgesia (Table 14.3).

Preoxygenation, also called *denitrogenation*, is the deliberate replacement of nitrogen in the patient's functional residual capacity (FRC) with oxygen. Eight vital capacity breaths of 100% oxygen over 60 seconds, or tidal volume breathing of 100% oxygen for 3 minutes, replaces roughly 80% of the FRC with oxygen. This provides a crucial margin of safety during periods of apnea or upper airway obstruction that can occur with induction of general anesthesia. Adequate preoxygenation can delay or eliminate the onset of hypoxemia during the period between the intravenous induction of anesthesia and the start of controlled ventilation.

An inhaled induction of anesthesia is often chosen for pediatric patients in whom preinduction placement of an intravenous catheter is impractical (also see Chapter 34). Also, it may be indicated in the patient who is anticipated to have a difficult airway to manage, because spontaneous respiratory efforts are preserved with an inhaled induction of anesthesia. However, inhaled anesthetics ablate protective airway reflexes and pharyngeal muscular tone, so this method will not be suitable for all patients in whom difficulties with airway management are anticipated. Sevoflurane is the most commonly used anesthetic for inhaled induction of anesthesia because of its low pungency, high potency (permitting delivery of high-inspired oxygen concentration), and rapidity of onset.

Intravenous induction of anesthesia is the most common technique in the adult patient. Pharmacologic options include propofol, thiopental, etomidate, ketamine, and a benzodiazepine–opioid combination (also see Chapters 8 and 9). After the patient loses consciousness,

Table 14.2 Sample Enhanced Recovery Protocol for Laparoscopic Surgery for Patient With Nonmetastatic Colorectal Cancer

	Protocol
Preoperative	No bowel preparation
	Preoperative carbohydrate loading (clear carbohydrate liquid) 2 hours before surgery
	Enoxaparin antithrombotic prophylaxis
Intraoperative	Laparoscopic approach to surgery
	Balanced IV fluids <2500 mL on day of surgery
	TAP block, standard anesthesia protocol for GA
	PONV prophylaxis: dexamethasone, ondansetron, metoclopramide
Postoperative	Avoiding opioids, multimodal analgesia (oral when possible, including acetaminophen, NSAIDs)
	No nasogastric tube postoperatively
	Postoperative oxygen 4–6 L/min
	Early oral feeding (oral nutritional supplement 4 hours postoperatively, light diet POD 1, full diet POD2)
	Urinary catheter removed POD 1
	Full mobilization POD 1

GA, General anesthesia; *NSAIDs*, nonsteroidal antiinflammatory drugs; *POD*, postoperative day; *PONV*, postoperative nausea and vomiting; *TAP*, transversus abdominis plane.
From Pisarska M, Torbicz G, Gajewska N, et al. Compliance with the ERAS protocol and 3-year survival after laparoscopic surgery for nonmetastatic colorectal cancer. *World J Surg.* 2019;43(10):2552–2560.

Table 14.3 General Anesthesia: Detailed Planning

	Premedication	Airway Management	Induction of Anesthesia	Maintenance of Anesthesia[a]	Postoperative Analgesia
Management options	- Anxiolysis - Disease-specific (e.g., nonparticulate antacid for active GERD symptoms, bronchodilator for symptomatic asthma)	- Facemask - SGA - Endotracheal intubation[a] 1. Awake 2. Postinduction	- Intravenous - Inhaled	- One-drug - Two-drug - Multimodal	- Nonopioid medications: acetaminophen, gabapentin, NSAIDs, ketamine, lidocaine infusion - Local anesthetic infiltration - Regional anesthesia - Opioids—IV and/or oral

[a]See text for details.
GERD; Gastroesophageal reflux disease; *NSAIDs*, nonsteroidal antiinflammatory drugs; *SGA*, supraglottic airway.

ventilation via a mask is initiated. The anesthesia provider may then choose to administer an inhaled anesthetic to increase the depth of anesthesia before airway instrumentation. If tracheal intubation is planned, a neuromuscular blocking drug is usually given to facilitate direct laryngoscopy (also see Chapter 11).

Sometimes an intravenous rapid-sequence induction (RSI) is indicated. RSI is performed in patients at increased risk for aspiration of gastric contents (e.g., clinically significant gastroesophageal reflux disease, delayed gastric emptying, unknown fasting state, or a known full stomach). The goal of RSI is to minimize the time between onset of unconsciousness and tracheal intubation and reduce the risk of regurgitation by applying cricoid pressure. The sequence of events involves (1) preoxygenation; (2) intravenous administration of a hypnotic (e.g., propofol); (3) immediate administration a of a rapid-onset neuromuscular blocking drug (e.g., succinylcholine 1.0 to 1.5 mg/kg or rocuronium 1.0 to 1.2 mg/kg); (4) application of cricoid pressure (using a force of 30 newtons, approximately 7 pounds); (5) avoidance of ventilation via a mask; (6) tracheal intubation; and (7) release of cricoid pressure after confirmation of correct endotracheal tube placement.

Though ventilation via a mask is generally avoided with RSI, the use of positive pressure less than 20 cm H_2O (called *modified RSI*) should minimize the risk of gastric insufflation and may be needed if the patient develops hypoxemia before tracheal intubation. Although RSI with cricoid pressure has been used for several decades and is a standard approach, a 2015 metaanalysis did not demonstrate a measurable impact of cricoid pressure on clinical outcomes during RSI.[10]

Airway management techniques (e.g., direct laryngoscopy, supraglottic airway placement) are implemented after the intravenous or inhaled induction of anesthesia. However, if the anesthesia provider anticipates difficulty with ventilation via a mask or tracheal intubation, then tracheal intubation should be initiated before induction of anesthesia (i.e., awake intubation) (also see Chapter 16).

After induction of anesthesia and appropriate airway management, anesthesia is maintained typically by administration of a combination of anesthetic drugs, each titrated to achieve the desired anesthetic goal while minimizing side effects.[1,2] In principle, one anesthetic (e.g., propofol or a potent inhaled agent) can be used for maintenance of anesthesia. However, a large dose is typically required to control ANS responses to surgical stimulation. For example, the minimum alveolar concentration (MAC) to block the adrenergic response to incision (heart rate and mean arterial pressure within 15% of preincision value), called *MAC-BAR,* is approximately 1.3 MAC for isoflurane and desflurane in 60% nitrous oxide (total MAC of 1.9).[11]

The use of two drugs to maintain anesthesia represents an approach called *balanced anesthesia.* Most commonly, an opioid is added to propofol or an inhaled anesthetic to provide control of ANS nociceptive responses to surgical stimulation. For example, when a patient receiving inhaled anesthesia with desflurane or isoflurane receives fentanyl 1.5 mcg/kg 5 minutes before surgical incision, the MAC-BAR decreases to 0.4 MAC plus 60% nitrous oxide (total MAC of 1). However, opioids have many side effects, including life-threatening respiratory depression (also see Chapter 9). The opioid epidemic provided additional incentive to examine perioperative opioid use, including intraoperative administration.

The concept of multimodal analgesia for acute postoperative pain management (also see Chapter 40) led to increased interest in multimodal general anesthesia, which involves simultaneously addressing multiple targets in the nociceptive system.[2] Table 14.4 summarizes a rational strategy to implement multimodal general anesthesia. A key goal is to make multimodal pain control a key objective postoperatively. Currently, there are no studies on the impact of multimodal general anesthesia on persistent postoperative opioid use or other clinical outcomes.

The postoperative disposition of the patient also influences anesthetic choice for maintenance and emergence from anesthesia. Patients undergoing outpatient surgery require special attention to the prevention of postoperative and postdischarge nausea and vomiting (also see Chapter 37). This may involve selection of a less emetogenic anesthetic maintenance drug (e.g., propofol) or administration of multiple antiemetic drugs (also see Chapter 39).

Regional Anesthesia

Superficial and deep operations on the extremities, particularly the distal extremities, may be amenable to peripheral nerve block (see Chapter 18). Because surgical anesthesia may be achieved without sedation, this technique is particularly attractive in patients for whom systemic disease (e.g., severe pulmonary disease, cardiovascular disease, or renal failure) may present a significant challenge during general anesthesia. Unlike neuraxial anesthesia, the localized sympathectomy resulting from peripheral nerve block rarely results in systemic hypotension. However, peripheral nerve blockade as the primary anesthetic technique requires patient cooperation and may be inappropriate in patients with dementia, acute intoxication, or other conditions associated with altered mental status. Peripheral nerve blockade may be difficult to accomplish or may result in an inadequate, "patchy" block. If surgical anesthesia is not achieved with a peripheral nerve block, the anesthesia provider is faced with the options of supplementing the block with local anesthesia, administering intravenous analgesics and hypnotics, postponing surgery and reattempting the block at a later time, or converting to general anesthesia.

Neuraxial anesthesia can provide excellent operating conditions in the lower extremities and lower abdomen. Higher levels of neuraxial blockade (e.g., midthoracic to high thoracic) with surgical anesthesia concentrations of local anesthetic (e.g., epidural 2% lidocaine) result in more profound sympathectomy and increased risk of hypotension, which may require infusion of vasoactive medications to maintain hemodynamic stability. However, analgesic concentrations of local anesthetic (e.g., epidural 0.1% ropivacaine) are commonly given via thoracic epidural catheter to provide postoperative analgesia after open thoracic surgery and abdominal surgery. The smaller concentration of local anesthetic required for analgesia (as opposed to surgical anesthesia) results in decreased incidence of hypotension.

Postoperative disposition of the patient also influences medication choice or type of regional anesthesia. Patients undergoing ambulatory surgery who receive spinal anesthesia may have a prolonged recovery time if they receive long-acting local anesthetics. Ambulatory surgical patients undergoing procedures associated with significant postoperative pain may benefit from a long-lasting peripheral nerve block or nerve catheter placement.[12]

The anesthesia provider may choose to administer sedation to improve patient comfort during a procedure performed with regional anesthesia, although the term

Table 14.4 Multimodal General Anesthesia Strategy

Component of Anesthesia	Primary Drug[a]	Secondary Drug[b]
Antinociception[c,d]	Opioids (e.g., remifentanil)	Propofol
	Ketamine (NMDA antagonist)	Sevoflurane
	Dexmedetomidine (α_2 agonist)	
	Lidocaine (antiinflammatory, sodium channel blockade)	
	NSAID (antiinflammatory)	
Unconsciousness (and amnesia)[e]	Propofol	Ketamine
	Sevoflurane (inhaled anesthetic)	Remifentanil
		Dexmedetomidine
		Magnesium (NMDA agonist)
		NMBA (decrease proprioception)
Immobility	NMBA	Magnesium (smooth muscle relaxant)
		Propofol (central muscle relaxation)
		Sevoflurane (central muscle relaxation)

[a]Primary: drug that explicitly maintains that component of anesthesia
[b]Secondary: drug that "implicitly" (i.e., additionally) contributes
[c]Simultaneous use of antinociceptive drugs creates opioid-sparing effect
[d]In the absence of an antinociception monitor heart rate and blood pressure changes are used as a measure of nociceptive response.
[e]Electroencephalogram (EEG) monitoring is essential to track the level of unconsciousness and guide the dose of hypnotics. *NMBA*, Neuromuscular blocking agent; *NMDA*, N-methyl-D-aspartic acid; *NSAIDs*, nonsteroidal antiinflammatory drugs.
Adapted from Brown EN, Pavone KJ, Naranjo M. Multimodal general anesthesia: Theory and practice. *Anesth Analg*. 2018;127(5):1246–1258, Table 1.

MAC would not be used if the primary anesthetic was a regional technique.

Monitored Anesthesia Care

Pharmacologic sedation using opioids or hypnotic medications is often provided as a component of MAC (also see Chapters 8 and 9). Nonpharmacologic approaches such as video or audio distraction or verbal reassurance can also complement a MAC technique. The ASA depth of sedation continuum can be used to choose the level of sedation that is most appropriate for the patient undergoing MAC. Local or topical anesthesia administered by the surgeon is commonly used during MAC to provide adequate analgesia for the procedure. The anesthesia provider must track the total dose of local anesthetic and be alert for signs of local anesthetic toxicity (also see Chapter 10). The injection of local anesthetic near sensitive areas (e.g., face, eyes) may initially require a deeper level of sedation until the injection is complete.

The most dangerous anesthetic risk during MAC is respiratory depression from excessive sedation. The manifestations of respiratory depression include upper airway obstruction, hypoventilation, and hypoxemia. During MAC, end-tidal capnography can be accomplished with a nasal cannula that has a dedicated sampling line

attached. However, capnography monitoring is less reliable in this setting, and the absence of increased end-tidal CO_2 does not guarantee the adequacy of ventilation. The medications typically used for sedation during MAC (benzodiazepines, opioids, propofol) produce dose-dependent respiratory depression. Ketamine and dexmedetomidine are less likely to cause hypoventilation but have other potential side effects and may have synergistic sedative effects with other hypnotic medications (also see Chapter 8).

A 2021 retrospective study examined over 1000 MAC cases that required conversion to general anesthesia.[13] Common reasons for conversion included patient intolerance (manifested by patient movement, disinhibition, patient discomfort), patient-related complications (e.g., hemodynamic instability, aspiration, coughing, hypoxemia), or procedural factors (e.g., change in procedure, surgical request, bleeding, extended surgical time).

ACKNOWLEDGMENT

The editors and publisher would like to thank Dr. Elizabeth Whitlock for contributing to this chapter in the previous edition of this work. It has served as the foundation for the current chapter.

REFERENCES

1. Egan TD, Svensen CH. Multimodal general anesthesia: A principled approach to producing the drug-induced, reversible coma of anesthesia. *Anesth Analg.* 2018 Nov;127(5):1104–1106. doi:10.1213/ANE.0000000000003743. PMID: 30335656.

2. Brown EN, Pavone KJ, Naranjo M. Multimodal general anesthesia: Theory and practice. *Anesth Analg.* 2018 Nov;127(5):1246–1258. doi:10.1213/ANE.0000000000003668. PMID: 30252709; PMCID: PMC6203428.

3. Cohen NA, McMichael JP. What's new in ... Definitions of monitored anesthesia care. *ASA Newsl.* 2004;68(6):22–26.

4. American Society of Anesthesiologists. Position on Monitored Anesthesia Care. Last Amended: October 17, 2018. https://www.asahq.org/standards-and-guidelines/position-on-monitored-anesthesia-care Accessed December 22, 2021

5. Bhananker SM, Posner KL, Cheney FW, et al. Injury and liability associated with monitored anesthesia care: A closed claims analysis. *Anesthesiology.* 2006;104(2):228–234.

6. Weinstein EJ, Levene JL, Cohen MS, Andreae DA, Chao JY, Johnson M, Hall CB, Andreae MH. Local anaesthetics and regional anaesthesia versus conventional analgesia for preventing persistent postoperative pain in adults and children. Cochrane Database Syst Rev. 2018 Jun 20;6(6):CD007105. doi: 10.1002/14651858.CD007105.pub4. PMID: 29926477; PMCID: PMC6377212.

7. Smith LM, Cozowicz C, Uda Y, Memtsoudis SG, Barrington MJ. Neuraxial and combined neuraxial/general anesthesia compared to general anesthesia for major truncal and lower limb surgery: A systematic review and meta-analysis. *Anesth Analg.* 2017 Dec;125(6):1931–1945. doi:10.1213/ANE.0000000000002069. PMID: 28537970.

8. Esper SA, Holder-Murray J, Subramaniam K, Boisen M, Kenkre TS, Meister K, Foos S, Wong H, Howard-Quijano K, Mahajan A. Enhanced recovery protocols reduce mortality across eight surgical specialties at academic and university-affiliated community hospitals. *Ann Surg.* 2020 Nov 18. doi:10.1097/SLA.0000000000004642. Epub ahead of printPMID: 33214486.

9. Pisarska M, Torbicz G, Gajewska N, Rubinkiewicz M, Wierdak M, Major P, Budzyński A, Ljungqvist O, Pędziwiatr M. Compliance with the ERAS Protocol and 3-year survival after laparoscopic surgery for non-metastatic colorectal cancer. *World J Surg.* 2019 Oct;43(10):2552–2560. doi:10.1007/s00268-019-05073-0 PMID: 31286185.

10. Algie CM, Mahar RK, Tan HB, et al. Effectiveness and risks of cricoid pressure during rapid sequence induction for endotracheal intubation. *Cochrane Database Syst Rev.* 2015;11:CD011656.

11. Daniel M, Weiskopf RB, Noorani M, Eger 2nd EI. Fentanyl augments the blockade of the sympathetic response to incision (MAC-BAR) produced by desflurane and isoflurane: Desflurane and isoflurane MAC-BAR without and with fentanyl. *Anesthesiology.* 1998 Jan;88(1):43–49. doi:10.1097/00000542-199801000-00009. PMID: 9447854.

12. Ilfeld BM. Continuous peripheral nerve blocks: An update of the published evidence and comparison with novel, alternative analgesic modalities. *Anesth Analg.* 2017 Jan;124(1):308–335. doi:10.1213/ANE.0000000000001581. PMID: 27749354.

13. Kim S, Chang BA, Rahman A, Lin HM, DeMaria Jr S, Zerillo J, Wax DB. Analysis of urgent/emergent conversions from monitored anesthesia care to general anesthesia with airway instrumentation. *BMC Anesthesiol.* 2021 Jun 29;21(1):183. doi:10.1186/s12871-021-01403-9 PMID: 34187367; PMCID: PMC8240303.

15 ANESTHESIA DELIVERY SYSTEMS

Stephen D. Weston

THE ANESTHESIA WORKSTATION

In the decades after the first public demonstration of ether anesthesia in 1846 the anesthesia delivery system consisted of handheld devices ranging from ether- or chloroform-soaked cloths to more sophisticated inhalers that could regulate the administered dose of anesthetic.[1] The modern anesthesia workstation remains at its core a device for delivering inhaled anesthesia, but incorporates many additional functions focused on safety and ease of use (Table 15.1). The sheer number of tasks and solutions for which the anesthesia workstation is designed explains its complexity. Many innovations in workstation design aim to enhance patient safety. American Society of Anesthesiologists (ASA) closed claims analysis of adverse anesthetic outcomes related to anesthetic gas delivery equipment shows a decrease in such claims from 4% in the 1970s to approximately 1% in 2000–2011.[2] Further, the severity of the events leading to the claims has decreased, with more reports of awareness under anesthesia and fewer involving death or permanent brain injury.

Table 15.1 Functions of the Modern Anesthesia Workstation

Function	Description	Safety Feature
Inhaled anesthetic delivery	Deliver volatile anesthetic gas at precise concentrations.	Continuously display inspired and exhaled anesthetic concentration.
	Allow rebreathing of the exhaled anesthetic gases after removing carbon dioxide.	Continuously display inspired and exhaled carbon dioxide concentration.
Oxygen delivery	Individually meter oxygen and two or more other breathing gases, while continuously enriching the inhaled gas with anesthetic vapors.	Continuously measure and display the inspired oxygen concentration. Prevent hypoxic gas mixtures caused by operator error or gas supply failure. Provide a breathing circuit manual oxygen flush feature. Possess a backup supply of oxygen. Display gas pipeline and backup tank supply pressures.
Facilitate ventilation of patient's lungs	Ventilate the patient manually ("bag" ventilation) with adjustable breathing circuit pressure. Ventilate the patient mechanically, with sophisticated ventilator modes comparable to the ICU.	Measure and display ventilatory parameters such as respiratory rate, tidal volume, and airway pressure.
Remove excess anesthetic gases	Eliminate ("scavenge") excess gas from the patient's breathing circuit and remove this gas from the room.	
Information display	Provide an integrated platform for displaying anesthetic, hemodynamic, and respiratory parameters and for collecting this data into an electronic medical record.	

ICU, Intensive care unit.

Anesthesia providers must be aware of the operational characteristics and "functional anatomy" of their anesthesia workstations. There is increased variation among anesthesia workstations, with operational and preuse checkout procedures becoming more divergent, thus mandating device-specific familiarity. Contemporary machines have automated preuse checkout procedures, but machines can pass automated checkouts despite the presence of unsafe conditions.[3]

Although providing a detailed description of each component of the anesthesia machine is beyond the scope of this chapter, starting with a generic approach provides a suitable foundation for understanding a specific workstation model. It is worth emphasizing that if there is any doubt about the correct functioning of an anesthesia workstation, and there is difficulty with ventilation or oxygenation, then ventilating the patient from an alternative source of oxygen such as an E-cylinder is often appropriate. Trouble-shooting of the anesthesia machine can commence once the patient is safe.

FUNCTIONAL ANATOMY OF THE ANESTHESIA WORKSTATION

Gas Supply System

Although modern anesthesia workstations are often largely electronically controlled, the interior of the anesthesia machine remains a pneumatic system, a place where breathing gases are delivered from their supply

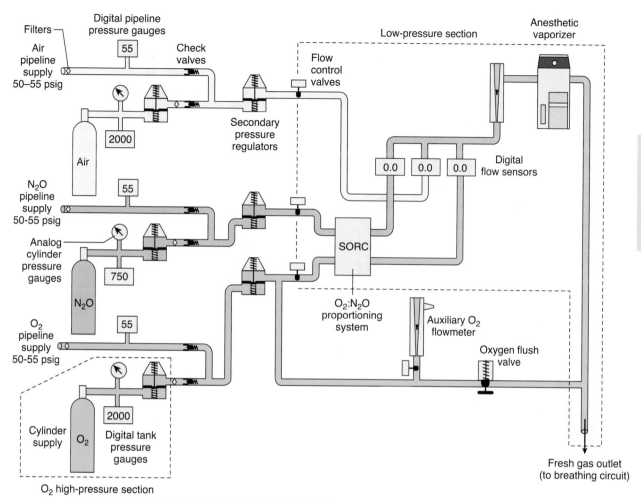

Fig. 15.1 Anesthesia workstation gas supply system represented by the Dräger Apollo anesthesia workstation. The high-pressure system extends from the gas cylinders to the high-pressure regulators (*dashed lines* around O_2 high-pressure section only). The intermediate-pressure section extends from the high-pressure regulators to the flow control valves and includes the tubing and components originating from the pipeline inlets. The low-pressure section (*dashed lines*) extends from the flow control valves to the breathing circuit. See text for additional details. (From Dräger Medical. *Instructions for Use: Apollo*. Telford, PA: Dräger Medical; 2012.)

sources, measured and mixed, passed through (or by) an anesthetic vaporizer, and delivered to the patient's breathing circuit. Although the details of this gas supply system may differ between the various manufacturers' anesthesia workstations, their overall schematic is similar. The gas supply system of a typical contemporary workstation with electronic controls is depicted in Fig. 15.1.

High-Pressure Section: Auxiliary E-Cylinder Inlet

During normal operation, the high-pressure section of the anesthesia machine is not active, because the hospital's central gas supply system serves as the primary gas source for the machine. However, it is a requirement to have at least one attachment for an oxygen cylinder to serve as a backup source of oxygen in case of failure of the hospital supply source. The cylinders are mounted to the anesthesia machine by the hanger yoke assembly. Each hanger yoke is also equipped with the Pin Index Safety System (PISS), which is a safeguard to reduce the risk of a medical gas cylinder error caused by interchanging cylinders (Fig. 15.2). Two metal pins on the yoke assembly are arranged to project precisely into corresponding holes on the cylinder head–valve assembly of the tank. Each gas or combination of gases has a specific pin arrangement.[4]

The maximum pressure in E-cylinders full of oxygen is approximately 2200 pounds per square inch gauge (psig).

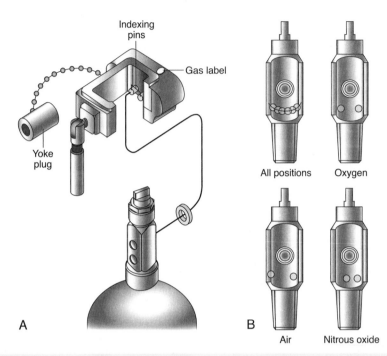

Fig. 15.2 E-cylinder hanger yoke assembly. (A) Standard E-cylinder hanger yoke assembly highlighting the gas-specific indexing pins, sealing gasket, and yoke plug. The yoke plug should be inserted when a tank is not in place. (B) Pin Index Safety System holes machined into the cylinder head–valve mechanism of the compressed gas cylinders. (From Yoder M. Gas supply systems. In: Understanding Modern Anesthesia Systems. Telford, PA: Dräger Medical; 2009.)

(The *gauge pressure* is the pressure above the ambient atmospheric pressure.) The full tank pressure is 750 psig for nitrous oxide and 2200 psig for air. These pressures are much higher than the normal hospital pipeline supply pressure of 50 to 55 psig. A *high-pressure regulator* therefore reduces the variable high pressure in the E-cylinder to a lower, nearly constant pressure output to the intermediate-pressure section of the anesthesia machine.

Three points about the safe use of the auxiliary oxygen E-cylinder system should be noted. First, checking the E-cylinders is *not* part of an automatic machine checkout. The anesthesia provider must manually open each cylinder and check the pressure gauges on the front of the machine. Second, it is imperative to keep the auxiliary E-cylinders closed during normal operation using pipeline gases, as an open oxygen cylinder may allow the anesthesia provider to be unaware of catastrophic pipeline failure. If the oxygen tank is *already open* when pipeline failure occurs, the "low oxygen pressure" alarm, which is a high-intensity alarm, will not sound until the auxiliary tank is already depleted. Finally, in case of known or suspected pipeline contamination or crossover (e.g., from nitrous oxide in the oxygen pipeline) leading to delivery of a hypoxic gas mixture, backup oxygen from the E-cylinder will not flow unless the anesthesia machine is disconnected from the pipeline, because the system is designed to preferentially draw from the pipeline as long as it is adequately pressured.[5,6]

Calculation of remaining gas volume in an oxygen E-cylinder based on its pressure has practical implications for patient care in the setting of failed pipeline oxygen supply in the operating room or for patient transport within the hospital. A full oxygen E-cylinder contains 650 L of oxygen at 2200 psig. Because oxygen is a compressed gas, the gauge pressure is directly proportional to the amount of oxygen in the tank. For example, at 1100 psig, there is half a tank left (325 L of oxygen) remaining. Because nitrous oxide is a compressed liquid, the relationship between its pressure and volume is different. A full nitrous oxide E-cylinder contains about 1600 L of gas at 750 psig. As the nitrous oxide gas flows out of the cylinder, further liquid is vaporized and the pressure in the tank remains unchanged. Therefore the pressure of a nitrous oxide tank remains at 750 psig until there is no more liquid in the tank, at which point the pressure begins to fall. By this point, at least 75% of the tank has been depleted.

Intermediate-Pressure Section

Gas Pipeline Inlet: Central Gas Supply Source

Three gases are typically piped into the operating room by the hospital's central gas supply system: oxygen, air, and nitrous oxide, all at 50 to 55 psig. The pipeline supply terminates with one of two types of connector: the Diameter Index Safety System (DISS) connector system or the quick coupler system. Within each type, the connectors for oxygen, air, and nitrous oxide are mutually incompatible. DISS connectors rely on matching diameters in the male and female connections to properly seat and thread the connection.[4] Quick couplers use pins and corresponding slots on the male and female ends, respectively, in order to ensure correct connections. Because these connectors can be plugged together or released with a simple twisting motion, they are especially appealing for equipment that needs to be moved between locations. In both systems the wall plates and hoses are color-coded for ease of identification: green for oxygen, yellow for air, and blue for nitrous oxide.

Oxygen Flush Valve

The oxygen flush valve allows manual delivery of a high flow rate of 100% oxygen directly to the patient's breathing circuit. The oxygen flush valve may be employed to overcome circuit leaks or to rapidly increase the inhaled oxygen concentration. Flow from the oxygen flush valve bypasses the anesthetic vaporizers and enters the low-pressure circuit downstream at a rate between 35 and 75 L/min.

Oxygen flushing during the inspiratory phase of positive-pressure ventilation can produce barotrauma if the anesthesia machine does not incorporate a fresh gas decoupling feature or an appropriately adjusted inspiratory pressure limiter. A defective or damaged valve can stick in the fully open position and result in barotrauma. Oxygen flow from a valve sticking in a partially open position can dilute the inhaled anesthetic agent concentration, potentially resulting in awareness under anesthesia.[7]

Pneumatic Safety Systems

Within the intermediate-pressure section of the machine there are two safety systems that minimize the risk of delivery of a hypoxic gas mixture in case the oxygen pressure decreases significantly. The oxygen supply failure alarm sensor provides an audible and visual warning to the clinician if the oxygen pressure drops below a manufacturer-specified minimum. This alarm cannot be silenced until the pressure is restored to the minimum value (e.g., by opening the oxygen E-cylinder on the machine). In addition, the oxygen supply failure protection device, sometimes called the "fail-safe valve," affects the flow of other gases when oxygen supply pressure is low. The fail-safe valve either shuts off (binary valve) or reduces (proportional valve) the flow of other gases such as nitrous oxide or air. The term *fail-safe* as it pertains to these valves is a misnomer: only the inspired oxygen concentration monitor in the breathing circuit and clinical acumen can protect the patient from hypoxic gas delivery.

Auxiliary Oxygen Flowmeter

Auxiliary oxygen flowmeters are commonly encountered on anesthesia workstations, serving as a convenience feature for low-flow oxygen. Because the flowmeter is usually operational even when the machine is off, the auxiliary oxygen flowmeter can also serve as a safety feature because it allows the use of an oxygen delivery source (e.g., a manual resuscitation bag) in the case of a system power failure. The source of oxygen for the auxiliary flowmeter is the same as for the other oxygen flow control valves. In cases of suspected hospital oxygen pipeline contamination or crossover switching to an E-cylinder that is not part of the anesthesia machine is imperative.

Low-Pressure Section

The purpose of the high- and intermediate-pressure sections of the anesthesia workstation is to deliver a reliable source of breathing gases at a stable and known working pressure to the low-pressure section of the gas supply system. The clinician interfaces with the low-pressure section of the gas supply system, shaping its output to deliver a known composition of gas and anesthetic to the breathing circuit. The low-pressure section of the gas supply system begins at the flow control valves and ends at the outlet of the fresh gas line (see Fig. 15.1). Key components include the flow control valves, the flowmeters or flow sensors, the vaporizer manifold, and the anesthetic vaporizers. The breathing circuit, including the circle system, breathing bag, and ventilator, will be treated separately.

Flow Control Assemblies

The flow control valves on the anesthesia workstation allow the operator to select a *total fresh gas flow* of known composition that enters the low-pressure section of the anesthesia workstation. These valves are therefore an important anatomic landmark: they separate the intermediate-pressure section from the low-pressure section. After leaving the flowmeters, the mixture of gases travels through a common manifold and may be directed through an anesthetic vaporizer if selected. The total fresh gas flow and the anesthetic vapor then travel toward the common gas outlet, or fresh gas outlet (see Fig. 15.1).

Newer anesthesia workstations are increasingly equipped with electronic flow sensors instead of flow tubes. These systems may employ conventional control knobs or an entirely electronic interface to control gas flow. Numerous flow sensor technologies can be applied, such as hot-wire anemometers, a differential pressure transducer method, or mass flow sensors. Regardless of the mechanism of flow measurement, these systems depend on electrical power to display the gas flow. When system electrical power is totally interrupted, some backup mechanical means usually exists.

Mechanical flow control and flow display remain common, even on some newer workstations, either as primary or especially as backup systems. The flow control valve assembly consists of a flow control knob, a tapered needle valve, a valve seat, and a pair of valve stops.[6] For safety, the oxygen flow control knob is typically distinctively fluted, larger in diameter, and may project beyond the control knobs of the other gases.

The flow control valve regulates the amount of flow that enters a tapered glass flow tube. A mobile indicator float inside the calibrated flow tube indicates the amount of flow passing through the annular space between the float and the flow tube. The indicator float hovers freely in an equilibrium position in the tube, where the upward force resulting from gas flow equals the downward force on the float resulting from gravity. The viscosity and density of the particular gas determine its behavior in the glass tube, and therefore the calibration on these flowmeters is gas-specific. The flow tube has historically been a very fragile component of the anesthesia workstation. Flow tube leaks are a potential hazard because the flowmeters are located downstream from hypoxia-preventing safety devices, except the breathing circuit oxygen analyzer.[6]

Proportioning Systems

On anesthesia workstations with electronically controlled gas flow, the machine is programmed to prevent the user from selecting a hypoxic gas mixture for delivery to the fresh gas outlet. For manually controlled flowmeters, the concern is that a user could mistakenly select oxygen and nitrous oxide flows that result in a hypoxic mixture. A proportioning system prevents this by means of a pneumatic-mechanical interface between the oxygen and nitrous oxide flows or a mechanical link between the oxygen and nitrous oxide flow control valves. Proportioning systems can override flows set by the anesthesia provider, either decreasing nitrous oxide flow or increasing oxygen flow in order to maintain a nonhypoxic fresh gas flow. The specific devices and designs used to accomplish this control vary among manufacturers. As always, the presence of a functioning oxygen analyzer in the patient's breathing circuit is the best and final protection against delivery of a hypoxic gas mixture.

Vaporizer Mount and Interlock System

The vaporizer mounts on modern anesthesia workstations allow for detachment and replacement of the anesthetic vaporizers by the workstation operator. The benefits of detachable vaporizer mountings include ease of maintenance, the need for fewer vaporizer positions on the workstation, and the ability to remove the vaporizer in the setting of malignant hyperthermia.[8] This ability to remove and reintroduce an element to the pneumatic structure of the low-pressure section of the anesthesia machine brings an increased potential for leaks or fresh gas flow obstruction as a result of an inappropriately seated vaporizer or other connection-related failures. After adding or changing a vaporizer on the anesthesia machine, the operator should make sure it is properly seated.

The vaporizer interlock device ensures that fresh gas cannot flow through more than one vaporizer at a time. The design of vaporizer interlock devices varies significantly. These devices are not immune from failure, with anesthetic overdose as a potential consequence.

Anesthetic Vaporizers

The inhaler used by William T. G. Morton in the first public demonstration of ether anesthesia was effective, but there was no way to regulate its output concentration or compensate for changes in temperature caused by the vaporization of the liquid anesthetic. Modern variable bypass–type vaporizers are temperature compensated and can maintain precise outputs accurately over a wide range of input gas flow rates. The introduction of desflurane to the clinical setting required an even more sophisticated vaporizer design to handle the unique physical properties of this agent (also see Chapter 7). Vaporizers incorporating computerized control technology emerged in "cassette" vaporizer systems. An injection-type vaporizer has also been introduced, spraying precise amounts of liquid anesthetic agent into the fresh gas stream. Before discussing any of these systems, certain physical chemical principles are briefly reviewed to facilitate an understanding of the operating principles, construction, and design of contemporary anesthetic vaporizers.

Physics

When a gas exists within a container, the gas molecules collide with the walls and exert a force. The pressure within the container is the force per unit area exerted on the walls. According to the ideal gas law, that pressure is directly proportional to the number of molecules of gas present within the space, directly proportional to the temperature, and inversely proportional to the volume of the container that confines a gas. When a mixture of ideal gases exists in a container, each gas creates its own pressure, which is the same pressure as if the individual gas occupied the container alone. The total pressure may be calculated by simply adding together the pressures of each gas—Dalton's law of partial pressures. At sea level, the ambient pressure is 760 mm Hg, which equals 1 atmosphere (atm) or 101.325 kilopascals (kPa).

In the clinical setting oxygen and anesthetic concentrations are typically specified as a *volume percent*. Volume percent is simply the percentage of volume occupied by the gas relative to the sum of all gases present, which is the same as the proportion of an individual gas by its *partial pressure* (mm Hg) as a percentage of the total pressure (under idealized conditions encountered in the operating room). Thus although the partial pressure of "room air" oxygen is lower at elevation (129 mm Hg in Denver, Colorado) than it is at sea level (160 mm Hg), it remains approximately 21% at both altitudes.

Volatile liquids such as inhaled anesthetic agents are characterized by a high propensity to evaporate, or *vaporize*. When a volatile liquid is exposed to air or other gases, molecules at the liquid surface with sufficient kinetic energy escape and enter the vapor phase. If a volatile anesthetic is placed within a contained space, such as an anesthetic vaporizer, molecules will continue to escape into the vapor phase until the rate at which molecules evaporate is equal to the rate of return to the liquid phase (a process known as *condensation*). When this equilibrium is reached, the composition of the vapor remains constant and it is said to be "saturated" with anesthetic, and the anesthetic molecules in the gas phase bombard the walls of the container, creating a partial pressure known as the *saturated vapor pressure,* or simply *vapor pressure*. Liquids with a higher tendency to evaporate and generate higher vapor pressures are described as "more volatile."

Vapor pressure is a physical property of a substance, with each substance having its own unique value at any given temperature (Fig. 15.3). Vapor pressure is temperature dependent and is *not* affected by changes in atmospheric pressure. Evaporation is diminished at colder temperatures because fewer molecules possess sufficient kinetic energy to escape into the vapor phase. Conversely, at warmer temperatures, evaporation is enhanced and vapor pressure increases. Because vapor pressure values are unique to each liquid anesthetic agent, anesthetic vaporizers must be constructed in an agent-specific manner.[8]

Energy is required for a molecule of volatile anesthetic to evaporate into the gas phase–that energy is absorbed from the surroundings in the form of heat. The amount of energy required to change 1 gram of a particular liquid into vapor at a constant temperature during evaporation is referred to as the *latent heat of vaporization*. In a well-insulated container the energy for vaporization must come from the liquid itself. In the absence of an outside heat source, the temperature of the remaining liquid decreases as vaporization progresses. This cooling effect can lead to significant reductions in vapor pressure, and therefore of volatile anesthetic molecules moving into the gas phase. Unless the evaporative cooling effect of the liquid anesthetic agent is mitigated and compensated for, vaporizer output will decrease.

The *boiling point* of a liquid is defined as the temperature at which vapor pressure equals atmospheric pressure and the liquid begins to boil. The boiling point of most contemporary volatile anesthetic agents is not relevant to vaporizer design under most clinical situations. Desflurane, however, boils at a temperature commonly encountered in clinical settings and has a high saturated vapor pressure (Table 15.2). These properties mandate a special vaporizer design to control agent delivery.

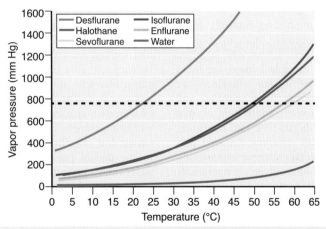

Fig. 15.3 Vapor pressure versus temperature curves for desflurane, isoflurane, halothane, enflurane, sevoflurane, and water. Note that the curve for desflurane differs dramatically from that of the other contemporary inhaled anesthetic agents. Also note that all inhaled agents are more volatile than water. *Dashed line* indicates 1 atm (760 mm Hg) of pressure, which illustrates the boiling point at sea level (normal boiling point). (From inhaled anesthetic package insert equations and Susay SR, Smith MA, Lockwood GG. The saturated vapor pressure of desflurane at various temperatures. Anesth Analg. 1996;83:864-866.)

Table 15.2 Physical Properties of Inhaled Volatile Anesthetic Agents

Property	Halothane	Isoflurane	Sevoflurane	Desflurane
SVP* @ 20°C (mm Hg)	243	238	157	669
SVC† @ 20°C at 1 atm‡ (v/v%)	32	31	21	88
MAC§ at age 40 yr (v/v%)	0.75	1.2	1.9	6.0
MAPP¶ (mm Hg)	5.7	9.1	14.4	45.6
Boiling point @1 atm (°C)	50.2 (122.4°F)	48.5 (119.3°F)	58.6 (137.3°F)	22.8 (73°F)

*SVP, Saturated vapor pressure. From anesthetic prescribing information.
†SVC, Saturated vapor concentration: the percentage of anesthetic agent relative to ambient pressure within an equilibrated (saturated) container (SVP/ambient pressure).
‡1 atm, 1 atmosphere = ambient pressure at sea level (760 mm Hg).
§MAC, Minimum alveolar concentration: the alveolar concentration that produces immobility in response to a noxious stimulus in 50% of subjects. The denominator is approximately sea level pressure (760 mm Hg).
¶MAPP, Minimum alveolar partial pressure. The alveolar partial pressure that produces immobility in response to a noxious stimulus in 50% of subjects (the numerator in the MAC calculation). Not affected by altitude. Calculated as MAC (fraction) × 760 mm Hg (i.e., for isoflurane = 0.012 × 760 mm Hg). × 760 mm Hg (i.e., for isoflurane = 0.012 × 760 mm Hg).
v/v%, Volume percent.

Modern Vaporizer Types

The saturated vapor pressure of volatile anesthetic agents, even at normal operating room temperatures, results in gas concentrations that greatly exceed those used clinically, so these concentrations must be diluted to safe ranges. Virtually all modern vaporizers are *out-of-circuit*, and their controlled output is introduced into the breathing circuit through a fresh gas line. Specific types of vaporizers currently include the *variable bypass vaporizer*, the *dual-circuit vaporizer*, the *cassette vaporizer*, and the *injection vaporizer*.

Variable Bypass Vaporizers

Variable bypass refers to the method of carefully regulating the concentration of vaporizer output by diluting gas fully saturated with anesthetic agent with a larger flow of gas. A diagram of a variable bypass vaporizer is shown in Fig. 15.4. Variable bypass vaporizers are *agent-specific, flow-over, temperature-compensated*, and *pressure-compensated*. The concentration control dial determines the ratio of the fresh gas flow that continues through the bypass chamber to the flow diverted into the vaporizing chamber. A temperature-compensating device, either an expansion element or temperature-sensitive bimetallic strip, further adjusts that ratio, for example, by increasing the amount of flow into the vaporizing chamber as the temperature falls. Vaporizer concentration control dials are labeled to set vaporizer output in terms of volume percent, and the vaporizers are calibrated at sea level. Because the physical properties and clinical concentrations of each agent are unique, the diverting ratios are specific to each agent and dial setting. Variable bypass vaporizers can be used to deliver halothane, isoflurane, sevoflurane, and older agents, but not desflurane, because of this agent's unique physical properties.

An ideal variable bypass vaporizer would maintain a constant concentration output at a given setting regardless of variables such as the fresh gas flow rate, temperature, intermittent backpressure from the breathing circuit, carrier gas composition, and barometric pressure. Modern vaporizers generally have excellent performance characteristics, with minimal variation in clinical performance in conditions encountered in an operating room.

Understanding the influence of barometric pressure on variable bypass vaporizer output can help to illustrate concepts regarding vaporizer function. Perhaps surprisingly, the "depth of anesthesia" administered at a given dial setting on a variable bypass vaporizer is relatively independent of atmospheric pressure. (This is not necessarily true with other vaporizer types.) A liquid's vapor pressure is independent of barometric pressure; therefore as altitude increases and barometric pressure declines, the partial pressure of anesthetic agent in the variable bypass vaporizing chamber remains constant despite a decline in the partial pressures of other constituent breathing gases and the total ambient pressure. The vaporizer output's *concentration* (volume percent) of anesthetic is significantly greater than the dial setting, but the *partial pressure* delivered is close to what it would be at that dial setting at sea level. And because anesthetic depth is determined by the *partial pressure* of volatile agents in the brain, the clinical impact is minor. Although inhaled anesthetics are rarely used in hyperbaric conditions, similar considerations would apply.

Contemporary variable bypass vaporizers incorporate many features to minimize or eliminate hazards once

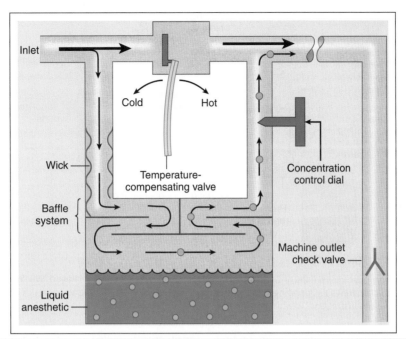

Fig. 15.4 Simplified schematic of a variable bypass vaporizer. Rotation of the concentration control dial diverts a portion of the total fresh gas flow through the vaporizing chamber, where wicks saturated with liquid anesthetic ensure a large gas–liquid interface for efficient vaporization. A temperature-compensating valve diverts more or less fresh gas flow through the vaporizing chamber to offset the effects of changes in temperature on the vapor pressure of the liquid anesthetic. Gases saturated with the vapor of the liquid anesthetic join gases that have passed through the bypass chamber for delivery to the machine outlet check valve (if present). When the concentration control dial is in the off position, no fresh gas inflow enters the vaporizing chamber. (Modified from Chakravarti S, Basu S. Modern anaesthesia vapourisers. *Ind J Anaesth*. 2013;57[S];464–471.)

associated with these devices. Misfilling of anesthetic vaporizers with the wrong agent can result in an overdose or underdose of volatile anesthetic. Agent-specific, keyed filling devices help prevent misfilling. Overfilling is minimized by locating the filler port at the maximum safe liquid level. Tipping of a variable bypass vaporizer can allow the liquid agent to enter the bypass chamber and cause an extremely high output. Modern vaporizers are firmly secured to a manifold on the anesthesia workstation to prevent tipping.

Vaporizers and the vaporizer–machine interface are potential sources of gas leaks that can result in patient awareness during inhaled anesthesia. Loose filler caps, filler plugs, and drain valves are probably the most common sources of leaks. Another common source of gas leak occurs at the junction of the vaporizer and the mounting bracket or manifold, where broken mounting assemblies or foreign bodies can compromise the seal between the vaporizer and its point of attachment. Gas leaks can also occur within the vaporizer itself as a result of mechanical failure. Assessment for low-pressure system leaks, including the vaporizer mount,

is addressed in the section "Checking Your Anesthesia Workstation."

Although rarely reported, contamination of anesthetic vaporizer contents has occurred, including organic contaminants and bacteria.[9]

Desflurane Dual-Gas Blender

Because of its unique physical characteristics, a variable bypass vaporizer cannot be used for desflurane. First, the vapor pressure of desflurane is 669 mm Hg at 20°C (68°F), nearly 1 atm, and significantly higher than all other contemporary inhaled anesthetic agents. If desflurane were placed in a variable bypass vaporizer, prohibitively high bypass chamber flow rates would be required to dilute the vaporizing chamber output to clinical concentrations. Second, desflurane's moderate potency means that the amount of desflurane vaporized over a given period is considerably greater than for other inhaled anesthetics. The concomitantly greater cooling would be difficult to compensate for without an external heat source. Finally, desflurane's boiling point of 22.8°C (73°F) at 1 atm can be encountered in normal operating

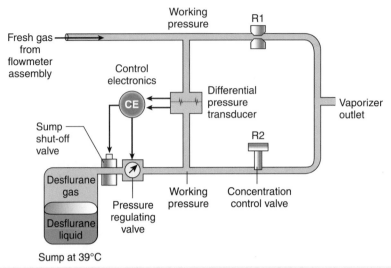

Fig. 15.5 Simplified schematic of Tec 6 desflurane vaporizer (Datex-Ohmeda, Madison, WI). See text for details. (From Andrews JJ. Operating Principles of the Ohmeda Tec 6 Desflurane Vaporizer: A Collection of Twelve Color Illustrations. Washington, DC: Library of Congress; 1996.)

room conditions. If the anesthetic agent were to boil within a variable bypass–type vaporizer, the output would be uncontrollable.

By outward appearance, the desflurane "vaporizer" is similar to variable bypass vaporizers, but its design and operating principles are radically different (Fig. 15.5). The desflurane vaporizers are electrically heated, thermostatically controlled, constant temperature, pressurized, electromechanically coupled, dual-circuit, gas vapor *blenders*. The desflurane sump is heated above the liquid's boiling point, providing a source of pressurized desflurane vapor that is the starting point of a second gas circuit parallel to the fresh gas flow. The vapor's pressure is then downregulated, and a conventional concentration control dial is used to control the flow of vapor to mix with the fresh gas.

The desflurane blender behaves differently from the variable bypass vaporizer at altitude. Because of its design, the delivered desflurane *concentration* is relatively stable as barometric pressure drops, and thus the delivered *partial pressure* of desflurane is lower. At altitude, therefore, the anesthesia provider must compensate by increasing the set desflurane concentration by a factor equal to the percentage decrease in barometric pressure compared with sea level. Furthermore, use of nitrous oxide at low flows can decrease the output from the desflurane blender independently of atmospheric pressure.

Cassette Vaporizers

Cassette vaporizer systems use a permanent control unit housed within the workstation and interchangeable cassettes containing anesthetic liquid to serve as vaporizing chambers. A variety of agent-specific cassettes are available; they are color-coded for the operator and also magnetically coded to allow the anesthesia machine to identify which cassette has been inserted. For anesthetics other than desflurane, the cassette vaporizing system acts as a computer-controlled variable bypass vaporizer. The flow through the vaporizing chamber is controlled by a central processing unit, such that compensation for temperature, carrier gas concentration, and flow rates can be carried out precisely. When the pressure inside the cassette's vaporizing chamber rises above the pressure in the bypass chamber, as when room temperature is above desflurane's boiling point of 22.8°C (73°F), then the function of the cassette changes to become a vapor injector. A check valve between the bypass chamber and the vaporizing chamber closes so that no fresh gas enters the vaporizing chamber and anesthetic vapor does not travel retrograde uncontrolledly into the fresh gas. Under computer control, pure desflurane vapor is injected to achieve the desired concentration.

Injection-Type Vaporizers

Some anesthesia workstations use injection-type vaporizers. Liquid anesthetic is injected into a heated vaporizing chamber that may also contain a heated evaporative surface. The vaporizing chamber may serve as a source of vapor that is metered into the fresh gas, or the fresh gas flow may transit the chamber to be enriched with anesthetic vapor. Design details differ by manufacturer. In all cases the process is under microprocessor control.

ANESTHETIC BREATHING CIRCUITS

Fresh gas departs from the supply system and enters the anesthetic breathing circuit through the fresh gas line. The primary functions of the breathing circuit are to deliver oxygen and other gases to the patient and to eliminate carbon dioxide (CO_2). The breathing system must contain a low-resistance conduit for gas flow, a reservoir that can meet the patient's inspiratory flow demand, and an expiratory port or valve to vent excess gas. Circle system breathing circuits have an absorber to eliminate CO_2 and are the most common circuits used in anesthesia. Circuits without CO_2 absorbers are variations on the Mapleson circuits; these are commonly used by anesthesia providers during patient transport, procedural sedation, airway management out of the operating room, and as "T-pieces" on intubated patients.

Circle Breathing Systems

The circle breathing system is so named because it allows circular, unidirectional flow of gas facilitated by one-way valves (Fig. 15.6). The main advantage of the circle system is that anesthetic gas is conserved and rebreathed. The capability to rebreathe exhaled gases is a unique aspect of circle systems as compared with intensive care unit (ICU) ventilators, in which the entirety of each exhaled breath is vented into the room. To allow safe rebreathing of exhaled gases, CO_2 must be efficiently removed. Waste gas, which is composed of excess carrier gas, anesthetic agent, and CO_2, must be scavenged and eliminated. The essential components that allow these functions are reviewed here.

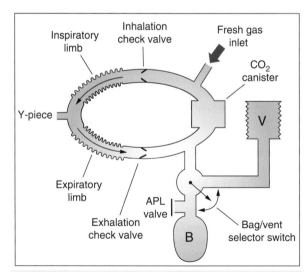

Fig. 15.6 Schematic diagram of the components of a circle anesthesia breathing system. Rotation of the bag/vent selector switch permits substitution of an anesthesia machine ventilator (V) for the reservoir bag (B). The volume of the reservoir bag is determined by the fresh gas inflow and adjustment of the adjustable press-limiting (APL) valve. (From Brockwell RC, Andrews JJ. Delivery systems for inhaled anesthetics. In: Barash PG, Cullen BF, Stoelting RK, eds. *Clinical Anesthesia*. Philadelphia, PA: Lippincott Williams & Wilkins; 2006:557–594).

Fresh Gas Inlet

Fresh gas, in the composition selected by the anesthesia provider as described earlier, flows into the circle system from the common gas outlet of the anesthesia machine. In "bag" mode when the mechanical ventilator is not selected, the fresh gas enters the circuit in a continuous fashion. During mechanical ventilation, various mechanisms exist to decouple the fresh gas during inspiration.

Unidirectional Valves

Two one-way valves are essential elements of the circle breathing system. The two limbs of the breathing circuit are connected to the valves, thereby creating an inspiratory and expiratory limb. The valves permit positive-pressure breathing and ensure that gas is not rebreathed until it has passed through the CO_2 absorber. If a unidirectional valve sticks in the open position, inappropriate rebreathing of CO_2 may occur. Capnography may help with diagnosis, as each valve demonstrates a characteristic CO_2 waveform when incompetent.[10] If the expiratory valve sticks shut, total occlusion of the circuit, with resultant breath stacking and barotrauma, can occur. Assessing for proper unidirectional valve function should be part of the anesthesia workstation preuse checkout procedure. Anesthesia workstations are constructed so that either valve function and motion can be visibly assessed, or malfunction is indicated by the workstation.

Corrugated Breathing Circuit Tubing

The breathing circuit tubing serves as a conduit for delivery of gases to and from the patient. This large-bore tubing, which accounts for most of the volume within the circle system, is designed to provide minimal resistance and resist kinking. These circuits are compliant, such that some of the volume intended for delivery to the patient is lost to distention of the tubing. Many modern workstations perform a compliance test to compensate for this effect. This compliance testing should be performed with the actual circuit that will be used for anesthesia delivery. If circuit length will be increased using an extension, the compliance, leak, and flow tests should be performed with the extension in place.

Y-Piece

The Y-piece is the most distal part of the breathing circuit (i.e., nearest the patient), the point at which the inspiratory and expiratory limbs merge. It has a 15-mm inner diameter to connect to an endotracheal tube or elbow connector and a 22-mm outer diameter to connect to a facemask. The dead space in the circle breathing system begins at the Y-piece and continues on the side connected to the patient. The gas sampling port is located at or near the Y-piece to allow monitoring of both inspiratory and expiratory gases.

Adjustable Pressure-Limiting Valve

The adjustable pressure-limiting (APL) valve, also known as a "pop-off" or pressure relief valve, is an operator-adjustable relief valve that vents excess breathing circuit gas to the scavenging system and provides control of the breathing system pressure during spontaneous and manual modes of ventilation. When fully open, the APL valve allows for spontaneous breathing at atmospheric pressure. When the APL valve is partially closed, the spontaneously breathing patient will receive continuous positive airway pressure (CPAP). At greater degrees of closure, the APL valve facilitates delivery of assisted or controlled breaths by manual compression of the reservoir bag. Switching to a ventilator mode excludes, or closes, the APL valve.

Anesthesia Reservoir Bag or "Breathing Bag"

The anesthesia reservoir bag, or "breathing bag," provides several important functions, including (1) serving as a reservoir for exhaled gas and excess fresh gas, (2) providing a means of delivering manual ventilation or assisting spontaneous breathing, (3) serving as a visual or tactile means of monitoring a patient's spontaneous breathing efforts, and (4) partially protecting the patient from excessive positive pressure in the breathing system. The reservoir bag is the most compliant part of the breathing system, and is designed to distend well beyond its nominal volume at a plateau pressure less than 60 cm H_2O. Classically, the reservoir bag was excluded from the breathing circuit when the ventilator was in use. On some contemporary workstations, however, the reservoir bag is integral to circuit function during mechanical ventilation, where it serves as an exhaled and fresh gas reservoir.

Carbon Dioxide Absorbent

Circle breathing systems require a means of CO_2 removal from the exhaled gases to avoid rebreathing and hypercapnia. Although increasing the fresh gas inflow to high levels can dilute out most CO_2 in the circle system, this is a very inefficient way to conduct an anesthetic. Characteristics of an ideal CO_2 absorbent include a lack of reactivity with common anesthetics, an absence of toxicity, low resistance to airflow, minimal dust production, low cost, ease of handling, and high efficiency. It should also be easy to assess for absorbent depletion (i.e., a diminished ability to remove CO_2). Finally, the container that houses the absorbent should be easy to remove and replace, should maintain breathing circuit integrity if quickly replaced during use, and should impose minimal risk of causing breathing system leaks or obstruction.

CO_2 is removed from the breathing circuit through a series of reactions in the absorber canister, transforming CO_2 into water, heat, and other by-products. Most absorbents use calcium hydroxide [$Ca(OH)_2$] to react with

---

BOX 15.1 Carbon Dioxide Absorber Reactions (Net and Sequential)

CO_2 Reaction With Soda Lime

Net reaction:

$$CO_2 + Ca(OH)_2 \rightarrow CaCO_3 + H_2O + \text{heat}$$

Sequential reactions:

1. $CO_{2\,(gas)} + H_2O_{(liquid)} \rightleftarrows H_2CO_{3\,(aqueous)}$
2. $H_2CO_3 + 2NaOH \text{ (or KOH)} \rightarrow Na_2CO_3 \text{ (or } K_2CO_3) + 2H_2O + \text{heat}$

3. $Na_2CO_3 \text{ (or } K_2CO_3) + Ca(OH)_2 \rightarrow CaCO_3 + 2NaOH^*$ (or KOH^*) + heat

  *Note: NaOH and KOH are catalysts in this reaction mechanism (they are neither created nor destroyed).

CO_2 Reaction With Lithium Hydroxide Monohydrate

$$2LiOH \cdot H_2O + CO_2 + \text{heat} \rightarrow Li_2CO_3 + 3H_2O$$

---

the exhaled CO_2, producing insoluble calcium carbonate ($CaCO_3$) (Box 15.1). However, because CO_2 does not react quickly with $Ca(OH)_2$, water and small amounts of stronger base catalysts are required to speed up the reaction.

Soda lime, a mixture of $Ca(OH)_2$, water, and small amounts of strong base, is a traditional absorbent. CO_2 reacts with liquid water to yield carbonic acid (H_2CO_3). Second, the strong base additives NaOH and KOH react quickly with H_2CO_3 to yield the soluble salts sodium carbonate (Na_2CO_3) and potassium carbonate (K_2CO_3). All available active strong base is quickly depleted. Third, the carbonates react with $Ca(OH)_2$ to yield insoluble $CaCO_3$. This step regenerates the strong base catalysts. By-products of the entire process are water and heat.

Volatile anesthetic agents can interact with the strong bases found in calcium hydroxide–based absorbents to form degradation products. Sevoflurane can undergo a base-catalyzed degradation into a substance known as *compound A,* which is nephrotoxic in rats at concentrations that can occur in the breathing circuit during clinical conditions. No human data show a relationship between sevoflurane use and postoperative renal dysfunction. The sevoflurane package insert states that patient exposure should not exceed 2 MAC-hours at flow rates between 1 and 2 L/min in order to minimize risk from compound A. Flow rates less than 1 L/min are not officially recommended, although these recommendations predate several studies demonstrating safety at lower flow rates.[11]

Strong-base-containing absorbents that are extremely dry (desiccated) can also degrade inhaled anesthetics to clinically significant concentrations of carbon monoxide (CO), reaching blood carboxyhemoglobin levels of 35% or greater.[12] A typical scenario would be the first case on a Monday morning, after high continuous gas flows had accidentally been left on throughout the weekend and desiccated the absorbent. Desiccation of absorbent is unlikely to occur during anesthesia delivery because CO_2 absorption produces water and patients exhale humidified gas.

Many newer absorbents have trace or no KOH or NaOH. Lithium hydroxide (LiOH)–based absorbents do not require these catalysts at all. LiOH is a strong base and reacts quickly with CO_2 (see Box 15.1). Although liquid water is not required to generate carbonic acid as in the classic Ca(OH)2 reaction, some water molecules are still required for the CO_2 reaction with LiOH. LiOH absorbent produces essentially no CO or compound A and maintains excellent CO_2 absorption.

Some chemical reactions within the absorbent canister are exothermic, and fires within the circle system circuit have been reported, though rarely.[13] Extreme heat has been especially noted with desiccated absorbents, particularly a now-discontinued formulation called Baralyme and sevoflurane. LiOH absorbents that are not hydrated before shipping (anhydrous) are also potentially a risk. The degree of desiccation cannot be ascertained by inspection.

Conventional absorbents contain an indicator dye, *ethyl violet,* that allows anesthesia personnel to visually assess the functional integrity of the absorbent. When the absorbent is fresh, the pH exceeds 10 and the dye is colorless. As the absorbent becomes exhausted, the pH drops below 10 and the dye becomes purple, indicating that the absorptive capacity of the material has been exhausted. Unfortunately, ethyl violet may not always be a reliable indicator. For example, color reversion (purple back to white) can occur with some absorbents because of the strong base catalysts. Many newer indicators are resistant to color reversion.

The size and shape of the absorptive granules are designed to maximize surface area while minimizing resistance to airflow. The smaller the granule size, the greater the surface area that is available for absorption. However, as particle size decreases, airflow resistance increases. As the absorbent granules settle in their canisters, small passageways inevitably form. These passages allow gas to flow preferentially through low-resistance areas. This phenomenon, known as *channeling,* may substantially decrease the functional absorptive capacity for CO_2.

Additional Components of the Circle Breathing Systems

Several additional components are added to the circle breathing system circuit. Although not conceptually essential to the function of the circle system, they are critical for patient safety.

Filters and Heat and Moisture Exchangers

The normal warming and humidifying function of the upper airway is often bypassed by an artificial airway during anesthesia. The use of heat and moisture exchangers (HMEs) within the anesthesia breathing circuit is a common practice. HMEs function by absorbing warmth and moisture as exhaled gas moves through in one direction and then returning that warmth and humidity to the next breath as the inspired gas moves through in the other direction. HMEs therefore only function when placed between the Y-connector and the patient.

Filters are used to prevent the transmission of microbes from the patient to the machine and hence potentially to other patients. The filter should have an efficiency rating higher than 95% for particle sizes of 0.3 μm. Such filters are often placed on the expiratory limb of the anesthesia circuit where it connects to the anesthesia machine, and many circuit manufacturers ship their circuits with this filter already in place. During the COVID-19 pandemic, the Anesthesia Patient Safety Foundation recommended the addition of a second filter at the Y-connector for COVID-positive patients.[14] This not only serves as an extra layer of protection against contaminating the interior of the anesthesia machine but also puts a filter near the patient, allowing for the patient's exhaled gases to be filtered during disconnects, for example, when moving the operating room table. The use of a heat and moisture exchanging filter (HMEF) at this site in the patient circuit achieves the functions of both HMEs and filters.

The disposition of the gas sampled by the gas analyzer via the gas sampling line may affect decision making about filter configuration. Some workstations send the sampled gas directly to the scavenge; for these, sampling at the patient Y-connector is appropriate. Other workstations return the sampled gas to the circle system. The advantage of returning the sampled gas to the circuit is that it reduces loss of volatile anesthetic to scavenge. However, in this configuration it is recommended that there be a filter between the patient and the gas sample port.[14] Degradation of the CO_2 waveform can occur, especially with pediatric patients. There is an additional filter at the machine side, typically as part of the sample gas line water trap. The efficiency of the filter should be verified with the manufacturer.

Heated Humidifiers

Active humidification systems, such as heated-wire circuits with vaporizers or a long water-saturated wick, are more commonly found in ICU ventilators, but also exist in circle-system configurations. These systems can help prevent intraoperative hypothermia; disadvantages include added cost and complexity. Generally, they are not commonly used except in pediatric patients or during longer surgeries. Appropriate filters must also be in place when heated humidifiers are used.

Inspired Oxygen Concentration Monitor

There must be an oxygen sensor monitoring the oxygen concentration in the inspiratory limb or at the Y-piece of the breathing circuit. A low oxygen concentration alarm must sound within 30 seconds if the inspired oxygen concentration drops below a set limit, which cannot be adjusted to less than 18%. The oxygen sensor is truly the patient's last line of defense from receiving a hypoxic gas mixture. *Galvanic cell oxygen analyzers* are often used for this purpose, but they require daily calibration. A common location for galvanic sensors is on the housing of the inspiratory unidirectional valve. Modern anesthesia workstations increasingly use *side-stream multigas analyzers* sampling from the Y-piece as the exclusive inspiratory oxygen monitor. *Paramagnetic oxygen analysis* is typically used in these monitors; these sensors require less frequent calibration.

Flow Sensors

At a minimum, an anesthesia workstation must have a sensor for exhaled gas flow and tidal volume. Some workstations also use flow sensor measurements as a feedback signal to maintain stable tidal volume delivery at varying fresh gas flow rates. A variety of technologies are used to achieve flow measurement.

Breathing Circuit Pressure Sensors

Anesthesia workstations must continuously display pressure in the breathing system. Operator-adjustable alarms must be present for *high pressure* and for *continuous positive pressure* lasting 15 seconds or longer. An alarm must also sound for sustained negative pressure. Finally, when automatic ventilation is in use, the machine must sound an alarm whenever the breathing pressure falls below a preset or adjustable *threshold pressure* for more than 20 seconds, alerting the operator to potential disconnection.

The location of pressure sensors in the breathing system varies. They are often located in the nondisposable portion of either the inspiratory or expiratory limb near one of the unidirectional valves. Breathing circuit pressure may not accurately represent the patient's airway pressure, as the pressure transduction occurs far from the patient.

Circle System Function

The circle system is designed to allow rebreathing of gases. The extent of rebreathing, and therefore the conservation of exhaled gases, depends on the fresh gas flow rate. A circle system operated in a *semiopen* manner connotes a high fresh gas flow rate with minimal rebreathing and high venting of waste gas through the APL valve or the waste gas valve of the ventilator. By contrast, contemporary circle systems are usually operated in a *semiclosed* manner, meaning that significant rebreathing occurs, but some waste flow is vented through the APL or waste gas valve of the ventilator. There is no universally accepted definition of *low-flow* anesthesia, but this is usually accepted to mean a technique where fresh gas flow is less than 1 to 2 L/min fresh gas flow. The advantages of low-flow anesthesia include the decreased

use of volatile anesthetic agents, improved temperature and humidity control, and reduced environmental pollution. The disadvantages include difficulty in rapidly adjusting anesthetic depth and the theoretical possibility of accumulating unwanted exhaled gases or anesthetic degradation products.

A *closed* system is one in which the rate of oxygen inflow exactly matches metabolic demand, rebreathing is complete, and no waste gas is vented (APL valve remains closed). A volatile anesthetic agent is added to the breathing circuit in liquid form in precise amounts or is initially introduced through the vaporizer. Closed-circuit anesthesia maximizes the advantages of low-flow anesthesia. However, the technical demands of the technique relative to the benefits make it impractical for routine use with contemporary equipment; thus it is rarely employed.

In the circle system the concentration of the patient's inspired gases can differ significantly from the concentration of the gases in the fresh gas flow. The volume of the circle system is filled with a combination of the patient's exhaled gases (after removal of CO_2) plus the fresh gas flow that is added. As the fresh gas flow rate decreases, the proportion of the circuit that is made up of the patient's exhaled gas increases. For example, the patient's exhaled gas will have a lower oxygen concentration than the inhaled, and at low fresh gas flow, this exhaled oxygen concentration will have a greater contribution to the circuit concentration than the fresh gas concentration. Therefore the inspired oxygen concentration reaching the patient will be lower than the fresh gas oxygen concentration that is first entering the circuit. This phenomenon is most obvious at low fresh gas flows and low oxygen concentration in the fresh gas flow. In addition, at low fresh gas flows, any changes in the oxygen or anesthetic concentrations by the provider will be slow to take effect, because of the lesser relative contribution of the fresh gas to the total circuit volume.

Oxygen has a relatively constant uptake (related to metabolism) compared with volatile anesthetics, whose uptake depends on the gradient between the alveolar and blood levels of anesthetic. Early in an inhaled anesthetic, a large proportion of the volatile agent in the inspired breath will be taken up by the patient, with little exhaled back into the circuit (also see Chapter 7). To maintain the desired level of anesthetic, the anesthesia provider will either select a higher concentration of anesthetic vapor in the fresh gas flow to reach the desired concentration of inspired anesthetic or use higher fresh gas flows so that the effect of the exhaled gas on inspired concentration is minimized. As the tissues become saturated with anesthetic, the uptake of anesthetic agent decreases, and the exhaled concentration of agent is similar to the fresh gas concentration of agent.

Circle breathing systems have several disadvantages. They have a complex design that may consist of ten or more individual connections, setting the stage for misconnections, disconnections, obstructions, and leaks. The patient's work of breathing can be increased by the various valves and circuit components. The large and compliant circle breathing system may compromise tidal volume delivery during controlled ventilation because of compressible volume. Finally, there are the complications associated with the CO_2 absorbers as outlined earlier.

Because of this complexity, troubleshooting anesthesia workstation ventilation issues can be difficult. If there are concerns about the adequacy of patient ventilation (e.g., hypoventilation, circuit disconnection, elevated breathing circuit pressures), prepare to immediately switch to manual ventilation with a self-inflating resuscitation bag. After reestablishing ventilation (and considering administration of intravenous [IV] anesthesia if inhaled anesthesia was the primary anesthetic), troubleshooting of the anesthesia workstation can commence.

Mapleson Breathing Systems

Mapleson described and analyzed five different breathing circuits, designated A through E, that are classically referred to by his name (Fig. 15.7). The Mapleson F system, more commonly referred to as the *Jackson–Rees system,* and the Bain system (a modification of the Mapleson D, Fig. 15.8) were added later. The Mapleson systems share certain features with the circle breathing system: they accept fresh gas flow, supply the patient with gas from a reservoir to meet inspiratory flow and volume requirements, and eliminate CO_2. They differ from the circle system by having bidirectional gas flow and lacking an absorber. To eliminate CO_2 and prevent rebreathing, these systems depend on an appropriate rate of fresh gas inflow. All the circuits except for the Mapleson E version use a bag as an additional reservoir.

Even though the components and their arrangement are simple, functional analysis of the Mapleson systems is complex. The amount of CO_2 rebreathing with each system is affected by multiple factors, including the fresh gas inflow rate, minute ventilation, and ventilation mode (spontaneous or controlled). For example, in spontaneous ventilation the Mapleson A is most efficient (requires the least fresh gas flow to prevent rebreathing), but it is the least efficient in controlled ventilation. The other Mapleson systems do not exhibit such a marked difference between spontaneous and controlled ventilation. The summary of relative efficiencies in spontaneous ventilation is A > DFE > CB, whereas during controlled ventilation it is DFE > BC > A.[15]

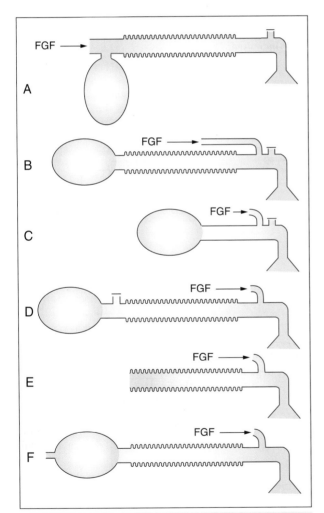

Fig. 15.7 Schematic diagrams of the Mapleson breathing systems A through F. *FGF,* Fresh gas flow. (Modified from Willis BA, Pender JW, Mapleson WW. Rebreathing in a T-piece: Volunteer and theoretical studies of Jackson-Rees modification of Ayre's T-piece during spontaneous respiration. *Br J Anaesth.* 1975;47:1239-1246.)

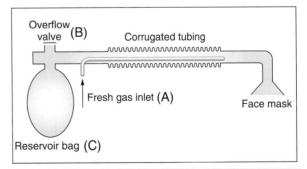

Fig. 15.8 Schematic diagram of the Bain breathing system. Fresh gas flow (FGF) enters a narrow tube (A) located within the larger corrugated expiratory limb. The overflow valve (B) is an adjustable pressure-limiting valve located near the FGF inlet and reservoir bag (C). (Modified from Bain JA, Spoerel WE. A streamlined anaesthetic system. *Can Anaesth Soc J.* 1972;19:426–435.)

Mapleson systems have low resistance to gas flow because they are small and contain few parts. Changes in the fresh gas flow composition result in similar rapid changes in the breathing circuit. In addition, the volatile anesthetic agents within a Mapleson breathing circuit have no chance of degradation because of the absence of a CO_2 absorber. However, given their need for higher gas flows to prevent rebreathing, they are not as economical with regard to carrier gas and volatile anesthetic usage as the circle system. Conservation of heat and humidity is less efficient. Finally, scavenging of waste gas can be challenging.

Self-Inflating Manual Resuscitators

Although rarely used for delivery of inhaled anesthetics in modern practice, the self-inflating manual resuscitation bag is an essential part of every anesthesia workstation. The key feature of this device is a compressible reservoir, typically made of silicone, that automatically expands upon release (Fig. 15.9). Unlike the Mapleson circuits, the self-inflating manual resuscitator may be used for hand ventilation in the absence of a pressurized oxygen or air source. These devices are ubiquitous for patient transport, cardiopulmonary resuscitation, and emergency back-up should the anesthesia workstation ventilator or pressurized oxygen supply fail.

The manual resuscitator possesses two one-way valves. A *nonrebreathing valve* located between the bag and the patient is closed during exhalation to direct exhaled gas flow out of the expiratory port. An *inlet valve* between the reservoir and the oxygen source is open during exhalation (bag recoil) to allow the bag to refill with oxygen or room air. Depending on design, a *pop-off* valve may be present to limit the peak inspiratory pressure, which can easily reach high levels with these devices. *Oxygen tubing* and *oxygen reservoirs* exist in a variety of designs, but generally allow the delivered fraction of inspired oxygen to be increased.

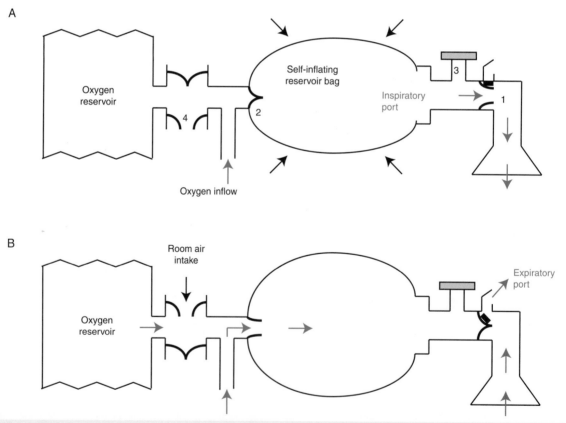

Fig. 15.9 Self-inflating manual resuscitator. (A) Flow of gas during inspiration. *(1)* Nonrebreathing valve, *(2)* bag inlet valve, *(3)* pop-off or pressure-limiting valve (standard for pediatric and infant devices), and *(4)* outflow or excess-oxygen venting valve. (B) Flow of gas during expiration. See text for details. (Redrawn after Dorsch JA, Dorsch SE. The anesthesia machine. In: Dorsch JA, Dorsch SE, eds. Understanding Anesthesia Equipment. 5th ed. Baltimore, MD: Williams & Wilkins; 2008:83, Chapter 10 Manual Resuscitators; and Lien S, Verreault DJ, Alston TA. Sustained airway pressure after transient occlusion of a valve venting a self-inflating manual resuscitator. *J Clin Anesth*. 2013;25[5]:424–425.)

ANESTHESIA VENTILATORS

Today's anesthesia workstation ventilators incorporate many capabilities of ICU ventilators, including a multiplicity of ventilation modes and the ability to allow for patient triggering of the ventilator. ICU ventilators are open circuit, using entirely fresh gas for each breath, and venting all exhaled gas into the patient's room. The anesthesia workstation, on the other hand, must also incorporate a means of collecting and redelivering the patient's exhaled gas in the semiclosed circle breathing system, presenting unique engineering challenges in the design and control of the anesthesia ventilator. Historically the most common solution to this challenge has been the inclusion of a bellows in the anesthesia workstation. Alternatives to the bellows design will be discussed as well.

Bellows Ventilators

In bellows ventilators the bellows serves as a volume reservoir for breathing gas, and the ventilator uses "a bag in a bottle" design to deliver breaths. The bellows are housed in a rigid, airtight housing, and pressurized gas flows into the housing, thereby compressing the bellows.

As the bellows is compressed, the breathing gas is delivered to the patient. A mixture of the patient's exhalation and fresh gas flowing into the breathing circuit refill the bellows. Once the bellows is refilled, excess circuit gas is vented to the scavenging system during the expiratory pause. Figs. 15.10 and 15.11 illustrate the inspiratory and expiratory phases of mechanical ventilation with an ascending bellows ventilator. Note that the bellows ventilator uses pressurized gas from the intermediate-pressure section of the anesthesia machine to drive the bellows. Even though the ventilator is pneumatically driven, all modern anesthesia ventilators are under electronic control.

Standing or *ascending* bellows rise on exhalation; in case of circuit leak or disconnection, the bellows will fall, alerting the anesthesia provider. *Hanging* or *descending* bellows ventilators are less commonly used because the bellows appear to rise and fall normally even with a complete circuit disconnect. The source of the drive gas for the bellows may be either oxygen or air, depending on the design of the workstation. Knowing the type of gas used to drive the bellows ventilator can be important in oxygen failure emergencies or austere conditions. If oxygen

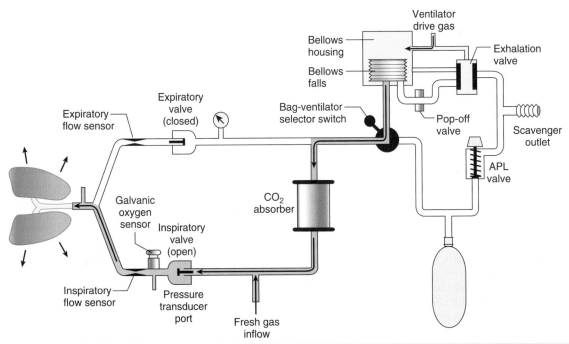

Fig. 15.10 Inspiratory phase of ventilation with an ascending bellows ventilator. The ventilator drive gas circuit is located outside the bellows, and the patient's breathing circuit is inside the bellows. During the inspiratory phase, the electronically controlled ventilator driving gas enters the bellows chamber and causes the pressure to increase, thereby compressing the bellows, which delivers gas to the patient's lungs. The drive gas also closes the exhalation valve and prevents the breathing gas from escaping into the scavenging system. Compensation for the impact of fresh gas flow on tidal volume accuracy is accomplished by monitoring the inhaled tidal volumes and adjusting ventilator drive gas volumes accordingly. *APL,* Adjustable pressure-limiting; *CO₂,* carbon dioxide. (Image courtesy Dr. Michael A. Olympio, modified with his permission; Adapted from Datex-Ohmeda. Aisys Anesthesia Machine: Technical Reference, Madison, Wis., 2005, Datex-Ohmeda.)

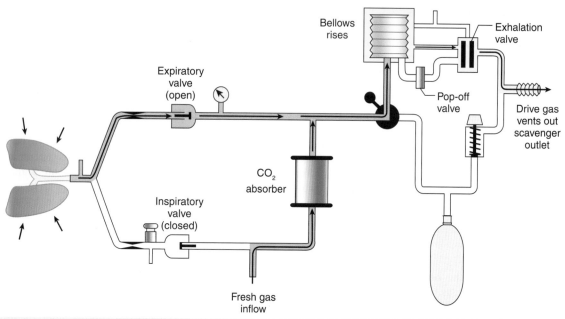

Fig. 15.11 Expiratory phase of ventilation with an ascending bellows ventilator. In the early expiratory phase the patient is able to exhale into the bellows because the ventilator exhalation valve is now open, thus allowing the drive gas in the bellows housing to vent through the scavenger outlet. The pop-off or ventilator relief valve prevents bellows gas from escaping at this point so the bellows can fill. In the late expiratory phase positive end-expiratory pressure (PEEP) is provided by pressurization of the bellows housing and pressure modulation of the expiratory valve. (Courtesy Dr. Michael A. Olympio; modified with his permission. Adapted with permission from Datex-Ohmeda. Aisys Anesthesia Machine: Technical Reference. Madison, WI: Datex-Ohmeda; 2005.)

is used as the drive gas, then the amount of oxygen consumed by the anesthesia machine will equal the amount of oxygen selected for fresh gas flow *plus* an amount approximately equal to the minute ventilation being delivered by the ventilator. Whereas a full E-cylinder (650 L capacity) can provide 10 hours of use with oxygen fresh gas flow of 1 L per minute and manual ventilation through the circle system, that same E-cylinder will provide less than a 2-hour supply in an adult patient when oxygen is used as the ventilator drive gas.

Mechanically Driven Piston Ventilators

Mechanically driven, electronically controlled piston-type ventilators use a computer-controlled stepper motor instead of compressed drive gas to deliver tidal volume. The piston operates much like the plunger of a syringe in a cylinder of essentially zero compliance. The ventilator has primary control over the volume displaced in the circuit and uses the data from pressure sensors to create pressure control breaths; the computerized controls can support a variety of ventilator modes.

In a bellows ventilator the breathing bag is excluded from the circuit during mechanical ventilation. In contrast, with a piston ventilator, the breathing bag acts as the reservoir for rebreathing. The ventilator employs a *fresh gas decoupling valve* to exclude fresh gas from being added to the tidal volume during inspiration. During

inspiration, the fresh gas is added to the breathing bag. During the expiratory phase, the breathing bag initially fills with exhaled gas; then, as the piston returns to its starting position, the fresh gas decoupling valve opens, and fresh gas flow plus gas from the breathing bag refill the piston chamber. Although the piston tends to be fully or partially concealed from view, the movement of the breathing bag can provide visual feedback of circuit disconnect or leak.

Other Anesthesia Ventilator Systems

There are other approaches to mechanical ventilation among anesthesia workstation manufacturers. One workstation uses a novel device called a *volume reflector* (essentially a long plastic tube with a volume of a little more than 1 L) coiled compactly to fit in the anesthesia workstation.[16] The volume reflector is functional and "in-circuit" during all modes of ventilation. It is interposed between the patient and the breathing bag or ventilator, acting as a volume reservoir while simultaneously preventing mixing between the gas at the two ends of the tube.

A number of newer ICU ventilators use turbine technology to generate mechanical ventilation. Turbine ventilators use mechanical energy to spin a small turbine (fan) at very high speeds to create pressure and flow. One manufacturer has designed an anesthesia workstation around a turbine mechanical ventilator.[16] The major advantage of the turbine is that it can be placed directly within the circle system. Unlike piston-driven ventilation, the turbine is primarily a pressure generator. The ventilator uses flow sensors and electronic controls to generate a number of modes of mechanical ventilation, including volume and pressure control, pressure support, and airway pressure release ventilation.

Target-Controlled Inhalational Anesthesia

Traditionally, anesthesia providers directly control the composition and rate of the fresh gas flow. That is, they do *not* control the inspired concentration of oxygen, anesthetic vapor, or other gases; nor do they control the expired concentration of these gases. Rather, they control only that portion of gas that is added to the circle system every minute, namely, the fresh gas flow. The fresh gas mixes with the gases already in the circle breathing system, and thus there may be a significant difference between the composition of the fresh gas flow and the composition of the inspired (or expired) gases. As the fresh gas flow is decreased, there is potentially a greater difference between the fresh gas composition and the actual inspired composition.

On anesthesia workstations where the flow control valves and the anesthetic vaporizers are under electronic control, it is possible to implement *target-controlled inhalational anesthesia*. The targets subject to control are the end-tidal anesthetic agent and the end-tidal oxygen concentration. Currently, several major manufacturers have target-controlled systems available. The major advantage of the target control is reduced consumption of anesthetic agent. These systems rely on proprietary algorithms, and depending, for example, on how fast the algorithm tries to achieve the desired anesthetic depth, the target-controlled system might actually prioritize rapid achievement of a set anesthetic agent (requiring high initial fresh gas flow with high anesthetic agent use) over reducing fresh gas flow and anesthetic agent consumption.[17] The benefits of low-flow anesthesia could be realized by a vigilant anesthesia provider, but at the expense of significant manipulation of the anesthesia machine's settings.

Although the target-controlled modes of inhalational anesthesia seem likely to reduce anesthetic agent use and to provide an additional layer of patient safety in low-flow anesthesia, none are currently approved by the U.S. Food and Drug Administration.

Fresh Gas Flow Compensation and Fresh Gas Decoupling

On older bellows-type anesthesia workstations, the portion of fresh gas flow that occurred during an inspiratory cycle was added to the set tidal volume, leading to variation in tidal volume depending on the set fresh gas flow. Newer workstations have engineering features that provide compensation of fresh gas flow to maintain stable tidal volume

delivery. Broadly speaking, the workstation will either exclude the fresh gas from the inspiratory limb of the circuit during inspiration or it will use electronic controls to compensate for the fresh gas flow's contribution. The precise manner in which this is accomplished accounts for much of the variation in breathing system design.

SCAVENGING SYSTEMS

Scavenging is the collection and subsequent removal of waste anesthetic gases from both the anesthesia machine and the anesthetizing location. Scavenging is required because the fresh gas flow rates used during most anesthetic regimens deliver more volatile anesthetic agents and nitrous oxide than necessary, in addition to more oxygen than is being consumed. Without scavenging, therefore, operating room personnel could be exposed to anesthetic gases, and there could be an increased risk of an oxygen-rich environment supporting combustion.

Scavenging systems may be *active* or *passive*. In active systems the scavenging system is connected to a vacuum source, such as the hospital's suction system. Passive systems simply vent the waste gas into a heating, ventilation, and air conditioning (HVAC) system or through a hose to the building's exterior. Passive systems are less common in contemporary operating rooms and will not be discussed further here. Scavenging systems may also be *open* or *closed*. An open scavenging system allows for room air to be entrained into the flow of waste gas, whereas a closed system does not.[18]

Waste anesthetic gases are vented from the anesthesia system either through the APL valve or through a ventilator relief valve. However, the following circumstances can lead to waste anesthetic gases entering the operating room: poor facemask fit, endotracheal tube leak, or breathing circuit or anesthesia workstation leak. Ventilator drive gas in contemporary bellows-type ventilators (in addition to the flow from the reflector gas module on volume reflector machines) is vented via the scavenging system as well. This is significant because under conditions of high fresh gas flow and high minute ventilation, the gases flowing into the scavenging interface may overwhelm the evacuation system and pollute the room.

An *open, active* scavenging interface uses a reservoir, typically a canister, that is open to the operating room atmosphere. Waste anesthesia gas is discharged into the bottom of the canister, and waste gas vacuum is used to create a continuous flow from the canister into the hospital central vacuum system (Fig. 15.12). The continuous flow rate must be higher than the overall rate at which gas is discharged from the machine, but because of the reservoir, the system can tolerate intermittent discharges into the waste gas system that briefly exceed that rate. When the amount of waste gas being discharged from the anesthesia workstation is less than the continual flow

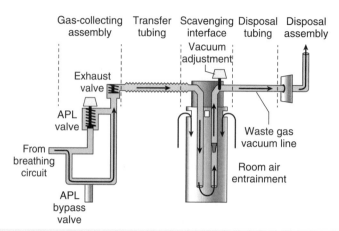

Fig. 15.12 Schematic of an open, active acavenging system. Waste gas is intermittently discharged into the bottom of the canister. The waste gas vacuum line terminates at the bottom of the canister as well. The canister acts as a reservoir when the instantaneous rate of waste gas discharge into the canister exceeds the instantaneous rate of waste gas removal, as during patient exhalation. But the vacuum is set high enough that room air is entrained through most of the respiratory cycle, ensuring clearance of all waste gas. *APL*, Adjustable pressure-limiting. (From Brockwell RC, Andrews JJ. Delivery systems for inhaled anesthetics. In: Barash PG, Cullen BF, Stoelting RK, eds. Clinical Anesthesia. Philadelphia, PA: Lippincott Williams & Wilkins; 2006:557–594.)

in the scavenging system, then the balance of that flow is obtained from entrained room air. Daily workstation preuse checkout must ensure adequate vacuum flow so that waste gas does not spill out into the room through the relief ports. The open system does not require positive- or negative-pressure relief valves because the canister is open to the atmosphere.

In a *closed, active* scavenging system the waste gas is discharged from the anesthesia machine into a reservoir bag. The bag is connected to continuous suction and discharges waste gas to the evacuation system. With peak discharge of waste gas (as at patient exhalation), the bag will expand, subsequently emptying during the inspiratory phase. The operator must adjust the vacuum control valve so that the reservoir bag remains properly inflated, neither overdistended nor completely deflated. A closed, active scavenging system requires at least two valves. If the scavenging system pressure exceeds a preset pressure, gas is vented to the operating room through the positive-pressure relief valve. If the scavenging system pressure is too negative, then room air is entrained through the negative-pressure relief valve. Some systems have additional backup valves.

Scavenging systems minimize operating room pollution, yet they add complexity to the anesthesia system. Excessive vacuum applied to a scavenging system can cause undesirable negative pressures within the breathing system. Obstruction of scavenging pathways can cause excessive positive pressure in the breathing circuit. Even when the patient is protected from barotrauma by positive-pressure relief valves, alarm conditions can contribute to potentially unsafe conditions, in addition to provider stress and case delay. Inadequate vacuum

to the interface can cause venting of waste gas into the operating room.

CHECKING YOUR ANESTHESIA WORKSTATION

A complete preanesthesia checkout procedure (PAC) must be performed each day before the anesthesia workstation is first used, and an abbreviated version should be performed before each subsequent case. Evidence suggests that anesthesia providers frequently do not perform a complete PAC and may miss faults even when explicitly looking for them on a sabotaged machine.[19,20] Furthermore, all contemporary anesthesia workstations have automated checkout procedures, none of which can assure that the basic safety requirements for safe delivery of anesthetic care have been met. In their 2008 *Recommendations for Pre-Anesthesia Checkout Procedures*[21] the ASA suggests that many anesthesia providers are not fully aware of what elements are checked by the automated procedures. Even review of user's manuals does not always make it obvious.

The ASA's *Recommendations for Pre-Anesthesia Checkout Procedures* is summarized in Table 15.3. These recommendations focus on ensuring the *availability* of key equipment and assessing the *function* of that equipment. There are 15 items that must be completed daily or whenever the anesthesia workstation is moved to a new location. An eight-item subset of these must be repeated before each subsequent anesthetic procedure. *The importance of these items for the safe delivery of anesthesia care cannot be overemphasized.*

Table 15.3 Summary Recommendations of the *2008 Pre-anesthesia Checkout Procedures*

Items to Be Completed Daily

Item #	Task
1	Verify that auxiliary oxygen cylinder and self-inflating manual ventilation device are available and functioning
2	Verify that patient suction is adequate to clear the airway
3	Turn on the anesthesia delivery system and confirm that AC power is available
4	Verify the availability of required monitors, including alarms
5	Verify that pressure is adequate on the spare oxygen cylinder mounted on the anesthesia machine
6	Verify that the piped gas pressures are ≥50 psig
7	Verify that vaporizers are adequately filled and, if applicable, that the filler ports are tightly closed
8	Verify that the gas supply lines have no leaks between the flowmeters and the common gas outlet
9	Test the scavenging system function
10	Calibrate, or verify the calibration of, the oxygen monitor, and check the low-oxygen alarm
11	Verify that carbon dioxide absorbent is not exhausted
12	Perform breathing system pressure and leak testing
13	Verify that gas flows properly through the breathing circuit during both inspiration and exhalation
14	Document the completion of checkout procedures
15	Confirm the ventilator settings, and evaluate readiness to deliver anesthesia care (anesthesia time-out)

Items to Be Completed Before Each Procedure

Item #	Task
2	Verify that patient suction is adequate to clear the airway
4	Verify the availability of required monitors, including alarms
7	Verify that vaporizers are adequately filled and, if applicable, that the filler ports are tightly closed
11	Verify that carbon dioxide absorbent is not exhausted
12	Perform breathing system pressure and leak testing
13	Verify that gas flows properly through the breathing circuit during both inspiration and exhalation
14	Document the completion of checkout procedures
15	Confirm the ventilator settings, and evaluate readiness to deliver anesthesia care (anesthesia time-out)

Modified from Sub-Committee of American Society of Anesthesiologists Committee on Equipment and Facilities. *Recommendations for Pre-anesthesia Checkout Procedures.* 2008.

Item 1: Verify Auxiliary Oxygen Cylinder and Self-Inflating Manual Ventilation Device Are Available and Functioning (Daily)

The anesthesia provider must always be prepared to keep the patient alive without the assistance of the anesthesia machine. The most important safety check in any anesthesia location before commencing the day's procedures is the presence of a self-inflating manual ventilation device and a source of oxygen that is separate from the anesthesia workstation and hospital pipeline oxygen supply. These items must be present at every anesthetizing location. Note that the presence of a non–self-inflating Mapleson-type breathing circuit is *not* adequate to meet this item. The auxiliary oxygen tank, typically an E-cylinder, should be checked to make sure it is full and also for the presence of an attached flowmeter and a means to open the cylinder valve.

Item 2: Verify Patient Suction Is Adequate to Clear the Airway (Every Case)

Adequate suction with tubing of appropriate length and an oral suctioning tool are necessary before the start of any case. Although this is often changed by an anesthesia technician or other personnel during room turnovers, the provider must verify this item before commencing the anesthetic.

Item 3: Turn On Anesthesia Delivery System and Confirm That AC Power Is Available (Daily)

Contemporary anesthesia workstations have backup battery power if wall power should fail. If a case is inadvertently started on battery backup power, the first obvious sign of power failure can be catastrophic system shutdown when the backup batteries are exhausted. Before commencing the day's anesthetic procedures, functioning AC power should be verified.

Item 4: Verify Availability of Required Monitors and Check Alarms (Every Case)

The ASA *Recommendations* include in this item both the presence of monitoring supplies (blood pressure cuffs of appropriate sizes, pulse oximetry probes, etc.), functional tests of critical monitoring equipment (pulse oximeter and capnography), and functional tests of alarm conditions. The importance of an audible alarm is emphasized.

The ASA *Recommendations* include functional tests of alarm conditions that may be difficult to carry out. Before commencing an anesthetic, one should ensure the presence of a pulse oximeter signal and an end-tidal CO_2 signal *and* the presence of an audible alarm when that signal is discontinued. This may be done by placing the pulse oximeter on the anesthesia provider to check for function and then removing to check for alarm, and similarly by blowing into the circuit sample line to test capnometry function and for alarm condition when discontinued. In practice, many anesthesia providers assess the function of these critical monitors by placing them on the patient and do not necessarily test for the alarm function before each case.

Item 5: Verify That Pressure Is Adequate on the Spare Oxygen Cylinder Mounted on the Anesthesia Machine (Daily)

In addition to verifying the presence of a separate source of cylinder oxygen, the anesthesia provider should verify the presence of an adequately filled oxygen cylinder mounted on the anesthesia workstation. Verification of oxygen cylinder pressure is accomplished by opening the oxygen cylinder or cylinders on the back of the machine and evaluating the tank gauge pressure.

As discussed earlier, if the tank is to be used in the setting of a suspected oxygen pipeline contamination, the pipeline supply must be disconnected from the machine for tank gas to flow into the gas supply system. Furthermore, the spare oxygen tank should remain closed when using pipeline oxygen to prevent inadvertent emptying of this important emergency supply. In situations where there is no pipeline oxygen and the cylinder is to

be the primary source of oxygen for the anesthetic then oxygen supply sufficient for the entire expected duration of the anesthetic is required.

Item 6: Verify That Piped Gas Pressures Are 50 psig or Higher (Daily)

A daily check of adequate pipeline pressures is specified in the *Recommendations for Pre-Anesthesia Checkout Procedures*. A more detailed daily preuse check of the pipeline system may be part of institutional protocols. For example, a quick daily inspection of connections, supply hoses, gas pressures, and the presence of more than 90% oxygen in the inspiratory limb greatly minimizes risk. An important safety item on all machines is an audible and visual alarm that warns the operator of diminishing oxygen supply pressure. The only way to evaluate this safety device is to disconnect the wall oxygen supply and shut off the oxygen supply tank in order to generate the alarm condition. The 2008 *Recommendations* do not mandate this maneuver.

Item 7: Verify That Vaporizers Are Adequately Filled and, If Applicable, That the Filler Ports Are Tightly Closed (Every Case)

The anesthesia provider should verify that there is an adequate supply of anesthetic agent in the vaporizer if an inhaled anesthetic is planned. High and low agent alarms are recommended when providing an inhaled anesthetic. Loose filler caps on the vaporizer may introduce a breathing system leak that is missed during other parts of the precheck.

Item 8: Verify That No Leaks Are Present in the Gas Supply Lines Between the Flowmeters and the Common Gas Outlet (Daily)

The anesthesia workstation should be thoroughly investigated daily for the possibility of leaks in the low-pressure system, from the flow control valves, through the vaporizers, and to the common gas outlet. Unfortunately, the procedures for performing this item, sometimes called the low-pressure leak test, are different for different anesthesia workstations, emphasizing the importance of machine familiarity and local protocols.

Two areas of the low-pressure leak test deserve emphasis. First, some anesthesia workstations include an outlet check valve. The implication of this check valve is that positive pressure in the breathing circuit *cannot* be used to check for leaks upstream in the low-pressure system (internal to the machine), because the pressure will not be transmitted past the check valve. On these machines, a negative pressure test must be performed, as described in the user's manuals. Second, most vaporizer leaks are not detected unless the vaporizer is set to *on*. Therefore a thorough low-pressure leak test can require testing multiple vaporizers, depending on machine configuration. Some automated machine checks may have the ability to test for leaks in the vaporizer, but many do not.

Item 9: Test Scavenging System Function (Daily)

For every anesthesia machine, the evaluation of the scavenging system is a manual maneuver. No automated checks are conducted. Given the multiplicity of scavenge configurations, local protocols and provider familiarity are necessary.

Item 10: Calibrate, or Verify Calibration of, the Oxygen Monitor and Check the Low Oxygen Alarm (Daily)

The oxygen concentration analyzer is one of the most important monitors on the anesthesia workstation. It is the only monitor positioned to detect oxygen delivery problems downstream from the flow control valves and the only monitor that detects the actual oxygen concentration delivered to the patient. Whether or not the oxygen sensor requires calibration, the function of the low-oxygen concentration alarm should be tested daily. This may be done by manually setting the low oxygen concentration alarm limit to more than 21% while exposing the analyzer to room air, thereby generating the alarm condition.

Item 11: Verify Carbon Dioxide Absorbent Is Not Exhausted (Every Case)

Before each anesthetic, the absorbent should be assessed for color change characteristic of absorbent exhaustion. Some exhausted absorbents may pass visual inspection. The presence of *inspired* CO_2 on capnography during the case is an important indicator for identifying exhausted absorbent.

Item 12: Perform Breathing System Pressure and Leak Testing (Every Case)

This PAC item verifies that positive pressure can be developed and sustained in the breathing circuit and that the APL ("pop-off") valve properly relieves pressure in the circuit. It is not rare for either the disposable breathing circuit components or the fixed anesthesia machine components to leak. Therefore a leak check of the breathing system is of paramount importance before every case. This test can be easily performed manually by occluding

the Y-piece on an assembled circuit, closing the APL valve, and using the O_2 flush button to pressurize the circuit. The circuit passes the leak test if it holds pressure for at least 10 seconds. The flow into the circuit during this test must be off.

On many modern anesthesia machines, breathing circuit leak testing is an automated feature, although manual steps are still required for test preparation. Circuit compliance is also automatically assessed on some machines during this phase to guide ventilator tidal volume delivery. Therefore the test should be performed with the circuit that is going to be used. The APL valve should also be assessed at this time by opening it widely after the pressure test and ensuring that the breathing circuit pressure decreases rapidly to zero.

Item 13: Verify That Gas Flows Properly Through the Breathing Circuit During Both Inspiration and Exhalation (Every Case)

Problems with unidirectional valves are difficult to discover during the PAC. A functional test has been described whereby a test lung is placed at the Y-piece, and the anesthesia provider assesses inspiratory and expiratory flow by alternately compressing the breathing bag and the test lung. The valves can be visually inspected during this so-called *flow test*. Obstructed valves can also be felt during the to-and-fro breathing. Undetected circuit obstructions are particularly ominous and can manifest dramatically and sometimes immediately after induction. Subtle circuit obstruction may not be appreciable except by capnometry.

Automated machine checks may not assess for (or detect) obstruction to flow within the breathing circuit. A number of complications and near-misses involving an obstructed breathing circuit have been reported despite the performance of the automated circuit check.[3]

A full checkout procedure with a test lung is uncommon in this era of automated machine checks. If this test is omitted, providers must be cognizant of the fact that unidirectional valve malfunction and breathing circuit obstruction have not been ruled out before starting the case.

Item 14: Document Completion of Checkout Procedures

Documentation of completion of the anesthetic checkout procedure by *providers* should occur within the anesthetic record. Currently, no guidance is available regarding where anesthesia or biomedical technician documentation of checkout procedures should occur. However, it would be prudent to maintain a detailed departmental log as a quality assurance tool.

Item 15: Confirm Ventilator Settings and Evaluate Readiness to Deliver Anesthesia Care (Anesthesia Time-Out)

The last step in the PAC is an "anesthesia time-out," during which the anesthesia provider confirms the following six items before the induction of anesthesia: (1) monitors are functional; (2) capnogram tracing is present; (3) oxygen saturation by pulse oximetry is being measured; (4) flowmeter and ventilator settings are properly working; (5) manual/ventilator switch is set to manual; and (6) vaporizer is adequately filled.

The final preinduction checklist focuses on the anesthesia workstation and does not include everything the provider might wish to verify immediately before induction of anesthesia, such as medications, equipment for an anticipated difficult airway, and so on. Some providers rely on other final check mnemonic devices. Regardless of the specific steps, a final checklist that verifies the presence and function of key safety items is fundamental to the safe delivery of anesthesia.

ACKNOWLEDGMENT

The editor and publisher would like to thank Dr. Patricia Roth for contributing a chapter on this topic in the prior edition of this work. It has served as the foundation of the current chapter.

REFERENCES

1. Thompson PW, Wilkinson DJ. Development of anaesthetic machines. *Br J Anaesthesia*. 1985;57(7):640–648.
2. Mehta SP, Eisenkraft JB, Posner KL, Domino KB. Patient injuries from anesthesia gas delivery equipment: A closed claims update. *Anesthesiology*. 2013;119:788–795. https://doi.org/10.1097/ALN.0b013e3182a10b5e.
3. Yang KK, Lewis IH. Mask induction despite circuit obstruction: An unrecognized hazard of relying on automated machine check technology. *A & A Case Rep*. 2014;2:143–146. https://doi.org/10.1213/XAA.0000000000000026.
4. Malayaman SN, Mychaskiw G II, Ehrenwerth J. Medical gases: Storage and Supply. In: Ehrenwerth J, Eisenkraft JB, Berry JM, eds. *Anesthesia Equipment: Principles and Applications, 2nd ed*. Philadelphia, PA: Saunders; 2013:3–24.
5. Anderson WR, Brock-Utne JG. Oxygen pipeline supply failure: A coping strategy. *J Clin Monit*. 1991;7:39–41.
6. Eisenkraft JB. The anesthesia machine and workstation. In: Ehrenwerth J, Eisenkraft JB, Berry JR, eds. *Anesthesia Equipment: Principles and Applications, 2nd ed*. Philadelphia, PA: Saunders; 2013:25–63.
7. Mun SH, No MY. Internal leakage of oxygen flush valve. *Korean J Anesthesiol*. 2013;64:550–551. https://doi.org/10.4097/kjae.2013.64.6.550.
8. Eisenkraft JB. Anesthesia vaporizers. In: Ehrenwerth J, Eisenkraft JB, Berry JM, eds. *Anesthesia Equipment: Principles and Applications, 2nd ed*. Philadelphia, PA: Elsevier Saunders; 2013:64–94.
9. Wallace AW. Sevoflurane contamination: Water accumulation in sevoflurane vaporizers can allow bacterial growth in the vaporizer. *A&A Case Rep*. 2016;6:399–401. https://doi.org/10.1213/XAA.0000000000000330.
10. Kaczka DW, Chitilian HV, Vidal Melo MF. Respiratory monitoring. In: Gropper MA, ed. *Miller's Anesthesia, 9th ed*. Philadelphia, PA: Elsevier; 2020:1298–1339.
11. Feldman JM, Hendrickx J, Kennedy RR. Carbon dioxide absorption during inhalation anesthesia: A modern practice. *Anesth Analg*. 2020. https://doi.org/10.1213/ANE.0000000000005137.
12. Berry PD, Sessler DI, Larson MD. Severe carbon monoxide poisoning during desflurane anesthesia. *Anesthesiology*. 1999;90:613–616. https://doi.org/10.1097/00000542-199902000-00036.
13. Laster M, Roth P, Eger EI. Fires from the interaction of anesthetics with desiccated absorbent. *Anesth Analg*. 2004;99:769–774. Table of contents. https://doi.org/10.1213/01.ANE.0000136553.69002.C9.
14. Feldman J, Loeb R, Philip J. FAQ on anesthesia machine use, protection, and decontamination during the COVID-19 pandemic. *Anesth Patient Safety Found*. 2020. https://www.apsf.org/faq-on-anesthesia-machine-use-protection-and-decontamination-during-the-covid-19-pandemic/ accessed 1.15.21.
15. Kaul T, Mittal G. Mapleson's breathing systems. *Indian J Anaesth*. 2013;57:507. https://doi.org/10.4103/0019-5049.120148.
16. Bokoch MP, Weston SD. Inhaled anesthetics: Delivery systems. In: Gropper MA, ed. *Miller's Anesthesia, 9th ed*. 9th edition Philadelphia, PA: Elsevier; 2020. 572–637.
17. Wetz AJ, Mueller MM, Walliser K, Foest C, Wand S, Brandes IF, Waeschle RM, Bauer M. End-tidal control vs. manually controlled minimal-flow anesthesia: A prospective comparative trial. *Acta Anaesthesiol Scand*. 2017;61:1262–1269. https://doi.org/10.1111/aas.12961.
18. Eisenkraft JB, McGregor DG. Waste anesthetic gases and scavenging systems. In: Ehrenwerth J, Eisenkraft JB, Berry JM, eds. *Anesthesia Equipment: Principles and Applications, 2nd ed*. Philadelphia, PA: Elsevier Saunders; 2013:125–147.
19. Larson ER, Nuttall GA, Ogren BD, Severson DD, Wood SA, Torsher LC, Oliver WC, Marienau MES. A prospective study on anesthesia machine fault identification. *Anesth Analg*. 2007;104:154–156. https://doi.org/10.1213/01.ane.0000250225.96165.4b.
20. O'Shaughnessy SM, Mahon P. Compliance with the automated machine check. *Anaesthesia*. 2015;70:1005–1006. https://doi.org/10.1111/anae.13159.
21. American Society of Anesthesiologists, 2008. Recommendations for Pre-Anesthesia Checkout Procedures.

16 AIRWAY MANAGEMENT

Maytinee Lilaonitkul, Andrew Infosino

Expertise in airway management is the cornerstone of safe anesthesia practice. The past decades have seen an evolution of airway management, notably with the adoption of supraglottic airway (SGA) devices in the early 1990s and, more recently, the rapid uptake of video laryngoscopy as a first-line technique in the management of both routine and difficult airways and as an educational training tool for novice learners. The recognition of the significant role of human factors and nontechnical skills in difficult and emergent airway management has also led to the increased use of cognitive aids, checklists, and simulation-based training to enhance patient safety.

Difficult or failed airway management is a major factor in anesthesia-related morbidity and mortality.[1,2] Expertise in safe airway management requires (1) knowledge of the anatomy and physiology of the airway, (2) a thorough history and physical examination focused on the airway, (3) proficiency with the range of airway devices, (4) individualized primary and backup airway management plans, (5) effective team communication, and (6) application of cognitive aids and guidelines such as the American Society of Anesthesiologists (ASA) difficult airway algorithm (Fig. 16.1).[1]

ANATOMY AND PHYSIOLOGY OF THE UPPER AIRWAY

Nasal Cavity

Air is warmed and humidified as it passes through the nares during normal breathing before it enters the larynx, the trachea, and then the lower airways. Resistance to airflow through the nasal passages is twice that through the mouth and accounts for approximately 50% to 75% of total airway resistance.[3]

The majority of the sensory innervation of the nasal cavity is derived from the ethmoidal branch of the ophthalmic nerve and branches of the maxillary division of the trigeminal nerve from the sphenopalatine ganglion.[3]

Oral Cavity and Pharynx

The oral cavity is bordered superiorly by the hard and soft palates, posteriorly by the faucial arches just anterior to the tonsils, and laterally by the buccal mucosa. The tongue occupies the majority of the floor of the oral cavity. The pharynx connects the nasal and oral cavities to the larynx and esophagus. The pharynx is composed of the nasopharynx, oropharynx, and hypopharynx. The nasopharynx is separated from the oropharynx by the soft palate. The epiglottis demarcates the border between the oropharynx and the hypopharynx (Fig. 16.2). Airway resistance may be increased by prominent lymphoid tissue in the nasopharynx. The tongue is the predominant cause of airway resistance in the oropharynx. Obstruction by the tongue is increased by relaxation of the genioglossus muscle during anesthesia.

Branches of the maxillary division of the trigeminal nerve that innervate the mouth include the greater and lesser palatine nerves and the lingual nerve. The greater and lesser palatine nerves provide most of the sensation to the superior border of the oral cavity and the tonsils, and the lingual nerve provides sensation to the anterior two-thirds of the tongue. The posterior third of the tongue, the soft palate, and the oropharynx are innervated by the glossopharyngeal nerve (cranial nerve IX). The internal branch of the superior laryngeal nerve, which is a branch of cranial nerve X (vagus), provides sensory innervation to the hypopharynx, including the base of the tongue, posterior surface of the epiglottis, aryepiglottic folds, and arytenoids.[3]

Larynx

The adult larynx is located at the level of the third to sixth cervical vertebrae. One of its primary functions is to protect the distal airways by closing during swallowing to prevent aspiration. This protective mechanism, when exaggerated, becomes laryngospasm. The larynx is composed of a cartilaginous framework connected by fascia, muscles, and ligaments. There are three unpaired and three paired cartilages. The unpaired cartilages are the epiglottis, thyroid, and cricoid, and the paired cartilages are the arytenoids, corniculates, and cuneiforms. The cricoid cartilage is shaped like a signet ring, wider in the cephalocaudal dimension posteriorly, and is the only cartilage that is a full ring structure. The vocal cords are formed by the thyroarytenoid ligaments and are the narrowest portion of the

Fig. 16.1 Difficult airway algorithm: Adult patients. (1) The airway manager's choice of airway strategy and techniques should be based on their previous experience; available resources, including equipment, availability, and competency of help; and the context in which airway management will occur. (2) Low- or high-flow nasal cannula and head elevated position throughout procedure. Noninvasive ventilation during preoxygenation. (3) Awake intubation techniques include flexible bronchoscope, video laryngoscopy, direct laryngoscopy, combined techniques, and retrograde wire-aided intubation. (4) Other options include but are not limited to alternative awake technique, awake elective invasive airway, alternative anesthetic techniques, induction of anesthesia (if unstable or cannot be postponed) with preparations for emergency invasive airway, and postponing the case without attempting the previous options. (5) Invasive airway techniques include surgical cricothyrotomy, needle cricothyrotomy with a pressure-regulated device, large-bore cannula cricothyrotomy, or surgical tracheostomy. Elective invasive airway techniques include the previous options and retrograde wire-guided intubation and percutaneous tracheostomy. Also consider rigid bronchoscopy and extracorporeal membrane oxygenation (ECMO). (6) Consideration of size, design, positioning, and first- versus second-generation supraglottic airways may improve the ability to ventilate. (7) Alternative difficult intubation approaches include but are not limited to video-assisted laryngoscopy, alternative laryngoscope blades, combined techniques, intubating the supraglottic airway (with or without flexible bronchoscopic guidance), flexible bronchoscopy, introducer, and lighted stylet or lightwand. Adjuncts that may be employed during intubation attempts include tracheal tube introducers, rigid stylets, intubating stylets, or tube changers and external laryngeal manipulation. (8) Includes postponing the case or postponing the intubation and returning with appropriate resources (e.g., personnel, equipment, patient preparation, awake intubation). (9) Other options include but are not limited to proceeding with procedure using facemask or supraglottic airway ventilation. Pursuit of these options usually implies that ventilation will not be problematic. (From Apfelbaum JL, Hagberg CA, Connis RT, et al. 2022 American Society of Anesthesiologists practice guidelines for management of the difficult airway. Anesthesiology. 2021. doi: 10.1097/ALN.0000000000004002. Epub ahead of print. PMID: 34762729.)

ASA DIFFICULT AIRWAY ALGORITHM: ADULT PATIENTS

Pre-Intubation: Before attempting intubation, choose between either an awake or post-induction airway strategy. Choice of strategy and technique should be made by the clinician managing the airway.[1]

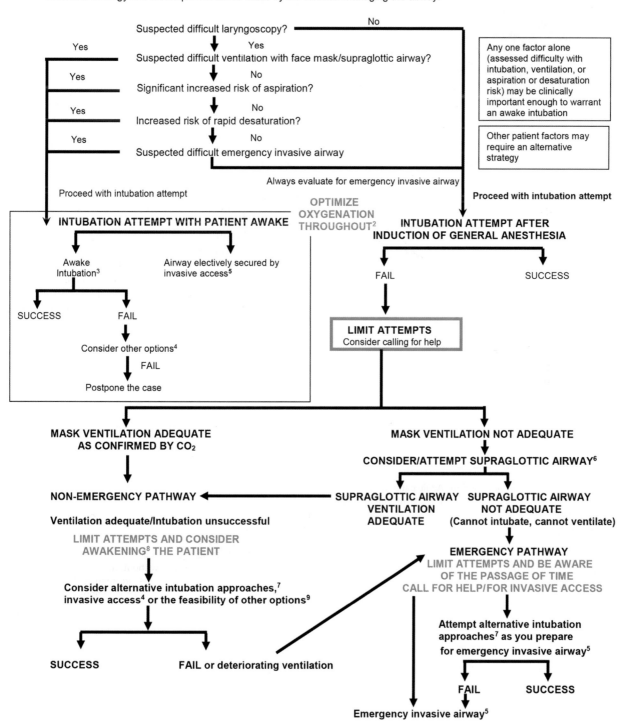

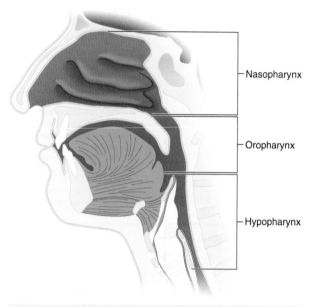

Nasopharynx

Oropharynx

Hypopharynx

Fig. 16.2 Functional anatomy of the upper airway: Sagittal section through the head and neck showing the subdivisions of the pharynx. (From Redden RJ. Anatomic considerations in anesthesia. In: Hagberg CA, ed. *Handbook of Difficult Airway Management.* Philadelphia: Churchill Livingstone; 2000:7, Fig. 1.6.)

adult airway (Fig. 16.3A and B). An understanding of the motor and sensory innervation of the nasal, oropharyngeal, and laryngeal structures is important for performing anesthesia of the upper airway (Table 16.1).

Trachea

The trachea extends from the larynx to the carina, which overlies the fifth thoracic vertebra. An adult trachea is

10 to 15 cm long and supported by 16 to 20 horseshoe-shaped cartilages. The sensory innervation of the trachea is from the recurrent laryngeal nerve, a branch of cranial nerve X (vagus).

AIRWAY ASSESSMENT

History and Anatomic Examination

Airway assessment is the first step to formulate an airway management plan.[4] A comprehensive assessment consists of a medical and surgical history of the patient's airway, a review of previous anesthetic and medical records, and a physical examination of the airway.[1] History of worsening airway symptoms or pathology, obstructive sleep apnea, and the risk of aspiration should be elicited in detail.[5,6] Various congenital and acquired disease states are associated with difficult airway management (Tables 16.2 and 16.3). Of note, a history of neck irradiation is the most significant predictor of inability to mask ventilate.[7] Patients who have a history of difficult airway management may have been informed by their previous anesthesia provider. Patients' difficult airway specifics should be documented in the medical record, and the patient should be given written documentation and/or a notification bracelet. The anesthetic record should contain a description of the airway difficulties, the grade of laryngeal view, and the airway management techniques used.[1]

Physical Examination Findings

Single physical examination features and bedside airway evaluation tests have a low sensitivity and specificity for predicting a difficult airway (Table 16.4). Evaluating the tests in combination offers greater predictive value.[8–10] Examination of the oropharyngeal space, submandibular

Table 16.1	Motor and Sensory Innervation of Larynx	
Nerve	**Sensory**	**Motor**
Superior laryngeal, internal division	Epiglottis	None
	Base of tongue	
	Supraglottic mucosa	
	Thyroepiglottic joint	
	Cricothyroid joint	
Superior laryngeal, external division	Anterior subglottic mucosa	Cricothyroid muscle
Recurrent laryngeal	Subglottic mucosa	Thyroarytenoid muscle
		Lateral cricoarytenoid muscle
		Interarytenoid muscle
		Posterior cricoarytenoid muscle

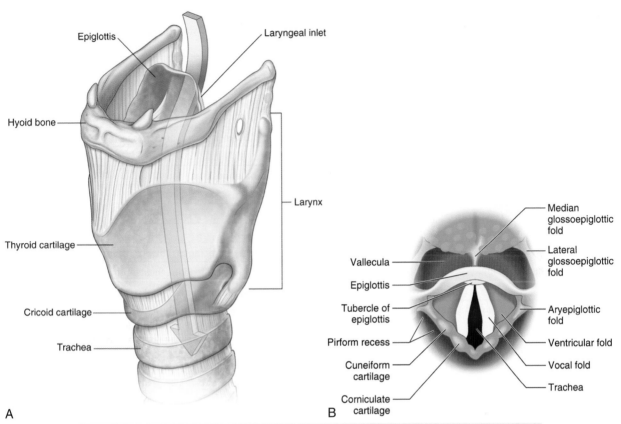

Fig. 16.3 (A) Lateral view of the larynx. (B) Superior view through the laryngeal inlet. (A from *Gray's Anatomy for Students*, 4th ed. 1049. 1041, Fig. 8.209B. B from *Miller's Anesthesia*, 9th ed, vol. 1. p. 1377, Fig. 44.6, from Redden RJ. Anatomic considerations in anesthesia. In: Hagberg CA, ed. *Handbook of Difficult Airway Management*. Philadelphia: Churchill Livingstone; 2000, p. 8, Fig. 1.8.)

Table 16.2	Congenital Syndromes Associated With Difficult Laryngoscopy and Endotracheal Intubation
Syndrome	**Description**
Trisomy 21	Small mouth, large tongue, small subglottic diameter
	Laryngospasm is common
Goldenhar (oculoauriculovertebral anomalies)	Mandibular hypoplasia and cervical spine abnormality
Klippel-Feil	Reduced neck mobility resulting from cervical vertebral fusion
Pierre Robin	Small mouth, large tongue, and mandibular hypoplasia
Treacher Collins (mandibular dysostosis)	Severe facial deformity, relative macroglossia, and mandibular hypoplasia
Turner	Reduced neck mobility, high arched palate, mandibular hypoplasia, temporomandibular joint contracture, and short trachea

Table 16.3 Pathologic States That Influence Airway Management

Pathologic State	Difficulty
Infection	
Epiglottitis (infectious)	Laryngoscopy may worsen obstruction
Abscess (submandibular, retropharyngeal, Ludwig angina)	Distortion of the airway renders mask ventilation or endotracheal intubation extremely difficult
Croup, bronchitis, pneumonia	Airway irritability with a tendency for cough, laryngospasm, bronchospasm
Papillomatosis	Airway obstruction
Tetanus	Trismus renders oral endotracheal intubation impossible
Trauma	
Traumatic foreign body	Airway obstruction
Cervical spine injury	Neck manipulation may traumatize the spinal cord
Basilar skull fracture	Nasotracheal intubation attempts may result in intracranial tube placement
Maxillary or mandibular injury	Airway obstruction, difficult facemask ventilation, and endotracheal intubation
	Cricothyroidotomy may be necessary with combined injuries
Laryngeal fracture	Airway obstruction may worsen during instrumentation
	Endotracheal tube may be misplaced outside the larynx
Laryngeal edema (after intubation)	Irritable airway
	Narrowed laryngeal inlet
Soft tissue neck injury (edema, bleeding, subcutaneous emphysema)	Anatomic distortion of the upper airway
	Airway obstruction
Neoplasia	
Neoplastic upper airway tumors (pharynx, larynx)	Inspiratory obstruction with spontaneous ventilation
Lower airway tumors (trachea, bronchi, mediastinum)	Airway obstruction may not be relieved by endotracheal intubation
	Lower airway is distorted
Radiation therapy	Fibrosis can make mask ventilation and laryngoscopy difficult
Immune disorder	
Inflammatory rheumatoid arthritis	Mandibular hypoplasia, temporomandibular joint arthritis, immobile cervical vertebrae, laryngeal rotation, and cricoarytenoid arthritis make laryngoscopy difficult
Ankylosing spondylitis	Fusion of the cervical spine may make direct laryngoscopy difficult
Temporomandibular joint syndrome	Limited mouth opening
Scleroderma	Tight skin and temporomandibular joint involvement make mouth opening difficult
Sarcoidosis	Airway obstruction (lymphoid tissue)
Angioedema	Obstructive swelling can make ventilation and endotracheal intubation difficult
Endocrine	
Acromegaly	Large tongue and overgrown mandible can make mask ventilation and laryngoscopy difficult
Diabetes mellitus	Decreased mobility of the atlanto-occipital joint may make laryngoscopy difficult
Hypothyroidism	Large tongue and abnormal soft tissue (myxedema) make ventilation and laryngoscopy difficult
Thyromegaly	Goiter may produce extrinsic airway compression or deviation
Obesity	Increased upper airway soft tissue can make mask ventilation and laryngoscopy difficult

space and compliance, and cervical spine mobility, in addition to evaluation of patients' body habitus can help to identify increased risk of difficult airway management. Recognition of patients who may be difficult in terms of laryngoscopy and intubation, in addition to difficult mask, SGA placement, or surgical airway can highlight the need for further evaluation and preparation.[1]

Oropharyngeal Space

The Mallampati test is used to evaluate the oropharyngeal space and its predicted effect on ease of direct laryngoscopy and endotracheal intubation.[11] For the modified Mallampati score, the observer should be at eye level with the patient holding the head in a neutral position, opening the mouth maximally, and protruding the tongue without phonating. The airway is classified according to what structures are visible (Fig. 16.4).[12] There is a correlation between a modified Mallampati score of 3 and 4 with difficult laryngoscopy.

Class I: The soft palate, fauces, uvula, and tonsillar pillars are visible.
Class II: The soft palate, fauces, and uvula are visible.
Class III: The soft palate and base of the uvula are visible.
Class IV: The soft palate is not visible.

In conjunction with the Mallampati examination, the interincisor gap, the size and position of the maxillary and mandibular teeth, and the conformation of the palate can be assessed.[1] An interincisor gap of less than 3 to 4.5 cm correlates with difficulty achieving a line of view on direct laryngoscopy.[10] Maxillary prominence or a receding mandible also correlates with a poor laryngoscopic view. Overbite results in a reduction in the effective interincisor gap when the patient's head and neck are optimally positioned for direct laryngoscopy. A narrow or highly arched palate is another airway examination finding that is associated with a potential difficult airway.[1]

The submandibular space is the area into which the soft tissues of the pharynx must be displaced to obtain a line of vision during direct laryngoscopy. Anything that limits the submandibular space or compliance of the tissue will decrease the amount of anterior displacement that can be achieved. Micrognathia limits the pharyngeal space (tongue positioned more posterior) and the space in which the soft tissues need to be displaced. This causes the glottic structures to be anterior to the line of vision during direct laryngoscopy.

The extent of an individual's ability to prognath the mandible is another correlate of the visualization of glottic structures on direct laryngoscopy. The upper lip bite test (ULBT) classification system is as follows (class III is associated with a difficult intubation)[10]:

Class I: Lower incisors can bite above the vermilion border of the upper lip.
Class II: Lower incisors cannot reach vermilion border.
Class III: Lower incisors cannot bite the upper lip.[13]

Ludwig angina, tumors or masses, radiation scarring, burns, and previous neck surgery are conditions that can decrease submandibular compliance.[1]

Table 16.4 Preoperative Airway Physical Examination Findings Associated With Difficult Airway Management

Physical Exam Findings	Mask Ventilation	SGA Ventilation	Intubation	Cricothyroid Membrane Access
High BMI (>30 kg/m²) and increased neck circumference (>40 cm)	•	•	•	•
Male sex	•	•		
Female sex				•
Edentulous	•	•		
Prominent upper incisors		•	•	
Reduced interincisor gap (<3 cm)		•	•	
Mallampati class III or IV	•		•	
Limited ability to protrude lower mandible	•		•	
Limited cervical spine mobility	•		•	•
Reduced neck tissue compliance secondary to previous irradiation	•		•	•
Thyromental distance <6 cm			•	
Beard	•			

BMI, Body mass index

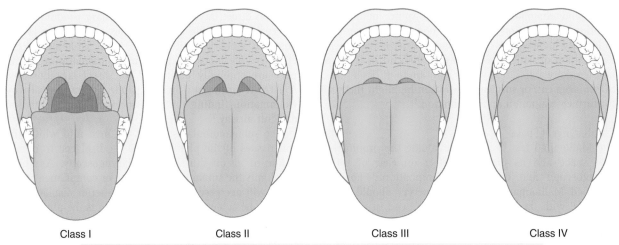

| Class I | Class II | Class III | Class IV |

Fig. 16.4 Mallampati classification. (From Samsoon GLT, Young JRB. Difficult tracheal intubation: A retrospective study. *Anaesthesia.* 1987;42:487–490, used with permission.)

Thyromental/Sternomental Distance

A thyromental distance (mentum to thyroid cartilage) less than 6 to 7 cm correlates with a poor laryngoscopic view. This is typically seen in patients with a receding mandible or a short neck, which creates a more acute angle between the oral and pharyngeal axes and limits the ability to bring them into alignment. This distance is often estimated in fingerbreadths. Three ordinary fingerbreadths approximate this distance. The sternomental distance can also be used—it should measure more than 12.5 to 13.5 cm.[10]

Atlanto-occipital Extension/Cervical Spine Mobility

Extension of the head on the atlanto-occipital joint is important for aligning the oral and pharyngeal axes to obtain a line of vision during direct laryngoscopy (Fig. 16.5). Flexion of the lower neck, by elevating the head approximately 10 cm, aligns the laryngeal and pharyngeal axes. These two maneuvers place the head in the "sniffing" position and bring the three axes into optimal alignment. In this position the patient's ear canal is aligned with the sternal notch. Atlanto-occipital extension is quantified by the angle traversed by the occlusal surface of the maxillary teeth when the head is fully extended from the neutral position. More than 30% limitation of atlanto-occipital joint extension from a norm of 35 degrees, or less than 80 degrees of extension/flexion, is associated with an increased incidence of difficult endotracheal intubation.[14,15]

Body Habitus/Other Examination Findings

A retrospective analysis of almost 700 patients with difficult mask ventilation combined with difficult laryngoscopy identified 12 independent risk factors: Mallampati III or IV, neck radiation changes or neck mass, male sex, limited thyromental distance, presence of teeth, body mass index (BMI) ≥30 kg/m², age ≥46 years, presence of beard, thick neck, unstable cervical spine or limited neck extension, and limited jaw protrusion.[16,17]

Cricothyroid Membrane

When routine airway management techniques have failed, ventilation is not adequate, and endotracheal intubation is unsuccessful, invasive airway control through the cricothyroid membrane is indicated (see Fig. 16.1).[1] Correctly identifying the cricothyroid membrane before airway instrumentation is important, especially in patients with difficult airways. The cricothyroid membrane can be identified by first locating the thyroid cartilage, then sliding the fingers down the neck to the membrane, which lies just below. Alternatively, in patients who do not have a prominent thyroid cartilage identification of the cricoid cartilage can be achieved by palpating the neck at the sternal notch and sliding the fingers cephalad until a cartilage that is wider and higher (cricoid cartilage) than those below is felt. The superior border of the cricoid cartilage demarcates the inferior border of the cricothyroid membrane. Ultrasound imaging can help to identify the cricothyroid membrane and any overlying vascular structures.[18,19] Predictors of difficulty identifying the cricothyroid membrane include female sex, age less than 8 years, presence of large neck circumference, reduced cervical spine mobility, a displaced airway, overlying neck malformation, irradiated neck, and previous tracheostomy.[19,20]

Additional Airway Investigations

Further imaging can be helpful, especially for patients with known upper airway pathologies. Plain radiograph may identify the size, shape, and location of foreign bodies in the airway and tracheal compression or deviation. Computed tomography (CT) and magnetic resonance

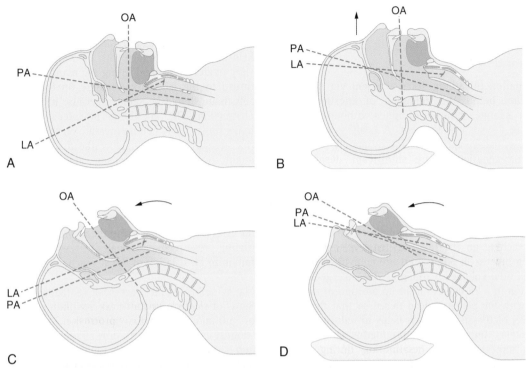

Fig. 16.5 Schematic diagram showing alignment of the oral axis (*OA*), pharyngeal axis (*PA*), and laryngeal axis (*LA*) in four different head positions. Each head position is accompanied by an inset that magnifies the upper airway (the oral cavity, pharynx, and larynx) and superimposes, as a variously bent *bold dotted line*, the continuity of these three axes with the upper airway. (A) The head is in a neutral position with a marked degree of nonalignment of the OA, PA, and LA. (B) The head is resting on a large pad that flexes the neck on the chest and aligns the LA with the PA. (C) Extension of the head on the neck without concomitant elevation of the head. (D) Combination of the head resting on a pad (which flexes the neck on the chest) and extension of the head on the neck, which brings all three axes into alignment (sniffing position).

imaging (MRI) can offer a more detailed evaluation of complex airway pathologies and allow for multidisciplinary airway planning with the surgeon.

Preoperative nasal endoscopy can help to assess the degree of airway swelling, the nature of periglottic lesions, and the extent of anatomy distortion caused by airway pathologies.[4]

AIRWAY MANAGEMENT TECHNIQUES

Facemask Ventilation

Ventilation via a facemask is a vital airway management skill. Prospectively identifying patients at risk for difficult facemask ventilation and developing proficient facemask ventilation skills are fundamental to the practice of anesthesia. Facemasks are available in a variety of sizes. When a facemask is properly sized, the top will sit on the bridge of the nose and the bottom will sit between the lower lip and the chin.

The incidence of difficult facemask ventilation ranges from 1% to 8%, depending on the definition used.[1,20,21] Causes include inadequate mask seal, excessive gas leak, or excessive resistance to the ingress or egress of gas. In addition, difficult facemask ventilation can develop after multiple laryngoscopy attempts. Patients with difficult facemask ventilation can develop hypoxemia, hypercarbia, and aspiration of gastric contents, resulting in hypoxic brain damage or death.[2,21] Independent variables associated with difficult facemask ventilation include (1) age older than 55 years, (2) BMI higher than 30 kg/m², (3) a beard, (4) lack of teeth, (5) a history of snoring or obstructive sleep apnea, (6) Mallampati class III to IV, (7) history of neck radiation, (8) male sex, (9) limited ability to protrude the mandible, and (10) history of an airway mass or tumor.[20,21] Another analysis, using more stringent criteria for "impossible" mask ventilation (defined as inability to establish face mask ventilation despite multiple airway adjuvants and two-hand mask ventilation), identified five independent predictors: (1) neck radiation changes,

(2) male sex, (3) sleep apnea, (4) Mallampati III or IV, and (5) presence of a beard.[7]

Preoxgenation

Preoxygenation (breathing 100% oxygen) via facemask is important before the induction of anesthesia and allows for a longer duration of apnea without desaturation during airway management. A healthy adult, who is not obese, can be apneic for approximately 9 minutes after preoxygenation before significant desaturation occurs. Obesity, pregnancy, and other conditions that significantly decrease functional residual capacity (FRC) or increase oxygen consumption decrease the time to desaturation (Fig. 16.6).[22]

Several techniques of preoxygenation can achieve the goal of reaching an end-tidal oxygen level above 90%. Eight deep breaths in 60 seconds are equivalent to three minutes of tidal volume breathing of 100% oxygen.[23] Preoxygenation in a 25-degrees head-up position or ramping position with the patient's head raised so that the ear is at the level of the sternal notch helps to reduce dependent atelectasis, improve ventilation/perfusion matching, decrease time to oxygen desaturation during apnea, and improve the direct laryngoscopy view, especially in obese patients (Fig 16.7).[24,25] The addition of noninvasive positive-pressure ventilation is another technique that can improve preoxygenation, especially in obese patients.[26]

After induction of anesthesia, the facemask should be held to the patient's face with the fingers of the anesthesia provider's left hand lifting the mandible (chin lift, jaw thrust) to the facemask. Pressure on the submandibular soft tissue should be avoided because it can cause airway obstruction. The anesthesia provider's left thumb and index finger apply counterpressure on the facemask. Anterior pressure on the angle of the mandible (jaw thrust), atlanto-occipital joint extension, and chin lift combine to maximize the pharyngeal space. Differential application of pressure with individual fingers can improve the seal attained with the facemask. The anesthesia provider's right hand is used to generate positive pressure by squeezing the reservoir bag of the anesthesia breathing circuit. Ventilating pressure should ideally be less than 20 cm H_2O to minimize insufflation of the stomach.

Managing Inadequate Facemask Ventilation

Signs of inadequate facemask ventilation include absent or minimal chest rise, absent or inadequate breath sounds, cyanosis, insufflation of the stomach, low oxygen saturation, absent or inadequate exhaled carbon dioxide, and hemodynamic changes associated with hypoxemia or hypercarbia.[1]

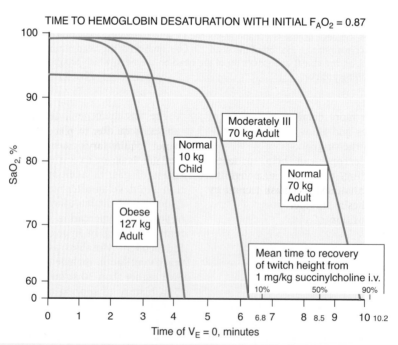

Fig. 16.6 The oxygen saturation (SaO_2) versus time of apnea of various types of patients. The time to reach an SaO_2 of 80% was 8.7 minutes in a healthy 70-kg adult but was 3.1 minutes in an obese patient. F_AO_2, Alveolar fraction of oxygen; V_E, minute ventilation. (From Benumof JL, Dagg R, Benumof R. Critical hemoglobin desaturation will occur before return to an unparalyzed state following 1 mg/kg intravenous succinylcholine. *Anesthesiology.* 1997;87[4]:979-982.)

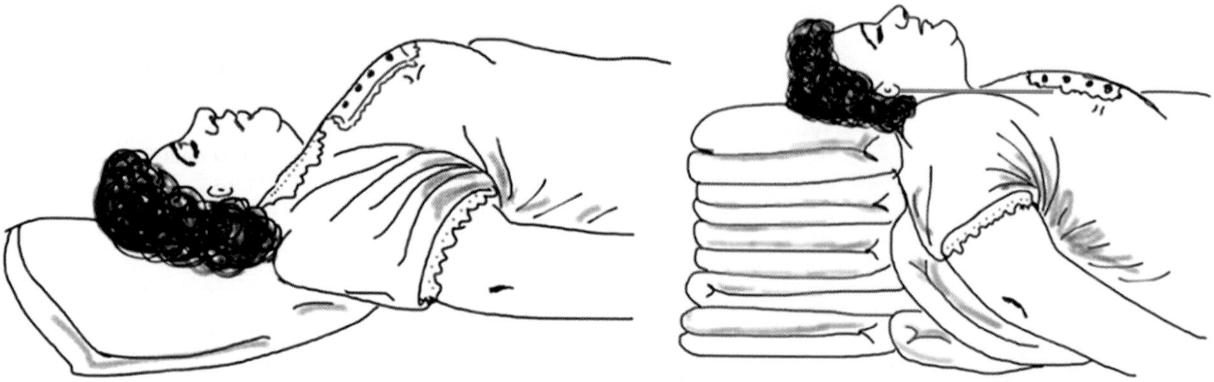

Fig. 16.7 A comparison between supine and ramped position in an obese patient. In a supine position (*left*) the ear is below the level of the sternal notch. In a ramped position (*right*), the *red line* indicates that the ear canal is at the same level as the sternal notch, and the face is parallel with the ceiling.

Inadequate facemask ventilation is usually the result of decreased compliance and increased resistance. Oral and nasal airways are designed to create an air passage by displacing the tongue from the posterior pharyngeal wall. The distal tip of the oral and nasal airway should be at the angle of the mandible when the proximal end is aligned with the mouth or the nose, respectively. An oral airway may generate a gag reflex or cause laryngospasm in an awake or lightly anesthetized patient. Nasal airways are better tolerated during lighter levels of anesthesia, but are relatively contraindicated in patients who have coagulation or platelet abnormalities or have basilar skull fractures.

Presence of a beard or lack of teeth may result in an inadequate seal between the patient's face and the mask, making it difficult to deliver positive pressure. If the patient is amenable, shaving or trimming a beard can improve facemask seal. If a patient's dentures are well adhered, allowing them to be left in place or use of an oral airway can improve facemask seal in edentulous patients.

If oral and nasal airways do not optimize ventilation with a facemask, a two-handed facemask technique should be used. The anesthesia provider uses the right hand to mirror the hand position of the left to improve facemask seal and jaw thrust. A second person can assist by ventilating the patient with the reservoir bag. In spite of corrective measures, if difficult or impossible facemask ventilation continues, intubation or placement of an SGA should be attempted.[1]

Supraglottic Airways

SGAs have become central to airway management in anesthesia practice. SGAs consist of a mask-like cuff connected to an airway tube, which can be connected to the anesthesia breathing circuit. The distal tip of the cuff should be against the upper esophageal sphincter (cricopharyngeus muscle), the lateral edges rest in the piriform sinuses, and the proximal end seats posterior to the base of the tongue (Fig. 16.8). Newer SGAs have additional built-in features such as bite blocks, conduits for orogastric tube placement, enhanced cuff designs to improve seal, and in some cuff pressure monitors. Other features that may differ between types of SGAs include the location (perilaryngeal or pharyngeal) and mechanism of seal (inflatable cuff or preshaped cuffless device). SGAs are sized according to the patient's weight, and sizes vary by manufacturer (Tables 16.5–16.7).

SGAs can be used as the primary mode of airway management, especially in ambulatory surgery, or as a conduit for endotracheal intubation or for rescue ventilation during difficult airway management. SGAs are easier and quicker to place than endotracheal tubes and do not require laryngoscopy. The majority of SGAs are available in sizes for infant, pediatric, and adult patients. Advantages include fewer hemodynamic changes with insertion and removal, less coughing and bucking with removal, no need for muscle relaxants, preserved laryngeal competence and mucociliary function, and less laryngeal trauma.[27]

Many of the factors that result in difficult mask ventilation and intubation do not overlap with those that influence SGA success (see Table 16.4). SGAs may still be successful when other oxygenation or ventilation techniques have failed.[28] Difficult SGA placement or failure has been associated with small mouth opening, supraglottic or extraglottic disease, fixed cervical spine deformity, use of cricoid pressure, poor dentition/edentulous or large incisors, male sex, surgical table rotation, and increased BMI.[28a,29] The incidence of failed SGA placement, defined as an airway event requiring LMA Unique removal and tracheal intubation, is 1.1%.[29]

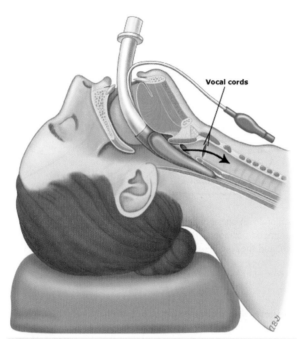

Vocal cords

Fig. 16.8 Proper positioning of supraglottic airways within the oropharynx. The distal tip of the supraglottic airway cuff should rest on the upper esophageal sphincter, the lateral edges rest in the piriform sinuses, and the proximal end seats posterior to the base of the tongue. (From https://www.uptodate.com/contents/supraglottic-devices-including-laryngeal-mask-airways-for-airway-management-for-anesthesia-in-adults?search=supraglottic%20airway&source=search_result&selectedTitle=1~150&usage_type=default&display_rank=1)

Table 16.6	Appropriate-Size Air-Q Masked Intubating Laryngeal Airway Size Recommendations and Maximum Cuffed Oral Endotracheal Tube Sizes	
Air-Q Size	**Weight (kg)**	**Maximum Oral Endotracheal Tube Size**
0.5	<4	4.0
1	4–7	4.5
1.5	7–17	5.0
2.0	17–30	5.5
2.5	30–50	6.5
3.5	50–70	7.5
4.5	70–100	8.5

Table 16.7	Appropriate-Size i-gel Supraglottic Airways and Maximum Oral Endotracheal Tube Sizes	
i-gel Size	**Weight (kg)**	**Maximum Oral Endotracheal Tube Size (mm)**
1	2–5	N/A
1.5	5–12	N/A
2	10–25	N/A
2.5	25–35	N/A
3	30–60	6.0
4	50–90	7.0
5	>90	8.0

Table 16.5	Appropriate-Size Laryngeal Mask Airway (LMA) Based on Patient Weight and Maximum Oral Endotracheal Tube Sizes	
LMA Size	**Weight (kg)**	**Maximum Oral Endotracheal Tube Size (mm)**
1	<5	3.0 uncuffed
1.5	5–10	4.0 uncuffed, 3.5 cuffed
2	10–20	4.5 uncuffed, 4.0 cuffed
2.5	20–30	4.5 cuffed
3	30–50	5.5 cuffed
4	50–70	5.5 cuffed
5	70–100	6.5 cuffed
6	>100	6.5 cuffed

Despite rapid advances in the design of SGAs, aspiration remains a concern, and their use is contraindicated in patients at high risk for regurgitation of gastric contents. Although there have been numerous studies where SGAs have been successfully used in nonsupine positions, obesity, long surgical time, and intraabdominal or airway procedures, one must consider the risk versus benefit of use in these situations.[27] After placement of an SGA, it is important to confirm correct positioning by observing normal capnograph trace, auscultation of breath sounds, and ensuring adequate tidal volume is achieved with minimal oropharyngeal leak at positive-pressure breaths under 20 cm H_2O.

Unsuccessful placement may result from inadequate depth of anesthesia, downfolding of the epiglottis blocking the airway passage, or excessive air leak caused by inadequate seal. Maneuvers such as increasing depth of anesthesia during insertion, repositioning the patient's head or SGA, adjusting the amount of air in the cuff, and upsizing or downsizing the SGA can help to overcome these problems. One should consider converting to an endotracheal tube if problems persist despite these maneuvers. Intubation through these devices can be facilitated by use of an intubation catheter or a fiberoptic bronchoscope.

About 20% to 25% of patients report a sore throat after SGA placement, which is usually self-resolving.[30] Other reported complications from using SGAs in patients with difficult airways include bronchospasm, postoperative swallowing difficulties, respiratory obstruction, laryngeal nerve injury, edema, and hypoglossal nerve paralysis.[1] The risk of pulmonary aspiration increases with gastric inflation, high airway pressures, and poor SGA positioning over the glottis.[6]

Laryngeal Mask Airways (LMAs)

LMA Unique

The LMA Unique is the single-use version of the reusable LMA Classic. The LMA Unique consists of a flexible shaft connected to a polyvinylchloride (Unique) oval-shaped mask that seals around the laryngeal inlet (Fig. 16.9). Before placement, the cuff should be deflated, the device should be lubricated, and the patient's head should be positioned in the sniffing position. The LMA Uniques are designed to be inserted by holding the shaft between the index finger and thumb, with the tip of the index finger at the junction of the mask and the tube. Upward pressure against the hard palate is applied as they are advanced toward the larynx until resistance is felt. The LMA Unique can be used as a conduit for endotracheal intubation. Table 16.5 lists the largest endotracheal tubes that can be used for each size of the LMA Unique.

LMA Fastrach

The LMA Fastrach is available in reusable and single-use models. It was designed to obviate the problems encountered when attempting to blindly intubate the trachea through the LMA Unique or Classic. The LMA Fastrach is used with a specialized endotracheal tube that exits the laryngeal mask at a different angle than a standard

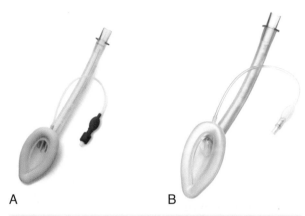

Fig. 16.9 (A) Reusable LMA Airway. (B) Single-use LMA Unique. (Image courtesy Teleflex Incorporated. © [2021] Teleflex Incorporated. All rights reserved.)

endotracheal tube and results in better alignment with the airway.

LMA ProSeal/LMA Supreme

The reusable LMA ProSeal and single-use LMA Supreme are modifications of the LMA Classic (Fig. 16.10). They both have an improved oropharyngeal seal without increasing mucosal pressure, which allows for ventilation with higher airway pressures when compared with the LMA Classic/Unique.[31] They both also have a second lumen that opens at the distal tip of the mask to act as an esophageal vent to keep gases and fluid separate from the airway and facilitate placement of an orogastric tube.

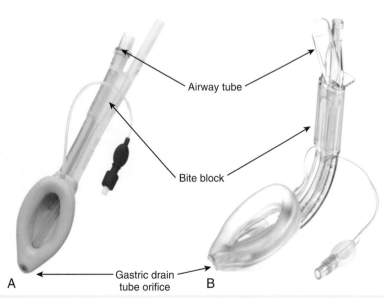

Airway tube

Bite block

Gastric drain tube orifice

Fig. 16.10 (A) Reusable LMA Proseal Airway. (B) Single-use LMA Supreme Airway. Features include a gastric drain, built-in bite block, and modified cuffs for improved airway seal. (Image courtesy Teleflex Incorporated. © [2021] Teleflex Incorporated. All rights reserved.)

This is designed to decrease the risk of regurgitation and aspiration of gastric contents. The LMA Supreme also has an added seal at the esophageal sphincter to help reduce risk of gastric insufflation during ventilation. The placement of an orogastric tube can help to confirm proper placement of these devices. Both devices also have a built-in bite block to decrease the chance of obstruction of the airway tube.

LMA Flexible

The LMA Flexible has a wire-reinforced, flexible airway tube that allows it to be positioned away from the surgical field while minimizing loss of seal. This can be useful for procedures involving the head and neck. Insertion of the LMA Flexible can be more difficult compared with other SGAs. Using a stylet or introducer may help with insertion of this device.

Air-Q Intubating Laryngeal Airways

The Air-Q intubating laryngeal airways (ILAs) are SGAs that can be used either as a primary airway or as an intermediary channel for intubation of the trachea (Fig. 16.11). They have an elliptical, inflatable, cuffed mask and a slightly curved airway tube with a detachable connector and an incorporated bite block. Several features serve to aid intubation: a short shaft, no aperture bars within the mask, a detachable connector so that the wide lumen of the shaft can be used for intubation, and a distal airway tube shaped to direct an endotracheal tube toward the larynx.[27] When used as a conduit for intubation, each size of the Air-Q laryngeal airway has a corresponding maximum cuffed endotracheal tube size (see Table 16.6). After an endotracheal tube is placed, removal of the Air-Q device is aided by a removal stylet. A newer model called Air-Q Self-Pressurizing (AirQsp) also has an added feature of a self-pressurizing cuff that inflates during positive-pressure ventilation and deflates during exhalation.

i-gel Supraglottic Airways

The i-gel is a single-use SGA device composed of a soft, gel-like, noninflatable cuff that is designed to form an anatomic seal over the laryngeal inlet. One advantage of the i-gel is a lower reported incidence of postoperative sore throat.[32] It has a widened, flattened stem with a rigid bite block that acts as a buccal stabilizer to reduce rotation and malpositioning and a port for gastric tube insertion (Fig. 16.12). The i-gel has a wide-bore airway channel designed to facilitate endotracheal intubation with fiber-optic guidance.[27,32] Adult sizes can accommodate endotracheal tube sizes from 6.0 to 8.0 mm (see Table 16.7).

Endotracheal Intubation

Endotracheal intubation by direct laryngoscopy is the most common method of securing the airway during general anesthesia (Box 16.1). Equipment and drugs used for endotracheal intubation include a properly sized endotracheal tube, laryngoscope, functioning suction catheter, appropriate anesthetic drugs, monitoring equipment, and equipment for providing positive-pressure ventilation of the lungs with oxygen.

Proper positioning is crucial to successful direct laryngoscopy. Alignment of the oral, pharyngeal, and laryngeal axes is necessary for creating a line of vision from the lips to the glottic opening (see Fig. 16.5). Elevation of the patient's head 8 to 10 cm with pads under the occiput (shoulders remaining on the table) and extension of the head at the atlanto-occipital joint serve to align these axes. The height of the operating table should be adjusted so that the patient's face is near the level of the standing anesthesia provider's xiphoid cartilage.

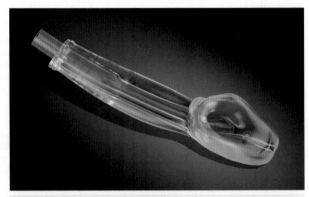

Fig. 16.12 The i-gel ® is a single-use supraglottic airway device composed of a soft, gel-like, noninflatable cuff that is designed to form an anatomic seal over the laryngeal inlet. It has a widened, flattened stem with a rigid bite block that acts as a buccal stabilizer to reduce rotation and malpositioning, and a port for gastric tube insertion. (From Gabbott DA, Beringer R. The iGEL supraglottic airway: A potential role for resuscitation? *Resuscitation.* 200773[1]:161–162.)

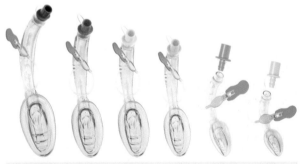

Fig. 16.11 Air-Q ® disposable supraglottic airways in adult and pediatric sizes. The removable color-coded connector allows for intubation with a standard endotracheal tube. (Image courtesy Cookgas, St. Louis, MO.)

> **Box 16.1** Indications for Endotracheal Intubation
>
> - Provide a patent airway
> - Prevent inhalation (aspiration) of gastric contents
> - Need for frequent suctioning
> - Facilitate positive-pressure ventilation of the lungs
> - Operative position other than supine
> - Operative site near or involving the upper airway
> - Airway maintenance by mask difficult

The laryngoscopic view obtained is classified according to the Cormack and Lehane classification system. Grade III or IV views are associated with difficult intubation (Fig. 16.13).[33]

Rapid-Sequence Induction of Anesthesia With Cricoid Pressure

Rapid-sequence induction with cricoid pressure should be considered in patients with increased risk for regurgitation of gastric contents. Rapid-sequence induction involves the rapid induction of anesthesia and neuromuscular blockade followed immediately by direct laryngoscopy and intubation. Cricoid pressure (Sellick maneuver) is used to prevent spillage of gastric contents into the pharynx during the period from induction of anesthesia to successful placement of a cuffed endotracheal tube. It can be applied by an assistant exerting downward external pressure with the thumb and index finger on the cricoid cartilage to displace the cartilaginous cricothyroid ring posteriorly and thus compress the underlying upper esophagus against the cervical vertebrae (Fig. 16.14). The magnitude of downward external pressure (30 newtons is recommended) that needs to be exerted on the cricoid cartilage to reliably occlude the esophagus is difficult to judge. The use of cricoid pressure has been questioned for several reasons, including the following: (1) there is a lack of validation in models other than cadavers; (2) aspiration can occur despite the use of cricoid pressure; (3) cricoid pressure can cause relaxation of the lower esophageal sphincter, which can favor regurgitation; (4) cricoid pressure may increase the difficulty of mask ventilation or worsen the laryngoscopic view; and (5) MRI has shown that the esophagus may be lateral and not directly posterior to the cricoid cartilage in patients, resulting in inadequate esophageal compression.[34,35] Other MRI studies have suggested that although the esophagus is laterally displaced in some patients, the hypopharynx is the structure that is being compressed by cricoid pressure, and the cricoid and hypopharynx move together as a unit. Even if lateral movement occurs, there is compression of this structure. The use of cricoid pressure remains controversial.[35] Cricoid pressure can be released if it impedes oxygenation, ventilation, or visualization of the glottis.

Difficult Airway Management

Difficult airway management includes difficult mask or SGA ventilation, laryngoscopy, or endotracheal intubation. Difficult laryngoscopy is defined as the inability to visualize any portion of the vocal cords; difficult endotracheal intubation is defined as the inability to intubate despite multiple attempts and has been reported to occur in up to 7% of patients.[20] Failed intubation of the trachea occurs in about 1 in 2000 patients in an elective setting and can result in catastrophic patient outcome.[2]

Closed malpractice claims related to difficult intubation between 2000 and 2012 showed that inadequate airway planning and inappropriate management (73%) were the main factors leading to patient harm. Large studies indicate that the most common failures included perseveration on failed techniques, failure to use an SGA for rescue oxygenation, delay in calling for help, and delay in attempting a surgical airway.[6,36] These studies highlight the importance of nontechnical skills such as situational awareness, communication, and teamwork in managing the difficult

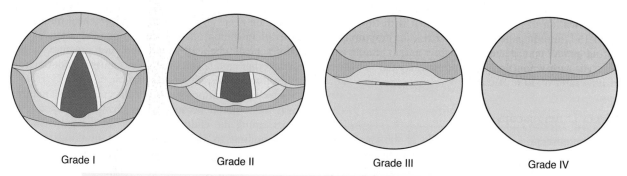

| Grade I | Grade II | Grade III | Grade IV |

Fig. 16.13 Four grades of laryngoscopic view. Grade I: Most of the glottis is visible. Grade II: Only the posterior portion of the glottis is visible. Grade III: The epiglottis but no part of the glottis can be seen. Grade IV: No airway structures are visualized. (From Cormack RS, Lehane J. Difficult tracheal intubation in obstetrics. *Anaesthesia*. 1984;39[11]:1105–1111.)

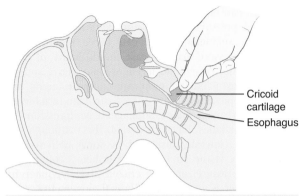

— Cricoid
cartilage

— Esophagus

Fig. 16.14 Cricoid pressure is provided by an assistant exerting downward pressure with the thumb and index finger on the cricoid cartilage (approximately 5-kg pressure) so that the cartilaginous cricothyroid ring is displaced posteriorly and the esophagus is thus compressed (occluded) against the underlying cervical vertebrae.

airway. Cognitive aids such as difficult airway algorithms should be used (see Fig. 16.1). The communication and teamwork necessary for managing difficult airways can be improved using role-playing exercises or simulation.

A comprehensive airway history and assessment is crucial for developing an airway management plan for each patient. The following management options in patients with anticipated or history of difficult airway should be considered: (1) awake endotracheal intubation, (2) noninvasive initial intubation techniques, (3) video laryngoscopy as an initial approach to intubation, and (4) maintaining spontaneous ventilation.[1] A patient's risk of aspiration and ability to cooperate with airway management should be considered when making an initial plan, and a difficult airway cart should be immediately available. In addition to routine preoxygenation and optimal patient positioning, the use of apneic oxygenation techniques after induction of anesthesia can delay the onset of hypoxia and allow more time for safe airway manipulation in patients with difficult airways. One approach is the application of nasal cannula oxygen with flow rates up to 15 L/min. In patients at higher risk for desaturation during airway management high-flow nasal cannula can be used, with warmed and humidified oxygen delivered at flow rates of 30 to 70 L/min.[37]

Direct Laryngoscopy

The laryngoscope is traditionally held in the anesthesia provider's left hand. If not opened by extension of the head, the patient's mouth may be manually opened by counterpressure of the right thumb on the mandibular teeth and right index finger on the maxillary teeth ("scissoring"). Simultaneously with insertion of the laryngoscope blade, the patient's lower lip can be rolled

away with the anesthesia provider's left index finger to prevent damage by the laryngoscope blade. The blade is then inserted on the right side of the patient's mouth and then moved to the midline, and the tongue is shifted to the left. Pressure on the teeth or gums must be avoided as the blade is advanced forward and centrally toward the epiglottis. The anesthesia provider's wrist is held rigid as the laryngoscope is lifted along the axis of the handle to cause anterior displacement of the soft tissues and bring the laryngeal structures into view. The handle should not be rotated as it is lifted to prevent damaging the patient's upper teeth or gums. Manipulation of the patient's thyroid cartilage externally on the neck, commonly using backward upward rightward pressure (BURP), may facilitate exposure of the glottic opening.[20]

The endotracheal tube is held in the anesthesia provider's right hand like a pencil and introduced into the right side of the patient's mouth with the natural curve directed anteriorly. The endotracheal tube should be advanced toward the glottis from the right side of the mouth, as midline insertion usually obscures visualization of the glottic opening. The tube is advanced until the proximal end of the cuff is 1 to 2 cm past the vocal cords, which should place the distal end of the tube midway between the vocal cords and carina. Some endotracheal tubes also have a vocal cord marker to guide optimal depth of insertion. At this point, the laryngoscope blade is carefully removed from the patient's mouth. The cuff of the endotracheal tube is inflated with air to create a seal against the tracheal mucosa. This seal facilitates positive-pressure ventilation of the lungs and decreases the likelihood of aspiration of pharyngeal or gastric contents. A cuff manometer can be used to confirm cuff pressures between 20 and 30 cm H_2O to minimize the likelihood of mucosal ischemia resulting from prolonged pressure on the tracheal wall (Fig. 16.15).

After endotracheal cuff inflation, the anesthesia provider must rapidly confirm correct placement in the trachea. Detecting end-tidal CO_2 with capnography is the gold standard for confirming endotracheal intubation rather than inadvertent esophageal intubation. Symmetric chest rise with manual ventilation and bilateral breath sounds are necessary to confirm endotracheal intubation rather than endobronchial intubation. Palpation of the endotracheal tube cuff while applying pressure in the suprasternal notch can also help confirm endotracheal rather than endobronchial intubation.

After confirmation of correct placement, the endotracheal tube should be secured in position with tape. In adults taping the endotracheal tube at the patient's lips corresponding to the 21- to 23-cm markings on the endotracheal tube usually places the distal end of the endotracheal tube in the mid-trachea.

The success rate of endotracheal intubation using direct laryngoscopy in patients without a predicted difficult intubation is higher than 99%, and in patients with predicted difficult intubation is 84%.[38,39]

directly elevates the epiglottis to expose the glottic opening.

Laryngoscope blades are numbered according to their size. A Macintosh 3 and Miller 2 are the standard intubating blades for adult patients. The Macintosh 4 and Miller 3 blades can be used for larger adult patients.

Video Laryngoscopy

Video laryngoscopy plays an important role in both routine and difficult airway management. Video laryngoscopy is now often used as the initial approach for patients with predicted difficult airways. Studies have demonstrated higher first-pass intubation success rates when compared with direct laryngoscopy.[40] This has led to its rapid adoption in the emergency and critical care settings. The ability to view the intubation process in real time on a remote screen also makes video laryngoscopy an invaluable tool for teaching and as a means of communication and raising situational awareness among team members in the operating room.

Video laryngoscopy can help obtain a view of the larynx by providing indirect visualization of the glottic opening without alignment of the oral, pharyngeal, and tracheal axes and enable endotracheal intubation in patients who have conditions that can make traditional laryngoscopy difficult or impossible (e.g., limited mouth opening, inability to flex or extend the neck).

Video laryngoscopes consist of a handle, a light source, and a blade with a video camera at the distal end to enable the glottis to be visualized indirectly on a video monitor. Depending on the model and manufacturer, the video monitor may be a stand-alone unit or a smaller screen that is attached directly to the handle. Manufacturers are now offering single-use models that eliminate the need for reprocessing. Some video laryngoscopes offer a disposable blade that fits over a reusable handle/camera.

Video laryngoscopes are also recommended for intubating patients with respiratory infections that are transmissible via aerosol or respiratory droplets such as tuberculosis or coronavirus disease 2019 (COVID-19). Video laryngoscopy allows the intubator to be farther away from the patient's face when compared with direct laryngoscopy. This reduces the intubator's risk of exposure to airway secretions, contamination, and potential infection.[41,42]

Video laryngoscope blades are offered in curved Macintosh-style blades, straight Miller-style blades, and angulated blades. The Macintosh-style or Miller-style blades can be used for direct laryngoscopy or by viewing the monitor. These blades are inserted using the standard direct laryngoscopy techniques with or without a stylet in the endotracheal tube. The view obtained by looking at the monitor usually offers a slightly improved view compared with looking directly in the patient's mouth because the camera is more distally located and provides

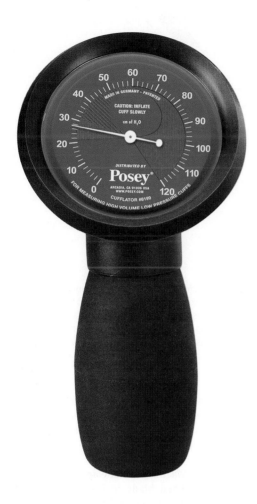

Fig. 16.15 Posey ® 8199 Cufflator endotracheal tube inflator and manometer. (Image courtesy Posey Company, Arcadia, CA.)

Choice of Direct Laryngoscope Blade

The major advantages of a curved laryngoscope blade, such as a Macintosh blade, is that the larger flange improves the ability to shift the tongue to the left, thereby improving visualization of the glottic inlet and creating more space to pass the endotracheal tube. The major advantage of a straight blade, such as a Miller blade, is that it has a smaller profile, which can be beneficial in patients with a smaller mouth opening.

The tip of the curved blade is advanced into the space between the base of the tongue and the pharyngeal surface of the epiglottis into the vallecula, which elevates the epiglottis and exposes the glottic opening (Fig. 16.16A). The tip of the straight blade is passed beneath the laryngeal surface of the epiglottis (see Fig. 16.16B). Forward and upward movement of the blade exerted along the axis of the laryngoscope handle

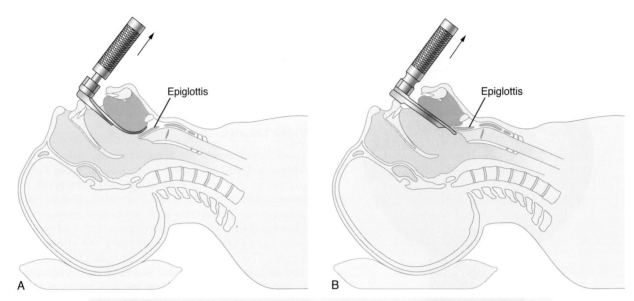

Fig. 16.16 Schematic diagram depicting the proper position of the laryngoscope blade for exposure of the glottic opening. (A) The distal end of the curved blade is advanced into the space between the base of the tongue and the pharyngeal surface of the epiglottis. (B) The distal end of the straight blade is advanced beneath the laryngeal surface of the epiglottis. Regardless of blade design, forward and upward movement exerted along the axis of the laryngoscope handle, as denoted by the *arrows*, serves to elevate the epiglottis and expose the glottic opening.

a wider visual field. The advantage of these blades is user familiarity with the blade type and a display that can be used for instructional purposes.[40]

The angulated blades allow for visualization of the glottic structures with minimal flexion or extension of the patient's head and neck. They are also useful in patients with anterior larynxes.[40] The tip of the laryngoscope blade may be placed in the vallecula or be used to lift the epiglottis directly. These blades usually require a preshaped stylet that matches the curvature of the blade and are usually inserted midline in the mouth. An endotracheal tube with the preshaped stylet is advanced using direct visualization in the pharynx until it can be seen on the monitor, after which the tube is advanced into the trachea close to the blade, based on the image on the monitor. A limitation of these devices is difficulty directing the endotracheal tube into the glottis despite good glottic visualization. This usually occurs when the video laryngoscope is inserted too deeply. Withdrawing the blade slightly, although often giving a poorer laryngoscopic view, can improve the ability to direct the endotracheal tube through the glottic opening.

Video laryngoscopy can be performed on awake patients with difficult airways after topical application of local anesthetic to the airway.[43] Selected video laryngoscopes are described in the following sections.

GlideScope

GlideScope offers both a reusable Titanium line and a single-use Spectrum line of video laryngoscopes handles and blades. The Titanium line comes with curved Macintosh-style blade in a MAC T3 and MAC T4 size, comparable to a typical Macintosh 3 or 4 blade, in addition to angulated blades in LoPro T3 and T4 sizes. The GlideScope Spectrum is a single-use line that comes with a typical curved Macintosh blade in a DVM S3 and S4 size and an angulated blade in LoPro S3 and S4 sizes (Fig. 16.17). These angulated blades are anatomically shaped with a fixed (60-degree) angle and should be used with the GlideRite rigid stylet, as this stylet matches the shape of the blade. The blades have a fog-resistant video camera embedded in the undersurface that transmits the digital image to a high-resolution color monitor that can be mounted on a pole. Recommended GlideScope blades for pediatric and adult patients are listed in Table 16.8.

The GlideScope is associated with improved glottic visualization compared with direct laryngoscopy, especially in patients with potential difficult airways.[38,44] One study showed the overall success rate with the GlideScope to be 96% in patients with predicted difficult airways and 94% when used as a rescue device for failed direct laryngoscopy, suggesting the advantage of GlideScope for use in these situations.[45]

C-MAC

The C-MAC (KARL STORZ Endoscopy) comes in a reusable model with a variety of stainless steel blades, with a camera located on the distal end of the blade that displays on a high-definition monitor. The reusable blades

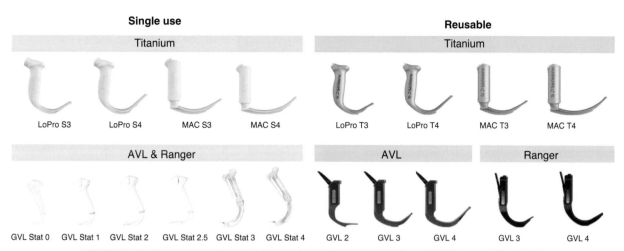

Fig. 16.17 Comparison of the single-use and reusable GlideScope® blades in different sizes and styles. (Used with permission, ©Verathon Inc.)

Table 16.8	Video Laryngoscopes Suitable for Infants, Children, Teenagers, and Adults	
Age Group	**Weight**	**Model**
Premature infants	<2.5 kg	GlideScope GVL 0 C-MAC Miller 0
Neonates	2.5-5 kg	GlideScope GVL 1 C-MAC Miller 1
Infants/ toddlers	5-15 kg	GlideScope GVL 2 C-MAC Miller 1
Small children	15–30 kg	GlideScope GVL 2.5 C-MAC Macintosh 2 McGrath MAC 2
Children/ teenagers	30–70 kg	GlideScope GVL 3 GlideScope Titanium S3/T3 C-MAC Macintosh 3 C-MAC D Blade Pediatric McGrath MAC 3
Teenagers/ adults	>70 kg	GlideScope GVL 4 GlideScope Titanium S4/T4 C-MAC Macintosh 4 C-MAC D Blade Adult McGrath MAC 4

In difficult airway situations using the D-blade improves the glottic view and has intubation success rates similar to the GlideScope when compared with direct laryngoscopy.[44,46] Recommended C-MAC blades for pediatric and adult patients are listed in Table 16.8.

McGrath Scope
The McGrath video laryngoscope is a portable device that consists of a reusable handle and light source with a small color display that can rotate and swivel that is directly attached to the handle. The handle and camera fit into single-use polycarbonate blades. These blades are available in Macintosh 3, Macintosh 4, and an angulated

come in several sizes and styles, including a Macintosh 3, Macintosh 4, and adult angulated D-blade for difficult airways (Fig. 16.18). They have a lateral guide for an oxygen or suction catheter. The interface between the laryngoscope blade and the monitor allows for easy interchange of different blades. There is also a newer C-MAC Five S single-use line of video laryngoscopes with a C-MAC S Imager Camera that fits inside a single-use plastic handle/blade. The single-use C-MAC comes in Macintosh 3, Macintosh 4, and angulated adult D-blades.

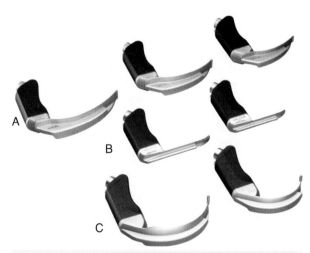

Fig. 16.18 Comparison of the different C-MAC® blade types. (A) Macintosh-style blade, (B) Miller-style blade, and (C) D-blade. (© KARL STORZ SE & Co. KG, Germany.)

adult-sized X-blade. Recommended McGrath blades for pediatric and adult patients are listed in Table 16.8.

Endotracheal Tube Stylets, Introducers, and Airway Exchange Catheters

A variety of endotracheal tube stylets, introducers, and airway exchange catheters (AECs) may be used in selected patients to facilitate difficult endotracheal intubation, endotracheal tube exchange, and SGA exchange for an endotracheal tube. In addition, AECs can provide an airway conduit to assist with reintubation. Some of the devices have a hollow lumen and connectors to allow jet ventilation. Ventilation through the lumen should be used only in emergency situations because of the high risk of complications, including barotrauma, pneumothorax, pneumomediastinum, and subcutaneous emphysema. When using intubating stylets in a patient with a difficult airway, intubation is successful in 78% to 100% of patients.[1] Complications of intubating stylets include bleeding, oropharyngeal trauma, tracheal trauma, and sore throat. Complications of endotracheal tube exchangers include tracheal/bronchial laceration and gastric perforation.[1]

Stylet

Stylets are made from plastic-coated, malleable metal that is used to stiffen and provide curvature to an endotracheal tube. Stylets can help facilitate placement of the endotracheal tube through the glottis. The tip of the stylet should not protrude past the end of the endotracheal tube to minimize the potential for airway trauma. The stylet should be carefully removed after successful intubation. Endotracheal tube stylet sizes are listed in Table 16.9.

Gum Elastic Bougie

A gum elastic bougie is a solid, 60-cm long, 15 Fr introducer with a 40-degree curve approximately 3.5 cm from the distal tip. It is used to facilitate intubation in patients with a poor laryngoscopic view. It is passed under the epiglottis and into the glottis. A characteristic bumping or clicking is felt in most tracheal placements as the bougie is advanced down the tracheal cartilages, but is not felt in esophageal placements. An endotracheal tube is then advanced over the bougie and into the airway and the bougie is removed.

Frova Intubating Introducer

The Frova Intubating Introducer has a distal angulated tip and an internal channel to accommodate a stiffening rod or allow jet ventilation. It is available in a pediatric (35 cm long, 8 Fr) and an adult (65 cm long, 14 Fr) size. The pediatric introducer can be used with endotracheal tubes from 3.0 mm to 5.5 mm. The adult introducer can be used with endotracheal tubes 6.0 mm and larger. The Frova Intubating Introducer is inserted in a similar

Table 16.9	Endotracheal Tube, Suction Catheter, and Stylet Size Based on Age and Weight			
Age (yr)	Weight (kg)	Endotracheal Tube ID (mm)	Suction Catheter (Fr)	Stylet (Fr)
Premature	<1.5	2.5	6	6
Premature	1.5–2.5	3.0	6	6
Newborn	3.5	3.5	8	6
1	10	4.0	8	6
2–3	15	4.5	10	6
4–6	20	5.0	10	10
7–9	30	5.5	12	10
10–12	40	6.0	14	10
13–15	50	6.5	14	14
>16	>60	7.0	18	14

Fr, French; ID, internal diameter.

manner to the gum elastic bougie for patients with poor laryngoscopic views (Fig. 16.19A).

Aintree Intubation Catheter

The Aintree Intubation Catheter (AIC) is 56-cm long, 19 Fr diameter, and has a large 4.7-mm lumen. It comes with two Rapi-Fit adapters. One is for jet ventilation, and the other for connection to an anesthesia circuit or Ambu bag.

The AIC can also be used to exchange SGAs for endotracheal tubes size 7.0 mm or larger. The AIC is threaded onto a fiber-optic bronchoscope and then placed in the lumen of the SGA and advanced as a unit through the vocal cords into the trachea. The fiber-optic bronchoscope is then removed from the AIC. With the AIC in the trachea, the SGA is carefully removed, and an endotracheal tube is then placed over the AIC into the trachea. Finally, the AIC is removed (see Fig. 16.19B).

Cook Airway Exchange Catheter

Cook AECs are 83 cm in length and are available in 11, 14, and 19 Fr sizes. They are designed for endotracheal tube exchange. These catheters are hollow and can allow for jet ventilation or oxygenation through an anesthesia circuit or Ambu bag using Rapi-Fit adapters in emergency situations.[47] For orotracheal intubation, AEC insertion of 20 to 22 cm depth, and for nasotracheal intubation, insertion of 27 to 30 cm depth is sufficient for tube exchange and can help avoid complications. If placed deeper, there is a risk of bronchial perforation or pneumothorax. To help with placement of an endotracheal tube over an AEC, laryngoscopy can displace tissues. Using a smaller endotracheal tube may also facilitate the use of AECs. They can also be left in the trachea

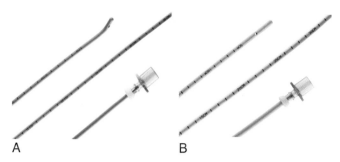

Fig. 16.19 (A) Frova Intubating Introducer. (B) Aintree Intubation Catheter. (Images courtesy Cook Medical, Bloomington, IN.)

after endotracheal tube removal to help with reintubation if necessary in patients with difficult airways. The Cook extra-firm, soft-tip AEC is designed for double-lumen tube exchange. It is 100 cm in length and available in 11 or 14 Fr sizes.

Flexible Fiber-Optic Endotracheal Intubation

Fiber-optic intubation can be useful for difficult airway management. Fiber-optic intubation can be performed through the nose or mouth in awake, sedated, or anesthetized patients. The decision to perform fiber-optic endotracheal intubation in an awake versus an anesthetized patient is dependent on the risk of a difficult airway and the cooperation of the patient. Fiber-optic endotracheal intubation may be advantageous in patients with unstable cervical spines. The technique does not require movement of the patient's neck and can be performed in an awake patient, thereby allowing for evaluation of the patient's neurologic function after endotracheal intubation and surgical positioning.

Patients who have sustained an injury to the upper airway from either blunt or penetrating trauma are at risk for the endotracheal tube creating a false passage by exiting the airway through the disrupted tissue during direct laryngoscopy. By performing a fiber-optic intubation, not only can the injury be assessed but the endotracheal tube can also be placed beyond the level of the injury, thus minimizing the risk of subcutaneous emphysema.

A disadvantage of fiber-optic endotracheal intubation is that it requires time to set up and prepare the patient's airway. Blood and secretions can easily obscure the view of the fiber-optic bronchoscope; therefore administration of an antisialagogue is recommended, and suctioning may be necessary. Infections, hematomas, edema, or masses in the upper airway may make fiber-optic intubation more difficult. Inflating the cuff of the endotracheal tube to hold the pharyngeal walls open may be helpful. An SGA may be an effective conduit by providing a direct channel to the glottis and minimizing the blood

and secretions that may be obscuring the fiber-optic bronchoscope.

Awake Fiber-Optic Endotracheal Intubation

Awake fiber-optic intubation should be considered if there is a history of a difficult airway or an unstable cervical spine. Performing intubation before induction of anesthesia allows for continuation of spontaneous breathing, preservation of muscle tone, preservation of airway reflexes, and assessment of neurologic function after intubation. This is especially important in patients who are at risk for difficult mask ventilation or pulmonary aspiration of gastric contents. Patient cooperation is critical to this technique.

Awake fiber-optic intubation can be performed through the nose or mouth. In general, the nasal route is easier because the angle of curvature of the endotracheal tube naturally approximates that of the patient's upper airway. The risk of inducing bleeding is more frequent when the nasal route is used and therefore relatively contraindicated in patients at risk for bleeding, such as those with platelet abnormalities or coagulation disorders.

Patient Preparation
The procedure should be fully explained to the patient, and an antisialagogue should be administered (glycopyrrolate 0.2–0.4 mg intravenously). The patient should be monitored throughout the procedure, and sedation can be carefully administered.

Airway Anesthesia
Airway anesthesia is achieved by topical application of a local anesthetic or by specific nerve blocks. Topical airway anesthesia can be achieved by spraying (atomizing or nebulizing) or direct application (ointment, gels, or gargling solutions). Several commercial devices are available to assist with topical application of local anesthetic. The larger particle size of a spray tends to cause it to be deposited in the pharynx, with only a small proportion reaching the trachea. The small particle

size of a nebulized spray is carried more effectively into the trachea and the smaller airways. Lidocaine is the preferred topical local anesthetic because of its broad therapeutic window. Usually, 1% and 2% solutions are used for nerve blocks and infiltration, whereas 4% solutions are used topically.[48] Benzocaine is less preferred, as it can cause methemoglobinemia even in therapeutic doses. Tetracaine has a very narrow therapeutic window, and the maximum allowable dose (1.2 mg/kg) can easily be exceeded.

Nose and Nasopharynx

To minimize the potential risk of bleeding from the nasal mucosa, 0.05% oxymetazoline hydrochloride (HCl) spray should be administered for vasoconstriction. Phenylephrine nasal spray should be avoided because of the potential for systemic absorption and phenylephrine toxicity. Topical anesthesia of the nasal mucosa can be achieved using lidocaine solution applied directly on soaked cotton-tipped swabs or pledgets or by nasal airways covered in lidocaine ointment.

Tongue and Oropharynx

Topical anesthesia can be achieved by spraying, direct application, or bilateral blocks of the glossopharyngeal nerve at the base of each anterior tonsillar pillar. The patient can gargle with 2% viscous lidocaine solution, or 4% lidocaine solution can be atomized or nebulized to the oropharynx. Care should be taken to ensure that the total dose of lidocaine is less than 7 mg/kg to minimize the risk of local anesthetic toxicity. Approximately, 2 mL of 2% lidocaine injected at a depth of 0.5 cm is sufficient to block the glossopharyngeal nerves on each side. Aspiration with the syringe before injecting the local anesthetic solution is necessary to ensure that the needle is not intravascular or through the tonsillar pillar.

Larynx and Trachea

Anesthesia of the larynx and trachea to prevent coughing during the procedure may be achieved by atomizing or nebulizing lidocaine as described earlier or by superior laryngeal nerve block or transtracheal block.

Superior Laryngeal Nerve Block

The superior laryngeal nerves lie between the greater cornu of the hyoid bone and the superior cornu of the thyroid cartilage as they traverse the thyrohyoid membrane to the submucosa of the piriform sinus. Blockade of these nerves, which must be done bilaterally, begins with cleaning the overlying skin with antiseptic solution. The cornu of the hyoid bone or the thyroid cartilage may be used as a landmark. A 22- to 25-G needle is "walked" off the cephalad edge of the thyroid cartilage or the caudal edge of the hyoid bone, and approximately 2 to 3 mL of 2% lidocaine is injected on each side.

Transtracheal Block

For a transtracheal block, the skin is prepared with antiseptic solution and a 20-G intravenous (IV) catheter is advanced through the cricothyroid membrane while simultaneously aspirating with an attached syringe filled with 4 mL of 2% lidocaine. When air is aspirated, the catheter is advanced into the trachea and the needle is withdrawn. The syringe is reattached to the catheter, aspiration of air is reconfirmed, and the local anesthetic solution is rapidly injected at end expiration to enhance spread in the trachea and proximal bronchial trees during inspiration.

Fiber-Optic Intubation Techniques

Nasal fiber-optic intubation of the trachea involves the use of a lubricated endotracheal tube. The diameter of the fiber-optic bronchoscope should be at least 1.5 mm smaller than the internal diameter of the endotracheal tube. Softening the endotracheal tube in warm water before use makes it less likely to cause mucosal trauma or submucosal tunneling. The endotracheal tube is advanced through the nose into the pharynx by aiming posteriorly. If resistance is met at the back of the nasopharynx, 90 degrees of counterclockwise rotation allows the endotracheal tube to pass less traumatically because the bevel then faces the posterior pharyngeal wall. Suction should be immediately available throughout the procedure to minimize secretions.

For oral fiber-optic intubation, using a channeled oral airway that fits an endotracheal tube can help keep the fiber-optic scope midline and create space in the oropharynx. Having an assistant gently extend the tongue out of the patient's mouth can help by elevating the epiglottis. The endotracheal tube can either be advanced in the mouth with the fiber-optic bronchoscope or can be secured at the top of the scope and advanced after the fiber-optic bronchoscope has entered the trachea. Inflation of the endotracheal tube cuff during advancement of the fiber-optic bronchoscope in the pharynx can create an enlarged pharyngeal space and help keep the optics of the fiber-optic bronchoscope from being obscured. The inflated cuff can also angle the tip of the endotracheal tube more anteriorly to facilitate advancing the bronchoscope through the vocal cords. If this technique is used, it is important to deflate the cuff before advancing the endotracheal tube into the trachea.

After the fiber-optic bronchoscope has passed through the vocal cords, the tracheal rings and carina should be identified. The scope should be placed 4 to 5 cm above the carina, and the endotracheal tube should be advanced into the trachea over the bronchoscope. Resistance to advancement often means that the endotracheal tube is impacted on an arytenoid, and the endotracheal tube should be rotated and gently advanced. The fiber-optic bronchoscope can be used to confirm the appropriate depth of endotracheal tube placement before it is withdrawn. Resistance to removing the fiber-optic bronchoscope may indicate that the bronchoscope has inadvertently passed through the Murphy eye of the endotracheal tube or kinked in the pharynx. In both instances the endotracheal tube and the scope must be withdrawn together to avoid damaging the fiber-optic bronchoscope.

Fiber-Optic Endotracheal Intubation After Induction of General Anesthesia

Asleep fiber-optic intubation technique is employed when the patient is not cooperative or when mask ventilation is not anticipated to be difficult. Fiber-optic intubation during general anesthesia can be done either through the nose or the mouth and with the patient breathing spontaneously or under controlled ventilation. Supplemental oxygen can be delivered via nasal cannula or a nasal airway connected to the anesthesia breathing circuit with a 15-mm connector during the procedure.

In anesthetized patients the soft tissues of the pharynx are relaxed and limit space for visualization with the fiber-optic bronchoscope, which can be overcome by using jaw thrust, specialized oral airways, inflating the endotracheal tube cuff in the pharynx, or applying traction on the tongue. It is helpful to have a second anesthesia provider available to assist during fiber-optic intubation.

Endoscopy Mask

The single-use endoscopy mask is designed with a port that will accommodate an endotracheal tube and a fiber-optic bronchoscope through a diaphragm. This device allows for spontaneous or controlled ventilation while fiber-optic nasal or oral intubation is being performed.

Rigid Fiber-Optic Intubating Stylets

Both the Bonfils (Karl Storz) and Levitan FPS (Clarus Medical) are rigid intubating stylets with an incorporated fiber-optic imaging, allowing visualization of the glottis from the tip of the endotracheal tube via an attached eyepiece or video screen. Endotracheal tubes are loaded onto the shaft and advanced into the trachea. The Bonfils has a 40-cm, nonmalleable, metal shaft with a 40-degree curve at the distal end (Fig. 16.20). The Levitan FPS is a 30-cm, semimalleable intubating stylet that was developed for use in the emergency department. Both devices can be used with or without the aid of direct laryngoscopy in the management of normal and difficult airways. Their slim profiles make them advantageous for use in patients with limited mouth opening or cervical spine mobility. Studies indicate that both the Bonfils and Levitan are comparable in terms of success rate and time to intubation but demonstrate a high failure rate among novice users.[49,50]

INVASIVE AIRWAY ACCESS

In situations when intubation is not successful and it is not possible to ventilate or oxygenate via mask or SGA, emergency invasive airway access should be used per the difficult airway algorithm (see Fig. 16.1).[1] Invasive airway access consists of percutaneous or surgical cricothyrotomy or transtracheal jet ventilation via the cricothyroid membrane. Relative contraindications to these techniques include disease of the anterior aspect of the neck (tumors, infection, stenosis), laryngeal or tracheal disruption, or coagulopathy.

Cricothyrotomy

An emergency cricothyrotomy can be a lifesaving procedure when one is unable to intubate and ventilate. A planned cricothyrotomy can also be used as a first-line technique to secure an airway when a noninvasive technique is not possible because of factors such as facial trauma, upper airway bleeding, or upper airway obstruction. A cricothyrotomy is best performed with the patient in the sniffing position to optimize the ability to identify the cricothyroid membrane. A percutaneous cricothyrotomy uses the Seldinger technique. A needle is advanced at a 90-degree angle through the cricothyroid membrane while aspirating with an attached syringe. A change in resistance is felt as a pop when the needle enters the trachea and air is aspirated. The needle should be directed caudally at a 30- to 45-degree angle. A guidewire is then advanced through the needle, followed by removal of the needle, a small incision adjacent to the wire, and placement of a combined dilator and airway of adequate caliber (>4 mm). Finally, the wire and dilator are removed, leaving the airway in place.

The surgical cricothyrotomy involves a vertical or horizontal skin incision, followed by a horizontal incision through the cricothyroid membrane through which a standard endotracheal tube or tracheostomy tube is placed. A tracheal hook, dilator, AEC, or bougie can assist in placement of the airway. A surgical cricothyrotomy can also be valuable as a rescue technique if a percutaneous cricothyrotomy is unsuccessful. Commercial percutaneous and surgical cricothyrotomy kits are available that require minimal assembly for use in emergency circumstances.

Both percutaneous and surgical cricothyrotomies have similar success rates, and the choice of technique should be based on the individual practitioner's knowledge and proficiency.[51,52]

When one is unable to intubate and ventilate, it is important to make the decision to perform cricothyroidotomy early. Potential complications include bleeding; infection; subglottic stenosis; and injury to the larynx, trachea, or esophagus.[17,52]

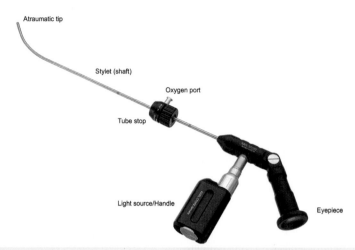

Atraumatic tip

Stylet (shaft)

Oxygen port

Tube stop

Light source/Handle

Eyepiece

Fig. 16.20 The Bonfils intubation endoscope with incorporated fiber-optic imaging, allowing visualization of the glottis from the tip of the endotracheal tube via an attached eyepiece. (© KARL STORZ SE & Co. KG, Germany.)

Transtracheal Jet Ventilation

Transtracheal jet ventilation via the cricothyroid membrane is another potentially lifesaving procedure when one is unable to intubate and ventilate. The cricothyroid membrane is identified and punctured at a 90-degree angle with a catheter over a needle connected to a syringe. When air is aspirated, the catheter should be advanced off the needle into the trachea at a 30- to 45-degree angle caudally. After reconfirming correct placement by aspiration of air, the catheter is then connected to a high-pressure oxygen source. Commercially available products contain kink-resistant catheters and specialized tubing for high-pressure (50 psi) ventilation. Potential complications include pneumothorax, pneumomediastinum, bleeding, infection, and subcutaneous emphysema.

Retrograde Endotracheal Intubation

Retrograde endotracheal intubation can be performed without identification of the glottic inlet. It has been used in cases of anticipated and unanticipated difficult airway management, particularly when there is bleeding, airway trauma, decreased mouth opening, or limited neck movement.

The cricothyroid membrane is punctured with a needle with a syringe attached as described earlier. After confirming that the needle is in the trachea, the syringe is detached and a guidewire is threaded through the needle in a cephalad direction and then retrieved from the mouth with a forceps. An endotracheal tube is threaded over the wire until it stops on impact with the anterior wall of the trachea. Tension on the guide can be relaxed to allow the endotracheal tube to pass farther into the trachea before removing the wire. Commercially available kits have improved this technique by adding a guiding catheter that fits over the wire and inside the endotracheal tube.

Endotracheal Extubation

Endotracheal extubation after general anesthesia requires skill and judgment. It is generally safest to extubate when the patient is fully awake. Any residual neuromuscular blockade should be reversed, and 100% O_2 should be administered before extubation. The oropharynx should be suctioned and a bite block placed to prevent the patient from biting and occluding the endotracheal tube. Extubation criteria include spontaneous respirations with adequate minute ventilation, satisfactory oxygenation and acid-base status, hemodynamic stability, and the ability to follow commands. Endotracheal extubation during a light level of anesthesia (as evidenced by disconjugate gaze, breath-holding, or coughing) increases the risk of laryngospasm. Patients who are obese or have a history of obstructive sleep apnea may benefit from positioning with the head-of-bed elevated for extubation.[53,54] Before extubation, the endotracheal tube cuff should be deflated. Immediately after endotracheal extubation, 100% O_2 should be delivered by facemask, and confirmation of adequate ventilation and oxygenation should be assessed by clinical signs and capnography.

Deep endotracheal extubation, before the return of protective airway reflexes, is generally associated with less coughing and attenuated hemodynamic effects on emergence. This may be preferred in patients at risk from adverse effects of increased intracranial or intraocular pressure, bleeding into the surgical wound, or wound dehiscence. The relative contraindications to deep extubation include previous difficult facemask ventilation or endotracheal intubation; high risk of aspiration; restricted access to the airway; obstructive sleep apnea or morbid obesity; and a surgical procedure that may have resulted in airway edema, bleeding, or irritability. Deep extubation may also predispose to airway obstruction from decreased upper airway tone from anesthetic agents.

A plan for reintubation should be made in patients at risk of failed extubation and those with difficult airways (Fig. 16.21). High-risk patients include those with airway edema, morbid obesity, and respiratory insufficiency.[17] Deflating the endotracheal tube cuff and confirming the presence or absence of a cuff leak can help determine if significant airway edema is present. Extubation over an AEC or insertion of SGA before extubation provides a conduit to reintubation and allows for oxygenation and/or ventilation if necessary.[1,54] Extubation of the trachea is always elective, and postponing extubation may be appropriate in some cases when the patient has increased risk for requiring reintubation.

COMPLICATIONS

Complications of endotracheal intubation are rare and can be categorized as those occurring (1) during laryngoscopy and endotracheal intubation, (2) while the endotracheal tube is in place, and (3) after endotracheal extubation (Box 16.2).

Complications During Laryngoscopy and Endotracheal Intubation

Laryngoscopy and intubation can lead to a sore throat in up to 40% of patients.[55] Care should be taken during laryngoscopy to minimize trauma. Use of larger endotracheal tubes and overinflating endotracheal tube cuffs may also increase the likelihood of sore throat. Sore throat is usually self-limiting and resolves in 24 to 72 hours.

One of the most common complications of laryngoscopy is dental damage (incidence 1 in 4500 patients).[56] Patients at increased risk for dental damage include those with preexisting poor dentition or fixed dental work. Use of a plastic shield placed over the upper teeth may help in selected patients but will decrease the interincisor distance and may make laryngoscopy more difficult. Other possible complications from laryngoscopy include oral or pharyngeal injury; lip lacerations and bruises;

and laryngeal, arytenoid, esophageal, or tracheal damage. The risk for airway trauma is increased in patients with difficult airways that require multiple laryngoscopies for intubation.

Laryngoscopy and intubation cause stimulation of the sympathetic nervous system, which can cause systemic hypertension, tachycardia, and increased intracranial pressure. These physiologic responses can cause adverse effects, especially in patients with preexisting hypertension, ischemic heart disease, or certain neurologic conditions.

Aspiration is another potential complication that can occur during laryngoscopy. Patients at greater risk for aspiration include those who have not fasted, have symptomatic gastroesophageal reflux, have delayed gastric emptying, or are morbidly obese. Notably, aspiration is the most common cause of death among major anesthesia airway complications.[6]

Accidental esophageal intubation, if unrecognized, can result in the inability to oxygenate and ventilate the patient and can lead to significant morbidity and mortality. This highlights the importance of using capnography to confirm correct placement of the endotracheal tube immediately after intubation. If the endotracheal tube is inserted too deep, this will result in endobronchial intubation. This can lead to ventilation of only one lung and result in increased shunting and inadequate oxygenation. Kinking of the endotracheal tube or obstruction from secretions or blood in the endotracheal tube can lead to inadequate oxygenation and ventilation. The risk of accidental extubation intraoperatively can be minimized by noting the proper insertion depth and adequately securing the endotracheal tube. When the position of the patient (e.g., turning prone or lateral) is changed, the correct position of the endotracheal tube should be reconfirmed.

Complications After Endotracheal Extubation

One-third of adverse airway events occur during emergence or recovery from anesthesia.[6] Many are the result of inadequate oxygenation and ventilation after extubation. Causes include laryngeal edema, laryngospasm, or bronchospasm. Most laryngospasm episodes can be treated with the application of positive pressure through a facemask and jaw thrust. Severe laryngospasm may require the administration of propofol or muscle relaxants such as rocuronium or succinylcholine. Excessive endotracheal cuff pressures can cause damage to the tracheal mucosa and result in airway edema. This may progress to destruction of cartilaginous rings and subsequent fibrous scar formation and tracheal stenosis, especially if there is prolonged endotracheal intubation with excessive cuff pressures. Using high-volume, low-pressure cuffs and keeping cuff pressures less than 25 cm H_2O can help prevent these complications.

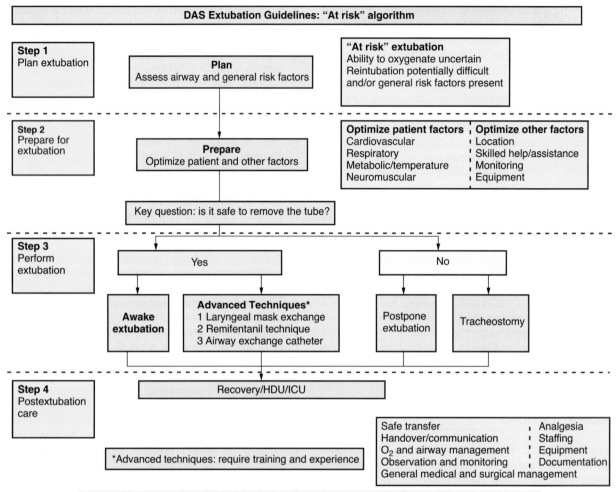

Fig. 16.21 The Difficult Airway Society (DAS) extubation guidelines for at-risk patients. *HDU,* High-dependency unit; *ICU,* intensive care unit. (From Mitchell V, Dravid R, Patel A, et al. Difficult Airway Society guidelines for the management of tracheal extubation. *Anaesthesia.* 2012;67[3]:318–340.)

AIRWAY MANAGEMENT IN INFANTS AND CHILDREN (ALSO SEE CHAPTER 34)

Airway Management Differences Between Infants and Adults

Understanding the differences between the infant and adult airway is critical to proper airway management in pediatric anesthesia (Box 16.3). The anatomic and physiologic differences between the infant airway and the adult airway decrease as children grow and resolve by about 12 to 14 years of age.

The larynx in infants is located higher in the neck than in adults. In infants the larynx is typically at the level of C3–C4, and in adults the larynx is usually at the level of C4–C5. The higher larynx in infants causes the tongue to shift more superiorly, closer to the palate. As a result, the tongue more easily apposes the palate, which can cause airway obstruction. An infant's tongue is also larger in proportion to the size of the mouth than in adults. The relatively large size of the tongue makes direct laryngoscopy more difficult and can contribute to obstruction of the upper airway during sedation, inhalation induction of anesthesia, and emergence from anesthesia. Jaw thrust or an oral airway can shift the tongue to a more anterior position and resolve upper airway obstruction. A nasal airway can also be beneficial in these situations.

The epiglottis in an infant's airway is often described as relatively larger, stiffer, and more omega-shaped than an adult epiglottis. More importantly, an infant's epiglottis is typically angled in a more posterior position, thereby blocking the view of the vocal cords during

---

Box 16.2 Complications of Endotracheal Intubation

During Direct Laryngoscopy and Endotracheal Intubation
Dental and oral soft tissue trauma
Systemic hypertension and tachycardia
Cardiac dysrhythmias
Myocardial ischemia
Inhalation (aspiration) of gastric contents

While the Endotracheal Tube Is in Place
Endotracheal tube obstruction
Endobronchial intubation
Esophageal intubation
Endotracheal tube cuff leak
Pulmonary barotrauma
Nasogastric distention
Accidental disconnection from the anesthesia breathing circuit
Tracheal mucosa ischemia
Accidental extubation

Complications After Endotracheal Extubation
Laryngospasm
Inhalation (aspiration) of gastric contents
Pharyngitis (sore throat)
Laryngitis
Laryngeal or subglottic edema
Laryngeal ulceration with or without granuloma formation
Tracheitis
Tracheal stenosis
Vocal cord paralysis
Arytenoid cartilage dislocation

Box 16.3 The Infant Airway Versus the Adult Airway

- Larynx positioned higher in the neck
- Tongue larger relative to mouth size
- Epiglottis larger, softer, and angled more posteriorly
- Head and occiput larger relative to body size
- Short neck
- Narrow nares
- Cricoid ring is the narrowest region

---

direct laryngoscopy. In infants and small children it is often necessary to lift the epiglottis with the tip of the blade of the laryngoscope to visualize the vocal cords in order to successfully intubate the trachea.

An infant's airway is funnel-shaped, with a relatively large thyroid cartilage above and a relatively narrow cricoid cartilage below. The cricoid cartilage is the narrowest portion of an infant's airway, whereas the vocal cords are the narrowest portion of an adult's airway. The cricoid cartilage is circular, allowing correctly sized uncuffed endotracheal tubes to successfully seal and protect the airway from aspiration.

An infant's head and occiput are proportionally larger than an adult's. The proper position for direct

laryngoscopy and endotracheal intubation in an adult is often described as the sniffing position with the head elevated and the neck flexed at C6–C7 and extended at C1–C2 (see Fig. 16.5). An infant or small child, on the other hand, requires a shoulder or neck roll to prevent the hyperflexion caused by their relatively larger occiput in order to establish an optimal position for facemask ventilation and direct laryngoscopy. An infant's nares are relatively smaller than an adult's and can offer significant resistance to airflow and increase the work of breathing, especially when there are secretions, edema, or bleeding.

Oxygen consumption per kilogram is much higher in infants than in adults. This results in a much shorter allowable time for intubation before the infant desaturates, even after adequate preoxygenation. This can be a significant issue, especially in difficult intubations.

Managing the Normal Airway in Infants and Children

A complete history and a focused physical examination are the first steps in managing the pediatric airway.

History

The history should include whether there were any problems with previous anesthetics; prior anesthetic records should be reviewed if they are available. A history of snoring should prompt additional questioning about whether the infant or child has obstructive sleep apnea. Obstructive sleep apnea can lead to respiratory obstruction during the induction and emergence phases of anesthesia and in the postoperative period, especially if opioids are used for pain management. Syndromes involving mandibular hypoplasia can make aligning the oral, pharyngeal, and laryngeal axes difficult during direct laryngoscopy and may require alternative approaches to airway management. Syndromes involving cervical spine abnormalities can limit flexion and extension and can also make laryngoscopy and intubation challenging (see Table 16.2).

Physical Examination

It is often difficult to perform a complete physical examination on infants and children, as they may be afraid or unwilling to cooperate. Asking a child to look up at the sky and then down at the floor is one way of assessing neck extension and flexion. If there are any masses, tumors, or abscesses in the neck or upper airway that compromise neck flexion, extension, or breathing function, further evaluation is important and should include CT to evaluate the location and degree of any airway compromise. Children will often voluntarily open their mouths to enable determination of a Mallampati classification. If an infant or child is uncooperative, examining the profile of an infant or child can indicate whether the thyromental distance is short and whether the patient has micrognathia or a hypoplastic mandible.

The parent(s) and the child should be directly asked whether there are any loose teeth. If loose teeth are identified, care should be taken to avoid dislodging these teeth during airway management. Very loose teeth can be removed before proceeding with airway management to prevent accidental dislodgement and possible aspiration.

Preanesthetic Medication and Parental Presence During Induction of Anesthesia

Parental presence during induction of anesthesia is increasingly becoming the standard approach for pediatric patients. Parental presence can minimize the need for preanesthetic medication in infants and children. If parental presence during induction of anesthesia is used, it is important to designate a member of the perioperative team to escort the parents from the operating room to the waiting area after the induction of anesthesia is completed and to address any worries parents may have after witnessing the induction.

Anxious parents can transfer their anxiety to their children. Thus preoperative anxiety in either the child or the parents can result in a child that is uncooperative, upset, or crying during the induction of anesthesia. Preoperative anxiety has been associated with posthospitalization behavioral changes, including nightmares, separation anxiety, enuresis, eating disorders, and temper tantrums. The "unpleasant" induction experience can also result in increased anxiety during subsequent anesthetics.[57,58]

Preoperative clinic visits or telephone consultations should spend adequate time addressing any questions or concerns about anesthesia. The anesthesia provider should also assess and address any anxiety in the child or the parents during the preoperative consultation on the day of surgery. Child-life services can be extremely useful preoperatively by using age-appropriate play therapy and preoperative instruction. Older children and teenagers can be coached to reduce their anxiety and taught coping skills. The goal is to decrease anxiety and prepare both pediatric patients and their parents for their perioperative anesthesia experience.

Preanesthetic medication can facilitate the induction of anesthesia in very anxious children. Preanesthetic medication is often not necessary in infants younger than 6 months because stranger anxiety does not usually develop until 6 to 9 months of age. If the child has an IV catheter in place, midazolam can be administered in small doses and titrated to effect.

If the child does not have an IV catheter in place, midazolam syrup can be given orally in a dose of about 0.5 mg/kg up to a maximum dose of about 20 mg. If the child is uncooperative with taking midazolam orally, it

can also be given intranasally, intramuscularly, or rectally. In cases in which older children are uncooperative, agitated, or violent it may be necessary to administer intramuscular ketamine in a dose of about 3 mg/kg to facilitate IV catheter placement and the induction of anesthesia.

Induction of Anesthesia

IV induction of anesthesia with propofol is usually safer and quicker than an inhaled induction of anesthesia. After the infant or child loses consciousness and the ability to ventilate with a facemask is verified, either an SGA device can be inserted or a neuromuscular blocking drug can be given to facilitate direct laryngoscopy and endotracheal intubation. Although it is possible to perform laryngoscopy on infants and children without a neuromuscular blocking drug by using higher doses of sevoflurane or propofol, using a neuromuscular blocking drug such as rocuronium can facilitate laryngoscopy and intubation, decrease the incidence of laryngospasm, and decrease the amount of anesthetic agents required for laryngoscopy.

When the infant or child does not have an IV catheter in place, inhaled induction of anesthesia can be performed. Beginning the induction of anesthesia with the odorless mixture of nitrous oxide and oxygen through a facemask then slowly increasing the concentration of sevoflurane is a common approach in a cooperative child. Young children who are uncooperative and crying can be induced with 8% sevoflurane. When the infant or child becomes unconscious, the nitrous oxide should be turned off to administer 100% oxygen to adequately preoxygenate before inserting an SGA or an endotracheal tube. An IV catheter should then be placed. Once the ability to ventilate the patient has been confirmed, either an SGA device can be inserted or a neuromuscular blocking drug can be given to facilitate laryngoscopy and endotracheal intubation.

Direct Laryngoscopy and Endotracheal Intubation

When performing direct laryngoscopy and endotracheal intubation in infants and children, it is important to appropriately position the infant or child with a roll under the neck or shoulders. The oropharynx should be visualized as divided into three compartments: (1) the tongue swept to the left by the laryngoscope blade, (2) the laryngoscope blade in the middle of the mouth, and (3) the endotracheal tube entering from the right side of the mouth. External pressure at the level of the thyroid or cricoid cartilage is sometimes necessary to bring the vocal cords into view.

Once the trachea is intubated, correct positioning of the endotracheal tube should be confirmed by end-tidal

CO_2, by watching the chest rise and fall, and by auscultation of both right and left lungs. Because the trachea in infants and children is short, it is easy to accidentally intubate a main bronchus. The correct depth of a cuffed endotracheal tube can be estimated by palpating the endotracheal tube cuff in the suprasternal notch. The correct tracheal depth of an uncuffed endotracheal tube can be estimated by placing the double line at the distal end of the endotracheal tube at the vocal cords while performing direct laryngoscopy. In infants and children it is especially important to reconfirm that the endotracheal tube is correctly positioned by listening for equal bilateral breath sounds after securing the endotracheal tube and whenever there is a change in the patient's position.

Airway Equipment

Nasal and Oral Airways

Nasal and oral airways can sometimes be useful in pediatric patients to relieve airway obstruction, especially during facemask ventilation at the beginning or end of anesthesia. The nasal airway should be carefully placed through one of the nares after lubricating its exterior. The nasal airway must be long enough to pass through the nasopharynx but short enough that it still remains above the glottis.

Oral airways relieve airway obstruction by displacing the tongue anteriorly. Too large an oral airway will either obstruct the glottis or may cause coughing, gagging, or laryngospasm in a patient who is not deeply anesthetized. Too small an oral airway will push the tongue posteriorly and make the airway obstruction worse. Oral airways should be placed with care to prevent trauma to the teeth and oropharynx.

Supraglottic Airways

SGAs are placed in the patient's oropharynx to facilitate oxygenation and ventilation; they can also deliver inhalational anesthetics. They can be used for both routine airway management and difficult airway situations. In difficult airway situations they can be used as rescue devices to oxygenate/ventilate and can be used as conduits for fiber-optic intubation. Although SGAs are ideally suited for situations in which the patient is breathing spontaneously, they can also be used to deliver positive-pressure ventilation. Care must be taken when using positive-pressure ventilation when using SGAs to minimize peak inspiratory pressure. Patients who have lung disease or whose peak inspiratory pressures are higher than normal are poor candidates for an SGA. In these patients air may leak into the esophagus, resulting in distention of the stomach and increase the risk for emesis and aspiration. As SGAs do not protect the airway from aspiration, they should not be routinely used in patients with full stomachs or those at increased risk for aspiration. Many types of SGAs are available for infants and children, including the LMA, air-Q ILAs, i-gel, Portex Soft Seal, and Ambu AuraStraight.

Laryngeal Mask Airways

LMA Unique SGAs are available in seven sizes (1, 1.5, 2, 2.2, 3, 4, 5, and 6) appropriate for a range of pediatric patients. The LMA Supreme has an additional lumen that is designed to vent the esophagus and is available in the same seven sizes. The appropriate size LMA is most easily determined by using the weight of the infant or child, and the recommended weight is listed on the package and on the shaft of the LMA (see Table 16.5). An LMA that is too large will be more difficult to place. An LMA that is too small will not form a good seal, making positive-pressure ventilation more challenging.

After the LMA has been inserted and its cuff has been inflated, correct positioning should be confirmed by auscultation of breath sounds and by end-tidal CO_2. Ideally, the cuff of the LMA should be inflated with just enough air to allow positive-pressure ventilation. Overinflation of the LMA cuff has been associated with mucosal damage and postoperative sore throat and may not decrease the leak pressure. Ideally, the pressure in the cuff of the LMA should be adjusted and measured with a manometer (see Fig. 16.15).[59] A cuff pressure of 30 to 40 cm H_2O may be necessary to prevent a circuit leak with positive-pressure ventilation.

Air-Q Intubating Laryngeal Airways

Air-Q ILAs are another type of SGA device used for infants and children. Their major advantage is a design that facilitates endotracheal intubation with standard oral endotracheal tubes. The Air-Q airway shaft has a large diameter allowing for easier intubation with the appropriately sized endotracheal tube. The Air-Q single-use ILA is available in six sizes (1, 1.5, 2, 2.5, 3.5, and 4.5) appropriate for a range of pediatric patients. The air-Q Blocker has an additional lumen that is designed to vent the esophagus and is available in sizes 2.5, 3.5, and 4.5. Determining the appropriate size is most easily estimated by using the weight of the infant or child (see Table 16.6).

i-gel Supraglottic Airways

i-gel SGAs are made from a thermoplastic elastomer and have a soft, gel-like, noninflatable cuff. They have an integral bite block and a gastric channel for protection against aspiration (except for size 1). i-gel SGAs are available in seven sizes (1, 1.5, 2, 2.5, 3, 4, and 5). The appropriate size is most easily estimated by using the weight of the infant or child (see Table 16.7).

Endotracheal Tubes

The appropriately sized endotracheal tube for infants and children can be estimated by using the following formula for uncuffed endotracheal tubes:

$$\frac{(Age + 16)}{4} = \text{endotracheal tube (ID) size}$$

To adapt this formula to cuffed endotracheal tubes, it is necessary to subtract half a size from the calculated size because the cuff is located on the outside of the endotracheal tube. Endotracheal tubes a half size larger and a half size smaller than calculated should also be available. An appropriately sized suction catheter should always be available to suction secretions, blood, or fluid from the endotracheal tube (see Table 16.9).

Cuffed Versus Uncuffed Endotracheal Tubes

Although uncuffed endotracheal tubes have historically been used in infants and smaller children, cuffed endotracheal tubes are being increasingly used, especially for short-term intubation in the operating room setting. Cuffed endotracheal tubes have the cuff on the outside, which adds to the external diameter and may necessitate using a 0.5-mm internal diameter smaller than using an uncuffed tube. The smaller internal diameter cuffed tube has more resistance to airflow and increases the work of breathing. This is less significant today, as modern ventilators are better able to accurately deliver tidal volumes at appropriate pressures for small infants and decrease their work of breathing. Using cuffed endotracheal tubes minimizes the need for repeated laryngoscopy, allows for lower fresh gas flows, decreases the amount of inhalational anesthetic used, and decreases the concentrations of anesthetic gases detectable in operating rooms. Using cuffed endotracheal tubes does not increase the incidence of postextubation croup when compared with the use of uncuffed endotracheal tubes.[60,61]

When cuffed endotracheal tubes are used in infants and children, the cuff pressure should be measured and adjusted to maintain a cuff pressure of approximately 20 to 25 cm H_2O. A leak pressure may be used to approximate a cuff pressure, but ideally the cuff pressure should be measured directly with a manometer (see Fig. 16.15), as this will most closely correlate with the pressure of the cuff on the tracheal mucosa. If the cuff pressure is too low, it will be difficult to ventilate the patient with positive pressure. If the cuff pressure is too high, this can cause tracheal mucosal injury, postoperative sore throat, and postextubation croup.[61] In rare cases, often involving prolonged intubation, cuff pressures that are too high can result in tracheal stenosis. If nitrous oxide is used during the case, or in cases in which there is the potential for significant airway edema the cuff pressure should be monitored periodically during the case. The cuff pressure should be measured and recorded in the anesthesia record.

When uncuffed endotracheal tubes are used in infants and children, the leak pressure should be checked. The correct size uncuffed endotracheal tube is one that results in a leak pressure of approximately 20 to 25 cm H_2O. If the uncuffed tube is too large, the leak pressure will be too high. In this situation the endotracheal tube should be replaced with a smaller one to prevent tracheal mucosal injury, postextubation croup, and the possibility of subsequent tracheal stenosis. If the uncuffed tube is too small, the leak pressure will be too low. In this situation it will be difficult to ventilate the patient with positive pressure, and the endotracheal tube should be replaced with a larger one or with a cuffed endotracheal tube. The leak pressure should be measured and documented in the anesthesia record.

Microcuff Endotracheal Tubes

Microcuff pediatric endotracheal tubes offer several distinct advantages over conventional pediatric cuffed endotracheal tubes. Microcuff endotracheal tubes have a cuff made from a microthin polyurethane membrane that is 10 μm thick. The cuff is also cylindrical, rather than round or oval. These tubes seal the airway at lower cuff pressures than conventional endotracheal tubes, reducing the potential for tracheal mucosal edema and postextubation croup; however, using Microcuff endotracheal tubes does not eliminate the incidence of postextubation croup. The appropriately sized endotracheal tube must be used, and the inflation pressure should be measured.[62] The cuff on the Microcuff endotracheal tube is also shorter and placed closer to the tip of the endotracheal tube, which decreases the chances of the cuff herniating above the vocal cords. The Microcuff endotracheal tube has an intubation depth mark indicating the correct depth for insertion, increasing the probability of correct placement. Microcuff endotracheal tubes are available in sizes ranging from 3.0 to 7.0 mm, in 0.5-mm increments.

Stylets

Using a stylet stiffens the endotracheal tube and makes it easier to manipulate during direct laryngoscopy and endotracheal intubation. The appropriately sized stylet should always be immediately available (see Table 16.9).

Laryngoscopes

In general, a straight-blade laryngoscope is easier to use in infants and small children than a curved blade because of its smaller profile. The smaller tip of the straight blade more effectively lifts the epiglottis than the curved blade. However, curved blades have a larger flange that retracts the tongue to the left more effectively and may be useful in patients with larger-than-normal tongues (e.g., Beckwith–Wiedemann syndrome, trisomy 21).

In infants younger than 1 year a Miller 1 straight laryngoscope blade is most useful. In children between 1 and 3 years of age a size 1.5 straight laryngoscope blade, such as a Wis-Hipple, is recommended. A longer straight laryngoscope blade such as a Miller 2 is appropriate for most children between 3 and 10 years of age. The tracheas of children older than 11 years are often more easily intubated with a curved laryngoscope blade, such as a Macintosh 2 or 3. Both straight and curved laryngoscope blades of various sizes should be available.

Video Laryngoscopy

Video laryngoscopes are useful tools for managing both the unexpected and expected difficult pediatric intubation. Video laryngoscopes have a camera and a light source near the tip of the blade and a separate video display. Although direct laryngoscopy requires a direct line of sight to the glottic opening and vocal cords, video laryngoscopy allows the anesthesia provider to view the glottic opening indirectly, without the need for aligning the oral, pharyngeal, and laryngeal axes (see Fig. 16.5). Thus the major advantage of video laryngoscopy over direct laryngoscopy is the ability to see "around the corner" to view the glottic opening and vocal cords, even in patients with limited neck extension, hypoplastic mandibles, or "anterior" airways.

Video laryngoscopy is easier to learn than fiber-optic bronchoscopy because it mimics the skills of direct laryngoscopy. Video laryngoscopy is an excellent tool for teaching laryngoscopy for both routine and difficult airways because both the learner and instructor can view the monitor at the same time.

Video laryngoscopy requires adequate mouth opening to allow space both for placing the video laryngoscope for an optimal view and for manipulating the endotracheal tube so that it is able to pass through the vocal cords. Video laryngoscopy has been shown in studies to improve the ability to see the glottic opening and vocal cords in pediatric patients with both normal and difficult airways and is associated with higher first-attempt success rates and shorter median intubation times than direct laryngoscopy, without increasing complication rates.[63,64]

GlideScope Video Laryngoscopes

The GlideScope video laryngoscopes are available in both reusable and single-use models (see Fig. 16.17). Digital cameras are mounted at the tips of the blades, and the video image is viewed on a separate high-resolution monitor. Recommended reusable GlideScopes for pediatric patients are the Titanium models because of their excellent optics. The reusable Titanium GlideScopes include Macintosh-style curved blades (MAC T3 and MAC T4) and angulated blades (LoPro T2, T3, and T4). The smallest reusable Titanium blade (LoPro T2) can be used in infants as small as 3 kg. The single-use Spectrum GlideScopes are available in a wide variety of pediatric-sized blades, including straight blades (Miller S0 and Miller S1), Macintosh-style curved blades (DVM S3 and S4), and angulated blades (LoPro S1, S2, S3, and S4). The Miller S0 blade can even be used in premature infants under 3 kg. See Table 16.8 for recommended GlideScopes based on patient weight.

C-MAC Video Laryngoscopes

The C-MAC video laryngoscope is also available in both reusable and single-use models. The reusable model consists of a camera with a wide-angle lens mounted at the tip of a reusable stainless steel blade, with a video display on a separate high-resolution monitor. Recommended reusable C-MAC blades for pediatric patients include straight blades (Miller 0 and Miller 1), Macintosh-style curved blades (MAC 0, 2, 3, and 4) and angulated D-blades (pediatric D and adult D) (see Fig 16.18). The pediatric D-blade is designed for children but is too large for small infants. The newer C-MAC Five S single-use line of video laryngoscopes consists of a video display, a light source, and the C-MAC S Imager Camera that fits inside a single-use plastic handle and blade. The single-use C-MAC Five S laryngoscopes come in fewer blade sizes and are currently available with Miller 0, Miller 1, Macintosh 3, Macintosh 4, and angulated adult D-blades. See Table 16.8 for recommended C-MAC video laryngoscope blades based on patient weight.

McGrath MAC Video Laryngoscopes

The McGrath MAC video laryngoscope consists of a reusable video laryngoscope that is inserted into a single-use, plastic, curved blade, with a video display mounted on the handle of the laryngoscope. The McGrath video laryngoscope blades are available in Macintosh-style curved blades (MAC 1, MAC 2, MAC 3, and MAC 4) and in an angulated X3 blade. See Table 16.8 for recommended McGrath video laryngoscopes based on patient weight.

Fiber-Optic Bronchoscopy

A flexible fiber-optic bronchoscope is another tool for managing a difficult pediatric airway. It is particularly valuable when the patient's mouth opening or neck mobility is limited. Disadvantages of a fiber-optic bronchoscope include a limited field of vision and the potential for blood or secretions to obscure the view. The smallest fiber-optic bronchoscopes are 2.2 mm in diameter and can be used for endotracheal tubes as small as 3.0 mm internal diameter. These small bronchoscopes do not have a suction channel and have fewer fiber-optic bundles and inferior optics compared with larger bronchoscopes. In general, the fiber-optic bronchoscope should be at least 1 mm smaller in outside diameter than the internal diameter of the endotracheal tube.

Infants and children are unlikely to be able to cooperate with an awake fiber-optic intubation. Therefore it is often easier to perform an asleep fiber-optic intubation. Some anesthesia providers prefer to maintain spontaneous ventilation during fiber-optic intubation, especially if there is concern about the ability to ventilate the patient's lungs with a facemask. Oxygenation via nasal cannula in infants and children can increase the time available for fiber-optic intubation. Neuromuscular blockade can provide better viewing conditions, as there is no movement, less fogging of the bronchoscope, and less chance of laryngospasm. Using a swivel adaptor with a bronchoscopy port allows either continued spontaneous ventilation or assisted positive-pressure ventilation through the facemask.

For nasal fiber-optic laryngoscopy and endotracheal intubation, a vasoconstrictor, such as oxymetazoline hydrochloride 0.05% nasal spray, should be administered to the nasal mucosa to prevent or minimize nasal bleeding, which makes viewing the glottis and vocal cords more challenging. Phenylephrine should not be administered for vasoconstriction to the nasal mucosa of infants and small children because of the risk of phenylephrine toxicity.

For oral fiber-optic laryngoscopy and endotracheal intubation, an SGA can provide an excellent channel directly to the vocal cords by shielding the bronchoscope from secretions and blood. It is recommended to select the largest endotracheal tube that will easily fit through the SGA and the largest bronchoscope that will fit through the endotracheal tube. If an SGA is used as a conduit for oral fiber-optic laryngoscopy and endotracheal intubation, it can be left in place until the end of the procedure.

Managing the Difficult Airway in Infants and Children

The same general principles for managing a normal pediatric airway apply to managing both an unexpected and an expected difficult pediatric airway. Anesthesia providers should be familiar with algorithms for managing difficult pediatric airways.[65,66] It is unlikely that infants and children will cooperate with procedures such as an awake fiber-optic endotracheal intubation. Therefore, it is often necessary to induce anesthesia and manage the airway with the patient asleep. Infants and children desaturate much more rapidly than adults because their oxygen consumption per kilogram is much higher than adults. This time constraint presents an additional challenge when managing difficult airways in infants and children.

Unexpected Difficult Airway

When an unexpected difficult airway occurs in pediatric patients, the most important first step is to call for an additional anesthesia colleague to help (Fig. 16.22). A surgeon adept in surgical airway management should also be called, as an emergent surgical airway may be necessary. A pediatric difficult airway cart should be obtained, which should include appropriately sized video laryngoscopes; fiber-optic bronchoscopes; and supraglottic, nasal, and oral airways. It is critical that the anesthesia provider not persist with repeated attempts at direct laryngoscopy. This can result in trauma to the upper

Fig. 16.22 Difficult airway infographic: Pediatric patient example. (A) Time out for identification of the airway management plan. A team-based approach with identification of the following is preferred: the primary airway manager and backup manager and role assignment, the primary equipment and the backup equipment, and the person(s) available to help. Contact an ECMO team/otolaryngologic surgeon if noninvasive airway management is likely to fail (e.g., congenital high airway obstruction, airway tumor). (B) Color scheme. The colors represent the ability to oxygenate/ventilate: green, easy oxygenation/ventilation; yellow, difficult or marginal oxygenation/ventilation; and red, impossible oxygenation/ventilation. Reassess oxygenation/ventilation after each attempt, and move to the appropriate box based on the results of the oxygenation/ventilation check. (C) Nonemergency pathway (oxygenation/ventilation adequate for an intubation known or anticipated to be challenging): deliver oxygen throughout airway management; attempt airway management with the technique/device most familiar to the primary airway manager; select from the following devices: supraglottic airway, video laryngoscopy, flexible bronchoscopy, or a combination of these devices (e.g., flexible bronchoscopic intubation through the supraglottic airway); other techniques (e.g., lighted stylets or rigid stylets may be used at the discretion of the clinician); optimize and alternate devices as needed; reassess ventilation after each attempt; limit direct laryngoscopy attempts (e.g., one attempt) with consideration of standard blade video laryngoscopy in lieu of direct laryngoscopy; limit total attempts (insertion of the intubating device until its removal) by the primary airway manager (e.g., three attempts) and one additional attempt by the secondary airway manager; after four attempts, consider emerging the patient and reversing anesthetic drugs if feasible. Clinicians may make further attempts if the risks and benefits to the patient favor continued attempts. (D) Marginal/emergency pathway (poor or no oxygenation/ventilation for an intubation known or anticipated to be challenging): treat functional (e.g., airway reflexes with drugs) and anatomic (mechanical) obstruction; attempt to improve ventilation with facemask, tracheal intubation, and supraglottic airway as appropriate; if all options fail, consider emerging the patient or using advanced invasive techniques. (E) Consider a team debrief after all difficult airway encounters: identify processes that worked well and opportunities for system improvement and provide emotional support to members of the team, particularly when there is patient morbidity or mortality. Developed in collaboration with the Society for Pediatric Anesthesia and the Pediatric Difficult Intubation Collaborative: John E. Fiadjoe, MD, Thomas Engelhardt, MD, PhD, FRCA, Nicola Disma, MD, Narasimhan Jagannathan, MD, MBA, Britta S. von Ungern-Sternberg, MD, PhD, DEAA, FANZCA, and Pete G. Kovatsis, MD, FAAP. (From Apfelbaum JL, Hagberg CA, Connis RT, et al. 2022 American Society of Anesthesiologists practice guidelines for management of the difficult airway. *Anesthesiology*. 2021. doi: 10.1097/ALN.0000000000004002. Epub ahead of print. PMID: 34762729.)

airway, edema, and bleeding. In most situations an SGA should be inserted for rescue oxygenation and ventilation while allowing time to obtain additional personnel and airway equipment. If blood or significant secretions are in the airway, a video laryngoscope is a better option than a pediatric fiber-optic bronchoscope for viewing the glottis and intubating the trachea. SGAs can serve as a conduit for fiber-optic intubation by providing a channel that prevents blood and secretions from obscuring the view.

Expected Difficult Airway

An expected difficult airway in pediatric patients should be approached with caution. Only preanesthetic medications that have minimal ventilatory depressant effects, such as midazolam or dexmedetomidine, should be used. These preanesthetic medications should be administered in a location with pulse oximetry monitoring and

appropriate airway equipment, including suction and a method of delivering oxygen with positive pressure.

An additional anesthesia colleague and a surgeon capable of establishing a surgical airway should be in the operating room before beginning the induction of anesthesia. In certain patients it may be more appropriate to proceed directly to a strategy other than direct laryngoscopy for managing the airway (i.e., SGA, fiber-optic intubation, video laryngoscopy, or surgical airway). The history and physical examination may indicate situations in which direct laryngoscopy will not be successful, such as a patient in halo traction.

Tracheal Extubation in Infants and Children

Deep Versus Awake Extubation

There is no consensus as to whether deep or awake extubation is the better approach in pediatric patients. The

DIFFICULT AIRWAY INFOGRAPHIC: PEDIATRIC PATIENTS

Deliver oxygen/optimize oxygenation

Ensure Appropriate Anesthetic Depth

A — TIME OUT
Airway Management, Backup & Help Plans
Consider ECMO/Elective Invasive Airway

AIRWAY PLAN SUCCESFUL? — YES → Continue as planned

NO

OXYGENATION/VENTILATION ADEQUATE?

YES — CONSIDER CALL FOR HELP
MARGINAL — CALL FOR HELP
NO — CALL FOR HELP

B

C

D — Treat Anatomical & Functional Obstruction

Oxygenation/Ventilation Adequate After Each Attempt? — YES / NO

3+1 Attempts? — YES → Consider Emerging Patient

Failure? — YES

Failure? — YES → Advanced Techniques (E.g., Rigid Bronchoscopy, Emergency Invasive Airway, ECMO)

DEBRIEF E

- Select preferred technique in the Box
- Alternate & Optimize Techniques, Limit Attempts
- Reassess Ventilation After Each Attempt
- Evaluate for Task Fixation, Loss aversion

Facemask   Videolaryngoscopy   Tracheal Tube   Flexible Intubation Scope   Supraglottic Airway

limited number of studies support that deep extubation may decrease the risk of overall airway complications, including cough and desaturation, but may increase airway obstruction compared with awake extubation in pediatric patients after general anesthesia.[67-69]

Postextubation Stridor

Infants and small children are at higher risk than adults for stridor after endotracheal extubation. Postextubation stridor occurs most commonly when an uncuffed endotracheal tube that is too large or a cuffed endotracheal tube that is overinflated is used. The resulting pressure on the tracheal mucosa causes venous congestion and edema. In severe cases the arterial blood supply can be compromised, causing mucosal ischemia. As resistance to flow through the airway is inversely proportional to the radius of the lumen to the fourth power, 1 mm of edema in a pediatric airway is much more significant than 1 mm of edema in an adult airway. Other risk factors for postextubation stridor include multiple endotracheal intubation attempts, unusual positioning of the head during surgery, increased duration of surgery, and procedures involving the upper airway, such as rigid bronchoscopy. Of note, patients with trisomy 21 tend to have narrower subglottic areas and tracheas and are at higher risk for postextubation stridor. Smaller endotracheal tubes should be used for these patients.

An infant or child with postextubation stridor usually presents with respiratory distress in the postanesthesia care unit. Nasal flaring, retractions, an increased respiratory rate, audible stridor, and decreased oxygen saturation are common clinical findings.

Treatment of postextubation stridor depends on the degree of respiratory distress. Mild symptoms can be managed with humidified oxygen and prolonged observation in the postanesthesia care unit. Severe cases may require aerosolized racemic epinephrine and postoperative observation in an intensive care unit. Patients whose respiratory distress is severe and not relieved with these measures may need to be emergently reintubated with a smaller endotracheal tube.

Obstructive Sleep Apnea

Infants and children with obstructive sleep apnea are at significant risk for airway obstruction and respiratory distress in the postoperative period. At baseline, these infants and children hypoventilate, resulting in hypercapnia and often arterial hypoxemia when they sleep. Residual inhaled anesthetics or residual neuromuscular blockade can depress airway reflexes, decrease skeletal muscle tone, and reduce respiratory drive. Opioids must be carefully titrated both intraoperatively and postoperatively, as they can depress ventilatory drive and decrease upper airway tone.

Awake, rather than deep, tracheal extubation in patients with obstructive sleep apnea is safer. All infants and children with obstructive sleep apnea should be monitored postoperatively with pulse oximetry, and high-risk patients should be monitored in an intensive care unit setting.

Laryngospasm

Infants and children are more prone to laryngospasm than older children and adults. Laryngospasm most commonly occurs during either inhalational induction of anesthesia or emergence from anesthesia, often after extubation or removal of an SGA. Most laryngospasm episodes in pediatric patients can be treated successfully with continuous positive-pressure ventilation via facemask with 100% oxygen while applying a chin lift and jaw thrust. The positive pressure may have to be as high as 50 to 60 cm H_2O to successfully break the laryngospasm. If positive pressure is not successful and the infant or child is desaturating or bradycardic, further intervention is necessary. If there is IV access, laryngospasm can be treated with 0.6 to 1.0 mg/kg of IV propofol. If laryngospasm persists, 0.2 to 0.3 mg/kg of IV rocuronium can be administered. If there is no IV access, laryngospasm should be treated with 0.6 to 1.0 mg/kg of intramuscular rocuronium or 1.5 to 2.0 mg/kg of intramuscular succinylcholine.[70]

Extubation After a Difficult Intubation

Tracheal extubation of an infant or child after a difficult intubation should be considered carefully because reintubation can be more difficult than the initial intubation. These patients should be extubated fully awake and after neuromuscular blockade is fully reversed. Appropriate equipment and personnel for urgent reintubation should be available.

Postoperative factors that can further compromise respiratory function must also be considered when extubating infants or children with difficult airways. For example, postoperative pain, especially if there is splinting from an abdominal or thoracic incision, may compromise respiratory function. Postoperative pain requiring significant opioid use will also compromise breathing by decreasing respiratory drive. Regional anesthesia can decrease the use of opioids and may allow earlier extubation.

Edema of the airway from surgical trauma, positioning, or excessive fluid administration can significantly affect the ability to extubate infants and children with difficult airways and can make emergency reintubation more difficult. These patients should remain intubated until the edema has resolved. Fiber-optic laryngoscopy is an excellent tool for examining the SGA in the intubated infant or child for determining whether there is any significant residual airway edema.

ACKNOWLEDGMENT

The editors and publisher would like to thank Dr. Kerry Klinger for contributing to this chapter in the previous editions of this work. It has served as the foundation for the current chapter.

REFERENCES

1. Apfelbaum JL, Hagberg CA, Connis RT, et al. 2022 American Society of Anesthesiologists Practice Guidelines for Management of the Difficult Airway. *Anesthesiology.* 2021. doi:10.1097/ALN.0000000000004002 Nov 11Epub ahead of print. PMID: 34762729 Apfelbaum JL, Hagberg CA, Caplan RA, et al. Practice guidelines for management of the difficult airway: an updated report by the American Society of Anesthesiologists Task Force on Management of the Difficult Airway. Anesthesiology. 2013;118(2):251–270.

2. Cook TM, MacDougall-Davis SR. Complications and failure of airway management. *Br J Anaesth.* 2012;109(suppl1):i68–i85.

3. Sahin-Yilmaz A, Naclerio RM. Anatomy and physiology of the upper airway. *Proc Am Thorac Soc.* 2011;8(1):31–39.

4. Crawley SM, Dalton AJ. Predicting the difficult airway. *Br J Anaesth.* 2015;15(5):253–257.

5. Nagappa M, Wong DT, Cozowicz C, et al. Is obstructive sleep apnea associated with difficult airway? Evidence from a systematic review and meta-analysis of prospective and retrospective cohort studies. *PLoS One.* 2018;13(10):e0204904.

6. Cook TM, Woodall N, Frerk C. Fourth National Audit Project. Major complications of airway management in the UK: Results of the Fourth National Audit Project of the Royal College of Anaesthetists and the Difficult Airway Society. Part 1: Anaesthesia. *Br J Anaesth.* 2011;106(5):617–631.

7. Kheterpal S, Martin L, Shanks AM, et al. Predictors and outcomes of impossible mask ventilation: A review of 50,000 anesthetics. *Anesthesiology.* 2009;110(4):891–897.

8. Roth D, Pace NL, Lee A, et al. Bedside tests for predicting difficult airways: An abridged Cochrane diagnostic test accuracy systematic review. *Anaesthesia.* 2019;74(7):915–928.

9. Baker P. Assessment before airway management. *Anesthesiol Clin.* 2015;33(2):257–278.

10. Khan ZH, Mohammadi M, Rasouli MR, et al. The diagnostic value of the upper lip bite test combined with sternomental distance, thyromental distance, and interincisor distance for prediction of easy laryngoscopy and intubation: A prospective study. *Anesth Analg.* 2009;109(3):822–824.

11. Mallampati SR, Gatt SP, Gugino LD, et al. A clinical sign to predict difficult tracheal intubation: A prospective study. *Can Anaesth Soc J.* 1985;32(4):429–434.

12. Samsoon G, Young J. Difficult tracheal intubation: A retrospective study. *Anaesthesia.* 1987;42(5):487–490.

13. Khan ZH, Kashfi A, Ebrahimkhani E. A comparison of the upper lip bite test (a simple new technique) with modified Mallampati classification in predicting difficulty in endotracheal intubation: A prospective blinded study. *Anesth Analg.* 2003;96(2):595–599.

14. El-Ganzouri AR, McCarthy RJ, Tuman KJ, et al. Preoperative airway assessment: Predictive value of a multivariate risk index. *Anesth Analg.* 1996;82(6):1197–1204.

15. Bellhouse CP, Dore C. Criteria for estimating likelihood of difficulty of endotracheal intubation with the Macintosh laryngoscope. *Anaesth Intensive Care.* 1988;16(3):329–337.

16. Kheterpal S, Healy D, Aziz MF, et al. Incidence, predictors, and outcome of difficult mask ventilation combined with difficult laryngoscopy: A report from the Multicenter Perioperative Outcomes Group. *Anesthesiology.* 2013;119(6):1360–1369.

17. Law JA, Broemling N, Cooper RM, et al. The difficult airway with recommendations for management—part 2—the anticipated difficult airway. *Can J Anesth.* 2013;60(11):1119–1138.

18. Siddiqui N, Yu E, Boulis S, You-Ten KE. Ultrasound is superior to palpation in identifying the cricothyroid membrane in subjects with poorly defined neck landmarks: A randomized clinical trial. *Anesthesiology.* 2018;129(6):1132–1139.

19. Kristensen MS, Teoh WH, Rudolph SS. Ultrasonographic identification of the cricothyroid membrane: Best evidence, techniques, and clinical impact. *Br J Anaesth.* 2016;117(Suppl 1):i39–i48.

20. Law JA, Broemling N, Cooper RM, et al. The difficult airway with recommendations for management—part 1—difficult tracheal intubation encountered in an unconscious/induced patient. *Can J Anesth.* 2013;60(11):1089–1118.

21. El-Orbany M, Woehlck HJ. Difficult mask ventilation. *Anesth Analg.* 2009;109(6):1870–1880.

22. Benumof JL, Dagg R, Benumof R. Critical hemoglobin desaturation will occur before return to an unparalyzed state following 1 mg/kg intravenous succinylcholine. *Anesthesiology.* 1997;87(4):979–982.

23. Bouroche G, Bourgain JL. Preoxygenation and general anesthesia: A review. *Minerva Anestesiol.* 2015;81(8):910–920.

24. Dixon BJ, Dixon JB, Carden JR, et al. Preoxygenation is more effective in the 25 degrees head-up position than in the supine position in severely obese patients: A randomized controlled study. *Anesthesiology.* 2005(102):1110–1115.

25. Collins JS, Lemmens HJ, Brodsky JB, et al. Laryngoscopy and morbid obesity: A comparison of the "sniff" and "ramped" positions. *Obes Surg.* 2004;14(9):1171–1175.

26. Futier E, Constantin JM, Pelosi P, et al. Noninvasive ventilation and alveolar recruitment maneuver improve respiratory function during and after intubation of morbidly obese patients: A randomized controlled study. *Anesthesiology.* 2011;114(6):1354–1363.

27. Hernandez MR, Klock PA Jr, Ovassapian A. Evolution of the extraglottic airway: A review of its history, applications, and practical tips for success. *Anesth Analg.* 2012;114(2):349–368.

28. Timmermann A. Supraglottic airways in difficult airway management: Successes, failures, use and misuse. *Anaesthesia.* 2011;66(suppl 2):45–56.

28a. Law JA, Broemling N, Cooper RM, et al. The difficult airway with recommendations for management—part 2—the anticipated difficult airway. *Can J Anesth.* 2013;60(11):1119–1138.

29. Ramachandran SK, Mathis MR, Tremper KK, et al. Predictors and clinical outcomes from failed laryngeal mask airway unique: A study of 15,795 patients. *Anesthesiology.* 2012;116(6):1217–1226.

30. L'Hermite J, Dubout E, Bouvet S, et al. Sore throat following three adult supraglottic airway devices: A randomised controlled trial. *Eur J Anaesthesiol.* 2017;34(7):417–424.

31. Wong DT, Yang JJ, Jagannathan N. Brief review: The LMA supreme supraglottic airway. *Can J Anesth J.* 2012;59(5):483–493.

32. de Montblanc J, Ruscio L, Mazoit JX. Benhamou D. A systematic review and meta-analysis of the i-gel(®) vs laryngeal mask airway in adults. *Anaesthesia.* 2014;69(10):1151–1162.

33. Cormack R, Lehane J. Difficult tracheal intubation in obstetrics. *Anaesthesia.* 1984;39(11):1105–1111.

34. Smith KJ, Dobranowski J, Yip G, et al. Cricoid pressure displaces the esophagus: An observational study using magnetic resonance imaging. *Anesthesiology.* 2003;99(1):60–64.

35. Salem MR, Khorasani A, Zeidan A, Crystal GJ. Cricoid pressure controversies: Narrative review. *Anesthesiology.* 2017;126(4):738–752.

36. Joffe AM, Aziz MF, Posner KL, Duggan LV, Mincer SL, Domino KB. Management of difficult tracheal intubation: A

closed claims analysis. *Anesthesiology.* 2019;131(4):818–829.

37. Patel A, Nouraei SA. Transnasal Humidified Rapid-Insufflation Ventilatory Exchange (THRIVE): A physiological method of increasing apnoea time in patients with difficult airways. *Anaesthesia.* 2015;70(3):323–329.

38. Griesdale DE, Liu D, McKinney J, Choi PT. Glidescope® video-laryngoscopy versus direct laryngoscopy for endotracheal intubation: A systematic review and meta-analysis. *Can J Anesth.* 2012;59(1):41–52.

39. Aziz MF, Dillman D, Fu R, Brambrink AM. Comparative effectiveness of the C-MAC video laryngoscope versus direct laryngoscopy in the setting of the predicted difficult airway. *Anesthesiology.* 2012;116(3):629–636.

40. Paolini J, Donati F, Drolet P. Review article: Video-laryngoscopy: Another tool for difficult intubation or a new paradigm in airway management? *Can J Anesth.* 2013;60(2):184–191.

41. De Jong A, Pardo E, Rolle A, Bodin-Lario S, Pouzeratte Y, Jaber S. Airway management for COVID-19: A move towards universal videolaryngoscope? *Lancet Respir Med.* 2020;8(6):555.

42. Zeidan A, Bamadhaj M, Al-Faraidy M, Ali M. Videolaryngoscopy intubation in patients with COVID-19: How to minimize risk of aerosolization? *Anesthesiology.* 2020;133:481–483.

43. Rosenstock CV, Thogersen B, Afshari A, et al. Awake fiberoptic or awake video laryngoscopic tracheal intubation in patients with anticipated difficult airway management: A randomized clinical trial. *Anesthesiology.* 2012;116(6):1210–1216.

44. Serocki G, Neumann T, Scharf E, et al. Indirect videolaryngoscopy with C-MAC D-blade and GlideScope: A randomized, controlled comparison in patients with suspected difficult airways. *Minerva Anestesiol.* 2013;79(2):121–129.

45. Aziz MF, Healy D, Kheterpal S, et al. Routine clinical practice effectiveness of the Glidescope in difficult airway management: An analysis of 2,004 Glidescope intubations, complications, and failures from two institutions. *Anesthesiology.* 2011;114(1):34–41.

46. Hoshijima H, Mihara T, Maruyama K, et al. C-MAC videolaryngoscope versus Macintosh laryngoscope for tracheal intubation: A systematic review and meta-analysis with trial sequential analysis. *J Clin Anesth.* 2018;49:53–62.

47. Duggan LV, Law JA, Murphy MF. Brief review: Supplementing oxygen through an airway exchange catheter: Efficacy, complications, and recommendations. *Can J Anesth.* 2011;58(6):560–568.

48. Simmons ST, Schleich AR. Airway regional anesthesia for awake fiberoptic intubation. *Reg Anesth Pain Med.* 2002;27(2):180–192.

49. Webb A, Kolawole H, Leong S, Loughnan TE, Crofts T, Bowden C. Comparison of the Bonfils and Levitan optical stylets for tracheal intubation: A clinical study. *Anaesth Intensive Care.* 2011;39(6):1093–1097.

50. Thong SY, Wong TG. Clinical uses of the Bonfils Retromolar Intubation Fiberscope: A review. *Anesth Analg.* 2012;115(4):855–866.

51. Kristensen MS, Teoh WH, Baker PA. Percutaneous emergency airway access; prevention, preparation, technique and training. *Br J Anaesth.* 2015;114(3):357–361.

52. Hamaekers A, Henderson J. Equipment and strategies for emergency tracheal access in the adult patient. *Anaesthesia.* 2011;66(suppl 2):65–80.

53. Mitchell V, Dravid R, Patel A, et al. Difficult airway society guidelines for the management of tracheal extubation. *Anaesthesia.* 2012;67(3):318–340.

54. Cavallone LF, Vannucci A. Review article: Extubation of the difficult airway and extubation failure. *Anesth Analg.* 2013;116(2):368–383.

55. Hagberg C, Georgi R, Krier C. Complications of managing the airway. *Best Pract Res Clin Anaesthesiol.* 2005;19(4):641–659.

56. Warner ME, Benenfeld SM, Warner MA, et al. Perianesthetic dental injuries: Frequency, outcomes, and risk factors. *Anesthesiology.* 1999;90(5):1302–1305.

57. Kain ZN, Mayes LC, Caldwell-Andrews AA, Karas DE, McClain BC. Preoperative anxiety, postoperative pain, and behavioral recovery in young children undergoing surgery. *Pediatrics.* 2006;118(2):651–658.

58. Kain ZN, Caldwell-Andrews AA, Maranets I, et al. Preoperative anxiety and emergence delirium and postoperative maladaptive behaviors. *Anesth Analg.* 2004;99(6):1648–1654.

59. Wong JG, Heaney M, Chambers NA, Erb TO, von Ungern-Sternberg BS. Impact of laryngeal mask airway cuff pressures on the incidence of sore throat in children. *Paediatr Anaesth.* 2009;19(5):464–469.

60. Weiss M, Dullenkopf A, Fischer JE, et al. European Paediatric Endotracheal Intubation Study Group. Prospective randomized controlled multi-centre trial of cuffed or uncuffed endotracheal tubes in small children. *Br J Anaesth.* 2009;103(6):867–873.

61. Liu J, Zhang X, Gong W, et al. Correlations between controlled endotracheal tube cuff pressure and postprocedural complications: A multicenter study. *Anesth Analg.* 2010;111(5):1133–1137.

62. Sathyamoorthy M, Lerman J, Lakshminrusimha S, Feldman D. Inspiratory stridor after tracheal intubation with a MicroCuff(R) tracheal tube in three young infants. *Anesthesiology.* 2013;118(3):748–750.

63. Smereka J, Madziala M, Dunder D, Makomaska-Szaroszyk E, Szarpak L. Comparison of Miller laryngoscope and UEScope videolaryngoscope for endotracheal intubation in four pediatric airway scenarios: A randomized, crossover simulation trial. *Eur J Pediatr.* 2019;178(6):937–945.

64. Park R, Peyton JM, Fiadjoe JE, et al. PeDI Collaborative Investigators; PeDI Collaborative Investigators. The efficacy of GlideScope® videolaryngoscopy compared with direct laryngoscopy in children who are difficult to intubate: An analysis from the paediatric difficult intubation registry. *Br J Anaesth.* 2017 Nov 1;119(5):984–992.

65. Krishna SG, Bryant JF, Tobias JD. Management of the difficult airway in the pediatric patient. *J Pediatr Intensive Care.* 2018;7(3):115–125.

66. Weiss M, Engelhardt T. Proposal for the management of the unexpected difficult pediatric airway. *Paediatr Anaesth.* 2010;20(5):454–464.

67. Koo CH, Lee SY, Chung SH, Ryu JH. Deep vs. awake extubation and LMA removal in terms of airway complications in pediatric patients undergoing anesthesia: A systemic review and meta-analysis. *J Clin Med.* 2018 Oct 14;7(10):353.

68. Von Ungern-Sternberg BS, Davies K, Hegarty M, Erb TO, Habre W. The effect of deep vs. awake extubation on respiratory complications in high-risk children undergoing adenotonsillectomy: A randomised controlled trial. *Eur J Anaesthesiol.* 2013;30(9):529–536.

69. Baijal RG, Bidani SA, Minard CG, Watcha MF. Perioperative respiratory complications following awake and deep extubation in children undergoing adenotonsillectomy. *Paediatr Anaesth.* 2015;25(4):392–399.

70. Orliaguet GA, Gall O, Savoldelli GL, Couloigner V. Case scenario: Perianesthetic management of laryngospasm in children. *Anesthesiology.* 2012;116(2):458–471.

17 SPINAL, EPIDURAL, AND CAUDAL ANESTHESIA

Alan J.R. Macfarlane, David W. Hewson, Richard Brull

PRINCIPLES

Spinal, epidural, and caudal blocks are collectively referred to as *central neuraxial blocks*. Significant procedural, physiological, and pharmacological differences exist between the techniques, but all blocks result in some combination of sympathetic, sensory, and motor blockade. Spinal anesthesia requires a small amount of drug to produce rapid, profound, reproducible, but finite neuraxial blockade. In contrast, epidural anesthesia typically progresses more slowly, is commonly prolonged using a catheter, and requires a comparatively larger volume of local anesthetic, which may be associated with systemic side effects and complications unknown to spinal anesthesia. Combined spinal and epidural techniques blur some of these differences but add flexibility to clinical care.

[1]The editors and publisher would like to thank Drs. Kenneth Drasner, Merlin D. Larson, and Vincent Chan for contributing to this chapter in previous editions of this work. It has served as the foundation for the current chapter.

PRACTICE

Central neuraxial blocks are widely used in surgery, obstetrics, acute postoperative pain management, and the field of chronic pain. A single-injection spinal or epidural is commonly used to provide anesthesia for surgery to the lower abdomen, pelvic organs (e.g., prostate), and lower limbs, as well as for cesarean deliveries. Continuous catheter-based epidural infusions are most often used for obstetric labor analgesia and to provide postoperative pain relief after major thoracoabdominal or lower limb surgery. When epidural analgesia is used as a component of enhanced recovery after surgery protocols, this must be balanced against possible motor block and a reduction in mobility. Caudal blocks are mostly performed for surgical anesthesia and analgesia in children (also see Chapter 34) and for therapeutic analgesia in adults with chronic pain (also see Chapter 44). Indwelling long-term spinal catheters may be inserted for chronic malignant and nonmalignant pain.

EVIDENCE

The impact of neuraxial anesthesia and analgesia on perioperative morbidity and mortality is a challenging and ongoing matter of investigation. In brief, when compared with systemic opioid analgesia, epidural analgesia is superior and improves respiratory outcomes in adults undergoing noncardiac surgery.[1] However, recent evidence suggests cardiovascular complications such as myocardial infarction may be increased when epidural analgesia is combined with general anesthesia.[2] Overall, all outcome benefits appear to be greatest when neuraxial anesthesia is used alone rather than combined with general anesthesia.[2]

ANATOMY

The spinal cord is continuous with the medulla oblongata proximally and terminates distally in the conus medullaris as the filum terminale (fibrous extension) and cauda equina (neural extension) (Fig. 17.1). This distal termination varies from L3 in infants to the lower border of L1 in adults.

The spinal cord lies within the bony vertebral canal and is surrounded by three membranes: from innermost to outermost, the pia mater, the arachnoid mater, and the dura mater (Fig. 17.2). The pia mater is a highly vascular

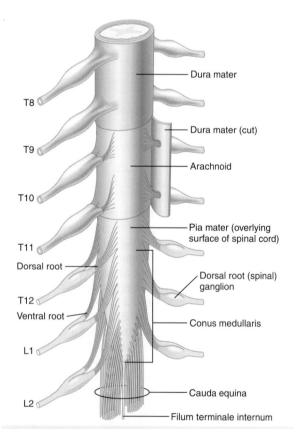

Fig. 17.1 Terminal spinal cord and cauda equina. (From Bridenbaugh PO, Greene NM, Brull SJ. Spinal [subarachnoid] blockade. In Cousins MJ, Bridenbaugh PO, eds. Neural Blockade in Clinical Anesthesia and Management of Pain. Philadelphia: Lippincott-Raven; 1998:203–242.)

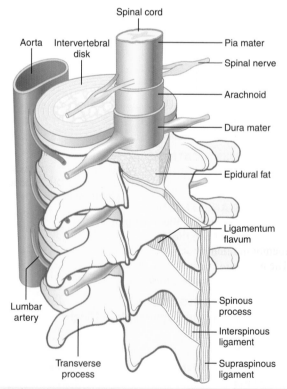

Fig. 17.2 The spine in an oblique view. (From Afton-Bird G. Atlas of regional anesthesia. In Miller RD, ed. Miller's Anesthesia. Philadelphia: Elsevier; 2005.)

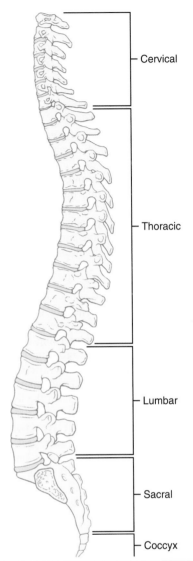

Fig. 17.3 The vertebral column from a lateral view exhibits four curvatures. (From Covino BG, Scott DB, Lambert DH. Handbook of Spinal Anaesthesia and Analgesia. Philadelphia: WB Saunders; 1994:12–24.)

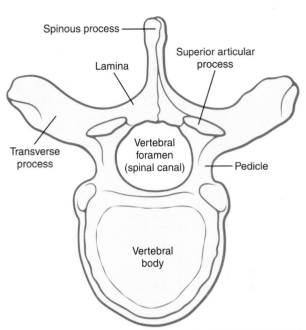

Fig. 17.4 Typical thoracic vertebra. (From Covino BG, Scott DB, Lambert DH. Handbook of Spinal Anaesthesia and Analgesia. Philadelphia: WB Saunders; 1994.)

membrane that closely invests the spinal cord and brain. The arachnoid mater is a delicate, nonvascular membrane and is the principal barrier to drugs crossing into (and out of) the cerebrospinal fluid (CSF). The dura mater is a tough fibroelastic membrane. CSF resides in the subarachnoid (or *intrathecal*) space between the pia mater and the arachnoid mater.

Surrounding the dura from the foramen magnum to the sacral hiatus is the epidural space. The epidural space is bounded anteriorly by the posterior longitudinal ligament, laterally by the pedicles and intervertebral foramina, and posteriorly by the ligamentum flavum. Contents include nerve roots, fat, areolar tissue, lymphatics, and blood vessels.

The ligamentum flavum (Latin for "yellow ligament") also extends from the foramen magnum to the sacral hiatus and is composed of right and left ligamenta flava, which join to form an acute midline angle (see Fig. 17.2).[3] At some vertebral levels (particularly in the cervical and high thoracic spine), midline gaps in the continuity of the ligamentum flavum may exist.[4] Ligament thickness, distance from the ligament to the dura, and skin-to-dura distance also show significant interindividual variability. The vertebral canal is triangular and largest in cross-sectional area at the lumbar levels, whereas it is circular and smallest in area at the thoracic levels. Immediately posterior to the ligamentum flavum are either the lamina of vertebral bodies or the interspinous ligaments (which connect the spinous processes). Finally there is the supraspinous ligament, which extends from the seventh cervical vertebra to the sacrum and attaches to the vertebral spinous processes (see Fig. 17.2).

There are 7 cervical, 12 thoracic, and 5 lumbar vertebrae and a sacrum (Fig. 17.3). The vertebral arch, spinous process, pedicles, and laminae form the posterior elements of the vertebra, and the vertebral body forms the anterior element (Fig. 17.4). The vertebrae are joined anteriorly by fibrocartilaginous joints with central discs containing the nucleus pulposus and posteriorly by the zygapophyseal (facet) joints. Thoracic spinous processes are angulated more steeply caudad as opposed to the almost horizontal angulation of the lumbar spinous processes. These differences are clinically important for needle insertion and advancement (Fig. 17.5).

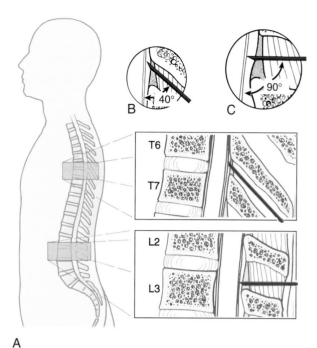

A

Fig. 17.5 Lumbar and thoracic epidural technique. The cephalad (acute) angle of needle insertion during thoracic epidural cannulation may provide a slightly longer distance of "needle travel" before entering the epidural space (A). In contrast, during lumbar epidural cannulation (B) the distance traveled is modified by a more perpendicular angle of needle insertion (C). (From Brull R, Macfarlane AJR, Chan VWS. Spinal, epidural and caudal anesthesia. In Miller RD, Cohen NH, Eriksson LI, et al, eds. Miller's Anesthesia. 8th ed. Philadelphia: Saunders Elsevier; 2015:Fig. 56.9.)

The sacral canal contains the terminal portion of the dural sac, which typically ends at S2 in adults and lower in children. The sacral canal also contains a venous plexus.

Spinal Nerves

Dorsal (afferent) and ventral (efferent) nerve roots merge distal to the dorsal root ganglion to form spinal nerves (Fig. 17.6). There are 31 pairs of spinal nerves (8 cervical, 12 thoracic, 5 lumbar, 5 sacral, and 1 coccygeal). The nerves pass through the intervertebral foramen, ensheathed by the dura, arachnoid, and pia, which, respectively, become the epineurium, the perineurium, and the endoneurium. Preganglionic sympathetic fibers originate in the intermediolateral gray columns between T1 and L2 and pass via the ventral nerve root to the paravertebral sympathetic ganglia and more distant plexuses (Fig. 17.7).

Blood Supply

Two posterior spinal arteries supply the posterior one-third of the spinal cord, whereas the anterior two-thirds of the spinal cord are supplied by a single anterior spinal artery (Fig. 17.8). One of the largest anastomotic feeder arteries to the anterior system is the artery of Adamkiewicz, which arises from the aorta and enters an intervertebral foramen between T7 and L4 on the left. Infarction in the territory of the anterior spinal artery leads to *anterior spinal artery syndrome,* classically manifesting as motor weakness and loss of pain and temperature sensation below the affected spinal level, but with retention of proprioception and vibratory sense because of the

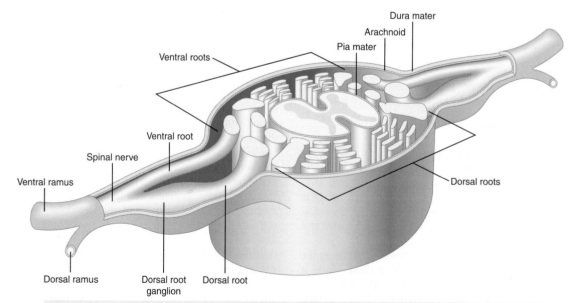

Fig. 17.6 The spinal cord and nerve roots. (From Covino BG, Scott DB, Lambert DH. Handbook of Spinal Anaesthesia and Analgesia. Philadelphia: WB Saunders; 1994:19.)

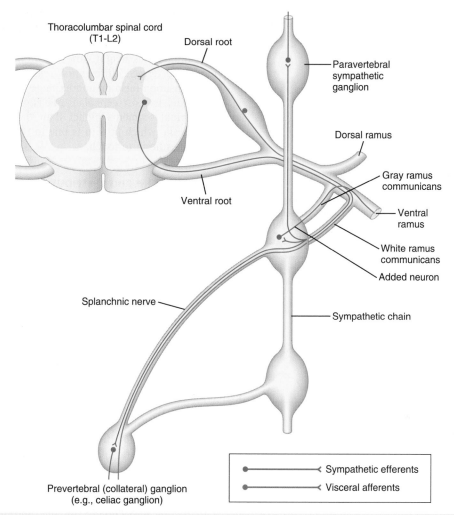

Thoracolumbar spinal cord (T1-L2)

Dorsal root

Paravertebral sympathetic ganglion

Dorsal ramus

Gray ramus communicans

Ventral ramus

Ventral root

White ramus communicans

Added neuron

Splanchnic nerve

Sympathetic chain

Prevertebral (collateral) ganglion (e.g., celiac ganglion)

Sympathetic efferents

Visceral afferents

Fig. 17.7 Cell bodies in the thoracolumbar portion of the spinal cord (T1–L2) give rise to the peripheral sympathetic nervous system. Preganglionic efferent fibers travel in the ventral root and then via the white ramus communicans to paravertebral sympathetic ganglia or more distant sites such as the celiac ganglion. Afferent fibers travel via the white ramus communicans to join somatic nerves, which pass through the dorsal root to the spinal cord.

preserved blood supply to the dorsal columns. Ischemia and infarction may result from profound systemic hypotension, thrombosis or emboli, vasculopathy, trauma, or as a consequence of surgery to the aorta.

Longitudinal anterior and posterior spinal veins communicate with segmental anterior and posterior radicular veins before draining into the internal vertebral venous plexus in the medial and lateral components of the epidural space. These drain into the azygous system.

Anatomic Variations

Variations exist in size and structure of the spinal nerve roots and CSF volume, both of which may contribute to variability in spinal block quality, height, and regression

time. Similarly, the epidural space is more segmented and less uniform than previously believed, which may be a factor in the unpredictability of drug spread. Finally, contents of the epidural space also vary and can influence the volume of local anesthetic required.

MECHANISM OF ACTION

Administration of local anesthetics to the neuraxis disrupts nerve transmission within the spinal cord, the spinal nerve roots, and the dorsal root ganglia. Nerves in the subarachnoid space are easily anesthetized, even with a small dose of local anesthetic, compared with the extradural nerves, which are often ensheathed by dura

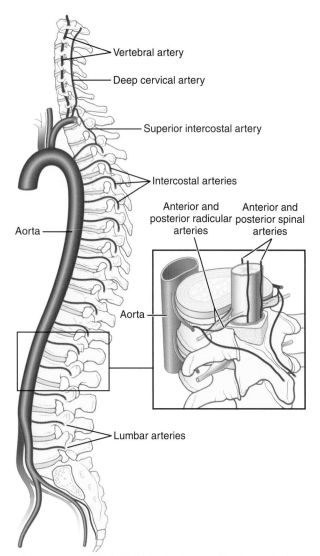

Vertebral artery

Deep cervical artery

Superior intercostal artery

Intercostal arteries

Anterior and posterior radicular arteries

Anterior and posterior spinal arteries

Aorta

Aorta

Lumbar arteries

Fig. 17.8 Arterial blood supply to the spinal cord. (Modified from Covino BG, Scott DB, Lambert DH. Handbook of Spinal Anaesthesia and Analgesia. Philadelphia: WB Saunders; 1994:24.)

mater (the "dural sleeve"). The speed of neural blockade depends on the size, surface area, and degree of myelination of the nerve fibers exposed to the local anesthetic. Small preganglionic sympathetic fibers (B fibers, 1 to 3 μm, moderately myelinated) are most sensitive to local anesthetic blockade. Unmyelinated polymodal ("slow" pain) C fibers (0.3 to 1 μm) are blocked more readily than the myelinated A-delta pinprick sensation fibers (1 to 4 μm) responsible for cold sensation, which in turn are blocked more readily than heavily myelinated A-beta fibers (5 to 12 μm) conducting touch sensation. Large myelinated A-alpha motor fibers (12 to 20 μm) are

the most resistant to local anesthetic blockade. Clinical onset of spinal blockade usually follows this pattern, with block regression occurring in the reverse order.[5] Maximum block height varies according to each sensory modality, termed *differential sensory block.* Therefore cold sensation (also an approximate level of sympathetic blockade) is most cephalad and is, on average, one to two spinal segments higher than the level of pinprick anesthesia, which in turn is one to two segments higher than anesthesia to touch.

Drug Uptake and Distribution

Local anesthetic injected directly into the CSF diffuses from areas of high concentration toward other segments of the spinal cord.[6] Local anesthetic diffuses through the pia mater and penetrates through the spaces of Virchow-Robin (extensions of the subarachnoid space accompanying the blood vessels that invaginate the spinal cord from the pia mater) to reach the deeper dorsal root ganglia. A portion of the subarachnoid drug diffuses outward to enter the epidural space, and some is taken up by the blood vessels of the pia and dura maters.

Drug penetration and uptake are directly proportionate to the drug mass, CSF drug concentration, contact surface area, lipid content (high in spinal cord and myelinated nerves), and local tissue vascular supply, but inversely related to nerve root cross-sectional area.

Epidural drug uptake and distribution are more complex. Some of the injected local anesthetic (<20%) traverses the dura into the CSF[7] and some is absorbed into the plasma compartment, but the majority spreads by bulk flow longitudinally and circumferentially within the epidural space and is taken up by epidural fat. Factors that may enhance the distribution of local anesthetic within the epidural space are small epidural space cross-sectional area (resulting in greater spread in the thoracic levels), decreased epidural space compliance, decreased epidural fat content, decreased local anesthetic leakage through the intervertebral foramina (e.g., in the elderly and those with spinal stenosis), and increased epidural venous engorgement (e.g., during pregnancy).[8] The direction of drug spread also varies with the vertebral level. Spread is mostly cephalad in the lumbar and low thoracic region, but caudad after a high thoracic injection.[8]

Drug Elimination

No local anesthetic drug metabolism takes place in the CSF. Regression of neural blockade arises primarily from a decline in CSF and/or epidural drug concentration resulting from vascular absorption. Local anesthetics with higher lipid solubility (e.g., bupivacaine) form a depot within epidural fat, thereby slowing this process.

PHYSIOLOGIC EFFECTS

Neuraxial anesthesia causes blockade of the sympathetic and somatic (sensory and motor) nervous systems. The physiologic effects of epidural anesthesia are similar to those of spinal anesthesia, with the exception that local anesthetic blood levels reach concentrations sufficient enough to produce systemic effects on their own.

Cardiovascular

Blockade of the peripheral (T1–L2) and cardiac (T1–T4) sympathetic fibers reduces systemic vascular resistance (SVR) and, to a much lesser extent, cardiac output, commonly resulting in arterial hypotension after spinal or epidural blockade. The degree to which arterial blood pressure decreases with either spinal or epidural technique depends on multiple factors.

Systemic Vascular Resistance

The vasodilatory changes depend on both baseline sympathetic tone (i.e., higher baseline sympathetic nervous system activity in older patients equates to a greater SVR reduction and consequent hypotension compared with younger patients)[9] and the extent of the sympathectomy (i.e., the height of the block). The sympathectomy typically extends two to six dermatomes cephalad to the sensory block level with spinal anesthesia but the same level with epidural anesthesia.[10]

Cardiac Output

Cardiac output is the product of heart rate and stroke volume, and it is generally either maintained or slightly decreased during the onset of spinal anesthesia. Venous and arterial vasodilation reduces preload (venous return) and afterload (SVR), respectively. Because 75% of the total blood volume resides in the venous system, the venodilation effect predominates and stroke volume is reduced. Despite a compensatory baroreceptor-mediated sympathetic response (vasoconstriction and increased heart rate) above the level of blockade, the reduction in venous return and right atrial filling reduce signal output from intrinsic atrial and great vein chronotropic stretch receptors,[10] thereby increasing parasympathetic activity. The two opposing responses result in a minimal change in heart rate unless neuraxial anesthesia is extended to the T1 level when blockade of the cardioaccelerator fibers (in addition to a marked reduction in venous return) may result in severe bradycardia and even asystole. The Bezold-Jarisch reflex can also cause profound bradycardia and circulatory collapse after spinal anesthesia, especially in the presence of hypovolemia, when a small end-systolic left ventricular volume may trigger a mechanoreceptor-mediated bradycardia.[11]

Central Nervous System

Spinal anesthesia–induced hypotension may decrease cerebral blood flow (CBF) in older patients and those with preexisting hypertension. However, in studies that demonstrated a decrease in cerebral perfusion[12] there was no postoperative change in cognitive function in any of the patients. Nevertheless avoiding hypotension would seem prudent. Spinal anesthesia has been shown to result in significant patient sedation in the absence of systemic sedatives caused by decreased afferent stimulation of the reticular activating system.[13] Intravenous sedative and hypnotic drug doses should be reduced accordingly in the context of concomitant neuraxial blockade.

Respiratory

Alterations in pulmonary variables during lumbar and low thoracic neuraxial block are usually of little clinical importance. A decrease in vital capacity follows a reduction in expiratory reserve volume related to paralysis of the abdominal muscles necessary for forced exhalation and cough rather than a decrease in phrenic or diaphragmatic function. These changes are more marked in obese patients and those with severe respiratory disease.[14] In the postoperative setting of thoracoabdominal surgery the analgesic benefits of neuraxial techniques render improvements in respiratory function that outweigh the modest changes described earlier arising from the blockade itself.[14]

Gastrointestinal

Neuraxial blockade from T5 to L1 disrupts splanchnic sympathetic innervation to the gastrointestinal tract, resulting in increased colonic mucosal blood flow and motility because of unopposed parasympathetic (vagal) activity. These local effects may be opposed by the direct arterial blood pressure–dependent effect on intestinal perfusion caused by thoracic epidural-induced hypotension.[15] Correction of systemic hypotension by vasopressor therapy (e.g., norepinephrine) reverses impaired colonic perfusion. The impact of neuraxial analgesia on clinically relevant gastrointestinal outcomes such as anastomotic healing and postoperative ileus remains an area of ongoing research and some controversy.

Renal

Despite a predictable decrease in renal blood flow accompanying neuraxial blockade, this decrease is of little physiologic importance. The belief that neuraxial blocks frequently cause urinary retention is questionable (see "Complications").

INDICATIONS

Neuraxial Anesthesia

Single-injection spinal anesthesia is useful for procedures of known duration involving the lower limbs, perineum, pelvis, or lower abdomen. It is especially useful when patients wish to remain conscious or when one or more comorbid conditions, such as severe respiratory disease or an airway that may be difficult to manage, increases the risks of general anesthesia. Epidural anesthesia allows for more prolonged surgical anesthesia by catheter-based local anesthetic delivery. Indwelling catheter-based spinal anesthesia is less conventional, but may be useful when insertion of an epidural catheter is challenging or in the setting of severe cardiac disease when the reliability of a single-shot spinal anesthetic must be combined with the hemodynamic stability of low-dose incremental adminstration.

Neuraxial Analgesia

Spinal or epidural local anesthetics, along with other additives such as opioids, provide excellent-quality, long-lasting intraoperative and postoperative analgesia for labor and delivery[16] (also see Chapter 33), hip[17] or knee replacement[18] (also see Chapter 32), laparotomy,[19] thoracotomy (also see Chapter 27),[20] and even after cardiac surgery (also see Chapter 26).[21] Neuraxial local anesthetics may also be used in the management of chronic pain (also see Chapter 44).

CONTRAINDICATIONS

Absolute

Absolute contraindications to neuraxial blockade are patient refusal, localized infection at the needle insertion site and allergy to any of the drugs to be administered. A patient's inability to maintain stillness during needle puncture (which could expose neural structures to traumatic injury),[22] as well as increased intracranial pressure (which may predispose to brainstem herniation)[23] are also considered strong contraindications to a neuraxial technique.

Relative

Relative contraindications can be approached by system and must be weighed against the potential benefits of neuraxial blockade.

Neurologic
Myelopathy or Peripheral Neuropathy
Although preexisting central or peripheral neurologic deficit has never been definitively demonstrated to increase susceptibility to injury after neuraxial anesthesia or analgesia (the double-crush phenomenon), the risk-benefit ratio of performing neuraxial techniques should be considered carefully in patients with preexisting central or peripheral neurologic diseases. Chronic low back pain without neurologic deficit is not a contraindication to neuraxial blockade.

Spinal Stenosis
There is an association between the presence of spinal stenosis and nerve injury after neuraxial techniques.[24] When suspected nerve injury occurs in patients with underlying spinal stenosis, the relative causative contributions of neuraxial needling, local anesthetic maldistribution, surgical positioning, and natural history of cord or nerve root impingement from the stenosis itself are often unclear. Asymptomatic and undiagnosed spinal stenosis is relatively common in the elderly, and the vast majority undergo neuraxial blockade without incident.

Previous Spine Surgery
Previous spine surgery does not predispose patients to an increased risk of neurologic complications.[24] However, in the presence of scar tissue, adhesions, hardware, or bone grafts, needle access to the CSF or epidural space and epidural catheter insertion may be challenging or impossible. In addition, the resultant spread of local anesthetic in the CSF or epidural space in particular can be unpredictable and incomplete.

Multiple Sclerosis
Because of the demyelinating pathology, patients with multiple sclerosis (MS) may be more sensitive to neuraxial local anesthetics and exhibit a prolonged motor and sensory blockade. There is no conclusive evidence that neuraxial blockade itself worsens MS symptoms, and neuraxial techniques are not absolutely contraindicated in this patient group.[25]

Spina Bifida
Depending on the severity of the neural tube defect, the potential for traumatic needle injury to the spinal cord may be increased. The spread of local anesthetic in the CSF and epidural space (if present) can also be markedly variable. In any of these circumstances a careful evaluation of neurologic status must first be undertaken and noted along with documentation of the discussion of the risks and benefits.

Cardiac (Also See Chapter 26)
Aortic Stenosis or Fixed Cardiac Output
The potential rapid and significant reduction in SVR after spinal anesthesia risks dangerous decreases in coronary perfusion in afterload-dependent patients.[26] In the presence of aortic stenosis, neuraxial anesthesia

must be considered on an individual patient basis in the context of disease severity, left ventricular function, and case urgency. Invasive continuous blood pressure monitoring, concurrent vasopressor infusion, and/or a catheter-based neuraxial anesthetic with repeated small doses of local anesthetic facilitate hemodynamic control.

Hypovolemia

An exaggerated hypotensive response because of vaso-dilatory effects may occur, and euvolemia should be targeted before and during neuraxial anesthesia to minimize relative hypotension.

Hematologic

Thromboprophylaxis and Antithrombotic and Thrombolytic Therapy

Catastrophic cases of epidural (or subdural) hematoma and permanent paralysis after neuraxial techniques in patients on various anticoagulant medications, including low-molecular-weight heparin (LMWH), have occurred. The American Society of Regional Anesthesia and Pain Medicine (ASRA) guidelines regarding neuraxial techniques (including catheter removal) in patients receiving antiplatelet, heparin, anti–factor Xa, and direct oral anticoagulation agents should be consulted before practitioners undertake a neuraxial technique.[27] Herbal medications can have an impact on coagulation pathways, and the time from herbal discontinuation to normal hemostasis is 24 hours for ginseng, 36 hours for ginkgo, and 7 days for garlic.[27] It is not currently deemed necessary to discontinue these medications before surgery or anesthesia, although they may have a confounding impact if other anticoagulant medications are administered.

Patients who have received therapeutic fibrinolytic or thrombolytic therapy within the preceding 48 hours should not undergo spinal or epidural techniques because of the risk of epidural hematoma.

Inherited Coagulopathy

Hemorrhagic complications after neuraxial techniques in patients with known hemophilia, von Willebrand disease, or idiopathic thrombocytopenic purpura are infrequent when factor levels are more than 0.5 IU/mL for factor VIII, von Willebrand factor, and ristocetin cofactor activity, or when the platelet count is more than 50×10^9/L before block performance. The minimum safe factor levels and platelet count for neuraxial blockade remain undefined in both the obstetric and general populations, and an individual risk–benefit assessment is required in all cases.[28]

Infection

Concerns exist regarding iatrogenic seeding of active systemic infection to the neuraxis, particularly if a catheter is left *in situ*. This concern, along with the risk of profound hypotension secondary to vasodilation from sympathectomy, may be sufficient reason to avoid neuraxial techniques in patients with significant fever, evidence of ongoing bacteremia, or septic shock. Patients with evidence of systemic infection may safely undergo neuraxial anesthesia once a response to antibiotic therapy has been demonstrated.[29]

SPINAL ANESTHESIA

Factors Affecting Block Height

The dermatomal levels required for various surgical procedures are outlined in Fig. 17.9. Intraabdominal structures such as the peritoneum (T4), bladder (T10), and uterus (T10) have a spinal segment innervation more cephalad than the corresponding skin incision used to operate on these structures. Drug, patient, and procedural factors can all affect the distribution of local anesthetic spread within the intrathecal space,[30] but not all are controllable by the anesthesia provider, leading to significant interpatient variability (Table 17.1). Ultimately baricity, dose, and patient positioning are most important.

Drug Factors
Baricity

Baricity is the ratio of the density of a local anesthetic solution to the density of CSF. It is conventionally defined at 37°C because density varies inversely with temperature. Plain bupivacaine 0.5%, for example, may be isobaric at 24°C but is slightly hypobaric at 37°C. The density of CSF is 1.00059 g/mL. Local anesthetic solutions that have the same density as CSF are termed *isobaric,* those that have a higher density than CSF are termed *hyperbaric,* and those with a lower density are termed *hypobaric.* Dextrose and sterile water are commonly added to render local anesthetic solutions either hyperbaric or hypobaric, respectively. Hyperbaric solutions have a more predictable spread,[31] preferentially moving to the dependent regions of the intrathecal space. Hypobaric solutions spread to nondependent regions, whereas isobaric solutions tend not to be influenced by gravity. The administration of hyperbaric local anesthetic to patients in the lateral decubitus position will therefore preferentially affect the dependent side. The natural curvatures of the vertebral column influence local anesthetic spread in patients placed in the horizontal supine position immediately after intrathecal administration. Hyperbaric local anesthetics injected at the L3–L4 or L4–L5 interspace will spread from the height of the lumbar lordosis down toward the trough of the thoracic kyphosis, resulting in a higher level of anesthetic effect than isobaric or hypobaric solutions.[30]

III

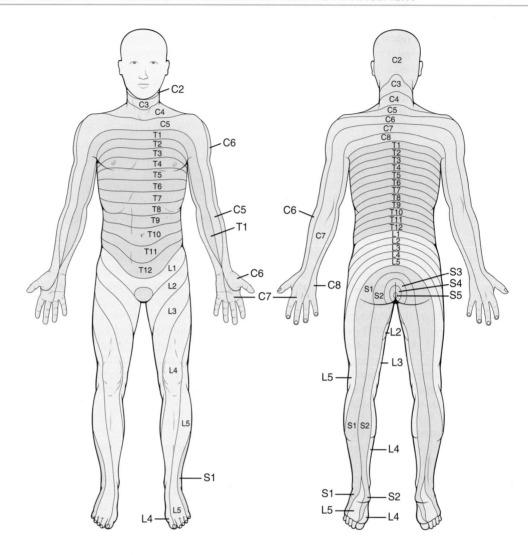

Sensory level anesthesia necessary for surgical procedures

Sensory level	Type of surgery
S2-S5	Hemorrhoidectomy
L2-L3 (knee)	Foot surgery
L1-L3 (inguinal ligament)	Lower extremity surgery
T10 (umbilicus)	Hip surgery Transurethral resection of the prostate Vaginal delivery
T6-T7 (xiphoid process)	Lower abdominal surgery Appendectomy
T4 (nipple)	Upper abdominal surgery Cesarean section

Fig. 17.9 Areas of sensory innervation by spinal nerves and the sensory level required for various surgical procedures. Note that the thoracic nerves supply the thorax and abdomen and the lumbar and sacral nerves supply the lower limb. (Modified from Veering BT, Cousins MJ. Epidural neural blockade. In Cousins MJ, Bridenbaugh PO, Carr DB, et al., eds. Neural Blockade in Clinical Anesthesia and Management of Pain. Philadelphia: Lippincott-Raven; 2009:241–295.)

Table 17.1	Factors Affecting Spinal Local Anesthetic Distribution and Block Height		
Factors	**More Important**	**Less Important**	**Not Important**
Drug factors	Dose Baricity	Volume Concentration Temperature of injection Viscosity	Additives other than opioids
Patient factors	CSF volume Advanced age Pregnancy	Weight Height Spinal anatomy Intraabdominal pressure	Menopause Gender
Procedure factors	Patient position Epidural injection following spinal injection	Level of injection (hypobaric more than hyperbaric) Fluid currents Needle orifice direction Needle type	

CSF, Cerebrospinal fluid.
Modified from Greene NM. Distribution of local anesthetic solutions within the subarachnoid space. *Anesth Analg.* 1985;64(7):715–730.

Dose

Dose (i.e., mass), volume, and concentration are inextricably linked (volume × concentration = dose), but dose is the most reliable determinant of local anesthetic spread (and thus block height) of isobaric and hypobaric solutions.[32] Hyperbaric local anesthetic injections are primarily influenced by baricity.

The choice of local anesthetic or additive drugs (other than opioids) does not influence spread if all other factors are controlled. Opioids may increase the extent of spread,[30] possibly as a result of pharmacologic enhancement at the extremes of the spread, where the local anesthetic effect alone would have been subclinical.[33]

Patient Factors

Many patient factors can influence the number of spinal levels anesthetized from a spinal anesthetic. These factors include height, weight, age, and gender.

Although lumbosacral CSF pressure is fairly constant, the CSF volume varies between patients, which influences peak block height and regression.[34] Although block height varies inversely with CSF volume, CSF volume itself does not correlate well with simple anthropomorphic measurements other than body weight.[34] The increased abdominal mass in obese patients and possible increased epidural fat may decrease CSF volume and therefore increase the spread of local anesthetic and block height.[35]

CSF density varies with gender, menopausal status, and pregnancy (also see Chapter 33), but the clinical relevance of these factors is probably unimportant.

Advanced age is associated with increased block height (also see Chapter 35). In older patients CSF volume decreases, whereas its specific gravity increases. Furthermore, neuronal sensitivity to local anesthetics increases with age.[36]

In the lateral position the broader shoulders of males relative to their hips make this position slightly more head-up, whereas the reverse is true in females. Despite this, whether males actually have reduced cephalad spread as compared with females in the lateral position is not clear.

Variations of the spine such as scoliosis can make needle insertion more difficult but have little effect on local anesthetic spread if the patient is turned supine. Kyphosis, however, in a supine patient may affect the spread of a hyperbaric solution.

During pregnancy, spread of local anesthetic is enhanced by changes in the lumbar lordosis and by the volume and density of CSF, by twin pregnancies compared with singletons, by intraabdominal pressure increases (possibly), and by a progesterone-mediated increase in neuronal sensitivity (also see Chapter 33).

Procedure Factors

The spread of local anesthetic within the subarachnoid space appears to stop 20 to 25 minutes after injection; thus positioning of the patient is most important during this period, particularly in the initial few minutes. A head-up tilt can reduce the cephalad spread of hyperbaric solutions, whereas flexion of the hips and Trendelenburg positioning flatten the lumbar lordosis and increase cephalad spread in most circumstances.[37] A "saddle block" in which only the sacral nerve roots are anesthetized can be achieved with a small dose of hyperbaric local anesthetic while the patient remains sitting for up to 30 minutes. Block height is more extensive with hypobaric solutions if they are administered to patients who are in the sitting position.

The specific needle design and orifice orientation may affect block characteristics. With hypobaric solutions, cephalad alignment of the orifice of Whitacre, but not Sprotte, needles produces higher spread.[38] The orientation of the needle orifice does not appear to affect the spread of hyperbaric solutions. When directing the needle orifice to one side (and using hyperbaric anesthetic), a more marked unilateral block is achieved, again when using a Whitacre rather than a Quincke needle.[39]

The level of injection does not affect block height with hyperbaric solutions. With isobaric solutions, the block height is generally higher the more cephalad the injection.[40] Injection rate and barbotage (repeated aspiration and reinjection of CSF) of isobaric and hyperbaric solutions have not consistently been shown to affect block height. The injection of local anesthetic or even saline into the epidural space after a spinal anesthetic increases the block height and is discussed later.

Duration of the Block

Duration is affected primarily by the dose,[41] the intrinsic properties of the local anesthetic (which affect elimination from the subarachnoid space), and the use of additives (if applicable). Hyperbaric solutions have a shorter duration of action than isobaric solutions.[41]

Pharmacology

The clinical effects of intrathecal local anesthetics are mediated by drug uptake, distribution, and elimination from the CSF. These variables in turn are dictated in part by the pKa (dissociation ionization constant), lipid solubility, and protein binding of the local anesthetic solution. The choice and dose of local anesthetic depend on both the required duration and location of surgery. Table 17.2 shows a range of local anesthetics commonly used for spinal anesthesia with corresponding doses, onset times, and durations of action.

Short- and Intermediate-Acting Local Anesthetics

Procaine is an ester local anesthetic and one of the oldest spinal anesthetics. It is not commonly used because of a more frequent failure rate than lidocaine, significantly more nausea, and a slower time to recovery.

Chloroprocaine is an ultra–short-acting ester that is rapidly metabolized by pseudocholinesterase with minimal systemic or fetal effects. Preservative-free chloroprocaine is of interest in ambulatory surgery because of its reliable, short-duration spinal anesthesia,[42] with a faster recovery time than procaine, lidocaine, and bupivacaine. Transient neurologic symptoms (TNS; discussed later, under "Complications") can occur, albeit at a considerably lesser rate (0.6%) than lidocaine (14%).[43]

Articaine is an ester metabolized by nonspecific cholinesterases and has been widely used for dental nerve blocks. It has not been used in spinal anesthesia.

Lidocaine is a hydrophilic, relatively poorly protein-bound amide local anesthetic with a rapid onset and intermediate duration. Because of an association with both permanent nerve injury and TNS, the use of intrathecal lidocaine has declined.

Table 17.2 Dose, Block Height, Onset Times, and Duration of Commonly[a] Used Spinal Anesthetics

Local Anesthetic Mixture	Dose (mg)		Duration (min)		Onset (min)
	To T10	To T4	Plain	Epinephrine (0.2 mg)	
Lidocaine 5% (with/without dextrose)	40–75	75–100	60–150[b]	20%–50%	3–5
Mepivacaine 1.5% (no dextrose)	30–45[c]	60–80[d]	120–180[e]	–	2–4
Chloroprocaine 3% (with/without dextrose)	30–40	40–60	40–90[f]	N/R	2–4
Bupivacaine 0.5%–0.75% (no dextrose)	10–15	12–20	130–230[g]	20%–50%	4–8
Levobupivacaine 0.5% (no dextrose)	10–15	12–20	140–230[g]	–	4–8
Ropivacaine 0.5%–1% (with/without dextrose)	12–18	18–25	80–210[h]	–	3–8

Note that duration depends on how the regression of the block is measured, which varies widely between studies.
[a]Lidocaine is not commonly used now.
[b]Regression to T12.
[c]Note peak with these doses was T12 and not in all cases.
[d]Median peak block height in this study with 60 mg was T5, not T4.
[e]Regression to S1 for block duration.
[f]Regression to L1.
[g]Regression to L2.
[h]Regression to S2.
From Brull R, Macfarlane AJR, Chan VWS. Spinal, epidural and caudal anesthesia. In Miller RD, Cohen NH, Eriksson LI, et al., eds. Miller's Anesthesia. 8th ed. Philadelphia: Saunders Elsevier; 2015:1696, Table 56.4.
N/R, Not recommended.

Prilocaine is an amide local anesthetic with an intermediate duration of action. It is rarely associated with TNS and may be used in the ambulatory surgery setting (also see Chapter 37). In large doses (>600 mg; not used in spinal anesthesia) prilocaine can result in methemoglobinemia.

Mepivacaine is an amide local anesthetic, but the incidence of TNS after hyperbaric mepivacaine was similar to that of lidocaine.[43] TNS occur less frequently with the isobaric preparation.

Long-Acting Local Anesthetics

Tetracaine is an ester packaged either as niphanoid crystals or as an isobaric 1% solution. A 0.5% hyperbaric preparation can be created for perineal and abdominal surgery. Tetracaine is usually combined with a vasoconstrictor additive because the duration of tetracaine alone can be unreliable. Although such combinations can provide up to 5 hours of anesthesia, the addition of phenylephrine in particular has been associated with TNS.

Bupivacaine is a highly protein-bound amide with a slow onset because of its relatively high pKa and a duration of action of 2.5 to 3 hours.[44] Doses as low as 4 to 5 mg of bupivacaine are used in ambulatory procedures.[45] Bupivacaine is rarely associated with TNS.

Levobupivacaine is the pure S(−) enantiomer of racemic bupivacaine. Although levobupivacaine's potency appears to be slightly less than bupivacaine, the majority of clinical studies using identical doses of levobupivacaine and bupivacaine have found no significant difference in clinical efficacy for spinal anesthesia. Levobupivacaine is less cardiotoxic than bupivacaine, but this is only a theoretical risk in spinal anesthesia.

Ropivacaine is another highly protein-bound amide local anesthetic. With the same pKa (8.1) as bupivacaine, it has a medium speed of onset and a long duration of action, but is less potent. The proposed advantages of spinal ropivacaine are less cardiotoxicity and greater motor-sensory block differentiation, resulting in less motor block. When given in an equivalent dose to bupivacaine, there is slightly less motor block and earlier recovery with ropivacaine.[46]

Spinal Additives

A variety of medications may exert a direct analgesic effect on the spinal cord and nerve roots or prolong the quality and/or duration of sensory and motor blockade. The coadministration of such drugs often allows a reduction in the dose of local anesthetic, with the advantage of reducing motor blockade with faster recovery while still producing the same degree of analgesia.

The pharmacology of intrathecal opioid administration is complex because of a combination of direct spinal cord dorsal horn opioid receptor activation, cerebral opioid receptor activation after CSF transport, and peripheral and central systemic opioid effects after vascular uptake. The effect at each site depends on both the dose administered and the physicochemical properties of the opioid, particularly lipid solubility. Highly lipid-soluble drugs such as fentanyl and sufentanil have a more rapid onset and shorter duration of action than more hydrophilic opioids. Greater lipid solubility also results in rapid uptake into both blood vessels (with a resultant systemic effect) and fatty tissue. The spread of lipophilic opioids within the CSF is therefore more limited than hydrophilic opioids such as (preservative-free) morphine, which demonstrate greater spread as a result of slower uptake and elimination from the CSF. As a result, hydrophilic opioids have a more frequent risk of late respiratory depression. The extent of neural tissue and vascular uptake also affects the potency of intrathecal opioids. For example, the relative intrathecal to intravenous potency of morphine is 200:1 to 300:1, whereas for fentanyl and sufentanil it is only 10:1 to 20:1.[47] Other side effects of intrathecal opioids are discussed under "Complications."

Hydrophilic Opioids

Preservative-free morphine is widely used, providing analgesia for up to 24 hours.[48] Analgesic benefit with minimal side effects is achieved with 100 µg for cesarean delivery (also see Chapter 33). The most efficacious dose for major orthopedic surgery is less clear,[49] but side effects increase without improvement in analgesia with doses of 300 µU or more, and in fact it has been suggested to avoid spinal opioids in arthroplasty surgery to reduce adverse effects. Spinal opioids alone are commonly given as a simple alternative to epidural local anesthetic–based analgesia. For major abdominal surgery or thoracotomies, 500 µg or more may be used, but the optimal dose that balances analgesia versus the risk of adverse effects remains unclear.

Diamorphine is a lipid-soluble prodrug that crosses the dura faster than morphine and is cleared from the CSF more quickly than morphine. It is converted to morphine and 6-monoacetyl morphine, both of which are µ-agonists with a relatively long duration of action.

Hydromorphone is not commonly used for spinal analgesia and does not provide any advantage compared with morphine.

Meperidine is an opioid of intermediate lipid solubility, but it also has some local anesthetic properties. Although it has been administered as the sole intrathecal anesthetic in both obstetric and general surgery, it is rarely used. The neurotoxicity profile is unclear.

Lipophilic Opioids

Fentanyl and sufentanil are used frequently in obstetrics for labor analgesia and cesarean delivery (see Chapter 33). Fentanyl is useful in ambulatory surgery because of its rapid onset time of 10 to 20 minutes and relatively short duration of 2 to 3 hours. It is also preferred to longer-acting opioids in the elderly or patients at risk of late respiratory depression.

Vasoconstrictors

Epinephrine and phenylephrine can prolong sensory and motor blockade when added to local anesthetics. The α_1-adrenergic-mediated vasoconstriction reduces systemic local anesthetic uptake, and epinephrine may also enhance analgesia via a direct α_2-adrenergic-mediated effect. Tetracaine, lidocaine, and bupivacaine spinal anesthesia can all be prolonged by epinephrine. Although there are no human data to support the theory, there is a concern that potent vasoconstrictive action places neural blood supply at risk.

α_2-Agonists

Intrathecal clonidine, dexmedetomidine, and epinephrine all act on prejunctional and postjunctional α_2-adrenergic receptors in the dorsal horn of the spinal cord. Clonidine prolongs sensory and motor blockade by approximately 1 hour and improves analgesia. It can cause non–dose-related hypotension and sedation lasting up to 8 hours, however. Dexmedetomidine is approximately 10-fold more α_2-receptor selective than clonidine and appears to prolong motor and sensory block without hemodynamic compromise.

Other Drugs

Intrathecal neostigmine prolongs motor and sensory blockade and reduces postoperative analgesic requirements, but its benefits are limited by nausea, vomiting, bradycardia, and, in higher doses, lower extremity weakness. Midazolam also prolongs sensory and motor blockade. However, animal data suggest that midazolam may be neurotoxic. Intrathecal ketamine, adenosine, tramadol, magnesium, and nonsteroidal antiinflammatory drugs are unlikely to have any clinical value.

Technique

Technique can be classified into a series of steps: preparation, position, projection, and puncture (i.e., the four Ps).

Preparation

Informed consent must be obtained and thoroughly documented, including disclosure of proposed benefits, relevant risks, and possible alternative techniques. Resuscitation equipment must be immediately available, intravenous access should be secured, and noninvasive monitoring is necessary.

The most important characteristics of a spinal needle are the shape of the tip and the needle diameter. Needle tips either cut (Pitkin and Quincke-Babcock) or spread (Whitacre, Sprotte, and Pencan) the dura (Fig. 17.10). In the latter group needles have a conical, pencil-point tip that provides better tactile sensation and reduces the incidence of post–dural puncture headache. Using smaller-gauge cutting, but not pencil point, needles appears to reduce the incidence of post–dural puncture headache.[50]

The failure rate is increased with 29-gauge needles,[51] so pencil-point needles of 25 gauge, 26 gauge, or 27 gauge probably represent the optimal needle choice.

Strict aseptic technique is of utmost importance. One of the most common organisms responsible for bacterial meningitis after spinal anesthesia is the oral commensal *Streptococcus viridans,* emphasizing the purpose of wearing a mask during the performance of spinal anesthesia. A combination of chlorhexidine and alcohol together is the most effective skin cleanser.[52] Chlorhexidine must be allowed to dry completely before skin puncture because chlorhexidine is profoundly neurotoxic and may cause arachnoiditis.

Current consensus guidelines recommend that neuraxial blocks be performed with the patient awake,[22] because general anesthesia or heavy sedation prevent a patient from expressing warning signs of pain or paresthesia if the needle is in close proximity to nerve tissue. In circumstances when the risks of performing the technique awake outweigh the benefits (for example, in a patient with severe movement disorder risking accidental and sudden needle-to-nerve contact) the practitioner and patient may agree that the procedure is best performed asleep.

Position

The two most common patient positions to facilitate the performance of spinal anesthesia are lateral decubitus and sitting. The prone position is rarely used. The choice of a particular position depends on patient, procedural, and practitioner preferences. The lateral decubitus position facilitates coadministration of intravenous anxiolytic medication if required and may be more comfortable for certain patients. Patients are placed with their back parallel to the edge of the operating table, thighs flexed onto the abdomen, with the neck flexed to allow the forehead to be as close as possible to the knees in an attempt to widen the spaces between spinous processes and posterior vertebral elements. Whenever possible, the patient should be positioned such that spread of hypobaric, isobaric, or hyperbaric solution to the operative site is optimized.

Identification of the midline may be easier when the patient is placed in the sitting position, especially when obesity or scoliosis render midline anatomy difficult to examine. An assistant helps maintain the patient in a vertical plane while asking the patient to comfortably flex their neck, relax their shoulders, and curve or "push out" their back in an attempt to widen the spaces between spinous processes and posterior vertebral elements. Hypotension may be more common in the sitting position.

Projection and Puncture

The spinal cord terminates at the level of L1–L2, so needle insertion above this level should be avoided. The intercristal line is the line drawn between the two iliac crests and corresponds, with imperfect reliability, to the level of the L4 vertebral body or the L4–L5 interspace.[53]

Front view

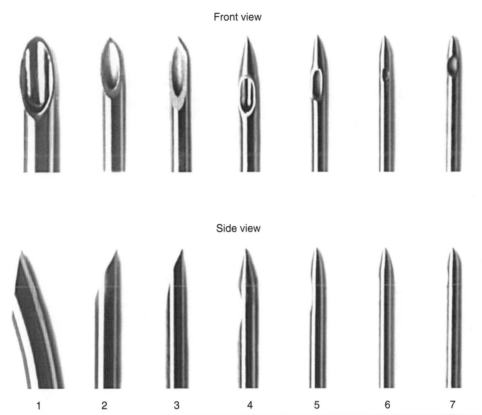

Side view

| 1 | 2 | 3 | 4 | 5 | 6 | 7 |

Fig. 17.10 Comparative needle configuration for (1) 18-gauge Tuohy, (2) 20-gauge Quincke, (3) 22-gauge Quincke, (4) 24-gauge Sprotte, (5) 25-gauge Polymedic, (6) 25-gauge Whitacre, and (7) 26-gauge Gertie Marx. (From Schneider MC, Schmid M. Postdural puncture headache. In Birnbach DJ, Gatt SP, Datta S, eds. Textbook of Obstetric Anesthesia. Philadelphia: Churchill Livingstone; 2000:487–503.)

Once the appropriate space (usually L3–L4, L2–L3, or L4–L5) has been selected, subcutaneous local anesthetic is infiltrated and an introducer needle is inserted at a slight cephalad angle of 10 to 15 degrees through the skin, subcutaneous tissue, and supraspinous ligament to reach the interspinous ligament. Depending on the habitus of the patient, the introducer needle may not be sufficiently long to reach the interspinous ligament, or conversely in slender patients, it may directly puncture the dura if inserted to the hub. The spinal needle, with its bevel parallel to the midline, is advanced slowly through the introducer until the characteristic change in resistance is noted as the needle tip passes through the ligamentum flavum and dura into the intrathecal space, when a subtle "click" or "pop" sensation often occurs. The stylet is then removed, and clear CSF should appear at the needle hub. If the CSF does not flow, the needle might be obstructed, and rotation in 90-degree increments can be undertaken until CSF appears. If CSF does not appear in any quadrant, the needle should be advanced a few millimeters and rechecked. If CSF still has not appeared, the needle should be withdrawn and the insertion steps repeated. A

common reason for failure is insertion of the needle off the midline. After CSF is freely obtained, the anesthetic dose is injected at a rate of approximately 0.2 mL/sec. After completion of the injection, CSF can be aspirated into the syringe and reinjected into the subarachnoid space to reconfirm needle tip location.

The paramedian approach may be useful in the setting of diffuse calcification of the interspinous ligament. A skin wheal is raised 1 cm lateral and 1 cm caudad to the corresponding spinous process. The spinal introducer and needle are inserted 10 to 15 degrees off the sagittal plane in a cephalomedial plane (Fig. 17.11). If the needle contacts bone, it is redirected slightly in a cephalad direction and the needle "walked up" the lamina. The characteristic feel of the ligamentum flavum and dura is possible, but with this approach the needle is not passing through the supraspinous and interspinous ligaments.

Use of Ultrasonography
Ultrasonography of the lumbar spine can accurately identify the intervertebral levels, the midline spinous process, the midline interspinous window, the paramedian

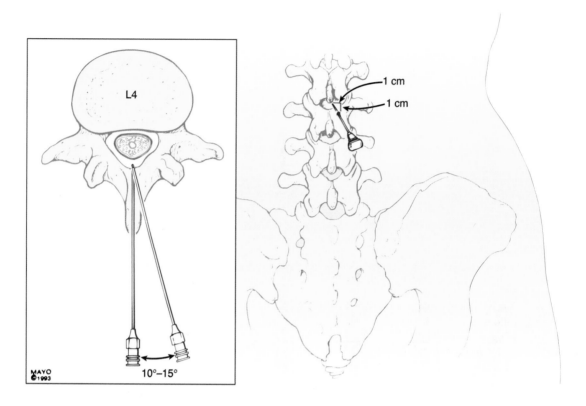

L4

1 cm

1 cm

10°–15°

MAYO
©1993

Fig. 17.11 Vertebral anatomy of the midline and paramedian approaches to central neuraxis blocks. The midline approach highlighted in the inset requires anatomic projection in only two planes: sagittal and horizontal. The paramedian approach shown in the inset and in the posterior view requires an additional oblique plane to be considered, although the technique may be easier in patients who are unable to cooperate in minimizing their lumbar lordosis. The paramedian needle is inserted 1 cm lateral and 1 cm caudad to the caudad edge of the more superior vertebral spinous process. The paramedian needle is inserted approximately 15 degrees off the sagittal plane, as shown in the inset. (Courtesy the Mayo Foundation, Rochester, MN.)

interlaminar window, and the depth to the intrathecal space.[53] Ultrasound facilitates identification of the optimal location for spinal needle insertion and estimation of the skin-to-intrathecal space distance and thereby can reduce procedural failure rates.[54] Ultrasound is most useful in patients with difficult surface landmarks (e.g., obesity), spine disorders (e.g., scoliosis), or previous spine surgery.

Special Spinal Techniques

Continuous spinal anesthesia allows incremental dosing of local anesthetic to achieve (or maintain) spinal anesthesia at a desired vertebral level with better hemodynamic stability than a single-shot spinal injection.[55] This approach is useful in controlling arterial blood pressure in patients with severe aortic stenosis or pregnant women with complex cardiac disease. It may also be used in prolonged cases rather than the combined spinal-epidural

(CSE) technique or when previous spinal surgery may hinder reliable epidural spread. Spinal microcatheters exist, but small-gauge catheters (less than 24 g in particular) have been associated with cauda equina syndrome,[56] probably because of lumbosacral pooling of local anesthetic. Catheter-over-the-needle devices are also available for use with continuous spinal anesthesia, with the advantage of minimizing leakage of CSF around the catheter, but they may be more difficult to insert.

The terms *unilateral spinal anesthesia* and *selective spinal anesthesia* overlap slightly, but both refer to small-dose techniques that capitalize on baricity and patient positioning to hasten recovery. For example, 4 to 5 mg of hyperbaric bupivacaine with unilateral positioning can be adequate for knee arthroscopy. In selective spinal anesthesia minimal local anesthetic doses are used with the goal of anesthetizing only the sensory fibers to the specific surgical site.[57]

Box 17.1 Modified Bromage Scale

0 No motor block
1 Inability to raise extended leg; able to move knees and feet
2 Inability to raise extended leg and move knee; able to move feet
3 Complete block of motor limb

From Brull R, Macfarlane AJR, Chan VWS. Spinal, epidural and caudal anesthesia. In Miller RD, Cohen NH, Eriksson LI, et al., eds. *Miller's Anesthesia*. 8th ed. Philadelphia: Saunders Elsevier; 2015. Box 56.1.

Monitoring of the Block

Once the spinal anesthetic has been administered, the onset, extent, and quality of the sensory and motor blocks must be assessed, and heart rate and arterial blood pressure should be monitored due to resultant sympathetic blockade. Cold sensation and pinprick representing C fibers and A-delta fibers, respectively, are used most often to assess sensory block. Loss of sensation to cold usually occurs first, verified using ethyl chloride spray, ice, or alcohol, followed by the loss of sensation to pinprick, verified using a needle that does not pierce the skin. Finally, loss of sensation to touch occurs. The modified Bromage scale (Box 17.1) is most commonly used to measure motor block, although this represents only lumbosacral motor fibers.[58] Confirming that the level of loss of sensation to cold or pinprick is two to three segments above the expected level of surgical stimulus and the presence of a motor block are commonly considered indicators of adequate surgical anesthesia.

EPIDURAL ANESTHESIA

Factors Affecting Epidural Block Height

Drug Factors

The volume and total dose of local anesthetic injected into the epidural space are the most important drug-related factors that affect block height. As a general principle, 1 to 2 mL of solution should be injected per segment to be blocked. Bicarbonate, epinephrine, and opioids influence the onset, quality, and duration of analgesia and anesthesia, but do not affect spread (Table 17.3).

Patient Factors

Age can influence epidural block height. Up to 40% less volume may be required in thoracic epidurals in the elderly, possibly because of decreased leakage of local anesthetic through intervertebral foramina, decreased compliance of the epidural space, or an increased sensitivity of the nerves (also see Chapter 35). Only the extremes of patient height influence local anesthetic spread in the epidural space. Weight is not well correlated with epidural block height. Less local anesthetic is required to produce

Table 17.3 Factors Affecting Epidural Local Anesthetic Distribution and Block Height

Factors	More Important	Less Important	Not Important
Drug factors	Volume Dose	Concentration	Additives
Patient factors	Elderly age Pregnancy	Weight Height Pressure in adjacent body cavities	
Procedure factors	Level of injection	Patient position	Speed of injection Needle orifice direction

From Visser WA, Lee RA, Gielen MJM. Factors affecting the distribution of neural blockade by local anesthetics in epidural anesthesia and a comparison of lumbar versus thoracic epidural anesthesia. *Anesth Analg*. 2008;107(2):708-721.

the same epidural spread of anesthesia in pregnant patients, in part because of engorgement of epidural veins secondary to increased abdominal pressure (also see Chapter 33). Continuous positive airway pressure increases the spread of a thoracic epidural block, although the influence of intermittent positive pressure ventilation is unclear.

Procedure Factors

The level of injection is the most important procedural factor that affects epidural block height. In the upper cervical region spread of injectate is mostly caudal; in the midthoracic region spread is equally cephalad and caudal; and in the low thoracic region, spread is primarily cephalad.[59] After a lumbar epidural, spread is more cephalad than caudal. Some studies suggest that the total number of segments blocked is less in the lumbar region compared with thoracic levels for a given volume of injectate. Patient position affects lumbar epidural injections, with preferential spread and faster onset to the dependent side in the lateral decubitus position. The Trendelenburg position increases cephalad spread in obstetric patients. Needle bevel direction and speed of injection do not appear to significantly influence the spread of a bolus injection.

Pharmacology

Local anesthetics for epidural use may be classified into short-, intermediate- and long-acting drugs. A single bolus dose of local anesthetic can provide surgical anesthesia ranging from 45 minutes up to 4 hours depending on the type administered and the use of any additives (Table 17.4). Most commonly, however, an epidural catheter is left *in situ* so that additional local anesthetic can be administered to extend, strengthen, or titrate the anesthesia or analgesia.

Table 17.4	Comparative Onset Times and Analgesic Durations of Local Anesthetics Administered Epidurally in 20- to 30-mL Volumes			
Drug	**Conc. (%)**	**Onset (min)**	**Duration - Plain (min)**	**Duration - 1:200,000 Epinephrine (min)**
Chloroprocaine	3	10-15	45-60	60-90
Lidocaine	2	15	80-120	120-180
Mepivacaine	2	15	90-140	140-200
Bupivacaine	0.5-0.75	20	165-225	180-240
Etidocaine	1	15	120-200	150-225
Ropivacaine	0.75-1.0	15-20	140-180	150-200
Levobupivacaine	0.5-0.75	15-20	150-225	150-240

Data from Cousins MJ, Bromage PR. Epidural neural blockade. In Cousins MJ, Bridenbaugh PO, eds. *Neural Blockade in Clinical Anesthesia and Management of Pain*. Philadelphia: JB Lippincott; 1988:255; Brown DL. Spinal, epidural and caudal anesthesia. In Miller RD, Cohen NH, Eriksson LI, et al., eds. *Miller's Anesthesia*. 7th ed. Philadelphia: Saunders Elsevier; 2010:1611-1638.

Short-Acting and Intermediate-Acting Local Anesthetics

Procaine is not commonly used because the resultant block can be unreliable and of poor quality.

Chloroprocaine is available in 2% and 3% preservative-free solutions. Before preservative-free preparations, large volumes of chloroprocaine had been associated with deep, burning lumbar back pain.[60] This was thought to be secondary to the ethylenediaminetetraacetic acid that chelated calcium and caused a localized hypocalcemia.

Articaine is not widely used for epidural anesthesia and has not been studied extensively.

Lidocaine is available in 1% and 2% solutions. Unlike spinal anesthesia, TNS is not commonly associated with epidural lidocaine.

Prilocaine is available in 2% and 3% solutions. The 2% solution produces a sensory block with minimal motor block. In large doses prilocaine is associated with methemoglobinemia.

Mepivacaine is available as 1%, 1.5%, and 2% preservative-free solutions. The 2% preparation has an onset time similar to that for lidocaine of approximately 15 minutes, but a slightly longer duration (up to 200 minutes with epinephrine).

Long-Acting Local Anesthetics

Tetracaine is not widely used because of unreliable block height and, in larger doses, systemic toxicity.

Bupivacaine is available in 0.25%, 0.5%, and 0.75% preservative-free solutions. More dilute concentrations such as 0.125% to 0.25% can be used for analgesia. However, disadvantages include cardiac and central nervous system toxicity and potential motor block from larger doses.

Levobupivacaine administered epidurally has the same clinical characteristics as bupivacaine but is less cardiotoxic. Liposomal bupivacaine is not licensed for epidural use.

Ropivacaine is available in 0.2%, 0.5%, 0.75%, and 1.0% preservative-free preparations. It is associated with a superior safety profile compared with bupivacaine, with a higher seizure threshold and less cardiotoxicity.

Epidural Additives
Vasoconstrictors

Epinephrine reduces vascular absorption of local anesthetics in the epidural space. The effect is greatest with lidocaine,[61] mepivacaine, and chloroprocaine (up to 50% prolongation); less with bupivacaine and levobupivacaine; and limited with ropivacaine, which already has intrinsic vasoconstrictive properties (see Table 17.4). Epinephrine itself may also have some analgesic benefits because of absorption into CSF and dorsal horn α_2-receptor activation. Phenylephrine is used less widely and is less effective than epinephrine.

Opioids

Opioids synergistically enhance the analgesic effects of epidural local anesthetics without prolonging motor block. A combination of local anesthetic and opioid reduces the dose-related adverse effects of each drug independently. Opioid-related side effects are dose-dependent, and there appears to be a therapeutic ceiling effect above which only side effects increase. Opioids may also be administered to the epidural space without local anesthetic. Epidural opioids cross the dura and arachnoid membrane to reach the CSF and spinal cord dorsal horn. Lipophilic opioids, such as fentanyl and sufentanil, partition into epidural fat and therefore are found in lower concentrations in CSF than hydrophilic opioids, such as morphine and hydromorphone. Fentanyl and sufentanil are also readily absorbed into the systemic circulation, which may be their principal analgesic mechanism.

Epidural morphine can be administered as a bolus (duration of up to 24 hours) or continuously. The optimal bolus analgesic dose that minimizes side effects is 2.5 to 3.75 mg.[62] Hydromorphone is more hydrophilic than fentanyl but more lipophilic than morphine and has a duration of 18 hours. Epidural fentanyl and sufentanil have a faster onset but a shorter duration (only 2 to 3 hours). Diamorphine is available in the United Kingdom. An extended-release liposomal formulation of morphine is available for single-shot epidural administration and offers prolonged analgesia compared with morphine, potentially avoiding the need for continuous local anesthetic infusion via indwelling catheter.

α₂-Agonists

Epidural clonidine prolongs sensory block to a longer extent than motor block and reduces both epidural local anesthetic and opioid requirements. Clonidine may also reduce immune stress and cytokine response, but side effects include hypotension, bradycardia, dry mouth, and sedation. Epidural dexmedetomidine can reduce intraoperative anesthetic requirements, improve postoperative analgesia, and prolong both sensory and motor block.

Other Drugs

Ketamine, neostigmine, midazolam, tramadol, dexamethasone, and droperidol have all been studied but are not commonly used.

Carbonation and Bicarbonate

Both carbonation of the solution and adding bicarbonate increase the solution pH and therefore the nonionized free-base proportion of local anesthetic. Although this increases the speed of epidural block onset by producing more rapid intraneural diffusion, this apparent advantage must be weighed against the risk of drug error when mixing solutions for epidural administration and the extra preparation time this inevitably incurs.[63–65]

Technique

Preparation

Patient preparation as previously described for spinal anesthesia must equally be applied to epidural anesthesia, namely consent, monitoring, resuscitation equipment, and intravenous access. Sterility is arguably even more important than spinal anesthesia because a catheter is often left *in situ*. The nature and the duration of surgery must be understood so that the epidural may be inserted at the appropriate level (Table 17.5) and the appropriate drugs chosen. The risks and benefits will vary depending on the severity of patient comorbid conditions. Tuohy needles are most commonly used (see Fig. 17.10). They are usually 16 or 18g and have a shaft marked in 1-cm intervals with a 15- to 30-degree curved, blunt Huber needle tip designed to both reduce the risk of accidental

| Table 17.5 | Suggested Epidural Insertion Sites for Common Surgical Procedures |

Nature of Surgery	Suggested Level of Insertion	Remarks
Hip surgery Lower extremity Obstetric analgesia	Lumbar L2-L5	
Colectomy, anterior resection Upper abdominal surgery	Lower thoracic T6-T8	Spread more cranial than caudal
Thoracic	T2-T6	Midpoint of surgical incision

Modified from Visser WA, Lee RA, Gielen MJM. Factors affecting the distribution of neural blockade by local anesthetics in epidural anesthesia and a comparison of lumbar versus thoracic epidural anesthesia. *Anesth Analg.* 2008;107(2):708-721.

dural puncture and guide the catheter cephalad. The catheter is made of a flexible, calibrated, radiopaque plastic with either a single end hole or multiple side orifices near the tip. Multiple orifice catheters improve analgesia and lead to fewer catheter reinsertions compared with single-orifice devices.[66]

Position

The sitting and lateral decubitus positions necessary for epidural puncture are the same as those for spinal anesthesia, and success rates are comparable. As with spinal anesthesia, epidurals are ideally performed with the patient awake.[22]

Projection and Puncture

Important surface landmarks include the intercristal line (corresponding to the L4–L5 interspace), the inferior angle of the scapula (corresponding to the T7 vertebral body), the root of the scapular spine (T3), and the vertebra prominens (C7) (Fig. 17.12). Ultrasonography may be useful to identify the desired level.

A variety of needle approaches to the epidural space exist: midline, paramedian, modified paramedian (Taylor approach), and caudal. A midline approach, in which the angle of approach is only slightly cephalad, is commonly chosen for lumbar and low thoracic approaches. In the midthoracic region the approach should be more cephalad because of the significant downward angulation of the spinous processes (see Fig. 17.5). The needle should be advanced in a controlled fashion with the stylet in place through the supraspinous ligament and into the interspinous ligament, at which point the stylet can be removed and the loss-of-resistance syringe attached. This method may increase the chance of a false loss of resistance, possibly because of midline defects in the interspinous ligament.

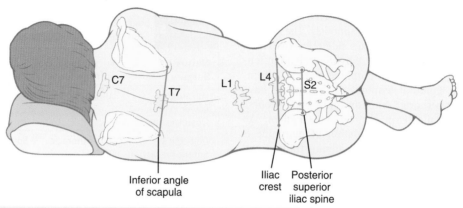

Fig. 17.12 Surface landmarks are a guide to the vertebral level. (From Brown DL, ed. *Atlas of Regional Anesthesia.* Philadelphia: WB Saunders; 1992.)

Air or saline (or a combination) is commonly used to detect a loss of resistance when identifying the epidural space (Fig. 17.13). Each involves intermittent or constant gentle pressure applied to the plunger of the syringe while the needle tip is advanced in a controlled manner though the ligamentum flavum. Usually the ligamentum flavum is identified as a tougher structure with increased resistance, and when the epidural space is subsequently entered, the pressure applied to the syringe plunger allows the fluid to flow with minimal resistance into the epidural space. Air is considered less reliable in identifying the epidural space, resulting in a higher chance of inadequate block,[67] and may cause both pneumocephalus (which can result in headaches) and even venous air embolism in rare cases. Fluid inserted through the epidural needle before catheter insertion can also reduce the risk of epidural vein cannulation by the catheter.[68] However, saline injection can make it more difficult to detect an accidental dural puncture because the appearances of saline and CSF may be similar to the naked eye (although they can be distinguished on glucose or protein testing).

With the hanging-drop technique, a drop of solution such as saline is placed within the hub of the needle after the needle is placed in the ligamentum flavum. When the needle tip reaches the epidural space, the solution is "sucked in" as a result of subatmospheric pressure inside the epidural space.

When a lumbar midline approach is used, the depth from skin to the ligamentum flavum in most patients is between 3 and 6 cm. Ultrasonography can predict this depth before needle insertion. When the epidural space is identified, the depth should be noted, the syringe removed from the Tuohy needle, and a catheter gently threaded to leave 4 to 6 cm in the space. The catheter should be easy to thread, and some patients experience a very transient "pop" or "click" as the catheter is advanced within the epidural space. Less than 4 cm in length in the epidural space may increase the risk of catheter dislodgement and inadequate analgesia. Threading more catheter increases the likelihood of catheter malposition,

unilateral blockade, or complications.[69] The Tsui test can be used to confirm catheter tip location using a special electrically conducting catheter.[70] This stimulates the spinal nerve roots with a low electrical current resulting in twitches of the corresponding muscles.

Paramedian Approach

The paramedian approach is particularly useful in the mid- to high-thoracic region, where the angulation of the spinous processes is steeper and the posterior spaces between vertebrae narrower. The Tuohy needle should be inserted 0.5 to 1 cm lateral to the inferior tip of the spinous process corresponding to the vertebra above the desired interspace. The needle is then advanced perpendicular in all planes to the skin until the lamina is contacted and then redirected medially and cephalad to enter the ligamentum flavum and, after loss of resistance, the epidural space. The Taylor approach is a modified paramedian approach via the L5–S1 interspace, which may be useful in trauma patients who cannot tolerate or are not able to maintain a sitting position. The needle is inserted 1 cm medial and 1 cm caudad to the posterior superior iliac spine and is angled medially and cephalad at a 45- to 55-degree angle.

Before initiating an epidural local anesthetic infusion, the catheter should be aspirated gently to check for blood or CSF and a test dose administered to exclude intrathecal or intravascular catheter placement. A test dose typically consists of a very small dose of local anesthetic that otherwise would produce evidence of motor or sensory blockade if injected intrathecally, but does not readily produce evidence of somatic blockade when injected into the epidural space. Some practitioners advocate the addition of epinephrine to the test dose because a resultant tachycardia may warn of intravascular catheter placement.

Use of Ultrasonography

As with spinal anesthesia, preprocedural ultrasound imaging can assist in the siting of epidural anesthesia in patients whose surface landmarks are difficult to discern

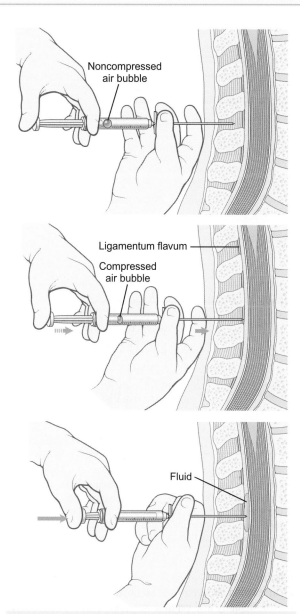

Fig. 17.13 Loss-of-resistance technique. The needle is inserted into the ligamentum flavum, and a syringe containing saline and an air bubble is attached to the hub. After compression of the air bubble is obtained by applying pressure on the syringe plunger, the needle is carefully advanced until its entry into the epidural space is confirmed by the characteristic loss of resistance to syringe plunger pressure and the fluid enters the space easily. (From Afton-Bird G. Atlas of regional anesthesia. In Miller RD, ed. *Miller's Anesthesia*. Philadelphia: Elsevier; 2005.)

or who have spinal deformities. Sonographic imaging of the thoracic spine is more challenging than that of the lumbar spine because of narrower interspinous and interlaminar windows. Nonetheless, ultrasound scanning before needle insertion (i.e., prescanning) can help identify the optimal site for needle insertion, predict the

skin-to-dura distance, and reduce the rate of lumbar epidural block failure rate.[54] Moreover, neuraxial ultrasonography by experienced practitioners may improve block efficacy.[71] Real-time guidance is a more challenging technique. Real-time ultrasound-guided epidural needle insertion is relatively easier in the pediatric population because of limited ossification of the vertebral column. The epidural catheter tip, dural displacement, and extent of cranial spread of a fluid bolus can all be visualized.

COMBINED SPINAL-EPIDURAL ANESTHESIA

CSE anesthesia allows the flexibility of a rapid-onset spinal block, and the epidural catheter allows anesthesia or analgesia to be extended as the spinal block resolves. This is particularly useful in obstetrics (also see Chapter 33). Another advantage is the ability to administer a low dose of intrathecal local anesthetic and, if necessary, use the epidural catheter to extend the block. Adding either local anesthetic or saline alone to the epidural space via the catheter compresses the dural sac and increases the block height. This latter technique of epidural volume extension (EVE) allows smaller doses of intrathecal local anesthetic to be used while significantly hastening motor recovery.[72] This sequential technique also provides greater hemodynamic stability for high-risk patients.

Technique

Most commonly the epidural needle is placed first, followed by either a "needle-through-needle" technique using specific needle equipment (Fig. 17.14) or a separate spinal needle insertion at the same or a different interspace. The separate needle insertion technique[73] has the advantage of being able to confirm that the epidural catheter is functional before spinal anesthesia is administered but does theoretically risk shearing the *in situ* epidural catheter.

CAUDAL ANESTHESIA

Caudal anesthesia involves the deposition of medication into the epidural space via the sacral hiatus. Caudal anesthesia is popular in pediatric anesthesia (also see Chapter 34). In adults the extent of cephalad spread of local anesthetic from the sacral hiatus is mostly limited to the lumbosacral roots; therefore caudal anesthesia is most useful when sacral anesthetic spread is desired (e.g., perineal procedures), where a spinal surgery scar may prevent a lumbar anesthetic technique, or more commonly, in chronic pain and cancer pain management (also see Chapter 44). Both fluoroscopy and ultrasonography can help guide correct needle placement.

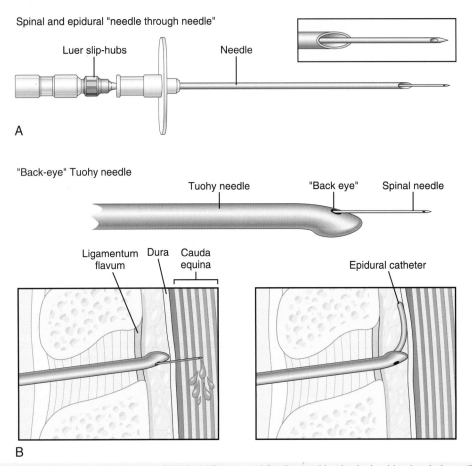

Fig. 17.14 (A) A spinal needle and epidural needle are used for the combined spinal-epidural technique. (B) Tuohy needle with a "back eye" that permits placement of the spinal needle directly into the subarachnoid space *(left panel)* and subsequent threading of the epidural catheter into the epidural space after removal of the spinal needle. (Modified from Veering BT, Cousins MJ. Epidural neural blockade. In Cousins MJ, Bridenbaugh PO, Carr DB, et al., eds. *Neural Blockade in Clinical Anesthesia and Management of Pain.* Philadelphia: Lippincott-Raven; 2009:241–295.)

Pharmacology

The local anesthetics used for caudal anesthesia are similar to those described for epidural anesthesia and analgesia. In adults approximately twice the lumbar epidural dose is required to achieve a similar block with the caudal approach.

Technique

Patient preparation as described before applies equally to caudal anesthesia. The prone position, lateral decubitus position, and the knee–chest position may be used. Caudal anesthesia requires identification of the sacral hiatus, where the two sacral cornua are joined by the sacrococcygeal ligament (an extension of the ligamentum flavum). The hiatus can be approximated as the apex of an equilateral triangle whose base is formed by the two posterior superior iliac spines (Fig. 17.15).

After the sacral hiatus is identified, subcutaneous local anesthetic is infiltrated and the caudal needle (or Tuohy needle if a catheter is to be placed) is inserted at an angle of approximately 45 degrees to the sacrum. A decrease in resistance to needle insertion (or loss of resistance if a Tuohy needle is used) should be appreciated as the needle tip passes through the sacrococcygeal ligament and enters the caudal epidural space. The needle tip should be advanced no more than approximately 1 to 2 cm into the caudal epidural space and, in adults, never beyond the S2 level (approximately 1 cm inferior to the posterior superior iliac spine), which is the level to which the dural sac extends. Additional needle advancement increases the risk of dural puncture and intrathecal injection of medication. Before injection of any drugs, aspiration to see if CSF can be withdrawn should be performed and a test dose administered to exclude intravascular or intrathecal placement.

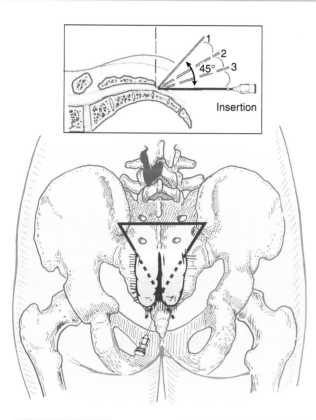

Fig. 17.15 Caudal technique. Palpating fingers locate the sacral cornua by using the equilateral triangle. Needle insertion is completed by insertion and withdrawal in a stepwise fashion (inset, so-called "1-2-3 insertion") until the needle can be advanced into the caudal canal and the solution can be injected easily (without creation of a subcutaneous "lump" of fluid). (From Brull R, Macfarlane AJR, Chan VWS. Spinal, epidural and caudal anesthesia. In Miller RD, Cohen NH, Eriksson LI, et al., eds. *Miller's Anesthesia.* 8th ed. Philadelphia: Saunders Elsevier; 2015:Fig. 56.10.)

COMPLICATIONS

Clear distinction should be made between the physiological effects of the neuraxial technique and complications, which imply some harm to the patient.[74] The material risks associated with neuraxial anesthesia must be intimately understood and respected because catastrophic injury is not unknown.

Neurological

Serious neurological complications associated with neuraxial anesthesia are rare, but suspected nerve injury arising from neuraxial techniques should prompt immediate attention and risk stratification to guide further investigation, including emergent imaging if necessary. The reported incidence of nerve injury after neuraxial techniques varies greatly depending on the presence or absence of specific patient or procedural risk factors, such as anticoagulation medication or poor aseptic technique. Epidural (including CSE) anesthesia is associated with a more frequent rate of nerve injury compared with spinal anesthesia.[75] Further, neuraxial anesthesia performed in adults for the purposes of perioperative anesthesia or analgesia is associated with an increased likelihood of neurological complications compared with that performed in the obstetric, pediatric, and chronic pain settings.[76] Radicular pain or paresthesia occurring during any neuraxial procedure should warn the practitioner of possible needle-to-nerve contact and prompt immediate needle withdrawal.

Paraplegia

The overall frequency of paraplegia after neuraxial anesthetic techniques is reported to be approximately 2 to 4.2 per 100,000, but there are markedly different incidences depending on individual procedural risk factors.[76] A variety of mechanisms can lead to paraplegia after neuraxial blockade, including direct needle trauma, vertebral canal hematoma, epidural abscess, periprocedural hypotension of the spinal cord circulation, adhesive arachnoiditis, or maladministration of neurotoxic medications. Disruption of normal cord blood supply and resultant ischemic injury are thought to be the final common pathway for many of these injuries.

Epidural Hematoma

Bleeding within the vertebral canal resulting in an epidural (or subdural) hematoma can cause ischemic compression of the spinal cord or nerve roots and lead to permanent neurologic deficit if not recognized and evacuated expeditiously. In the 2009 UK national audit the incidence of epidural hematoma was found to be 1 in 19,500 epidural anesthetics, but there were no cases of hematoma after 360,000 spinals.[76] Overall, the incidence of epidural hematoma is approximately 0.7 per 100,000 neuraxial anesthetics.[76] Many risk factors have been associated with the development of an epidural hematoma, including difficult or traumatic needle or catheter insertion, use of larger needles (the risk is higher with epidural than with spinal techniques), coagulopathy, female sex, and advanced age. Radicular back pain, prolonged blockade longer than the expected duration of the neuraxial technique, and bladder or bowel dysfunction are features commonly associated with a space-occupying lesion within the vertebral canal and should prompt immediate clinical review and magnetic resonance imaging on an urgent basis, given that surgical hematoma evacuation is a time-critical intervention to prevent permanent harm.

Epidural Abscess

Staphylococcal infections arising from organisms on the patient's skin are one of the most common epidural-related infections, which usually present with insidious back pain, tenderness, progressive neurological deficit, and systemic symptoms of infection. The presence of a concomitant systemic infection, diabetes, immuno-compromised states, and prolonged maintenance of an epidural (or spinal) catheter are risk factors. The rate of serious neuraxial infection is less than 3 per 100,000[77] for spinal anesthesia, whereas infectious complications after epidural techniques may be at least twice as common.[76] Obstetric patients appear less likely to develop deep infections related to epidural analgesia. Chlorhexidine in an alcohol base solution is the most effective antiseptic for the purposes of neuraxial techniques, and scrupulous attention to aseptic technique is a prerequisite for all neuraxial procedures.

Post-Dural Puncture Headache

Headache is relatively common and results from unintentional or intentional puncture of the dura membrane. The incidence is approximately 0.5% in spinal anesthesia and is minimized by using smaller-gauge, noncutting-tip spinal needles and orientating the needle bevel parallel with the axis of the spine. In obstetrics accidental dural puncture during epidural insertion may occur in around 1.5% of patients, with approximately two-thirds of these patients subsequently developing a post–dural puncture headache.[78] Additional risk factors for post–spinal puncture headache are listed in Box 17.2.

The loss of CSF through the dura may cause traction on pain-sensitive intracranial structures as the brain loses support and sags (Fig. 17.16). This loss of CSF may also initiate compensatory yet painful intracerebral vasodilation to offset the decreased intracranial pressure.[79] The characteristic feature of a post–dural puncture headache is a frontal or occipital headache that worsens with the upright or seated posture and is relieved by lying supine. Associated symptoms can include nausea, vomiting, neck pain, dizziness, tinnitus, diplopia, hearing loss, cortical blindness, cranial nerve palsies, and even seizures. Symptoms usually

---

Box 17.2 Relationships Among Variables and Post-Dural Puncture Headache

Factors That Can Increase the Incidence of Headache After Spinal Puncture
- Age: Younger, more frequent
- Sex: Females > males
- Needle size: larger > smaller
- Needle bevel: less when the needle bevel is placed in the long axis of the neuraxis
- Pregnancy: more when pregnant
- Dural punctures: more with multiple punctures

Factors That Do Not Increase the Incidence of Headache After Spinal Puncture
- Continuous spinal infusion
- Timing of ambulation

From Brull R, Macfarlane AJR, Chan VWS. Spinal, epidural and caudal anesthesia. In Miller RD, Cohen NH, Eriksson LI, et al., eds. Miller's Anesthesia. 8th ed. Philadelphia: Saunders Elsevier; 2015:Box 56.2.

---

begin within 3 days of the procedure, and approximately two-thirds start within the first 48 hours. Spontaneous resolution usually occurs within 7 days in the majority of cases, but a minority of patients still have symptoms at 6 months.

Conservative management for post–dural puncture headache includes supine positioning, hydration, caffeine, and oral analgesics. The use of sumatriptan has varying effects. Epidural blood patch is the definitive therapy,[80] with a single patch resulting in a 90% initial improvement rate and persistent resolution of symptoms in 61% to 75% of cases. A blood patch is ideally performed 24 hours after dural puncture and subsequent to the development of classic post–dural puncture headache symptoms. Prophylactic bedrest or epidural blood patching are not efficacious. It is recommended to insert the blood patch needle at or caudad to the level of the dural puncture, with 20 mL of blood being a reasonable starting target volume.[81] A second epidural blood patch may be performed 24 to 48 hours later if the first is ineffective.

Total Spinal Anesthesia

Total spinal anesthesia is characterized by rapidly progressive bradycardia, hypotension, loss of consciousness, apnea, and cardiac arrest caused by inadvertent spread of local anesthetic to the cervical nerve roots and brainstem. Although rare, total spinal anesthesia can occur after any inadvertent intrathecal injection of large volumes of local anesthetic. Management is supportive of the resulting respiratory and cardiovascular compromise.

Transient Neurological Symptoms

TNS are characterized by bilateral or unilateral pain in the buttocks radiating to the legs or, less commonly, isolated buttock or leg pain. Symptoms occur within 24 hours of the resolution of an otherwise uneventful spinal anesthetic and are not associated with any neurological deficits or laboratory abnormalities. Pain can be mild or severe but typically resolves spontaneously in less than 1 week. TNS are more likely after intrathecal lidocaine and mepivacaine and are far less frequent with bupivacaine.[82] The phenomenon is related to the concentration of lidocaine, the addition of dextrose or epinephrine, and solution osmolarity. TNS are less commonly associated with epidural procedures. The risk also appears more likely in the lithotomy position for surgery. Nonsteroidal antiinflammatory drugs are the first line of treatment, but opioids may be required.

Cardiovascular

Hypotension

Hypotension is more likely with peak block height higher than or equal to T5, age of 40 years or older, baseline systolic blood pressure less than 120 mm Hg, combined spinal and general anesthesia, spinal puncture at or above the L2–L3 interspace, and the addition of phenylephrine

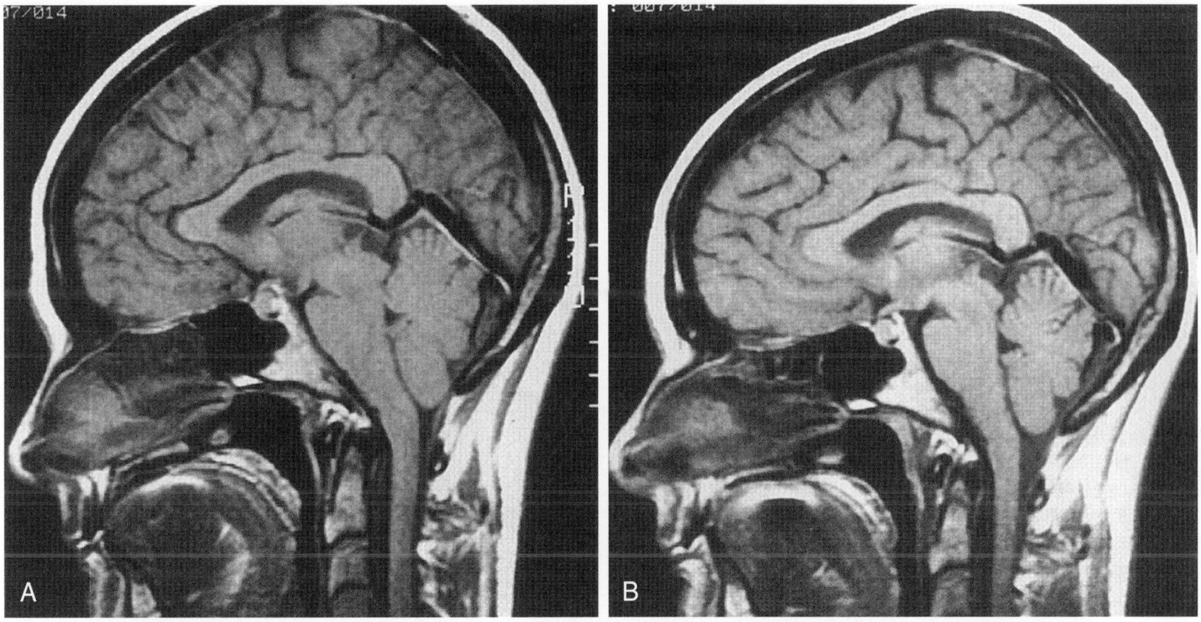

Fig. 17.16 Anatomy of a "low-pressure" headache. (A) A T1-weighted sagittal magnetic resonance image demonstrates a "ptotic brain" manifested as tonsillar herniation below the foramen magnum, forward displacement of the pons, absence of the suprasellar cistern, kinking of the chiasm, and fullness of the pituitary gland. (B) A comparable image of the same patient after an epidural blood patch and resolution of the symptoms demonstrates normal anatomy. (From Drasner K, Swisher JL. In Brown DL, ed. *Regional Anesthesia and Analgesia*. Philadelphia: WB Saunders; 1996.)

to the local anesthetic. Hypotension is also independently associated with chronic alcohol consumption, history of hypertension, body mass index (BMI), and the urgency of surgery.[83] Nausea is a common symptom of hypotension in the setting of neuraxial anesthesia; other symptoms include vomiting, dizziness, and dyspnea.

Bradycardia
The mechanism has been described earlier, but factors that may increase the likelihood of exaggerated bradycardia include baseline heart rate less than 60 beats/min, age of 40 years or younger, male sex, nonemergency status, β-adrenergic blockade and prolonged duration of surgery.[84]

Respiratory

The risk of respiratory depression associated with neuraxial opioids is dose-dependent, with a reported frequency that can be as high as 3% after the administration of 0.8 mg of intrathecal morphine.[85] Respiratory depression may stem from rostral spread of opioids within the CSF to the chemosensitive respiratory centers in the brainstem. With lipophilic anesthetics, respiratory depression is generally an early phenomenon occurring within the first 30 minutes (and has not been reported after 2 hours), whereas with intrathecal morphine, late respiratory depression may occur up to 24 hours after injection. Monitoring, including

respiratory rate and sedation score, for the first 24 hours after the administration of intrathecal morphine is recommended. A low oxygen saturation can be a late sign, particularly if supplemental oxygen is being used. Respiratory depression is reduced with use of intrathecal morphine doses less than 0.3 mg.[86] Patients with sleep apnea can be particularly sensitive, and considerable caution must be exercised in this group.[87] Older patients also have a more frequent risk of respiratory depression, and therefore the dose of neuraxial opioids should be reduced (also see Chapter 35). Coadministration of systemic sedatives also increases this risk.

Infection

Bacterial meningitis is a rare but potentially catastrophic complication, most commonly arising after intrathecal transmission of oral bacteria such as *S. viridans* during spinal anesthesia. Facemasks should therefore be worn during all neuraxial procedures. Epidural abscess is described earlier.

Wrong-Route Drug Delivery

Small-bore medical connection syringe systems carry an inherent risk of inadvertent wrong-route drug administration by the administration of a drug intended for the

313

intravascular compartment into the epidural or intrathecal space or vice versa. Such errors can have catastrophic consequences, including death. The International Organization for Standardization (ISO) has published a group of standards for medical small-bore connectors, including ISO 80369-6:2016, which addresses connectors (so-called NR-Fit) for neuraxial applications and peripheral nerve blocks.

Backache

There is no association between epidural analgesia and new-onset back pain up to 6 months postpartum.

Nausea and Vomiting

Nausea and vomiting may be secondary to either direct exposure of the chemoreceptor trigger zone in the brain to emetogenic drugs (e.g., opioids), hypotension, or gastrointestinal hyperperistalsis secondary to unopposed parasympathetic activity. Nausea or vomiting after spinal anesthesia is more likely with the addition of phenylephrine or epinephrine to the local anesthetic, peak block height of T5 or higher, baseline heart rate more rapid than 60 beats/min, history of motion sickness, and the development of hypotension during spinal anesthesia. Intrathecal morphine has the highest risk of opioid-induced nausea or vomiting, whereas fentanyl and sufentanil carry the lowest risk.[88] Again these side effects are dose-dependent. Using less than 0.1 mg morphine reduces the risk without compromising the analgesic effect.

Urinary Retention

Urinary retention can occur in as many as one-third of patients after neuraxial anesthesia. Local anesthetic blockade of the S2, S3, and S4 nerve roots inhibits urinary function as the detrusor muscle is weakened. Neuraxial opioids can further complicate urinary function by suppressing detrusor contractility and reducing the sensation of urge.[89] Spontaneous return of normal bladder function is expected once the sensory level regresses to less than S2–S3. Along with male sex and age (possibly the result of sex and age-specific pathologies such as benign prostatic hypertrophy), long-acting local anesthetics and intrathecal morphine are also linked to urinary retention after neuraxial anesthesia.[90]

Pruritus

Pruritus can be distressing and is the most common side effect related to the intrathecal administration of opioids, with rates between 30% and 100%.[91] Parturients are at particular risk.[92] The incidence is not dependent on the type of

opioid administered, although reducing the dose reduces the likelihood of pruritus, and lipophilic agents (such as fentanyl) will result in a shorter duration of itching. Naloxone, naltrexone, or the partial agonist nalbuphine can be used for treatment. Ondansetron and propofol are also useful antipruritic therapies.

Shivering

The rate of shivering is as frequent as 55%[93] and is more related to epidural than to spinal anesthesia. One postulated cause is the relatively cold temperature of the epidural injectate, which can affect the thermosensitive basal sinuses. The addition of neuraxial opioids, specifically fentanyl and meperidine, reduces the likelihood of shivering.[93] Prewarming the patient with a forced air warmer and avoiding the administration of cold epidural and intravenous fluids also reduce the incidence of shivering.

Complications Unique to Epidural Anesthesia

Intravascular Injection

Epidural anesthesia can produce local anesthetic systemic toxicity (LAST, see Chapter 10), primarily through the unintentional administration of drug into an epidural vein. The frequency of vascular puncture by needle or catheter is approximately 10%, with rates highest in the obstetric population, in whom these vessels are relatively dilated.[94] Seizures related to epidural anesthesia may be as frequent as 1%.[77] In obstetrics (also see Chapter 33) the likelihood of intravascular injection is decreased by placing the patient in the lateral position during needle and catheter insertion, administering fluid through the epidural needle before catheter insertion, using a single-orifice rather than multiorifice catheter or a wire-embedded polyurethane compared with polyamide epidural catheter, and advancing the catheter less than 6 cm into the epidural space. The paramedian approach and the use of a smaller-gauge epidural needle or catheter does not reduce the risk of epidural vein cannulation.

Using epinephrine mixed with local anesthetic as a test dose can be unreliable, and so prevention of LAST should always involve observation for blood flow through the epidural catheter under the influence of gravity when first inserted and both aspiration of the catheter and incremental administration of the local anesthetic before every dose.

Subdural Injection

The subdural extraarachnoid space is a potential space between the arachnoid and dura mater.[95] Infrequently (and unbeknown to the provider and patient) the Tuohy needle tip and/or catheter tip can enter into the subdural space, with subsequent local anesthetic administration resulting in a higher-than-expected block developing 15 to 30 minutes after injection. With a subdural block, the motor block will be modest compared with the extent of sensory blockade, because the subdural space is relatively more capacious in the posterior and lateral aspects, leading to sparing of the anterior motor nerve roots.[96]

Sympathetic blockade may also be relatively spared for the same reason, although cases are described with hypotension from partial sympathectomy. The treatment is symptomatic, and the catheter should be removed and resited.

REFERENCES

1. Pöpping DM, Elia N, Van Aken HK, et al. Impact of epidural analgesia on mortality and morbidity after surgery. *Ann Surg.* 2014;259:1056–1067.
2. Smith LM, Cozowicz C, Uda Y, Memtsoudis SG, Barrington MJ. Neuraxial and combined neuraxial/general anesthesia compared to general anesthesia for major truncal and lower limb surgery: A systematic review and meta-analysis. *Anesth Analg.* 2017;125:1931–1934.
3. Reina MA, Lirk P, Puigdellívol-Sánchez A, Mavar M, Prats-Galino A. Human lumbar ligamentum flavum anatomy for epidural anesthesia. *Anesth Analg.* 2016;122:903–907.
4. Lirk P, Kolbitsch C, Putz G, et al. Cervical and high thoracic ligamentum flavum frequently fails to fuse in the midline. *Anesthesiology.* 2003;99:1387–1390.
5. Liu S, Kopacz DJ, Carpenter RL. Quantitative assessment of differential sensory nerve block after lidocaine spinal anesthesia. *Anesthesiology.* 1995;82:60–63.
6. Greene NM. Distribution of local anesthetic solutions within the subarachnoid space. *Anesth Analg.* 1985;64:715–730.
7. Clement R, Malinovsky JM, Le Corre P, Dollo G, Chevanne F, Le Verge R. Cerebrospinal fluid bioavailability and pharmacokinetics of bupivacaine and lidocaine after intrathecal and epidural administrations in rabbits using microdialysis. *J Pharmacol Exp Ther.* 1999;289:1015–1021.
8. Visser WA, Lee RA, Gielen MJM. Factors affecting the distribution of neural blockade by local anesthetics in epidural anesthesia and a comparison of lumbar versus thoracic epidural anesthesia. *Anesth Analg.* 2008;107:708–721.
9. Rooke GA, Freund PR, Jacobson AF. Hemodynamic response and change in organ blood volume during spinal anesthesia in elderly men with cardiac disease. *Anesth Analg.* 1997;85:99–105.
10. Greene NM. *Physiology of spinal anesthesia.* Baltimore: Williams & Wilkins; 1981. 3rd ed.
11. Crystal GJ, Salem MR. The Bainbridge and the "reverse" Bainbridge reflexes: History, physiology and clinical relevance. *Anesth Analg.* 2012;114:520–532.
12. Minville V, Asehnoune K, Salau S, et al. The effects of spinal anesthesia on cerebral blood flow in the very elderly. *Anesth Analg.* 2009;108:1291–1294.
13. Pollock J, Neal JM, Liu SS, Burkhead D, Polissar N. Sedation during spinal anesthesia. *Anesthesiology.* 2000;93:728–734.
14. Groeben H. Epidural anesthesia and pulmonary function. *J Anesth.* 2006;20:290–299.
15. Freise H, Fischer LG. Intestinal effects of thoracic epidural anesthesia. *Curr Opin Anaesthesiol.* 2009;22:644–648.
16. Hawkins JL. Epidural analgesia for labor and delivery. *N Engl J Med.* 2010;362:1503–1510.
17. Macfarlane AJR, Prasad GA, Chan VWS, Brull R. Does regional anaesthesia improve outcome after total hip arthroplasty? A systematic review. *Br J Anaesth.* 2009;103:335–345.
18. Macfarlane AJR, Prasad GA, Chan VWS, Brull R. Does regional anesthesia improve outcome after total knee arthroplasty?. *Clin Orthop Relat Res.* 2009;467:2379–2402.
19. Nishimori M, Low JHS, Zheng H, Ballantyne JC. Epidural pain relief versus systemic opioid-based pain relief for abdominal aortic surgery. *Cochrane Database Syst Rev.* 2012(7):CD005059.
20. Joshi GP, Bonnet F, Shah R, et al. The comparative effects of postoperative analgesic therapies on pulmonary outcome: Cumulative meta-analyses of randomized, controlled trials. *Anesth Analg.* 2008;107:1026–1040.
21. Svircevic V, van Dijk D, Nierich AP, et al. Meta-analysis of thoracic epidural anesthesia versus general anesthesia for cardiac surgery. *Anesthesiology.* 2011;114:271–282.
22. Neal JM, Barrington MJ, Brull R, et al. The Second ASRA Practice Advisory on Neurologic Complications Associated With Regional Anesthesia and Pain Medicine: Executive summary 2015. *Reg Anesth Pain Med.* 2015;40(5):401–430.
23. Hilt H, Gramm HJ, Link J. Changes in intracranial pressure associated with extradural anaesthesia. *Br J Anaesth.* 1986;58:676–680.
24. Hebl JR, Horlocker TT, Kopp SL, Schroeder DR. Neuraxial blockade in patients with preexisting spinal stenosis, lumbar disk disease, or prior spine surgery: Efficacy and neurologic complications. *Anesth Analg.* 2010;111:1511–1519.
25. Perlas A, Chan VWS. Neuraxial anesthesia and multiple sclerosis. *Can J Anaesth.* 2005;52:454–458.
26. McDonald SB. Is neuraxial blockade contraindicated in the patient with aortic stenosis?. *Reg Anesth Pain Med.* 2004;29:496–502.
27. Horlocker TT, Vandermeulen E, Kopp SL, Gogarten W, Leffert LR, Benzon HT. Regional anesthesia in the patient receiving antithrombotic or thrombolytic therapy: American Society of Regional Anesthesia and Pain Medicine Evidence-Based Guidelines (fourth edition). *Reg Anesth Pain Med.* 2018;43:263–309.
28. Choi S, Brull R. Neuraxial techniques in obstetric and non-obstetric patients with common bleeding diatheses. *Anesth Analg.* 2009;109:648–660.
29. Wedel DJ, Horlocker TT. Regional anesthesia in the febrile or infected patient. *Reg Anesth Pain Med.* 2006;31:324–333.
30. Hocking G, Wildsmith JAW. Intrathecal drug spread. *Br J Anaesth.* 2004;93:568–578.
31. Tetzlaff JE, O'Hara J, Bell G, et al. Influence of baricity on the outcome of spinal anesthesia with bupivacaine for lumbar spine surgery. *Reg Anesth.* 1995;20:533–537.
32. Van Zundert AA, Grouls RJ, Korsten HH, Lambert DH. Spinal anesthesia: Volume or concentration—what matters? *Reg Anesth.* 1996;21:112–118.
33. Sarantopoulos C, Fassoulaki A. Systemic opioids enhance the spread of sensory analgesia produced by intrathecal lidocaine. *Anesth Analg.* 1994;79:94–97.
34. Carpenter RL, Hogan QH, Liu SS, et al. Lumbosacral cerebrospinal fluid volume is the primary determinant of sensory block extent and duration during spinal anesthesia. *Anesthesiology.* 1998;89:24–29.
35. Taivainen T, Tuominen M, Rosenber PH. Influence of obesity on the spread of spinal analgesia after injection of plain 0.5% bupivacaine at the L3-4 or L4-5 interspace. *Br J Anaesth.* 1990;64:542–546.
36. Veering BT. The role of ageing in local anaesthesia. *Pain Rev.* 1999;6:167–173.
37. Kim JT, Shim JK, Kim SH, et al. Trendelenburg position with hip flexion as a rescue strategy to increase spinal anaesthetic level after spinal block. *Br J Anaesth.* 2007;98:396–400.
38. Urmey WF, Stanton J, Bassin P, Sharrock NE. The direction of the Whitacre needle aperture affects the extent and duration of isobaric spinal anesthesia. *Anesth Analg.* 1997;84:337–341.

III

39. Casati A, Fanelli G, Cappelleri G, et al. Effects of spinal needle type on lateral distribution of 0.5% hyperbaric bupivacaine. *Anesth Analg.* 1998;87:355–359.
40. Sanderson P, Read J, Littlewood DG, et al. Interaction between baricity (glucose concentration) and other factors influencing intrathecal drug spread. *Br J Anaesth.* 1994;73:744–746.
41. Malinovsky JM, Renaud G, Le Corre P, et al. Intrathecal bupivacaine in humans: Influence of volume and baricity of solutions. *Anesthesiology.* 1999;91:1260–1266.
42. Goldblum E, Atchabahian A. The use of 2-chloroprocaine for spinal anaesthesia. *Acta Anaesthesiol Scand.* 2013;57:545–552.
43. Zaric D, Pace NL. Transient neurologic symptoms (TNS) following spinal anaesthesia with lidocaine versus other local anaesthetics. *Cochrane Database Syst Rev.* 2009(2):CD003006.
44. Casati A, Vinciguerra F. Intrathecal anesthesia. *Curr Opin Anaesthesiol.* 2002;15:543–551.
45. Nair GS, Abrishami A, Lermitte J, Chung F. Systematic review of spinal anaesthesia using bupivacaine for ambulatory knee arthroscopy. *Br J Anaesth.* 2009;102:307–315.
46. Whiteside JB, Burke D. Comparison of ropivacaine 0.5% (in glucose 5%) with bupivacaine 0.5% (in glucose 8%) for spinal anaesthesia for elective surgery. *Br J Anaesth.* 2003;90:304–308.
47. Hamber EA, Viscomi CM. Intrathecal lipophilic opioids as adjuncts to surgical spinal anesthesia. *Reg Anesth Pain Med.* 1999;24:255–263.
48. Meylan N, Elia N, Lysakowski C, Tramèr MR. Benefit and risk of intrathecal morphine without local anaesthetic in patients undergoing major surgery: Meta-analysis of randomized trials. *Br J Anaesth.* 2009;102:156–167.
49. Murphy PM, Stack D, Kinirons B, Laffey JG. Optimizing the dose of intrathecal morphine in older patients undergoing hip arthroplasty. *Anesth Analg.* 2003;97:1709–1715.
50. Zorrilla-Vaca A, Healy RZ-VC. Finer gauge of cutting but not pencil-point needles correlate with lower incidence of post-dural puncture headache: A meta-regression analysis. *J Anesth.* 2016;30:855–863.
51. Flaatten H, Rodt SA, Vamnes J, et al. Postdural puncture headache. A comparison between 26- and 29-gauge needles in young patients. *Anaesthesia.* 1989; 44:147–149.
52. Hebl JR. The importance and implications of aseptic techniques during regional anesthesia. *Reg Anesth Pain Med.* 2006;31:311–323.
53. Chin KJ, Karmakar MK, Peng P. Ultrasonography of the adult thoracic and lumbar spine for central neuraxial blockade. *Anesthesiology.* 2011;114:1459–1485.
54. Perlas A, Chaparro LE, Chin KJ. Lumbar neuraxial ultrasound for spinal and epidural anesthesia: A systematic review and meta-analysis. *Reg Anesth Pain Med.* 2016;41:251–260.
55. Moore JM. Continuous spinal anesthesia. *Am J Ther.* 2009;16:289–294.
56. Rigler ML, Drasner K, Krejcie TC, et al. Cauda equina syndrome after continuous spinal anesthesia. *Anesth Analg.* 1991;72:275–281.
57. Vaghadia H, Viskari D, Mitchell GW, Berrill A. Selective spinal anesthesia for outpatient laparoscopy. I: characteristics of three hypobaric solutions. *Can J Anaesth.* 2001;48:256–260.
58. Bromage PR. A comparison of the hydrochloride and carbon dioxide salts of lidocaine and prilocaine in epidural analgesia. *Acta Anaesthesiol Scand Suppl.* 1965;16:55–69.
59. Visser WA, Liem TH, van Egmond J, Gielen MJ. Extension of sensory blockade after thoracic epidural administration of a test dose of lidocaine at three different levels. *Anesth Analg.* 1998; 86:332–335.
60. Stevens RA, Urmey WF, Urquhart BL, Kao TC. Back pain after epidural anesthesia with chloroprocaine. *Anesthesiology.* 1993;78:492–497.
61. Marinacci AA. Neurological aspects of complications of spinal anesthesia, with medicolegal implications. *Bull Los Angeles Neurol Soc.* 1960;25:170–192.
62. Sultan P, Gutierrez MC, Carvalho B. Neuraxial morphine and respiratory depression: Finding the right balance. *Drugs.* 2011;71:1807–1819.
63. Hillyard SG, Bate TE, Corcoran TB, Paech MJ, O'Sullivan G. Extending epidural analgesia for emergency Caesarean section: A meta-analysis. *Br J Anaesth.* 2011;107:668–678.
64. Covino BG, Scott DB, McClure JH. *Handbook of Epidural Anaesthesia and Analgesia.* Fribourg, Switzerland: Mediglobe; 1999.
65. Morison DH. Alkalinization of local anaesthetics. *Can J Anaesth.* 1995;42:1076–1079.
66. Segal S, Eappen S, Datta S. Superiority of multi-orifice over single-orifice epidural catheters for labor analgesia and cesarean delivery. *J Clin Anesth.* 1997;9:109–112.
67. Murphy JD, Ouanes JPP, Togioka BM, et al. Comparison of air and liquid for use in loss-of-resistance technique during labor epidurals: A meta-analysis. *J Anesth Clin Res.* 2011;2:175.
68. Mhyre JM, Lou VH, Greenfield M, et al. A systematic review of randomized controlled trials that evaluate strategies to avoid epidural vein cannulation during obstetric epidural catheter placement. *Anesth Analg.* 2009;108:1232–1242.
69. Afshan G, Chohan U, Khan FA, et al. Appropriate length of epidural catheter in the epidural space for postoperative analgesia: Evaluation by epidurography. *Anaesthesia.* 2011;66:913–918.
70. Tsui BC, Gupta S, Finucane B. Confirmation of epidural catheter placement using nerve stimulation. *Can J Anaesth.* 1998;45:640–644.
71. Grau T, Leipold RW, Conradi R, Martin E, Motsch J. Efficacy of ultrasound imaging in obstetric epidural anesthesia. *J Clin Anesth.* 2002;14:169–175.
72. Lew E, Yeo SW, Thomas E. Combined spinal-epidural anesthesia using epidural volume extension leads to faster motor recovery after elective cesarean delivery: A prospective, randomized, double-blind study. *Anesth Analg.* 2004; 98:810–814.
73. Rawal N. Combined spinal-epidural anaesthesia. *Curr Opin Anaesthesiol.* 2005;18:518–521.
74. Mackey D. Physiologic effects of regional block. In: Brown DL, ed. *Regional Anesthesia and Analgesia.* Philadelphia: WB Saunders; 1996.
75. Brull R, McCartney CJL, Chan VWS, El-Beheiry H. Neurological complications after regional anesthesia: contemporary estimates of risk. *Anesth Analg.* 2007;104:965–974.
76. Cook TM, Counsell D, Wildsmith JAW. Royal College of Anaesthetists Third National Audit Project. Major complications of central neuraxial block: Report on the Third National Audit Project of the Royal College of Anaesthetists. *Br J Anaesth.* 2009;102:179–190.
77. Auroy Y, Benhamou D, Bargues L, et al. Major complications of regional anesthesia in France. *Anesthesiology.* 2002;97:1274–1280.
78. Choi PT, Galinski SE, Takeuchi L, et al. PDPH is a common complication of neuraxial blockade in parturients: A meta-analysis of obstetrical studies. *Can J Anaesth.* 2003;50:460–469.
79. Turnbull DK, Shepherd DB. Post-dural puncture headache: Pathogenesis, prevention and treatment. *Br J Anaesth.* 2003;91:718–729.
80. Harrington BE. Postdural puncture headache and the development of the epidural blood patch. *Reg Anesth Pain Med.* 2004;29:136–163.
81. Paech MJ, Doherty DA, Christmas T, Wong CA. Epidural Blood Patch Trial Group. The volume of blood for epidural blood patch in obstetrics: A randomized, blinded clinical trial. *Anesth Analg.* 2011;113:126–133.
82. Gozdemir M, Muslu B, Sert H, et al. Transient neurological symptoms after spinal anaesthesia with levobupivacaine

5 mg/ml or lidocaine 20 mg/ml. *Acta Anaesthesiol Scand.* 2010;54:59–64.

83. Hartmann B, Junger A, Klasen J, et al. The incidence and risk factors for hypotension after spinal anesthesia induction: An analysis with automated data collection. *Anesth Analg.* 2002;94:1521–1529.

84. Lesser JB, Sanborn KV, Valskys R, Kuroda M. Severe bradycardia during spinal and epidural anesthesia recorded by an anesthesia information management system. *Anesthesiology.* 2003;99:859–866.

85. Gwirtz KH, Young JV, Byers RS, et al. The safety and efficacy of intrathecal opioid analgesia for acute postoperative pain: Seven years' experience with 5969 surgical patients at Indiana University Hospital. *Anesth Analg.* 1999;88:599–604.

86. Gehling MTM. Risks and side-effects of intrathecal morphine combined with spinal anaesthesia: A meta-analysis. *Anaesthesia.* 2009;64:643–651.

87. Horlocker TT, Burton AW, Connis RT, et al., American Society of Anesthesiologists Task Force on Neuraxial Opioids Practice guidelines for the prevention, detection and management of respiratory depression associated with neuraxial opioid administration. *Anesthesiology.* 2009;110:218–230.

88. Borgeat A, Ekatodramis G, Schenker CA. Postoperative nausea and vomiting in regional anesthesia: A review. *Anesthesiology.* 2003;98:530–547.

89. Kuipers PW, Kamphuis ET, van Venrooij GE, et al. Intrathecal opioids and lower urinary tract function: A urodynamic evaluation. *Anesthesiology.* 2004;100:1497–1503.

90. Baldini G, Bagry H, Aprikian A, Carli F. Postoperative urinary retention: Anesthetic and perioperative considerations. *Anesthesiology.* 2009;110:1139–1157.

91. Rathmell JP, Lair TR, Nauman B. The role of intrathecal drugs in the treatment of acute pain. *Anesth Analg.* 2005;101(5 suppl):S30–SS4.

92. Kumar K, Singh SI. Neuraxial opioid-induced pruritus: An update. *J Anaesthesiol Clin Pharmacol.* 2013;29:303–307.

93. Crowley LJ, Buggy DJ. Shivering and neuraxial anesthesia. *Reg Anesth Pain Med.* 2008;33:241–252.

94. Bell DN, Leslie K. Detection of intravascular epidural catheter placement: A review. *Anaesth Intensive Care.* 2007;35:335–341.

95. Reina MA, Collier CB, Prats-Galino A, Puigdellívol-Sánchez A, Machés FDAJ. Unintentional subdural placement of epidural catheters during attempted epidural anesthesia: An anatomic study of spinal subdural compartment. *Reg Anesth Pain Med.* 2011;36:537–541.

96. Ralph C, Williams M. Subdural or epidural?. *Anaesthesia.* 1996;51:175–177.

18 PERIPHERAL NERVE BLOCKS

Edward N. Yap, Andrew T. Gray

INTRODUCTION

The Role of Regional Anesthesia

Peripheral nerve blocks can provide surgical anesthesia and postoperative pain relief (Table 18.1). The main emphasis of this chapter will be on ultrasound guidance for peripheral nerve blocks. However, paresthetic-based techniques and nerve stimulation also are possible for nerve localization. In addition, ultrasound guidance and nerve stimulation technologies can be combined for some regional blocks.

Preparation to Perform a Regional Nerve Block

Foundation of Knowledge
To perform safe and effective peripheral nerve blocks, an understanding of peripheral neuroanatomy, ultrasound technology, local anesthetic pharmacology, and risks associated with peripheral nerve blocks is needed.

Patient and Surgeon Factors
The willingness of the patient and the surgeon, in addition to the anatomic location of the surgery, must be taken into consideration when incorporating peripheral nerve blocks into an anesthetic plan. A thorough preoperative review of the patient's medical history, including any comorbid diseases, allergies, prior neuropathy, and concurrent anticoagulation medications, must be performed to rule out any contraindications in providing a peripheral nerve block.

Monitors and Equipment
Peripheral nerve blocks may be performed preoperatively in a dedicated block area or in the operating room. The patient must have a functional peripheral intravenous line and monitoring equipment, including pulse oximetry, electrocardiogram (ECG), and noninvasive blood pressure machine. Supplemental oxygen, emergency medications, and airway equipment must be readily accessible. Sedation

may be indicated, depending on the patient's anxiety and magnitude of pain.

The patient, ultrasound machine, and anesthesia provider must be positioned in a way to optimize the nerve block being performed. For most blocks, the provider is positioned on the ipsilateral side and the ultrasound on the contralateral side of the block region. The choice of the ultrasound probe (Fig. 18.1) and needle is dependent on the location of the peripheral nerve block; the addition of placing a catheter will depend on the type of surgery being performed, the duration of hospital stay, and patient and surgeon preference.

Choice of Local Anesthetic

The choice of local anesthetic for peripheral nerve blockade depends on several factors, including the desired onset, duration, and degree of conduction block (see Chapter 10). Lidocaine and mepivacaine, 1% to 1.5%, produce surgical anesthesia in 10 to 20 minutes that lasts 2 to 3 hours. Ropivacaine 0.5% and bupivacaine 0.375% to 0.5% have a slower onset and produce less motor blockade, but the effect lasts for at least 6 to 8 hours. The addition of epinephrine 1:200,000 (5 μg/mL) can serve as a marker for intravascular injection and can increase the duration of a conduction block. In addition, through a decrease in the rate of systemic absorption, epinephrine can reduce peak plasma levels of local anesthetic. Practitioners may also add perineural steroids (e.g., preservative-free dexamethasone) to local anesthetics to prolong regional blocks.[1] Considerations for the choice of local anesthetic solution for intravenous regional anesthesia are different from those for peripheral nerve blocks (see the later discussion under "Intravenous Regional Anesthesia [Bier Block]").

Regional Block Checklist

A standardized regional block checklist should be reviewed before performing a peripheral nerve block to improve safety.[2,3] The checklist should include surgical consent, site marking, allergies, anticoagulation status, proposed peripheral nerve block, local anesthetic dose, side of the block, monitors implemented, emergency equipment available, and sedation plan.

Risks and Prevention

Infection

Infectious risk associated with a peripheral nerve block or placement of a peripheral nerve catheter is rare.[4] However, an infection can cause significant morbidity and may lead to permanent neurologic injury. By performing proper hand hygiene, using maximal barriers during nerve block and catheter placement, and providing antiseptic solution at the site of insertion, the rate of infection can be reduced.

Hematoma

The risk of developing a hematoma depends on the location of the peripheral nerve block being performed, the proximity to vascular structures, and vascular compressibility. With the use of ultrasound and proper aspiration technique, vascular puncture can be reduced.[5] A review of the patient's medical history with an emphasis on any anticoagulation medications is important. The American Society of Regional Anesthesia and Pain Medicine provides guidelines on anticoagulation management.[6]

Local Anesthetic Systemic Toxicity (Also See Chapter 10)

Local anesthetic systemic toxicity (LAST) secondary to local anesthetic absorption can range from mild symptoms to major neurologic and cardiovascular toxicity.

Table 18.1 Examples of Peripheral Nerve Blocks

Origin	Specific Block
Cervical plexus	Superficial
Brachial plexus	Interscalene Supraclavicular Infraclavicular Axillary
Lumbar plexus	Lateral femoral cutaneous[a] Femoral Adductor canal Saphenous Obturator[a]
Sacral plexus	Proximal sciatic Popliteal sciatic

[a]Not covered in this chapter.

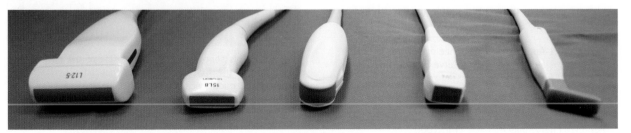

Fig. 18.1 Ultrasound transducers for regional blocks. (From Gray AT. *Atlas of Ultrasound-Guided Regional Anesthesia*. 3rd ed. Philadelphia: Elsevier-Saunders; 2018:21.)

A variety of factors, including patient risk factors, concurrent medications, total local anesthetic dose, and anatomic location of the peripheral nerve block, play a role in the risk of LAST. There is no single measure to prevent LAST; however, using the smallest effective dose, an incremental injection, aspiration before injection, an intravascular marker (i.e., epinephrine), and ultrasound guidance may decrease the risk. Lipid emulsion resuscitation remains the cornerstone of therapy to treat patients with LAST.[7,8]

Nerve Injury

Nerve injury may result from direct needle trauma, inadvertent intraneural injection, or drug neurotoxicity. Serious neurologic injury from a peripheral nerve block is rare; however, the rate of transient paresthesia that resolves within days to weeks postoperatively is substantially higher.[9-11] The use of ultrasound to identify nerves, limiting the injection pressure, and patient feedback may help decrease the rate of nerve injury, although clinical outcome data are limited.

Wrong-Sided Block

Wrong site, wrong procedure, and wrong patient peripheral nerve blocks are potentially serious medical errors that are inherent risks in performing any medical procedure.[12] Although rare, this complication can be reduced by having a universal protocol that includes a checklist to ensure the correct patient, the proper surgery site, and correct laterality (Table 18.2).

ULTRASOUND BASICS

An understanding of ultrasound imaging and transducer manipulation is important in providing safe and effective peripheral nerve blocks.

Basic Ultrasound Physics

Ultrasound imaging uses sound waves with frequency greater than 20 kHz. The use of ultrasound for medical purposes was first recognized in the 1930s. Since then, improvements in technology have paved the way to produce real-time images to help in diagnostics and interventions. Medical ultrasound machines use piezoelectric crystals in the transducer that convert electrical currents into mechanical pressure waves and vice versa, sending and receiving ultrasound echoes to thereby generate images.

As ultrasound waves pass through different body tissues, the resistance to the propagation of ultrasound waves, or acoustic impedance, changes depending on the density of the tissue. Solid tissues have denser particles that effectively reflect waves that will be received by the transducer, displayed as brighter or hyperechoic structures. Less dense tissue does not reflect ultrasound waves as effectively, displayed as darker or hypoechoic structures. Tissues that do not reflect any ultrasound waves are considered anechoic.

Improving image resolution, or the ability to distinguish one structure from another, will optimize performance of peripheral nerve blocks. Increasing the frequency of the ultrasound wave will improve resolution of the image but will decrease the penetration of the ultrasound waves. Decreasing the frequency will lower the resolution but will improve the penetration to deeper tissue because there is less attenuation. Increasing the receiver gain (i.e., amplification of the returning echo signal) can to some extent compensate for attenuation.

Echogenic Properties of Nerves and Tissue

Peripheral nerves can be recognized on ultrasound scans by their fascicular echotexture. Central nerves (such as the cervical ventral rami) and very small nerves (such as the phrenic nerve) have a monofascicular or oligofascicular appearance (Fig. 18.2). Most peripheral nerves have a

Table 18.2	Approximate Incidence of Adverse Events During Peripheral Nerve Blocks
Adverse Event	**Approximate Incidence**
Anesthetic systemic toxicity	1 in 2000[5]
Peripheral nerve injury	1 in 1000
Wrong side/site block	1 in 10,000

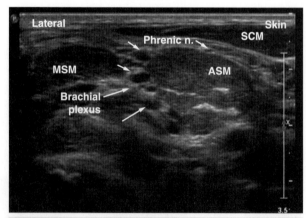

Fig. 18.2 This sonogram of the right side of the neck shows the roots of the brachial plexus as they pass between the anterior and middle scalene muscles. The core of these large peripheral nerves is less echogenic than the surrounding muscle. The phrenic nerve is a small hypoechoic structure seen on the anterior surface of the anterior scalene muscle. *ASM*, Anterior scalene muscle; *MSM*, middle scalene muscle; *SCM*, sternocleidomastoid muscle.[20]

polyfascicular appearance, which consists of a collection of small round hypoechoic dots (from the nerve fascicles or nerve fiber content) surrounded by hyperechoic stroma (from the nerve connective tissue). This pattern can be referred to as "honeycomb" or "bunch of grapes." Although we use the term *nerve fascicles,* it is understood that only a subset of the total number of fascicles will be evident on an ultrasound scan because thin layers of connective tissue that divide fascicles cannot be resolved on the image.[13] Nerves have a relatively constant cross-sectional area along their course, which helps distinguish these anatomic structures from adjacent tendons.

Ergonomics and Transducer Manipulation

Proper ergonomics are essential for ultrasound-guided interventions. It is important to maintain proper posture and position to reduce anesthesia provider fatigue (e.g., optimize patient position, bed height, and position of the display). A comfortable grip on the ultrasound transducer and resting the ulnar aspect of the transducer hand on the patient will promote stability. There are five basic transducer manipulation techniques to help optimize the ultrasound image: sliding, tilting, rocking, rotation, and compression. Peripheral nerves exhibit anisotropy, which means that the reflected echoes depend on the angle of insonation.[14] The transducer can be tilted to maximize the returning echoes from the peripheral nerve. Slide and rotate the transducer to find the needle tip while maintaining nerve visibility. For some regional blocks, the soft tissue will allow the transducer to rock back and reduce the angle of insonation, thereby improving needle tip visibility. Visual inspection is a good technique before using ultrasound guidance or if needle lineups are difficult.[15] Most practitioners compress adjacent veins while introducing the needle to reduce the chance of venous puncture.

Regional Block Technique

There are multiple approaches to peripheral nerve blocks. Most blocks can be performed with a short-axis view of the nerve to be blocked. This view is stable for nerves with a relatively straight path. The in-plane technique, with the entire needle shaft and tip within the plane of imaging, is often used to guide needle placement (Fig. 18.3). Alternatively, the out-of-plane approach can be used so that the needle tip crosses the plane of imaging as an echogenic dot. The quality of imaging and identification of structures are more important than approach. Differences in outcomes have been difficult to show when comparing various approaches to blocks in clinical studies.

Peripheral Nerve Catheters

Catheters can be placed adjacent to peripheral nerves for postoperative analgesia by infusion of dilute local anesthetic solutions. Continuous peripheral nerve blocks

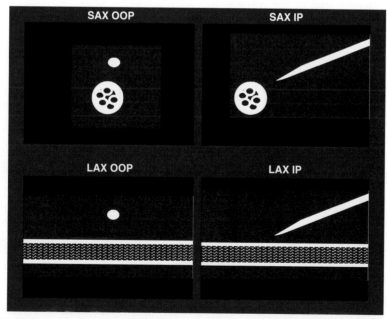

Fig. 18.3 Approaches to regional block with ultrasound. *LAX IP,* Long-axis imaging, in-plane needle approach; *LAX OOP,* long-axis imaging, out-of-plane needle approach; *SAX IP,* short-axis imaging, in-plane needle approach; *SAX OOP,* short-axis imaging, out-of-plane needle approach. (From Gray AT. *Atlas of Ultrasound-Guided Regional Anesthesia.* 3rd ed. Philadelphia: Elsevier; 2018:30.)

can be used in the hospital setting to facilitate vigorous early joint mobilization after orthopedic surgery. They can also be used to provide potent analgesia for outpatient surgery. For placement of these catheters, the peripheral nerve should be located with an ultrasound in a fashion similar to that for a single-injection block. A large-bore needle (e.g., 17-gauge Tuohy) is used for the block and placed at the desired location, and then the catheter is threaded through the needle. Injection of a local anesthetic or dextrose solution immediately before catheter placement can be useful by creating more space adjacent to the nerve. Similar to an intravenous catheter, there are some catheter systems that thread the catheter over the needle after placement of the catheter–needle system at the desired location. Peripheral nerve catheters are more prone to dislodgment than epidural catheters because movement of skin near the catheter entry point is more likely.

CERVICAL PLEXUS BLOCK

The cervical plexus is formed by the second, third, and fourth cervical nerves. With the patient's head turned to the opposite side, the superficial cervical plexus can be blocked by infiltration of local anesthetic solution just deep to the platysma and investing fascia of the neck along the posterior lateral border of the sternocleidomastoid muscle (Fig. 18.4). The anesthesia produced by a cervical plexus block includes the area from the inferior surface of the mandible to the level of the clavicle. A cervical plexus block is used most often to provide anesthesia in conscious patients undergoing carotid endarterectomy. Although combined superficial and deep cervical plexus blocks have traditionally been used for this surgical procedure, a superficial block alone is often sufficient.

UPPER EXTREMITY BLOCKS

Brachial Plexus

The brachial plexus is a network of nerves that is composed of five nerve roots (C5, C6, C7, C8, and T1) that provide both motor control and sensory input for almost the entire upper extremity (Fig. 18.5). The skin over the shoulder is supplied by the supraclavicular nerves of the cervical plexus, and the medial aspect of the arm is supplied by the intercostobrachial branch of the second intercostal nerve (Fig. 18.6). The C5–T1 nerve roots form ventral rami and trunks in the space between the anterior and middle scalene muscles in the cervical region and then pass over the first rib and under the clavicle. The trunks form three anterior and three posterior divisions, which recombine to create three cords in the infraclavicular region. These cords divide into terminal branches in the axillary region. The location of the surgery, experience of the anesthesia provider, and patient factors, such as body habitus, help determine where along the brachial plexus a peripheral nerve block should be performed (Table 18.3).

Interscalene Block

An interscalene block targets the ventral rami of the brachial plexus (derived from C5, C6, C7, C8, and T1 nerve roots) and is therefore suited for surgeries that involve the distal clavicle, shoulder, and upper arm.[16–18] The interscalene block can spare the inferior trunk (from C8 and T1, partly the ulnar distribution of the brachial plexus) and thus is not always suitable for distal forearm and hand surgeries.

An interscalene block is traditionally performed near the C6 vertebral level, where the brachial plexus emerges in between the anterior and middle scalene muscles. The patient's head is turned toward the contralateral side of the block to help expose the interscalene groove. A linear ultrasound probe is placed in a transverse plane at the C6 vertebral level, providing a short-axis view of the brachial plexus. Anatomic structures that are identified should be the middle scalene muscle, anterior scalene muscle, sternocleidomastoid muscle, and brachial plexus (Fig. 18.7). The obtained view has a "stoplight" appearance of the brachial plexus that refers typically to a monofascicular C5 and bifascicular C6[19] ventral rami as aligned in a parallel fashion from superficial to deep.

Using the in-plane technique, the needle is inserted from the lateral to medial direction through the middle

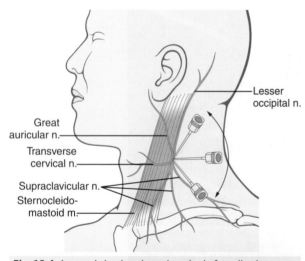

Great auricular n.

Transverse cervical n.

Supraclavicular n.

Sternocleido-mastoid m.

Lesser occipital n.

Fig. 18.4 Anatomic landmarks and method of needle placement for a superficial cervical plexus block. With the patient's head turned to the side, local anesthetic is infiltrated along the posterolateral border of the sternocleidomastoid muscle. (Modified from Brown DL, Factor DA, eds. *Regional Anesthesia and Analgesia*. Philadelphia: WB Saunders; 1996:245.)

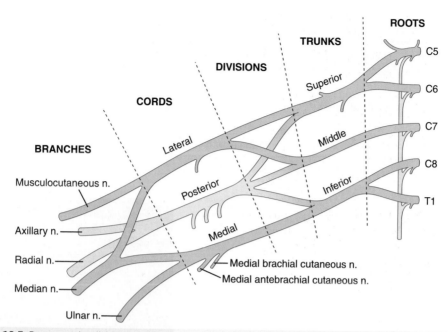

Fig. 18.5 Roots, trunks, divisions, cords, and branches of the right brachial plexus. (Modified from Johnson RL, Kopp SL, Kessler J, Gray AT. Peripheral nerve blocks and ultrasound guidance for regional anesthesia. In Gropper MA, ed. *Miller's Anesthesia*. 9th ed. Philadelphia: Elsevier; 2020:1459.)

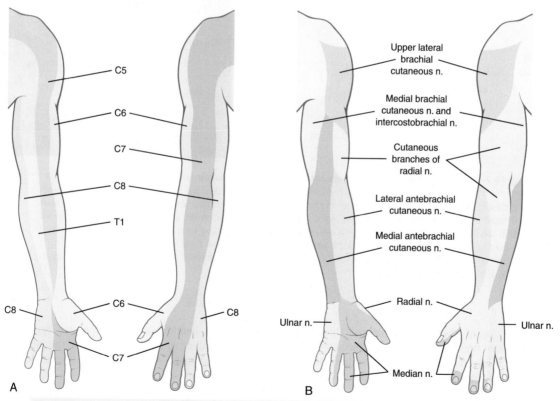

Fig. 18.6 (A) Cutaneous distribution of the cervical and thoracic roots of the upper extremity. (B) Cutaneous distribution of the peripheral nerves of the upper extremity. (Modified from Johnson RL, Kopp SL, Kessler J, et al. Peripheral nerve blocks and ultrasound guidance for regional anesthesia. In Gropper MA, ed. *Miller's Anesthesia*. 9th ed. Philadelphia: Elsevier; 2020:1724, 1459.

Table 18.3 Techniques for Brachial Plexus Block

Technique	Level	Advantage	Potential Drawback(s)
Interscalene	Roots/trunks	Shoulder coverage	Hemidiaphragmatic paresis Inferior trunk sparing
Supraclavicular	Trunks/divisions	Overall completeness	Pneumothorax risk
Infraclavicular	Cords	Catheter placement	Deep to pectoral muscles
Axillary	Branches	Shallow block	Musculocutaneous nerve sparing

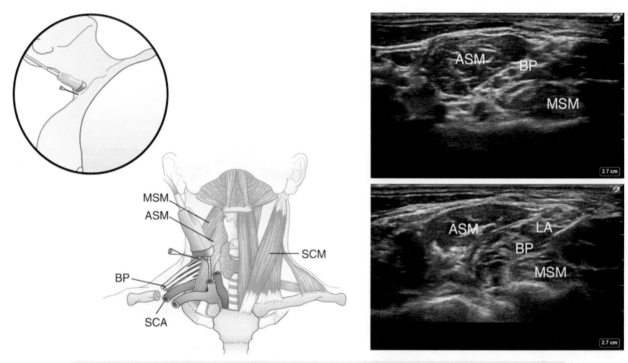

Fig. 18.7 The brachial plexus passes between the anterior and middle scalene muscles and joins the subclavian artery as it passes over the first rib (*left, lower drawing*). Interscalene block of the brachial plexus is performed with the patient supine and the head turned to the contralateral side (*left, upper drawing*). The interscalene groove is imaged with high-frequency ultrasound (*right, upper sonogram*). The needle advances from lateral to medial within the plane of imaging. Interscalene block is performed by infiltrating local anesthetic around the roots of the brachial plexus as they pass between the anterior and middle scalene muscles (*right, lower sonogram*). *ASM*, Anterior scalene muscle; *BP*, brachial plexus; *LA*, local anesthetic; *MSM*, middle scalene muscle; *SCA*, subclavian artery; *SCM*, sternocleidomastoid muscle.

scalene muscle toward the brachial plexus. Once the needle passes into the brachial plexus fascia sheath, local anesthetic is injected. To ensure an adequate block, spread of the local anesthetic should be seen along the cervical ventral rami.

The interscalene block has the potential risk of Horner syndrome, recurrent laryngeal nerve block, epidural or subarachnoid injection, vertebral artery injection, and pneumothorax. The risk of transient phrenic nerve block

and resultant hemidiaphragmatic paresis can be reduced with interscalene injections lower in the neck with a smaller volume and lower concentration of local anesthetic.[20,21]

Supraclavicular Block

Supraclavicular block of the brachial plexus is achieved by injecting 20 to 30 mL of local anesthetic solution around the brachial plexus, where it is usually tightly bundled and adjacent to the subclavian artery, just cephalad to the clavicle. Pneumothorax is the most common serious complication of a supraclavicular block (about a 1% incidence) and can be manifested initially as cough, dyspnea, or pleuritic chest pain. Block of the phrenic nerve occurs frequently (50% of procedures) but generally causes no clinically significant symptoms. Bilateral supraclavicular blocks are not recommended for fear of bilateral pneumothorax or phrenic nerve paralysis. Likewise, patients with chronic obstructive pulmonary disease may not be ideal candidates for a supraclavicular block. Advantages of a supraclavicular block are rapid onset and ability to perform the block with the arm at the side of the patient. The increased risk for pneumothorax may limit the use of supraclavicular block for outpatients. Because of these risks, many practitioners have advocated the use of ultrasound imaging to guide supraclavicular blocks.

The supraclavicular block can be performed with a similar technique to interscalene blocks described previously. The ultrasound probe is moved closer to the clavicle and faces caudally to facilitate imaging of the brachial plexus adjacent to the subclavian artery and over the first rib. The broad first rib serves as a backstop to prevent advancement of the needle toward the thorax. In this location almost all practitioners utilize the in-plane technique because of the proximity of the pleura. The goal is to have local anesthetic distribute underneath the inferior trunk of the brachial plexus, although evidence now suggests that multiple injections are necessary for complete brachial plexus anesthesia.

Infraclavicular Block

The infraclavicular block targets the medial, lateral, and posterior cords of the brachial plexus and is suitable for surgeries of the arm below the shoulder. The cords of the brachial plexus are named in relation to the axillary artery as the plexus travels underneath the clavicle toward the axilla.

The infraclavicular block is performed with the short-axis in-plane approach (Fig. 18.8). A linear or curvilinear ultrasound transducer with a small footprint may be used. The choice of needle is dependent on the patient's body habitus and whether a continuous catheter will be placed. The patient is positioned supine with the arm abducted, elbow flexed, and arm externally rotated if possible. This will retract the clavicle and straighten the neurovascular bundle. The ultrasound transducer is placed medial to the coracoid process in a parasagittal plane (about halfway between the supraclavicular and axillary regions). Key structures to identify on the ultrasound image are the pectoral major and minor muscles, axillary artery and vein, and cords of the brachial plexus. Although the cords of the brachial plexus may be visualized around the axillary artery, they can be difficult to delineate on the ultrasound image.

The needle approaches in plane from cephalad to caudad (lateral to medial) for an infraclavicular block. After a skin wheal of local anesthetic is placed, the needle is directed toward the space between the lateral cord and the axillary artery. The goal of the infraclavicular block is to spread the local anesthetic around the axillary artery in a U-shape, as this will assure blockade of all three wall-hugging cords of the brachial plexus.

The advantages of the infraclavicular block are the close proximity of the brachial plexus to the artery, relatively consistent anatomy, and a stable site for placement of a continuous peripheral nerve catheter. Because of the close proximity to the clavicle and the depth of the block, performing this block can be challenging in some patients.

Axillary Block

The axillary block targets the terminal branches of the brachial plexus in the axilla: the median, ulnar, radial, and musculocutaneous nerves. The axillary block is suitable for surgeries of the elbow, forearm, wrist, and hand.

The axillary block is typically performed with a linear transducer using a short-axis view of the nerves and vessels in the axilla and an in-plane approach (Fig. 18.9). The patient is positioned supine with the arm to be blocked abducted and externally rotated. The ultrasound image should display the axillary artery and vein(s); terminal branches of the brachial plexus; conjoint tendon; and the biceps, triceps, and coracobrachialis muscles.[22] The relation of the terminal branches to the axillary artery is usually as follows: median (superficial), ulnar (medial), radial (posterior), and musculocutaneous (lateral, traversing through the coracobrachialis muscle). The block is performed with a 5- to 7-cm needle, approaching in plane from cephalad to caudad (lateral to medial) toward the branches of the brachial plexus. The goal is to surround each terminal branch of the brachial plexus with local anesthetic, often leading to local anesthetic spread circumferentially around the axillary artery. The musculocutaneous nerve can be targeted separately after block of the other branches of the brachial plexus.[23]

The advantages of this block include a lower risk of complications when compared with other brachial plexus blocks (e.g., no risk of concomitant phrenic nerve block or pneumothorax). The axillary block is also a simpler block to perform, given its superficial nature. The disadvantages include the potential risk of intravascular injection and hematoma, given the proximity of the axillary artery and veins, unsuitability for a peripheral nerve catheter, and lack of coverage for the upper arm and shoulder.

Intercostobrachial Nerve Block

The intercostobrachial nerve is a thoracic nerve (derived from T2 and T3) that provides cutaneous innervation to the medial half of the arm. This block may be used as a

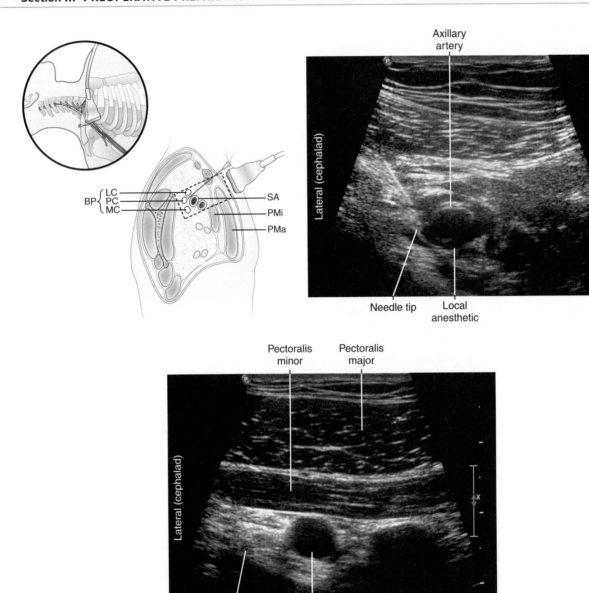

Fig. 18.8 Technique of infraclavicular block. (*Left*) With the patient supine and the arm abducted and externally rotated, an ultrasound transducer is placed inferior to the clavicle to visualize the subclavian artery and adjacent cords of the brachial plexus. A needle is advanced caudally within the plane of imaging until its tip lies within the fascial sheath that surrounds the brachial plexus deep to the axillary artery. In the sonograms (*right*) the needle tip passes between the lateral and medial cords of the brachial plexus and injects local anesthetic that surrounds the three cords. *BP*, Brachial plexus; *LC*, lateral cord; *MC*, medial cord; *PC*, posterior cord; *PMa*, pectoralis major muscle; *PMi*, pectoralis minor muscle; *SA*, subclavian artery. (Sonograms from Gray AT. *Atlas of Ultrasound-Guided Regional Anesthesia*. 3rd ed. Philadelphia: Elsevier; 2018:97, 98.)

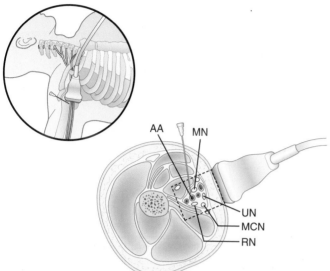

Fig. 18.9 Axillary block. The arm is abducted 90 degrees. Key structures in the right axilla are visualized with a high-frequency ultrasound transducer. The arrangement of the branches of the brachial plexus around the axillary artery is shown in the inset. The sonogram shows the block needle advancing from lateral within the plane of imaging. The needle tip passes deep to the artery and injects local anesthetic that surrounds the radial nerve. Additional injections ensure local anesthetic spread around the ulnar and median nerves. *A* and *AA*, Axillary artery; *LA*, local anesthetic; *MCN*, musculocutaneous nerve; *MN*, median nerve; *RN*, radial nerve; *UN*, ulnar nerve.

supplement to brachial plexus blocks to improve tolerance of an arm tourniquet or to improve surgical conditions for proximal arm surgery. The intercostobrachial nerve can be blocked by subcutaneous infiltration in the medial half of the arm with 2 to 3 mL of local anesthetic.

LOWER EXTREMITY BLOCKS

The lower extremity nerves originate from the lumbar and sacral plexuses (Fig. 18.10). The lumbar plexus is composed of the first four lumbar nerves (L1–L4). Lower extremity nerves that arise from the lumbar plexus include the lateral femoral cutaneous, femoral, and obturator nerves. The sacral plexus is composed of the first four sacral nerves (S1–S4) and receives contributions from L4 and L5. This plexus gives rise to the sciatic nerve.

Femoral Nerve

Femoral Nerve Block
The femoral nerve is the largest branch of the lumbar plexus and derives from the ventral rami of L2–L4. This nerve provides motor innervation to the quadriceps and sensation from the anterior thigh and medial leg. The femoral nerve descends through the psoas muscle and then travels between the psoas and iliacus muscles,

exiting the pelvis under the inguinal ligament. Femoral nerve block is suitable for surgeries of the anterior thigh (e.g., quadriceps tendon surgery) and provides analgesia for hip, femur, and knee surgeries.

The femoral nerve block is typically performed distal to the point at which the femoral nerve passes under the inguinal ligament (Fig. 18.11). The nerve block is performed with a 5- to 7-cm echogenic needle with a linear transducer and short-axis in-plane approach. The patient is positioned supine, and the transducer is placed in a transverse plane 1 to 2 cm distal to the inguinal ligament. Important structures to identify in the ultrasound image are the femoral artery and vein, femoral nerve, sartorius and iliopsoas muscles, and the fascia lata and fascia iliaca (which can be difficult to delineate). The femoral nerve is lateral to the femoral artery and is a flat oval or triangular polyfascicular structure under both the fascia lata and fascia iliaca. The needle is advanced from lateral to medial toward the lateral corner of the femoral nerve, and typically two "pops" can be felt as the needle is advanced through the fascia lata and fascia iliaca. Once the needle tip is under the fascia iliaca and adjacent to the femoral nerve, local anesthetic is injected to surround the nerve.

The advantage of femoral nerve block is its reliability in providing analgesia to the anterior thigh and medial leg. It is a good location for a peripheral nerve catheter because it is away from the thigh tourniquet and surgical

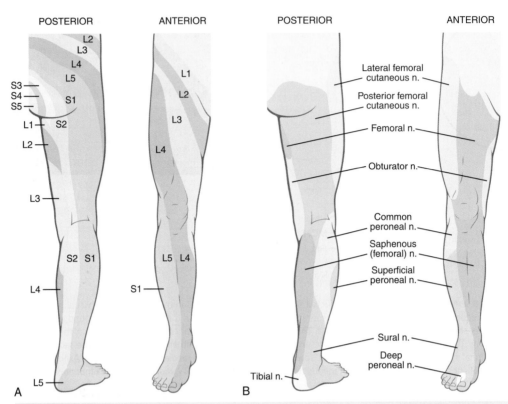

Fig. 18.10 (A) Cutaneous distribution of the lumbosacral nerves. (B) Cutaneous distribution of the peripheral nerves of the lower extremity. Note that the cutaneous distribution of the obturator nerve is highly variable but shown here on the medial aspect of the thigh. (Modified from Horlocker TT, Kopp SL, Wedel DJ. Nerve blocks. In Miller RD, ed. *Miller's Anesthesia*. 8th ed. Philadelphia: Elsevier; 2015:1738.)

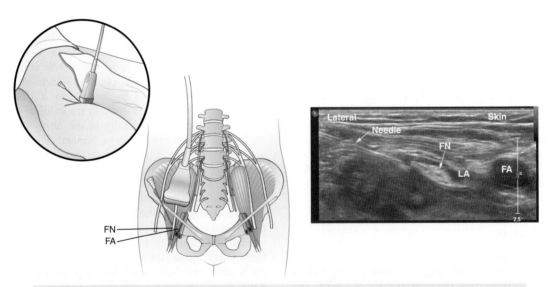

Fig. 18.11 Femoral nerve block. The femoral nerve runs over the surface of the iliopsoas muscle as it passes under the inguinal ligament. The iliac fascia invests the femoral nerve and iliopsoas muscle, which is anatomically separate from the femoral sheath. Femoral nerve block is performed with short-axis imaging of the femoral nerve and artery. In the sonogram the block needle passes from lateral to medial, deep to the fascia iliaca, and injects local anesthetic that surrounds the femoral nerve. *FA*, Femoral artery; *FN*, femoral nerve; *LA*, local anesthetic.

site. Its predictable and shallow anatomy makes it a relatively easy block to master. However, femoral nerve block does cause quadriceps muscle weakness, which may not be favorable for early mobilization and may increase the risk of falls postoperatively.[24]

Adductor Canal and Saphenous Nerve Blocks

The adductor canal block targets distal branches of the femoral nerve as they travel deep to the sartorius muscle in the thigh. Sensory nerves from the femoral nerve are still present near the adductor canal (e.g., the saphenous nerve and infrapatellar nerve). However, many motor nerves have already branched off and innervated their corresponding muscles (all except the nerves to the vastus medialis muscle). Therefore the advantage of the adductor canal block includes analgesia for knee surgery, with minimal quadriceps muscle weakness.[25,26]

The patient is positioned supine with the leg to be blocked slightly externally rotated and bent at the knee (Fig. 18.12). A short-axis in-plane approach with a linear transducer is used. A 5- to 7-cm echogenic needle is appropriate for this block. The adductor canal block is performed midthigh, where the superficial femoral artery is near the middle of the undersurface of the sartorius muscle belly. The subsartorial nerves may be visible just lateral to the superficial femoral artery; however, in many cases these nerves are difficult to discern. The goal is to direct the needle from lateral to medial and anterior to posterior and achieve local anesthetic spread under the thick fascia that covers the posterior surface of the sartorius muscle, lateral to the superficial femoral artery.

The saphenous nerve is a terminal branch of the femoral nerve that carries sensory nerve fibers from the medial aspect of the leg, ankle, and foot. Depending on the desired location of blockade, the saphenous nerve can be blocked at the thigh, leg, or ankle. Many practitioners use the adductor canal approach described earlier to block the saphenous nerve in the thigh.

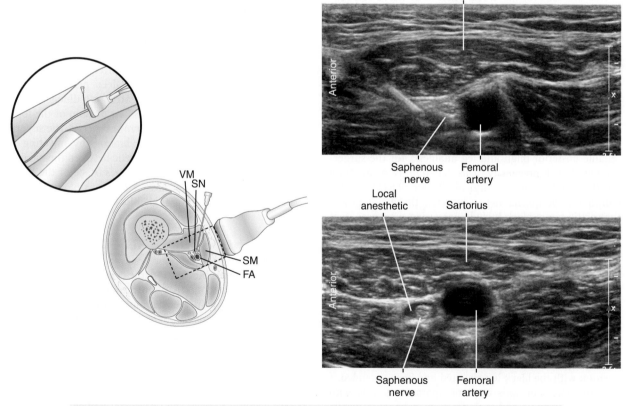

Fig. 18.12 Saphenous nerve block near the adductor canal. With the patient supine and leg externally rotated, the medial thigh is scanned in axial section with high-frequency ultrasound. The needle advances from anterior to posterior within the plane of imaging. The saphenous nerve is not always visible, but it courses with the superficial femoral artery, deep to the sartorius muscle. Local anesthetic surrounds the saphenous nerve. *FA*, Femoral artery; *SM*, sartorius muscle; *SN*, saphenous nerve; *VM*, vastus medialis muscle. (Sonograms from Gray AT. *Atlas of Ultrasound-Guided Regional Anesthesia.* 2nd ed. Philadelphia: Elsevier; 2012.)

Sciatic Nerve

Proximal Sciatic Nerve Block

The sciatic nerve is the largest branch of the sacral plexus and consists of the L4, L5, and S1–S4 spinal nerves. It provides motor and sensory innervation of the posterior thigh and most of the leg. As the sciatic nerve exits the pelvis via the greater sciatic foramen, it travels along the posterior thigh anterior to the gluteus maximus and biceps femoris and posterior to the adductor magnus muscles. The sciatic nerve block is suitable for surgeries involving the posterior thigh, lower leg, foot, and ankle and can also improve analgesia after knee surgery.

There are three main approaches to the sciatic nerve block: the anterior, the transgluteal, and the subgluteal approaches. Only the transgluteal approach will be described here. For the transgluteal approach, the patient is placed in the lateral position with the block leg up and the leg slightly flexed at the hip (Fig. 18.13). A transverse, short-axis in-plane approach with a low-frequency linear or curvilinear transducer and a 10-cm echogenic needle are used for the block. The sciatic nerve can reliably be located traveling halfway between the greater trochanter of the femur and the ischial tuberosity, deep to the gluteus maximus muscle. The nerve at this level appears as a hyperechoic, polyfascicular triangular structure. The needle is directed lateral to medial and posterior to anterior toward the lateral border of the sciatic nerve. The goal is to place the needle below the fascial plane of the gluteus maximus muscle and have the local anesthetic spread around the nerve.

The advantages of the sciatic nerve block are the reliable posterior thigh and leg analgesia for the surgeries mentioned previously. This location is away from the thigh tourniquet or surgical site for placement of a continuous peripheral nerve catheter. Disadvantages of the sciatic nerve block include hamstring weakness, foot drop, and potential procedural discomfort and difficulty caused by the depth of the block.

Popliteal Block of the Sciatic Nerve

The popliteal block targets the sciatic nerve as it enters the popliteal fossa, at which point the nerve divides into its common peroneal and tibial nerve components. This block is commonly used for foot and ankle surgery, usually combined with a saphenous nerve block to cover the medial aspect of the leg. The patient is placed in lateral position with the block leg elevated and knee extended.[27] A transverse, short-axis in-plane approach is used with a linear transducer and a 5- to 7-cm echogenic needle (Fig. 18.14). The ultrasound transducer is placed in the popliteal fossa, locating the sciatic nerve posterior to the popliteal vein and artery. The nerve is blocked at the bifurcation of the sciatic nerve into the tibial and common peroneal nerves, which can be located by sliding the ultrasound transducer along the course of the nerves. The needle is advanced from lateral to medial, with the goal of local anesthetic distribution around both components of the sciatic nerve, creating a "donut" of local anesthetic around each nerve. After injection, the transducer can be slid distally to verify tracking of the local anesthetic with the common peroneal and tibial nerves as they separate in the distal popliteal fossa.

Ankle Block

All five peripheral nerves that supply the foot can be blocked (ankle block) at the level of the malleoli (Fig. 18.15). The tibial nerve is the major nerve to the sole of the foot. This nerve lies on the heel side of the posterior tibial artery and can be blocked by infiltrating 3 to 5 mL of local anesthetic solution in a fanning pattern around this artery. The sural nerve innervates the lateral side of the foot and can be blocked by injecting 5 mL of local anesthetic solution in the groove between the lateral malleolus and the calcaneus near the small saphenous vein. The saphenous nerve innervates the medial aspect of the foot. Infiltration of 5 mL of local anesthetic solution anterior to the medial malleolus near the great saphenous vein blocks this nerve. The deep peroneal nerve innervates the webbing between the first and second toes and is blocked by injecting 5 mL of local anesthetic solution adjacent to the anterior tibial artery. Alternatively, if arterial pulsation is absent, the deep peroneal nerve can also be blocked deep to the extensor hallucis longus tendon and extensor retinaculum. The dorsum of the foot is innervated by the superficial peroneal nerve. The superficial branches of this nerve are blocked by injecting a subcutaneous ridge of local anesthetic between the medial and lateral malleoli over the anterior surface of the foot. Because the foot does not have a generous blood supply, systemic toxicity after an ankle block is rare.

CHEST AND ABDOMEN BLOCKS

Peripheral nerve blocks for the chest and abdomen can provide intraoperative and postoperative analgesia, reduce systemic pain medications, improve patient satisfaction, and improve patient discharge times from the postanesthesia care unit.

Intercostal Nerve Block

Intercostal nerve blocks target the ventral rami of the thoracic spinal nerves. The intercostal nerves travel inferior to the associated rib within the subcostal groove and inferior to the accompanying intercostal vein and artery. At the angle of the ribs, these nerves travel in the space between the internal intercostal and innermost intercostal muscles. These blocks are beneficial for thoracic and upper abdominal surgery, in addition to after chest wall

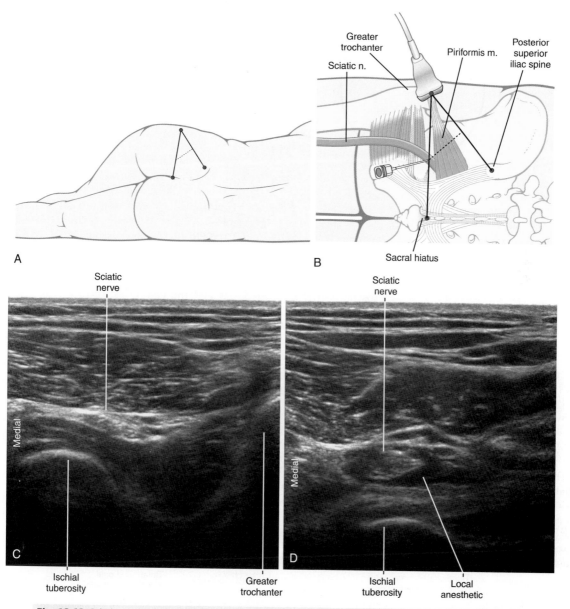

Fig. 18.13 Sciatic nerve block. (A) Patient positioning. (B) Anatomic landmarks. (C and D) The sciatic nerve lies beneath a point 5 cm caudad along a perpendicular line that bisects a line joining the posterior iliac spine and the greater trochanter of the femur. This point is also usually the intersection of that perpendicular line with a line joining the greater trochanter and the sacral hiatus. (C and D from Gray AT. *Atlas of Ultrasound-Guided Regional Anesthesia.* 3rd ed. Philadelphia: Elsevier; 2018:188.)

trauma. However, because of the proximity of the pleura, there is a potential risk of a pneumothorax. LAST is possible because of the high-peak plasma levels after injection, in addition to the need for multiple nerve blocks for adequate dermatomal coverage of the surgical incision.

For this block, the patient is positioned prone, and a linear transducer placed in a short-axis parasagittal plane is used at the midscapular line. A 5-cm echogenic needle is used to inject 3 to 5 mL of local anesthetic at

each level, proceeding in a caudad to cephalad direction. The ultrasound image should demonstrate the intercostal muscles, pleura, and adjacent ribs and their acoustic shadows. The goal of the block is to have spread of local anesthetic in between the innermost and internal intercostal muscles along the inferior border of the rib. Intercostal nerves also can be blocked more centrally by injecting just deep to the erector spinae muscle at the lateral edge of the transverse process.[28,29]

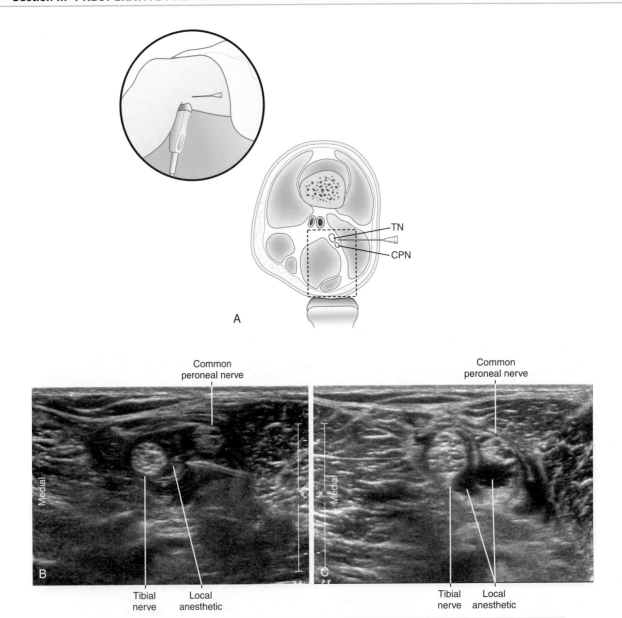

Fig. 18.14 Popliteal block of the sciatic nerve. (A) The patient is positioned supine with the leg elevated to allow the popliteal fossa to be scanned from below with high-frequency ultrasound. (B and C) The block needle passes from the lateral thigh through the biceps femoris muscle and injects local anesthetic around the tibial and common peroneal nerves. *CPN,* Common peroneal nerve; *TN,* tibial nerve. (B and C from Gray AT. *Atlas of Ultrasound-Guided Regional Anesthesia.* 3rd ed. Philadelphia: Elsevier; 2018:197.)

Transversus Abdominis Plane Block

The transversus abdominis plane (TAP) block is an abdominal wall field block targeting the ventral rami of the thoracic and lumbar spinal nerves (T7–L1) as they travel in the plane between the transversus abdominis and internal oblique muscles. The block provides analgesia for lower abdominal surgery and may help with laparoscopic surgery. Because the block relies on a large volume of local anesthetic for appropriate spread, there is some risk of local anesthetic toxicity. There also is a small potential for intraperitoneal and intrahepatic injection.

For this block, the patient is positioned supine, and a linear transducer is placed in a transverse plane at the midaxillary line (Fig. 18.16). The ultrasound image should demonstrate the external oblique, internal oblique, and transversus abdominis muscles. A 7- to 10-cm echogenic needle is used to inject at least 20 mL of local anesthetic per

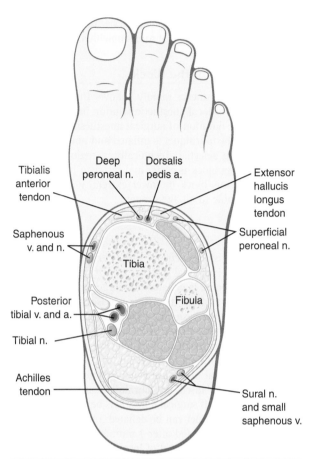

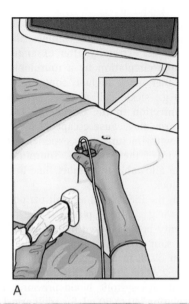

A

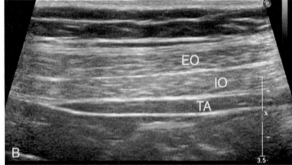

B

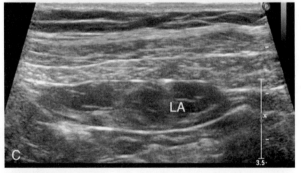

C

Fig. 18.15 Cross-sectional anatomy for an ankle block. An ankle block is performed by injecting local anesthetic solution at five separate nerve locations. The superficial peroneal nerve, sural nerve, and saphenous nerve are usually blocked by subcutaneous infiltration because they may have already branched as they cross the ankle joint. The tibial and deep peroneal nerves require deeper injection adjacent to the accompanying blood vessels (the posterior tibial and anterior tibial arteries, respectively). Because the block needle approaches the ankle from many angles, it is convenient to elevate the foot by supporting the calf. (Modified from Brown DL, Factor DA, eds. *Regional Anesthesia and Analgesia*. Philadelphia: WB Saunders; 1996.)

Fig. 18.16 Transversus abdominis plane (TAP) block. (A) For the classic posterior TAP block, the patient is in the supine position with the transducer placed near the midaxillary line between the costal margin and pelvic brim. (B and C) The needle travels through the external oblique and internal oblique muscles to enter the fascial plane between the internal oblique and underlying transversus abdominis muscles. The injection should be performed near the posterior border of the transversus abdominis muscle so that the injection distributes with well-defined margins where the nerves enter the plane. *EO*, external oblique; *IO*, internal oblique; *LA*, local anesthetic; *TA*, transversus abdominis. (A, Redrawn from Gray AT. *Atlas of Ultrasound-Guided Regional Anesthesia*. 3rd ed. Philadelphia: Elsevier; 2018:273.)

side. The needle is directed in the anterior to posterior direction, with the goal of local anesthetic distribution between the transversus abdominis and internal oblique muscles.

INTRAVENOUS REGIONAL ANESTHESIA (BIER BLOCK)

Intravenous regional anesthesia (or Bier block, named after August Bier) is a method of producing anesthesia of the arm or leg. This anesthetic technique is used for surgical procedures with minimal postoperative pain and duration of 2 hours or less. The technique involves intravenous injection of large volumes of dilute local anesthetic into an extremity after exsanguination and isolation of the circulation by a tourniquet. Contraindications to Bier block include contraindications to a tourniquet (e.g., sickle cell disease, ischemic vascular disease, or infection in the extremity). Lacerations to the blocked arm may cause escape of local anesthetic, and patients with fractures may experience pain during exsanguination of the extremity. Tourniquet pain and the maximum allowable tourniquet time limit the duration of the block.

To perform the Bier block, a small peripheral intravenous catheter (e.g., 22 g) is placed in the distal portion of the extremity being blocked (Fig. 18.17). The extremity is then exsanguinated by wrapping with an Esmarch bandage from distal to proximal, and then a tourniquet is inflated to 250 to 275 mm Hg (at least 100 mm Hg above the patient's systolic blood pressure). Plain local anesthetic solution (40 to 50 mL for adult arms) is injected through the intravenous catheter and then the catheter is removed. Patients may begin experiencing pain at the tourniquet site after 45 minutes; a double-tourniquet technique may be employed to help mitigate this. With a double tourniquet, the proximal cuff is initially inflated, and once the patient experiences pain, the distal cuff is inflated over the anesthetized arm and the proximal cuff deflated.

Selection of Local Anesthetic

Commonly used local anesthetic solutions for intravenous regional anesthesia are 0.5% lidocaine or chloroprocaine (plain solutions without epinephrine). Bupivacaine is avoided because of potential systemic toxicity, which can include malignant ventricular cardiac dysrhythmias leading to refractory cardiac arrest. Preservative-free solutions of local anesthetic are recommended because preservatives have been associated with thrombophlebitis.

Characteristics of the Block

The onset of anesthesia rapidly follows the intravenous administration of local anesthetic solution into the isolated extremity. The duration of surgical anesthesia depends on the time that the tourniquet is inflated and not on the local anesthetic drug selected. Technically, a regional intravenous anesthesia block is easier and faster to perform than a brachial plexus block or lower extremity block and is readily applicable to all age groups.

Risks

The principal risk associated with intravenous regional anesthesia is the potential systemic toxicity that may occur when the tourniquet is deflated and large amounts of local anesthetic solution from the previously isolated part of the extremity enter the systemic circulation. Local anesthetic levels peak approximately 2 to 5 minutes after tourniquet deflation. One approach to reducing the risk of toxicity is to keep the tourniquet inflated for at least 20 minutes, even if the surgical procedure is completed in less time. If 40 minutes have elapsed, the tourniquet can be deflated in a single maneuver. If surgical duration is between 20 and 40 minutes, the tourniquet can be deflated, reinflated immediately, and finally deflated after 1 minute. This method will reduce the peak plasma level of local anesthetic. Limitation of extremity movement (including avoidance of extremity elevation) after release of the tourniquet is also useful for minimizing local anesthetic blood levels.

If the extremity is not adequately exsanguinated, the skin will have a blotchy appearance after injection of the local anesthetic. In this situation the quality of the block and surgical field will be poor.

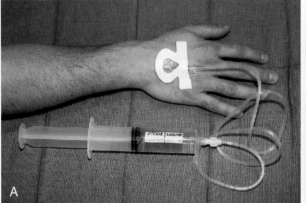 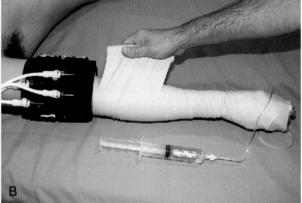

Fig. 18.17 (A) Placement and securing of a small intravenous catheter. (B) Exsanguination of the arm with an Esmarch bandage before inflation of the tourniquet and injection of the local anesthetic solution through the catheter.

REFERENCES

1. Albrecht E, Reynvoet M, Fournier N, Desmet M. Dose-response relationship of perineural dexamethasone for interscalene brachial plexus block: A randomised, controlled, triple-blind trial. *Anaesthesia.* 2019;74(8):1001–1008. PMID: 30973188.

2. Mulroy MF, Weller RS, Liguori GA. A checklist for performing regional nerve blocks. *Reg Anesth Pain Med.* 2014;39:195–199.

3. Henshaw DS, Turner JD, Dobson SW, et al. Preprocedural checklist for regional anesthesia: Impact on the incidence of wrong site blockade (an 8-year perspective). *Reg Anesth Pain Med.* 2019 Jan 13.

4. Alakkad H, Naeeni A, Chan VW, et al. Infection related to ultrasound-guided single-injection peripheral nerve blockade: A decade of experience at Toronto Western hospital. *Reg Anesth Pain Med.* 2015;40:82–84.

5. Barrington MJ, Kluger R. Ultrasound guidance reduces the risk of local anesthetic systemic toxicity following peripheral nerve blockade. *Reg Anesth Pain Med.* 2013;38:289–297.

6. Horlocker TT, Vandermeulen E, Kopp SL, Gogarten W, Leffert LR, Benzon HT. Regional anesthesia in the patient receiving antithrombotic or thrombolytic therapy: American Society of Regional Anesthesia and Pain Medicine Evidence-Based Guidelines (fourth edition). *Reg Anesth Pain Med.* 2018;43(3):263–309. PMID: 29561531.

7. Weinberg GL. Lipid emulsion infusion: Resuscitation for local anesthetic and other drug overdose. *Anesthesiology.* 2012;117:180–187.

8. Fettiplace MR, Weinberg G. The mechanisms underlying lipid resuscitation therapy. *Reg Anesth Pain Med.* 2018;43(2):138–149. PMID: 29356774.

9. Sites BD, Taenzer AH, Herrick MD, et al. Incidence of local anesthetic systemic toxicity and postoperative neurologic symptoms associated with 12,668 ultrasound-guided nerve blocks: An analysis from a prospective clinical registry. *Reg Anesth Pain Med.* 2012;37:478–482.

10. Neal JM, Barrington MJ, Brull R, et al. The Second ASRA Practice Advisory on Neurologic Complications Associated With Regional Anesthesia and Pain Medicine: Executive summary 2015. *Reg Anesth Pain Med.* 2015;40(5):401–430.

11. Lam KK, Soneji N, Katzberg H, et al. Incidence and etiology of postoperative neurological symptoms after peripheral nerve block: A retrospective cohort study. *Reg Anesth Pain Med.* 2020;45(7):495–504. PMID: 32471926.

12. Hudson ME, Chelly JE, Lichter JR. Wrong-site nerve blocks: 10 yr experience in a large multihospital health-care system. *Br J Anaesth.* 2015;114:818–824.

13. Silvestri E, Martinoli C, Derchi LE, et al. Echotexture of peripheral nerves: Correlation between US and histologic findings and criteria to differentiate tendons. *Radiology.* 1995;197:291–296.

14. Soong J, Schafhalter-Zoppoth I, Gray AT. The importance of transducer angle to ultrasound visibility of the femoral nerve. *Reg Anesth Pain Med.* 2005;30:505.

15. Lam NC, Fishburn SJ, Hammer AR, et al. A randomized controlled trial evaluating the see, tilt, align, and rotate (STAR) maneuver on skill acquisition for simulated ultrasound-guided interventional procedures. *J Ultrasound Med.* 2015;34(6):1019–1026.

16. Kapral S, Greher M, Huber G, et al. Ultrasonographic guidance improves the success rate of interscalene brachial plexus blockade. *Reg Anesth Pain Med.* 2008;33:253–258.

17. Kim DH, Lin Y, Beathe JC, et al. Superior trunk block: A phrenic-sparing alternative to the interscalene block: A randomized controlled trial. *Anesthesiology.* 2019;131(3):521–533. PMID: 31283740.

18. Auyong DB, Hanson NA, Joseph RS, et al. Comparison of anterior suprascapular, supraclavicular, and interscalene nerve block approaches for major outpatient arthroscopic shoulder surgery: A randomized, double-blind, noninferiority trial. *Anesthesiology.* 2018;129(1):47–57. PMID: 29634491.

19. Franco CD, Williams JM. Ultrasound-guided interscalene block: Reevaluation of the "stoplight" sign and clinical implications. *Reg Anesth Pain Med.* 2016;41(4):452–459. PMID: 27203394.

20. Kessler J, Schafhalter-Zoppoth I, Gray AT. An ultrasound study of the phrenic nerve in the posterior cervical triangle: Implications for the interscalene brachial plexus block. *Reg Anesth Pain Med.* 2008;33:545–550.

21. Gautier P, Vandepitte C, Ramquet C, et al. The minimum effective anesthesia volume of 0.75% ropivacaine in ultrasound-guided interscalene brachial plexus block. *Anesth Analg.* 2011;113:951–955.

22. Gray AT. The conjoint tendon of the latissimus dorsi and teres major: An important landmark for ultrasound-guided axillary block. *Reg Anesth Pain Med.* 2009;34:179–180.

23. Schafhalter-Zoppoth I, Gray AT. The musculocutaneous nerve: Ultrasound appearance for peripheral nerve block. *Reg Anesth Pain Med.* 2005;30:385–390.

24. Ilfeld BM. Single-injection and continuous femoral nerve blocks are associated with different risks of falling. *Anesthesiology.* 2014;121:668–669.

25. Andersen HL, Gyrn J, Møller L, et al. Continuous saphenous nerve block as supplement to single-dose local infiltration analgesia for postoperative pain management after total knee arthroplasty. *Reg Anesth Pain Med.* 2013;38:106–111.

26. Machi AT, Sztain JF, Kormylo NJ, et al. Discharge readiness after tricompartment knee arthroplasty: Adductor canal versus femoral continuous nerve blocks—A dual-center, randomized trial. *Anesthesiology.* 2015;123(2):444–456.

27. Gray AT, Huczko EL. Schafhalter-Zoppoth I. Lateral popliteal nerve block with ultrasound guidance. *Reg Anesth Pain Med.* 2004;29:507–509.

28. Forero M, Adhikary SD, Lopez H, Tsui C, Chin KJ. The erector spinae plane block: A novel analgesic technique in thoracic neuropathic pain. *Reg Anesth Pain Med.* 2016;41(5):621–627. PMID: 27501016.

29. Nielsen MV, Moriggl B, Hoermann R, Nielsen TD, Bendtsen TF, Børglum J. Are single-injection erector spinae plane block and multiple-injection costotransverse block equivalent to thoracic paravertebral block?. *Acta Anaesthesiol Scand.* 2019;63(9):1231–1238. PMID: 31332775.

19 PATIENT POSITIONING AND ASSOCIATED RISKS

Kristine E.W. Breyer

Patient positioning in the operating room facilitates surgical procedures; however, positioning can be a source of patient injury and can alter intraoperative physiology. Positioning injuries during surgery remain a significant source of perioperative morbidity. Anesthesia providers share a critical responsibility for the proper positioning of patients in the operating room.[1] This chapter will review general physiologic changes during positioning, commonly used intraoperative positions, specific positioning concerns, and common intraoperative positioning-related injuries. Most literature regarding positioning injuries focuses on peripheral nerve injuries and pressure-related injuries.

PHYSIOLOGIC ASPECTS OF POSITIONING

Physiologic responses play an essential role in blunting hemodynamic changes that would otherwise occur from positional changes in our day-to-day lives. Central, regional, and local mechanisms are involved. When a person reclines from an upright to a supine position, venous return to the heart increases and this increases preload, stroke volume, and cardiac output. These changes cause a brief increase in arterial blood pressure, which in turn activates afferent baroreceptors from the aorta (via the vagus nerve) and within the walls of the carotid sinuses (via the glossopharyngeal nerve) to decrease sympathetic outflow and increase parasympathetic impulses to the sinoatrial node and myocardium. This parasympathetic outflow counters the increase in arterial blood pressure from increased preload, and as a result, systemic arterial blood pressure is maintained within a narrow range during postural changes in the nonanesthetized setting.

Central, regional, and local physiologic responses are important in maintaining hemodynamics when changing positions during the course of daily activities. During various types of anesthesia, some of these responses can be blunted, which can change a patient's hemodynamic responses to positional changes.

Pulmonary physiology is also altered by positional changes, which are further exaggerated during anesthesia. For example, when nonanesthetized people lie down, their functional residual capacity (FRC) decreases as a result of the diaphragm shifting upward. In anesthetized patients, the decrease in FRC is more dramatic, and often closing capacity exceeds FRC, leading to increases in ventilation-perfusion ($\dot{V}/\dot{Q}$) mismatching and hypoxemia. Furthermore, positioning that limits diaphragmatic movement pushes on the chest wall or abdomen, causing intrapulmonary shunting from atelectasis.

GENERAL POSITIONING PRINCIPLES

Proper positioning requires the cooperation of anesthesia providers, surgeons, and nurses to ensure patient well-being and safety while permitting surgical exposure. Positioning also involves maintaining spine and extremity neutrality, proper padding, and securing the patient to prevent inadvertent changes in position. Patients often remain in the same position for long periods; therefore prevention of positioning-related complications often requires compromise and judgment. During normal sleep, we change positions, which prevents prolonged compression and excessive stretch. During anesthesia, patients lose the ability to both sense injury and change position, increasing their risk for injury.[2]

General principles for intraoperative positioning include maintaining anatomic neutrality whenever possible and limiting more extreme positions. Padding is an essential part of injury prevention but not always successful for pressure injury prevention. Excess padding can exert pressure on tissues. Maintaining neutrality of the patient's spine and extremities prevents undue stretch. Tissues overlying bony prominences, such as the heels and sacrum, must be padded to prevent soft tissue ischemia caused by pressure. Pay attention to pressure created by equipment such as retractors, stop-cocks, nasal probes and tubes, esophageal probes and tubes, and equipment that enters and exits the sterile field, such as x-ray fluoroscopy equipment.

The American Society of Anesthesiologists (ASA) published a 2011 Practice Advisory for Prevention of Peripheral Neuropathies that was updated in 2018 to reflect a synthesis of updated literature and expert opinion.[3] ASA practice advisories are not intended as standards or absolute requirements and may be modified based on clinical needs and patient factors.

Risk assessment for perioperative nerve injury begins with the preoperative history and physical (Box 19.1). Ideally, patients are placed in a surgical position that they can tolerate when awake. The duration of more extreme positions, when necessary, should be limited

> **Box 19.1** Preoperative History and Physical to Assess Risk of Nerve Injury
>
> - Review a patient's preoperative history and perform a physical examination to identify body habitus, preexisting neurologic symptoms, diabetes mellitus, peripheral vascular disease, alcohol dependency, arthritis, and sex (e.g., male sex and its association with ulnar neuropathy).
> - When judged appropriate, ascertain whether patients can comfortably tolerate the anticipated operative position.

Advisory recommendations from Practice Advisory for the Prevention of Perioperative Peripheral Neuropathies 2018: An Updated Report by the American Society of Anesthesiologists Task Force on Prevention of Perioperative Peripheral Neuropathies. *Anesthesiology*. 2018;128(1):11-26.

as much as possible. Preexisting neuropathies should also be documented, as these may place patients at greater risk of "double crush syndrome," a phenomenon in which two subclinical nerve insults occur and result in clinically apparent neuropathy.[4] The ASA advisory recommends documenting intraoperative positioning actions to facilitate continuous improvement processes; however, the advisory does not specify time intervals for documentation of positioning. Postoperative assessment in the recovery room and documentation of injury is also recommended.[3]

Supine

The supine position, also called the *dorsal decubitus position,* is the most common position for surgery (Fig. 19.1A). In the classic supine position the head, neck, and spine all retain neutrality. One or both arms can be abducted or adducted alongside the patient. Arm abduction should be limited to less than 90 degrees in order to prevent brachial plexus injury from the head of the humerus pushing into the axilla. The ASA advisory recommends against elbow flexion to reduce the risk of ulnar neuropathy but noted a lack of consensus on the acceptable degree of flexion during the perioperative period.[3] Elbow extension must be limited to protect the median nerve from stretching.

With the arm on an arm board, the hands and forearms should remain in a supinated position or a neutral position with the palm toward the body to reduce external pressure on the ulnar nerve (see Fig. 19.1B). When the arms are adducted, they are usually held alongside the body with a "draw sheet" that passes under the body and over the arm and is then tucked directly under the torso (not the mattress) to ensure that the arm remains properly placed next to the body. Finally, padding should be placed to protect all bony prominences in addition to stopcocks or intravenous lines that may exert pressure on the skin during the operation (see Fig. 19.1C).[3]

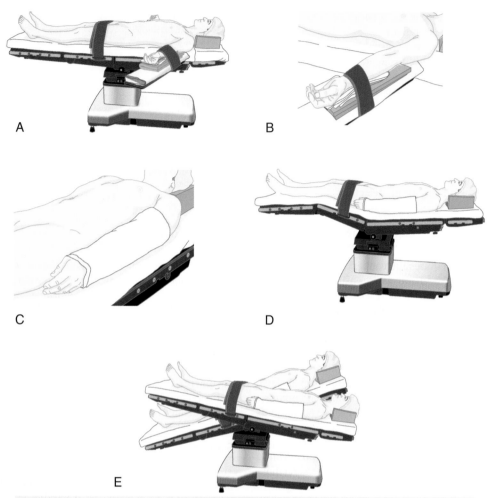

Fig. 19.1 (A) Supine positioning. Note the asymmetry of the base of the table, placing the patient's center of gravity over the base if positioned in the usual direction. (B) Arm position on the arm board. Abduction of the arm should be limited to less than 90 degrees whenever possible. The arm is supinated, and the elbow is padded. (C) Arm tucked at patient's side. Arm in neutral position with palm to hip. The elbow is padded, and one needs to ensure that the arm is supported. (D) Lawn-chair position. Flexion of the hips and knees decreases tension on the back. (E) Trendelenburg position (head tilted down) and reverse Trendelenburg position (head tilted up). Shoulder braces should be avoided to prevent brachial plexus compression injuries.

Variations of the Supine Position

Frequently used variations of the supine position include the lawn-chair, frog-leg, and Trendelenburg positions. The lawn-chair position (see Fig. 19.1D) flexes the hips and knees slightly, which reduces stress on the back, hips, and knees. This modified supine position is often better tolerated by patients who are awake or undergoing monitored anesthesia care. The legs are placed slightly above the level of the heart, which facilitates venous drainage from the lower extremities. Furthermore, the xiphoid to pubic distance is decreased, reducing tension on the abdominal musculature. Typically the back of the bed is raised, the legs below the knees are lowered to an equivalent angle, and a slight Trendelenburg tilt is used to level the hips with the shoulders.

The frog-leg position, in which the hips and knees are flexed and the hips are externally rotated with the soles of the feet facing each other, facilitates procedures to the perineum, medial thighs, genitalia, and rectum. The knees must be supported in order to minimize stress or dislocation of the hips.

Tilting a supine patient head-down with the pubic symphysis as the highest part of the trunk is called the

Trendelenburg position (see Fig. 19.1E). It is named after a 19th-century German surgeon who first described its use for abdominal surgery. Walter Cannon, a Harvard physiologist, is credited with popularizing the use of Trendelenburg positioning to improve hemodynamics for patients in hypovolemic shock during World War I. Trendelenburg positioning is commonly used today to increase venous return during hypotension, improve exposure during abdominal and laparoscopic surgery, and prevent air emboli during central line placement.

The Trendelenburg position does produce hemodynamic and respiratory changes. Initially, placement of the patient head-down causes an autotransfusion from the legs with about a 9% from baseline increase in cardiac output in 1 minute. However, these changes are not sustained, and within 10 minutes, many hemodynamic variables, including cardiac output, return to baseline values. Nevertheless, Trendelenburg positioning is still part of the initial resuscitative efforts to treat hypovolemia. The abdominal contents are displaced toward the diaphragm, which decreases FRC and can also decrease pulmonary compliance, necessitating higher airway pressures during mechanical ventilation. Intraocular pressure and intracranial pressure (ICP) can also increase. In patients with increased ICP and impaired cerebral autoregulation Trendelenburg positioning should be avoided. For patients receiving general anesthesia who will be placed in the Trendelenburg position, endotracheal intubation is strongly recommended over supraglottic airways because of the risk of pulmonary aspiration of gastric contents. A prolonged head-down position can lead to swelling of the face, conjunctivae, larynx, and tongue, with an increased potential for postoperative upper airway obstruction. An air leak should be verified around the endotracheal tube or the larynx visualized before extubation.[5]

Because of gravity, a patient in a steep Trendelenburg position may shift or slide excessively. Several measures can be used to reduce this risk, including use of nonsliding mattresses beneath the patient. Caution should be applied when shoulder braces are used because of considerable risk of compression or stretch injury to the brachial plexus; the ASA practice advisory recommends against the use of shoulder braces in the steep Trendelenburg position whenever possible.[3]

Conversely, the reverse Trendelenburg position (see Fig. 19.1E) tilts the supine patient upward so that the head is higher than any other part of the body. This position is most often used to facilitate upper abdominal surgery. Again, patients must be prevented from slipping on the table. Patients in reverse Trendelenburg, particularly those patients who are hypovolemic, are at risk for hypotension caused by decreased venous return. Invasive arterial blood pressure monitoring should be calibrated (i.e., zeroed) at the level of the external auditory meatus in order to optimize cerebral perfusion.

Complications

Backache may occur in the supine position, as the normal lumbar lordotic curvature is lost during general anesthesia with muscle relaxation or a neuraxial blockade. Consequently, patients with extensive kyphosis, scoliosis, or a previous history of back pain may require extra padding of the spine or slight flexion at the hip and knee.

The base of the operating room table is asymmetric; usually, the patient's torso is placed over the pedestal of the table (see Fig 19.1). However, patients are sometimes positioned with their torso over the other end of the table (so-called *reverse orientation*) to improve surgical access or to permit passage of equipment under the nonpedestal end of the table, such as C-arm x-ray devices. This places the patient's center of gravity farther away from the most stable portion (fulcrum) of the operating room table. This shift can cause the operating room table to tilt and tip over, especially if bed-lengthening extensions are used or the bed is tilted in the Trendelenburg position. In addition, the act of unlocking an operating room table to reposition its location can change the fulcrum point and lead to table tipping and resultant fall risk for the patient. For patients with large body mass, caution is advised when placing them in reverse orientation on an operating room table. Operating room table weight limits should be strictly observed, as they differ substantially with normal versus reverse orientation.

Lithotomy

The lithotomy position (Fig. 19.2A–C) is frequently used during gynecologic, rectal, and urologic surgeries. The legs are abducted 30 to 45 degrees from the midline, the knees are flexed, and the legs are held by supports. The patient's hips are flexed to varying degrees depending on the type of lithotomy required for the procedure: standard, low, or high lithotomy. The legs should be raised and lowered simultaneously to prevent spine torsion. The lower extremities should be padded to prevent compression against the leg rests. The common peroneal nerve wraps around the head of the fibula on the lateral leg and is at significant risk of injury. The ASA practice advisory recommends avoiding prolonged pressure on the peroneal nerve at the fibular head.[3]

The foot section of the operating room table is usually lowered or taken away to facilitate the procedure. If the arms are on the operating table alongside the patient, the hands and fingers may lie near the open edge of the lowered section of the table. When the foot of the bed is raised again at the end of the procedure, the hand position must be verified to avoid a potentially disastrous crush injury to the fingers (see Fig. 19.2D). For this reason, positioning the arms on armrests far from the table hinge point is always recommended when patients are in the lithotomy position.

The lithotomy position causes several physiologic changes. When the legs are elevated, preload increases,

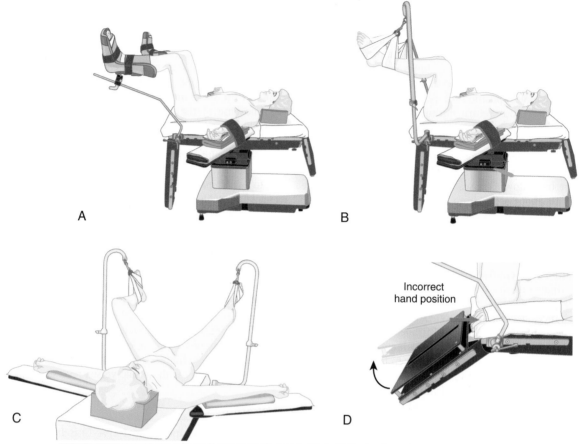

A

B

C

D

Fig. 19.2 (A) Lithotomy position. Hips are flexed 80 to 100 degrees with the lower leg parallel to the body. Arms are on armrests away from the hinge point of the foot section. (B) Lithotomy position with "candy cane" supports. (C) Lithotomy position with correct position of "candy cane" stirrups away from lateral fibular head. (D) Improper position of arms in lithotomy position with fingers at risk for compression when the lower section of the bed is raised.

In the figure D there is a label: Incorrect hand position

causing a transient increase in cardiac output. In addition, the lithotomy position causes the abdominal viscera to displace the diaphragm cephalad, reducing lung compliance and potentially resulting in a decreased tidal volume. Again, the normal lordotic curvature of the lumbar spine is lost in this position, potentially aggravating any previous lower back pain.

Lower extremity compartment syndrome is a rare but devastating complication associated with the lithotomy position. It occurs when perfusion to an extremity is inadequate because of either restricted arterial flow (from leg elevation) or obstructed venous outflow (from direct limb compression or excessive hip flexion). This results in ischemia, edema, and rhabdomyolysis from increased tissue pressure within a fascial compartment. In a large retrospective review of over 500,000 surgeries the incidence of compartment syndromes was markedly higher in the lithotomy (1 in 8720) and lateral decubitus (1 in 9711) positions as compared with the supine

(1 in 92,441) position. Long surgical procedure time was the only distinguishing characteristic of the surgeries in which patients developed lower extremity compartment syndromes.[6] In a retrospective multicenter review of 185 urologic patients who were placed in high lithotomy position the overall complication rate because of positioning was 10%. Neurapraxia was the most common positioning-related complication (12 of 18 patients). Two patients from this cohort had compartment syndrome, and for both patients the time in high lithotomy exceeded 5 hours.[7] Therefore it is recommended to periodically lower the legs to the level of the body if surgery extends beyond several hours.

Lateral Decubitus

In the lateral decubitus position the patient lies on the nonoperative side to facilitate surgery in the thorax, retroperitoneum, or hip (Fig. 19.3A). The patient must be

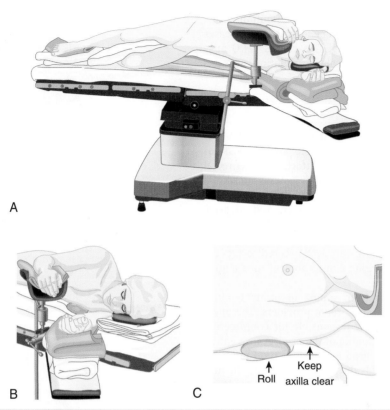

Fig. 19.3 (A) Lateral decubitus position. Note flexion of the lower leg, padding between the legs, and proper support of both arms. (B) Lateral decubitus position showing placement of arms and head. Note additional padding under headrest to ensure alignment of head with spine. Headrest should be kept away from the dependent eye. (C) Use of axillary roll in lateral decubitus position. The roll, in this case a bag of intravenous fluid, is placed well away from the axilla to prevent compression of the axillary artery and brachial plexus.

well secured to avoid falling or tilting forward or backward. Often a beanbag or bedding roll is used to provide stability. A kidney rest can also be used to help secure the patient.

The extremities must be carefully positioned to prevent injury. The dependent leg should be somewhat flexed, with a pillow or other padding between the knees to minimize excessive pressure on bony prominences, reduce back strain, and minimize stretch of lower extremity nerves. The dependent arm is placed in front of the patient on a padded arm board. The nondependent arm is often supported over folded bedding or suspended with an armrest or foam cradle (see Fig. 19.3B). Neither arm should be abducted more than 90 degrees to prevent injury to the brachial plexus from the humeral head. Additionally, an axillary roll should be placed underneath the patient just caudal to the axilla—*not* placed in the axilla itself. The axillary roll prevents compression injury to the dependent brachial plexus and dependent axillary vascular structures (see Fig. 19.3C). Sometimes

an axillary roll is not used if an inflatable beanbag is being used for positioning; however, the team must ensure that there is no compression in the axilla. With invasive arterial monitoring, consider placing the catheter in the dependent arm to detect positioning compression of the axillary neurovascular structures.

The patient's head must be kept in a neutral position to prevent excessive lateral rotation of the neck and stretch injuries to the brachial plexus. This positioning may require additional head support (see Fig. 19.3B). The dependent ear should be checked to avoid folding and undue pressure. The eyes should be securely taped before repositioning if the patient is asleep. The dependent eye must be checked frequently for external compression.

Lastly, the lateral decubitus position changes pulmonary function. In a patient who is mechanically ventilated the combination of the lateral weight of the mediastinum and disproportionate cephalad pressure of abdominal contents on the dependent diaphragm decreases compliance of the dependent lung and favors ventilation of the nondependent lung. Simultaneously, pulmonary blood flow to the dependent lung increases because of the effect of gravity. This causes V̇/Q̇ mismatching and can affect alveolar ventilation and gas exchange.

Prone

The prone or ventral decubitus position (Fig. 19.4A) is used primarily for surgical access to the posterior fossa of the skull, the posterior spine, the buttocks and perirectal area, and the lower extremities. When general anesthesia is required in the prone position, endotracheal intubation, intravenous access, Foley catheter, and invasive hemodynamic access should all be obtained in the supine position first while the patient is still on a gurney. Make sure all lines and tubes are very well secured to prevent dislodgement during turning and to prevent tube migration during the case.

Turning the patient from supine to prone requires coordination of all operating room providers. The anesthesia provider is primarily responsible for coordinating the move and for repositioning of the head. An exception is in cases in which the head is placed in rigid pin fixation and the surgeon holds the pin frame. During the turn to prone, the head, neck, and spine are maintained in a neutral position. Some patients requiring prone positioning have unstable spines necessitating surgical operation. There are also reports in the literature of cerebrovascular events occurring from presumed carotid and vertebral artery injury during turning. For some cases when neuromonitoring will be used for the surgical procedure "preflip," baseline recordings are obtained before turning the patient prone for safety documentation.

To minimize risk of dislodgement, disconnect as many monitors and lines as is safe and possible before turning the patient from supine to the prone position. This is particularly helpful for lines and monitors on the side that rotates the farthest (the outside arm). Many anesthesia providers disconnect the endotracheal tube immediately before turning and reconnect it immediately after prone positioning to reduce the risk of inadvertent extubation.

The position of the head is very important for the prone position. In most cases the head is maintained in a neutral position using a surgical pillow, horseshoe headrest, or Mayfield rigid head pins. Several commercially available pillows are specially designed for the prone position. Most, including disposable foam versions, support the forehead, malar regions, and chin with a cutout for the eyes, nose, and mouth. The prone position is a risk factor for perioperative visual loss, which is discussed later. Mirror systems are available to facilitate checking face positioning (see Fig. 19.4B). The anesthesia provider must ensure that the eyes and nose are free from pressure and document these findings at regular intervals

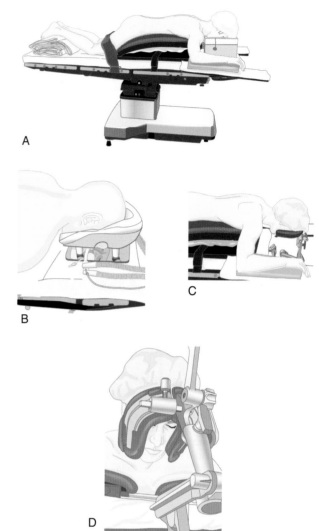

Fig. 19.4 (A) Prone position with Wilson frame. Arms are abducted less than 90 degrees whenever possible. Pressure points are padded, and the chest and abdomen are supported away from the bed to minimize abdominal pressure and preserve pulmonary compliance. A foam head pillow has cutouts for the eyes and nose and a slot to permit the endotracheal tube to exit. Eyes must be checked frequently. (B) Mirror system for prone position. Bony structures of the head and face are supported, and monitoring of eyes and airway is facilitated with a plastic mirror. (C) Prone position with horseshoe adapter. Head height is adjusted to position the neck in a neutral position. (D) Prone position, face seen from below. Horseshoe adapter permits superior access to airway and visualization of eyes. Width may be adjusted to ensure proper support by facial bones.

throughout the case. Facial pressure wounds are a complication of prone positioning. The horseshoe headrest supports only the forehead and malar regions and allows excellent access to the airway (see Fig. 19.4C and D).

Rigid fixation pins support the head without any direct pressure on the face, allow access to the airway, and hold the head firmly in one position that can be finely adjusted for optimal neurosurgical exposure (Fig. 19.5A). Patient movement must be prevented when the head is held in

rigid pins; slipping out of the pins can result in scalp lacerations, skull fractures, and even cervical spine injury.

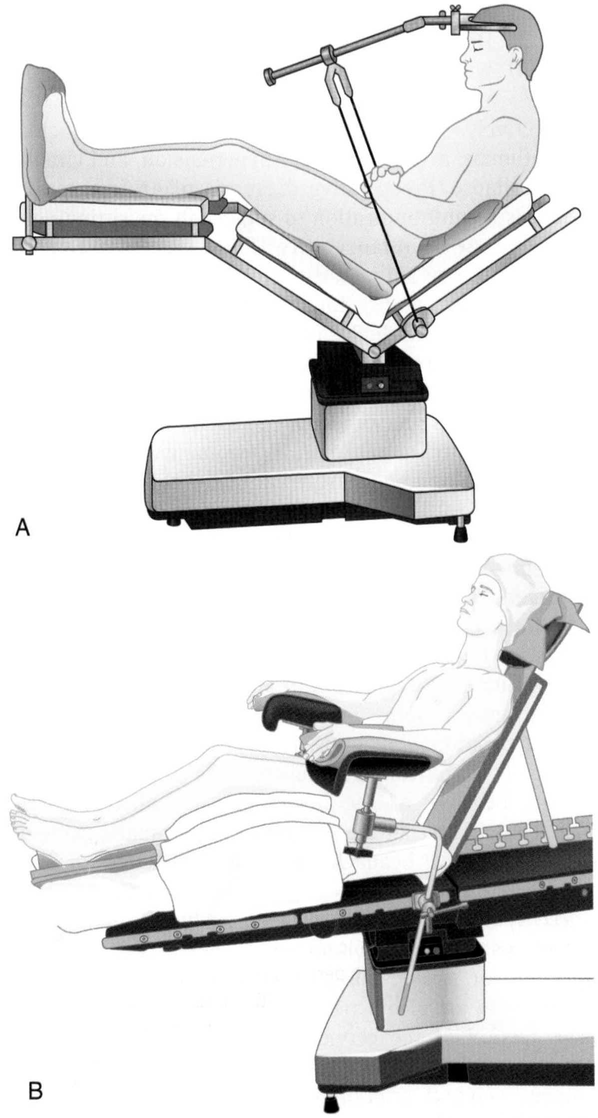

Legs should be padded and flexed slightly at the knees and hips. Both arms may be positioned to the patient's sides, tucked in the neutral position as described for the supine patient, or placed next to the patient's head on arm boards. Again, the arms should not be abducted greater than 90 degrees to prevent excessive stretching of the brachial plexus. Extra padding under the elbow will be needed to prevent compression of the ulnar nerve. Recommendations from the ASA practice advisory on protective padding are noted in Box 19.2.

The abdomen should hang relatively freely for patients in the prone position. This alleviates external pressure on the abdomen, which can otherwise cause problems with ventilation and hypotension by compressing the inferior vena cava and reducing venous return. The thorax should be supported by firm rolls or bolsters placed along each side from the clavicle to the iliac crest. Multiple commercial rolls and bolsters are available, including the Wilson frame (see Fig. 19.4A), Jackson table, Relton frame, and Mouradian/Simmons modification of the Relton frame. All devices and special operating room tables for the prone position serve to minimize abdominal compression. To prevent tissue injury, pendulous structures (e.g., male genitalia and female breasts) should be clear of compression; the breasts should be placed medial to the bolsters. The lower portion of each roll or bolster must be placed under its respective iliac crest to prevent pressure injury to the genitalia and to avoid pressure on femoral vasculature.

Similar to the supine position, hemodynamics are well maintained, and pulmonary function is actually superior to the supine position. The FRC is improved compared with supine positioning, leading to improved oxygenation. For obese patients, pulmonary compliance

A

B

Fig. 19.5 (A) Sitting position with Mayfield head pins. The patient is typically semirecumbent rather than sitting, as the legs are kept as high as possible to promote venous return. Arms must be supported to prevent shoulder traction. Note that the head holder support is preferably attached to the back section rather than the thigh section of the table so that the patient's back may be adjusted or lowered emergently without first detaching the head holder. (B) Sitting position adapted for shoulder surgery. Note the absence of pressure over the ulnar area of the elbow.

Box 19.2 Recommendations for Protective Padding

- Padded arm boards may be used to decrease the risk of upper extremity neuropathy.
- Chest rolls in the laterally positioned patient may be used to decrease the risk of upper extremity neuropathy.
- Padding at the elbow may be used to decrease the risk of upper extremity neuropathy.
- Specific padding to prevent pressure of a hard surface against the peroneal nerve at the fibular head may be used to decrease the risk of peroneal neuropathy.
- Avoid the inappropriate use of padding (e.g., padding too tight) to decrease the risk of perioperative neuropathy.

Advisory recommendations from Practice Advisory for the Prevention of Perioperative Peripheral Neuropathies 2018: An Updated Report by the American Society of Anesthesiologists Task Force on Prevention of Perioperative Peripheral Neuropathies. *Anesthesiology*. 2018;128(1):11–26.

is improved in the prone position with the abdomen hanging freely. The prone position has been used to improve respiratory function and mortality rate in patients with acute respiratory distress syndrome[8](also see Chapter 41).

Proper prone positioning of patients relies on a secure table and correct secure attachment of headrest equipment. Horseshoe and rigid fixation pin headrests attach to adjustable articulating supports; any slippage or failure of this bracketing device may lead to complications if the head suddenly drops. Jackson tables can actually tilt or flip 180 degrees as a result of disengagement of the turning locking mechanisms.

Sitting

In the sitting position (see Fig. 19.5B) the patient's head and the operative field are located above the level of the heart. The sitting position can provide excellent surgical exposure for some cervical spine and neurosurgical procedures, particularly of the posterior fossa and superior cervical spine. Blood loss may also be reduced owing to decreased venous pressure in the operative field.[9] A variation of the sitting position, the "beach chair" position, has been increasingly used for shoulder surgeries, including arthroscopic procedures. This position offers access to the shoulder from both the anterior and posterior aspect and potential for great mobility of the arm at the shoulder joint.

In the sitting position the patient's head must be adequately fixed. This can be done either with a head strap, tape, or rigid fixation. The arms should be supported and padded. The anesthesia provider should ensure that the shoulders are even or very mildly elevated in order to avoid stretch injury between the neck and shoulders. The knees are usually slightly flexed for balance and to reduce stretching of the sciatic nerve, and the feet are also supported and padded.

The most significant complication from the sitting position is risk of venous air embolism (VAE). During intracranial procedures, a significant amount of air can be entrained through the open dural venous sinuses. Low venous pressure in the operative field creates a gradient for air entry into the venous system, similar to the risk of venous air entry during central line placement. The important fear is the occurrence of a paradoxical air embolism. Patients undergoing planned surgery in the sitting position should be first evaluated to rule out anatomic intracardiac shunts. If an intracardiac shunt is present, even small amounts of entrained venous air may result in a stroke or myocardial infarction. Transesophageal echocardiography (TEE) studies have documented some degree of venous air in most patients undergoing neurosurgery in the sitting position, with incidence as high as 100%. Clinically significant VAE has a much smaller incidence of 0.5% to 3%.[9,10] Currently TEE is the

gold standard for detection of intracardiac shunts. Even with screening, contrast echocardiography septal patency may not always be detected. A 2014 metaanalysis assessing accuracy of TEE for detection of intracardiac shunts compared with autopsy, cardiac catheterization, or surgery found a sensitivity of 89% and specificity of 91% for TEE.[11]

Other means of evaluating for intracardiac shunts include transthoracic echocardiography (TTE) and transcranial Doppler (TCD). Recent studies comparing TTE or TCD with TEE reveal sensitivities and specificities of 46% and 99% for TTE and 97% and 93% for TCD, respectively.[10-13] Other complications of VAE include arrhythmias, acute pulmonary hypertension, and circulatory collapse. Preoperative diagnosis of an intracardiac shunt is a contraindication to surgery in the sitting position. The use of intraoperative TEE or precordial Doppler ultrasound may aid in early detection of entrained air.[14]

Patients are at risk for hypotension from pooling of blood in the lower body. The lower extremities are often wrapped in Ace bandages or compression stockings. Intravenous fluids and vasopressors are usually required in order to raise mean arterial pressure. Invasive arterial blood pressure monitoring is recommended for these cases and should be measured at the level of the external auditory meatus in order to optimize cerebral perfusion pressure. Central venous catheter (CVC) access is also recommended for these cases. Long-arm CVCs provide intravenous access without being near the surgical field. Multiorifice CVCs offer an advantage over conventional CVCs for improved aspiration of air should a VAE occur.

Pneumocephalus occurs in almost all patients undergoing cervical spine or posterior fossa surgery in the sitting position if diagnosed on postoperative imaging. Clinically significant pneumocephalus is more rare and occurs because of the lower pressure of cerebrospinal fluid in the sitting position. Symptomatic patients may experience headache, confusion, seizures, or even temporary hemiparesis. Patients experiencing any of these symptoms need to also be evaluated to rule out other postoperative complications, such as intracranial bleeding or stroke. Complications from head and neck positioning are also a risk of the sitting position. Excessive flexion of the cervical spine can impede cerebral venous outflow, contributing to swelling, and can also impede cerebral arterial inflow, causing hypoperfusion of the brain. Macroglossia can also occur with excessive neck flexion. TEE monitoring combined with neck flexion can cause compression of laryngeal structures and the tongue. A minimum distance of two fingerbreadths between the mandible and the sternum is recommended for a normal-sized adult in order to prevent these complications. If preoperative examination reveals that the patient has a further decreased range of motion, then intraoperative positioning should not extend beyond the patient's normal limitations.[15]

POSITIONING FOR ROBOTIC-ASSISTED SURGERY

Robotic-assisted surgery (RAS) came into use around 1999 and has quickly become the norm for many urologic operations.[13,14,16,17] RAS is quickly expanding its use. A 2020 study analyzed laparoscopic surgical procedures and found an increase in robotic assistance from 2% in 2012 to 15% in 2018.[18] For surgeons, RAS offers advantages regarding range of motion and accuracy of laparoscopic instrumentation. RAS is now used widely, including in operations for hernia repair, colorectal, cholecystectomy, video-assisted thoracoscopic surgery, and even some cardiac and head and neck operations.

RAS does introduce some new safety and positioning challenges. Laparoscopic instruments are placed through ports in the patient and then the robot is docked. Docking is the process of physically attaching the robot arms to the laparoscopic instruments. This is a critical safety concern. Traditional, or standard, operating tables *cannot* be repositioned once the robot is docked to the laparoscopic instruments. Moving a traditional operating table risks dislodgement of the laparoscopic instruments in relationship to the patient. At our institution, where traditional operating tables are used in conjunction with a robotic-assist device, our practice is to power off the operating table, unplug the bed, and turn off the bed remote control to prevent inadvertent bed movement while the robot is docked. Some institutions have specialized robotic operating beds that communicate with the robotic operating system. These beds can allow for safe movement of the bed while the robot is docked. Review the equipment at your institution and highlight safety concerns during your surgical timeout.

Once the robot is docked, direct access to the patient is limited. The anesthesia provider should place all monitors, intravenous lines, and invasive lines that might be required during the case before docking the robot. Many robotic urologic and gynecologic operations are performed with the patient in steep Trendelenburg (30–45 degrees) and lithotomy position, with the arms tucked in neutral position bilaterally to the sides. The patient must be very well secured to avoid slipping in steep Trendelenburg position. Many medical institutions use a nonslip mattress (such as a bean bag and foam) on the bed. To better secure the patient, chest straps are often placed in an X configuration over the chest. Use of shoulder braces can also help, although there are case reports of brachial plexus injuries because of stretch between the shoulder and neck. Consider testing the patient in the planned surgical position before the surgical start to ensure that the patient is properly positioned, does not slip, and can tolerate positioning from a physiologic standpoint. If shoulder braces are employed, monitor for excessive stretch at the patient's neck. The endotracheal tube should be well secured to avoid migration. Often a metal tray or table is placed above the patient's face in order to provide protection from laparoscopic equipment.[15–21]

Physiologic changes during robotic surgery are the result of both laparoscopic insufflation and the steep Trendelenburg positioning, when used. Hemodynamic changes are largely caused by laparoscopic insufflation, whereas changes in respiratory mechanics are also affected by positioning. FRC decreases with laparoscopy and the addition of steep Trendelenburg, which further decreases it. This is caused by the combination of the pressure of abdominal contents from laparoscopy and Trendelenburg positioning pushing up on the diaphragm. It can also be worsened by chest fixation that is applied to prevent the patient from slipping off the table. Peak and plateau airway pressures may increase as much as 50% above baseline. Between changes in pulmonary compliance, decreased FRC, and the need for increased minute ventilation with carbon dioxide insufflation, intraoperative mechanical ventilation can be quite challenging during these cases.[15–22]

Other complications from robotic laparoscopic surgeries include laryngeal edema and optic neuropathy. Consider checking for airway leak at the start and at the end of the surgical procedure before extubation.

PRESSURE INJURIES

Pressure injuries are caused by prolonged pressure that inhibits capillary blood flow over a bony prominence. In animal models damage has been shown to start within 2 hours with 70 mm Hg force. Classification of pressure ulcers is according to the consensus panel from the National Pressure Sore Advisory Panel. Stages range from intact, nonblanchable erythema (stage 1) to full-thickness tissue loss (stage 4). Muscle damage occurs before skin and subcutaneous tissue damage and is likely the result of increased oxygen requirements of muscle. In the supine position areas most at risk include the sacrum, heels, and occiput. In the prone position the chest and knees are at greatest risk for pressure injury. For patients in the sitting position, the ischial tuberosities are at greatest risk.[20,23]

Most intraoperative pressure injuries (>80%) are discovered within 72 hours of surgery and occur most often in operations lasting more than 3 hours. Prolonged surgical time is associated with greater incidence of pressure injury. Cardiac, thoracic, orthopedic, and vascular patients had the highest incidences.

Aside from pressure injuries over bony prominences, pressure injuries in the lips, tongue, and nasal alae can occur from endotracheal tubes, nasogastric tubes, and other medical devices. Ensure that pressure from medical devices is minimized. This is particularly important during hypotension or hypothermia when the tissue is more vulnerable to pressure-induced injuries.

BITE INJURIES

Transcranial motor-evoked potentials (Tc-MEPs) are becoming more commonly used for both spine surgical procedures and neurosurgical procedures (also see Chapter 32). Tc-MEPs involve contraction of the temporalis and masseter muscle, which has been implicated in tongue, lip, and even tooth injuries because of biting motion. A retrospective review of over 17,000 cases employing Tc-MEPs found an overall incidence of 0.14%. The tongue was most frequently injured (~80% of all associated injuries).[21,24] Severity of injury ranged from minor bruising to the necessity of laceration repair by suture in 25 of 111 patients. Some medical institutions use bite blocks between the right and left molars ("double-bite blocks") for these cases to prevent these injuries. Even so, approximately 50% of injured patients did have double-bite blocks in place. Commercial devices are available, but they often are of questionable additional benefit.

PERIPHERAL NERVE INJURIES

Peripheral nerve injury remains a serious perioperative complication and a significant source of professional liability despite its low incidence. The ASA Closed Claims Project database reported on nerve injury in 1990 and 1999.[1] However, malpractice claims cannot be used to determine the true incidence of nerve injury. A 2018 qualitative systematic review estimated the incidence of perioperative peripheral nerve injury in a general population of surgical patients as <1%, with a higher incidence in cardiac, neurosurgery, and some orthopedic procedures.[4] Injuries occur when peripheral nerves are subjected to compression, stretch, ischemia, metabolic derangement, and direct trauma/laceration during surgery.[25] Because sensation is blocked by unconsciousness or regional anesthesia, early warning symptoms of pain with normal spontaneous repositioning are absent.[1,22,26]

Peripheral nerve injury is a complex phenomenon with a multifactorial cause. Upper extremity neuropathies are more common than lower extremity neuropathies. A 2019 medicolegal analysis of perioperative nerve injuries cites brachial plexus injuries as the most common neuropathies, followed by injury to the ulnar nerve.[27] Interestingly the distribution of nerve injury claims has changed over time. Spinal cord injury and lumbosacral nerve root neuropathy were predominantly associated with regional anesthesia. Epidural hematoma and chemical injury represented 29% of the known mechanisms of injury among the claims filed. The injuries were probably related to the use of neuraxial block in patients who are receiving anticoagulation drugs and the increased usage of blocks for chronic pain management.[1,23,28,29]

There is no direct evidence that positioning or padding alone can prevent perioperative neuropathies. Most injuries, particularly injuries to nerves of the upper extremity such as the ulnar nerve and brachial plexus, occurred in the presence of adequate positioning and padding. Stretch injuries in peripheral nerves are caused by compromise of the vascular plexus (vasa nervorum) that runs alongside supplying these nerves. This can be the result of either an obstruction in venous outflow or an obstruction to arterial inflow. Compression injuries can manifest in several different ways. Neurapraxia is caused by a relatively short ischemia time and usually causes only a transient dysfunction. Axonotmesis is a demyelinating injury. Neurotmesis is caused by a severed or disrupted nerve, and usually deficits are permanent.[2]

The precise cause of peripheral nerve injuries is often not clear, making identification of modifiable factors difficult to ascertain. Generally, maintaining neutral positioning as much as possible is advised. Stretch, overflexion, and overextension should all be avoided. Superficial nerves, especially near bony prominences, should be padded (common peroneal at fibular head, ulnar nerve at elbow). Padding and support should distribute weight as evenly as possible. Ensure that equipment (such as laparoscopic equipment, C-arms, and other x-ray equipment) is never resting directly on the patient.

In a retrospective study of 1000 consecutive spine surgeries that used somatosensory evoked potential (SSEP) monitoring the incidence of position-related upper extremity SSEP changes was calculated and compared for five different surgical positions. A modification of arm position reversed 92% of upper extremity SSEP changes. The incidence of position-related upper extremity SSEP changes was significantly more frequent in the prone "superman" (7%) and lateral decubitus (7.5%) positions compared with the supine arms out, supine arms tucked, and prone arms tucked positions (1.8%–3.2%). Reversible SSEP changes were not associated with postoperative deficits.[30] The ASA practice advisory recommendations for positioning the upper and lower extremities are listed in Boxes 19.3 and 19.4.

Ulnar Nerve

The incidence of ulnar neuropathy from intraoperative positioning is estimated between 0.04% and 0.5%,[4] but the degree of morbidity can be severe. Ulnar deficits result in the inability to abduct the fifth finger and cause decreased sensation to the fourth and fifth fingers, giving the appearance of a "claw" hand.

Multiple studies have attempted to elucidate causes and risk factors for ulnar neuropathy. In a large retrospective review of perioperative ulnar neuropathy lasting longer than 3 months risk factors were patients who were either very thin or obese and those with prolonged postoperative bedrest. In this study there was no association with intraoperative patient position or anesthetic technique. In the ASA Closed Claims Project database

---

BOX 19.3 Recommendations for Positioning the Upper Extremities

Positioning Strategies to Reduce Perioperative Brachial Plexus Neuropathy

- When possible, limit arm abduction in a supine patient to 90 degrees.
  - The prone position may allow patients to comfortably tolerate abduction of their arms to greater than 90 degrees.

Positioning Strategies to Reduce Perioperative Ulnar Neuropathy

- Supine patient with arm on an arm board: Position the upper extremity to decrease pressure on the postcondylar groove of the humerus (ulnar groove).
  - Either supination or the neutral forearm position may be used to facilitate this action.
- Supine patient with arms tucked at side: Place the forearm in a neutral position.
- Flexion of the elbow: When possible, avoid flexion of the elbow to decrease the risk of ulnar neuropathy.[a]

Positioning Strategies to Reduce Perioperative Radial Neuropathy

- Avoid prolonged pressure on the radial nerve in the spiral groove of the humerus.

Positioning Strategies to Reduce Perioperative Median Neuropathy

- Avoid extension of the elbow beyond the range that is comfortable during the preoperative assessment to prevent stretching of the median nerve.

Periodic Assessment of Upper Extremity Position During Procedures

- Periodic perioperative assessments may be performed to ensure maintenance of the desired position.

[a]There is no consensus on an acceptable degree of flexion during the perioperative period. Advisory recommendations from Practice Advisory for the Prevention of Perioperative Peripheral Neuropathies 2018: An Updated Report by the American Society of Anesthesiologists Task Force on Prevention of Perioperative Peripheral Neuropathies. *Anesthesiology*. 2018;128(1):11–26.

BOX 19.4 Recommendations for Positioning the Lower Extremities

Positioning Strategies to Reduce Perioperative Sciatic Neuropathy

- Stretching of the hamstring muscle group: Positions that stretch the hamstring muscle group beyond the range that is comfortable during the preoperative assessment may be avoided to prevent stretching of the sciatic nerve.
- Limiting hip flexion: Because the sciatic nerve or its branches cross both the hip and the knee joints, assess extension and flexion of these joints when determining the degree of hip flexion.

Positioning Strategies to Reduce Perioperative Femoral Neuropathy

- When possible, avoid extension or flexion of the hip to decrease the risk of femoral neuropathy.

Positioning Strategies to Reduce Perioperative Peroneal Neuropathy

- Avoid prolonged pressure on the peroneal nerve at the fibular head.

Advisory recommendations from Practice Advisory for the Prevention of Perioperative Peripheral Neuropathies 2018: An Updated Report by the American Society of Anesthesiologists Task Force on Prevention of Perioperative Peripheral Neuropathies. *Anesthesiology*. 2018;128(1):11–26.

---

diabetes, alcohol use disorder, cigarette smoking, and cancer were found to be risk factors. In this study 9% of ulnar injury claims had an explicit mechanism of injury, and in 27% of claims, the padding of the elbows was explicitly stated.[1,25,31]

Brachial Plexus

The brachial plexus is susceptible to injury from stretching and compression because of its superficial course in the axilla and proximity to the humeral head. Motor and sensory deficits are wide-ranging, although sensory deficits in the ulnar nerve distribution are common. Injury is most associated with arm abduction more than 90 degrees, lateral rotation of the head, asymmetric retraction of the sternum for internal mammary artery dissection during cardiac surgery, and direct trauma. In cardiac surgery patients requiring median sternotomy brachial plexus injury has been specifically associated with the C8–T1 nerve roots. Patients should be positioned with the head midline, arms kept at the sides, the elbows mildly flexed, and the forearms supinated.

Other Upper Extremity Nerves

Isolated injuries to the radial and median nerves are rare. Injury to the radial nerve can cause wrist drop, the inability to abduct the thumb, and the inability to extend the fingers from the metacarpophalangeal joints. The most superficial portion of the radial nerve is in the lower one-third of the upper arm, where the nerve goes across the spiral groove of the humerus. The median nerve is relatively protected, with its most vulnerable location being in the antecubital fossa adjacent to veins used for intravenous access. The ASA practice advisory recommends avoiding the improper use of automated blood pressure cuffs on the arm (below the antecubital fossa), when possible, to reduce the risk of upper extremity neuropathy.[3]

Lower Extremity Nerves

Injuries to the sciatic and common peroneal nerves occur most often in the lithotomy position. The sciatic nerve can be injured with stretch from external rotation of the leg and also from hyperflexion at the hip. As previously mentioned, the common peroneal nerve is most at risk for injury as it wraps around the head of the fibula. Injury to the common peroneal nerve can cause footdrop, inversion of the foot, and sensory deficit. A femoral neuropathy will present with decreased flexion of the hip, decreased extension of the knee, or a loss of sensation over the superior aspect of the thigh and medial/anteromedial side of the leg. The obturator nerve can be injured during a difficult forceps delivery, in the lithotomy position, or by excessive flexion of the thigh to the groin. An obturator neuropathy will present with inability to adduct the leg and decreased sensation over the medial thigh. A cadaveric study revealed that abduction of the hips of greater than 30 degrees puts significant strain on the obturator nerve. This strain was significantly reduced or eliminated by adding at least 45 degrees of hip flexion.[26,32]

According to a prospective study of close to 1000 patients, the overall incidence of nerve injury in the lithotomy position is 1.5%. The obturator nerve was most frequently injured, followed closely by the lateral femoral cutaneous nerve and sciatic and peroneal nerves. Neuropathy was evident within 4 hours of the surgical end time. Symptoms were paresthesias and pain, and interestingly no motor weakness was found in this study. Length of surgery greater than 2 hours was the only risk factor found.[33] For 14 of 15 patients with nerve injury, the symptoms resolved within 4 months of surgery. In a previous retrospective study the same authors determined the incidence of lower extremity motor neuropathy (greater than 3 months' duration) in patients undergoing surgery in the lithotomy position to be 1 in 3608, with the common peroneal nerve being most affected.[34]

EVALUATION AND TREATMENT OF PERIOPERATIVE NEUROPATHIES

The ASA practice advisory recommends a simple postoperative assessment of extremity nerve function in the recovery room.[3] When a nerve injury becomes apparent postoperatively, it is essential that a directed physical examination be performed to correlate and document the extent of sensory or motor deficits with the preoperative examination in addition to any intraoperative events. A neurologic consultation can help define the neurogenic basis, localize the site of the lesion, and determine the severity of injury for guiding prognostication. With proper diagnosis and management, most injuries resolve, but months to years may be required.

Most sensory neuropathies are transient and require only reassurance to the patient with follow-up, whereas most motor neuropathies include demyelination of peripheral fibers of a nerve trunk (neurapraxia) and generally take 4 to 6 weeks for recovery. Injury to the axon within an intact nerve sheath (axonotmesis) or complete nerve disruption (neurotmesis) can cause severe pain and disability. When reversible, recovery often takes 3 to 12 months. Interim physical therapy is recommended to prevent contractures and muscle atrophy.

If a new sensory or motor deficit is found postoperatively, electrophysiologic evaluation by a neurologist within the first week may provide useful information concerning the characteristic and temporal pattern of the injury. However, another examination after 4 weeks, when enough time has elapsed for the electrophysiologic changes to evolve, will provide more definitive information about the site, nature, and severity of the nerve injury. Regardless, electrophysiologic testing must be interpreted within the clinical content for which it was obtained. No single test can define the cause of injury.

PERIOPERATIVE EYE INJURY AND VISUAL LOSS

The incidence of perioperative eye injuries is approximately 0.05%, and they account for 3% of claims in the ASA Closed Claims Project database (also see Chapter 31). Greater monetary settlements were associated with ocular injuries as compared with nonocular injuries. Perioperative eye injuries include corneal abrasions and postoperative vision loss (POVL).[1,31,35]

Corneal abrasions are by far the most common type of perioperative ocular injury, with an incidence of 0.11% in a 2014.[36] During general anesthesia, the natural lid reflex is abolished and tear production is decreased, which places the cornea at risk. Symptoms most commonly manifest as sensation of a foreign body in the eye upon awakening from anesthesia, photophobia, blurry vision, and erythema. Risk factors include increased age, length of surgery, prone position, Trendelenburg position, and supplemental oxygen delivery in the postanesthesia care unit.[36] Precautionary measures to reduce the incidence of corneal abrasion include early and careful taping of the eyelids after induction of anesthesia, care regarding dangling objects when leaning over patients, and close observation as patients awaken. Ophthalmic ointments may add another layer of protection and combat dry eye. Patients often try to rub their eyes or nose with pulse oximeter probes, arm boards, and intravenous lines attached before they are fully awake.

POVL is a devastating complication that has been associated with specific surgeries and patient risk factors. The incidence is the lowest for noncardiac surgery and ranges up to 0.09% for patients undergoing spine surgery in the prone position.[31,35] Ischemic optic neuropathy (ION) and, to a lesser extent, central retinal arterial occlusion from direct retinal pressure are the conditions most cited as potential causes. Perioperative factors associated with an increased risk of ION include prolonged hypotension, long duration of surgery, large blood loss, large-volume crystalloid use, anemia or hemodilution, and increased intraocular or venous pressure from the prone position. Patient risk factors associated with ION include hypertension, diabetes, atherosclerosis, morbid obesity, and tobacco use. However, with the exception of obvious external compression of the eyes, the cause of POVL appears to be multifactorial in nature with no consistent underlying mechanism.[33,37]

In 1999 the ASA Committee on Professional Liability established the ASA Postoperative Visual Loss Registry to better understand the complication. By 2005 131 cases were reported to the registry; 73% of these reported cases involved patients undergoing spine surgeries and 9% involved cardiac surgery. In a 2006 report of 93 patients with POVL after prone spine surgery 89% were diagnosed with ION, predominantly posterior, and 11% with central retinal artery occlusion (CRAO).[38] In patients who were diagnosed with ION 66% had documented bilateral involvement, of which 42% had eventual improvement in vision, although often clinically insignificant. Compared with CRAO, patients with ION had significantly higher anesthetic duration (9.8 ± 3.1 vs. 6.5 ± 2.2 hours), estimated blood loss (median 2 vs. 0.75 L), and crystalloid infusion (9.7 ± 4.7 vs. 4.6 ± 1.7 L). Patients with ION were also relatively healthy (64% ASA I and II), and 72% were male. In 2006 the ASA issued a practice advisory for POVL associated with spine surgery (also see Chapter 32). Unfortunately, no definite recommendations were made concerning the issue of induced hypotension, use of vasopressors, or transfusion threshold owing to the multifactorial nature and the low incidence of the injury. Despite a lack of direct evidence, several suggestions were made for high-risk patients undergoing complex spine surgery.[34,35,38,39]

Until the causative factors of this devastating type of injury are better defined, patient management strategies will continue to be debated. With regard to patient positioning, the anesthesia provider should be aware that intraocular pressures are increased in the dependent eye in the lateral position and both eyes in the prone position in the absence of any external pressure. Eye checks should be frequently performed and documented. Time in the prone position should be limited whenever possible. Fortunately, in a retrospective review of 5.6 million patients in the National (Nationwide) Inpatient Sample the largest U.S. all-payer hospital inpatient care database, the rate of POVL decreased from 1996 to 2005, perhaps because of an increase in awareness of this complication.[36,40]

ANESTHESIA OUTSIDE THE OPERATING ROOM

Anesthesia care providers are increasingly involved with procedures performed in remote locations such as for gastrointestinal endoscopy, cardiac catheterization, interventional radiology, neuroradiology, magnetic resonance imaging/computed tomography, and office-based procedures (also see Chapter 38). Vigilance is particularly important outside the operating room to maintain patient safety because of the less familiar environment, relative lack of positioning equipment, and variability in staff and nursing training with regard to patient positioning. For example, many locations do not routinely have safety straps or arm supports available. In some settings, such as magnetic resonance imaging, radiation therapy, and computed tomography, the anesthesia provider is not continuously in direct proximity to the patient. In such an environment, where practice patterns have often evolved in the context of nonanesthetized patients, the anesthesia provider will be primarily responsible for verifying the safety of each patient's position and for implementing guidelines for patients receiving anesthesia.

CONCLUSION

The positioning of patients during anesthesia care is an essential aspect of intraoperative care. Each position has different physiologic effects on ventilation and circulation. Despite provider awareness, position-related complications, including peripheral nerve injuries, continue to remain a significant source of patient morbidity. The entire operative team, including anesthesia providers, must work together when positioning each patient to ensure the patient's comfort and safety in addition to the desired surgical exposure. Ideally, the final position should appear natural: a position that the patient would comfortably tolerate if awake and not sedated for the anticipated duration of the procedure.

REFERENCES

1. Cheney FW, Domino KB, Caplan RA, Posner KL. Nerve injury associated with anesthesia: A closed claims analysis. *Anesthesiology.* 1999;90(4):1062–1069.
2. Johnson RL, Warner ME, Staff NP, Warner MA. Neuropathies after surgery: Anatomical considerations of pathologic mechanisms. *Clin Anat.* 2015;28(5):678–682.
3. Practice Advisory for the Prevention of Perioperative Peripheral Neuropathies 2018: An updated report by the American Society of Anesthesiologists Task Force on Prevention of Perioperative Peripheral Neuropathies. *Anesthesiology.* 2018;128(1):11–26.
4. Chui J, Murkin JM, Posner KL, Domino KB. Perioperative peripheral nerve injury after general anesthesia: A qualitative systematic review. *Anesth Analg.* 2018;127(1):134–143.
5. Geerts BF, van den Bergh L, Stijnen T, et al. Comprehensive review: Is it better to use the Trendelenburg position or passive leg raising for the initial treatment of hypovolemia?. *J Clin Anesth.* 2012;24(8):668–674.

6. Warner ME, LaMaster LM, Thoeming AK, et al. Compartment syndrome in surgical patients. *Anesthesiology.* 2001;94(4):705–708.

7. Anema JG, Morey AF, McAninch JW, et al. Complications related to the high lithotomy position during urethral reconstruction. *J Urol.* 2000;164(2):360–363.

8. Guérin C, Reignier J, Richard JC, PROSEVA Study Group, et al. Prone positioning in severe acute respiratory distress syndrome. *N Engl J Med.* 2013;368(23):2159–2168.

9. Black S, Ockert DB, Oliver Jr WC, et al. Outcome following posterior fossa craniectomy in patients in the sitting or horizontal positions. *Anesthesiology.* 1988;69:49–56.

10. Ganslandt O, Merkel A, Schmitt H, et al. The sitting position in neurosurgery: Indications, complications and results. A single institution experience of 600 cases. *Acta Neurochir (Wien).* 2013;155(10):1887–1893.

11. Mojadidi MK, Bogush N, Caceres JD, et al. Diagnostic accuracy of transesophageal echocardiogram for the detection of patent foramen ovale: A meta-analysis. *Echocardiography.* 2014;31(6):752–758.

12. Mojadidi MK, Roberts SC, Winoker JS, et al. Accuracy of transcranial Doppler for the diagnosis of intracardiac right-to-left shunt: A bivariate meta-analysis of prospective studies. *JACC Cardiovasc Imaging.* 2014;7(3):236–250.

13. Mojadidi MK, Winoker JS, Roberts SC, et al. Accuracy of conventional transthoracic echocardiography for the diagnosis of intracardiac right-to-left shunt: A meta-analysis of prospective studies. *Echocardiography.* 2014;31(9):1036–1048.

14. Mammoto T, Hayashi Y, Ohnishi Y, et al. Incidence of venous and paradoxical air embolism in neurosurgical patients in the sitting position: Detection by transesophageal echocardiography. *Acta Anaesthesiol Scand.* 1998;42:643–647.

15. Warner M. Positioning the head and neck. In: Martin JT, Warner MA, eds. *Positioning in Anesthesia and Surgery.* 3rd ed. Philadelphia: WB Saunders; 1997.

16. Hu JC, Gu X, Lipsitz SR, et al. Comparative effectiveness of minimally invasive vs open radical prostatectomy. *JAMA.* 2009;302(14):1557–1564.

17. Wright JD, Ananth CV, Lewin SN, et al. Robotically assisted vs laparoscopic hysterectomy among women with benign gynecologic disease. *JAMA.* 2013;309(7):689–698.

18. Sheetz KH, Claflin J, Dimick JB. Trends in the adoption of robotic surgery for common surgical procedures. *JAMA Netw Open.* 2020 Jan 3;3(1):e1918911. PMID: 31922557; PMCID: PMC6991252. doi:10.1001/jamanetworkopen.2019.18911.

19. Gainsburg DM. Anesthetic concerns for robotic-assisted laparoscopic radical prostatectomy. *Minerva Anestesiol.* 2012;78(5):596–604.

20. Hsu RL, Kaye AD, Urman RD. Anesthetic challenges in robotic-assisted urologic surgery. *Rev Urol.* 2013;15(4):178–184.

21. Kalmar AF, De Wolf AM, Hendrickx JFA. Anesthetic considerations for robotic surgery in the steep Trendelenburg position. *Adv Anesth.* 2012;30:75–96.

22. Lestar M, Gunnarsson L, Lagerstrand L, et al. Hemodynamic perturbations during robot-assisted laparoscopic radical prostatectomy in 45 degrees Trendelenburg position. *Anesth Analg.* 2011;113(5):1069–1075.

23. Cushing CA, Phillips LG. Evidence-based medicine: Pressure sores. *Plast Reconstr Surg.* 2013;132(6):1720–1732.

24. Tamkus A, Rice K. The incidence of bite injuries associated with transcranial motor-evoked potential monitoring. *Anesth Analg.* 2012;115(3):663–667.

25. Winfree CJ, Kline DG. Intraoperative positioning nerve injuries. *Anesthesiology.* 2009;111:490–497.

26. Welch MB, Brummett CM, Welch TD, et al. Perioperative peripheral nerve injuries: A retrospective study of 380,680 cases during a 10-year period at a single institution. *Anesthesiology.* 2009;111(3):490–497.

27. Grant I, Brovman EY, Kang D, Greenberg P, Saba R, Urman RD. A medicolegal analysis of positioning-related perioperative peripheral nerve injuries occurring between 1996 and 2015. *J Clin Anesth.* 2019;58:84–90. Epub 2019 May 22. PMID: 31128482. doi:10.1016/j.jclinane.2019.05.013.

28. Fitzgibbon DR, Posner KL, Domino KB, et al. Chronic pain management: American society of Anesthesiologists Closed Claims Project. *Anesthesiology.* 2004;100(1):98–105.

29. Cheney FW. The American Society of Anesthesiologists Closed Claims Project: What have we learned, how has it affected practice, and how will it affect practice in the future? *Anesthesiology.* 1999;91(2):552–556.

30. Kamel IR, Drum ET, Koch SA, et al. The use of somatosensory evoked potentials to determine the relationship between patient positioning and impending upper extremity nerve injury during spine surgery: A retrospective analysis. *Anesth Analg.* 2006;102(5):1538–1542.

31. Warner MA, Warner ME, Martin JT. Ulnar neuropathy. Incidence, outcome, and risk factors in sedated or anesthetized patients. *Anesthesiology.* 1994;81(6):1332–1340.

32. Litwiller JP, Wells Jr RE, Halliwill JR, et al. Effect of lithotomy positions on strain of the obturator and lateral femoral cutaneous nerves. *Clin Anat.* 2004;17(1):45–49.

33. Warner MA, Warner DO, Harper CM, et al. Lower extremity neuropathies associated with lithotomy positions. *Anesthesiology.* 2000;93(4):938–942.

34. Warner MA, Martin JT, Schroeder DR, et al. Lower-extremity motor neuropathy associated with surgery performed on patients in a lithotomy position. *Anesthesiology.* 1994;81(1):6–12.

35. Roth S, Thisted RA, Erickson JP, et al. Eye injuries after nonocular surgery. A study of 60,965 anesthetics from 1988 to 1992. *Anesthesiology.* 1996;85(5):1020–1027.

36. Segal KL, Fleischut PM, Kim C, et al. Evaluation and treatment of perioperative corneal abrasions. *J Ophthalmol.* 2014;2014:901901.

37. Cheng MA, Todorov A, Tempelhoff R, et al. The effect of prone positioning on intraocular pressure in anesthetized patients. *Anesthesiology.* 2001;95(6):1351–1355.

38. Lee LA, Roth S, Posner KL, et al. The American Society of Anesthesiologists Postoperative Visual Loss Registry: Analysis of 93 spine surgery cases with postoperative visual loss. *Anesthesiology.* 2006;105(4):652–659 quiz 867–868.

39. American Society of Anesthesiologists Task Force on Perioperative Visual Loss. Practice advisory for perioperative visual loss associated with spine surgery: An updated report by the American Society of Anesthesiologists Task Force on Perioperative Visual Loss. *Anesthesiology.* 2012;116(2):274–285.

40. Shen Y, Drum M, Roth S. The prevalence of perioperative visual loss in the United States: A 10-year study from 1996 to 2005 of spinal, orthopedic, cardiac, and general surgery. *Anesth Analg.* 2009;109(5):1534–1545.

20 ANESTHETIC MONITORING

Ryan Paul Davis, Kevin K. Tremper*

INTRODUCTION

Anesthesiologists have long been at the forefront of patient monitoring. This has been of necessity because we are responsible for continuously assessing the patient's physiologic status and the effects of surgery and anesthetic agents. This chapter provides an introduction to the basic function and utility of the wide array of monitors employed in modern anesthesia care. Monitoring devices will be organized by organ system, not by physical property or technique on which that monitor derives its information. A detailed review of monitoring principles is available in a comprehensive text.[1]

Overview

In 1986 the American Society of Anesthesiologists established a set of basic monitoring standards, stating that the patient's oxygenation, ventilation, circulation, and temperature shall be continually evaluated.[2] These standards are periodically reviewed, affirmed, or updated, most recently in 2020. Many clinical situations will require additional monitoring. All of the organ systems monitored are perfused by the circulatory system (Fig. 20.1). Our monitoring of the patient attempts to continuously assess if the patient's state is "normal" or "abnormal" and to correct the cause of the abnormality, or at least treat the abnormal number generated by our monitor. We must understand the limitations of our monitors and how to use data from multiple devices to confirm our diagnosis and follow our treatment.

---

*Founder and equity holder in AlertWatch, Inc., a University of Michigan startup - a decision support alerting software system.

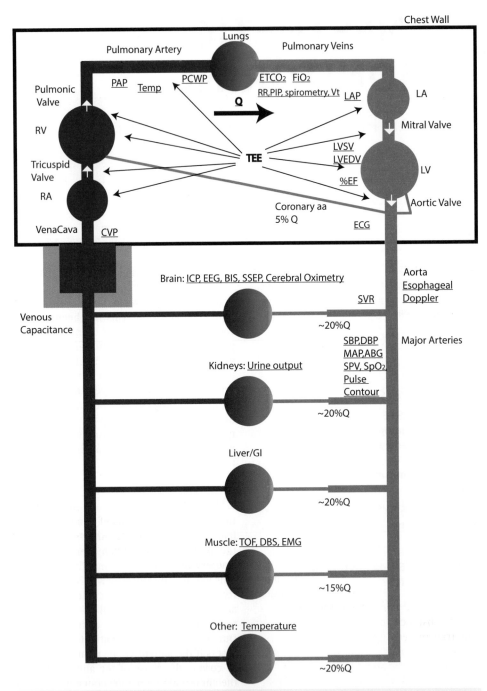

Fig. 20.1 A Summary of Monitors and the Circulation. Anatomic features are listed around the periphery, with monitored variables central and underlined (see Table 20.1 for normal values of monitored variables). The blood flows in a circuit with a cardiac output of roughly 20% each to the brain, kidneys, liver, GI tract, muscle mass, and other organs (skin, etc.). The systemic vascular resistance (*SVR*) is a calculated variable, reflecting the totality of blood flow and pressure. Roughly 70% of the blood is on the venous side. The venous capacitance is highly variable and acts as a buffer for changes in volume. Some variables may be measured or derived, depending on methodology. *aa,* Arteries; *ABG,* arterial blood gas; *BIS,* bispectral index scale; *CVP,* central venous pressure; *DBP,* diastolic blood pressure; *DBS,* double burst stimulation; *ECG,* electrocardiogram; *EEG,* electroencephalography; *EF,* ejection fraction; *EMG,* electromyography; *ETCO$_2$,* end-tidal CO$_2$; *FiO$_2$,* fraction of inspired oxygen; *GI,* gastrointestinal; *ICP,* intracranial pressure;

RESPIRATORY SYSTEM

Oxygen (O_2) is a colorless, odorless gas critical for cellular respiration. Lack of delivery of oxygen to tissues will result in cellular death. Carbon dioxide (CO_2) is a consequence of cellular metabolism and must be removed from the tissues to maintain acid–base homeostasis. This section will review monitors of patient oxygenation and ventilation.

Oxygenation

Inspired Oxygen
Inspired oxygen content, or fraction of inspired O_2 (FiO_2), can be measured by a variety of methods. Anesthesia machines most commonly use an amperometric sensor to measure O_2 in the fresh gas flow. Calibration is recommended, as the sensor, which is basically a fuel cell that consumes oxygen and generates current, has "drift" (i.e., the readings in a constant concentration of oxygen will not be constant). It is a slow responding device, meaning that it cannot be used to measure inspired/expired oxygen, as this rapidly changes. An alternative method of measuring inspired oxygen uses the fact that oxygen is paramagnetic. A paramagnetic oxygen sensor can be auto-calibrating, using room air as a source of 21% O_2. The gradient between the sample and the room air can be measured by a pressure transducer or a torsion wire. The fast response time allows the measurement of both inspired and expired oxygen content. Measuring expired O_2 (FeO_2) concentration during preinduction/preoxygenation also allows the determination of complete preoxygenation/denitrogenation, aiming for FeO_2 >85%, in addition to a rough estimate of O_2 consumption.

Pulse Oximetry
The pulse oximeter provides a continuous noninvasive estimate of arterial hemoglobin saturation (SaO_2) by analyzing light transmitted through living tissue, most commonly the finger or ear (Fig. 20.2).[3] The physical principle known as *Beer's law* relates the concentration of a dissolved substance to the log of the ratio of the incident and transmitted light intensity through a known distance. Oxyhemoglobin and reduced (deoxy) hemoglobin absorb red and infrared light differently. The pulse oximeter contains a light-emitting diode (LED) that emits two wavelengths of light (red, 660 nanometers, and

infrared, 940 nanometers) and a photodiode that measures light transmission. The device determines the signal related to arterial hemoglobin saturation by analyzing the pulsatile component of the light absorption tracing, hence the name pulse oximeter (Fig. 20.3). The following equation is calculated continuously by the device to determine the ratio of pulse-added red to pulse-added infrared light absorbance:

$$R = \frac{AC_{red}/DC_{red}}{AC_{IR}/DC_{IR}} \quad (Eq.\ 1)$$

This ratio (R) of absorbance is empirically calibrated to estimate SaO_2. That is, the device uses SaO_2 data derived from human volunteers to determine the relationship between the pulse oximeter saturation (SpO_2) and the ratio of light absorbance, R (Fig. 20.4).

Dyes and Dyshemoglobins
Standard pulse oximeters using two wavelengths of light can determine functional saturation, that is, the percentage of oxyhemoglobin, HbO_2 over HbO_2 plus reduced hemoglobin, Hb (two equations for two unknowns), using two equations:

$$SaO_2 = \frac{HbO_2}{HbO_2 + Hb} \quad (Eq.\ 2)$$

Functional Saturation

$$So_2 = \frac{HbO_2}{COHb + MetHb + HbO_2 + Hb} \quad (Eq.\ 3)$$

Fractional Saturation
Because pulse oximeters are calibrated using human volunteers who have little carboxyhemoglobin or methemoglobin, these forms of hemoglobin are not accounted for in a standard pulse oximeter's calculated SaO_2 (Eq. 2). Therefore if either carboxyhemoglobin (e.g., from carbon monoxide poisoning) or methemoglobin (e.g., from benzocaine or prilocaine toxicity) is present, the devices will produce an erroneous saturation value. These abnormal hemoglobins can be measured by use of a multiwavelength blood gas cooximeter, which requires a blood sample for accurate measurement (Eq. 3). Dyshemoglobinemias should be considered in patients with a discrepancy between PaO_2 on blood gas and SpO_2 or in specific clinical settings. Carboxyhemoglobin absorbs red light similarly to oxyhemoglobin, causing the pulse oximeter reading to

Fig. 20.1 (Cont.) *LA,* left atrium; *LAP,* left atrial pressure; *LV,* left ventricle; *LVEDV,* left ventricular end-diastolic volume; *LVSV,* left ventricular systolic volume; *MAP,* mean arterial pressure; *PAP,* pulmonary artery pressure; *PCWP,* pulmonary capillary wedge pressure; *PIP,* peak inspiratory pressure; *Q,* cardiac output; *RA,* right atrium; *RR,* respiratory rate; *RV,* right ventricle; *SBP,* systolic blood pressure; *SpO₂,* arterial O₂ saturation; *SPV,* systolic pressure variation; *SSEP,* somatosensory evoked potential; *TEE,* transesophageal echocardiography; *TOF,* train of four; *Vt,* tidal volume.

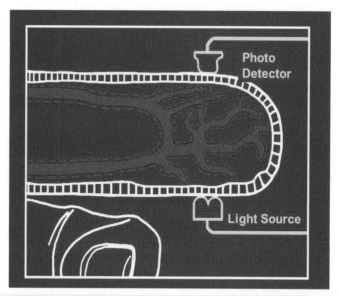

Fig. 20.2 Pulse Oximeter. Pulse oximeters (SpO_2) provide an estimate of arterial hemoglobin saturation (SaO_2) by analyzing the pulsatile absorbance of two frequencies of light (660 and 940 nanometers) emitted by light-emitting diodes (LEDs), the light source, and detected by a photodiode on the opposite side of the tissue bed of the finger. The photodiode generates a current when it detects any light: the red or infrared or room light. For that reason, the photodiode alternates a pulse of red light and room light with a pulse of infrared light and the room light. Then, when both LEDs are off, it measures room light alone, then subtracts the room light signal from the previous two signals, continuously correcting for changes in room light. It thereby derives a signal associated with the pulsing LED signals. The signal may be improved by decreasing ambient light by covering the probe with an opaque material.

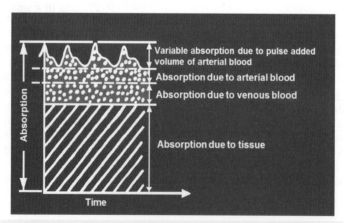

Fig. 20.3 Tissue Absorbances. As light is transmitted through tissues and detected by the photodiode, it is absorbed by all the tissues between the light source and the detector (i.e., skin, muscle, bone, and blood). Because the pulse oximeter is designed to determine a signal only related to arterial blood, it analyzes only the pulsatile absorbance noted at the top of the figure. The pulse oximeter therefore makes the assumption that whatever is pulsing must be arterial blood. In most cases this is true, but in some situations (e.g., patient motion) there can be large venous pulsations which can produce erroneously low saturation values.

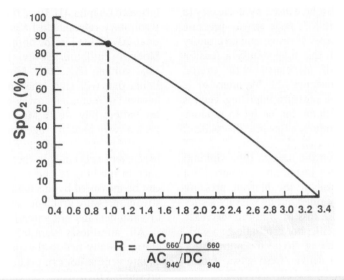

$$R = \frac{AC_{660}/DC_{660}}{AC_{940}/DC_{940}}$$

Fig. 20.4 Pulse Oximeter Calibration Curve. Because of all the absorbances between the light source and the photo detector, the concentrations of oxyhemoglobin and reduced hemoglobin cannot be measured specifically (i.e., the exact path length of the light is unknown). Using the pulse-added absorbance from both the infrared and red light source, a ratio of these pulse-added absorbances (Eq. 1) can be empirically related to SpO_2. That is, volunteer subjects breathe low inspired oxygen concentrations to produce hypoxemia while blood samples are obtained for SaO_2 measurement. These SaO_2 measurements are calibrated to the ratio of red to infrared pulsatile absorbance to develop the calibration curve shown, which is incorporated into the device. The ratio R ranges from approximately 0.4 to 3.4 as the saturation decreases from 100% to 0%. The volunteer data are only available from 100% saturation down to 75%. All values lower than that are extrapolated from the data. Note that at approximately an SpO_2 of 85%, the ratio of the two absorbances is 1.0. Therefore any condition that causes the ratio of pulse-added red to pulse-added infrared red light to tend toward 1.0 will produce a saturation of approximately 85%. This occurs with motion artifact, dyes, and methemoglobin toxicity.

equal the sum of carboxyhemoglobin and oxyhemoglobin, thus giving the impression the patient is adequately saturated with oxyhemoglobin even in the presence of severe carboxyhemoglobin toxicity. Methemoglobin has a dark appearance and absorbs both red and infrared light to a high degree, which causes the absorbance ratio R to tend toward 1. From the calibration curve, a ratio of 1 will produce an SpO_2 of 85% (see Fig. 20.4). Therefore an increasing amount of methemoglobin (especially >20%) will cause the pulse oximeter to display readings closer to 85%. That is, it will produce falsely low values when the patient has high SaO_2 and falsely high values of 85% when the patient is severely hypoxemic. Dyes produce similar errors as does methemoglobin (i.e., force the saturation towards 85%), although most are cleared from the circulation quickly and the error is only transient. Newer eight-wavelength pulse oximeters are available which can detect three saturations (oxy-, carboxy-, and methemoglobin).[4] Motion artifact will also cause the SpO_2 value to tend toward 85% because the motion artifact produces noise in the numerator and denominator of Equation 1. The ratio R is forced toward 1.0 like methemoglobin. In fact, any situation that results in a small signal-to-noise ratio may cause the SpO_2 to trend toward 85%.[3]

Ventilation

The respiratory rate, pattern, and depth are all important descriptors of ventilation. Qualitatively, ventilation depth and pattern can be observed by chest rise, auscultation, or reexpansion of the rebreathing bag on the anesthesia machine. In any acute situation where the adequacy of ventilation is an issue eliminating monitoring devices altogether and going to the source by listening for bilateral clear breath sounds with a stethoscope should be done immediately. This may rule out tension pneumothorax, acute bronchospasm, endobronchial intubation, pulmonary edema, or absence of ventilation altogether.

Airway Pressures

Increases in peak airway pressure merit investigation, as they imply an acute increase in airflow resistance, either in the circuit or the patient (e.g., from endotracheal tube [ETT] obstruction or bronchospasm). Increased peak airway pressure can also be caused by decreases in lung or chest wall compliance. If peak airway pressure is increased and simultaneously positive end-expiratory pressure (PEEP) is increased, this may signify a tension pneumothorax, especially if associated with arterial hypotension. In this circumstance the hypotension is caused by high intrathoracic pressure impeding venous return. The mechanical ventilator can be set to produce a brief pause at end inspiration, allowing the plateau pressure to be measured. External obstruction of an ETT (e.g., from a patient biting on the tube or tube kinking) can cause an increase in peak inspiratory pressure (PIP) with minimal or no increase in the plateau pressure (Fig. 20.5). This can be easily ruled out by passing a suction catheter down the ETT. A loss of or abrupt decrease in airway pressure is not specific, but can indicate a variety of major problems, including circuit disconnections, leaks, extubation, failure to deliver fresh gases, failure to set the ventilator properly, excess scavenging, and other anesthesia machine issues.[5] Airway pressure can be measured with analog gauges or electronic pressure transducers, analogous to those used for blood pressure measurements.

The difference between plateau pressure and PEEP is referred to as the "driving pressure." The static respiratory system compliance equals tidal volume divided by driving pressure. Increased focus on driving pressure is relevant to the treatment of acute respiratory distress syndrome (ARDS), as increases in driving pressure are associated with increased mortality.[6] In the operating room a metaanalysis of 17 randomized controlled trials of protective ventilation showed that increased driving pressure was associated with the development of postoperative pulmonary complications, whereas tidal volume and PEEP were not.[7] Other studies of mechanical ventilation in the operating room include titration of "best PEEP" in patients undergoing elective thoracic surgery[8] and open abdominal surgery.[9] In these studies the optimum PEEP is defined as the PEEP level resulting in the greatest respiratory system compliance or lowest driving pressure. Although driving pressure has shown promise as a variable to monitor and titrate ventilator settings, it cannot be viewed in isolation, given the multiple factors that affect the value, interpretation, and changes with time.[10] Driving pressure will remain a focus of interest in the management of mechanically ventilated patients inside and outside of the operating room; however, ventilator settings should be individualized to the patient.

Tidal Volume

A 2013 randomized trial of low tidal volume in adult patients undergoing abdominal surgery found better pulmonary outcomes associated with setting tidal volume at 6 to 8 cc/kg of ideal body weight, in addition to intraoperative recruitment maneuvers and PEEP.[11] This ventilation strategy is similar to that used in patients with ARDS

(also see Chapter 41). Once these tidal volumes are set, the respiratory rate should be adjusted to maintain an end-tidal CO_2 ($ETCO_2$) in the normal range of 35 to 40 mm Hg. Modern ventilators use a variety of modes to achieve this tidal volume (Fig. 20.6). Most ventilators have pressure limits that will alert when peak pressures are exceeded because of increased airway resistance in the circuit or in the patient (Fig. 20.7). Monitoring the tidal volume and peak airway pressure together will enable the practitioner to quickly detect any changes in resistance to airflow because of resistance in the system or decreased compliance in the lung or chest wall (Fig. 20.8). Tidal volumes can be measured by mechanical vanes rotating in the gas stream, pressure gradients across a flow restriction (fixed or variable), and hot wire anemometers.

All anesthesia ventilators require a "disconnect" alarm, usually tied to the airway pressure reading. Inadequate ventilation can occur despite a nominally normal pressure. When using pressure-controlled ventilation, a significant change in ventilator volume can occur without an alarm condition occurring. Mechanical alarms and indicators of ventilation do not ensure tracheal intubation. An esophageal intubation can return "adequate" pressures and volumes, and with transmission of sounds, appear to have bilateral breath sounds. With an intact circulation, measurement of expired CO_2 is the best monitor of ventilation, discussed in detail in the next section.

Capnography/End-Tidal CO_2

Capnography is the analysis of the continuous waveform of expired CO_2. Gas is continuously sampled from the ventilator circuit just on the patient side of the "Y" connector through a small tube into an infrared analyzer (also using Beer's law), and the CO_2 waveform is displayed on the physiologic monitor (Figs. 20.9 and 20.10). Carbon dioxide generated in the tissues is delivered to the right heart through the venous system into the lungs via the pulmonary arteries. Exchange of the CO_2 into the alveolar space is fairly efficient because CO_2 has 20 times the solubility in water as does oxygen. Therefore well-perfused alveoli achieve equilibrium with CO_2 in the blood. During expiration, alveolar gas leaves the lungs, exiting the trachea through the ETT, where the aspirated gas is sampled by the capnometer, producing a peak expired CO_2 close to the arterial carbon dioxide tension ($PaCO_2$). In healthy patients $ETCO_2$ is usually 3 to 5 mm Hg less than $PaCO_2$ during general anesthesia.

A patient's respiratory tidal volume is composed of alveolar gas volume and dead space volume. Dead space is defined as any portion of the tidal volume that does not participate in gas exchange. In healthy patients dead space is approximately one-third of the tidal volume. Dead space is composed of three subvolumes: apparatus dead space, anatomic dead space, and alveolar dead space (Fig. 20.9). Because the inspired gas contains no

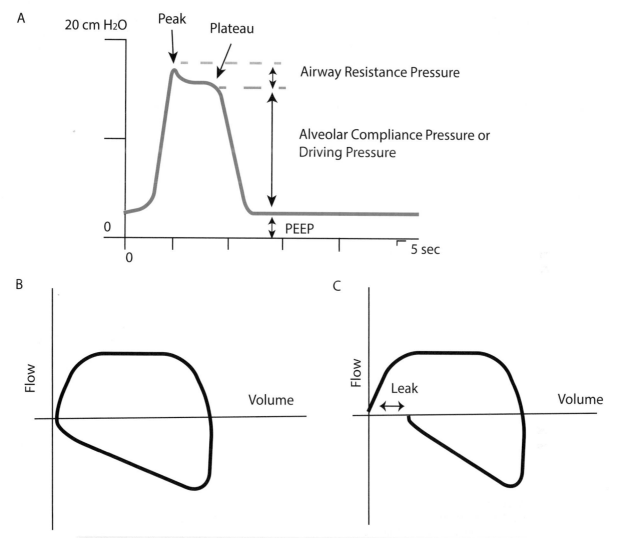

Fig. 20.5 Airway Pressure and Flow Volume. (A) Airway pressure in volume control ventilation with an expiratory pause demonstrates changes in airway pressure and can help determine the etiology of the obstruction. Peak airway pressure or peak inspiratory pressure (PIP) is the highest pressure that occurs inside the lung during inspiration. During an inspiratory pause, there is no air movement, so the airway pressure drops minimally in patients with normal airway resistance and results in a "plateau" in the airway pressure recording, called "plateau pressure." This plateau pressure reflects the airway pressure in the small airways and alveoli during a breath. The difference between plateau pressure and PEEP is called the "driving pressure." The difference between the peak and plateau pressure is caused by resistance within the breathing circuit and the patient's airways. When airway pressure increases because of increases in airway resistance, the PIP is affected greater than the plateau (e.g., with bronchospasm, endotracheal tube kinking). If the plateau pressure increases, other processes reducing lung or chest wall compliance (e.g., pulmonary edema, pneumothorax, increased tidal volume) may be the cause. Flow volume loops can also be evaluated for changes in ventilator parameters (B). For example, when there is a circuit leak (C), the expiratory portion of the flow volume loop will fail to return to the starting point.

CO_2 (unless the CO_2 absorber is malfunctioning and allowing rebreathing of CO_2 to occur), all these dead space gases will not contain CO_2. When expiration begins in the respiratory cycle, the sampling tube will first detect the apparatus dead space, followed by the anatomic dead space. Neither of these contains CO_2, so the capnogram will remain at zero during this initial phase I of the capnogram (Fig. 20.10). As the gas from the alveolar space (well-perfused with a CO_2 tension roughly the same as $PaCO_2$) and the alveolar dead space (with zero CO_2) mix

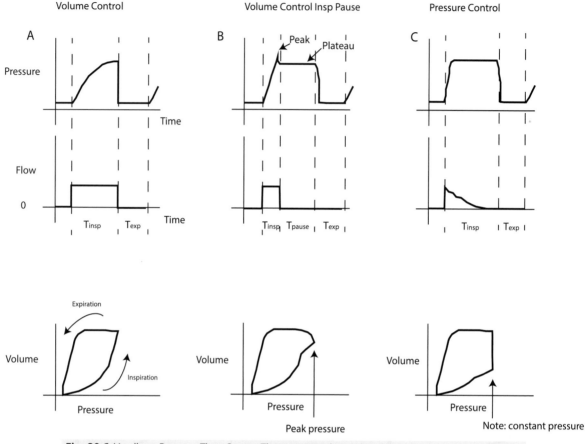

Fig. 20.6 Ventilator Pressure Time Curves. Three commonly employed modes of ventilation generate characteristic curves. (A) Volume control. (B) Volume control with inspiratory pause. (C) Pressure control. Only four variables determine mechanical ventilation: (1) inspiratory time (T_{insp}), (2) inspiratory pause time ($T_{insppause}$), (3) expiratory time (T_{exp}), and (4) inspiratory flow rate. In ventilators that have control loops faulty monitoring can lead to inadequate or hazardous ventilation. The compliance of the lung can be measured by dividing the tidal volume by the pressure. Dynamic compliance reflects the compliance during airflow, so it includes the resistance of the endotracheal tube and the compliance of the lungs. In volume control ventilation (A) the pressure and volume smoothly increase until expiration (which is passive). With an inspiratory pause (B), both the dynamic compliance and the static compliance of the lungs and chest wall can be measured by using either the peak pressure or the plateau pressure, respectively. In pressure control ventilation (C) the pressure is constant as volume increases, until expiration. The pressure–volume loops are different for the various ventilation modes as well.

and are detected at the sampling tube, the CO_2 waveform will rise from zero up to a plateau value, producing a rough square wave until inspiration begins and the CO_2 waveform immediately returns to zero. The final plateau value of the capnogram is the $ETCO_2$, which will approximately equal the $PaCO_2$ value if there is no alveolar dead space. The $ETCO_2$ value will almost always be lower than the $PaCO_2$ value. The size of this gradient will be in direct proportion to the amount of alveolar dead space in the expired volume, relative to the alveolar gas. The greater proportion of dead space, the lower the $ETCO_2$ value. For example, if the $PaCO_2$ was 40 mm Hg and half of the

alveoli that were ventilated were not perfused, the $ETCO_2$ would be 20 mm Hg. The phase II or upsloping portion of the capnogram, seen in Figs. 20.9 and 20.11B, can be slanted rightwards when the alveoli are emptying irregularly. This can occur in patients with chronic obstructive pulmonary disease or asthma, both of which are associated with obstruction to expired gas flow. In general, the increased slope of this phase of the capnogram is associated with greater airway resistance to expired gas flow.

Alveolar dead space may be increased in patients with chronic lung disease who have large emphysematous areas of the lung that increase alveolar dead space

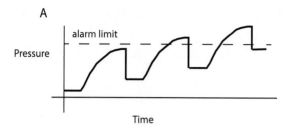

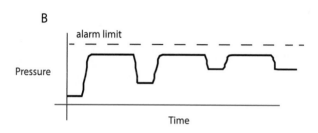

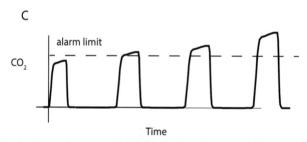

Fig. 20.7 Stacking Breaths. In both volume control (A) and pressure control (B) ventilation insufficient expiratory time leads to "stacking" of breaths and changes in the pressure waveform. In the case of volume control ventilation the pressure can increase, triggering an alarm. With pressure control ventilation, tidal volumes decrease and pressure remains constant. (This may trigger a high PEEP alarm.) The capnogram demonstrates decreased ventilation (increasing CO_2) and may change shape as well (C).

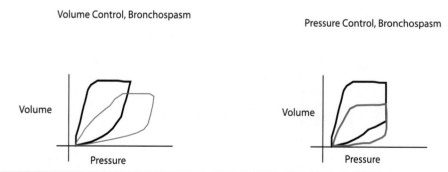

Fig. 20.8 Bronchospasm. With volume control ventilation (A), the set tidal volume is attempted to be delivered, with an increase in pressure. This results in the pressure volume loop being shifted to the right and flattened. In pressure control ventilation (B) the increased airway resistance of the lung results in a decreased tidal volume, without a change in the pressure (because that is the ventilator set point). Normal lungs, black tracing; bronchospasm, red tracing.

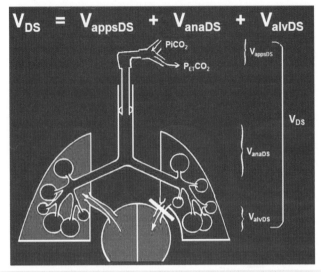

Fig. 20.9 Apparatus, Anatomic, and Alveolar Dead Space. To interpret the capnogram, one must first understand dead space and its components. This schematic shows the heart, lung, and ventilator circuit up to the Y-connector. Dead space volume (V_{DS}) is defined as any portion of the tidal volume that does not participate in gas exchange. It is further divided into three components: apparatus dead space (V_{appsDS}), anatomic dead space (V_{anaDS}), and alveolar dead space (V_{alvDS}). The apparatus dead space is the volume of gas between the Y-connector and the end of the endotracheal tube. The anatomic dead space is the dead space of the trachea and all conducting airways down to the alveoli. The alveolar dead space includes all nonperfused alveoli. In the figure the lung on the right has no blood flow, so all those alveoli are not perfused and therefore at the end of inspiration will have zero carbon dioxide. The lung on the left is well-perfused, and those alveoli can be assumed at the end of inspiration to equilibrate to the arterial carbon dioxide ($PaCO_2$) value.

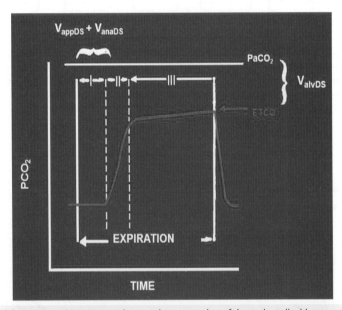

Fig. 20.10 Normal Capnogram. A capnogram is a continuous tracing of the carbon dioxide concentration sampled at the Y-connector on an intubated, ventilated patient and plotted versus time during the inspiratory and expiratory cycle. It can be divided into three phases. The first phase is the beginning of expiration when the apparatus and anatomic dead space are being sampled, both of which have zero carbon dioxide. Phase I starts when the mixed alveolar gases are detected and the capnogram rises up and reaches a plateau value, Phase III, which has only a slight rise as the mixed alveolar gases, are sampled during the end of the expiratory cycle. With the initiation of inspiration, the CO_2 value drops to zero and stays at zero until the next expiration. Note the end peak value is the $ETCO_2$.

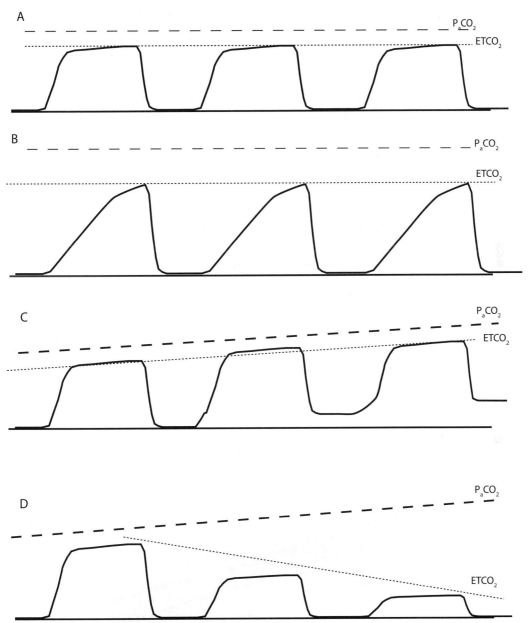

Fig. 20.11 Capnogram Abnormalities. (A) demonstrates a series of normal capnograms. The normal $PaCO_2$ to $ETCO_2$ gradient is 2 to 5 mm Hg. Note in (B) the slant of phase II of the capnogram is less steep. This rightward slant of the initiation of the alveolar gas detection can be observed in patients with asthma or chronic obstructive pulmonary disease. The greater the slant to the right (i.e., the lower the slope), the worse the expiratory airway resistance. The gradient of $PaCO_2$ to $ETCO_2$ has increased. The waveform in (C) shows a progressive rise in the baseline CO_2 value (i.e., there is a progressive increase in inspiratory carbon dioxide), noting a CO_2 rebreathing most commonly caused by an exhausted CO_2 absorber. (D) signifies a progressive drop in the $ETCO_2$ (i.e., a decrease in the height of the waveform). This is noted whenever there is an abrupt reduction in pulmonary blood flow (e.g., reduced cardiac output from pulmonary embolism or cardiac arrest).

and produce a large gradient between the $ETCO_2$ and $PaCO_2$. Acute changes in alveolar dead space occur in specific clinical situations. The classic case is pulmonary embolism, in which blood flow to some capillaries is completely obstructed by the emboli, causing an acute increase in alveolar dead space and an acute drop in the $ETCO_2$ value (see Fig. 20.11D). Increased dead space can also occur if there is a ventilation–perfusion mismatch causing less perfusion to well-ventilated areas of the lung. For example, when a patient is placed in the lateral position, the dependent lung is well perfused and ventilated but the nondependent lung is less well perfused and therefore has increased alveolar dead space. This combination can result in a decrease in the $ETCO_2$ value compared with the $PaCO_2$. Finally, there may be a progressive increase in alveolar dead space because of a global lack of lung perfusion when the cardiac output (CO) decreases (see Fig. 20.11D). For example, if a patient's CO is 5 L/min and for some reason acutely decreases to 2.5 L/min with unchanged alveolar ventilation, there will be less blood flowing per unit time to perfuse the same number of ventilated alveoli. The result is an increase in alveolar dead space and a drop in $ETCO_2$. For this reason, the $ETCO_2$ capnogram is often referred to as the "poor man's measure of cardiac output." Any significant decrease in CO will be associated with a drop in $ETCO_2$ (see Fig. 20.11D). In a patient with cardiac arrest the most important monitor of adequacy of chest compressions during cardiopulmonary resuscitation (CPR) is the capnogram. The presence of a capnogram tracing with every ventilated breath during CPR ensures there is both ventilation and perfusion of the lung. If there is no capnogram tracing during chest compressions (or if $ETCO_2$ <10 mm Hg), then there is no effective CO perfusing the patient's vital organs (also see Chapter 45). The other advantage of monitoring the capnogram during CPR is the lack of motion artifact, unlike other monitors used during CPR such as the electrocardiogram (ECG) and pulse oximeter. Because a normal continuous capnogram waveform reflects adequate ventilation and perfusion, one can argue that the capnogram is the most important monitor used during general anesthesia.

Although the sampling tube can be placed on nasal cannula or around the mouth in nonintubated patients, a reliable capnographic waveform is only achieved in an intubated patient or with a secure supraglottic airway. In nonclosed systems (where the sampling tube is placed by the airway under a mask or a nasal cannula) there may be aspiration of room air (which has no CO_2), which will dilute the capnographic sample.

CIRCULATORY SYSTEM

Multiple characteristics of the circulation can be measured, including the heart rate, ECG, blood pressure, urine output, central venous pressures, pulmonary artery pressures, CO, and systolic pressure variation (SPV) (Table 20.1). Some of these are difficult to measure, and all require interpretation. Many important variables cannot be measured, such as venous capacitance, organ blood flow/perfusion, and circulating blood volume. Other values are derived from combinations of measured values (e.g., stroke volume, vascular resistance). No single characteristic determines adequacy of perfusion, and a solid understanding of the underlying physiology is necessary to interpret even the simplest monitor.

Measurement of the Electrocardiogram

Continuous monitoring of the ECG, one of the American Society of Anesthesiologists (ASA) Basic Monitoring Standards, yields information on heart rate and rhythm. Simply, the ECG is a record of the electrical activity of the heart, measured at the body surface. Technically, it is the net dipole moment of the heart displayed on the vertical axis in millivolts versus time on the horizontal axis (Fig. 20.12). The operating room is an electrically noisy environment, and subtle ECG changes can be obscured by artifacts and by ECG filtering algorithms. ECG monitors used in the operating room have a filtering mode that reduces electrical interference, but may produce artifacts that look like concerning ECG changes (e.g., T-wave changes suggestive of myocardial ischemia). These monitors also have a "diagnostic mode," which removes all filtering and the artifacts it may induce. Therefore if the ECG on the monitor looks different from the preoperative ECG, it is best to switch the filters off, placing the monitor in the diagnostic mode to see if those changes are real. A three-lead system, which uses electrodes placed on both shoulders and the left abdomen below the ribcage, provides leads I, II, and III. The preferred method is a five-lead system, using a single precordial lead placed in the V_5 position, as V_5 is the most sensitive lead for detecting ischemia in patients receiving anesthesia[12,13] (Table 20.2, Fig. 20.13). Most of the dysrhythmias and ischemia seen during anesthesia can be detected by a combination of monitoring lead II and V_5.[13] ECG monitoring allows dysrhythmias, such as heart block, atrial fibrillation, ventricular fibrillation, bradycardia, asystole, and tachycardia, to be diagnosed and managed appropriately.

Blood Pressure and Flow

The primary function of the circulatory system is to maintain a constant supply of blood flow to all organs to allow them to maintain aerobic metabolism and their function. This system is composed of a basic pump, the heart; conduits, the blood vessels; and resistance as blood flows through the microcirculation. This is an Ohm's law system, $V = IR$, in which V is the blood pressure (perfusion pressure), I is the blood flow (cardiac output), and R is resistance (systemic vascular resistance). The pressure

Table 20.1 Normal Values

Measured Variable (Abbreviation)	Value (Units)
Systolic blood pressure (SBP)	90-140 mm Hg
Diastolic blood pressure (DBP)	60-90 mm Hg
Mean blood pressure (MAP)	70-105 mm Hg
Systolic pressure variation (SPV)[a]	3.9-6.0 mm Hg
Pulse pressure variation (PPV)[a]	5.0%-9.0%
Central venous pressure (CVP)	2-6 mm Hg
Right ventricular pressure	15-25/0-8 mm Hg
Pulmonary artery pressure (PAP)	15-25/8-15 mm Hg
Mean pulmonary artery pressure	10-20 mm Hg
Pulmonary capillary wedge pressure (PCWP)	6-12 mm Hg
Left atrial pressure (LAP)	6-12 mm Hg
Heart rate (HR)	60-90 beats/min
Arterial O_2 saturation (SpO$_2$)	95%-100%
Cardiac output (Q or CO)	4-8 L/m
Cardiac index (CI)	2.5-4.0 L/m/m^2
Ejection fraction (EF)	55%-70%
End diastolic volume	65-240 mL
Calculated Values	
Stroke volume (SV), stroke volume index (SVI)	60-100 mL/beat, 33-47 mL/m^2/beat
Systemic vascular resistance (SVR)	800-1200 dynes*sec/cm^5
Pulmonary vascular resistance (PVR)	<250 dynes*sec/cm^5
Respiratory Parameters	
Respiratory rate (RR)	12-20 breaths/min
Peak inspiratory pressure (PIP)	15-20 cm H_2O
Tidal volume (Vt)	6-8 mL/kg ideal body weight
End-tidal CO_2 (ETCO$_2$)	35-40 mm Hg
Cerebral Parameters	
Intracranial pressure (ICP)	5-15 mm Hg
Electroencephalogram (EEG)	Waveform varies by state of consciousness
Somatosensory evoked potential (SSEP)	Normal amplitude and latency
Bispectral index scale (BIS)	80-100 awake
Muscle Parameters	
Train-of-four (TOF)	4 twitches present
TOF ratio	>0.9
Double burst stimulation (DBS)	No fade
Tetany	No fade
Electromyography (EMG)	Depends on stimulus

From Mathis MR, Schechtman SA, Engoren MC, et al. Arterial pressure variation in elective noncardiac surgery: Identifying reference distribution and modifying factors. Anesthesiology. 2017;126:249-259.
[a]These are the range of normal values for monitored and measured variables in clinical practice. Indices are commonly obtained by dividing the value by the body surface area (BSA).

difference across the circulation of any organ is defined as the perfusion pressure, that is, the pressure on the upstream side of that system minus the pressure on the downstream side. For the systemic circulation, it is the mean arterial pressure (MAP) minus the central venous pressure (CVP); and for the pulmonary circulation, it is the mean pulmonary artery pressure (MPAP) minus the left ventricular end diastolic pressure, usually estimated by a pulmonary artery catheter wedge pressure (PAWP). Mean pressure is approximated by the following equations:

$$\text{Mean BP} = \frac{\text{Systolic BP} + 2 \times \text{Diastolic BP}}{3} \quad \text{(Eq. 4)}$$

or

$$\text{Mean BP} = \text{Diastolic BP} + \frac{1}{3}\left(\text{Systolic BP} - \text{Diastolic BP}\right) \quad \text{(Eq. 5)}$$

For the most vital of organs, the brain and heart, these perfusion pressures are slightly different. For the brain, it is the MAP minus the intracranial pressure (ICP)

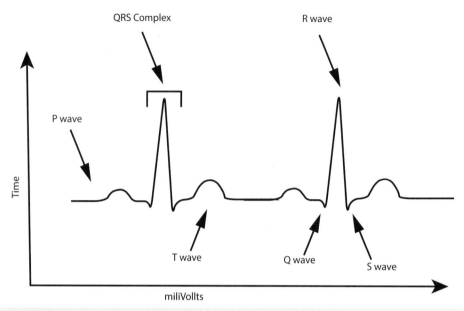

Fig. 20.12 ECG Waves. Electrical activity of the heart measured at the body surface. The net dipole moment of the heart is displayed on the vertical axis in millivolts versus time on the horizontal axis. The p wave represents atrial depolarization, the QRS complex represents ventricular depolarization (Q wave first downward wave of the QRS complex, R wave initial positive deflection, and S wave the negative deflection following the R wave), and the T wave represents ventricular repolarization. Changes in rate, rhythm, and electrical conductivity of the heart affect the timing and morphology of the ECG waveform. Interpreting these changes in a timely and accurate fashion can allow for quick implementation of lifesaving therapy by the vigilant anesthesia provider.

| **Table 20.2** | ECG Sensitivity for Detecting Ischemia |

	Landesberg et al.		**London et al.**	
	Single Leads		**Single Leads**	
	Infarct[a]	Ischemia		
V$_5$	75%	66%	V$_5$	75%
V$_4$	83%	79%	V$_4$	61%
V$_3$	75%	87%	V$_3$	24%
	Combination of Leads		**Combination of Leads**	
V$_3$ + V$_5$	100%	97%	II + V$_2$ + V$_3$ + V$_4$ + V$_5$	100%
V$_4$ + V$_5$	100%	92%	V$_4$ + V$_5$	90%
V$_3$ + V$_4$	83%	92%	II + V$_5$	80%
			II + V$_4$ + V$_5$	96%

[a]Percentages represent sensitivity of leads in patients (n = 12) who were subsequently diagnosed with myocardial infarct.
Landesberg and colleagues[12] and London and colleagues[13] evaluated the sensitivity of various leads for detecting ischemia in patients under anesthesia. Landesberg and colleagues focused on ST changes in the 12-lead ECG during and for 48 to 72 hours after surgery in patients undergoing vascular surgery. Leads had varying sensitivities in detecting ischemia or myocardial infarction. London and colleagues evaluated the use of intraoperative 12-lead ECG in patients with known or suspected coronary artery disease. The sensitivity for various leads in detecting ischemia was then estimated.

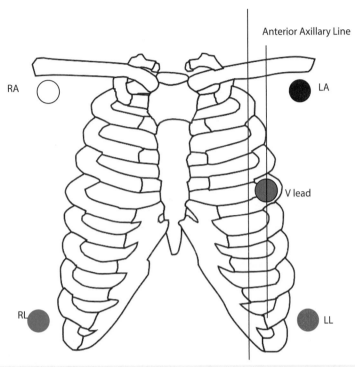

Fig. 20.13 ECG Lead Placement. The limb leads (*RA, LA, RL, LL*) are placed peripherally on the chest (or on the limbs if available). The V lead is placed in the fifth intercostal space in the anterior axillary line.

or CVP, whichever is higher, and for the left ventricle, it is the systemic diastolic pressure minus the right heart, or coronary sinus pressure. Because the left ventricle perfuses itself primarily during diastole, the diastolic pressure is used as the upstream pressure head. In all of these systems blood pressure correlates directly to blood flow, assuming the resistance is constant. Unfortunately, this cannot be guaranteed. In some situations the pressure may be normal but the flow may be reduced because of elevated resistance. The reverse is certainly true. With decreases in blood pressure, there will come a point at which the blood flow to that organ, or the body in general, will be insufficient. Therefore a primary goal of continual repeated measurements of blood pressure is to ensure that hypotension is not occurring. Fig. 20.14 presents a decision tree for the diagnosis of hypotension.

Blood Pressure: Hypotension

Intraoperative measurement and documentation of pulse and blood pressure were first done by the neurosurgeon Harvey Cushing in 1901. Documentation of pulse and blood pressure at least every 5 minutes is one of the ASA Basic Monitoring Standards. Despite this long history of measuring blood pressure at frequent intervals, the impact of hypotension and its duration on clinical outcomes had

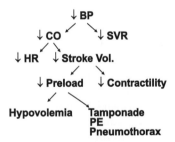

Fig. 20.14 Decision Tree Diagnosis of Acute Hypotension. Given that the cardiovascular system is a pressure = flows × resistance "circuit," the diagnosis and acute management of hypotension should follow the principles outlined earlier. This schematic does not account for increasing venous capacitance. If the blood pressure decreases, it must be because of a drop in either resistance or cardiac output. If there is no obvious reason for the acute drop in resistance (e.g., a sympathectomy from spinal anesthesia), then the cardiac output drop must be caused by a decrease in either heart rate or stroke volume. If the heart rate has not decreased, then the decrease in stroke volume must be because of a decrease in either preload or contractility. If there is no reason for a drop in contractility and the preload is decreased, the most common cause is a lack of relative volume, frequently caused by the increase in venous capacitance with anesthetics. One should always keep in mind the three acute mechanical obstructions to blood flow: cardiac tamponade, pulmonary embolism (PE), and tension pneumothorax.

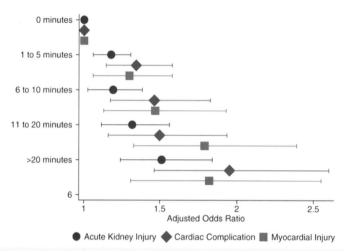

Fig. 20.15 Relationship Between Intraoperative Mean Arterial Pressure and Clinical Outcome After Noncardiac Surgery. This figure, from Walsh and colleagues,[15] demonstrates the adjusted odds ratio for acute kidney injury, cardiac complications, and myocardial injury by time spent with mean arterial pressure (MAP) <55 mm Hg. The cumulative time with a MAP <55 mm Hg was associated with a progressively increasing incidence of postoperative renal and cardiac injury.

not been determined until relatively recently. In 2009 a large prospective observational study found that an intraoperative MAP <50 mm Hg or a 40% decrease in MAP from the preoperative blood pressure for more than 10 minutes was associated with an increased incidence of postoperative adverse cardiac events.[14] A 2013 large database retrospective review noted that cumulative time with a MAP <55 mm Hg was associated with an increased incidence of postoperative renal injury and cardiac injury[15] (Fig. 20.15). Subsequently, a series of studies have confirmed these findings with respect to postoperative organ injury, including death[16] (Fig. 20.16). Classic anesthesia teaching has suggested keeping a patient's blood pressure within 20% of baseline values based on the theory that hypertensive patients require higher pressures to adequately perfuse organs habitually exposed to higher pressures. A 2017 retrospective cohort study evaluated both absolute blood pressure (i.e., MAP <65 mm Hg) and relative thresholds (20% below baseline) and found both were equally predictive of myocardial and kidney injury, with prolonged exposure associated with increased risk.[17] Additionally, there were no clinically important interactions with preoperative blood pressure, suggesting that anesthetic management can be based on intraoperative pressure regardless of preoperative pressure. A large 2020 multicenter observational study of patients undergoing noncardiac surgery divided patients into four risk categories based on factors such as ASA Physical Status, surgery type, and presence of chronic kidney disease. In the patients with higher preoperative risk scores intraoperative hypotension (MAP <60 mm Hg) was associated with increased risk of kidney injury.[18] Therefore intraoperative hypotension for adults can be defined as MAP

lower than 55 to 65 mm Hg depending on the patient's preoperative and procedural risk. Finally, patients require close blood pressure monitoring within the first 24 hours after surgery. A 2020 observational cohort study demonstrated that postoperative hypotension is common and is associated with myocardial injury.[19]

Noninvasive Blood Pressure (NIBP)

The use of an automatic noninvasive cuff, which measures blood pressure by the oscillometric method, is routine in anesthetic care. The cuff inflates beyond systolic pressure and slowly deflates until it detects pulsations, continues deflating until it detects maximal pulsations (the MAP), and further deflates until pulsatility is no longer detected. Although an oscillometric blood pressure system presents systolic and diastolic blood pressures, its most accurate measurement is the MAP (Fig. 20.17).[20] The size of the blood pressure cuff will influence the resultant blood pressure measurement. If the cuff is properly sized, its width will be approximately 40% of the circumference of the arm. If the cuff is too small, the blood pressure measurement will be too high; if it is too large, the measurements will be too low. The oldest noninvasive method of determining blood pressure is that of Riva-Rocci. In this approach a cuff with measuring capability (classically, a mercury sphygmomanometer) is used to occlude arterial flow distal to the cuff. The cuff is slowly deflated until arterial flow first returns, as determined by palpation. This pressure represents the systolic blood pressure. By using a Doppler probe, this method can be used to evaluate blood pressure in patients with severe hypotension or nonpulsatile flow (e.g., a patient with a left ventricular assist device [LVAD]).

Table 4 Summary of highest strength of associations of association of mortality and organ injury in noncardiac patients translated to risk categories. *Not statistically significant; †Hirsch (2015) performed a multivariable logistic regression model to analyse their data but did not report odds ratios, only P-values (P=0.409 for duration of mean blood pressure <50 mm Hg). HR, hazard ratio; MAP, mean blood pressure; OR, odds ratio; RR, relative risk.2

depth MAP/MAP	duration Minutes	mortality (≥80%)	mortality (≥80% & sig.)	acute kidney injury (≥80%)	acute kidney injury (≥80% & sig.)	myocardial injury (≥80%)	myocardial injury (≥80% & sig.)	stroke (≥80%)	stroke (≥80% & sig.)	delirium (≥80%)	delirium (≥80% & sig.)	overall organ injury (≥80%)	overall organ injury (≥80% & sig.)
< 80 mmHg	≥ 1												
	≥ 5	1.02	1.02									Low	Low
	≥ 10	1.04	1.04									Low	Low
	≥ 20												
< 75 mmHg	≥ 1	1.02	1.02									Low	Low
	≥ 5	1.09	1.09									Low	Low
	≥ 10												
	≥ 20												
< 70 mmHg	≥ 1	1.002*	1.002*					1.003*	1.003*			Low	Low
	≥ 5	1.01*	1.01*					1.015*	1.015*			Low	Low
	≥ 10	1.04	1.04					1.030*	1.030*			Low	Low
	≥ 20	1.09	1.09					1.062*	1.062*			Low	Low
< 65 mmHg	≥ 1	1.002*	1.002*	1.3*		1.01*		1.003*	1.003*			Moderate	Low
	≥ 5	1.01*	1.01*	1.6*		1.2*		1.015*	1.015*			Moderate	Moderate
	≥ 10	1.04	1.04	1.6*	1.3	1.3	1.3	1.030*	1.030*			Moderate	
	≥ 20	1.09	1.09	2.3	1.8	1.8	1.8	1.062*	1.062*			High	Moderate
< 60 mmHg	≥ 1	1.1*	1.1*	1.3*		1.1*		1.003*	1.003*			Low	Low
	≥ 5	1.1*	1.1*	1.6*		1.2*		1.015*	1.015*			Moderate	Moderate
	≥ 10	1.1*	1.2	1.8	1.8	1.5	1.5	1.030*	1.030*			Moderate	High
	≥ 20			2.3	2.3	2.5	1.8	1.062*	1.062*			High	High
< 55 mmHg	≥ 1	1.2*	1.2*	1.4*	1.2	1.3	1.3	1.003*	1.003*			Moderate	Low
	≥ 5	1.2	1.2	1.2	1.2	1.5	1.5	1.015*	1.015*			Moderate	Moderate
	≥ 10	1.4	1.4	2.3	2.3	1.8	1.8	1.030*	1.030*			High	High
	≥ 20	2.0	2.0	3.5	3.5	2.5	2.5	1.062*	1.062*			High	High
< 50 mmHg	≥ 1	1.2*	1.2*	1.6*	1.2	1.3	1.3	1.004*	1.004*	• p = 0.409*	• p = 0.409*	Moderate	Low
	≥ 5	2.4	2.4	2.3	2.3	4.4	4.4	1.020*	1.020*	• p = 0.409*	• p = 0.409*	High	High
	≥ 10	2.4	2.4	3.5	3.5	4.4	4.4	1.041*	1.041*	• p = 0.409*	• p = 0.409*	High	High
	≥ 20	2.4	2.4			4.4	4.4	1.083*	1.083*	• p = 0.409*	• p = 0.409*	High	High
< 45 mmHg	≥ 1	1.2*	1.2*	1.6*	1.2	1.3	1.3	1.013*	1.013*	• p = 0.409*	• p = 0.409*	Moderate	Low
	≥ 5	2.4	2.4	2.3	2.3	4.4	4.4	1.067*	1.067*	• p = 0.409*	• p = 0.409*	High	High
	≥ 10	2.4	2.4	3.5	3.5	4.4	4.4	1.138*	1.138*	• p = 0.409*	• p = 0.409*	High	High
	≥ 20	2.4	2.4			4.4	4.4	1.295*	1.295*	• p = 0.409*	• p = 0.409*	High	High
< 40 mmHg	≥ 1	1.2*	1.2*	3.8	3.8	1.3	1.3	1.013*	1.013*	• p = 0.409*	• p = 0.409*	High	High
	≥ 5	2.4	2.4	3.8		4.4	4.4	1.067*	1.067*	• p = 0.409*	• p = 0.409*	High	High
	≥ 10	2.4	2.4	5.1	5.1	4.4	4.4	1.138*	1.138*	• p = 0.409*	• p = 0.409*	High	High
	≥ 20	2.4	2.4	5.1	5.1	4.4	4.4	1.295*	1.295*	• p = 0.409*	• p = 0.409*	High	High

Low	1.0 < OR, RR or HR < 1.4
Moderate	1.4 ≤ OR, RR or HR < 2.0
High	OR, RR or HR ≥ 2.0
	evidence with quality score < 80%
	no evidence available

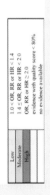

Fig. 20.16 Intraoperative Hypotension and the Risk of Postoperative Adverse Outcomes. This table from Wesselink and colleagues'16 demonstrates the risk of end-organ injury associated with different durations of blood pressure below given thresholds. Patients were divided into risk categories (low, medium, and high) based on the depth and duration of hypotension. The risk category tends to increase as the depth (degree of hypotension) and duration increased.

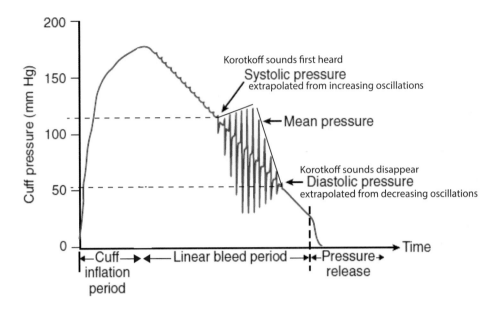

Fig. 20.17 Oscillometric Cuff and Korotkoff Sounds. Initial Korotkoff sounds correlate with the increasing cuff oscillations. The magnitude of the oscillations increases progressively to a peak and then decreases. The peak in oscillations is a measure of the mean arterial pressure, which is the most accurate measurement in an oscillometric cuff. The oscillometric systolic and diastolic pressures are inferred from the slope of the envelope around the oscillations. The decreasing oscillations correlate with the diastolic pressure and disappearance of Korotkoff sounds. (Adapted from Ehrenwerth J, Eisenkraft J, Berry J. Anesthesia Equipment: Principles and Applications. 2nd ed. Philadelphia: Saunders Elsevier; 2013.)

Invasive Arterial Blood Pressure Monitoring

Continuous monitoring of arterial blood pressure can be useful for patients with significant cardiovascular disease or for procedures associated with blood pressure lability or large fluid shifts. Placement of an arterial line is a sterile procedure, with many technical variations on placement. Some institutions have created protocols to be followed for any line placement. The most basic functions of an arterial line include beat-to-beat blood pressure measurement and a means of convenient blood sampling for intraoperative laboratory tests. In addition, arterial line waveform analysis facilitates assessment of the patient's intravascular status volume by measuring SPV and other measures of volume responsiveness. The radial artery is most commonly used because it has the least associated risk and is most easily palpable. Other placement sites include the brachial, femoral, or dorsalis pedis arteries. The risks and benefits of different blood pressure measurement techniques and sites of placement are listed in Table 20.3. Although all catheters are placed in the arterial circulation, the waveforms differ significantly, with systolic pressure rising as the monitoring site becomes more distal. Invasive blood pressures will not be identical to noninvasive oscillometric pressure because they assess pressures by completely different methods.

The arterial line is connected to a pressure transducer, which converts the mechanical energy of the arterial pulse into an electrical signal (Fig. 20.18). This fluid-filled tubing and transducer setup is an underdamped system, which can cause an amplification artifact of the systolic blood pressure. This artifact is worsened by increasing pulse rate and increasing amount of fluid (i.e., length of tubing) in the system; however, the MAP should remain accurate.[1]

Measures of Intravascular Volume Responsiveness

Systolic Pressure Variation

The gold standard for determining the adequacy of intravascular volume and cardiac function is transesophageal echocardiography (TEE). Although TEE can serve as a useful diagnostic and monitoring tool during surgery, it is not necessary or practical for most anesthetics. For procedures with large intravascular volume shifts and uncertainty about cardiac performance, traditional monitors of perfusion (e.g., blood pressure, heart rate, urine output) may not be enough. Substantial information can be derived from analyzing the variations of a continuous arterial pressure waveform in the setting of positive-pressure ventilation. For example, the transient

Table 20.3	Blood Pressure Measurement		
Method		**Advantage/Benefit/Indication**	**Disadvantage/Risk**
Riva-Rocci	Place cuff on upper arm. Palpate pulse, Inflate cuff, slowly deflate until pulse returns	Can be used without a stethoscope by palpation of pulse or Doppler flow detection	Only gives a systolic pressure, can work with nonpulsatile flow
Korotkoff	Place cuff on upper arm Auscultate over antecubital fossa, inflate cuff, slowly deflate, noting first and last auscultation sounds	Gives diastolic and systolic	Needs stethoscope, quiet environment
NIBP	Choose and apply correct cuff size, push start button	Automated, easy, independent of user, routine monitoring, measures mean pressure, interpolates systolic and diastolic	Does not work with hypotension, motion artifact, LVAD
Invasive	Connect intraarterial catheter to transducer	Wide range of pressure, measures a mean pressure and systolic and diastolic used when there is hemodynamic instability, vasopressor administration, need for beat-to-beat monitoring, additional benefit of access for blood draws	Invasive, potential for amplification artifact, dampening, hemorrhage, hematoma, infection, injury to artery or distal areas
	Radial	Accessible, most commonly used site	
	Brachial	Sometimes available when radial not	No redundant blood supply, uncomfortable, cannot flex arm
	Femoral	Large vessel, can give readings with profound vasoconstriction	Prone to infection, affected by prone positioning
	Dorsalis pedis	Can be accessible when radial artery is not (e.g., with arms tucked during surgery)	Some amplification of waveform

LVAD, Left ventricular assist device; *NIBP*, noninvasive blood pressure.

decrease in systolic blood pressure associated with a positive-pressure breath can predict the responsiveness of a patient to a fluid challenge.[21] If the decrease in systolic pressure is more than 10 mm Hg, the patient's CO is likely to increase with an intravenous (IV) fluid bolus. If this systolic pressure drop is less than 5 mm Hg, the patient's CO is not likely to improve with fluid bolus (Table 20.4). SPV may be manually calculated by freezing the arterial waveform on the physiologic monitor and measuring the systolic pressure differences, as shown in Fig. 20.19. In a patient with right ventricular overload the temporary decrease in venous return after a positive-pressure breath can actually improve right heart function by momentarily reducing right heart filling (overstretch), allowing the right heart volume to decrease to a point on the Starling curve with improved CO and subsequently arterial blood pressure. The SPV also provides an indirect assessment of the venous capacitance, which, when abnormal, indicates a potential of the blood pressure to improve with fluid administration (see Fig. 20.1).

One of the major limitations of SPV is that the patient must have a regular heart rate. For example, patients with atrial fibrillation will have irregular variations in systolic pressure even with normal blood volume. SPV values may also be affected by decreased lung or chest wall compliance, prone positioning, high PEEP, and surgical procedures with an open thoracic cavity. An evaluation of clinical modifying factors for SPV and pulse pressure variation (PPV) demonstrated that nonsupine position and preoperative β-blockers are independently associated with increased SPV and PPV, whereas tidal volumes greater than 8 mL/kg and PIPs greater than 16 cmH$_2$O are independently associated only with increased SPV.[22] The newer generation of physiologic monitors automatically calculate SPV and PPV.

Pulse Pressure Variation

Another method of analyzing arterial blood pressure during the positive pressure respiratory cycle is PPV. Calculation of PPV involves subtraction of minimum pulse pressure from maximum pulse pressure, dividing by the average pulse pressure, per the following equation:

$$PPV\% = \frac{PP_{max} - PP_{min}}{\dfrac{PP_{max} + PP_{min}}{2}} \times 100 \qquad (Eq.\ 6)$$

Because PPV is expressed as a percentage, the relative change in the pulse pressure may be more reliable over

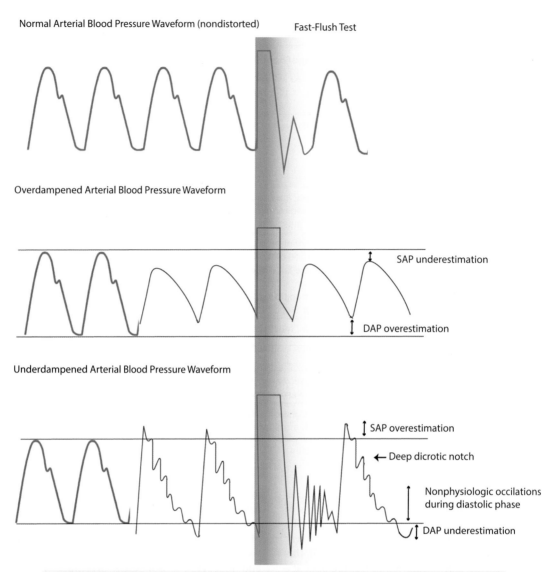

Fig. 20.18 Arterial Waveform Interpretation. The physical properties of arterial pressure transducers include natural frequency (how rapidly it oscillates in response to perturbation) and dampening coefficient (how rapidly it returns to the resting state). An overdampened system has a slurred upstroke, absent dicrotic notch, and loss of fine details (*middle figure*). If the natural frequency is too low, the pressure waveform will be an exaggerated or amplified version of intraarterial pressure. An underdampened system, by contrast, may show a systolic pressure overshoot and additional small, nonphysiologic pressure waves (*bottom figure*). The fast-flush test is a method for determining the system's dynamic response by analysis of the nature and duration of flush artifact. An adequate fast-flush test has a short oscillation cycle and amplitude that rapidly returns to rest (*top figure*). Despite differences in system characteristics, the MAP should remain accurate.

a wider range of blood pressures than the absolute value of SPV, which is measured in mm Hg (see Table 20.4 and Fig. 20.19).

Stroke Volume Variation

Analysis of stroke volume variation (SVV) is yet another technique using the arterial waveform to assess volume responsiveness (see Fig. 20.19). To determine SVV, a pulse contour algorithm is employed to estimate the stroke volume from the arterial pulse wave.[23] These estimates of arterial pulse volume are compared during the respiratory cycle in an analogous fashion with SPV and PPV. The percent reduction in estimated stroke volume associated with positive-pressure ventilation is used to assess

Table 20.4	Measures of Volume Responsiveness: SPV, PPV, and SVV	
	Fluid Responsive	**Not Fluid Responsive**
SPV	>10 mm Hg	<5 mm Hg
PPV	>15%	<7%
SVV	≥15%	<5%

These are three measures of volume responsiveness: systolic pressure variation (SPV), pulse pressure variation (PPV), stroke volume variation (SVV). There is a "gray zone" in which it is unclear if the patient would benefit from a fluid bolus.[13] If the patient is unlikely to suffer harm from the additional fluid, one option is to treat and reevaluate or to pursue additional monitoring of volume status, such as central venous pressure or transesophageal echo.

whether the patient's CO will improve after an IV fluid bolus. These measures of volume responsiveness (SPV, PPV, and SVV) are only accurate in patients with regular heart rhythm receiving closed-chest positive-pressure ventilation without excessively high levels of PEEP (see Table 20.4).

Central Venous Monitoring: CVP, PAP, and CO

As discussed earlier, blood pressure alone is not a sufficient variable to evaluate perfusion. Knowledge of CVP, pulmonary artery pressure (PAP), and CO may be helpful in guiding patient therapy. Additionally, central venous access may be necessary for administration of certain drugs and may act as secure access for large volumes of resuscitation fluids (Table 20.5).

Central Venous Pressure

Information obtained from a CVP line includes the CVP pressure and waveform. The CVP waveform has several components based upon the physiology of cardiac contraction, as described in Fig. 20.20. Despite the physiologic basis for the waveform, CVP monitoring is not a reliable measure to guide fluid therapy.[24] CVP placement is often performed at the internal jugular or subclavian vein. Femoral venous access provides a route for drug administration but does not readily provide the same waveform, as it is not in the thoracic cavity and is very distant from the heart. In measuring CVP we are attempting to infer the filling pressures in the right side of the

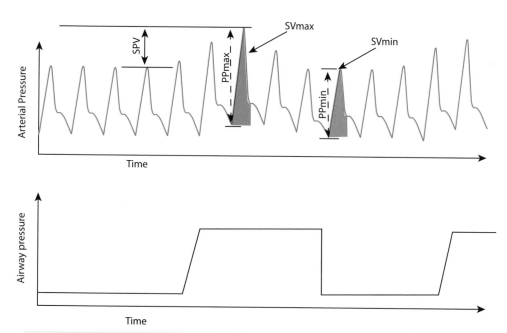

Fig. 20.19 Systolic Pressure Variation (*SPV*), Pulse Pressure Variation, and Stroke Volume Variation. A positive-pressure breath can result in a transient decrease in the systolic blood pressure, pulse pressure, and stroke volume. The mechanism is predominantly related to the positive intrathoracic pressure causing a decrease in venous return and subsequent decrease in right ventricular stroke volume, and ultimately left ventricular stroke volume, with resulting decrease in systolic pressure. Because of a delay in transit as blood moves between the right and left sides of the heart, the changes in stroke volume take several heartbeats to become evident on the arterial pressure waveform. The magnitude of the drop in systolic blood pressure and changes in pulse pressure (PPV) and stroke volume (SVV) can predict the responsiveness of a patient to an intravascular fluid challenge.

Table 20.5 Central Venous Access and Pressure Measurement

Route	Indications	Risk	Benefit
Any central venous catheter (CVC)	Unable to obtain peripheral access, route for potent vasoactive medications	Bleeding, infection	Stable intravenous (IV) access
Right internal jugular (RIJ)	Unable to obtain peripheral access, route for potent vasoactive medications	Carotid artery injury	Straight path to heart for pulmonary artery (PA) catheter
Left internal jugular (LIJ)	Unable to use RIJ	Carotid artery injury, thoracic duct injury, short distance to innominate vein	Can use if RIJ not available
Subclavian	Unable to use RIJ or LIJ	Pneumothorax risk, injury to brachial plexus, subclavian artery/vein	More comfortable for patient postop, can insert with cervical collar in place
Femoral	Disease of head and neck precluding use of neck access	Increased infection risk	Can apply pressure if bleeding
PA catheter	Unstable patient	In addition to central venous pressure (CVP) risks: PA rupture, dysrhythmias,	Can obtain cardiac output information, right and left heart pressures (CVP, PAPs, PCWP)

Practice guidelines for pulmonary artery (PA) catheterization have been published [Anesthesiology. 2003;99:988–1014]. These guidelines highlight considerations for their use: (1) Patient disease (does the patient have serious cardiac disease where knowledge of the cardiac output and filling pressures may alter treatment?). (2) Surgery (is the surgery a major one in which there will be fluid shifts or changes that will be reflected in the monitor?). (3) Setting (do the practitioners have the expertise to perform the procedure with minimum potential risk and maximum potential benefit?). Because these guidelines have been developed, other monitoring modalities such as transthoracic or transesophageal echocardiography and advanced analysis of arterial pressure tracings have seen increased use.

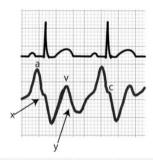

Fig. 20.20 CVP Waveform. The mean CVP value can be used to assess right heart filling pressure. The waveform can also be instructive. The "a-wave" represents atrial contraction against the closed tricuspid valve, the "c-wave" reflects tricuspid bulging as the ventricle contracts, the "x-descent" reflects atrial relaxation, the "v-wave" reflects atrial filling, and the "y-descent" is produced after atrial emptying.

heart. Because the compliance of the vascular space is determined by complex factors that can change rapidly, the relationship between venous pressures and volume status is also complex and unpredictable.

Although absolute CVP values are not predictive of intravascular volume status, they can be useful in the extremes. That is, a CVP <5 mm Hg suggests that an IV fluid bolus may improve cardiac filling, stroke volume,

and CO, whereas a CVP >16 mm Hg suggests that a fluid bolus is unlikely to improve CO.

This approach to assessing the utility of a physiologic variable has been described as a "gray zone analysis." That is, in the extremes the variable provides useful information, but in the range between those extremes (which one may have called the normal range) is an area where the utility of the variable is less valuable in assessing clinical status. However, even CVP values in the extremes are less predictive of fluid responsiveness than SPV and PPV.[24]

CVP Placement

Before performing central venous access, the anesthesia provider should discuss the risks and benefits with the patient and obtain informed consent. The ASA has published a practice guideline for central venous access.[25] The most common placement site is the internal jugular vein for reasons of access and safety. Subclavian vein catheterization has an increased risk of pneumothorax but is more comfortable in an awake patient. Femoral vein cannulation is the least common choice for reasons of sterility and deep venous thrombosis risk. Catheter size is determined by the desired number of lumens and need for rapid fluid administration. A large bore (>7 French) introducer cannula is capable of infusing blood or fluid at rapid rates (>750 mL/min) and provides a means to insert a pulmonary artery catheter or an additional

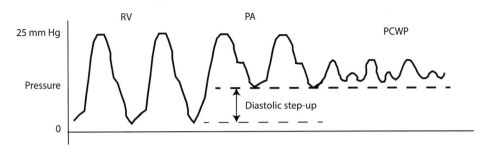

Fig. 20.21 The following is a trace of pressure versus distance as a pulmonary artery catheter is advanced from the right atrium through the right ventricle into the pulmonary artery and ultimately resting in a wedge position in the pulmonary artery. Note as the catheter is advanced from the right ventricle into the pulmonary artery the diastolic pressure is cut off and rises to the PA diastolic, which is only slightly higher than the pulmonary artery wedge pressure. If the pressure rises abruptly after the wedge is achieved and the balloon deflated, the catheter may be "overwedged" and should be immediately withdrawn a few centimeters until a pulmonary artery tracing is achieved.

multilumen catheter (PAC). However, catheter placement into an introducer sheath can significantly reduce fluid flow rate through the sheath.

Pulmonary Artery Pressure and Cardiac Output

A PAC is a 110-cm-long, balloon-tipped, right-heart-access catheter advanced from the right atrium (RA) to the right ventricle (RV) into a wedge position (PCWP) in the pulmonary artery (PA) by following the pressure waveforms noted in Fig. 20.21. Data from a PAC includes CO and pressures in the RA, RV, and PA. The PCWP serves as an estimate of left atrial pressure. This information can be used to diagnose a variety of conditions. Hemodynamic status can be grossly assessed by measuring wedge pressure and CO. Typical hemodynamic profiles associated with hypotension include hypovolemic shock (low PCWP, low CO), cardiogenic shock (high PCWP, low CO), and septic shock (low PCWP, high CO). Volume overload in a patient with normal cardiac function is associated with high PCWP and high CO. Under normal conditions, the pulmonary vascular system is a very low-resistance system, so the PCWP is only a few mm Hg lower than the PA diastolic pressure. In a patient with pulmonary embolism the resulting increase in pulmonary vascular resistance causes the PCWP to be significantly lower than the PA diastolic pressure. Table 20.6 describes a variety of acute causes of severe hypotension caused by mechanical disruption of the circulation and the typical PAC and airway pressures in each condition.

Methods of Measuring Cardiac Output

Thermodilution, the most common approach to measuring CO with a PAC, uses the dye dilution method of flow determination. A measured amount of "cold" (usually

Table 20.6 Differential Diagnosis for Hypotension Using Central Monitoring

Diagnosis	CVP	PAP	PCWP	Airway Pressure
Pneumothorax	↑	↑	↑	↑
Tamponade	↑	↑	↑	↔
PE	↑	↑	↓	↔

These are the changes in invasive hemodynamic and airway pressures associated with the three most common mechanical reasons for acute severe hypotension: pneumothorax, tamponade, and pulmonary embolism. To make these diagnoses, the patient must have a pulmonary artery catheter in place so that CVP, pulmonary artery pressure, and pulmonary artery capillary wedge pressure can be measured, along with airway pressure, in an intubated patient.

10 mL of crystalloid) is injected into the RA, and a thermistor measures the temperature distally. These temperature readings are recorded as a curve of change in temperature over time. The area under the curve (AUC) is proportional to the CO, with a small AUC associated with higher CO than a large AUC. Thermodilution is an intermittent measurement technique, but modified commercially available PA catheters can provide continuous CO data.

Despite all the hemodynamic data provided by the PAC, studies over the past 20 years have determined their benefits do not outweigh their risks in most patients.[26] These risks are substantial, including line sepsis, thrombosis, and PA rupture. Coincident with a decrease in PAC use has been an increase in TEE and transthoracic echocardiography for immediate diagnosis of cardiac pathology. If a PAC is used for the management of hemodynamic instability, it should be removed as soon as possible.

Alternative less invasive devices are increasingly available to estimate CO and assess patients' cardiovascular function. The Doppler effect (shift in frequency of the reflected signal versus the original) can be used to measure the velocity of blood flow. Esophageal Doppler, a CO measurement approach introduced in 1975, uses continuous-wave ultrasound directed through the esophagus and into the aorta to reflect off the blood moving back to the probe.[27] Stroke volume can then be derived by using an algorithm based on the beat-to-beat maximum velocity–time integral (or stroke distance), the cross-sectional area of the descending aorta, and a correction factor that transforms descending aortic blood flow into global CO. This can provide a noninvasive estimate of CO and detect hemodynamic changes in mechanically ventilated patients.[28]

More recently, devices have become available that analyze the pulse contour of an arterial waveform to estimate stroke volume.[29] Given the product of stroke volume and heart rate is CO, these devices provide a continuous estimate of CO without a PA catheter. This relies on transforming an arterial waveform pressure signal to CO and requires some assumptions be made on the dynamic characteristics of the arterial vasculature. Most systems use internal databases or nomograms based on demographics to accomplish this task. Some limitations include variable ability to detect changes in systemic vascular resistance (SVR) between systems, especially with large deviations from normal SVR (improved with newer systems); difficulty using in specific clinical scenarios, such as intraaortic balloon pump; and need for an accurate arterial waveform that is not overdamped or underdamped (see Fig. 20.18).

Other noninvasive monitoring systems, such as the ClearSight system (Edwards Lifesciences, Irvine, CA) are also gaining interest for monitoring. This system uses a finger cuff and two methods (volume clamp or vascular unloading) to provide continuous noninvasive blood pressure and other advanced hemodynamic information such as SVV and CO.[30] The cuff inflates in systole and deflates in diastole to keep the finger's vascular volume constant, as measured by a transmitted light signal. The pressure required to linearize flow is equivalent to the blood pressure. This has been examined in multiple settings and appears promising[31]; however, as with other technologies, it has limitations in certain settings (e.g., Raynaud disease, peripheral vascular disease, hypothermia, vasopressor use).

TEE Monitoring

One approach to rapid evaluation of the cardiac status is TEE. An ultrasound probe is inserted into the esophagus, and various views of the heart are obtained in real time. TEE views can reveal information about heart valves; chamber size (correlated with preload); contractile activity (e.g., ejection fraction); diastolic function; wall motion abnormalities; and signs of specific disease processes such as pulmonary embolism, cardiac tamponade, and aortic dissection. Limitations of TEE include the need for expertise in interpretation and access to the head of the patient. The most serious risks include esophageal trauma, bleeding, and perforation.

CENTRAL NERVOUS SYSTEM

Processed Electroencephalograph Monitoring

Although the electrical activity of the brain can be monitored with the multichannel electroencephalograph (EEG), processed EEG monitors focused on the frontal area have been developed for the sake of convenience. These devices have been developed through an empirical comparison of the awake and anesthetized EEG and output an index generated through a multistep process. EEG features are extracted, artifact is minimized, and an algorithm converts the EEG features to a numerical index, typically ranging from 100 (awake) to 0 (isoelectric EEG). These monitors are intended to assess anesthetic depth and reduce the incidence of awareness with postoperative recall (by avoiding subtherapeutic dosing) and minimize unnecessary anesthetic administration (by avoiding supratherapeutic dosing). The incidence of recall is between 1:500 and 1:1,000.[32,33] The most definitive work on these devices, in particular, the bispectral index scale (BIS) monitor, has demonstrated a reduction in the incidence of postoperative recall of intraoperative events when compared with no monitoring of anesthetic depth; however, BIS monitoring was not superior to the use of alerts based on the expired anesthetic concentrations.[32–34]

Minimum Alveolar Concentration Alert Monitoring

The minimum alveolar concentration (MAC) was developed as a method to assess and compare the relative potency of inhalation anesthetics. It is the end-expired concentration of an anesthetic at equilibrium at which 50% of the subjects move in response to a noxious stimulus.

Large randomized trials of patients receiving inhalation anesthetics have compared the use of alerts based on MAC with BIS monitoring on the incidence of awareness. Specifically, an alert based on age-adjusted MAC values of less than 0.7 was equivalent or superior to an alert based on BIS value in preventing awareness with postoperative recall.[32,33] These studies also noted that patients monitored by either method had a lower incidence of recall than patients without any anesthetic depth monitoring. When pure total intravenous anesthesia (TIVA) is used without any inhaled agent, no calculated MAC alert can be produced. In these patients the use of a neurologic monitor is recommended, especially if a nondepolarizing muscle relaxant is administered.[34] Newer decision support displays incorporate the combined age-adjusted MAC calculations used in this study to alert providers that the anesthetic level may be associated with postoperative recall.[35,36]

Earlier clinical data suggested that a combination of low BIS, low blood pressure, and low MAC (so-called "triple low") was associated with postoperative mortality, but a recent prospective trial of alerting for triple low did not demonstrate any difference in mortality.[37]

Intracranial Pressure Monitoring

Because the brain is enclosed in a fixed cranial vault, the perfusion pressure of the brain (cerebral perfusion pressure [CPP]) is defined as the MAP minus the ICP or CVP, whichever is higher. ICP is normally <20 mm Hg. When intracranial volume is increased (e.g., patients with intracranial tumor or hematoma), additional increases in volume (e.g., from cerebral edema, hemorrhage, increased cerebrospinal fluid from hydrocephalus) may dramatically increase the ICP. In these settings continuous monitoring of ICP may be useful to ensure brain perfusion (also see Chapter 30).

Two methods are commonly employed to monitor ICP. The first, ventriculostomy, requires a catheter inserted in a ventricle of the brain, with pressure transduced with a traditional disposable transducer, as used in arterial or central venous pressure monitoring. The transducer must be zeroed at the tragus of the ear (ear canal). An advantage of monitoring with a ventriculostomy is that cerebrospinal fluid may be removed to treat severe intracranial hypertension. A second technique of measuring ICP employs a device with a pressure transducer on the tip of a catheter inserted into the subdural space. These devices do not require zeroing.

Cerebral Oximetry

The oxygenation of a portion of the cerebral cortex can be monitored with a reflectance oximeter. This device uses near-infrared light in a fashion similar to a pulse oximeter. However, instead of using the pulsatile absorbance of light transmitted through tissue to estimate arterial saturation, the cerebral oximeter uses the reflected infrared light through the scalp and skull from a portion of the cerebral cortex beneath it. The measurement obtained is called *regional cerebral oxygen saturation (rSO₂)*. The light is reflected predominantly from the hemoglobin in the red blood cells within the vasculature of the cerebral cortex. The device presents a number between 1% and 100% saturation, again similar to a pulse oximeter. The algorithms for determining this saturation are proprietary to the manufacturers. These devices have been used in cardiac and vascular surgical procedures where there is a concern for impaired brain perfusion. rSO_2 values are usually around 70% (like mixed venous blood); rSO_2 values <50% or a 20% decrease from baseline values may be

associated with decreased cerebral oxygenation. A 2015 study suggested that cerebral oximetry may also be useful in the management of patients in the sitting position, such as shoulder surgery. In these patients rSO_2 changes may lead to adjustment of FiO_2 or minute ventilation.[38]

PERIPHERAL NERVOUS SYSTEM

Neuromuscular Monitoring

The use of neuromuscular blocking agents is an important part of many anesthetics. Monitoring the effects of drugs that block neuromuscular transmission at the synaptic junction is vital to prevent patient motion at inopportune times during the surgery and to prevent partial paralysis with risks of awareness, pulmonary aspiration, and hypoventilation at the end of surgery (also see Chapter 11).

Basic Physiology/Pharmacology

Normal neuromuscular transmission starts with a motor nerve impulse arriving at the end plate. Quanta of acetylcholine are released in response to the depolarization, diffuse across the neuromuscular synaptic cleft, bind to the postsynaptic nicotinic cholinergic receptor, trigger depolarization of the nerve, and open calcium channels with subsequent activation of actin–myosin chains and muscle contraction. Most of the acetylcholine is hydrolyzed enzymatically by acetylcholinesterase; the resulting choline is recycled into the nerve terminal. Nondepolarizing neuromuscular blocking drugs act by competitively inhibiting the binding of acetylcholine with the receptor. Because the blockade is competitive, it can be overcome with additional quanta of acetylcholine. The nondepolarizing blockers demonstrate fade with repeated stimulation, thought to be the result of presynaptic α3β2 acetylcholine receptor exhaustion.[39–41] Succinylcholine acts differently by binding to the receptor, activating it, resulting in prolonged depolarization and blockade of transmission.

Neuromuscular Blockade Monitor

The most common method to follow the effects of a nondepolarizing neuromuscular blocking agent is to use a twitch monitor and follow a train-of-four (TOF) count. The TOF monitor generates four supramaximal stimuli at 0.5-second intervals (2 Hz). As the degree of blockade deepens, the twitches first fade, then are progressively lost (Table 20.7). Assessment of very deep levels of blockade can be done by using a posttetanic count. The tetanic stimulus for 5 seconds primes the nerve terminal with more acetylcholine, allowing a posttetanic count to be done. Even low levels of neuromuscular blockade may be associated with adverse clinical outcomes. Succinylcholine induces a noncompetitive blockade (so-called *depolarizing block*), which can be followed by a single twitch. Traditionally, assessment of twitches is done by

Table 20.7 Assessment of Neuromuscular Blockade by Monitor Table

% Blockade	PTC	TOF	DBS	TOF Ratio	Tetany	Clinical
>100%	0	0/4	0	N/A	0	Flaccid
>100%	present	0	0	N/A		
90%	PTC >10	1 of 4	N/A	N/A		
80%		2 of 4		N/A		May breathe, maintain ETCO$_2$, but lack airway patency
75%		3 of 4		N/A		
0%–75%	N/A	4 of 4	Significant fade	0.2		
	N/A		Fade detectable	0.4		Risk of aspiration still present
	N/A		Some fade	0.7		Head lift >5 sec
	N/A			0.9	Fade at 50 Hz	
60%	N/A				No fade at 50 Hz, fade at 100 Hz	
30%	N/A				Fade at 200 Hz	
0%	N/A			1.0		

This table provides the responses of a neuromuscular blockade monitor as a function of block versus the stimulus posttetanic count (*PTC*), train-of-four (*TOF*), double-burst suppression (*DBS*), train-of-four ratio (*TOF ratio*), tetany, and the clinical response noted are given as a function of the percentage of neuromuscular blockade.

observation or palpation of the muscle stimulated by the twitch monitor. Newer monitors use more objective movement sensors (e.g., acceleromyography) to provide quantitative measurement of TOF ratio.[40,41]

Strict adherence to TOF criteria to determine "reversibility" of aminosteroid nondepolarizers (rocuronium and vecuronium) may be less necessary with the introduction of sugammadex; however, the importance of TOF monitoring is not diminished. TOF monitoring remains essential to determine appropriate dosing of sugammadex and adequacy of reversal after administration. Inattention to TOF can result in excessive or underdosing of neuromuscular blockade, resulting in inadequate relaxation, inadequate reversal, potentially adverse events, and increased costs. A 2020 study found that reversal with sugammadex is associated with a substantial reduction of postoperative pulmonary complications compared with traditional reversal with neostigmine.[42]

Evoked Potential

Evoked potential (EP) monitoring is indicated for procedures in which there may be neurologic injury caused by either mechanical trauma or ischemia (e.g., during spinal surgery, thoracic abdominal aneurysm surgery, or head and neck surgery). Monitoring of EPs requires constant attention of trained personnel. It is important for anesthesia providers to understand their use and limitations because these monitors affect the choice of anesthetic medications. The most commonly employed EPs are somatosensory evoked potentials (SSEPs) and motor evoked potentials (MEPs). Both involve a stimulating electrode and a sensing electrode continuously assessing the function of the sensory or motor nerve tract.

SSEPs involve delivering a small current to a sensory nerve and measuring the response on the sensory cortex with a scalp electrode. The response is viewed as voltage versus time plot. To reduce background noise, multiple responses are averaged to produce an SSEP waveform. Nerve injury or ischemia is associated with a decrease in amplitude and an increase in latency of the peaks in the waveform compared with the baseline waveform. Inhaled anesthetics (both halogenated agents and nitrous oxide) also produce marked decreases in amplitude and increases in latency at higher doses. Patients with preexisting compromise of brain or spinal cord integrity are especially susceptible to the effects of inhaled anesthetics on EP signals. Propofol is considered the drug of choice for maintenance of unconsciousness during EP monitoring. Dexmedetomidine has also been explored as an anesthetic adjunct because it causes minimal depression of EP signals in adults. A limitation of SSEPs for spine surgery is that they monitor sensory tracts (dorsal spinal cord), and not motor tracts (ventral spinal cord). A patient may undergo a procedure with intact SSEP signals when there is in fact damage to the motor tracts.

MEPs involve stimulating the motor cortex and detecting a response in muscle. MEPs therefore have the advantage of ensuring an intact ventral spinal cord and are more sensitive to both neural injury and anesthetic drugs. The disadvantage is that they require an intact neuromuscular junction, including avoidance of neuromuscular blocking drugs during MEP monitoring. MEPs are more profoundly affected by volatile anesthetics and nitrous oxide than SSEPs; therefore IV anesthetics are commonly employed. During EP monitoring, the anesthesia provider should communicate closely with the monitoring technician when adjusting the dose of anesthetic medications. Acute changes in MEP or SSEP signals require immediate discussion between the monitoring technician, surgeon, and anesthesia provider.

TEMPERATURE

General and neuraxial anesthetics interfere with normal thermoregulatory mechanisms and can result in perioperative hypothermia.[43] In the first hour after induction of general anesthesia the drop in core temperature is caused by redistribution of heat from the core to the periphery, not by heat loss. Malignant hyperthermia, although rare, can cause rapid increases in temperature. Therefore, we monitor temperature in our patients to manage intraoperative hypothermia (inadvertent or desired), prevent overheating when using perioperative warming techniques, and confirm and detect malignant hyperthermia (although increasing $ETCO_2$ is the earliest sign of this). Historically, core body temperature was measured orally or rectally with liquid thermometers. Although accurate, these devices were slow to respond, fragile, and cumbersome in an operating room environment. Infrared scanners directed at the tympanic membrane are used extensively preoperatively and postoperatively. The infrared response time is faster, but subject to errors because of cerumen and other obstructions to the optical path. Intraoperatively, the most common measurement device is a small thermistor located in a nasopharyngeal or esophageal probe. Changes in temperature cause a change in resistance in the thermistor, allowing rapid determination of temperature. The acceptable accuracy range is $\pm0.5°C$.

True core temperature is measured by probe placement in the PA, distal esophagus, tympanic membrane, or nasopharyngeal zones. Other sites that can approximate core temperature include oral, axillary, and bladder. Bladder temperature is highly affected by urine output, approaching true core temperature at high urine flows. Rectal and skin temperatures are highly variable relative to true core temperature (Table 20.8).

MAGNETIC RESONANCE IMAGING AND ADVERSE CONDITIONS

Magnetic resonance imaging (MRI) uses radiofrequency pulses to change the rotation of nuclei in atoms aligned in a very strong magnetic field. As the pulse is removed, the energy is released and can be imaged in multiple dimensions. The return of nuclei to their resting alignment is called "relaxation." Because different body tissues have different relaxation rates, better tissue differentiation (e.g., white vs. gray matter in the central nervous system [CNS]) can be obtained.

The static magnetic field decreases in strength with the square of the distance from the coil. MRI suites have

Table 20.8	Temperature Monitoring Sites	
Site	**Advantages**	**Disadvantages**
Pulmonary artery	Gives true blood temperature	Requires invasive procedure for placement
Tympanic	Gives "brain" temperature	May cause injury to tympanic membrane
Esophageal	Tends to reflect core temperature	Subject to cooling by respiratory gases
Nasopharyngeal	Gives "brain" temperature	Nosebleeds, ambient cooling/heating
Oral	Comfortable in awake patient	Not easily done in asleep patient
Bladder	Easily done if a urinary catheter is in place	Depends on urine output to reflect core temperature
Skin	Easy, noninvasive	Does not reflect core temperature, influenced by ambient temperature
Rectal		May not reflect true core temperature, uncomfortable placement in awake patient, nonsterile

All temperature readings are dependent on blood flow to the area. Alterations in blood flow will result in erroneous temperature readings. Surgical site can compromise monitoring (e.g., an open thorax can change esophageal temperature readings).

demarcation lines indicating the field strength at various distances. Better-designed suites have a series of rooms, so that direct access to the high magnetic environment is not possible without being screened. The hazards of providing anesthesia in this environment include equipment malfunction and physical danger to the patient and anyone present if metal objects become projectiles if brought close enough to the MRI scanner (also see Chapter 38).

All monitors are affected by the MRI environment.[44] Noise levels in an MRI suite can reach 95 dB, making auscultation of any sounds difficult (e.g., breath sounds, heart tones, Korotkoff sounds). The magnetic field will interfere with ECG monitoring as well. The rapidly changing magnetic field orientation can induce a current in any metal-containing loop (including standard pulse oximeters), causing heating and burns. Extended ventilation and sampling tubing help keep sensitive equipment away from the magnet.

MULTIFUNCTION DISPLAYS AND DECISION SUPPORT

The past decade has seen the progressive implementation of the complete electronic medical record (EMR) incorporating patient diagnoses (ICD-10 codes), laboratory results, and live monitored data flow sheets. This information is incorporated into anesthesia information management systems (AIMSs). Initially, AIMSs were developed to automate recording of patient monitor and anesthesia machine information. However, the true potential of this broad array of patient data is real-time integrated display and decision support analogous to systems developed for commercial aviation in the 1980s.[45] Clinical decision support (CDS) systems can be integrated into an AIMS or act as stand-alone systems.[46] Commercially available CDS systems include Talis Clinical and AlertWatch.

AlertWatch, like other CDS systems, allows for integration of clinical data in addition to live calculations to enhance the information.[36] The anesthesia provider can be notified in real time with calculated alerts, such as the cumulative time the MAP has been <60 mm Hg (Fig. 20.22). This type of live monitoring display attempts to reduce alarm fatigue by prioritizing them in the order they should be addressed.[36,47] Decision support systems such as AlertWatch that involve calculations are considered software devices and therefore require Food and Drug Administration (FDA) clearance as medical device data systems (MDDS) devices, similar to physiologic monitors. Relevant patient information such as net fluid balance can be automatically calculated and presented relative to the patient's estimated blood volume (BV). The BV equation uses a formula that includes height, weight, and gender and involves an exponent calculation, which can be difficult to determine without a computer.[48] Several studies have found that using AlertWatch can improve adherence to process measures such as glucose, ventilator, blood pressure, and fluid management.[47,49] There was also an association with reduced hospital charges and length of stay when AlertWatch users were compared with historical controls but not when compared with parallel controls.[47] A multi–operating room census view can be employed as a "control tower" to survey the activity in multiple operating rooms simultaneously[50] (Fig. 20.23). The future promise of systems such as AlertWatch is integration and processing of vast amounts of clinical data while promoting adherence to evidence-based guidelines and care management protocols, hopefully leading to better patient outcomes.

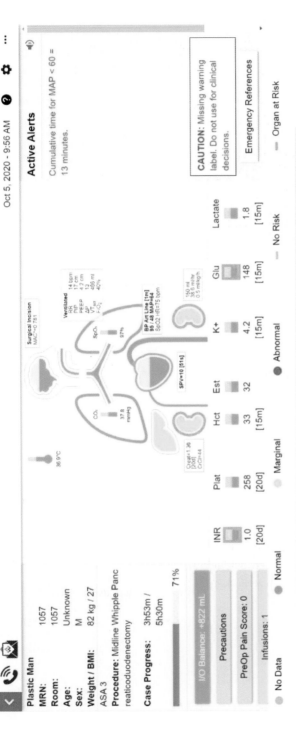

Fig. 20.22 AlertWatch Patient View. The patient view of this multisystem display. It is color coded, with green, yellow, and red designating normal range, slightly abnormal range, and abnormal range, respectively. The color orange designates comorbidities associated with that item. The display has three sections: patient information on the left, icon-based organ system view in the center, and active alerts on the right. Each icon and color-coded portion of the display have more information about that organ system or item displayed when the item is selected. There are multiple calculations being conducted in the background (see Ref. 3). For example, this patient has a +822 mL positive I/O balance with a green background, meaning this positive I/O balance volume is within 20% of the patient's estimated blood volume (on the right in patient information section) and a calculated age-adjusted MAC of 0.781 (noted as a green level in the Brain, in the middle patient icon section) and additionally the mean arterial blood pressure has been below 60 mm Hg for a total of 13 minutes (noted as an alert in the upper right in the Alerts section of the screen). This patient has heart and kidney disease and is on medications that affect international normalized ratio (INR) and has diabetes (all highlighted in orange).

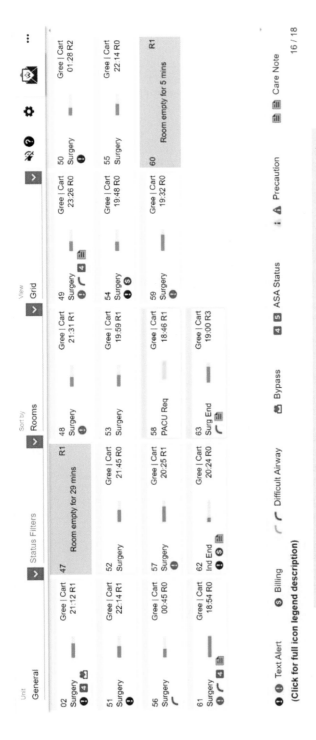

Fig. 20.23 Census View of AlertWatch. The census view of AlertWatch. Each rectangle represents a patient in an operating room (or critical care unit or labor and delivery). It shows the room number, the status of the case, (in operating room, induction end, etc.) and the anesthesia team in the room. If the bar in the middle is green, it means the case is on time; yellow means the case is longer than scheduled time; and red means the case is much longer than scheduled time. The colored circles with exclamation points come in three severities: black alerts (informational), red alert (more important information), and red flashing alerts (the issue needs immediate attention). A series of icons are defined at the bottom of the table. For example, a red elbow designates a history of difficult mask ventilation or difficult intubation.

REFERENCES

1. Szocik J, Barker SJ, Tremper KK. Fundamental Principles of Monitoring Instrumentation in Miller's Anesthesia. 8th ed. Vol. 1. Churchill Livingstone Elsevier; 2013.
2. American Society of Anesthesiologists Standards for Basic Anesthetic Monitoring, approved on October 21, 1986 and last amended on October 20, 2015 with an effective date of October 28, 2015. https://www.asahq.org/quality-and-practice-management/standards-and-guidelines. Accessed on September 29, 2020.
3. Tremper KK, Barker SJ. Pulse oximetry. *Anesthesiology.* 1989;70:98–108.
4. Barker SJ, Curry J, Redford D, Morgan S. Measurement of carboxyhemoglobin and methemoglobin by pulse oximetry. *Anesthesiology.* 2006;105:892–897.
5. Raphael DT. APSF Newsletter. 1998 Winter; 13(4).
6. Amato MBP, Meade MO, Slutsky AS, et al. Driving pressure and survival in the acute respiratory distress syndrome. *N Engl J Med.* 2015;372:747–755.
7. Neto AS, Hemmes SNT, Barbas CSV, et al. Association between driving pressure and development of postoperative pulmonary complications in patients undergoing mechanical ventilation for general anesthesia: A metal-analysis of individual patient data. *Lancet Respir Med.* 2016;4(4):272–280.
8. Park MH, Ahn HJ, Kim JA, et al. Driving pressure during thoracic surgery: A randomized clinical trial. *Anesthesiology.* 2019;130:385–393.
9. Ferrando C, Suarez-Sipmann F, Tusman G, et al. Open lung approach versus standard protective strategies: Effects on driving pressure and ventilatory efficiency during anesthesia–A pilot, randomized controlled trial. *PLoS One.* 2017;12(5):e0177399. May 11.
10. Meier A, Sell RE, Malhotra A. Driving pressure for ventilation of patients with acute respiratory distress syndrome. *Anesthesiology.* 2020;132:1569–1576.
11. Futier E, Constantin JM, Paugam-Burtz C, et al. A trial of intraoperative low-tidal-volume ventilation in abdominal surgery. *N Engl J Med.* 2013;369:428–437.
12. Landesberg G, Mosseri M, Wolf Y, Vesselov Y, Weissman C. Perioperative myocardial ischemia and infarction: Identification by continuous 12-lead electrocardiogram with online ST-segment monitoring. *Anesthesiology.* 2002;96:264–270.
13. London MJ, Hollenberg M, Wong MG, et al., Intraoperative myocardial ischemia: Localization by continuous 12-lead electrocardiography. *Anesthesiology.* 1988;69:232–241.
14. Kheterpal S, O'Reilly M, Englesbe MJ, et al. Preoperative and intraoperative predictors of cardiac adverse events after general, vascular, and urological surgery. *Anesthesiology.* 2009;110:58–66.
15. Walsh M, Devereaux PJ, Garg AX, et al. Relationship between intraoperative mean arterial pressure and clinical outcomes after noncardiac surgery. *Anesthesiology.* 2013;119:507–515.
16. Wesselink EM, Kappen TH, Torn HM, Slooter JC. Intraoperative hypotension and the risk of postoperative adverse outcomes: A systematic review. *British J of Anesthesia.* 2018;121(4):706–721.
17. Salmasi V, Maheshwari K, Yang D, et al. Relationship between intraoperative hypotension defined by either reduction from baseline of absolute thresholds, and acute kidney and myocardial injury after noncardiac surgery. A retrospective cohort analysis. *Anesthesiology.* 2017;126:47–65.
18. Mathis MR, Naik BI, Freundlich R, et al. Preoperative risk and the association between hypotension and postoperative acute kidney injury. *Anesthesiology.* 2020;132:461–475.
19. Liem VG, Hoeks SE, Mol KH, et al. Postoperative hypotension after noncardiac surgery and the association with myocardial injury. *Anesthesiology.* 2020;133:519–522.
20. Ehrenwerth J, Eisenkraft JB, Berry J. *Anesthesia Equipment: Principles and Applications.* 2nd ed. Philadelphia: Saunders an imprint of Elsevier; 2013.
21. Perel A, Minkovich L, Preisman S, et al. Assessing fluid-responsiveness by a standardized ventilatory maneuver (the respiratory systolic variation test). *Anesth Analg.* 2005;100:942–945.
22. Mathis MR, Schechtman SA, Engoren MC, et al. Arterial Pressure Variation in Elective Noncardiac Surgery: Identifying Reference Distribution and Modifying Factors. *Anesthesiology.* 2017;126:249–259.
23. Lahner D, Kabon B, Marscalek C, et al. Evaluation of stroke volume variation obtained by arterial pulse contour analysis to predict fluid responsiveness intraoperatively. *Br J Anaesth.* 2009;103(3):346–351.
24. Marik PE, Cavallazzi R. Does the central venous pressure predict fluid responsiveness? An updated meta-analysis and a plea for some common sense. *Crit Care Med.* 2013;41:1774–1781.
25. American Society of Anesthesiologists Practice Guidelines for Central Venous Access: An updated report by the American Society of Anesthesiologists Task Force on Central Venous Access. *Anesthesiology.* 2020;132:8–43.
26. Sandham JD, Hull RD, Brant RF, et al. A randomized, controlled trial of the use of pulmonary-artery catheters in high risk surgical patients. *N Engl J Med.* 2003;348:5–14.
27. Daigle RE, Miller CW, McLeod FD, Hokanson DE. Nontraumatic aortic blood flow sensing by use of an ultrasonic esophageal probe. *J Appl Physiology.* 1975;38(6):1153–1160.
28. Valteir B, Cholley BP, Belot JP, ed la Coussaye JE, Mateo J, Payen DM. Non-invasive monitoring of cardiac output in critically ill patients using transesophageal Doppler. *Am J Respir Crit Care Med.* 1998;158(1):77–83.
29. Grensemann J. Cardiac output monitoring by pulse contour analysis, the technical basics of less-invasive techniques. *Front Med.* 6;5:64
30. Chung E, Chen G, Alexander B, Cannesson M. Non-invasive blood pressure monitoring: A review of current applications. *Front Med.* 2003;7(1):91–101.
31. Chachula K, Lieb F, Hess Welter J, Graf N, Dullenkopf A. Non-invasive continuous blood pressure monitoring (ClearSight™ system) during shoulder surgery in the beach chair position: A prospective self-controlled study. 2020;20:217.
32. Avidan MS, Jacobsohn E, Glick D, et al. Prevention of intraoperative awareness in a high-risk surgical population. *N Engl J Med.* 2011;365:591–600.
33. Mashour GA, Shanks A, Tremper KT, et al. Prevention of intraoperative awareness with explicit recall in an unselected surgical population. A randomized comparative effectiveness trial. *Anesthesiology.* 2012;117:717–725.
34. Mashour GA, Orser BA, Avidan M. Intraoperative awareness from neurobiology to clinical practice. *Anesthesiology.* 2011;114:1218.
35. Mashour G, Esaki R, Vandervest J, et al. A novel electronic algorithm for detecting potentially insufficient anesthesia: Implications for the prevention of intraoperative awareness. *J Clin Monit Comput.* 2009;23:273–277.
36. Tremper KK, Mace JM, Gombert JM, et al. Design of a novel multifunction decision support display for anesthesia care: AlertWatch OR. *BMC Anesthesiology.* 2018. Feb 5.
37. Sessler D, et al. Triple-low alerts do not reduce mortality: A real-time randomized trial. *Anesthesiology.* 130:72–822019.
38. Picton P, Dering A, Alexander A, Neff M, Miller BS, Shanks A, Housey M, Mashour GA. Influence of ventilation strategies and anesthetic techniques on regional cerebral oximetry in the beach chair position: A prospective interventional study with a randomized comparison of two anesthetics. *Anesthesiology.* 2015. [Epub ahead of print].
39. Fagerlund MJ, Eriksson LI. Current concepts in neuromuscular transmission. *BJA.* 2009;103(1):108–114.
40. Murphy GS, Brull SJ. Residual neuromuscular block: Lessons unlearned.

Part I: Definitions, incidence, and adverse physiologic effects of residual neuromuscular block. *Anesth Analg.* 2010;111:120–128.

41. Brull SJ, Murphy GS. Residual neuromuscular block: Lessons unlearned. Part II: Methods to reduce the risk of residual weakness. *Anesth Analg.* 2010;111:129–140.

42. Kheterpal S, Vaughn MT, Dubovoy TZ. et al. Sugammadex versus neostigmine for reversal of neuromuscular blockade and postoperative pulmonary complications (STRONGER): A multicenter matched cohort analysis. *Anesthesiology.* 132,1371–1381.

43. Sessler D. Temperature monitoring and perioperative thermoregulation. *Anesthesiology.* 2008;109:318–338.

44. Patteson SK, Chesney JT. Anesthetic management for magnetic resonance imaging: Problems and solutions. *Anesth Analg.* 1992;74:121–128.

45. Tremper KK. Anesthesiology: From Patient Safety to Population Outcomes: The 49th Annual Rovenstine Lecture. *Anesthesiology.* 2011;114:755–770.

46. Nair BG, Gabel E, Hofer I, Schwid HA, Cannesson M. Intraoperative clinical decision support for anesthesia: A narrative review of available systems. *Anesth Analg.* 2017;124(2):603–617. PMID: 28099325. doi: 10.1213/ANE.0000000000001636.

47. Kheterpal S, Shanks A, Tremper KK. Impact of a novel decision support system on intraoperative process of care and postoperative outcomes. *Anesthesiology.* 2018;128:272–282.

48. Nadler SB, Hidalgo JU, Bloch T. Prediction of blood volume in normal human adults. *Surgery.* 1962;51:224–232.

49. Sathishkumar S, Lai M, Picton P, et al. Behavioral modification of intraoperative hyperglycemia management with a novel real-time audiovisual monitor. *Anesthesiology.* 2015;123:29–37.

50. Murray-Torres T, Casarella A, Bollini M, Wallace F, Avidan MS, Politi M. Anesthesiology Control Tower—Feasibility Assessment to Support Translation (ACTFAST): Mixed-methods study of a novel telemedicine-based support system for the operating room. *JMIR Hum Factors.* 2019; 2:e12155. Apr-Jun 6 Published online.

21 POINT-OF-CARE ULTRASOUND

Lindsey L. Huddleston, Kristine E.W. Breyer

Point-of-care ultrasound (POCUS) refers to the use of ultrasound at the patient's bedside for procedural guidance and/or aid in diagnosis. The use and application of POCUS has rapidly expanded over the past 20 years. POCUS is now routinely used by a number of different specialties within medicine. Increased use of ultrasound outside of the traditional radiology setting has been fueled by increasing portability, ease of use, ability to make rapid assessments, and ability to repeat examinations. In addition, there is mounting evidence demonstrating the value of ultrasound in various clinical settings. Multiple societies have published guidelines supporting the use of ultrasound by appropriately trained clinicians.[1,2] Anesthesiologists have long used ultrasound for both procedural (vascular access, nerve blocks) and diagnostic (transesophageal echocardiogram [TEE]) purposes. As POCUS has become more ubiquitous across many medical specialties, the scope in the perioperative setting has also expanded. Based on current Accreditation Council for Graduate Medical Education (ACGME) training requirements for anesthesiology residency, a new POCUS certificate program developed by the American Society of Anesthesiologists (ASA), and expert opinion regarding the use of perioperative POCUS,[3] this chapter will focus on the following applications for diagnostic ultrasound: basic cardiac ultrasound, lung ultrasound, and abdominal ultrasound.

REVIEW OF ULTRASOUND PHYSICS

Sound waves are mechanical longitudinal pressure waves that are characterized by frequency, amplitude, and wavelength. Sound waves with frequencies above 20,000 hertz (Hz) (or 20 kHz) are not audible by humans and are termed *ultrasound*. Medical ultrasound is usually in the 1 to 20 megahertz (MHz) range.

Ultrasound technology uses a principle called the *piezoelectric effect* (or pulse-echo principle) to generate and receive ultrasound waves using nonionizing radiation. Ultrasound transducers contain many piezoelectric crystals, and ultrasonic waves are received and transmitted by the transducer via the piezoelectric crystals. Electricity applied to the ultrasound transducer induces vibration and results in transmission of ultrasound waves (reverse piezoelectric effect). Sound waves that are reflected back create electrical charges in the crystal array (piezoelectric effect), and those charges are interpreted by the ultrasound machine to create an image.

How much an ultrasound wave is reflected back to the transducer and how much is propagated depends on *attenuation* and *acoustic impendence*. As ultrasound waves are transmitted through substances, the ultrasound wave undergoes attenuation—that is, the amplitude of the wave diminishes as it propagates through the tissue. Attenuation is caused by the reflection of waves back to the transducer, refraction (deflection) of sound waves to a different direction, scattering, and absorption, which produces heat. Most attenuation is caused by absorption. Acoustic impedance is the resistance to sound wave propagation through a medium. Acoustic impedance depends on and is directly proportional to the speed of the sound wave and the density of the medium. In medical ultrasound when an ultrasound wave is transmitted, the angle of transmission changes once a new tissue or medium is encountered, based upon the acoustic impedance of the two opposing substances; this results in reflection and refraction of the ultrasound waves. The difference in acoustic impedance between the two substances changes the reflection angles. Fluids generally have a low acoustic impedance, and therefore most sound waves are transmitted through the fluid and not reflected back to the transducer, producing a black or anechoic image. More solid substances (e.g., bone) generally have a higher acoustic impedance, causing more waves to be reflected back and producing a very bright white or hyperechoic signal. If two different tissues have exactly the same impedance, then no change will be observed.

Two-dimensional (2D) ultrasound, also called *B-mode* (for "brightness"), is the most commonly used ultrasound mode in POCUS. B-mode uses transducers with hundreds of piezoelectric crystals in a linear or phased array arrangement. Each piezoelectric crystal sends out pulses (transmits waves) less than 1% of the time, allowing for ultrasound signals to be received back over 99% of the time. This is known as *pulse wave ultrasonography*. Ultrasound waves are interpreted based on the amplitude of the returned wave and the timing and direction of the reflected wave. The intensity of the amplitude creates the grayscale for the image. The higher the amplitude of the reflected wave, the brighter (whiter) the interpreted image. The longer return times are interpreted as deeper structures. The horizontal axis of the image is determined by the location along the footprint of the probe at which the ultrasound wave is returned. The quality of a 2D image is determined by spatial resolution, temporal resolution, and field of view (FOV). The higher the frequency of the generated pulse waves, the better the resolution. However, higher-frequency waves also undergo more attenuation, resulting in poorer imaging of deeper structures. When acquiring images, operators can change transducer types (e.g., switching to a higher-frequency probe for better resolution of superficial structures) or make adjustments on the ultrasound machine (e.g., increasing the FOV size to capture more relevant structures) to create an optimal image.

M-mode (for "motion") is another ultrasound mode commonly used in POCUS. In this mode a single piezoelectric crystal along a single line within the transducer beam transmits waves, and the resulting image is displayed over time. M-mode has a very high sampling rate, which results in high resolution so that even rapid motion, such as the motion of the mitral valve, can be recorded. M-mode can also be useful to measure the changes in size and shape over time, such as the change in inferior vena cava (IVC) dimension with respiration.

ULTRASOUND TRANSDUCERS

Ultrasound transducers (commonly referred to as *probes*) used in medical ultrasound differ in their frequencies, arrangement of crystals, and mode of crystal excitation. Ultrasound transducers are generally classified as low frequency and high frequency. Low-frequency transducers produce longer wavelengths and have superior depth of penetration but decreased resolution. They are used to image deeper structures such as the heart or abdominal organs. High-frequency transducers produce shorter wavelengths and have greater resolution but achieve less depth of penetration. They are used to image more superficial structures, such as the internal jugular vein or radial artery. Three main transducers types are used in medical ultrasound: linear, curvilinear (convex), and phased array. Table 21.1 describes the properties and common clinical uses for each of these transducers.

PREPARING FOR THE EXAMINATION

As with any procedure performed in the perioperative setting, all necessary equipment must be gathered before starting the examination. This includes the ultrasound machine with proper probes attached, ultrasound gel, towels for removing the gel at the end of the examination, blankets for covering the patient to avoid unnecessary exposure, and potentially a second person to help with operating the machine controls during the examination. Proper patient positioning is also key to high-quality image acquisition. Other factors to consider include dimming lights and closing blinds to better see the ultrasound images and removing unnecessary equipment in the area so there is enough room for the ultrasound machine, operator, and any potential assistants.

Table 21.1 POCUS Transducers

Transducer Type	Frequency and Depth	Mode of Crystal Excitation	Clinical Applications
Linear	5–13 MHz 6 cm	Crystals activated in a sequential, linear fashion. Beams generated are parallel to each other and perpendicular to the probe's surface.	Best for superficial structures Vascular access Nerve blocks Pulmonary ultrasound (assessing for PTX) Gastric ultrasound (thin adults or pediatric patients)
Phased array	1–5 MHz 35 cm	A small number of crystals are activated simultaneously to create a large number of beams that are multidirectional and overlapping. Timing of stimulation of each crystal can vary, resulting in ability to evaluate motion and flow.	Optimal for movement Cardiac ultrasound (TTE/TEE) Lung ultrasound (pleural and parenchymal examination) Abdominal ultrasound (less commonly)
Curvilinear	2–5 MHz 30 cm	Crystals activated in a sequential, linear fashion. Beams generated diverge from each other because of the convex shape of the probe, creating a wider field of view.	Abdominal ultrasound Cardiac ultrasound (when no phased array probe available) Lung ultrasound (pleural examination)

PTX, Pneumothorax; TEE, transesophageal echocardiogram; *TTE,* transthoracic echocardiogram.

The ultrasound machine must be set up properly before any examination. Once the appropriate transducer is selected, the user should then select the appropriate "examination type" or "examination mode." The ultrasound machine will send out and interpret sound waves differently in different examination modes. For instance, imaging the heart using a low-frequency probe programmed for "abdominal examination" will yield a very difficult image to interpret. Appropriate depth should then be programmed so that the region of interest is centered and as large as possible. Because ultrasound waves do not travel well through air, ultrasound gel is critical to obtaining quality images for interpretation. The ultrasound gel acts as a conductive medium by preventing air space between the patient and the transducer. Ultrasound gel also facilitates probe movement during the examination. Lastly, it is important to know how to move the transducer to obtain an optimal image. Transducer movements include sliding, rocking, tilting (or fanning), and rotating (Fig. 21.1) (also see Chapter 18).

BASIC CARDIAC ULTRASOUND

The perioperative cardiac POCUS examination includes four basic views plus examination of the IVC. For the basic examination, the goal is to answer specific and mainly binary questions (e.g., "Is there a pericardial effusion?"). There are more advanced applications of perioperative cardiac ultrasound that may be applied by more experienced providers (e.g., evaluation of valves, noninvasive cardiac output measurements, evaluation of diastolic function); however, these require additional training that is beyond the scope of this chapter. The phased array ultrasound probe is favored for cardiac ultrasound, but the curvilinear probe can also be used.

Parasternal Long-Axis View

Patient positioning: For optimal image acquisition, patients should be positioned with their left side down. If patients are unable to position themselves, this can be accomplished by using pillows or towels below the patient's right side to help tilt them slightly left. If it is not possible to position the patient with their left side down, supine images can still be acquired; however, image quality may be poor, leading to limited or misinterpreted information.

Probe position and manipulation: Once the patient is positioned, the footprint of the ultrasound probe is placed between the third or fourth intercostal space, just to the left of the sternum. The indicator notch on the probe

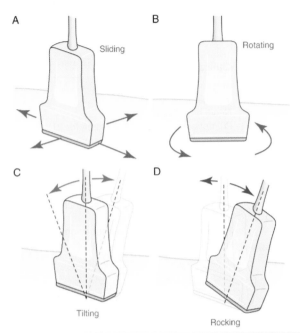

Fig. 21.1 Transducer movements. Four basic probe movements are used in POCUS image acquisition. These movements should be performed sequentially rather than simultaneously to optimize images with a systematic approach. (A) Sliding is relocation of the foot of the ultrasound probe to a new position on the skin surface. (B) Rotating is turning the ultrasound probe clockwise or counterclockwise along its central axis while maintaining contact with the skin surface. (C) Tilting (or fanning) is changing the angle of the probe interface along the short axis while maintaining a fixed position on the skin surface. (D) Rocking is motion along the long axis of the probe while maintaining a fixed position on the skin surface. (From Soni NJ, Arntfield R, Kory P. *Point of Care Ultrasound.* 2nd ed. Philadelphia: Elsevier; 2020:27, Fig. 3.8.)

acquisition and interpretation. Assessment of LV function should be done in a systematic way (similar to reading a chest radiograph or electrocardiogram) to avoid errors or misinterpretation. Box 21.1 describes the approach to LV function assessment in the PLAX view.

In addition to interpretation of LV function, a few other basic assessments can be made from the PLAX view. The first is evaluating for a pericardial effusion and distinguishing pericardial from pleural fluid. Fluid will appear black, or hypoechoic, on the screen. If fluid is noted anterior to the descending aorta (or above on the ultrasound screen), it is pericardial fluid. If the fluid is traveling behind the descending aorta (or below on the ultrasound screen), the fluid is in the pleural space (Fig. 21.4). The other assessment that can be made is chamber size relative to others. As a general rule, the RVOT, LVOT, and LA should have relatively the same anterior-to-posterior measurement. If one of them appears noticeably larger in the anterior-to-posterior dimension, that may suggest pathology but could also be a result of improper image acquisition and will require follow-up with formal imaging. For example, in the case of the LVOT appearing larger than the LA and RVOT this could suggest possible aortic aneurysm and/or dissection and will need to be followed up with formal echocardiography and/or computed tomography (CT) angiography of the chest depending on the patient's history and clinical presentation.

Parasternal Short-Axis View

Patient positioning: Patients should be positioned with their left side down.

Probe position and manipulation: Initial probe position is based on where the operator obtains the PLAX view. The key to obtaining an optimal parasternal short-axis (PSAX) view is to start from an optimal PLAX with the papillary muscles in the center of the screen. From this view, the probe is rotated approximately 90 degrees clockwise (the indicator notch points approximately to the patient's left shoulder) (see Fig. 21.2).

Image appearance and structures visualized: The PSAX should be a transverse view of the myocardium of the LV at the level of the papillary muscles. The LV should appear round, and both papillary muscles should be in view at approximately three and seven o'clock (see Fig. 21.3B). Although the septum and the right ventricle (RV) will be seen, the entire RV is not visualized in the PSAX, so assessment of RV size is not appropriate in this view.

Image interpretation: LV function can be assessed in the PSAX view; however, because the mitral valve is not visualized, only two of the four questions to assess LV function can be addressed (Box 21.2).

The presence of pericardial fluid can be detected on the PSAX view and will appear as hypoechoic material surrounding the heart. If the interventricular septum appears flat through any portion of the cardiac cycle

should be pointed toward the patient's right shoulder (Fig. 21.2). The operator may need to slide laterally or medially along the rib space or interrogate adjacent rib spaces to optimize image quality. In addition, the probe can be rotated and/or fanned until all structures desired are displayed on the ultrasound screen.

Image appearance and structures visualized: The heart should appear horizontal across the screen. An ideal parasternal long-axis (PLAX) image should include the following structures: (1) left ventricle (LV; the apex of the LV should *not* be seen); (2) left atrium (LA); (3) mitral valve with both the anterior and posterior leaflets and the annulus; (4) left ventricular outflow tract (LVOT), (5) aortic valve (at least two of the three leaflets), (6) right ventricular outflow tract (RVOT); and (7) descending aorta (Fig. 21.3A).

Image interpretation: The PLAX view is an ideal view for interpreting left ventricular systolic function. For the purposes of perioperative POCUS, this will likely be a qualitative rather than quantitative assessment (e.g., reduced LV systolic function). Quantitative assessments require more expertise and extensive training in image

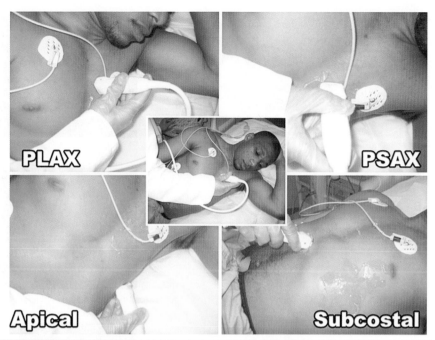

Fig. 21.2 Probe placement and patient position for basic cardiac views. For the PLAX, PSAX, and apical views, the patient is in the left lateral decubitus position *(center image)* for optimal imaging. The subcostal view is obtained with the patient in the supine position. (From Barnett CF, Sweeney DA, Huddleston LH. Ultrasonography: Advanced applications and procedures. In: Broaddus CV, et al. *Textbook of Respiratory Medicine*. Vol. 1, 7th ed. Philadelphia: Elsevier; 2022: e-Fig. 24.1.)

(leading to a "D-shaped" LV), this may indicate RV pressure or volume overload (Fig. 21.5). In this case the operator should attempt to obtain views of the RV in other views to confirm the finding or consider follow-up with a formal transthoracic echocardiogram or CT angiogram if there is concern for pulmonary embolus.

Apical Four-Chamber View

Patient positioning: The patient should be positioned with their left side down. The apical four-chamber (A4C) view is perhaps the most crucial view to ensure proper patient positioning because of the potential for foreshortening and misinterpretation of images acquired. Foreshortening occurs when the beam of the ultrasound does not pass through the true apex of the LV. This causes the apex of the LV to appear rounded and thick rather than thin and bullet shaped. Foreshortened images can lead to three important data misinterpretations: (1) any abnormalities of the LV apex will not be seen (e.g., LV thrombus); (2) LV function may appear better than it actually is; and (3) a normal, healthy RV may artifactually appear larger in size with reduced function.

Probe positioning and manipulation: To prevent foreshortening, the footprint of the ultrasound should be placed as close to the LV apex as possible. If possible, palpating the point of maximal impulse (PMI) can help the operator identify the LV apex. If the patient

is positioned correctly with their left side down, initial probe placement will be just anterior to the midaxillary line, usually one to two rib spaces below the nipple line. The indicator notch should be pointed out to the patient's left, and the ultrasound probe is often tilted so that the beam of the ultrasound is directed cephalad (see Fig. 21.2). The depth on the ultrasound machine will need to be increased when transitioning from the parasternal views to the A4C view.

Image appearance and structures visualized: All four chambers of the heart should be in view, and both the tricuspid and mitral valve should be clearly opening. In addition, the interventricular septum should be in the center of the ultrasound screen and be oriented vertically (see Fig. 21.3C). The LV apex should appear thin and not rounded (as discussed earlier).

Image interpretation: LV and RV function can be assessed in the A4C view (Box 21.3). However, the structures are farther away from the ultrasound probe, so wall thickening may be more difficult to determine because the endocardium is harder to visualize. Foreshortening can lead to inaccurate assessments of both LV and RV function. As with other views, pericardial fluid will be seen as hypoechoic fluid surrounding the heart in the A4C view. Because the right atrium (RA) and RV are clearly visualized in this view, collapse of the RA and/or RV may be seen, suggesting a hemodynamically significant pericardial effusion.

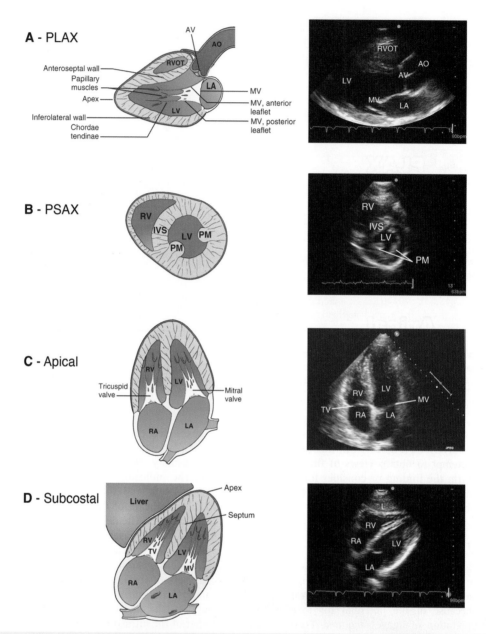

Fig. 21.3 Cross-sectional anatomy and ultrasound images for the four basic cardiac ultrasound views. (A) Parasternal long axis (PLAX). Note that on an optimal PLAX view, the apex is not fully visualized on the ultrasound image. (B) Parasternal short axis (PSAX) taken at the level of the papillary muscles. (C) Apical four-chamber view. (D) Subcostal four-chamber view. *AO,* Aorta; *AV,* aortic valve; *IVS,* intraventricular septum; *LA,* left atrium; *LV,* left ventricle; *MV,* mitral valve; *PM,* papillary muscle; *RA,* right atrium; *RV,* right ventricle; *RVOT,* right ventricular outflow tract; *TV,* tricuspid valve. (Modified from Soni NJ, Arntfield R, Kory P. *Point of Care Ultrasound.* 2nd ed. Philadelphia: Elsevier; 2020:115–122, Figs. 14.4, 14.5, 14.8, and 14.10.)

Subcostal and Inferior Vena Cava Views

Patient positioning: The subcostal and IVC views are obtained with the patient supine rather than with their left side down. If the patient can cooperate, having them bend their knees will help relax the abdominal muscles and aid in image acquisition. The subcostal view is the easiest view to obtain during cardiopulmonary resuscitation because the operator and probe position do not interfere with chest compressions.

Probe positioning and manipulation: To obtain the subcostal view, the ultrasound probe is placed on the patient's abdomen, 2 to 3 inches below the xyphoid process and just to the right of midline. The indicator notch is pointed toward the patient's left. The probe will be relatively flat on the abdomen, so the operator should keep their hand above the probe (see Fig. 21.2). To obtain the IVC view, the probe is rotated approximately 90 degrees counterclockwise from the subcostal view with the indicator notch now pointing toward the patient's head. For both views, the operator will likely need to apply gentle downward pressure on the abdomen to acquire images.

Image appearance and structures visualized: As in the A4C view, all four chambers of the heart and the mitral and tricuspid valves should be visualized. The right side of the heart will appear on the top of the screen with the left side of the heart deeper and toward the bottom of the screen (see Fig. 21.3D). In the IVC view, the liver will be seen with hepatic veins emptying into the IVC. The IVC will be in the longitudinal orientation and should be seen starting at the far left of the screen until it clearly empties into the RA (Fig. 21.6).

Image interpretation: LV function, RV size and function, and pericardial effusions can all be assessed in the subcostal view similarly to how they are assessed in the A4C view described earlier. The IVC view has been used to estimate right atrial pressure (RAP) and to aid with assessment of volume status. For both of these assessments, the absolute diameter and the change in diameter with respiration are measured. In a patient who is not undergoing positive-pressure ventilation a small IVC (<21 mm) that collapses significantly with respiration suggests a low RAP (<3 mm Hg), whereas a large IVC (>21 mm) that does not collapse with respiration suggests a high RAP (>10 mm Hg). Positive-pressure ventilation changes intrathoracic pressure; thus interpretation of the IVC differs between spontaneous ventilation and mechanical ventilation. Because of conflicting data in the existing literature, there is uncertainty about the accuracy of the IVC examination to predict fluid responsiveness.[4,5] In addition, pitfalls are associated with both acquiring images and interpreting the examination. For example, incorrectly identifying the aorta for the IVC can lead to the mistaken conclusion that there is an absence of respiratory variability. Finally, there are several clinical conditions where IVC size and respiratory variability may not accurately predict preload or volume responsiveness. This is the case in cardiac tamponade where the IVC appears large and noncollapsible but the patient is preload dependent.

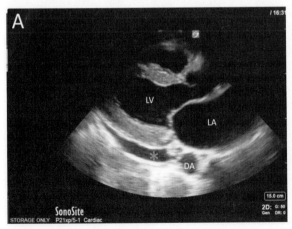
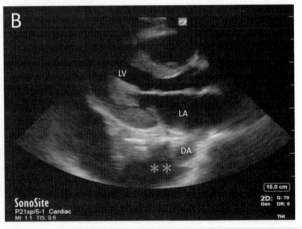

Fig. 21.4 Pericardial versus pleural fluid on PLAX view. (A) Pericardial fluid tracking anterior to the descending aorta compared with (B) pleural fluid tracking posterior to the descending aorta. *DA,* Descending aorta; *LA,* left atrium; *LV,* left ventricle; *asterisk,* pericardial fluid; *double asterisk,* pleural fluid.

> **Box 21.2** Left Ventricular (LV) Function Assessment in Parasternal Short-Axis (PSAX) View: Two Questions to Answer
>
> 1. Is the left ventricular chamber size (cavity) changing between systole and diastole?
>   - In the PSAX view if papillary muscles touch each other and/or the LV cavity seems to disappear during systole, this is suggestive of an underfilled LV cavity (similar to the transgastric view on transesophageal echocardiogram [TEE]).
> 2. Are the walls of the left ventricle getting thicker?
>   - If the LV is functioning normally, all of the walls of the LV myocardium should be moving equally to the center of the LV cavity.
>   - Regional wall motion abnormalities may be detected in this view; however, the PSAX is only one cross-section of the full LV myocardium and does not show the right ventricular (RV) myocardium well at all.
>   - To truly rule out wall motion abnormalities, a formal echocardiogram is needed to complete a thorough examination of all segments of the LV and RV myocardium.

> **Box 21.3** Left Ventricular (LV) and Right Ventricular (RV) Function Assessment in Apical Four-Chamber (A4C) View
>
> **LV function:** The four questions outlined in the PLAX section earlier can be used.
> **RV size:** Gross chamber size (particularly RV size relative to LV size) can be evaluated with the A4C view.
> - In a normal heart the RV should be approximately one-third the size of the LV and should not be apex forming.
> - If the RV appears large relative to the LV, ensure that the images are not foreshortened and then evaluate the RV in the subcostal view to confirm.
>
> **RV function:** Because of the shape of the RV, assessment of RV function is challenging with two-dimensional echocardiography, even with formal studies. For basic perioperative point-of-care ultrasound (POCUS), the main assessment is whether function is normal or abnormal—more advanced interpretation should be deferred. In the A4C view the following aspects of RV function should be evaluated:
> - Evaluation of the movement of the tricuspid annulus toward the apex, also known as tricuspid annular plane systolic excursion (TAPSE) on formal echocardiography. In a normally functioning RV the tricuspid annulus will move vigorously toward the apex of the heart.
> - Evaluation of the change in size of the RV cavity. A normal RV will have some decrease in cavity size in systole when compared with diastole.
> - Evaluation of the shape of the intraventricular septum. A flattened intraventricular septum suggests an abnormality of the RV.

Given these limitations, the IVC examination must be interpreted in the context of the entire clinical picture. The examination is most useful at extremes (e.g., very small, collapsing IVC) and when it can be repeated over time and after an intervention (such as fluid administration). Integrating the IVC examination with additional ultrasound findings from the cardiac, lung, and abdominal POCUS examinations is paramount. This practice will

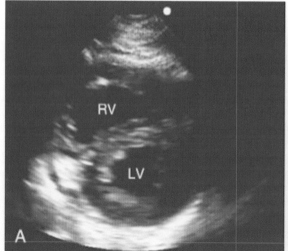
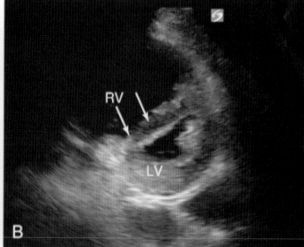

Fig. 21.5 Two PSAX images comparing a normal interventricular septum (A) with a "D-shaped," or flattened, interventricular septum in a patient with RV dysfunction (B). *LV,* Left ventricle; *RV,* right ventricle. (From Soni NJ, Arntfield R, Kory P. *Point of Care Ultrasound.* 2nd ed. Philadelphia: Elsevier; 2020:141, Fig. 16.12.)

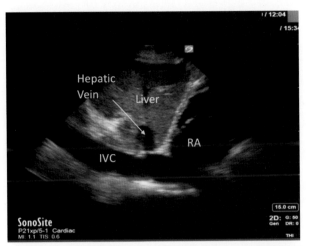

Fig. 21.6 Inferior vena cava ultrasound image showing the key sonographic characteristics of the hepatic vein emptying into the IVC and the junction of the IVC with the right atrium. *IVC*, Inferior vena cava; *RA*, right atrium.

help guide resuscitation and yield more accurate diagnoses in shock states.

PULMONARY ULTRASOUND

Ultrasound examination of the lungs can provide valuable information in the perioperative setting and pulmonary ultrasound can be used as a diagnostic tool to identify a number of pathologies in the acutely decompensating patient. Because ultrasound waves have poor penetration in air-filled structures, lung ultrasound relies on artifacts created by air/fluid or air/tissue interfaces. The lung examination can be divided into three separate components based on the different pathologies being evaluated: (1) evaluation for pneumothorax, (2) evaluation of interstitial and alveolar patterns, and (3) evaluation of the pleural space.

Normal Lung Examination

The appearance of a normal lung on ultrasound examination provides the basis for understanding the appearance of pulmonary pathology (Fig. 21.7). The first component of the normal lung examination is the presence of pleural sliding. The pleura appears as a bright, hyperechoic line. The visceral and parietal pleura slide against each other with respiration, creating the appearance of movement, sometimes referred to as "shimmering" or "ants crawling on a log." When using M-mode, the movement of the pleura against each other creates the appearance of a "sandy beach" (Fig. 21.8A). The second component of the normal lung examination is the presence of A-lines. A-lines are reverberation artifacts that appear as horizontal hyperechoic lines at equidistant

depths from the pleura. The last component of the normal lung examination is the presence of another ultrasound artifact called B-lines (also known as "comet tails"). B-lines originate from the pleural line and transverse to the bottom of the ultrasound screen. Although a few B-lines per intercostal space is normal, an abundance of B-lines indicates pathology.

Evaluation for Pneumothorax

Lung ultrasound is more sensitive than chest radiography for the detection of a pneumothorax.[6] Additionally, the examination is easy to perform and interpret rapidly, making it a useful tool to assess an unstable patient.

Patient positioning: The examination is easiest to perform in the supine (or near-to-supine) position; however, it is possible to perform the examination with patients in other positions as well.

Probe positioning and manipulation: Any of the commonly used ultrasound probes (linear, curvilinear, or phased array) are suitable to conduct the examination. Initial probe placement should be on the anterior chest wall at approximately the second intercostal space with the indicator notch of the probe pointing cephalad. Because air travels to the least dependent area of the chest, most pneumothoraces in supine patients will be identified in the anterior region of the chest between the second and fourth intercostal spaces. However, the operator should still perform a comprehensive and systematic examination imaging both lungs at multiple points on the chest wall and in multiple different rib spaces.

Image appearance and structures visualized: In each area or zone imaged the operator should adjust the probe until the landmarks of two ribs with shadowing behind them and the bright pleural line between them are identified.

Image interpretation: A suggested systematic algorithm for the interpretation of lung ultrasound for evaluation of pneumothorax is depicted in Fig. 21.10. The operator should assess for the sonographic signs of pneumothorax described in Box 21.4.

Evaluation of Interstitial and Alveolar Patterns

The presence of more than three B-lines per intercostal space is indicative of interstitial pathology. Several processes can lead to a diffuse B-line pattern, including pulmonary edema (noncardiogenic or cardiogenic), interstitial pneumonia, pulmonary fibrosis, contusion, tumor, and pneumonitis. The pattern of B-lines (spacing between B-lines, focal vs. diffuse) and the patient's clinical context will aid in narrowing the differential diagnosis. Although any of the commonly used ultrasound transducers are acceptable for the examination, the curvilinear or phased array probe may be needed to evaluate the deeper posterior lung fields. The operator should use the same approach for patient positioning, probe positioning and manipulation, and systematic interrogation

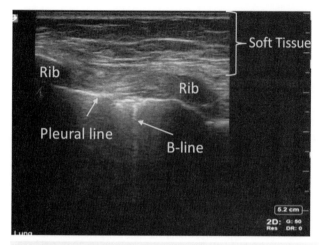
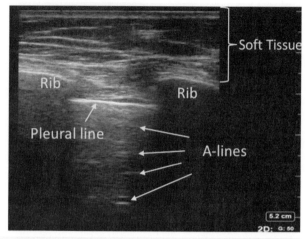

Fig. 21.7 Ultrasound images of normal lung. The pleural line is visualized as a bright line between the two rib spaces. B-lines are laser-like, hyperechoic vertical lines that arise from the pleural line and extend to the bottom of the ultrasound screen. A-lines are reverberation artifacts that appear as hyperechoic horizontal lines that are equidistant from the pleura.

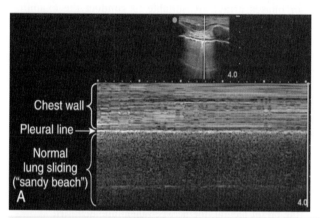
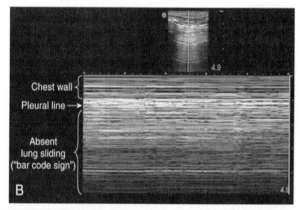

Fig. 21.8 (A) M-mode image of normal lung sliding with the normal aerated lung creating the appearance of a "sandy beach." (B) M-mode image of absent lung sliding where the "sandy beach" is replaced with horizontal lines throughout the image, resulting in a "bar-code" pattern. (Modified from Soni NJ, Arntfield R, Kory P. *Point of Care Ultrasound*. 2nd ed. Philadelphia: Elsevier; 2020:58, Fig. 8.5.)

of multiple zones of the chest wall, as described earlier in the pneumothorax examination.

Image interpretation: The presence of more than three B-lines in one intercostal space suggests the pathologic causes described earlier (Fig. 21.11). Focal patterns may be seen in areas of pneumonia, contusion, or tumor.

Evaluation of the Pleural Space

Pleural fluid is usually visible in the most dependent areas of the lung (typically, posterior-lateral). Lung ultrasound has a higher accuracy than chest radiography for detecting pleural fluid and can detect effusions as small as 20 mL.[7] Low-frequency probes (curvilinear or phased array) are preferred when evaluating the pleural

space because of the depth needed to visualize the key structures.

Patient positioning: Patients who are hemodynamically stable and able to position themselves can be in a seated upright position, resting their elbows on a surface in front of them. If patients are unstable or unable to sit upright, the examination can be performed in the supine or semi recumbent position, with the ipsilateral arm raised above the patient's head or positioned across the chest.

Probe positioning and manipulation: In a seated patient the operator should place the footprint of the ultrasound probe perpendicular to the skin on the lateral chest wall, just below the clavicle, with the indicator notch pointed toward the patient's head. In a supine or

Box 21.4 Four Sonographic Signs of Pneumothorax

1. **Absence of pleural sliding:**
   - If air is separating the visceral and parietal pleura, normal sliding is not seen and the bright pleural line will appear motionless. On M-mode, the "sandy beach" appearance will be replaced by straight lines throughout the entire image, often referred to as "bar code" (see Fig. 21.8B).
2. **Absence of B-lines:**
   - Detection of a few B-lines is a characteristic of normal lung ultrasound. B-lines originate from the visceral pleura and travel toward the edge of the ultrasound screen, erasing A-lines. Because the visceral pleura is not visualized in the presence of a pneumothorax, B-lines will be absent.
   - A-lines will be detected in both normal lung ultrasound and in the setting of a pneumothorax.
3. **Absence of lung pulse:**
   - The pleural motion with each heartbeat is referred to as "lung pulse" which is most easily recognizable in M-mode.
   - For a lung pulse to be detected, there has to be direct contact between the visceral and parietal pleura.
   - Thus if air is filling that potential space between the two pleura (pneumothorax), a lung pulse will not be present.
4. **Presence of lung point:**
   - The lung point is the interface where healthy lung starts and a pneumothorax ends.
   - Lung point is 100% specific for pneumothorax.
   - One side of the image will show normal pleura sliding, while the other side will show the absence of sliding. On M-mode, the "sandy beach" and "bar code" patterns appear to alternate over time (see Fig. 21.9).

semi recumbent patient the operator should place the probe in the midaxillary line with the indicator notch pointed toward the patient's head. The operator may need to move the probe to a more posterior position (where it is wedged between the patient and the bed) to visualize smaller pleural effusions. In both positions the operator should then move the probe systematically both in a craniocaudal and then lateral-to-medial direction to examine the entire space, identify the boundaries of the pleural effusions, and identify adjacent structures.

Image appearance and structures visualized: The diaphragm and liver or spleen (depending on which side of the patient is being examined) should be identified. In images acquired posteriorly the kidney may also come into view. Fluid will appear as an anechoic space between the visceral and parietal pleura. The presence of a pleural fluid collection will enhance the transmission of ultrasound waves, resulting in visualization of the vertebral bodies in the thoracic cavity above the diaphragm, also known as the "spine sign" (Fig. 21.12). Consolidated lung will appear hyperechoic and nearly identical to the liver in terms of density.

Image interpretation: Pleural fluid will be positively identified as an anechoic space between the visceral or parietal pleura and/or by identification of the "spine sign." Although quantification of pleural fluid volume

using sonographic measurements has been extensively studied, these formulas are not commonly used in clinical practice.[8] A qualitative assessment of small, moderate, or large volume is likely adequate for clinical decision making. Another useful descriptor is whether the effusion is simple or complex. Simple effusions appear anechoic and free flowing, whereas complex effusions can be characterized as homogenously or heterogeneously echogenic. Complex effusions may also have loculations, septations, or fibrinous stranding. Simple pleural effusions are often transudative, whereas complex effusions are more often exudative (e.g., from empyema, hemothorax, or malignancy).

An emerging body of literature has evaluated lung ultrasonography in the diagnosis of pneumonia in adults.[9,10] Lung consolidation may occur from atelectasis or pneumonia. Sonographic air bronchograms appear as hyperechoic lines and dots within the area of consolidated lung. These findings likely represent air-filled bronchi that are made visible by the surrounding consolidated lung. When they are immobile, they are called *static air bronchograms,* which can be seen in both atelectasis and pneumonia. However, when air bronchograms are mobile, they are called *dynamic,* and are highly specific for pneumonia as the cause of consolidation.

ABDOMINAL ULTRASOUND

FAST Examination

For patients who have sustained blunt or penetrating trauma, intraperitoneal bleeding can lead to hypovolemic shock and death. Historically, diagnostic peritoneal lavage was performed in the emergency department to detect hemoperitoneum. The Focused Assessment with Sonography in Trauma (FAST) examination was developed to quickly identify hemoperitoneum (free peritoneal fluid) and hemopericardium (fluid in the pericardial sac) in the trauma patient population. The FAST examination has four basic views: the right upper quadrant, left upper quadrant, pelvic, and subcostal cardiac views. The E-FAST (Extended-FAST) examination additionally surveys the anterior and lateral pleural spaces to evaluate for pneumothorax or hemothorax. Although the FAST and E-FAST examinations were originally used to evaluate and expedite care in unstable trauma patients, the FAST examination is a useful way to assess for free fluid in hypotensive patients at risk for intraperitoneal hemorrhage. A low-frequency probe is used for the FAST examination, as evaluated contents lie relatively deep to the anatomic surface. The curvilinear probe is excellent for abdominal examinations; however, the small footprint of the phased array can be advantageous as well.

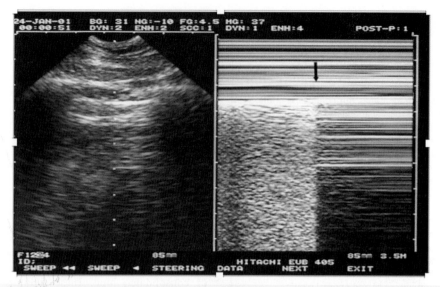

Fig. 21.9 A lung point is the boundary between aerated lung and air in the pleural space and is the most specific finding for a pneumothorax. The left image is two-dimensional ultrasound at the point where the pneumothorax begins. M-mode imaging *(right)* with arrowhead pointing to the transition point between normal aerated lung ("sandy beach") and pneumothorax ("barcode") pattern. (From Lichtenstein DA. Lung ultrasound in the critically ill. *Ann Intensive Care.* 2014;4:1, under Creative Commons license: https://creativecommons.org/licenses/by/2.0.)

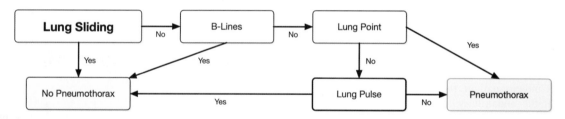

Fig. 21.10 Diagnostic algorithm for pneumothorax. The algorithm begins with assessment for lung sliding.

Right Upper Quadrant View

The right upper quadrant view evaluates the hepatorenal recess (Morrison pouch) and the space above and below the right diaphragm.

Patient positioning: For this examination, patients can lie in the supine position. Ideally, the arms are positioned slightly abducted from the patient's side.

Probe position and manipulation: Once the patient is positioned, the footprint of the ultrasound probe is placed around the right midaxillary line approximately at the level of the subxiphoid. The indicator notch on the probe should be pointed upward toward the patient's head. The operator may need to slide the probe dorsally along the rib space or interrogate adjacent rib spaces to optimize image quality. In addition, the probe can be rotated and/or fanned until all structures desired are displayed on the ultrasound screen.

Image appearance and structures visualized: An ideal right upper quadrant FAST image should include the following structures: (1) liver (coronal view), (2) right kidney, and (3) right diaphragm.

Image interpretation: A normal right upper quadrant FAST view will show the right diaphragm, liver, and right kidney adjacent to each other (Fig. 21.13A). An abnormal, or "positive," right upper quadrant FAST view will reveal a hypoechoic streak between these structures (see Fig. 21.13B). Hypoechoic streaks, which can be small or large, represent free fluid. It is critical to consider patient history and comorbidities when interpreting abdominal ultrasound imaging for free fluid. Patients with ascites, for instance, will have chronic free fluid.

Left Upper Quadrant View

The left upper quadrant view evaluates the splenorenal recess and the space above and below the left diaphragm.

Patient positioning: For this examination, patients can lie in the supine position. Ideally, the arms are positioned slightly abducted from the patient's side.

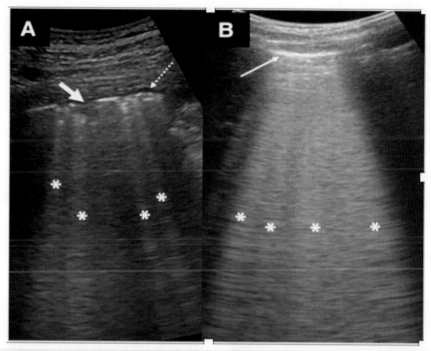

Fig. 21.11 Two examples of pathologic B-lines (indicated by *asterisks*) suggestive of interstitial edema. Arrows point to the pleural line. (Modified from Lee FC. Lung ultrasound: A primary survey of the acutely dyspneic patient. *J Intensive Care*, 2016;4[1]:57, under Creative Commons license: http://creativecommons.org/licenses/by/4.0.)

Probe position and manipulation: Once the patient is positioned, the footprint of the ultrasound probe is placed posteriorly (past the midaxillary line) approximately at the level of the subxiphoid. This recess is posterior, and a common description is for the operator to have the hand holding the ultrasound probe touching the patient's bed or knuckles to the gurney. The indicator notch on the probe should be pointed upward toward the patient's head. The operator may need to slide dorsally along the rib space or interrogate adjacent rib spaces to optimize image quality. In addition, the probe can be rotated and/or fanned until all structures desired are displayed on the ultrasound screen.

Image appearance and structures visualized: An ideal left upper quadrant FAST image should include the following structures: (1) spleen (coronal view), (2) left kidney, and (3) left diaphragm.

Image interpretation: A normal left upper quadrant FAST view will show the left diaphragm, spleen, and left kidney adjacent to each other (Fig. 21.14A). An abnormal, or "positive," left upper quadrant FAST view will reveal a hypoechoic streak between these structures, demonstrating free fluid (see Fig. 21.14B).

Pelvic View

The pelvic view evaluates for free fluid in the pelvis. In males the rectovesicular pouch is evaluated. In females the rectouterine (pouch of Douglas) and vesicouterine pouches are evaluated.

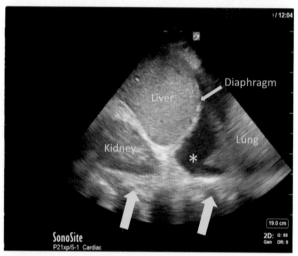

Fig. 21.12 Right-sided pleural effusion with anechoic pleural fluid (*asterisk*) and consolidated lung adjacent to the pleural fluid. Note that the spine shadow is seen both below and above the diaphragm (*arrows*). When the spine shadow is seen above the diaphragm, this is termed "spine sign" and is an indirect indicator of the presence of pleural fluid.

Positioning: For this examination, patients can lie in the supine position.

Probe position and manipulation: Once the patient is positioned, the footprint of the ultrasound probe is placed

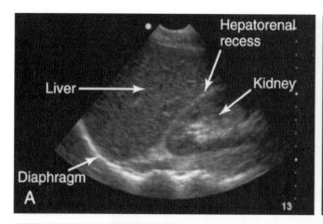
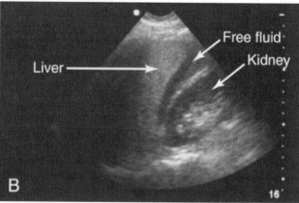

Fig. 21.13 (A) Normal right upper quadrant ultrasound image. (B) Right upper quadrant view with free fluid visualized between the liver and the kidney. The potential space between the liver and the kidney, also known as Morrison's pouch, is the most common place for free fluid to accumulate in the right upper quadrant view. (Modified from Soni NJ, Arntfield R, Kory P. *Point of Care Ultrasound*. 2nd ed. Philadelphia: Elsevier; 2020:221, Fig. 24.4.)

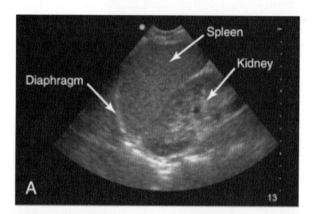
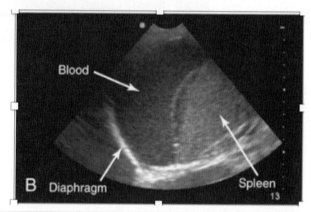

Fig. 21.14 (A) Normal left upper quadrant ultrasound image. (B) Left upper quadrant image showing free fluid between the spleen and the diaphragm. The subdiaphragmatic (or perisplenic) space is the most common place for free fluid to accumulate in the left upper quadrant view. (Modified from Soni NJ, Arntfield R, Kory P. *Point of Care Ultrasound*. 2nd ed. Philadelphia: Elsevier; 2020:221, Fig. 24.6.)

midline just above the pubic bone. The indicator notch on the probe should be pointed upward toward the patient's head for the long-axis view and toward the patient's right side for the short-axis view.

Image appearance and structures visualized: The bladder will be seen as a hypoechoic structure. In the short-axis view assess for hypoechoic streaks around the bladder and on the sides of the bladder. In the long-axis view assess for hypoechoic bands below and behind the bladder.

Image interpretation: A normal pelvic ultrasound will reveal a hypoechoic bladder without adjacent hypoechoic streaks or pockets (Fig. 21.15A and C). An abnormal pelvic ultrasound will reveal hypoechoic pockets either to the sides of the bladder or behind the bladder or uterus (see Fig. 21.15B and D). Once the bladder is decompressed (e.g., with a Foley catheter), the pelvic view can be difficult to interpret.

Gastric Ultrasound

Pulmonary aspiration causes significant morbidity in the perioperative setting and can lead to pneumonia, respiratory failure, acute lung injury, and potentially multiorgan failure and death. Point-of-care gastric ultrasound is an emerging tool that can aid in medical decision making when assessing aspiration risk. Although preoperative fasting guidelines are the mainstay for mitigation of aspiration risk before anesthesia, there are instances where adherence to these guidelines is unknown or where a patient's underlying medical conditions cause delayed gastric emptying. In these cases gastric ultrasound can be used to qualitatively and quantitatively assess gastric contents and enhance decision making with regard to delaying elective surgery.[11,12] Precautionary measures to decrease the risk and/or severity of aspiration include administration of antacids, decompression of the

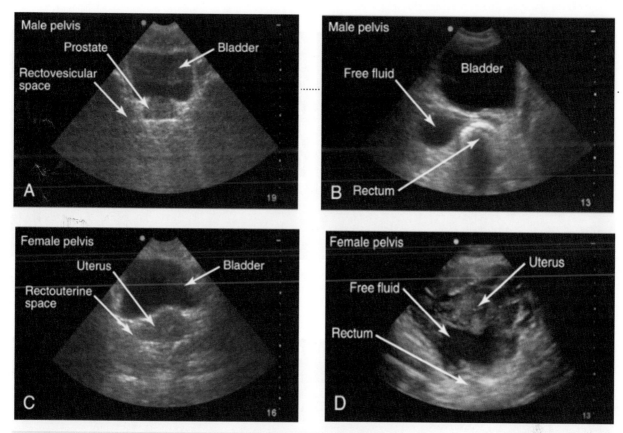

Fig. 21.15 Normal (A) and abnormal (B) male pelvis with free fluid collecting in the rectovesicular pouch. Normal (C) and abnormal (D) female pelvis with free fluid collecting in the rectouterine space (pouch of Douglas). In females the vesicouterine pouch should also be evaluated for the presence of free fluid. (Modified from Soni NJ, Arntfield R, Kory P. *Point of Care Ultrasound*. 2nd ed. Philadelphia: Elsevier; 2020:222, Fig. 24.8.)

stomach before induction, rapid-sequence intubation, and endotracheal intubation.

Patient positioning: For a complete and interpretable gastric ultrasound, images should be acquired first in the supine, then right lateral decubitus (RLD) position. In patients who are unable to be positioned in the RLD position the semi recumbent position is an acceptable alternative. The RLD position is considered superior to the semi recumbent position because in the RLD position, gastric contents are more likely to drain into the dependent antrum.

Probe positioning and manipulation: For most adults, the curvilinear probe should be used in the abdominal imaging setting. In pediatric patients a linear probe can also be used to provide greater resolution. The ultrasound transducer should be placed perpendicular to the skin in the epigastric region just below the subxiphoid margin. The probe should be in a sagittal plane with the indicator notch pointing cephalad. The operator should then slide the probe from left to right or right to left until the antrum is visualized in short axis at the level of the

abdominal aorta (Fig. 21.16). Rocking the ultrasound probe can help minimize obliquity of the antrum and optimize the final image.

Image appearance and structures visualized: The following structures should be identified and serve as anatomical landmarks to ensure an optimal image: liver, aorta (longitudinal), pancreas, and the superior mesenteric artery. The gastric antrum will be seen in short axis and can be differentiated from bowel by the thick, hypoechoic muscularis layer surrounding the hyperechoic serosa and mucosal layers.

Image interpretation: Assessment of gastric contents can be done both qualitatively and quantitatively. Qualitative assessment is broken down into three categories: empty, fluids present, or solids present. When empty, the antrum will either appear collapsed and flat or round to ovoid shape with thick walls, often described as a "bull's eye." Gastric secretions or clear liquids will appear anechoic or hypoechoic, and the antrum will distend and become thin walled when it contains fluid. Just after eating solid food, air ingested prevents visualization of the structures deep

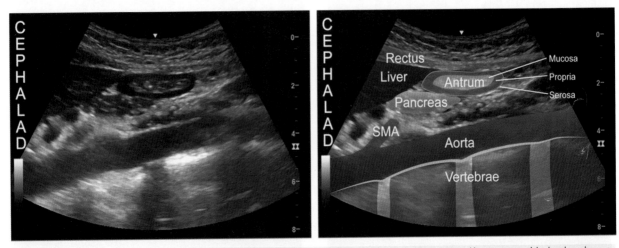

Fig. 21.16 Ultrasound image of an empty gastric antrum with the classic bull's-eye appearance. Key sonographic landmarks are identified in the right image. *SMA,* Superior mesenteric artery. (Modified from El-Boghdadly K, Wojcikiewicz T, Perlas A. Perioperative point-of-care gastric ultrasound. *BJA Educ.* 2019;19[7]:219–226.)

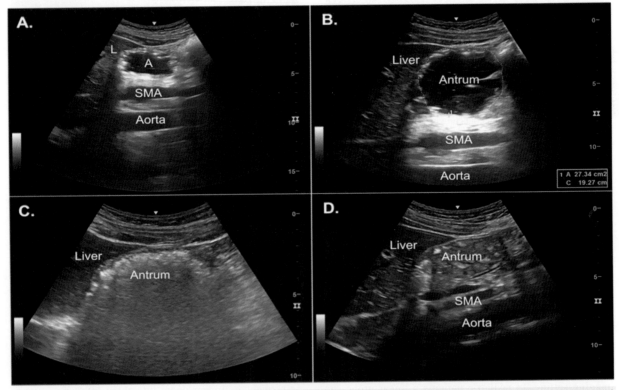

Fig. 21.17 Different stages of gastric filling by ultrasound imaging. (A) Gastric antrum beginning to dilate with small amount of anechoic fluid. (B) Dilated gastric antrum containing some air bubbles giving it a "starry night" appearance. Air bubbles can occur with ingestion of air from swallowing or with carbonated beverages. Both (A) and (B) are consistent with recent ingestion of clear fluids. Thick fluids (such as milk) will appear more echoic and homogenous within the antrum. (C) "Frosted glass" appearance of gastric antrum in the early stages after solid ingestion. Air ingested with chewing and swallowing prevents visualization of deeper structures. (D) Antrum filled with hyperechoic, heterogenous material representing ingestion of solid foods with varying consistencies. (Modified from El-Boghdadly K, Wojcikiewicz T, Perlas A. Perioperative point-of-care gastric ultrasound. *BJA Educ.* 2019;19[7]:219–226.)

to the antrum, creating a "frosted glass" appearance. The antrum then distends and appears to be full of contents with heterogenous echogenicity (Fig. 21.17). For quantitative assessment of gastric contents, the antral cross-sectional area (CSA) is measured in the RLD position. This can be done by measuring the craniocaudal and anterior-posterior diameters of the antrum from serosa to serosa and then calculating the area using the formula for the area of an eclipse (CSA = (AP × CC × π)/4). Alternatively, some ultrasound machines allow the operator to trace the circumference of the antrum at the level of the serosa and then automatically calculate the CSA. The volume of gastric content can be estimated from the CSA using mathematical models that stratify by patient age. Studies have found that a volume of <1.5 mL kg^{-1} (approximately 100 mL in an average-sized adult) is a normal finding in a fasted patient and carries a low risk of aspiration.[13,14] Volumes ≥1.5 mL kg^{-1} may indicate delayed emptying or a nonfasted state and are associated with a higher-than-baseline risk of aspiration.

CONCLUSIONS AND FUTURE DIRECTIONS

Perioperative POCUS is a rapidly expanding field and has become one of the core competencies of training in anesthesiology. It is essential for anesthesia providers to undergo training in POCUS and to incorporate diagnostic perioperative POCUS into their clinical practice. As the field continues to grow, it is important to recognize the limitations of each type of examination and to clearly define the scope of practice. POCUS is meant to be performed and interpreted by a clinician in real time. The examinations should be rapid, goal directed, easy to perform, and repeated over time as necessary. Clinicians must recognize when diagnostic accuracy is compromised by poor imaging, artifacts, or incomplete data and when to obtain formal imaging or seek consultation with a more experienced provider or specialist. There are many other applications for perioperative POCUS beyond the scope of this chapter (e.g., airway/tracheal ultrasound,

ultrasound for deep venous thrombosis, ocular ultrasound). As anesthesia providers become more proficient in perioperative POCUS, the scope of practice will expand and new applications for the use of ultrasound in the perioperative setting will emerge.

REFERENCES

1. Frankel HL, Kirkpatrick AW, Elbarbary M, et al. Guidelines for the appropriate use of bedside general and cardiac ultrasonography in the evaluation of critically ill patients—Part I. *Crit Care Med.* 2015;43(11):2479–2502.
2. Ultrasound guidelines: Emergency, point-of-care and clinical ultrasound guidelines in medicine. *Ann Emerg Med.* 2017;69(5).
3. Bronshteyn YS, Anderson TA, Badakhsh O, et al. American Society of Anesthesiologists Ad Hoc Committee on PoCUS. Diagnostic point-of-care ultrasound: Recommendations from an expert panel. *J Cardiothorac Vasc Anesth.* S1053-0770(21)00342-6, 2021.
4. Millington SJ. Ultrasound assessment of the inferior vena cava for fluid responsiveness: Easy, fun, but unlikely to be helpful. *Can J Anaesth.* 2019;66(6):633–638.
5. Bentzer P, Griesdale DE, Boyd J. Will this hemodynamically unstable patient respond to a bolus of intravenous fluids? *JAMA.* 2016;316(12):1298–1309.
6. Alrajhi K, Woo MY, Vaillancourt C. Test characteristics of ultrasonography for the detection of pneumothorax: A systematic review and meta-analysis. *Chest.* 2012;141(3):703–708.
7. Brogi E, Gargani L, Bignami E, et al. Thoracic ultrasound for pleural effusion in the intensive care unit: A narrative review from diagnosis to treatment. *Crit Care.* 2017;21(1):325.
8. Ibitoye BO, Idowu BM, Ogunrombi AB, Afolabi BI. Ultrasonographic quantification of pleura effusion: Comparison of four formulae. *Ultrasonograpy.* 2018;37(3):254–260.
9. Orso D, Guglielmo N, Copetti R. Lung ultrasound in diagnosing pneumonia in the emergency department: A systematic review and meta-analysis. *Eur J Emerg Med.* 2018;25(5):312–321.
10. Llamas-Álvarez AM, Tenza-Lozana EM, Latour-Pérez J. Accuracy of lung ultrasonography in the diagnosis of pneumonia in adults. *Chest.* 2017;151(2):374–382.
11. El-Boghdadly K, Wojcikiewicz T, Perlas A. Perioperative point-of-care gastric ultrasound. *BJA Educ.* 2019;19(7):219–226.
12. Gola W, Domagała M, Cugowski A. Ultrasound assessment of gastric emptying and the risk of aspiration of gastric contents in the perioperative period. *Anaesthesiol Intensive Ther.* 2018;50(4):297–302.
13. Lichtenstein DA. Lung ultrasound in the critically ill. *Ann Intensive Care.* 2014;4(1).
14. Lee FC. Lung ultrasound-a primary survey of the acutely dyspneic patient. *J Intensive Care.* 2016;4(1):57.

22 ACID–BASE BALANCE AND BLOOD GAS ANALYSIS

Linda L. Liu

The concentrations of hydrogen and bicarbonate ions in plasma must be precisely regulated to optimize enzyme activity, oxygen transport, and rates of chemical reactions within cells. Each day approximately 15,000 mmol of carbon dioxide (which can generate carbonic acid as it combines with water) and 50 to 100 mEq of nonvolatile acid (mostly sulfuric acid) are produced and must be eliminated safely. The body is able to maintain this intricate acid–base balance by utilizing buffers, pulmonary excretion of carbon dioxide, and renal elimination of acid. This chapter will define concepts important for understanding acids and bases, discuss clinical measurements of blood gases and their interpretation, and present a diagnostic approach to common acid–base disturbances.

DEFINITIONS

Acids and Bases

Bronsted and Lowry defined an acid as a molecule that can act as a proton (H^+) donor and a base as a molecule that can act as a proton acceptor. In physiologic solutions a strong acid is a substance that readily and irreversibly gives up an H^+, and a strong base avidly binds H^+. In contrast, biologic molecules are either weak acids or bases, which reversibly donate H^+ or reversibly bind H^+.

Acidemia and Acidosis

A blood pH less than 7.35 is called *acidemia,* and a pH greater than 7.45 is called *alkalemia,* regardless of the mechanism. The underlying process that lowers the pH is called an *acidosis,* and the process that raises the pH is known as an *alkalosis.* A patient can have a mixed disorder with both an acidosis and an alkalosis concurrently but can only be either acidemic or alkalemic. The last two terms are mutually exclusive.

Base Excess

Base excess (BE) is usually defined as the amount of strong acid (hydrochloric acid for BE greater than zero) or strong base (sodium hydroxide for BE less than zero) required to return 1 L of whole blood exposed in vitro to a P_{CO_2} of 40 mm Hg to a pH of 7.4.[1] Instead of an actual titration, the blood gas machine calculates the BE with algorithms utilizing plasma pH, blood P_{CO_2}, and hemoglobin concentration. The number is supposed to refer to the nonrespiratory or metabolic component of an acid–base disturbance. A BE less than zero (also called a *base deficit*) suggests the presence of a metabolic acidosis, and a value greater than zero suggests the presence of a metabolic alkalosis. In vitro, the number has been accurate but in the living organism, because ions do cross beyond vascular and cellular boundaries, a primary acute change in Pa_{CO_2} sometimes can cause the BE to move in the opposite direction, despite an unchanged metabolic acid–base status.[2] In clinical practice the BE is often used as a surrogate measure for lactic acidosis, which is one measurement to help determine adequacy of intravascular volume resuscitation.

REGULATION OF THE HYDROGEN ION CONCENTRATION

At 37°C, the normal hydrogen ion concentration in arterial blood and extracellular fluid is 35 to 45 nmol/L, which is equivalent to an arterial pH of 7.45 to 7.35, respectively. The normal plasma bicarbonate ion concentration is 24 ± 2 mEq/L. Physiologic changes to acid–base disturbances are corrected by three systems: buffers, ventilation, and renal response. The buffer systems provide an immediate chemical response, and the ventilatory response occurs in minutes whenever possible. The renal response can take days but can provide nearly complete restoration of the pH.

Buffer Systems

A buffer is defined as a substance within a solution that can prevent extreme changes in pH. A buffer system is composed of a base molecule and its weak conjugate acid. The base molecules of the buffer system bind excess hydrogen ions, and the weak acid protonates excess base molecules. The *dissociation ionization constant* (pK^a) indicates the strength of an acid and is derived from the classic Henderson-Hasselbalch equation (Fig. 22.1). The pK^a is the pH at which an acid is 50% protonated and 50% deprotonated. Hydrochloric acid, a strong acid, has a pK^a of −7, whereas carbonic acid, a weak acid, has a pKa of 6. The most important buffer systems in blood, in order of importance, are the (1) bicarbonate buffer system (H_2CO_3/HCO_3^-), (2) hemoglobin buffer system (HbH/Hb$^-$), (3) other protein buffer systems (PrH/Pr$^-$), (4) phosphate buffer system ($H_2PO_4^-/HPO_4^{2-}$), and (5) ammonia buffer system (NH_3/NH_4^+).

Bicarbonate Buffer System

Carbon dioxide, generated through aerobic metabolism, slowly combines with water to form carbonic acid, which spontaneously and rapidly deprotonates to form bicarbonate (Fig. 22.2). In this system the base molecule is bicarbonate and its weak conjugate acid is carbonic acid. Less than 1% of the dissolved carbon dioxide undergoes this reaction because it is so slow. However, the enzyme carbonic anhydrase, present in the endothelium, erythrocytes, and kidneys, catalyzes this reaction to accelerate the formation of carbonic acid and make this the most important buffering system in the human body when combined with renal control of bicarbonate and pulmonary control of carbon dioxide.

Hemoglobin Buffer System

The hemoglobin protein serves as an effective buffering system because it contains multiple histidine residues. Histidine is an effective buffer from pH 5.7 to 7.7 (pK^a 6.8) because of multiple protonatable sites on the imidazole side chains. Buffering by hemoglobin depends on the bicarbonate system to facilitate the movement of carbon dioxide intracellularly. (Fig. 22.3). At the lungs, the reverse process occurs. Chloride ions move out of the red blood cells as bicarbonate enters for conversion back to carbon dioxide. The carbon dioxide is released back into plasma and is eliminated by the lungs. This process allows a large fraction of extrapulmonary carbon dioxide to be transported back to the lungs as plasma bicarbonate.

Oxygenated and deoxygenated hemoglobin have different affinities for hydrogen ions and carbon dioxide. Deoxyhemoglobin takes up more hydrogen ions, which shifts the carbon dioxide/bicarbonate equilibrium to produce more bicarbonate and facilitates removal of carbon dioxide from peripheral tissues for release into the lungs. Oxyhemoglobin favors the release of hydrogen ions and shifts the equilibrium to more carbon dioxide formation. At physiologic pH, a small amount of carbon dioxide is

$$pH = pK_a + \log_{10} \frac{[Base]}{[Conjugate\ acid]}$$

Fig. 22.1 Henderson-Hasselbalch equation. *[Base]*, Concentration of base; *[Conjugate acid]*, concentration of conjugate acid.

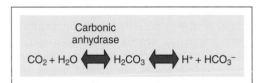

Fig. 22.2 Hydration of carbon dioxide results in carbonic acid, which dissociates into bicarbonate and hydrogen ions.

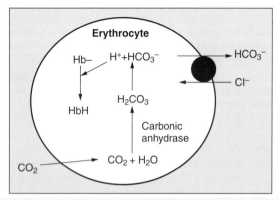

Fig. 22.3 Hemoglobin buffering system: Carbon dioxide freely diffuses into erythrocytes, where it combines with water to form carbonic acid, which rapidly deprotonates. The protons generated are bound up by hemoglobin. The bicarbonate anions are exchanged back into plasma with chloride.

also carried as carbaminohemoglobin. Deoxyhemoglobin has a greater affinity (3.5 times) for carbon dioxide, so venous blood carries more carbon dioxide than arterial blood (Haldane effect). These two mechanisms combine to account for the difference in carbon dioxide content of arterial versus venous plasma (25.6 mmol/L vs. 27.7 mmol/L, respectively).

Ventilatory Response

Central chemoreceptors lie on the anterolateral surface of the medulla and respond to changes in cerebrospinal fluid (CSF) pH. Carbon dioxide diffuses across the blood–brain barrier to elevate CSF hydrogen ion concentration, which activates the chemoreceptors and increases alveolar ventilation. The relationship between $Paco_2$ and minute ventilation is almost linear except at very high arterial $Paco_2$, when carbon dioxide narcosis develops, and at very low arterial $Paco_2$, when the apneic threshold is reached. There is a very wide variation in individual $Paco_2$/ventilation response curves, but minute ventilation generally increases 1 to 4 L/min for every 1 mm Hg increase in $Paco_2$. During general anesthesia, spontaneous ventilation will cease when the $Paco_2$ decreases to less than the apneic threshold, whereas in the awake patient, cortical influences prevent apnea, so the apneic threshold is not ordinarily observed.

Peripheral chemoreceptors are located at the bifurcation of the common carotid arteries and surrounding the aortic arch. The carotid bodies are the principal peripheral chemoreceptors and are sensitive to changes in Pao_2, $Paco_2$, pH, and arterial perfusion pressure. They communicate with the central respiratory centers via the glossopharyngeal nerves. Unlike the central chemoreceptors, which are more sensitive to hydrogen ions, the carotid bodies are most sensitive to Pao_2. Bilateral carotid endarterectomies abolish the peripheral chemoreceptor response, and these patients have almost no hypoxic ventilatory drive.

The stimulus from central and peripheral chemoreceptors to either increase or decrease alveolar ventilation diminishes as the pH approaches 7.4 such that complete correction or overcorrection is not possible. The pulmonary response to metabolic alkalosis is usually less than the response to metabolic acidosis. The reason is because progressive hypoventilation results in hypoxemia when breathing room air. Hypoxemia activates oxygen-sensitive chemoreceptors and limits the compensatory decrease in minute ventilation. Because of this, $Paco_2$ usually does not rise above 55 mm Hg in response to metabolic alkalosis for patients not receiving oxygen supplementation.

Renal Response

Renal effects are slower in onset and may not be maximal for up to 5 days. The response occurs via three mechanisms: (1) reabsorption of the filtered HCO_3^-, (2) excretion of titratable acids, and (3) ammonia (Fig. 22.4).[3] Carbon dioxide combines with water in the renal tubular cell. With the help of carbonic anhydrase, the bicarbonate produced enters the bloodstream while the hydrogen ion is exchanged with sodium and is released into the renal tubule. There, H^+ combines with filtered bicarbonate and dissociates into carbon dioxide and water with help from carbonic anhydrase located in the luminal brush border, and the carbon dioxide diffuses back into the renal tubular cell. The proximal tubule reabsorbs 80% to 90% of the bicarbonate this way, and the distal tubule takes care of the remaining 10% to 20%. Once the bicarbonate is reclaimed, further hydrogen ions can combine with HPO_4^{2-} to form $H_2PO_4^-$, which is eliminated in the urine. The last important urinary buffer is ammonia. Ammonia is formed from deamination of glutamine, an amino acid. The ammonia passively crosses the cell membrane to enter the tubular fluid. In the tubular fluid it combines with hydrogen ion to form NH_4^+, which is trapped within the tubule and excreted in the urine. All of these steps allow for the generation and return of bicarbonate into the bloodstream. The large amount of bicarbonate filtered by the kidneys allows for rapid excretion, if necessary, for compensation during alkalosis. The kidneys are highly effective in protecting the body against alkalosis except in association with sodium deficiency or mineralocorticoid excess.

ANALYSIS OF ARTERIAL BLOOD GASES

The ability to measure arterial blood gas (ABG) and venous blood gas has revolutionized patient care during anesthesia and in the intensive care unit (ICU). Although pulse oximetry and capnography can be monitored continuously, analysis of ABGs has increased our diagnostic ability and the accuracy of our measurements.

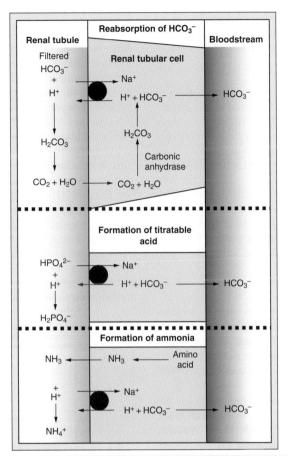

Fig. 22.4 Three mechanisms of renal compensation during acidosis to sequester hydrogen ions and reabsorb bicarbonate: (1) reabsorption of the filtered HCO_3^-, (2) excretion of titratable acids, and (3) production of ammonia.

Sampling

Arterial blood is most often obtained percutaneously from the radial, brachial, or femoral artery. In certain clinically stable situations venous pH, bicarbonate, and BE have sufficient agreement to be clinically interchangeable for arterial values and save an arterial puncture.[4] Venous pH is usually only 0.03 to 0.04 less than arterial values. Venous blood cannot be used for estimation of oxygenation for two reasons: venous Po_2 (Pvo_2) is significantly less than Pao_2 and depending on the site of the venous blood draw, differences in tissue metabolic activity may alter Pvo_2. Agreement between arterial and venous Pco_2 is too unpredictable to be clinically useful as a single test, but trends in Pco_2 may be helpful. Periodic correlations of arterial and venous measurements should be performed, especially when venous measurements are used for serial monitoring in critically ill patients.

A heparinized, bubble-free, fresh blood sample is required for blood gas analysis. Air bubbles should be removed because equilibration of oxygen and carbon dioxide in the blood with the corresponding partial pressures in the air bubble could influence the measured results. A delay in analysis can lead to oxygen consumption and carbon dioxide generation by the metabolically active white blood cells. Usually this error is small and can be reduced by placing the sample on ice. In some leukemia patients with a markedly increased white blood cell count this error can be large and lead to a falsely low Po_2 even though the patient's oxygenation is acceptable. This phenomenon is often referred to as *leukocyte larceny.*[5]

Temperature Correction

Decreases in temperature decrease the partial pressure of a gas in solution, even though the total gas content does not change. Both Pco_2 and Po_2 decrease during hypothermia, but serum bicarbonate is unchanged. This leads to an increase in pH if the blood could be measured at the patient's temperature. A blood gas with a pH of 7.4 and Pco_2 of 43 mm Hg at 37°C will have a pH of 7.5 and a Pco_2 of 31 mm Hg at 30°C.[6] Unfortunately, all blood gas samples are measured at 37°C, which raises the issue of how to best manage the ABG measurement in hypothermic patients. This has led to two management strategies: alpha-stat and pH-stat.

Alpha-Stat

Alpha-stat theory advocates measuring all blood gases at 37°C. Alpha refers to the protonation state of the imidazole side chain of histidine. The pKa of histidine changes with temperature so that its protonation state is relatively constant regardless of temperature. The term *alpha-stat* developed because as the patient's pH was allowed to drift with temperature, the protonation state of the histidine residues remained static. During cardiopulmonary bypass, an anesthesia provider using alpha-stat would manage the patient based on an ABG measured at 37°C and strive to keep that pH at 7.4, but the patient's true pH would be higher. No extra adjustments would be made for the patient's hypothermia.

pH-Stat

pH-stat is different from alpha-stat in that it requires keeping a patient's pH static at 7.4 based on the core temperature. During cardiopulmonary bypass, an anesthesia provider using pH-stat would manage the patient based on an ABG that is corrected for the patient's temperature. With hypothermia, this usually means adding carbon dioxide so that the patient's temperature-correct (hypothermic) blood gas has a pH of 7.4. In the ICU during targeted temperature management pH-stat management would mean lowering the patient's minute ventilation. The lower pH and higher P_{CO_2} maintained during pH-stat may improve cerebrovascular perfusion during hypothermia; however, there is still debate about which method provides better outcomes.[7]

Oxygenation

Decreases in temperature decrease the partial pressure of oxygen in solution. Because hypothermia causes the oxygen–hemoglobin dissociation curve to shift to the left, there is a higher affinity of hemoglobin to oxygen, making it easier for oxygen to attach to hemoglobin, but more difficult for it to diffuse to the tissues.

DIFFERENTIAL DIAGNOSIS OF ACID–BASE DISTURBANCES

Acid–base disturbances are categorized as respiratory or metabolic acidosis (pH less than 7.35) or alkalosis (pH more than 7.45). These disorders are further stratified into acute versus chronic based on their duration, which is gauged clinically by the patient's compensatory responses.[8] Patients may also have a mixed acid–base disorder. The approach to managing acid–base disorders should first involve searching for the causes rather than an immediate attempt to normalize the pH. Sometimes the treatment may be more detrimental than the original acid–base problem.

Adverse Responses to Acidemia and Alkalemia

Adverse responses can be associated with severe acidemia or alkalemia. Consequences of severe acidosis can occur regardless of whether the acidosis is of respiratory, metabolic, or mixed origin. Acidemia usually leads to decreased myocardial contractility and release of catecholamines. With mild acidosis, the release of catecholamines mitigates the myocardial depression. Patients with acute respiratory distress syndrome are typically managed with a lung-protective ventilation strategy with permissive hypercapnia and mild respiratory acidosis (also see Chapter 41). No significant impact on systemic vascular resistance, pulmonary vascular resistance, cardiac output, or systemic oxygen delivery has been seen.[9] With severe acidemia (pH <7.2), myocardial responsiveness to catecholamines decreases, so myocardial depression and hypotension predominate (Fig. 22.5). Respiratory acidosis may produce more rapid and profound myocardial dysfunction than metabolic acidosis because of the rapid

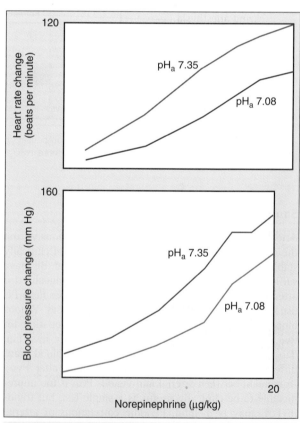

Fig. 22.5 Diminished hemodynamic response to intravenously administered norepinephrine in a canine model of lactic acidosis. *pH^a*, arterial pH. (From Ford GD, Cline WH, Fleming WW. Influence of lactic acidosis on cardiovascular response to sympathomimetic amines. *Am J Physiol.* 1968;215(5):1123-1129, used with permission.)

entry of carbon dioxide into the cardiac cell. In the brain this rapid increase in carbon dioxide can lead to confusion, loss of consciousness, and seizures.

Severe alkalemia (pH >7.6) can lead to decreased cerebral and coronary blood flow as a result of arteriolar vasoconstriction. The consequences of severe alkalosis are also more prominent with respiratory than with metabolic causes because of the rapid movement of carbon dioxide across cell membranes.[10] Acute hyperventilation can produce confusion, myoclonus, depressed consciousness, and seizures.

Respiratory Acidosis

Respiratory acidosis occurs when alveolar minute ventilation is inadequate relative to carbon dioxide production (Box 22.1). It can occur with a normal or increased minute ventilation if carbon dioxide production is increased or if there is decreased carbon dioxide elimination from lung disease. Decreased carbon dioxide elimination from a decreased minute ventilation can occur with volatile or intravenous anesthetics (see Chapter 8), neuromuscular blocking drugs (see Chapter 11), or neuromuscular disease. During anesthesia, increased rebreathing or absorption of carbon dioxide must also be considered.

Compensatory Responses and Treatment
Over the course of hours to days, the kidneys compensate for the respiratory acidosis by increasing hydrogen ion secretion and bicarbonate reabsorption. After a few days, the P_{CO_2} will remain increased but the pH will be near normal, which is the hallmark of a chronic respiratory acidosis. Respiratory acidosis with a pH of less than 7.2

indicates the need for increased ventilatory support. In patients with chronic respiratory acidosis the key approach is to avoid prolonged hyperventilation. The alkalosis from excessive ventilation and relative hypocapnia can result in central nervous system (CNS) irritability and cardiac ischemia. Also, the kidneys will now start to excrete bicarbonate. The increased serum bicarbonate has allowed the patient to maintain a normal pH with a relatively lower alveolar minute ventilation. After urinary excretion of bicarbonate, the patient's minute ventilation requirement will increase, which may affect weaning the patient from the ventilator.

Respiratory Alkalosis

Respiratory alkalosis occurs when alveolar minute ventilation is increased relative to carbon dioxide production. The increased alveolar minute ventilation can be related to a variety of causes (Box 22.2). Pa_{CO_2} is diminished relative to bicarbonate levels, resulting in a pH more than 7.45. The decreased Pa_{CO_2} and increased pH trigger the peripheral and central chemoreceptors to decrease the stimulus to breathe. During prolonged respiratory alkalosis, active transport of bicarbonate ions out of CSF causes the central chemoreceptors to reset to a lower Pa_{CO_2} level.

Compensatory Responses and Treatment
Respiratory alkalosis is compensated for by decreased reabsorption of bicarbonate ions from the renal tubules and increased urinary excretion of bicarbonate. Treatment of respiratory alkalosis is directed at correcting the underlying disorder. Mild alkalemia usually does not require treatment. In rare cases severe acute respiratory alkalosis (pH >7.6) may require sedation. During general anesthesia, acute respiratory alkalosis is easily remedied by decreasing total minute ventilation.

Metabolic Acidosis

Metabolic acidosis is present when accumulation of any acid in the body other than carbon dioxide results in a

---

Box 22.1 Causes of Respiratory Acidosis

Increased CO_2 production
Malignant hyperthermia
Hyperthyroidism
Sepsis
Overfeeding

Decreased CO_2 elimination
Intrinsic pulmonary disease (pneumonia, ARDS, fibrosis, edema)
Upper airway obstruction (laryngospasm, foreign body, OSA)
Lower airway obstruction (asthma, COPD)
Chest wall restriction (obesity, scoliosis, burns)
CNS depression (anesthetics, opioids, CNS lesions)
Decreased skeletal muscle strength (residual effects of neuromuscular blocking drugs, myopathy, neuropathy)

Increased CO_2 rebreathing or absorption
Exhausted soda lime
Incompetent one-way valve in breathing circuit
Laparoscopic surgery

ARDS, Acute respiratory distress syndrome; *CNS,* central nervous system; *CO_2,* carbon dioxide; *COPD,* chronic obstructive pulmonary disease; *OSA,* obstructive sleep apnea.

Box 22.2 Causes of Respiratory Alkalosis

Increased minute ventilation
Hypoxia (high altitude, low Fio_2, severe anemia)
Iatrogenic (mechanical ventilation)
Anxiety and pain
CNS disease (tumor, infection, trauma)
Fever, sepsis
Drugs (salicylates, progesterone, doxapram)
Liver disease
Pregnancy
Restrictive lung disease
Pulmonary embolism

CNS, Central nervous system; *Fio_2,* fractional concentration of inspired oxygen.

Box 22.3 Causes of Metabolic Acidosis

Anion Gap Acidosis
Methanol, ethylene glycol
Uremia
Lactic acidosis (e.g., from CHF, sepsis, cyanide toxicity)
Ethanol
Paraldehyde
Aspirin, INH
Ketones (e.g., starvation, diabetic ketoacidosis)

Nongap Acidosis
Excessive chloride administration (e.g., 0.9% saline infusion)
GI losses—diarrhea, ileostomy, neobladder, pancreatic fistula
Renal losses—RTA
Drugs—acetazolamide

CHF, Congestive heart failure; *GI*, gastrointestinal; *INH*, isoniazid; *RTA*, renal tubular acidosis.

Box 22.4 Causes of Elevated Lactate[12,21]

Type A—Perfusion Related
Distributive: sepsis, anaphylaxis
Cardiogenic/cardiac arrest
Hypovolemia: hemorrhagic
Obstructive: pulmonary embolism, cardiac tamponade
Tissue ischemia: mesenteric ischemia, burns, trauma, compartment syndrome, necrotizing soft tissue infections
Muscle activity: tonic-clonic seizures, increased work of breathing, disorders with acute muscle rigidity (e.g., serotonin syndrome, neuroleptic malignant syndrome, malignant hyperthermia)

Type B—Nonperfusion Related
Toxins: cyanide, carbon monoxide, cocaine, alcohol
Medications: metformin, linezolid, HIV reverse transcriptase inhibitors, epinephrine, inhaled β_2-agonists, propofol infusion syndrome
Malignancy
Liver failure

pH lower than 7.35 (Box 22.3). A compensatory increase in ventilatory elimination of carbon dioxide starts within minutes after the development of metabolic acidosis to provide a near-normal pH. Some patients, however, may not be able to sustain the increased minute ventilation and require mechanical ventilatory support.

Anion Gap

The best way to approach the differential diagnosis for a metabolic acidosis is to divide the causes into those that cause or do not cause an anion gap. The anion gap, defined as the difference between measured cations (sodium) and measured anions (chloride and bicarbonate), represents the concentration of anions in serum that are unaccounted for in this equation (Fig. 22.6). A normal anion gap value is 8 to 12 mEq/L and is mostly composed of anionic serum albumin.[11] A patient with a low serum albumin concentration will likely have a narrower anion gap value (each 1.0 g/dL decrease or increase in serum albumin less or more than 4.4 g/dL decreases or increases the actual concentration of unmeasured anions by approximately 2.5 mEq/L). An increase in the anion gap occurs when the anion replacing bicarbonate is not one that is routinely measured.

The most common unmeasured anions are lactic acid and keto acids. Lactic acid elevation may be caused by increased production, decreased clearance, or a combination of both. Skeletal muscles produce the greatest amount of

lactate among body tissues. The liver metabolizes approximately 60% of lactate produced, with the kidneys metabolizing 30%. A small amount of lactate is converted back to glucose via gluconeogenesis. Causes of an elevated lactate can be divided into those related to tissue hypoxia or systemic hypoperfusion, or etiologies not related to hypoperfusion.[12] (Box 22.4).

Nonanion Gap

Metabolic acidosis with a normal anion gap occurs when chloride replaces the lost bicarbonate, such as with a bicarbonate-wasting process in the kidneys (renal tubular acidosis) or gastrointestinal tract (diarrhea). Aggressive fluid resuscitation with normal saline (>30 mL/kg/h) will induce a nonanion gap metabolic acidosis secondary to excessive chloride administration, which impairs bicarbonate reabsorption in the kidneys.[13]

Strong Ion Difference

A second way to categorize metabolic acidoses is the strong ion difference (SID) approach, introduced by Peter Stewart in the 1980s.[14] His major tenet is that although serum bicarbonate and BE can be used to determine the extent of a clinical acid–base disorder, they do not help determine the mechanism of the abnormality. Instead, he proposed that the independent variables responsible for changes in acid–base balance are the SID (the difference between the completely dissociated cations and anions in plasma) (Fig. 22.7), the plasma concentration of nonvolatile weak acids (A_{TOT}), and the arterial carbon dioxide tension (Pa_{CO_2}). The strong ion approach distinguishes six primary acid–base disturbances (acidosis caused by decreased SID, alkalosis caused by increased SID, acidosis caused by increased A_{TOT}, alkalosis caused by decreased A_{TOT}, respiratory acidosis, or respiratory alkalosis) instead

$$\text{Anion gap} = [Na^+] - ([Cl^-] + [HCO_3^-])$$

Fig. 22.6 Calculation of the anion gap: The difference between the cations and the anions equals the concentration of unmeasured anions in serum.

$$SID = [\text{strong cations}] - [\text{strong anions}]$$
$$= [Na^+] + [K^+] + [Ca^{2+}] + [Mg^{2+}] - ([Cl^-] + [SO_4^{2-}] + [\text{organic acids}^-])$$
$$\approx [Na^+] + [K^+] - [Cl^-]$$

Fig. 22.7 Calculation of the strong ion difference (SID): The difference between the completely dissociated cations and anions in plasma.

of the four primary acid–base disturbances (respiratory acidosis or alkalosis, or metabolic acidosis or alkalosis), differentiated by the traditional Henderson-Hasselbalch equation. Under normal conditions, the SID is approximately 40 mEq/L. Processes that increase the SID increase blood pH, whereas processes that reduce it decrease pH. For instance, massive volume resuscitation with normal saline, which has a SID of 0, leads to an acidosis.

The major practical difference between the two theories (Stewart vs. Henderson-Hasselbalch) is the inclusion of the serum albumin concentration in the Stewart approach, which provides some increase in accuracy in certain clinical settings. If changes in serum albumin concentration are accounted for in measurement of the anion gap, the more complex Stewart approach does not appear to offer a clinically significant advantage over the traditional approach to acid–base disturbances.[15]

Compensatory Responses and Treatment

The compensatory responses for a metabolic acidosis include increased alveolar ventilation from carotid body stimulation and renal tubule secretion of hydrogen ions into urine. Chronic metabolic acidosis, as seen with chronic renal failure, is commonly associated with loss of bone mass because buffers present in bone are used to neutralize the nonvolatile acids.

Management of an anion gap metabolic acidosis is guided by diagnosis and treatment of the underlying cause in order to remove the nonvolatile acids from the circulation. Lactic acidosis related to hypoperfusion requires volume resuscitation, vasopressors, or inotropes, depending on the etiology of the shock, whereas other etiologies of elevated lactate require stopping offending drugs, removing the toxins, treating seizures, or improving the organ dysfunction. Diabetic ketoacidosis requires intravenous fluid and insulin therapy. Minute ventilation should be increased in a patient who is mechanically ventilated to compensate until more definitive treatment takes effect.

Bicarbonate therapy is more controversial and should be based on whether an anion gap is present or not. Administration of sodium bicarbonate is often given for a nongap metabolic acidosis because the problem is bicarbonate loss. Bicarbonate may be considered as a temporizing measure in the setting of an extreme anion gap acidosis, particularly when a patient is hemodynamically unstable. Sodium bicarbonate administration generates carbon dioxide, which,

unless eliminated by ventilation, can worsen any intracellular and extracellular acidosis. A common approach is to administer a small dose of sodium bicarbonate and then repeat the pH measurement and monitor hemodynamics to determine the impact of treatment.

Metabolic Alkalosis

Metabolic alkalosis is present when the pH is higher than 7.45 because of the gain of bicarbonate ions or loss of hydrogen ions. The loss of hydrogen ions is usually from the gastrointestinal tract or the kidney. The stimulus for bicarbonate reabsorption is usually from hypovolemia, hypokalemia, or hyperaldosteronism (Box 22.5). In hypovolemia associated with chloride loss (e.g., diuretics) bicarbonate is reabsorbed with sodium in the renal tubules. With the adoption of low tidal volumes and permissive hypercapnia for the ventilatory management of patients with acute respiratory distress syndrome (ARDS), a compensatory metabolic alkalosis is often a common finding for the critically ill patient (also see Chapter 41).

Compensatory Responses and Treatment

Compensatory responses for metabolic alkalosis include increased reabsorption or decreased secretion of hydrogen ions by renal tubule cells and alveolar hypoventilation. The efficiency of the renal compensatory mechanism is dependent on the presence of cations (sodium, potassium) and chloride. Lack of these ions impairs the ability of the kidneys to excrete excess bicarbonate and results in incomplete renal compensation. In contrast to metabolic acidosis the respiratory compensation for pure metabolic

---

Box 22.5 Causes of Metabolic Alkalosis

Chloride Responsive
Renal loss—diuretic therapy
GI loss—vomiting, NG suction
Alkali administration—citrate in blood products, acetate in
  TPN, bicarbonate

Chloride Resistant
Hyperaldosteronism
Refeeding syndrome
Profound hypokalemia

GI, Gastrointestinal; *NG*, nasogastric; *TPN*, total parenteral nutrition.

III

alkalosis is never more than 75% complete. As a result, the pH remains increased in patients with primary metabolic alkalosis. Treatment of metabolic alkalosis should be aimed at reducing the acid loss (e.g., by stopping gastric drainage) or fluid repletion with saline and potassium chloride, which allows the kidneys to excrete excess bicarbonate ions. Occasionally, a trial of acetazolamide may be useful in causing a bicarbonaturia. Life-threatening metabolic alkalosis is rarely encountered.

Diagnosis

The diagnosis of an acid–base disorder should occur in a structured fashion. Fig. 22.8 shows a stepwise algorithm for blood gas interpretation. Step 1, which determines oxygenation, will be discussed later in this chapter. Step 2 involves determining whether the patient is acidemic (pH <7.35) or alkalemic (pH >7.45). Step 3 looks at whether the cause is from a primary metabolic or respiratory process. Metabolic processes involve a change in bicarbonate concentration from 24 mEq/L, and respiratory processes involve a change in Pco_2 from 40 mm Hg. If the primary process is respiratory in origin,

> **Box 22.6** Determining Whether Respiratory Process Is Acute or Chronic
>
> **Acute Process**
> pH Δ0.08 for every 10 mm Hg Δ in Pco_2 from 40 mm Hg
> **Chronic Process**
> pH Δ 0.03 for every 10 mm Hg Δ in Pco_2 from 40 mm Hg

then step 4 assesses whether the abnormality is chronic or acute (Box 22.6). If a metabolic alkalosis is present, then the next step is to skip to step 7 and determine whether appropriate respiratory compensation is present (Box 22.7). If the measured Pco_2 is greater than expected, a concurrent respiratory acidosis is present. If the measured Pco_2 is less than expected, then a concurrent respiratory alkalosis is present. If a metabolic acidosis is present, then an anion gap should be calculated (step 5). If there is a gap, then a Δgap should be determined. The Δgap is the excess anion gap (anion gap minus 12) added back to the serum bicarbonate level. If the number is less than 22 mEq/L, then a concurrent nongap metabolic acidosis is present. If the number is more

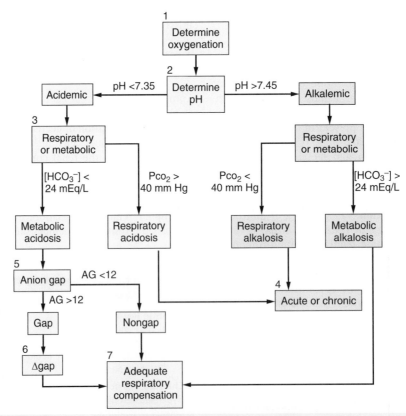

Fig. 22.8 Seven steps for acid–base diagnosis. Δgap, anion gap − 12 + [HCO$_3^-$]. If Δgap is less than 22 mEq/L, then concurrent nongap metabolic acidosis exists. If Δgap is greater than 26 mEq/L, then concurrent metabolic alkalosis exists. *AG*, Anion gap.

Box 22.7 Determining Appropriate Respiratory Compensation in Acid–Base Disorders

Metabolic Alkalosis

$Pco_2 = (0.7 \times HCO_3^-) + 21$

If measured Pco_2 > calculated Pco_2, then concurrent respiratory acidosis is present.

If measured Pco_2 < calculated Pco_2, then concurrent respiratory alkalosis is present.

Metabolic Acidosis

Winter formula:

$Pco_2 = (1.5 \times HCO_3^-) + 8$

If measured Pco_2 > calculated Pco_2, then concurrent respiratory acidosis is present.

If measured Pco_2 < calculated Pco_2, then concurrent respiratory alkalosis is present.

---

than 26 mEq/L, then a concurrent metabolic alkalosis is present. The last step, step 7, determines whether an appropriate respiratory compensation is present for the metabolic acidosis (see Box 22.7). If the measured Pco_2 is greater than expected, as calculated by Winter's formula:

$Pco_2 = (1.5 \times HCO_3^-) + 8$, then a concurrent respiratory acidosis is present. If the measured Pco_2 is less than calculated, then a concurrent respiratory alkalosis is present. See sample calculations in Fig. 22.9.

OTHER INFORMATION PROVIDED BY ANALYSIS OF ARTERIAL BLOOD GASES AND pH

Aside from acid–base problems, additional measurements and information available from a blood gas analysis include the patient's ability to ventilate and oxygenate, cardiac output estimates, and lactate measurement (also see Chapter 5).

Ventilation

$Paco_2$ reflects the adequacy of ventilation for removing carbon dioxide from blood. Increased dead space ventilation markedly decreases the efficiency of ventilation. The V_D/V_T ratio is the fraction of each tidal volume

---

A 23-year-old man with insulin-dependent diabetes presents to the emergency room with somnolence, influenza-like symptoms, nausea, vomiting, and anorexia.

Laboratory values: Na 130 mEq/L, Cl 80 mEq/L, HCO_3^- 10 mEq/L
ABG: pH 7.20, Pco_2 35 mm Hg, Po_2 68 mm Hg on room air

Step 1: Determine oxygenation:
A-a gradient $= [(P_B - P_{H_2O})F_{IO_2} - Paco_2/RQ] - Pao_2$
$= (150 - Paco_2/0.8) - Pao_2$
$= (150 - 35/0.8) - 68$
$= 38$
There is an A-a gradient, possibly from pneumonia or aspiration.

Step 2: Determine pH: pH <7.4, so there is an acidosis.

Step 3: $[HCO_3^-]$ <24 mEq/L and Pco_2 <40 mm Hg
Primary abnormality is from metabolic acidosis.

Step 4: Not applicable here since we are going down metabolic acidosis pathway.

Step 5: Determine anion gap
Anion gap $= [Na] - ([Cl] + [HCO_3^-])$ should be <12
$= 130 - (80 + 10)$
$= 40$ mEq/L
There is an anion gap, probably from starvation or diabetic ketoacidosis.

Step 6: Determine Δgap
Δgap $=$ anion gap $- 12 + [HCO_3^-]$
$= 40 - 12 + 10$
$= 38$ mEq/L
There is a concurrent metabolic alkalosis probably from vomiting.

Step 7: Is there appropriate respiratory compensation?
Winter's formula $= 1.5 [HCO_3^-] + 8 =$ expected Pco_2
$= 1.5 (10) + 8$
$= 23$ mm Hg
There is also a respiratory acidosis probably from somnolence.

Fig. 22.9 Example for calculating acid–base abnormalities. *ABG*, Arterial blood gas.

that is involved in dead space ventilation. This value is usually around 0.25 to 0.3 because of anatomic dead space. When minute ventilation is held constant during anesthesia, the gradient between $Paco_2$ and end-tidal CO_2 ($ETCO_2$) will increase if dead space is increased (e.g., pulmonary embolus or reduced cardiac output).

Oxygenation

Oxygenation is assessed by measurement of Pao_2. Arterial hypoxemia may be caused by (1) a low Po_2 in the inhaled gases (altitude, accidental occurrence during anesthesia), (2) hypoventilation, or (3) venous admixture with or without decreased mixed venous oxygen content. Acute hypoxemia causes activation of the sympathetic nervous system with endogenous catecholamine release, which augments blood pressure and cardiac output. The increased cardiac output will increase oxygen delivery from the lungs to peripheral tissues.

Alveolar Gas Equation

The alveolar gas equation estimates the partial pressure of alveolar oxygen by accounting for barometric pressure, water vapor pressure, and the inspired oxygen concentration (Fig. 22.10). Atmospheric oxygen is a constant 21% of barometric pressure; however, barometric pressure diminishes with altitude such that the decrease in inspired oxygen can become significant.

Hypoventilation leads to increased Pco_2, which encroaches on the space available in the alveolus for oxygen and dilutes the oxygen concentration. The alveolar gas equation estimates this decrease in alveolar oxygen concentration by subtracting an amount equal to the carbon dioxide divided by the respiratory quotient.[16]

Alveolar-Arterial Gradient

Calculation of the alveolar-arterial (A-a) gradient provides an estimate of venous admixture as the cause of hypoxemia (see Fig. 22.10). Venous admixture refers to deoxygenated venous blood mixing with oxygenated arterial blood through shunting. The A-a gradient formula calculates the difference in oxygen partial pressure between alveolar (Pao_2) and arterial (Pao_2) blood. Normally, the A-a gradient is less than 15 mm Hg while breathing room air as a result of shunting via the Thebesian and bronchial veins. Age increases the A-a gradient because of progressive increase in closing capacity relative to functional residual capacity (FRC). Increased fractional concentration of inspired oxygen (Fio_2) can lead to a larger gradient (up to 60 mm Hg while breathing Fio_2 1.0). Vasodilating drugs (nitroglycerin, nitroprusside, inhaled anesthetics), which inhibit hypoxic pulmonary vasoconstriction and increase ventilation/perfusion ($\dot{V}/\dot{Q}$ mismatch), can also increase the A-a gradient.

Larger A-a gradients suggest the presence of pathologic shunting, such as right-to-left intrapulmonary shunts (atelectasis, pneumonia, endobronchial intubation) or intracardiac shunts (congenital heart disease). The A-a gradient provides an assessment of the patient's

Alveolar gas equation: $Pao_2 = (Pb - P_{H_2O})Fio_2 - Paco_2/RQ$

Pao_2 = alveolar partial pressure oxygen (mm Hg)
Pb = barometric pressure (760 mm Hg at sea level)
P_{H_2O} = partial pressure of water vapor (47 mm Hg at 37°C)
Fio_2 = fraction inspired oxygen concentration
RQ = respiratory quotient (0.8 for normal diet)

A-a gradient = $Pao_2 - Pao_2$

For patient with Pao_2 of 363 mm Hg and $Paco_2$ of 40 mm Hg breathing Fio_2 1.0

$$Pao_2 = (760 - 47)(1.0) - 40/0.8$$
$$= (713) - 50$$
$$= 663 \text{ mm Hg}$$

A-a gradient = 663 - 363
           = 300 mm Hg

% shunt = 1% for every 20 mm Hg of A-a gradient
       = 300/20
       = 15%

Fig. 22.10 The alveolar gas equation, calculation of alveolar-arterial (A-a) gradient, and estimation of percentage of shunt.

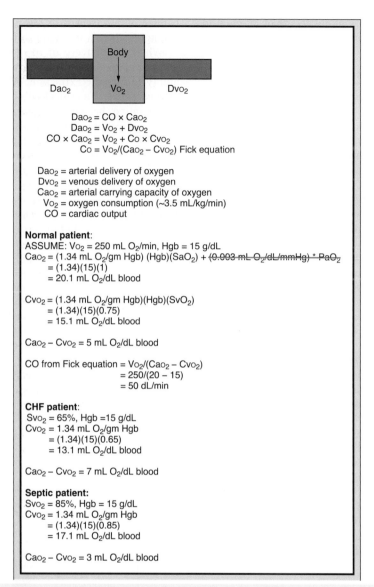

$$Dao_2 = CO \times Cao_2$$
$$Dao_2 = Vo_2 + Dvo_2$$
$$CO \times Cao_2 = Vo_2 + Co \times Cvo_2$$
$$Co = Vo_2/(Cao_2 - Cvo_2) \text{ Fick equation}$$

Dao_2 = arterial delivery of oxygen
Dvo_2 = venous delivery of oxygen
Cao_2 = arterial carrying capacity of oxygen
Vo_2 = oxygen consumption (~3.5 mL/kg/min)
CO = cardiac output

Normal patient:
ASSUME: Vo_2 = 250 mL O_2/min, Hgb = 15 g/dL
Cao_2 = (1.34 mL O_2/gm Hgb) (Hgb)(SaO_2) + ~~(0.003 mL O_2/dL/mmHg) * PaO_2~~
  = (1.34)(15)(1)
  = 20.1 mL O_2/dL blood

Cvo_2 = (1.34 mL O_2/gm Hgb)(Hgb)(SvO_2)
  = (1.34)(15)(0.75)
  = 15.1 mL O_2/dL blood

$Cao_2 - Cvo_2$ = 5 mL O_2/dL blood

CO from Fick equation = $Vo_2/(Cao_2 - Cvo_2)$
  = 250/(20 − 15)
  = 50 dL/min

CHF patient:
 SvO_2 = 65%, Hgb =15 g/dL
Cvo_2 = 1.34 mL O_2/gm Hgb
  = (1.34)(15)(0.65)
  = 13.1 mL O_2/dL blood

$Cao_2 - Cvo_2$ = 7 mL O_2/dL blood

Septic patient:
SvO_2 = 85%, Hgb = 15 g/dL
Cvo_2 = 1.34 mL O_2/gm Hgb
  = (1.34)(15)(0.85)
  = 17.1 mL O_2/dL blood

$Cao_2 - Cvo_2$ = 3 mL O_2/dL blood

Fig. 22.11 Calculation of cardiac output via Fick equation; arterial and mixed venous oxygen content; and arteriovenous difference in normal, septic, and heart failure patients. Amount of dissolved oxygen calculated by 0.003 mLO_2/dL/mm Hg *Po_2 can be ignored because of its small influence on Cao_2. *CHF*, Congestive heart failure.

shunt fraction and is more sensitive than pulse oximetry. A patient may have an Sao_2 of 100% but have a Pao_2 of only 90 mm Hg while breathing 100% oxygen. Significant shunting secondary to a pulmonary or cardiac process can occur despite the reassuring pulse oximeter reading. In patients with large shunts (>50%), administration of 100% oxygen will be unable to raise Pao_2.

To estimate the amount of shunt present, when Pao_2 is higher than 150 mm Hg, the shunt fraction is approximately 1% of cardiac output for every 20 mm Hg difference in the

A-a gradient. When Pao_2 is less than 150 mm Hg or when cardiac output is increased relative to metabolism, this guideline will underestimate the actual amount of venous admixture.

Pao_2/Fio_2 Ratio
The Pao_2/Fio_2 (P/F) ratio is a simple alternative to the A-a gradient to communicate the degree of hypoxemia. For patients with ARDS, the P/F ratio is used to categorize the severity of the disease (mild, moderate, severe); in

the "severe" patient the P/F ratio is less than or equal to 100 mm Hg (also see Chapter 41).[17]

Cardiac Output Estimates

Normal mixed PvO_2 is 40 mm Hg and is a balance between oxygen delivery and tissue oxygen consumption. A true PvO_2 should reflect blood from the superior and inferior vena cava and the heart. It is usually obtained from the distal port of an unwedged pulmonary artery (PA) catheter. Because of the complexity and risks of placing a PA catheter, many clinicians simply follow the trend from a central line placed in the superior vena cava.[18] If tissue oxygen consumption is unchanged, changes in PvO_2 reflect direct changes in cardiac output. The PvO_2 will decrease when there is inadequate cardiac output because the peripheral tissues have to increase oxygen extraction for aerobic metabolism. The PvO_2 will increase when there is high cardiac output (sepsis), peripheral shunting (arteriovenous fistulas), or impaired oxygen extraction (cyanide toxicity).

Fick Equation

If PaO_2, PvO_2, and hemoglobin are measured, the cardiac output can then be calculated by using the Fick equation (Fig. 22.11), which states that the delivery of oxygen in the veins must equal the delivery of oxygen in the arteries minus what is consumed (Vo_2). The delivery of oxygen is cardiac output multiplied by the amount of oxygen carried in the blood. The total amount of oxygen in the blood is the amount bound to hemoglobin and the amount dissolved in solution. Because the vast majority of the oxygen content in blood is bound to hemoglobin, the amount dissolved can often be left out of the equation in order to simplify calculations. The amount dissolved becomes important in situations such as severe anemia, when the amount carried by hemoglobin is low.[19]

Arteriovenous Difference

The difference between the arterial and mixed venous oxygen content (AV difference) is a good estimate of the adequacy of oxygen delivery (see Fig. 22.11). The normal AV difference is 4 to 6 mL/dL of blood. When tissue oxygen consumption is constant, a decreased cardiac output (congestive heart failure) leads to higher oxygen extraction, which increases the AV difference. An increased cardiac output (sepsis) or lower extraction (cyanide poisoning) leads to a lower AV difference.

When the delivery of oxygen is first reduced, oxygen consumption remains normal because of the body's ability to increase extraction. With further reductions in oxygen delivery, a critical point is reached when oxygen consumption becomes proportional to delivery. When oxygen consumption becomes supply dependent, cellular hypoxia occurs, which leads to progressive lactic acidosis and eventual death if uncorrected (Fig. 22.12).

Lactate Measurements

Arterial plasma lactate concentration is used as a marker of hypoperfusion and/or microcirculatory dysfunction and is a sensitive marker of disease severity. A value >2 mmol/L is considered significant, and its persistence predicts poor outcomes in critical illness.[20] Changes in lactate can provide early and objective information regarding the patient's response to therapy. For example, lactate measurement is a core element of the Hour-1 Surviving Sepsis 2016 Campaign bundle of care.[21] During anesthesia, an increasing lactate is usually associated with reduced tissue perfusion, but other causes of an increased lactate, such as medications or toxins, should be considered as well.

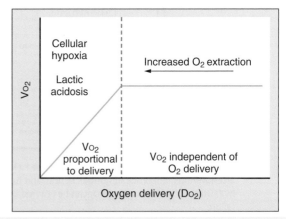

Fig. 22.12 Relationship of oxygen consumption (Vo_2) to oxygen delivery (Do_2): When oxygen consumption becomes supply dependent, cellular hypoxia occurs, which leads to progressive lactic acidosis and eventually death.

REFERENCES

1. Adrogue HJ, Gennari FJ, Galla JH, et al. Assessing acid-base disorders. *Kidney Int.* 2009;76:1239–1247.

2. Morgan TJ. The Stewart approach-one clinician's perspective. *Clin Biochem Rev.* 2009;30:41–54.

3. Koeppen. The kidney and acid-base regulation. *Adv Physiol Educ.* 2009;33:275–281.

4. Byrne AL, Bennett M, Chatterji R, et al. Peripheral venous and arterial blood gas analysis in adults: are they comparable? A systematic review and meta-analysis. *Respirology.* 2014;19:168–175.

5. Pardesi O, Bittner EA. Leukocyte larceny: a cause of pseudohypoxemia. *Can J Anaesth.* 2016;63:1374–1375.

6. Bisson J, Younker J. Correcting arterial blood gases for temperature: (when) is it clinically significant?. *Nurs Crit Care.* 2006;11:232–238.

7. Voicu S, Deye N, Malissin I, et al. Influence of α-stat and pH-stat blood gas management strategies on cerebral blood flow and oxygenation in patients treated with therapeutic hypothermia after our-of-hospital cardiac arrest: a crossover study. *Crit Care Med.* 2014;42:1849–1861.

8. Adrogue HJ, Madias NE. Secondary responses to altered acid-base status: the rules of engagement. *J Am Soc Nephrol.* 2010;21:920–923.

9. Acute Respiratory Distress Syndrome Network. Ventilation with lower tidal volumes as compared with traditional tidal volumes for acute lung injury and the acute respiratory distress syndrome. *N Engl J Med.* 2000;342:1301–1308.

10. Seifter JL, Chang HY. Disorders of acid-base balance: new perspectives. *Kidney Dis.* 2016;2:170–186.

11. Fidkowski C, Helstrom J. Diagnosing metabolic acidosis in the critically ill: bridging the anion gap, Stewart, and base excess methods. *Can J Anaesth.* 2009;56:247–256.

12. Anderson LW, Mackenhauer J, Roberts JC, et al. Etiology and therapeutic approach to elevated lactate. *Mayo Clin Proc.* 2013;88:1127–1140.

13. Lira A, Pinsky MR. Choices in fluid type and volume during resuscitation: impact on patient outcomes. *Ann Intensive Care.* 2014;4:1–13.

14. Stewart PA. Modern quantitative acid-base chemistry. *Can J Physiol Pharmacol.* 1983;61:1444–1461.

15. Masevicious FD, Dubin A. Has Stewart approach improved our ability to diagnose acid-base disorders in critically ill patients?. *World J Crit Care Med.* 2015;4:60–72.

16. Bigatello L, Pesenti A. Respiratory physiology for the anesthesiologist. *Anesthesiology.* 2019;130:1064–1077.

17. ARDS Definition Task Force. Acute respiratory distress syndrome: the Berlin definition. *JAMA.* 2012;307:2526–2533.

18. Dueck MH, Klimek M, Appenrodt S, et al. Trends but not individual values of central venous oxygen saturation agree with mixed venous oxygen saturation during varying hemodynamic conditions. *Anesthesiology.* 2005;103:249–257.

19. Wagner PD. The physiological basis of pulmonary gas exchange: implications for clinical interpretation of arterial blood gases. *Eur Respir.* 2015;45:227–243.

20. Bakker J, Postelnicu R, Mukherjee V. Lactate: where are we now?. *Crit Care Clin.* 2020;36:115–124.

21. Pino R, Singh J. Appropriate Clinical Use of Lactate Measurements. *Anesthesiology.* 2021. https://doi.org/10.1097/ALN.0000000000003655.

23 HEMOSTASIS

Anil K. Panigrahi

INTRODUCTION

Hemostasis is an ordered process involving cellular and biochemical components that functions to limit blood loss secondary to vascular injury, maintain intravascular blood flow, and promote revascularization after thrombosis. Normal physiologic hemostasis is a constant balance between procoagulant pathways responsible for generating localized hemostatic clot and counter-regulatory mechanisms that inhibit uncontrolled thrombus propagation or premature thrombus degradation. Vascular endothelium, platelets, plasma coagulation proteins, and fibrinolytic enzymes play equally important roles in this process. Derangements in this delicate system because of acquired or congenital disease states in addition to medications can lead to excessive bleeding or pathologic thrombus formation.

NORMAL HEMOSTASIS

Injury of the vascular endothelium results in platelet deposition at the injury site, a process often referred to as *primary hemostasis*. Although this initial platelet plug may prove adequate for a minor injury, control of more significant bleeding necessitates formation of a stable clot reinforced by crosslinked fibrin—a process mediated by activated plasma clotting factors and often referred to as *secondary hemostasis* (Fig. 23.1). Advances in our understanding of the cellular and molecular processes underlying hemostasis suggest a far more complex and nonlinear interplay between vascular endothelium, platelets, and clotting factors than is reflected in this model[1]; however, the terms primary and secondary hemostasis remain relevant for descriptive and diagnostic purposes.

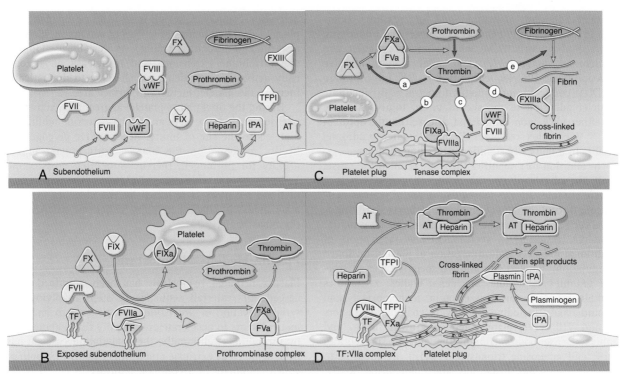

Fig. 23.1 Normal Hemostasis. (A) Normal endothelium. Procoagulants (factors [F] VII, VIII, IX, X, XIII, prothrombin), fibrinogen, and platelets circulate in their inactive forms. Anticoagulants (tissue factor pathway inhibitor [TFPI], heparin, and tissue plasminogen activator [tPA]) actively prevent endothelial spontaneous thrombus formation. (B) Vascular injury, initial phase. Subendothelial tissue factor (TF) exposed to circulating FVII forms a TF:VII complex. TF:VII activates FIX and FX. FIXa binds to platelets. FXa activates FV (FVa) to form prothrombinase complex, which converts localized, small amounts of prothrombin to thrombin. (C) Vascular injury, role of thrombin. Thrombin (a) activates FX and FV to form prothrombinase complexes that generate the secondary thrombin burst, (b) activates platelets, (c) separates FVIII from von Willebrand factor (vWF) and activates FVIII, (d) converts fibrinogen to fibrin, (e) activates factor XI, and (f) activates FXIII, the stabilizer of crosslinked fibrin. A stable clot is formed. (D) Control of coagulation and fibrin clot dissolution. Antithrombin (AT) binds heparin and potently inhibits thrombin activity. TFPI binds to FXa to inhibit the TF:VIIa complex. Plasminogen is activated to plasmin by tPA and cleaves fibrin into soluble fibrin split products. (From Huddleston LL, Liu LL. Hemostasis. In Miller RD, Pardo MC, eds. *Basics of Anesthesia*. 7th ed. Philadelphia: Elsevier; 2018. Figure 22.1.)

Vascular Endothelial Role in Hemostasis

The vascular endothelium serves an important role in reducing unprovoked thrombosis. Healthy endothelial cells possess antiplatelet and anticoagulant activity that functions to inhibit clot formation. The negatively charged vascular endothelium repels platelets, and endothelial cells produce potent platelet inhibitors such as prostacyclin (prostaglandin I₂) and nitric oxide that prevent adhesion of quiescent platelets. An adenosine diphosphatase (CD39) expressed on the surface of vascular endothelial cells also serves to block platelet activation through degradation of adenosine diphosphate (ADP), a potent platelet activator. The vascular endothelium also plays a pivotal anticoagulant role by expressing several inhibitors of plasma-mediated hemostasis. Endothelial cells can increase activation of protein C, an anticoagulant, via surface expression of thrombomodulin (TM), which acts as a cofactor for thrombin-mediated activation of protein C, making its activation 1000 times faster. Endothelial cells also produce tissue factor pathway inhibitor (TFPI), which inhibits the procoagulant activity of factor Xa and the TF–VIIa complex. Finally, the vascular endothelium synthesizes tissue plasminogen activator (tPA), which is responsible for activating fibrinolysis, a primary counter-regulatory mechanism limiting clot propagation.

Platelets and Hemostasis

Despite these natural defense mechanisms, upon injury the endothelium may shift the balance to promote platelet adhesion, activation, and aggregation.[2] Damage to vascular endothelial cells exposes the underlying extracellular matrix (ECM), which contains collagen, von Willebrand factor (vWF), and other platelet-adhesive glycoproteins. Platelet receptors for vWF (glycoprotein Ib-IX-V complex) and collagen (integrin $\alpha_2\beta_1$) facilitate platelet adhesion to the site of vessel injury. Absence of either vWF (von Willebrand disease) or glycoprotein Ib-IX-V complex receptors (Bernard–Soulier syndrome) results in a clinically significant bleeding disorder.

In addition to promoting their adhesion to the vessel wall, the platelet interaction with collagen serves as a potent stimulus for the subsequent phase of platelet activation. During the activation phase, platelets secrete agonists such as thromboxane A_2 (TxA_2) and release granular contents, resulting in recruitment and activation of additional platelets and propagation of plasma-mediated coagulation. Platelets contain two specific types of storage granules: α-granules and dense bodies. α-Granules contain numerous proteins essential to hemostasis and wound repair, including fibrinogen, coagulation factors V and VIII, vWF, platelet-derived growth factor, and others. Dense bodies contain the adenine nucleotides ADP and adenosine triphosphate (ATP), in addition to calcium, serotonin, histamine, and epinephrine. Redistribution of platelet membrane phospholipids during activation exposes newly activated platelet surface receptors and binding sites for calcium and coagulation factor

activation complexes, which is critical to propagation of plasma-mediated hemostasis. During activation, platelets also undergo structural changes to develop pseudopod-like membrane extensions and to release physiologically active microparticles, which serve to dramatically increase the platelet membrane surface area.

During the final phase, platelet aggregation, activators released during the activation phase recruit additional platelets to the site of injury. Newly active glycoprotein IIb/IIIa receptors on the platelet surface gain higher affinity for fibrinogen, thereby promoting crosslinking and aggregation with adjacent platelets. The importance of these receptors is reflected by the bleeding disorder associated with their hereditary deficiency, Glanzmann thrombasthenia.

Plasma-Mediated Hemostasis

Plasma-mediated hemostasis has been described as a cascade or waterfall sequence of steps involving the serial activation of proenzymes (zymogens) to enzymes and cofactors to accelerate and amplify fibrin generation by thrombin. Traditionally, the coagulation cascade has been depicted as extrinsic and intrinsic pathways, both of which culminate in a common pathway in which fibrin generation occurs (Fig. 23.2). This cascade model has proven to be an oversimplification, as it does not fully reflect in vivo hemostasis; however, it remains a useful

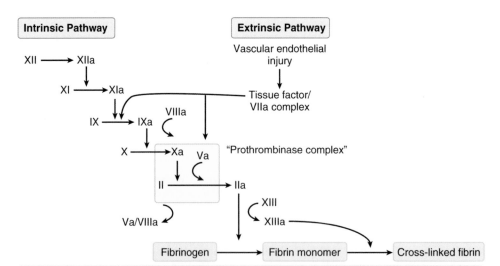

Fig. 23.2 Classic Coagulation Cascade. The coagulation cascade has been depicted as extrinsic (initiated by vascular injury) and intrinsic (because of contact activation) pathways, both of which culminate in a common pathway of thrombin (factor II) activation, which then converts fibrinogen to fibrin. The extrinsic pathway begins with exposure of blood plasma to tissue factor (TF) after injury to the vascular wall. The TF/factor VIIa complex activates factor IX of the intrinsic pathway, binds to factor VIIIa, and forms intrinsic tenase, which activates factor X. The intrinsic pathway then subsequently amplifies and propagates the hemostatic response to increase overall thrombin generation. (From Slaughter TF. The coagulation system and cardiac surgery. In: Estafanous FG, Barasch PG, Reves JG, eds. *Cardiac Anesthesia: Principles and Clinical Practice.* 2nd ed. Philadelphia: Lippincott Williams & Wilkins; 2001: 320.)

descriptive tool for organizing discussions of plasma-mediated hemostasis and interpreting in vitro coagulation tests.

The extrinsic pathway of coagulation is now understood to represent the initiation phase of plasma-mediated hemostasis and begins with exposure of blood plasma to tissue factor (TF). TF is prevalent in subendothelial tissues surrounding the vasculature; however, after vascular injury, small concentrations of factor VIIa circulating in plasma form phospholipid-bound activation complexes with TF, factor X, and calcium to promote conversion of factor X to Xa. Additionally, the TF/factor VIIa complex activates factor IX of the intrinsic pathway, further demonstrating the key role of TF in initiating hemostasis. Recent cell-based models of coagulation suggest that thrombin generation by way of the extrinsic pathway is limited by a natural inhibitor, TFPI; however, the small quantities of thrombin generated do activate factor XI and the intrinsic pathway. The intrinsic pathway then subsequently amplifies and propagates the hemostatic response to increase overall thrombin generation.

The final pathway, common to both extrinsic and intrinsic coagulation cascades, depicts thrombin generation and subsequent fibrin formation. Signal amplification results from activation of factor X by both intrinsic (FIXa, FVIIIa, Ca^{2+}) and extrinsic (TF, FVIIa, Ca^{2+}) tenase complexes. The tenase complexes in turn facilitate formation of the prothrombinase complex (FXa, FII [prothrombin], FVa [cofactor], and Ca^{2+}), which mediates a surge in thrombin generation from prothrombin. Thrombin proteolytically cleaves fibrinogen molecules to generate fibrin monomers, which polymerize into fibrin strands to form a clot. Finally, factor XIII is activated by thrombin and acts to covalently crosslink fibrin strands, producing an insoluble fibrin clot resistant to fibrinolytic degradation.

Regulation of Coagulation

Once activated, regulation of hemostasis proves essential to limit clot propagation beyond the injury site. Four major counterregulatory pathways have been identified that appear particularly important for downregulating hemostasis: fibrinolysis, TFPI, the protein C system, and serine protease inhibitors (SERPINs). The fibrinolytic system comprises a series of amplifying reactions that ultimately convert plasminogen to plasmin, a serine protease, which is responsible for the degradation of fibrin and fibrinogen (Fig. 23.3).[3] In vivo, plasmin generation is most often accomplished by release of tPA or urokinase from the vascular endothelium. Activity of tPA and urokinase is accelerated in the presence of fibrin, thereby limiting fibrinolysis to areas of clot formation. In addition to enzymatic degradation of fibrin and fibrinogen, plasmin inhibits coagulation by degrading essential cofactors V and VIII and reducing platelet glycoprotein surface receptors essential to adhesion and aggregation. As the fibrin clot is broken down, fibrinolytic activity is reduced by the rapid inhibition of free plasmin. Furthermore, excessive fibrinolysis is prevented by the function of two key SERPINs, namely plasmin-activator inhibitor-1 (PAI-1) and α_2-antiplasmin. PAI-1 serves as the primary inhibitor of tPA and urokinase, thereby decreasing plasmin generation, whereas α_2-antiplasmin directly inactivates circulating plasmin.

TFPI binds and inhibits factor Xa through the formation of membrane-bound complexes. These factor Xa–TFPI complexes also act to inhibit TF/factor VIIa

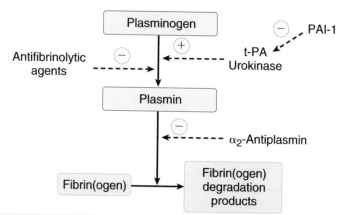

Fig. 23.3 The Fibrinolytic System. A series of amplifying reactions that ultimately convert plasminogen to plasmin, which degrades fibrin and fibrinogen.[3] Tissue plasminogen activator (tPA) and urokinase are principal activators of plasmin in vivo, and their function is reduced plasmin-activator inhibitor-1 (PAI-1), while α_2-antiplasmin directly inactivates circulating plasmin. (From Slaughter TF. The coagulation system and cardiac surgery. In: Estafanous FG, Barasch PG, Reves JG, eds. *Cardiac Anesthesia*: Principles and Clinical Practice. 2nd ed. Philadelphia: Lippincott Williams & Wilkins; 2001: 320.)

complexes, thereby downregulating the extrinsic coagulation pathway. The protein C system proves particularly important in regulating coagulation through inhibition of thrombin and the essential cofactors Va and VIIIa. After binding to thrombomodulin on the surface of the endothelial cell, thrombin's procoagulant function decreases and instead its ability to activate protein C is augmented. Activated protein C (APC), complexed with the cofactor protein S, degrades both factors Va and VIIIa. Loss of these critical cofactors limits formation of tenase and prothrombinase complexes essential to formation of factor Xa and thrombin, respectively. One of the most significant SERPINs regulating hemostasis is antithrombin (AT, formerly antithrombin III). AT inhibits thrombin in addition to factors IXa, Xa, XIa, and XIIa. Heparin binds AT, causing a conformational change that accelerates AT-mediated inhibition of targeted enzymes by over 100-fold.

BLEEDING DISORDERS

Certain hereditary or acquired disorders, systemic diseases, and environmental conditions can predispose a patient to excessive bleeding after tissue injury, including surgery. Given the complexity of the hemostatic system, bleeding can result from defects in or deficiency of coagulation factors, platelets, fibrinolysis, and vascular integrity. Patients with less than 20% to 30% of normal coagulation factor activity or platelet counts of less than 50,000/μL are more likely than patients with normal values to have uncontrolled intraoperative bleeding. Bleeding diatheses vary in clinical presentation depending on what component of the hemostatic system is affected.

Inherited Bleeding Disorders

Von Willebrand Disease
Inherited disorders of hemostasis include those involving platelet quantity and function, coagulation factor deficiencies, or disorders of fibrinolytic pathways. Among these inherited bleeding disorders, von Willebrand disease (vWD) is the most common, affecting up to 1% of the population. vWD is categorized into three main types (type 1, 2, and 3), with most cases demonstrating an autosomal dominant inheritance pattern (Table 23.1). vWF is synthesized by megakaryocytes and endothelial cells and once released from these cells, it circulates as a series of multimers formed from a basic dimer subunit. Under normal conditions vWF plays a critical role in platelet adhesion to the ECM and prevents degradation of factor VIII by serving as a carrier molecule. vWD is characterized by quantitative or qualitative deficiencies of vWF resulting in defective platelet adhesion and aggregation. Classically, patients with vWD describe a history of easy bruising, recurrent epistaxis, and menorrhagia, which are

characteristic of defects in platelet-mediated hemostasis. In more severe cases (i.e., type 3 vWD), concomitant reductions in factor VIII may lead to serious spontaneous hemorrhage, including hemarthroses.

Routine coagulation studies are generally not helpful in the diagnosis of vWD, as the platelet count and prothrombin time (PT) will be normal in most patients and the activated partial thromboplastin time (aPTT) may demonstrate mild-to-moderate prolongation depending on the level of factor VIII reduction. Initial screening tests for vWD involve measurement of vWF levels (vWF antigen) and vWF platelet binding activity in the presence of the ristocetin cofactor, which leads to platelet agglutination. Mild cases of vWD often respond to desmopressin acetate (DDAVP), which results in the release of vWF from endothelial cells. Use of vWF:factor VIII concentrates (e.g., Humate-P) may be indicated in the perioperative period if there is a significant bleeding history.[4]

Hemophilias
Hemophilia A (factor VIII deficiency) and hemophilia B (factor IX deficiency) are both X-linked inherited bleeding disorders most frequently presenting in childhood as spontaneous hemorrhage involving joints and/or deep muscles. Hemophilia A is more common with an incidence of 1:5000 males, whereas hemophilia B occurs in 1:30,000 males. The severity of the disease is dependent on an individual's baseline factor activity level. Severe disease, defined by less than 1% of coagulation factor activity, occurs in approximately two-thirds of patients with hemophilia A and one half of patients with hemophilia B. Classically, laboratory testing in patients with hemophilia reveals prolongation of the aPTT, whereas the PT, bleeding time, and platelet count remain within normal limits. However, a normal aPTT may also be seen in mild forms of hemophilia, and it is important to exclude vWD as a cause of factor VIII deficiency.

An increasingly common complication of hemophilia is the development of alloantibodies to factors VIII or IX, which block exogenous factor activity. This can occur in up to 30% of patients with severe hemophilia A and 3% to 5% of those with severe hemophilia B. Several approaches to reduce bleeding in these patients include substitution of porcine factor VIII, administration of activated factor VIII bypass activity (FEIBA) or nonactivated prothrombin complex concentrates (PCCs), or treatment with recombinant factor VIIa (rFVIIa).

Other Factor Deficiencies
Less common inherited factor deficiencies include deficiencies of factors VII, XI, XII, and XIII. Factor VII deficiency (prevalence: 1 in 500,000) most commonly presents with excessive bleeding after invasive procedures; heavy menstrual bleeding; or mucosal tract, joint, and muscle bleeding. Bleeding is uncommon with factor VII activity levels >10% and can be managed with

Table 23.1 Classification of von Willebrand Disease

Type	Characteristic	Inheritance	Prevalence	Diagnosis	Treatment
1	Partial quantitative deficiency of VWF	AD	Up to 1%	↓ vWF:Ag	DDAVP
				↓ vWF:RCo	FVIII/vWF concentrate
2	Qualitative defect of vWF (subtypes below)				
2A	↓ binding of vWF to platelets	AD	Uncommon	↓ vWF:Ag	DDAVP
				↓↓↓ vWF:RCo	FVIII/vWF concentrate
	↓ large multimers			↓ large multimers	
2B	↑ binding of vWF to platelets	AD	Uncommon	↑↑↑ LD-RIPA	FVIII/vWF concentrate
	↓ large multimers				
2M	↓ vWF function despite normal large multimers	AD	Uncommon	↓ vWF:Ag	DDAVP
				↓↓ vWF:RCo	FVIII/vWF concentrate
				↓ RIPA	
2N	↓ binding of VWF to FVIII	AR	Uncommon	↓↓ FVIII	DDAVP
					FVIII/vWF concentrate
3	Absent vWF	AR	Rare (1:250,000–1:1,000,000)	Absent vWF:Ag	FVIII/vWF concentrate
					Factor VIII concentrate
					Platelet transfusion

AD, Autosomal dominant; *AR*, autosomal recessive; *DDAVP*, desmopressin acetate; *FVIII*, coagulation factor VIII; *LD-RIPA*, low-dose ristocetin-induced platelet aggregation; *RIPA*, ristocetin-induced platelet aggregation; *vWF*, von Willebrand factor; *vWF:Ag*, von Willebrand factor antigen; *vWF:RCo*, von Willebrand factor ristocetin cofactor activity; ↓, ↓↓, ↓↓↓, relative decrease; ↑, ↑↑, ↑↑↑ relative increase.
Adapted from Nichols WL et al. von Willebrand disease (VWD): Evidence-based diagnosis and management guidelines, the National Heart, Lung, and Blood Institute (NHLBI) Expert Panel report (USA). *Haemophilia*. 2008;14(2):171-232, Table 5 and Figure 5.

rFVIIa. Factor XI deficiency, known as *hemophilia C* or *Rosenthal syndrome* (prevalence: 1 in 1,000,000), is characterized by isolated prolongation in aPTT and variable bleeding severity. Factor XI activity levels, however, do not correlate well with bleeding risk.[5] Most individuals do not experience spontaneous bleeding, hemarthrosis, or muscle hematomas, though bleeding episodes can occur under situations of hemostatic challenge such as trauma, surgery, or childbirth. Factor XII deficiency (prevalence: 1 in 1,000,000) can cause marked prolongation of aPTT but is associated with clotting rather than bleeding. Factor XIII is involved in stabilizing the fibrin clot. Factor XIII deficiency (prevalence: 1 in 2,000,000) presents with delayed bleeding after hemostasis, impaired wound healing, and, occasionally, pregnancy loss. Laboratory evaluation in these patients will demonstrate normal aPTT and PT, but the diagnosis can be confirmed by measurement of factor XIII activity levels.

Acquired Bleeding Disorders

Drug Induced

Medications represent the most significant cause of acquired coagulopathy in perioperative patients. In addition to anticoagulants such as heparin and warfarin, the increasing number of direct oral anticoagulants (DOACs) and antiplatelet drugs has further complicated perioperative management. Additionally, several classes of medications may unintentionally increase bleeding risk because of side effects, primarily through inhibition of platelet aggregation. These drugs include β-lactam antibiotics, nitroprusside, nitroglycerin, nitric oxide, and selective serotonin reuptake inhibitors (SSRIs), all of which can result in clinically significant bleeding in individuals with higher baseline risk. These medications should be considered in patients with an otherwise unexplained coagulopathy.

Vitamin K Deficiency

Vitamin K is an essential fat-soluble vitamin that is required for the carboxylation of factors II, VII, IX, and X and proteins C and S. Without carboxylation, these factors cannot bind to the phospholipid membrane of platelets and participate in hemostasis. Vitamin K is present in dietary sources (leafy greens) and also synthesized by bacteria in the gastrointestinal tract. Patients who are fasting, have poor dietary intake, or are receiving total parenteral nutrition and those with fat malabsorption (obstructive jaundice, intestinal ileus or obstruction, or bowel resection) are prone to vitamin K deficiency. As gut microbiota are a source of vitamin K, newborns, who have not yet developed normal microbiota, and patients undergoing oral antibiotic therapy are also susceptible to vitamin K deficiency.

Liver Disease

The liver is the primary site for production of procoagulant factors, including fibrinogen; prothrombin (factor II); factors V, VII, IX, X, XI, and XII; the anticoagulants protein C and S; and AT. Severe liver disease impairs synthesis of coagulation factors, produces quantitative and qualitative platelet dysfunction, and impedes clearance of activated clotting and fibrinolytic proteins. Laboratory findings commonly associated with liver disease include a prolonged PT and possible prolongation of the aPTT, suggesting that these individuals are at increased risk of bleeding. However, these abnormal values only reflect decreases in procoagulant factors and do not account for parallel decreases in anticoagulant factors (protein C, protein S, and AT). As a result, patients with chronic liver disease are thought to have a rebalanced hemostasis and actually generate amounts of thrombin equivalent to healthy individuals.[6]

Similarly, thrombocytopenia from platelet sequestration in the spleen is often observed in patients with liver disease and portal hypertension. However, levels of the plasma metalloprotease ADAMTS13, responsible for cleaving vWF multimers, are also decreased in chronic liver disease and result in high circulating levels of large vWF multimers, which promote platelet aggregation. Consequently, this increase in vWF may partially correct for thrombocytopenia and platelet dysfunction but can also result in a prothrombotic state and increase clotting risk.

Fibrinolysis of a formed clot is also aberrant in patients with liver disease. Excessive fibrinolysis is prevented by thrombin-activatable fibrinolysis inhibitor (TAFI), which blocks activation of plasmin from plasminogen. TAFI is synthesized by the liver, and because levels are decreased in patients with chronic liver disease, it was believed that such individuals are at increased bleeding risk because of hyperfibrinolysis. However, levels of PAI-1, an inhibitor of tPA and urokinase, are also increased in liver disease and may serve to normalize fibrinolytic activity. Thus, in patients with chronic liver disease, hemostatic mechanisms are rebalanced, but decreases in procoagulant and anticoagulant factors create a tenuous equilibrium that is easily disrupted. As a result, these patients are at risk for both bleeding and inappropriate clotting.

Renal Disease

Platelet dysfunction commonly occurs in association with chronic renal failure and uremia and has primarily been attributed to decreased platelet aggregation and adhesion to injured vessel walls. Impaired adhesion is likely the result of defects of glycoprotein IIb/IIIa, which facilitates platelet binding of fibrinogen and vWF. Additionally, accumulation of guanidinosuccinic acid and the resulting increase in endothelial nitric oxide synthesis further decrease platelet responsiveness. Red blood cell (RBC) concentration has also been suggested to contribute to impaired platelet activity, as correction of anemia shortens bleeding times. This is thought to be the result of the increased RBC mass displacing platelets from the center of the vessel and bringing them into close proximity of the endothelium, thereby promoting adhesion.

Disseminated Intravascular Coagulation

Disseminated intravascular coagulation (DIC) is a pathologic hemostatic response to TF/factor VIIa complex that leads to excessive activation of the extrinsic pathway, which overwhelms natural anticoagulant mechanisms and generates intravascular thrombin. Numerous underlying disorders may precipitate DIC, including sepsis, trauma, amniotic fluid embolus, malignancy, or incompatible blood transfusions (Table 23.2). Most often, DIC presents clinically as a diffuse bleeding disorder associated with consumption of coagulation factors and platelets during widespread microvascular thrombotic activity resulting in multiorgan dysfunction. Laboratory findings typical of DIC include reductions in platelet count; prolongation of the PT, aPTT, and thrombin time (TT); and elevated concentrations of soluble fibrin and fibrin degradation products (D-dimers). However, DIC is both a clinical and laboratory diagnosis, so laboratory data alone do not provide sufficient sensitivity or specificity to confirm a diagnosis.

Cardiopulmonary Bypass–Associated Coagulopathy

Institution of cardiopulmonary bypass (CPB) by directing blood flow through an extracorporeal circuit causes significant perturbations to the hemostatic system.[7] Initial priming of the bypass circuit results in hemodilution and thrombocytopenia. Adhesion of platelets to the synthetic surfaces of the bypass circuit further decreases platelet counts and contributes to platelet dysfunction. During CPB, expression of platelet surface receptors important for adhesion and aggregation (GPIb, GPIIb/IIIa) are downregulated and the number of vWF-containing α-granules are decreased, thereby impairing platelet function. Furthermore, induced hypothermia during CPB results in reduced platelet aggregation and plasma-mediated coagulation by decreasing clotting factor production and enzymatic activity. Increased plasmin generation may also occur during CPB, a process that accelerates clot lysis. Thus, antifibrinolytic drugs are often administered to decrease intraoperative blood loss.

PREOPERATIVE AND INTRAOPERATIVE MANAGEMENT

Table 23.2 Conditions Associated With Disseminated Intravascular Coagulation

Category	Conditions
Infections	Bacterial (gram-negative bacilli, gram-positive cocci) Viral (CMV, EBV, HIV, VZV, hepatitis) Fungal (histoplasma) Parasites (malaria)
Malignancy	Hematologic (AML) Solid tumors (prostate cancer, pancreatic cancer) Malignant tumors (mucin-secreting adenocarcinoma)
Obstetric causes	Amniotic fluid embolism Preeclampsia/eclampsia Placental abruption Acute fatty liver of pregnancy Intrauterine fetal demise
Massive inflammation	Severe trauma Burns Traumatic brain injury Crush injury Severe pancreatitis
Toxic/immunologic	Snake envenomation Massive transfusion ABO blood type incompatibility Graft versus host disease
Other	Liver disease/fulminant hepatic failure Vascular disease (aortic aneurysms, giant hemangiomas) Ventricular assist devices

AML, Acute myelogenous leukemia; *CMV*, cytomegalovirus; *EBV*, Epstein-Barr virus; *HIV*, human immunodeficiency virus; *VZV*, varicella zoster virus.
From Huddleston LL, Liu LL. Hemostasis. In Miller RD, Pardo MC, eds. *Basics of Anesthesia*. 7th ed. Philadelphia: Elsevier; 2018. Table 22.2.

Trauma-Induced Coagulopathy (also see Chapter 43)

Uncontrolled hemorrhage is a frequent cause of trauma-related deaths. Coagulopathy in this setting may be the result of acidosis, hypothermia, and hemodilution from resuscitation; however, an independent trauma-induced coagulopathy (TIC) is also experienced by these individuals.[8] The anticoagulant effect of APC is thought to play a primary role in TIC by decreasing thrombin generation via inhibition of factor Va and VIIIa and promoting fibrinolysis through inhibition of PAI-1. Hypoperfusion subsequent to traumatic injury is thought to be the stimulus for APC activation. Additionally, tissue damage results in shedding of the endothelial glycocalyx (EG), a gel-like matrix with anticoagulant properties that lines the vascular endothelium. The EG contains proteoglycans such as syndecan-1, hyaluronic acid, heparan sulfate, and chondroitin sulfate, that when shed during endothelial injury, result in an "autoheparinization" phenomenon that contributes to TIC. Impaired platelet responsiveness also contributes to increased bleeding in TIC. Although platelet counts appear to be normal, response to various agonists, including ADP, arachidonic acid (AA), and collagen, is reduced and thought to be the result of "platelet exhaustion" resulting from activation caused by widespread release of ADP from injured tissues. This diffuse activation renders platelets unresponsive to subsequent stimulation. Platelet insensitivity to ADP is also associated with increased susceptibility of clots to tPA-mediated fibrinolysis. The importance of early treatment to reduce hyperfibrinolysis in trauma is supported by the findings of the Clinical Randomisation of an Antifibrinolytic in Significant Haemorrhage 2 (CRASH-2) trial, which demonstrated a mortality benefit from early administration of the antifibrinolytic tranexamic acid.[9]

Treatment of Bleeding Disorders

von Willebrand Disease

Mild cases of vWD often respond to DDAVP, which causes the release of vWF from endothelial cells. One dose of DDAVP (0.3 µg/kg IV) will produce a complete or near-complete response in the majority of patients with type 1 vWD. DDAVP is contraindicated in type 2B vWD, as it may precipitate thrombocytopenia, which could worsen bleeding. In the setting of more significant surgical bleeding, use of plasma-derived vWF:factor VIII concentrate (Humate-P) or recombinant vWF (Vonvendi) is indicated. If vWF concentrates are not available, cryoprecipitate, which contains high levels of vWF, can be used, but its use is considered second line, as most cryoprecipitate has not undergone the pathogen inactivation processes used in preparing vWF concentrates.

Hemophilia

In most cases, perioperative management of patients with hemophilia A or B necessitates consultation with a hematologist and administration of recombinant or purified factor VIII or factor IX concentrates, respectively. Mild cases of hemophilia A may be treated with desmopressin. An increasingly common complication of hemophilia, particularly in the case of hemophilia A, has been the development of alloantibodies directed against the factor VIII protein. Administration of factor VIII concentrates will fail to control bleeding in patients with high-titer antibodies. Several approaches to reduce bleeding in these patients include substitution of porcine factor VIII, administration of activated FEIBA or nonactivated PCCs, or treatment with rFVIIa.

Disseminated Intravascular Coagulation

Management of DIC requires correction of the underlying condition precipitating hemostatic activation. Otherwise, treatment is mostly supportive and includes selective blood component transfusions to replete coagulation factors and platelets consumed in the process. The use of anticoagulants such as heparin remains controversial with recommendations that its use be limited to conditions with the highest thrombotic risk. Antifibrinolytic therapy generally is contraindicated in DIC owing to the potential for catastrophic thrombotic complications.

Platelet Disorders

In the nonbleeding patient, treatment of thrombocytopenia in the form of platelet transfusion is usually withheld until the platelet count is less than 10,000/μL. In the patient who is actively bleeding or requires surgical intervention, platelet transfusion is recommended to a goal of 50,000/μL, or in some cases, such as intracranial hemorrhage or neurosurgery, 100,000/μL.[10] Individuals who receive repeated platelet transfusions are at increased risk of forming antibodies to human leukocyte antigens (HLAs) or human platelet antigens. If such platelet alloimmunization develops, transfusion of standard platelet units may not increase platelet counts appropriately and use of HLA-matched units may be required.

Treatment of platelet dysfunction related to chronic renal disease includes administration of DDAVP (0.3 μg/kg IV), which stimulates release of vWF from endothelial cells. Additionally, conjugated estrogens (0.6 mg/kg/day intravenously for 5 days) have been demonstrated to shorten bleeding times, perhaps via decreased generation of nitric oxide. Transfusion of cryoprecipitate (rich in vWF and fibrinogen) may also be used to correct uremic platelet dysfunction; however, its use is often limited to patients with life-threatening bleeding because of the risks associated with transfusion of allogeneic blood products.

PROTHROMBOTIC STATES

Thrombophilia, a propensity for thrombotic events, commonly manifests clinically in the form of venous thrombosis (deep venous thrombosis [DVT] or pulmonary embolus [PE]). The pathogenesis of thrombosis is thought to be caused by the Virchow triad (blood stasis, endothelial injury, and hypercoagulability).[11] In the majority of cases, a risk factor or precipitating event is identified; however, a single factor generally does not result in clinically significant thrombosis. Instead, multiple factors act synergistically to increase risk. For example, thrombotic complications often occur after surgery or during pregnancy in association with an inherited thrombophilia; underlying malignancy; or other clinical risk factors such as obesity, smoking, or oral contraceptive use.

Inherited Thrombotic Disorders

Factor V Leiden and Prothrombin Gene Mutation

Because of more specific testing, an inheritable thrombotic predisposition is identified in as many as 50% of patients presenting with venous thromboembolism (VTE). The most common inherited prothrombotic conditions include single-point mutations in genes for factor V (factor V Leiden) or prothrombin (prothrombin G20210A). In the case of factor V Leiden, the mutation results in APC resistance whereby factor Va is no longer susceptible to APC-mediated degradation. This inability of APC to counterregulate the coagulation system results in a prothrombotic state that is found in approximately 5% of the Caucasian population. The prothrombin G20210A gene mutation causes increased plasma concentrations of prothrombin resulting in a hypercoagulable state. Individuals with factor V Leiden or the prothrombin gene mutation are at increased risk of developing DVTs, with homozygotes having the highest risk. Despite the increased relative risk, the absolute risk of blood clots in these patients remains low in the absence of other risk factors for hypercoagulability.

Protein C and Protein S Deficiency

Protein C deficiency is an autosomal dominant trait affecting approximately 1 in 500 individuals in the general population. Deficiency can be the result of reduced concentrations or function of protein C and may result in VTE, warfarin-induced skin necrosis, neonatal purpura (in homozygous neonates), and fetal loss.

As discussed earlier, protein S functions as a cofactor of protein C and functions to accelerate APC's ability to inactivate factors Va and VIIIa. Individuals with protein S deficiency present similarly to those with other inherited thrombophilias and are at increased risk of VTE and PE.

Both protein C and protein S deficiencies can be acquired secondary to underlying disease. Acquired protein C deficiency can be seen in DIC, liver disease, severe infection (especially meningococcemia), uremia, and those on vitamin K antagonist (VKA) anticoagulation. Acquired protein S deficiency has been associated with pregnancy, oral contraceptive use, DIC, human immunodeficiency virus (HIV) infection, nephrotic syndrome, and liver disease.

Acquired Thrombotic Disorders

Antiphospholipid Syndrome

Antiphospholipid syndrome (APS) describes an acquired autoimmune disorder characterized by venous and/or arterial thromboses and recurrent pregnancy loss. This syndrome may occur in association with autoimmune disorders such as systemic lupus erythematosus or rheumatoid arthritis, or it may occur in isolation. APS results from development of autoantibodies directed against phospholipid-binding proteins, which affect the coagulation system, and is associated with up to 10% of cases of DVT and 6% of cases of pregnancy-associated morbidity. In rare instances, a severe form of APS, termed *catastrophic APS*, can occur resulting in coagulopathy, ischemic necrosis of the extremities, and multiorgan failure and is associated with a mortality rate of up to 30%.[12]

Characteristically, APS results in mild prolongation of the aPTT and positive testing for antiphospholipid antibodies (aPLs), such as lupus anticoagulant, anticardiolipin, or anti-β_2-glycoprotein I antibodies. aPLs interfere with phospholipids common to many laboratory-based tests of coagulation. However, despite the prolonged aPTT, APS poses no increased bleeding risk. Instead, patients have greater risk for thrombosis. Isolated prolongation of an aPTT in a preoperative patient merits consideration of the diagnosis of APS. Patients with this syndrome who have experienced a thrombotic complication are at increased risk for recurrent thrombosis and most often are managed by lifelong anticoagulation.

Heparin-Induced Thrombocytopenia

Heparin-induced thrombocytopenia (HIT) describes an autoimmune-mediated drug reaction occurring in as many as 5% of patients receiving heparin therapy.[13] Patients with HIT experience a mild to moderate thrombocytopenia. However, unlike other drug-induced thrombocytopenias, HIT results in platelet activation and increased risk of venous and arterial thromboses. Evidence suggests that HIT is mediated by immunoglobulin G (IgG) antibodies, which bind to platelet factor 4 (PF4). Complexes composed of antibody, PF4, and heparin bind to platelet Fcγ receptors, thereby activating them. Risk factors for the development of HIT include patient population, gender, and heparin formulation used. Women are at increased risk of HIT, as are patients undergoing major surgical procedures compared with medical patients. Additionally, use of unfractionated heparin (UFH) carries a greater risk of HIT development than low-molecular-weight heparin (LMWH).

HIT manifests clinically as thrombocytopenia occurring 5 to 14 days after initiating heparin therapy. With prior heparin exposure, thrombocytopenia or thrombosis may occur within 1 day. A diagnosis of HIT should be considered for any patient experiencing thrombosis or thrombocytopenia (absolute or relative ≥50% reduction in platelet count) during or after heparin administration. Although HIT remains a clinical diagnosis, HIT antibody testing should be undertaken to confirm the diagnosis. The enzyme-linked immunosorbent assay (ELISA) is sensitive, but not as specific as the serotonin release assay (SRA), because the SRA indicates heparin-induced platelet activation. For many intensive care unit (ICU) patients, a positive ELISA test does not lead to a positive SRA, which means these patients are unlikely to have HIT.

Treatment of Thrombotic Disorders

Inherited Thrombophilias

Inherited thrombophilias are relatively rare in the general population, and screening for the presence of these diseases in the absence of VTE is not recommended. In the absence of coexisting precipitating conditions, presence of a family history, or history of thrombosis, risks associated with long-term preventive anticoagulation may outweigh potential benefits. Patients who present with VTE and test positive for an inherited thrombophilia are anticoagulated for their acute presentation. Continuation of anticoagulation after resolution of acute VTE is determined by severity of presentation, presence of more than one thrombophilia, and homozygosity or heterozygosity for thrombophilia.[14] In the case of pregnant patients with known thrombophilia, anticoagulation is often recommended in the antepartum and postpartum setting.

Antiphospholipid Syndrome

Patients with APS who have experienced a thrombotic complication are at increased risk for recurrent thrombosis and most often are managed by lifelong anticoagulation. Standard treatments involve VKAs, such as warfarin, and aspirin may be added for patients who experience arterial thromboses. Individuals who are or may become pregnant are commonly treated with LMWH during the antepartum period.[15]

Heparin-Induced Thrombocytopenia

In cases where HIT is suspected, heparin must be discontinued immediately (including UFH, LMWH, heparin-bonded catheters, and heparin flushes). Alternative nonheparin anticoagulation must be administered concurrently, as patients who develop HIT are at risk of thrombosis and may also require anticoagulation for the condition for which heparin was originally administered. In most cases, a direct thrombin inhibitor (e.g., bivalirudin, lepirudin, or argatroban) is substituted for heparin until adequate prolongation of the international normalized ratio (INR) can be achieved with warfarin. Initiation of warfarin alone is contraindicated for HIT treatment because the initial decreased synthesis of proteins C and S enhances the patient's prothrombotic state. Platelet transfusions should be held unless the patient is severely thrombocytopenic ($<20 \times 10^9$/L) with signs of bleeding. Use of DOACs (e.g., rivaroxaban, apixaban, dabigatran, edoxaban) is being investigated.[16] If possible, patients experiencing HIT should avoid future exposure to UFH; however, several reports describe subsequent limited perioperative re-exposure to UFH after laboratory testing ensures an absence of PF4/heparin immune complexes.

LABORATORY EVALUATION OF HEMOSTASIS

Preoperative Evaluation

The perioperative period presents significant challenges to the hemostatic system; therefore, identification and correction of hemostatic disorders can be of vital

Table 23.3 Common Tests of Hemostasis and Normal Ranges

Platelet Tests	Coagulation Tests	Fibrinolysis Tests
Count: 150–400 K/uL	Prothrombin time: 11.5–14.7 sec[a]	Thrombin time: 14.7–18.0 sec
Bleeding time: <11 min	Activated partial thromboplastin time: 23.8–35.7 sec[a]	Fibrinogen-fibrin degradation products: <5 µg/dL
Aggregometry (response to aggregating agents: collagen, adenosine diphosphate, epinephrine, and ristocetin)	Anti-factor Xa activity (calibrated to specific anticoagulant medication)	Fibrin D-dimer assay: <250 µg/mL
Platelet function analysis	Fibrinoge: 234–395 mg/dL	
Collagen/epinephrine: 94–193 sec	Activated clotting time: 70–140 sec	
Collagen/adenosine diphosphate: 71–118 sec		

From Huddleston LL, Liu LL. Hemostasis. In Miller RD, Pardo MC, eds. *Basics of Anesthesia*. 7th ed. Philadelphia: Elsevier; 2018. Table 22.3.
[a]The normal range varies with reagent lots.

importance. Unfortunately, assessment of bleeding risk continues to be a challenge, and the optimal methods for preoperative evaluation remain controversial. Although routine preoperative coagulation testing of all surgical patients may seem prudent, such an approach is costly and lacks predictive value for the detection of hemostatic abnormalities. Standard coagulation tests such as PT and aPTT were designed as diagnostic tests to be used when a bleeding disorder is suspected based on clinical evaluation (Table 23.3). As a result, when used as screening tests, these in vitro assays are limited in their ability to reflect the in vivo hemostatic response.[17]

Consequently, a carefully performed bleeding history remains the single most effective predictor of perioperative bleeding. In particular, patients should be asked whether they have experienced excessive bleeding after hemostatic challenges such as dental extractions, surgery, trauma, or childbirth and whether blood transfusions or reoperation were required to control the bleeding. Common presentations suggestive of a bleeding disorder may include frequent epistaxis necessitating nasal packing or surgical intervention. Oral surgery and dental extractions prove particularly good tests of hemostasis because of increased fibrinolytic activity on the mucous membranes of the oral cavity. Women with platelet disorders or vWD may experience menorrhagia, and postpartum hemorrhage commonly occurs in those with underlying disorders of hemostasis. A careful medication history, including direct questions relating to consumption of aspirin and nonsteroidal antiinflammatory drugs (NSAIDs), in addition to supplements such as ginkgo and vitamin E, should be included.[18]

For most patients, a thoughtfully conducted bleeding history will eliminate the need for preoperative laboratory-based coagulation testing. Should the preoperative history or physical examination reveal signs or symptoms suggestive of a bleeding disorder, further laboratory testing is indicated. Preoperative coagulation screening tests may be indicated, despite a negative history, in cases in which the planned surgery is commonly associated with significant bleeding (e.g., CPB). Finally, preoperative testing may prove justified in settings in which the patient is unable to provide an adequate preoperative bleeding history. Should evidence of a bleeding disorder be detected, underlying etiologies should be clarified if possible before proceeding with surgery.

Laboratory-Based Measures of Coagulation

Prothrombin Time

PT assesses the integrity of the extrinsic and common pathways of plasma-mediated hemostasis. It measures time required in seconds for fibrin clot formation to occur after mixing a sample of patient plasma with TF (thromboplastin) and calcium. It is sensitive to deficiencies in fibrinogen and factors II, V, VII, or X. As three of these factors have vitamin K–dependent synthesis (factors II, VII, and X), the PT assay has been used to monitor anticoagulation with VKAs such as warfarin. Heparin, LMWH, and fondaparinux inhibit thrombin and therefore should prolong the PT. However, most PT reagents contain heparin-binding chemicals that block this effect; thus, the PT remains normal in the setting of these medications.

The thromboplastin reagent, derived from animal or recombinant sources, can vary in its ability to bind factor VII and initiate coagulation, which limits interlaboratory comparisons. Given the importance of monitoring PT results for patients on long-term warfarin therapy, the INR was introduced by the World Health Organization as a means of normalizing PT results among different laboratories.

Any prolongation of the PT should be assessed further with mixing studies to determine whether delayed clot formation is attributable to a coagulation factor deficiency or an inhibitor (i.e., APL, fibrin degradation products). The mixing study is performed by mixing the patient's plasma sample with "normal" donor plasma. In the case of a coagulation factor deficiency, time to clot formation will correct, whereas it will remain prolonged in the presence of an inhibitor.

Activated Partial Thromboplastin Time

aPTT assesses integrity of the intrinsic and common pathways of plasma-mediated hemostasis. It measures the time required in seconds for fibrin clot formation to occur after mixing a sample of patient plasma with phospholipid, calcium, and an activator of the intrinsic pathway of coagulation (e.g., celite, kaolin, silica, or ellagic acid). It can detect low levels of prekallikrein; high-molecular-weight kininogen; factors XII, XI, IX, and VIII (intrinsic pathway); and low levels of factors II, V, and X and fibrinogen (common pathway). The aPTT is more sensitive to deficiencies in factors VIII and IX than other factors in the intrinsic and common pathways. In most cases, coagulation factor levels below 30% to 40% of normal are detectable; however, aPTT reagents vary in their sensitivity and may not be prolonged until levels drop below 15% for some factors. Both hemophilias A and B and vWD (because of potentially low levels of factor VIII) will prolong aPTT. UFH therapy and anticoagulation with parenteral direct thrombin inhibitors (DTIs) (e.g., argatroban) are monitored with aPTT levels. Unlike with the PT assay, there is no reference standard reagent for the aPTT, so individual institutions must set their own normal ranges, and aPTT values cannot be compared between laboratories.

Anti-Factor Xa Activity

The anti–factor Xa activity assay or factor Xa inhibition test is being used with increasing frequency to monitor heparin anticoagulation instead of, or in addition to, the aPTT assay. The assay involves combining patient plasma with reagent factor Xa and an artificial substrate that releases a colorimetric signal after factor Xa cleavage, thereby providing a functional assessment of heparin anticoagulant effect. Although aPTT values can be affected by several patient factors such as coagulation factor deficiencies, factor inhibitors, or the presence of lupus anticoagulant, measurement of the heparin-bound AT inhibition of factor Xa activity is not influenced by these variables. Anti–factor Xa testing can also be used to measure the effect of other anticoagulants such as LMWH, fondaparinux, and factor Xa inhibitors. Data supporting the use of anti–factor Xa over aPTT is sparse; however, it may be helpful to use anti–factor Xa testing in combination with the aPTT to monitor heparin effect.[19]

Thrombin Time

The TT measures the final step of the clotting pathway where fibrinogen is converted to fibrin. It measures the time required in seconds for fibrin clot formation to occur after mixing a sample of patient plasma with calcium and thrombin. Conditions that prolong the thrombin time include therapy with anticoagulants (including heparin and DTIs), hypofibrinogenemia (<100 mg/dL), dysfibrinogenemia (presence of abnormal fibrinogen), DIC, liver disease, high concentrations of serum proteins (multiple myeloma, amyloidosis), and circulating bovine thrombin antibodies (formed after exposure to topical bovine thrombin used for hemostasis during surgery).

Fibrinogen Level

A number of methods are available for measuring fibrinogen. The most common method reports functional fibrinogen activity and incorporates the Clauss method, in which diluted plasma is exposed to a high concentration of thrombin. The time to fibrin clot formation is compared with a standard calibration curve, and the fibrinogen concentration is extrapolated. Immunologic fibrinogen assays are used when clotting-based fibrinogen assays suggest hypofibrinogenemia in the absence of an obvious clinical explanation or when dysfibrinogenemia is suspected.

Tests of Platelet Function

Platelet Count

The platelet count continues to be used as a first-line test of platelet function. A platelet count is determined as part of a complete blood count and is performed by automated machines that use optical, impedance, or flow cytometric methods. Platelet clumping (which results from minimal platelet activation) and the presence of large platelets (as occurs in immune thrombocytopenic purpura) can lead to artificially decreased platelet counts. Conversely, if samples contain cellular debris (e.g., patients with thalassemias, leukemias, thrombotic thrombocytopenic purpura [TTP]), the platelet count may be overestimated by some methods.

Bleeding Time

The bleeding time test was the first in vivo assay of platelet function. To perform the test, a blood pressure cuff is inflated on the upper part of the arm to 40 mm Hg and a standardized 9-mm long and 1-mm deep incision is made on the volar surface of the forearm. Blood is blotted away every 30 seconds with filter paper until bleeding stops. A prolonged bleeding time (>11 minutes) can signify either platelet dysfunction or thrombocytopenia (<100,000/µL). The bleeding time has benefits of assessing natural hemostasis, does not require specialized equipment, and is not susceptible to artifacts from anticoagulant medications. However, the assay is invasive, time consuming, and poorly reproducible. Furthermore, a normal bleeding time does not predict adequate hemostasis during surgery, nor does an abnormal bleeding time predict abnormal surgical bleeding. As a result, the bleeding time may be used to help with diagnosis of inherited platelet disorders, but is not recommended as a preoperative screening test.[20]

Platelet Aggregometry

The technique for platelet aggregometry was developed in the 1960s and soon became the gold standard for assessment of platelet function. The classic method involves centrifugation of patient blood to obtain platelet-rich plasma, which is then analyzed in a cuvette at 37°C placed between a light source and photocell. Addition of platelet agonists such as ADP, epinephrine, collagen, and ristocetin stimulate platelet aggregation, which in turn results in a decrease in turbidity of the solution and an increase in light transmission. Newer systems involve the use of platinum electrodes upon which aggregated platelets adhere, thereby increasing impedance that is measured over time. Patterns based upon the kinetics and amplitude of response to these various agonists are associated with specific platelet disorders (e.g., Glanzmann thrombasthenia, Bernard–Soulier syndrome, vWD) and aid in their diagnosis. Platelet aggregometry can also be used for monitoring antiplatelet therapy.

Point-of-Care Measures of Coagulation

Although laboratory-based measures of coagulation remain the mainstay of preoperative coagulation testing, increasing availability of sensitive and specific point-of-care coagulation monitoring may soon offer opportunities to direct blood component and hemostatic drug therapy more specifically without the delays inherent to standard laboratory testing.

Activated Clotting Time

ACT measures the time in seconds for formation of a clot after a contact activation initiator (e.g., celite, kaolin) is added to a sample of freshly drawn whole blood. Because the ACT measures fibrin clot formation by way of intrinsic and common pathways, heparin and other anticoagulants prolong time to clot formation. Although the aPTT assay has replaced it in most clinical situations, the ACT's simplicity, low cost, and linear response at high heparin concentrations make it a popular perioperative coagulation monitor during surgical cases requiring high doses of heparin (e.g., cardiac and vascular surgery).

Viscoelastic Measures of Coagulation

Viscoelastic monitors measure the entire spectrum of clot formation in whole blood from early fibrin strand generation through clot retraction and fibrinolysis. The early thromboelastograph (TEG) developed by Hartert in 1948 has evolved into two independent viscoelastic

monitors available today: the modern TEG5000 and rotational thromboelastometry (ROTEM). In the case of TEG, a small (0.35 mL) sample of whole blood is placed into a rotating cup. A sensor pin is lowered into the cup, and as the fibrin clot begins to form, the pin meets increased resistance and begins to rotate with the cup. This movement is transferred via the pin to an attached torsion wire and electronic recorder (Fig. 23.4). A similar mechanism of movement and detection is employed in the ROTEM; however, in this system the cup remains stationary and the pin rotates. More recently, alternative viscoelastic measurement devices have been developed (Sonoclot Analyzer and TEG6s) in which a rapidly vibrating probe is immersed into a small sample of whole blood. As clot formation proceeds, impedance to probe movement increases, which in turn generates an electrical signal and characteristic clot signature.

Although variables derived from viscoelastic tracings do not coincide directly with laboratory-based tests of coagulation, various parameters describing clot formation and lysis are identified and measured (Fig. 23.5). Improvements in technique have led to easier use and the ability to perform point-of-care testing with rapid results. The addition of various trigger reagents provides further information on the extrinsic pathway, levels of fibrinogen, effects or presence of heparin, and resistance to lysis. Although viscoelastic monitors may detect

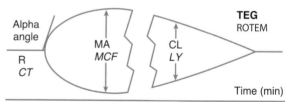

Variable	TEG	ROTEM
From start to 2-mm amplitude (clot initiation)	R (reaction time)	CT (clotting time)
From 2-mm to 20-mm amplitude (clot kinetics)	K (kinetics)	CFT (clot formation time)
Alpha angle	Slope between R and K	Angle of tangent at 2-mm amplitude
Maximum strength (clot strength)	MA (maximum amplitude)	MCF (maximum clotting time)
Clot lysis (at minutes)	CL 30, CL 60	LY 30, LY 60

Fig. 23.4 Measurements Derived From Viscoelastic Testing. Comparison of common variables for the global coagulation assays *TEG* (thromboelastography) and *ROTEM* (rotational thromboelastometry). *CL,* Clot lysis; *LY,* lysis. (From Huddleston LL, Liu LL. Hemostasis. In Miller RD, Pardo MC, eds. *Basics of Anesthesia.* 7th ed. Philadelphia: Elsevier; 2018. Figure 22.2.)

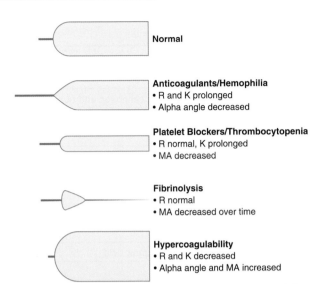

Fig. 23.5 Interpretation of Viscoelastic Tracings. Common thromboelastography examples with analysis. *K*, Kinetics; *MA*, maximum amplitude; *R*, reaction time. (From Huddleston LL, Liu LL. Hemostasis. In Miller RD, Pardo MC, eds. *Basics of Anesthesia.* 7th ed. Philadelphia: Elsevier; 2018. Figure 22.3.)

platelet dysfunction, the sensitivity and specificity are limited. Incorporation of a platelet mapping assay into TEG provides a method for viscoelastic measurement of drug-induced platelet inhibition with reasonable correlation to optical aggregometry.

One of the more common applications for viscoelastic monitoring has been real-time detection of excess fibrinolysis during trauma, liver transplantation, or cardiac surgery. Additionally, viscoelastic monitoring may prove beneficial in differentiating surgically related bleeding from that caused by a coagulopathy. Furthermore, when viscoelastic testing is incorporated in perioperative diagnostic algorithms to guide transfusion, they have been found to reduce overall blood product administration.[21]

Platelet Function Analysis
Several platelet function assays specifically designed as point-of-care instruments are becoming available. The platelet function analyzer (PFA-100) subjects citrated whole blood to high-shear stress within a capillary tube. The tube contains a membrane coated with collagen and platelet agonists, such as epinephrine or ADP. As platelets begin to adhere to the membrane and form a plug, the capillary aperture is occluded, which is recorded as the closure time. Prolonged closure times indicate platelet dysfunction; however, the result is not specific to a particular disorder, and results may be inaccurate in the setting of thrombocytopenia or anemia. Nevertheless, because the test is simple, rapid, and does not require special training, it may be useful as a screening tool to assess for platelet dysfunction.

ANTITHROMBOTIC AND PROCOAGULANT DRUGS

Throughout the surgical period patients may be administered medications to decrease or increase clot formation. An understanding of these medications, in addition to potential reversal strategies, is crucial for appropriate perioperative management. Antithrombotic drugs are usually used to reduce the formation of blood clots in the setting of coronary or cerebral atherosclerosis or after vascular thrombosis. They can be further subdivided into antiplatelet agents, anticoagulants, and thrombolytics (Table 23.4).

Antiplatelet Agents

Antiplatelet agents inhibit thrombus formation by inhibiting platelet adhesion to damaged endothelium and/or aggregation. Most common antiplatelet agents target the cyclooxygenase (COX) enzyme, P2Y12 receptor, or the platelet GPIIb/IIIa receptor.

Cyclooxygenase Inhibitors
There are two primary COX isozymes: COX-1 and COX-2. COX-1 maintains the integrity of the gastric lining and renal blood flow and initiates the formation of TxA2, which is important for platelet aggregation and secretion. COX-2 is responsible for synthesizing the prostaglandin mediators in pain and inflammation.

Small doses of aspirin irreversibly inhibit COX-1; however, COX-2 is 170 times less sensitive than COX-1 to aspirin, so only at high doses can aspirin irreversibly inhibit both COX-1 and COX-2. Because platelets have no deoxyribonucleic acid (DNA), they are unable to synthesize new COX-1 once aspirin has irreversibly inhibited the enzyme. As a result, despite its short half-life (15 to 20 minutes), aspirin's platelet-inhibitory effect persists for 7 to 10 days, which is the expected lifetime of anucleated platelets. The recovery of platelet function after aspirin requires generation of new platelets. Generally, megakaryocytes produce 10% to 12% of circulating platelets daily, so near-normal hemostasis is expected in 2 to 3 days after the last dose of aspirin, assuming normal platelet turnover. Otherwise, immediate reversal can only be achieved with platelet transfusions.

Most NSAIDs are nonselective, reversible COX inhibitors. Platelet function returns to normal 3 days after discontinuing the use of NSAIDs. Selective COX-2 antagonists such as celecoxib were developed to provide pain relief without the gastrointestinal bleeding complications, but several clinical trials with selective COX-2 antagonists reported increased risks for cardiovascular complications. Although COX-2 is not expressed by platelets, the increased thrombotic risk is thought to be caused, in part, by inhibition of prostacyclin (PGI_2) without inhibition of TxA_2, thus tipping the balance toward

Table 23.4 Common Classes of Antithrombotic, Thrombolytic, and Procoagulant Medications

Category	Subcategory	Generic Drug Names
Antiplatelet agents	Cyclooxygenase inhibitors	Aspirin, NSAIDS
	P2Y12 receptor antagonists	Ticlopidine, clopidogrel, prasugrel, cangrelor, and ticagrelor
	Platelet GPIIb/IIIa antagonists	Abciximab, eptifibatide, and tirofiban
Anticoagulants	Vitamin K antagonists	Warfarin
	Heparin	UFH, LMWH, fondaparinux
	Direct thrombin inhibitors	Argatroban, bivalirudin (IV), desirudin (SQ), dabigatran (PO)
	Factor Xa inhibitors	Rivaroxaban, apixaban, edoxaban
Thrombolytics	Fibrin-specific agents	Alteplase, reteplase, tenecteplase
	Non–fibrin-specific agents	Streptokinase
Antifibrinolytics	Lysine analogs	Tranexamic acid, epsilon-aminocaproic acid
Factor replacements	Recombinant factor VIIa	
	Factor VIII:vWF	
	Prothrombin complex concentrates	Three-factor PCC; four-factor PCC, activated PCC, FEIBA
	Fibrinogen concentrates	

FEIBA, Factor VIII bypass activity; *IV,* intravenous; *LMWH,* low-molecular-weight heparin; *NSAID,* nonsteroidal antiinflammatory drug; *PCC,* prothrombin complex concentrate; *PO,* per os, by mouth; *SQ,* subcutaneous; *UFH,* unfractionated heparin; *vWF,* von Willebrand factor.
From Panigrahi AK, Liu LL. Patient blood management: Coagulation. In Gropper MA, ed. *Miller's Anesthesia.* 9th ed. Philadelphia: Elsevier; 2020. Table 50.1.

thrombosis.[22] Consequently, it is now recommended to use COX-2 inhibitors only when necessary and with the lowest effective dose possible after weighing the risks and benefits.

P2Y12 Receptor Antagonists

Thienopyridines (e.g., clopidogrel, ticlopidine, and prasugrel) and nucleoside analogs (e.g., ticagrelor and cangrelor) interfere with platelet function as antagonists of the P2Y12 receptor. Both classes prevent binding of ADP by the P2Y12 receptor, which impairs platelet adhesion and aggregation by preventing the expression of GP IIb/IIIa on the surface of activated platelets. Thienopyridines are prodrugs requiring hepatic metabolism to generate the active metabolite that then irreversibly inactivates the ADP-binding site of the P2Y12 receptor. Ticagrelor and cangrelor function as reversible inhibitors that change the conformation of the P2Y12 receptor. Platelet function normalizes 7 days after discontinuing clopidogrel and 14 to 21 days after discontinuing ticlopidine.

Clopidogrel, the most commonly prescribed medication in this class, requires metabolism by CYP2C19 for activation and as a result has wide interindividual variability in inhibiting ADP-induced platelet function. Although many factors may be involved in this variability, genetic polymorphism of CYP2C19 along with ABCB1, which affects the intestinal permeability and oral bioavailability of clopidogrel, are thought to play a significant role. Patients treated with clopidogrel who have

decreased CYP2C19 activity were shown to have significantly increased risk of major cardiovascular events. The Food and Drug Administration (FDA) issued a black box warning on clopidogrel to make patients and health care providers aware that patients who are CYP2C19-poor metabolizers, who represent up to 14% of patients, are at high risk of treatment failure and that genotype testing may be helpful.

Ticagrelor has much lower interindividual variability because it binds to a separate site on the P2Y12 receptor, and both the parent drug and the active metabolite have antiplatelet effects. Because it is much shorter acting than clopidogrel, ticagrelor must be dosed twice daily, which may be of benefit before surgery. Cangrelor is the only P2Y12 inhibitor available for intravenous administration and exhibits rapid onset (seconds) and offset, with platelet function normalizing within 60 minutes of discontinuation. This rapid offset may allow for bridging therapy in patients with drug-eluting stents who require surgery.

GPIIb/IIIa Inhibitors

Glycoprotein IIb/IIIa inhibitors (GPIs) (e.g., abciximab, eptifibatide, and tirofiban) prevent platelet aggregation by decreasing the binding of fibrinogen and vWF to glycoprotein IIb/IIIa receptors on the surface of activated platelets. They are administered intravenously in order to limit ongoing arterial thrombosis or to prevent formation of occlusive thrombi and restenosis in diseased vessels. Abciximab is a noncompetitive, irreversible inhibitor of

GPIIb/IIIa, whereas eptifibatide and tirofiban are competitive, reversible GPIIb/IIIa antagonists. The inhibition provided by abciximab continues at various levels for several days after the infusion has been discontinued; however, platelet aggregation normalizes within 24 to 48 hours. Platelet aggregation returns to normal 8 hours after discontinuing eptifibatide and tirofiban. All of these medications can cause thrombocytopenia, but the effect is strongest with abciximab (incidence of about 2.5%).

Anticoagulants

Vitamin K Antagonists

Warfarin, the most frequently used oral VKA, inhibits the synthesis of factors II, VII, IX, and X and proteins C and S. Without vitamin K, these proteins do not undergo γ-carboxylation and therefore are unable to bind to phospholipid membranes during hemostasis. Warfarin has a long half-life (~36 hours), and the complete anticoagulant effect can take 3 to 4 days to emerge because of the long half-lives of the preexisting coagulation factors. Prothrombin (factor II) has the longest half-life (~60 hours), whereas factor VII and protein C have the shortest half-lives (3 to 6 hours). During the initiation of warfarin therapy, early reductions in the anticoagulant protein C relative to other coagulation factors can produce a hypercoagulable state, resulting in thrombosis or warfarin-induced skin necrosis. As a result, patients at high risk for thromboembolism must be bridged with another anticoagulant (usually heparin) until warfarin's full anticoagulant effect is achieved.

Warfarin is monitored using the INR, and the therapeutic range for warfarin anticoagulation is generally an INR of 2.0 to 3.0, except for patients with mechanical heart valves, where higher values are necessary (INR 2.5 to 3.5). The INR is not calibrated to evaluate nonwarfarin factor deficiencies such as from liver disease and should not be used to evaluate therapeutic effects of other anticoagulants. Warfarin has a very narrow therapeutic window, which can be easily affected by other medications, foods, and alcohol. Warfarin's pharmacokinetics are also affected by genetic variations in cytochrome P450 (CYP2C9 gene), which can result in altered metabolism. As a result, frequent laboratory monitoring is required when initiating warfarin therapy. If the target INR is not achieved in the usual time frame, pharmacogenetic testing for polymorphisms that affect the metabolism of warfarin may be considered.

Unfractionated Heparin

UFH is a mixture of different-length polysaccharides with a high molecular weight. UFH indirectly inhibits thrombin (factor IIa) and factor Xa by binding to AT. The benefits of heparin are its short half-life and ability to be fully reversed with protamine, a positively charged protein isolated from salmon. Patients may be resistant to UFH if they have hereditary insufficiency of AT or an acquired deficiency of AT from prolonged heparin administration. Treatment should be with recombinant or plasma-derived AT concentrates. If not available, plasma transfusions may be used, but this increases the risk of transfusion-associated circulatory overload (TACO) or other transfusion reactions (also see Chapter 25).

Heparin therapy is monitored with the aPTT or ACT. Full-dose heparin for cardiac surgery is administered as an intravenous bolus of 300 to 400 U/kg. An ACT greater than 400 seconds is usually considered safe for initiation of CPB. One mg protamine to 100 units of heparin is the reversal dose used at the conclusion of CPB.

Low-Molecular-Weight Heparin and Fondaparinux

LMWH is produced by cleaving UFH into shorter fragments, which results in greater indirect (AT-mediated) inhibition of factor Xa compared with that of thrombin (factor IIa). Similarly, fondaparinux, a synthetic pentasaccharide of the AT binding region of heparin, selectively inhibits factor Xa via AT. LMWH and fondaparinux cannot be monitored using the aPTT assay, but routine laboratory monitoring is usually not needed. However, in patients with renal failure, which affects drug excretion, or in pregnant women, obese patients, and neonates for whom drug levels are less certain after subcutaneous injection, drug levels can be assessed using anti–factor Xa activity assays.

LMWH and fondaparinux have longer half-lives than heparin and can be administered subcutaneously either once or twice daily. Protamine is only partially effective in reversing LMWH and not effective for fondaparinux. LMWH is contraindicated in patients with HIT. Although fondaparinux does not interact with PF4 to form the antigen responsible for HIT, data supporting its use in HIT are limited.

Direct Thrombin Inhibitors

DTIs bind directly to thrombin and do not require a cofactor such as AT to exert their effect. As their name implies, DTIs (e.g., lepirudin, argatroban, bivalirudin) bind directly to thrombin and do not require a cofactor such as AT to inhibit their activity. All DTIs inhibit thrombin in its free and fibrin-bound states, unlike heparin, which only has an effect on free thrombin. Clinical effects can be monitored with aPTT or ACT assays. Hirudin is a naturally occurring DTI found in leeches. Lepirudin is a recombinant hirudin analog, whereas argatroban and bivalirudin are synthetic agents. Argatroban, which has a half-life of 45 minutes, is the preferred DTI in patients with renal insufficiency because it is hepatically eliminated. Bivalirudin is a reversible DTI and is metabolized by plasma proteases and renally excreted. Bivalirudin is often chosen in patients with both renal and hepatic dysfunction because of its short half-life of 25 minutes, although dose adjustments are still necessary. There are no antidotes for any of the DTIs, so reversal depends on their clearance. All DTIs will interfere with the INR, but argatroban has the greatest effect, which can complicate the transition to long-term warfarin anticoagulation.

Direct Oral Anticoagulants

Several new DOACs have been introduced into the market over the past 10 years. DOACs are appealing alternatives to traditional VKAs, as they have more predictable pharmacokinetics and pharmacodynamics and fewer drug–drug interactions, allowing them to be dosed without daily laboratory monitoring. Until recently, a significant limitation has been the lack of specific antidotes for DOAC reversal. Agents such as idarucizumab and andexanet alfa have been introduced; however, their use remains costly and availability limited.

Most DOACs are approved for prevention of VTE after hip or knee replacement surgery, treatment and secondary prevention of VTE, and prevention of stroke in nonvalvular atrial fibrillation. They are not approved for use in patients with mechanical heart valves and are contraindicated in pregnancy. In studies comparing DOACs with warfarin for stroke prevention in atrial fibrillation, DOACs were found to have decreased rates of stroke, intracranial hemorrhage, and mortality, with similar rates of major bleeding events but increased gastrointestinal bleeding.[23] DOACs were also found to be of similar efficacy to VKAs in the treatment of acute symptomatic VTE, but significantly decreased the risk of major bleeding.[24]

DOACs can be divided into two broad categories: (1) those that inhibit thrombin and (2) those that inhibit factor Xa. Dabigatran (Pradaxa), a DTI, was the first new oral antithrombotic agent approved for the prevention of ischemic stroke in patients with nonvalvular atrial fibrillation since warfarin. Dabigatran is predominantly eliminated by the kidneys; therefore dosing should be reduced in patients with a CrCl <30 mL/min. Direct Xa inhibitors (rivaroxaban [Xarelto], apixaban [Eliquis], edoxaban [Savaysa], and betrixaban Bevyxxa]) are agents whose activity is directed against the active site of factor Xa. Most direct Xa inhibitors undergo some renal clearance, and half-lives may be prolonged in individuals with renal impairment and in older patients. Apixaban, however, has been approved for use in patients with end-stage renal disease requiring hemodialysis.[25]

Because of their predictable pharmacokinetics, routine monitoring of DOAC therapy is not required. However, testing may be necessary in the setting of suspected overdose, uncontrolled bleeding, or need for urgent/emergent surgery. Monitoring of dabigatran therapy is difficult, as the aPTT assay is nonlinear until dabigatran concentrations are quite high (>200 ng/mL). The TT is very sensitive to dabigatran, so although it is useful to detect any presence of the drug, it cannot be used to quantify the amount of drug present. Instead, if available, dilute TT or ecarin clotting time are both linear at clinically relevant dabigatran concentrations and are the tests of choice if monitoring is necessary.[26] For direct Xa inhibitors, anti-factor Xa activity assays are best suited for monitoring but must be specifically calibrated for each drug.

Thrombolytics

Thrombolytic therapy is used to break up or dissolve blood clots. These medications are most commonly used during acute myocardial infarctions, strokes, massive PE, arterial thromboembolism, and venous thrombosis. Thrombolytics may be given through an intravenous catheter systemically or directly to the site of blockage. Most thrombolytic agents are serine proteases that work by converting plasminogen to plasmin (plasminogen activators). Plasmin then degrades fibrinogen, fibrin, and crosslinked fibrin (found in the clot), thereby generating fibrin-degradation products.

Thrombolytic drugs are often divided into two categories: (1) non–fibrin-specific agents or (2) fibrin-specific agents. Streptokinase, produced by β-hemolytic streptococci, is a non–fibrin-specific thrombolytic and was the first clinically used thrombolytic agent. Because streptokinase is a bacterial protein, it can elicit an immune response, including allergic or anaphylactic reactions. Fibrin-specific thrombolytic drugs include recombinant tPAs such as alteplase, reteplase, and tenecteplase. The ability of a thrombolytic agent to selectively recognize plasminogen bound to fibrin surfaces rather than plasminogen in the circulation dictates its fibrin specificity. Fibrin-specific thrombolytic agents may confer a lower risk of hemorrhagic complications by limiting lysis to the site of thrombosis; however, data regarding such a benefit are conflicting.[27]

In addition to lysing clots, tPAs function as anticoagulants through the liberation of fibrin degradation products during fibrinolysis. These degradation products include fragment X (from fibrinogenolysis) and D-dimer (from crosslinked fibrin), which inhibit platelet aggregation.[28] Surgery or puncture of noncompressible vessels is contraindicated within a 10-day period after the use of thrombolytic drugs.

Procoagulant Drugs

Perioperative bleeding can be the result of surgical bleeding but also because of hemostatic deficiency resulting in microvascular bleeding. Although transfusion of blood products is the primary therapy used to correct hemostatic defects (see Chapter 25), anesthesia providers may use procoagulant drugs as adjuncts to reduce blood loss. These drugs can be divided into two different classes: antifibrinolytics and factor replacements (see Table 23.4).

Antifibrinolytics

There are two types of antifibrinolytics: the lysine analogs (epsilonaminocaproic acid [EACA] and tranexamic acid [TXA]) and a serine protease inhibitor, aprotinin. Aprotinin was removed from the U.S. market because of concerns of renal and cardiovascular toxicity and is now only available in Europe and Canada. The lysine analogs act to impair fibrinolysis by competitively inhibiting the binding site on plasminogen, leading to inhibition of plasminogen activation in addition to preventing plasminogen binding of fibrin. TXA and EACA likely have equivalent efficacy and decrease perioperative blood loss in cardiac surgery, liver transplantation, and orthopedic surgery.

The use of TXA in trauma patients was studied in the CRASH-2 trial and was associated with a reduction in all-cause mortality (14.5% vs. 16%, $P = 0.0035$), including the risk of death because of bleeding (4.9% vs. 5.8%, $P = 0.0077$), without an increase in vascular occlusive events.[9] Early administration of TXA was key in improving outcomes, however, as those who received the drug after 3 hours experienced increased risk of death from bleeding (relative risk [RR] of 1.44; 95% confidence interval [CI] 1.12 to 1.84; $P = 0.004$).[29] Similarly, the World Maternal Antifibrinolytic (WOMAN) Trial found that administration of TXA reduced death caused by bleeding in women with postpartum hemorrhage, especially if given within 3 hours of birth and was not associated with an increase in adverse effects.[30]

Overall, TXA and EACA appear to be inexpensive and low-risk adjunctive agents that should be considered for use in major surgery or critical bleeding. Administration of lysine analogs perioperatively does not appear to increase the risk of thrombosis, but further studies are necessary before this can be definitively concluded. However, there are reports of high-dose TXA causing seizures in patients undergoing cardiac surgery.[31] This is thought to be the result of TXA binding to $GABA_A$ receptors, which in turn reduces $GABA_A$-mediated inhibition in the central nervous system (CNS). Because of this effect, it is recommended that doses for cardiac surgery be limited to a loading dose of 10 mg/kg followed by an infusion of 1 mg/kg/hr.[32]

Recombinant Factor VIIa

rFVIIa increases the generation of thrombin via the intrinsic and extrinsic pathways to enhance hemostasis. rFVIIa binds TF, which accelerates the activation of factor X; however, rFVIIa is also thought to activate factor X in a TF-independent manner.[33] Both mechanisms result in a "burst" of thrombin and fibrin generation, which leads to clot formation. The halflife of rFVIIa is relatively short at only 2 to 2.5 hours, so it may require repeat dosing until the bleeding is controlled.

rFVIIa was originally FDA approved for use in hemophilia patients with inhibitors, and its successful use generated a great deal of interest in its potential to promote hemostasis in hemorrhaging patients without a preexistent coagulation disorder. Consequently, there has been increased off-label use of rFVIIa in cardiac surgery, trauma, and liver transplantation and in patients with intracranial hemorrhage and traumatic brain injury. Overall, trials have demonstrated decreased rates of blood product transfusion when rFVIIa was used; however, there were no significant improvements in mortality rates.[34] Furthermore, rates of venous and arterial thromboses (including coronary events) were increased. As a result, guidelines now recommend that rFVIIa no longer be used for the off-label indications of prevention and treatment of bleeding in patients without hemophilia.[35] Thus, given the lack of formal assessment, the thromboembolic risk of rFVIIa should be carefully weighed against the potential benefit as a "last ditch" treatment of refractory bleeding.

Prothrombin Complex Concentrate

PCCs are purified formulations of varying amounts of vitamin K–dependent coagulation factors. Three-factor PCCs differ from four-factor PCCs in that they do not contain significant amounts of factor VII. Most of the factors are preserved in the inactive state, with the aim of decreasing thrombogenic risk; however, FEIBA is a four-factor PCC that contains activated factor VII. Although PCCs are derived from human plasma, they are treated with at least one viral reduction process, which reduces the risk for infectious and noninfectious transfusion reactions. Because of their improved safety profile and small volume of administration compared with plasma, PCCs are the first-line treatment for emergent reversal of VKAs.

Fibrinogen Concentrate

Fibrinogen concentrate (FC) carries FDA approval for the correction of congenital fibrinogen deficiency but is increasingly used to correct acquired hypofibrinogenemia with the goals of reducing coagulopathy, bleeding, and transfusion requirements. FC is produced from pooled human plasma and undergoes solvent/detergent and viral inactivation steps during the manufacturing process. As a result, FC offers benefits over plasma and cryoprecipitate in terms of standardized fibrinogen content, low infusion volume, decreased infectious risk, and faster time to administration because of rapid reconstitution. Alternatively, cryoprecipitate and plasma are less costly and provide additional procoagulant factors (e.g., factors VIII and XIII and vWF) that could be beneficial during massive bleeding. Large-scale, randomized controlled trials comparing FC with cryoprecipitate are lacking; however, some hospitals have incorporated FC into viscoelastic test-based transfusion algorithms with the goal of reducing blood product transfusion rates.

PERIOPERATIVE MANAGEMENT OF ANTI-THROMBOTIC THERAPY

The perioperative management of patients who require chronic anticoagulation or antiplatelet therapy involves balancing the risk of surgical bleeding against the risk of developing postoperative thromboembolism. Preoperative evaluation should be performed by a multidisciplinary team with sufficient time before elective surgery in order to thoroughly review surgical risk factors and the medical indication for antithrombotic therapy and to develop a consensus plan for the discontinuation and reinstitution of anticoagulation or antiplatelet agents.

Vitamin K Antagonists

For patients taking VKAs, the current recommendation is to stop VKAs 5 days before surgery for those who are at low risk for perioperative thromboembolism (Table 23.5).[36] VKAs should be restarted 12 to 24 hours postoperatively if there is adequate hemostasis. Patients at high risk of thromboembolism should be placed on bridging anticoagulation with UFH or LMWH after discontinuation of VKAs. For patients at intermediate thromboembolic risk, there is no definitive guidance regarding bridging therapy, so the approach chosen should be based on individual patient and surgical risk factors.[37]

Heparins

For those patients receiving bridging therapy with UFH, the infusion should be stopped 4 to 6 hours before

Table 23.5	Perioperative Risk Stratification	
Risk	**Indication**	
High	Mechanical heart valve	
	Rheumatic valvular heart disease	
	CHADS score ≥5	
	VTE within 3 months or history of VTE when VKAs are discontinued	
Moderate	CHADS score of 3 or 4	
	VTE between 3 and 12 months or history of recurrence	
	Active cancer	
Low	CHADS score 0–2	
	VTE >12 months prior and no other risk factors	

CHADS: Congestive heart failure, hypertension, age ≥75, diabetes mellitus, prior stroke; *VKA,* vitamin K antagonist; *VTE,* venous thromboembolism.
From Panigrahi AK, Liu LL. Patient blood management: Coagulation. In Gropper MA, ed. *Miller's Anesthesia.* 9th ed. Philadelphia: Elsevier; 2020. Table 50.3.)

surgery and resumed without a bolus dose no sooner than 12 hours postoperatively. In surgeries with high postoperative bleeding risk, resumption of UFH should be delayed 48 to 72 hours until adequate hemostasis has been achieved. In patients receiving bridging therapy with LMWH, the last dose of LMWH should be administered 24 hours before surgery and dosing should be resumed 24 hours postoperatively in low-bleeding-risk surgery and delayed until 48 to 72 hours postoperatively for surgeries with high bleeding risk.[37]

Antiplatelet Agents

For patients receiving nonreversible antiplatelet agents (e.g., aspirin, clopidogrel, ticlopidine, and prasugrel), decisions regarding changes in therapy are based on the following factors: (1) the patient's risk of a perioperative cardiovascular event; (2) whether the surgery is a minor procedure, major procedure, or cardiac procedure; and (3) the timing and type of stent placement for those patients who have undergone recent percutaneous coronary intervention. Low-dose acetylsalicylic acid (ASA) has been shown to reduce the risk of stroke and myocardial infarction by 25% to 30%,[38] and continuation of perioperative ASA therapy may confer a significant reduction in myocardial infarction and other major cardiovascular events.[39] However, concerns remain that continuation of ASA therapy increases the risk of major bleeding.[40]

Consequently, current recommendations are to continue ASA for patients who are at moderate to high risk for cardiovascular events requiring noncardiac surgery and only stop ASA 7 to 10 days before surgery for patients at low risk for cardiovascular events. Patients on dual antiplatelet therapy (DAPT)—most commonly, ASA and clopidogrel—should discontinue the clopidogrel 5 days before cardiac or noncardiac surgery. Antiplatelet management of patients who have recently undergone percutaneous coronary procedures is unique because of the increased risk of stent thrombosis. If possible, surgery should be delayed for 30 days after bare-metal stent placement and ideally up to 6 months after drug-eluting stent placement.[41] If surgery is required before this time has passed, DAPT should be continued unless the risk of bleeding is thought to outweigh the risk of thrombosis. If a DAPT after stent implantation has been held before a surgical procedure, therapy should be restarted as soon as possible, given the substantial thrombotic risks.

Neuraxial Anesthesia and Anticoagulation

Many patients who are receiving anticoagulant or antiplatelet therapy may require procedures that could benefit from neuraxial anesthetics. Given the wide variety of antithrombotic medications being used by perioperative patients, anesthesia providers must be aware of the risks of bleeding and neurologic injury

Table 23.6 Recommended Time Intervals Before and After Neuraxial Puncture or Catheter Removal

	Time Before Puncture/ Catheter Manipulation or Removal	Time After Puncture/ Catheter Manipulation or Removal	Laboratory Tests
UFHs (for prophylaxis, ≤15,000 IU/day)	4–6 hr	1 hr	Platelet count for treatment >5 days
UFHs (for treatment)	IV 4–6 hr	1 hr	aPTT, ACT, platelet count
	SQ 24 hr	1 hr	
LMWH (for prophylaxis)	12 hr	4 hr	Platelet count for treatment >5 days
LMWH (for treatment)	24 hr	4 hr	Platelet count for treatment >5 days
Fondaparinux (for prophylaxis, 2.5 mg/day)	36–42 hr	6–12 hr	Anti–factor Xa, standardized for specific agent
Rivaroxaban	72 hr	6 hr	Anti–factor Xa, standardized for specific agent
Apixaban	72 hr	6 hr	Anti–factor Xa, standardized for specific agent
Dabigatran	5 days	6 hr	dTT
Warfarin	5 days and INR ≤1.4	After catheter removal	INR
Argatroban	Contraindicated		
Acetylsalicylic acid	None	None	
Clopidogrel	7 days	After catheter removal	
Ticlopidine	10 days	After catheter removal	
Prasugrel	7–10 days	After catheter removal	
		6 hr with loading dose	
Ticagrelor	5–7 days	After catheter removal	
		6 hr with loading dose	
NSAIDs	None	None	

ACT, Activated clotting time; *aPTT,* activated partial thromboplastin time; *dTT,* dilute thrombin time; *INR,* international normalized ratio; *IU,* international unit; *IV,* intravenous; *LMWH,* low-molecular-weight heparin; *NSAID,* nonsteroidal antiinflammatory drug; *SQ,* subcutaneous; *UFH,* unfractionated heparin; *vWF,* von Willebrand factor.
Adapted from Gogarten W et al.; European Society of Anaesthesiology. Regional anaesthesia and antithrombotic agents: Recommendations of the European Society of Anaesthesiology. *Eur J Anaesthesiol.* 2010;27(12):999–1015, with permission. Table 2.

associated with each therapy. Unfortunately, data from randomized controlled trials to guide the timing and management of antithrombotic therapy for neuraxial anesthesia in the perioperative setting are lacking. However, societies, including the American Society of Regional Anesthesia and Pain Medicine (ASRA) and the European Society of Anaesthesiology (ESA), have reviewed the available data and published guidelines to assist in management (Table 23.6).[42] These recommendations will continue to be updated as evidence on the bleeding risk of newer anticoagulants emerges and can be accessed at the point-of-care via smart device apps (e.g., ASRA Coags).

Emergent Reversal of Anticoagulants

Management of perioperative anticoagulation is becoming increasingly more complex with the advent of the DOACs and the number of patients who are now receiving chronic anticoagulation (Table 23.7). For those patients on VKA who are experiencing life-threatening bleeding or require emergency surgery, four-factor PCC is now the drug of choice for emergent reversal of oral VKA in place of plasma. Concomitant administration of vitamin K is required to restore carboxylation of vitamin K–dependent factors by the liver and provide a more sustained correction after the factors in the PCC infusion have been metabolized.

| Table 23.7 | Common Anticoagulants Along With the Required Laboratory Monitoring and Possible Reversal Agents for Emergencies |

Antithrombotic Agent	Drug Name	Stop Before Procedure	Monitoring	Reversal Agents
Antiplatelet agents	ASA	7 days	None	Platelet transfusion
	P2Y12 receptor antagonists	7–14 days		
	GPIIb/IIIa antagonists	24–72 hr		
Vitamin K antagonists	Warfarin	2–5 days	INR	PCC, FFP, vitamin K
Heparins	UFH	6 hr	aPTT, anti–factor Xa	Protamine
	LMWH	12–24 h	None required, but anti–factor Xa activity can monitor levels	Partially reversed by protamine
Pentasaccharide	Fondaparinux	3 days (prophylactic dosing)	None required, but anti–factor Xa activity can monitor levels	None
Direct thrombin inhibitors	Argatroban	4–6 hr	aPTT or ACT	None
	Bivalirudin	3 h		
	Dabigatran	2–4 days (longer if renal impairment)	None required, dTT can monitor levels	Idarucizumab
FXa inhibitors	Rivaroxaban	2–3 days	None required, but anti–factor Xa activity can monitor levels	PCC
	Apixaban	2–3 days		Andexanet alfa for rivaroxaban and apixaban
	Edoxaban	2–3 days		

ACT, Activated clotting time; *aPTT*, activated partial thromboplastin time; *ASA*, acetylsalicylic acid; *dTT*, dilute thrombin time; *FFP*, fresh frozen plasma; *INR*, international normalized ratio; *IV*, intravenous; *PCC*, prothrombin complex concentrate; *PT*, prothrombin time.
From Panigrahi AK, Liu LL. Patient blood management: Coagulation. In Gropper MA, ed. *Miller's Anesthesia*. 9th ed. Philadelphia: Elsevier; 2020. Table 50.5.

There are no direct reversal agents for intravenous DTIs; however, their half-lives are relatively short, so time and supportive medical care are often sufficient to manage their anticoagulant effect in acute clinical situations. For DOACs, several novel reversal agents are becoming available. Idarucizumab is a humanized antibody fragment that binds to dabigatran with an affinity 350 times greater than thrombin. The drug received FDA approval in 2015 and can completely reverse the anticoagulant effect of dabigatran in minutes.[43] For patients taking oral direct factor Xa inhibitors, andexanet alfa was approved in 2018 for the emergent reversal of rivaroxaban or apixaban.[44] Andexanet alfa is a recombinant derivative of factor Xa that acts as a decoy, binding away factor Xa inhibitors and thereby reversing their effect. However, to date, andexanet alfa has not been carefully studied in surgical patients, and there is a concern that the duration of its effect may be too limited or it may complicate procedures requiring CPB

by contributing to heparin resistance.[45,46] Alternatively, PCC has shown promise as a strategy for reversing factor Xa inhibitors in surgical patients.[47] Ultimately, when assessing the need for medication reversal, not only should the agent to be reversed be considered but also its pharmacokinetics, the patient's renal function, and the specifics regarding whether surgery is truly emergent or can wait for further drug clearance and level assessment.

CONCLUSION

Ongoing research has continued to reveal the complexity of the coagulation system, but an understanding of the fundamental principles of hemostasis will assist the anesthesia provider in identifying patients at risk of bleeding preoperatively and safely managing blood loss and treating acquired coagulopathy both intraoperatively and postoperatively. Careful preoperative assessment of patients receiving antithrombotic therapy and a multidisciplinary team approach between the patient, primary care physician, hematologist, surgeon, and anesthesia provider are essential to ensure the perioperative safety of these patients.

ACKNOWLEDGMENT

The author, editors, and publisher would like to thank Drs. Lindsey L. Huddleston and Linda L. Liu for contributing to this chapter in the previous edition of this work. Excerpts of their chapter were incorporated and serve as the foundation for the current chapter.

REFERENCES

1. Furie B, Furie BC. Mechanisms of thrombus formation. *N Engl J Med*. 2008;359:938–949.
2. Broos K, Feys HB, De Meyer SF, Vanhoorelbeke K, Deckmyn H. Platelets at work in primary hemostasis. *Blood Rev*. 2011;25:155–167.
3. Longstaff C, Kolev K. Basic mechanisms and regulation of fibrinolysis. *J Thromb Haemost*. 2015;13(Suppl 1):S98–105.
4. O'Donnell JS, Lavin M. Perioperative management of patients with von Willebrand disease. *Hematology Am Soc Hematol Educ Program*. 2019;2019:604–609.
5. Peyvandi F, et al. Coagulation factor activity and clinical bleeding severity in rare bleeding disorders: results from the European Network of Rare Bleeding Disorders. *J Thromb Haemost*. 2012;10:615–621.
6. Tripodi A, Mannucci PM. The coagulopathy of chronic liver disease. *N Engl J Med*. 2011;365:147–156.
7. Sniecinski RM, Chandler WL. Activation of the hemostatic system during cardiopulmonary bypass. *Anesth Analg*. 2011;113:1319–1333.
8. Chang R, Cardenas JC, Wade CE, Holcomb JB. Advances in the understanding of trauma-induced coagulopathy. *Blood*. 2016;128:1043–1049.
9. collaborators C-t, et al. Effects of tranexamic acid on death, vascular occlusive events, and blood transfusion in trauma patients with significant haemorrhage (CRASH-2): a randomised, placebo-controlled trial. *Lancet*. 2010;376:23–32.
10. American Society of Anesthesiologists Task Force on Perioperative Blood, M. Practice guidelines for perioperative blood management: an updated report by the American Society of Anesthesiologists Task Force on Perioperative Blood Management*. *Anesthesiology*. 2015;122:241–275.
11. Wolberg AS, Aleman MM, Leiderman K, Machlus KR. Procoagulant activity in hemostasis and thrombosis: Virchow's triad revisited. *Anesth Analg*. 2012;114:275–285.
12. Lim W. Antiphospholipid syndrome. *Hematology Am Soc Hematol Educ Program*. 2013:675–680 2013.
13. Greinacher A. CLINICAL PRACTICE. Heparin-Induced Thrombocytopenia. *N Engl J Med*. 2015;373:252–261.
14. De Stefano V, Rossi E. Testing for inherited thrombophilia and consequences for antithrombotic prophylaxis in patients with venous thromboembolism and their relatives. A review of the Guidelines from Scientific Societies and Working Groups. *Thromb Haemost*. 2013;110:697–705.
15. Bates SM, et al. VTE, thrombophilia, antithrombotic therapy, and pregnancy: Antithrombotic Therapy and Prevention of Thrombosis, 9th ed: American College of Chest Physicians Evidence-Based Clinical Practice Guidelines. *Chest*. 2012;141:e691S–e736S.
16. Warkentin TE, Pai M, Linkins LA. Direct oral anticoagulants for treatment of HIT: update of Hamilton experience and literature review. *Blood*. 2017;130:1104–1113.
17. Levy JH, Szlam F, Wolberg AS, Winkler A. Clinical use of the activated partial thromboplastin time and prothrombin time for screening: a review of the literature and current guidelines for testing. *Clin Lab Med*. 2014;34:453–477.
18. Wang CZ, Moss J, Yuan CS. Commonly Used Dietary Supplements on Coagulation Function during Surgery. *Medicines (Basel)*. 2015;2:157–185.
19. Zehnder J, Price E, Jin J. Controversies in heparin monitoring. *Am J Hematol*. 2012;87(Suppl 1):S137–S140.
20. Peterson P, et al. The preoperative bleeding time test lacks clinical benefit: College of American Pathologists' and American Society of Clinical Pathologists' position article. *Arch Surg*. 1998;133:134–139.
21. Karkouti K, et al. Point-of-Care Hemostatic Testing in Cardiac Surgery: A Stepped-Wedge Clustered Randomized Controlled Trial. *Circulation*. 2016;134:1152–1162.
22. Funk CD, FitzGerald GA. COX-2 inhibitors and cardiovascular risk. *J Cardiovasc Pharmacol*. 2007;50:470–479.
23. Ruff CT, et al. Comparison of the efficacy and safety of new oral anticoagulants with warfarin in patients with atrial fibrillation: a meta-analysis of randomised trials. *Lancet*. 2014;383:955–962.
24. van Es N, Coppens M, Schulman S, Middeldorp S, Buller HR. Direct oral anticoagulants compared with vitamin K antagonists for acute venous thromboembolism: evidence from phase 3 trials. *Blood*. 2014;124:1968–1975.
25. Wang X, et al. Pharmacokinetics, pharmacodynamics, and safety of apixaban in subjects with end-stage renal disease on hemodialysis. *J Clin Pharmacol*. 2016;56:628–636.
26. Douxfils J, et al. Laboratory testing in patients treated with direct oral anticoagulants: a practical guide for clinicians. *J Thromb Haemost*. 2018;16:209–219.
27. Ouriel K. Comparison of the safety and efficacy of the various thrombolytic agents. *Rev Cardiovasc Med*. 2002;3(Suppl 2):S17–S24.
28. Verni CC, Davila A, Sims CA, Diamond SL. D-Dimer and Fibrin Degradation Products Impair Platelet Signaling: Plasma D-Dimer Is a Predictor and Mediator of Platelet Dysfunction During Trauma. *J Appl Lab Med*. 2020;5:1253–1264.
29. collaborators C-, et al. The importance of early treatment with tranexamic acid in bleeding trauma patients: an exploratory analysis of the CRASH-2 randomised controlled trial. *Lancet*. 2011;377:1096–1101 1101 e1091–1092.
30. Collaborators WT. Effect of early tranexamic acid administration on mortality, hysterectomy, and other morbidities in women with postpartum haemorrhage (WOMAN): an international, randomised, double-blind, placebo-controlled trial. *Lancet*. 2017;389:2105–2116.
31. Murkin JM, et al. High-dose tranexamic Acid is associated with nonischemic clinical seizures in cardiac surgical patients. *Anesth Analg*. 2010;110:350–353.
32. Lecker I, Orser BA, Mazer CD. Seizing" the opportunity to understand antifibrinolytic drugs. *Can J Anaesth*. 2012;59:1–5.
33. Shibeko AM, Woodle SA, Lee TK, Ovanesov MV. Unifying the mechanism of recombinant FVIIa action: dose dependence is regulated by tissue factor and phospholipids. *Blood*. 2012;120:891–899.
34. Simpson E, et al. Recombinant factor VIIa for the prevention and treatment

of bleeding in patients without hae-mophilia. *Cochrane Database Syst Rev.* 2012:CD005011.

35. Lin Y, Moltzan CJ, Anderson DR. National Advisory Committee on, B. & Blood, P. The evidence for the use of recombinant factor VIIa in massive bleeding: revision of the transfusion policy framework. *Transfus Med.* 2012;22:383–394.

36. Douketis JD, et al. Perioperative management of antithrombotic therapy: Antithrombotic Therapy and Prevention of Thrombosis, 9th ed: American College of Chest Physicians Evidence-Based Clinical Practice Guidelines. *Chest.* 2012;141:e326S–e350S.

37. Hornor MA, et al. American College of Surgeons' Guidelines for the Perioperative Management of Antithrombotic Medication. *J Am Coll Surg.* 2018;227:521–536 e521.

38. Antithrombotic Trialists C. Collaborative meta-analysis of randomised trials of antiplatelet therapy for prevention of death, myocardial infarction, and stroke in high risk patients. *BMJ.* 2002;324:71–86.

39. Oscarsson A, et al. To continue or discontinue aspirin in the perioperative period: a randomized, controlled clinical trial. *Br J Anaesth.* 2010;104:305–312.

40. Devereaux PJ, et al. Aspirin in patients undergoing noncardiac surgery. *N Engl J Med.* 2014;370:1494–1503.

41. Levine GN, et al. 2016 ACC/AHA Guideline Focused Update on Duration of Dual Antiplatelet Therapy in Patients With Coronary Artery Disease: A Report of the American College of Cardiology/American Heart Association Task Force on Clinical Practice Guidelines. *J Am Coll Cardiol.* 2016;68:1082–1115.

42. Horlocker TT, et al. Regional Anesthesia in the Patient Receiving Antithrombotic or Thrombolytic Therapy: American Society of Regional Anesthesia and Pain Medicine Evidence-Based Guidelines (Fourth Edition). *Reg Anesth Pain Med.* 2018;43:263–309.

43. Pollack CV Jr, et al. Idarucizumab for Dabigatran Reversal - Full Cohort Analysis. *N Engl J Med.* 2017;377:431–441.

44. Connolly SJ, et al. Full Study Report of Andexanet Alfa for Bleeding Associated with Factor Xa Inhibitors. *N Engl J Med.* 2019;380:1326–1335.

45. Levy JH, Connors JM. Andexanet Alfa Use in Cardiac Surgical Patients: A Xa Inhibitor and Heparin Reversal Agent. *J Cardiothorac Vasc Anesth.* 2021;35:265–266.

46. Levy JH, Welsby I. Andexanet Alfa Use in Patients Requiring Cardiopulmonary Bypass: Quo Vadis? *A A Pract.* 2019;13:477.

47. Levy JH, Douketis J, Steiner T, Goldstein JN, Milling TJ. Prothrombin Complex Concentrates for Perioperative Vitamin K Antagonist and Non-vitamin K Anticoagulant Reversal. *Anesthesiology.* 2018;129:1171–1184.

FLUID MANAGEMENT

Catherine Chiu, Matthieu Legrand

INTRODUCTION

Perioperative fluid administration has two goals: to ensure adequate intravascular volume to maintain cardiac output and tissue perfusion and to prevent electrolyte and acid–base disturbances. Intravenous fluid therapy represents a core element of anesthesia practice, a companion to the classic triad of unconsciousness, pain relief, and muscle relaxation.[1] The anesthesia provider must select appropriate intravenous fluids and decide the appropriate timing and volume to be administered. This chapter will review the physiology of fluid balance, types of fluids available, and strategies to achieve optimal fluid balance in the perioperative setting.

PHYSIOLOGY OF FLUID BALANCE

Approximately 60% of body weight is composed of total body water. This total body water can then be divided into intracellular (~55%) and extracellular (~45%) components (Fig. 24.1). Intravascular fluid represents only 7.5% of total body water.

Transcapillary fluid shifts are driven by competing Starling forces across the endothelial membrane (Fig. 24.2), in addition to endothelial permeability. Hydrostatic pressure is the strongest driver of fluid movement. As fluid traverses a capillary bed, capillary hydrostatic pressure (P_c) decreases relative to interstitial hydrostatic pressure (P_i), whereas capillary oncotic pressure increases relative to interstitial oncotic pressure. A thin, gel-like layer known as the *glycocalyx* coats the endothelial membrane and is involved in the regulation of endothelial permeability.[2] Intravenous fluid resuscitation and other causes of increased intravascular hydrostatic pressure can degrade the glycocalyx layer, especially in patients with sepsis or other disease processes associated with microcirculatory dysfunction.[3,4]

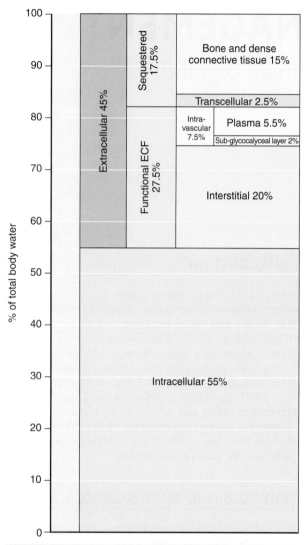

Fig. 24.1 Distribution of total body water. (From Edwards MR, Grocott MPW. Perioperative fluid and electrolyte therapy. In Gropper MA, et al, ed. Miller's Anesthesia. 8th ed. Philadelphia: Elsevier; 2015)

Because electrolytes can move freely across endothelial membranes, they do not produce significant osmotic forces in transcapillary fluid equilibrium under most circumstances. However, electrolytes do play a critical role in fluid shifts between the intracellular and extracellular compartments. Knowledge of normal electrolyte composition in the intravascular, intracellular, and extracellular compartments facilitates the choice of replacement fluids that help maintain the relative electrolyte balance and water distribution between compartments (Table 24.1).[5]

FLUID REPLACEMENT SOLUTIONS

Although many crystalloid and colloid replacement fluids are available for administration, the ideal fluid remains a source of debate. An understanding of individual fluid compositions facilitates an informed choice of replacement fluids (Table 24.2).

Crystalloids

Crystalloid solutions, a mixture of electrolytes and water, can be classified by composition (balanced vs. unbalanced) and tonicity (hypotonic, isotonic, and hypertonic). Balanced crystalloid solutions contain electrolytes in a ratio similar to plasma, unlike unbalanced solutions such as normal saline. Crystalloid solutions do not contribute to oncotic pressure because they diffuse out of the intravascular space shortly after administration.[6] Tonicity of a solution will affect osmolar equilibrium via the movement of water. To maintain equal intracellular and extracellular compartment osmolarity, hypotonic fluids will shift water toward the intracellular compartment, whereas hypertonic fluids will shift water toward the extracellular compartment.

Normal Saline

Normal saline (0.9% NaCl) is a slightly hypertonic solution with supraphysiologic concentrations of sodium and chloride. Stewart's approach to acid–base equilibrium (Fig. 24.3) allows a deeper understanding of normal saline's physiologic effects (also see Chapter 22). According to Stewart's approach, the plasma acid–base status is based on three parameters: the strong ion difference (SID), the arterial partial pressure of carbon dioxide ($PaCO_2$), and the total anion charge of all weak plasma acids (Atot). In this approach bicarbonate does not define acid–base disturbances. SID is a simple calculation of the difference in charge between the strong cations (i.e., Na^+, K^+, Ca^{++}, Mg^{++}) and strong anions (i.e., Cl^-, lactate, ketoacids, sulfates). Whereas the SID of plasma is around 40, the SID of normal saline is 0. Infusion of a solution with SID lower than plasma will lead to a decrease in plasma SID and metabolic acidosis because of the relative increase in [Cl^-] concentration at the expense of [HCO_3^-]. As such, resuscitation with low-SID solutions such as normal saline will inevitably lead to a hyperchloremic metabolic acidosis. Further consequences of normal saline–induced acidosis include the risk of increased plasma potassium because of cellular shifts. Potassium levels have been reported to be similar or higher than baseline using normal saline compared with balanced solutions, even if the balanced solutions contain a low concentration of potassium.[7,8] The use of normal saline has also been associated with a higher incidence of major

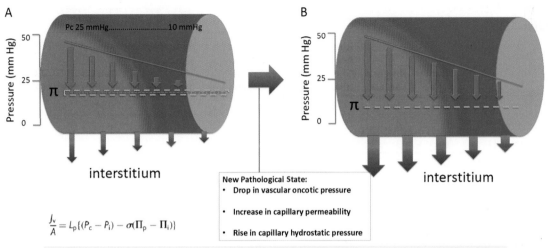

$$\frac{J_v}{A} = L_p\{(P_c - P_i) - \sigma(\Pi_p - \Pi_i)\}$$

Fig. 24.2 Starling forces governing transcapillary fluid shifts. Capillary hydrostatic forces decrease as plasma oncotic pressure increases across a capillary. *Red arrows* indicate intravascular hydrostatic pressure, *dotted line* indicates oncotic pressure, and *blue arrows* indicate transcapillary fluid shifts. Panel A represents normal physiologic states, and Panel B represents a pathologic state with contributing factors (in box) leading to increased fluid shift from the intravascular to the interstitial compartment. *A*, Surface area for filtration; J_v, net capillary flow rate; L_p, filtration coefficient; P_c, capillary hydrostatic pressure; P_i, interstitial hydrostatic pressure; Π_p, plasma protein oncotic pressure; Π_i, interstitial oncotic pressure; σ, reflection coefficient.

| **Table 24.1** Normal Fluid Composition |||||

Electrolyte	Plasma Fluid (mEq/L)	Intracellular Fluid (mEq/L)	Extracellular Fluid (mEq/L)
Sodium	142	10	140
Potassium	4	150	4.5
Magnesium	2	40	2
Calcium	5	1	5
Chloride	103	103	117
Bicarbonate	25	7	28

Modified from Frost E. Fluid management. In Pardo M, Miller RD, eds. *Basics of Anesthesia.* 7th ed. Philadelphia; Elsevier; 2018, Table 23.1.

adverse kidney morbidity in acutely and critically ill patients, increased coagulopathy, increased inflammation, and higher postoperative morbidity.[9] The increase in plasma chloride concentration after infusion of normal saline has been proposed as a mechanism for increased risk of acute kidney injury because of chloride-inducing vasoconstriction of the glomerular afferent arteriole and potentially decreased renal blood flow.

Balanced Crystalloid Solutions

Balanced solutions, such as Ringer's lactate and Plasma-Lyte, contain differing amounts of electrolytes to mimic plasma concentration. Most solutions contain an anion buffer, such as lactate, acetate, or gluconate, to maintain the electroneutrality of the solution. Metabolism of lactate and acetate results in plasma conversion to bicarbonate. Ringer's lactate and Plasma-Lyte have a higher SID (27 and 50, respectively) because of this alkalinizing effect.[10] With large-volume infusions, accumulation of these anion buffers has been a concern. For example, rapid acetate accumulation has been associated in some studies with hypotension and decreased cardiac contractility.[11,12] However, in a clinical trial of critically ill burn patients randomized to receive either lactated Ringer's or Plasma-Lyte there was no significant difference in mean arterial pressure, cardiac index, or acid–base disturbances between the two groups.[10] Their findings revealed only a transient increase in plasma acetate in the Plasma-Lyte group. Notably, patients in the Plasma-Lyte group had significantly lower ionized calcium levels, likely caused by the chelating effects of acetate. Close monitoring of ionized calcium is required when large volumes of Plasma-Lyte are being infused.

Other Crystalloid Solutions

Hypertonic saline (i.e., 3% NaCl) should only be administered to patients with intracranial hypertensive emergencies or acute symptomatic hyponatremia. Although the osmolarity of hypertonic saline is high, the resulting

Table 24.2 Composition of Common Replacement Fluids

	Normal Saline	Ringer's Lactate	Ringer's Acetate-Gluconate (Plasma-Lyte)	Ringer's Acetate-Malate (Isofundine)	Hydroxyethyl Starch 6% 130/0.4 (Voluven)	Gelatin (Gelofusine)	Albumin 4% (Albumex 4)
Sodium (mmol/L)	154	130	140	140	154	154	148
Potassium (mmol/L)	0	4	5	4			
Calcium (mmol/L)	0	3	0	2.5			
Magnesium (mmol/L)	0	0	3	1			
Chloride (mmol/L)	154	109	98	127	154	120	128
Bicarbonate (mmol/L)	0	0	0	0			
Lactate (mmol/L)	0	28	0	28			
Gluconate (mmol/L)	0	0	23	0			
Acetate (mmol/L)	0	0	27	24			
Osmolarity (mOsm/L)	308	275	294	304	308	274	250
SID	0	27	50	20	0	34	20

Adapted from Table 24.1 in Heming et al.[6] and Noritomi et al.[43]

intravascular fluid shifts are temporary. The risks of hypertonic saline include hypernatremia and peripheral vein thrombophlebitis.

Five percent dextrose is often used as a parenteral alternative to enteral free water replacement. Intravenous dextrose is immediately metabolized. The risk of hyperglycemia and hyponatremia makes the use of this solution suitable only for correcting symptomatic hypernatremia (i.e., intracellular dehydration) in patients unable to receive enteral water.

Colloids

Colloid solutions contain substances with large molecular weights, such as albumin or synthetic starches. Because of their greater plasma oncotic pressure, colloid solutions

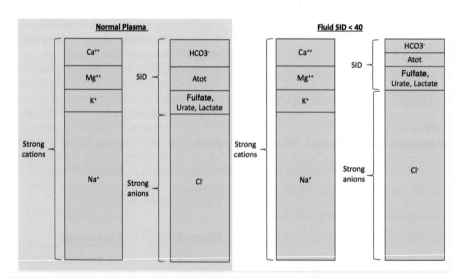

Fig. 24.3 Stewart's approach to plasma acid–base equilibrium. *Left*, Normal plasma. Plasma SID is normally around 40. *Right*, SID <40, which can result after resuscitation with a solution that has SID <40, such as normal saline. *SID*, Strong ion difference.

are expected to maintain intravascular volume longer than crystalloid solutions. Similarly, a smaller volume of colloid solution would be needed to maintain the same amount of intravascular volume compared with crystalloid solutions. However, in patients with critical illness and increased vascular permeability the intravascular half-life of colloids may be lower than expected.[13] For example, in one large trial of critically ill patients randomized to receive crystalloid or colloid fluid resuscitation the total amount of fluid given in the colloid arm was statistically less, but only by 100 mL per day over 4 days.[14] Another study of patients with severe sepsis or septic shock randomized to crystalloid versus colloid fluids found no difference in the total amount of fluids administered daily between the two groups.[15] There is a risk–benefit decision to choosing not only between crystalloids and colloids but also among colloid solutions themselves, as described later.

Albumin

Albumin accounts for up to 50% of the total plasma protein content and up to 70% to 80% of plasma oncotic pressure.[16] Commonly available preparations of albumin as a resuscitation fluid include 5% and 25% albumin. Although albumin is considered a physiologic plasma expander, the largest absolute amount of albumin resides in the interstitial fluid compartment. The interstitial albumin concentration ranges from 1.5 to 3 g/dL in most tissues, compared with 3.5 to 5 g/dL in plasma. Infused albumin will still be able to move into the interstitial compartment, and transfer is more rapid when the glycocalyx layer is degraded and vascular permeability is increased.

Several studies of albumin replacement compared with crystalloids in critically ill patients did not find a mortality difference.[15,17] Although a lower mortality rate was observed in a subgroup analysis of patients with septic shock, a randomized controlled trial is being performed for further evaluation. The potential benefit of albumin administration in the surgical population is largely unknown, and the acquisition cost is much higher than with crystalloids. Finally, because albumin is processed from human blood components, it may not be accepted as a resuscitation fluid by some Jehovah's Witness patients.

Synthetic Colloids

The high cost of albumin led to synthesis of large molecules with a base of starch, dextran, or gelatin that would remain intravascular for longer than crystalloid fluids. Many synthetic colloids are available for administration. They differ in molecular weight and molar substitutions to alter solubility.[18] The hydroxyethyl starch (HES) products can be identified by three characteristics: concentration (%), molecular weight, and molar substitution (e.g., 6% HES 130/0.4). The choice of synthetic colloids for fluid replacement therapy remains controversial for a number of reasons. In critically ill patients use of HES was associated with increased mortality and increased renal injury compared with the use of crystalloids.[14,19] In a 2020 trial of patients undergoing major abdominal surgery deemed at high risk of developing postoperative acute kidney injury (AKI) there was no mortality benefit in patients receiving HES compared with normal saline, but patients receiving HES had a higher risk of developing AKI. The authors' findings do not support the use of HES as a replacement fluid in this surgical population.[20] A systematic review of the safety and side effects of the different synthetic colloid solutions found increased incidence of anaphylactoid reactions and pruritis compared with albumin administration.[21] In cardiac surgery patients receiving HES there was a higher association with postoperative coagulopathy and clinical bleeding, and HES administration has been implicated in the development of coagulopathy in healthy volunteers, critically ill patients, and postsurgical patients.[21-24] This effect is likely caused by a reduction in circulating factor VIII and von Willebrand factors and impaired platelet function.

HEMODYNAMIC MONITORING FOR FLUID RESPONSIVENESS

An intravenous fluid bolus is typically administered with the goal of improving a patient's stroke volume and cardiac output. If the increase in stroke volume or cardiac output after the fluid bolus is greater than 10% to 15% of the prebolus values, the patient is considered "fluid responsive." Many factors can affect fluid responsiveness, including cardiac rhythm, patient positioning, intrathoracic pressure, and respiratory effort.[25] The impact of positive pressure ventilation on intrathoracic pressure and cardiac preload can be extremely useful in assessing fluid responsiveness. Specifically, when a patient receives a positive pressure mechanical ventilation breath, venous return will transiently decrease, causing the stroke volume to decrease a few seconds later. Commonly used surrogates of stroke volume include pulse pressure variation (PPV) and systolic pressure variation (SPV), which are easily measured with an intraarterial catheter (also see Chapter 20). SPV values of greater than 10 mm Hg and PPV values of greater than 13% have been used to predict fluid responsiveness in mechanically ventilated, critically ill patients.[26] SPV and PPV are most accurate in predicting fluid responsiveness in patients with a regular electrocardiogram (ECG) rhythm, mechanical ventilator tidal volume of 8 to 10 mL/kg, supine positioning, and without conditions that alter intrathoracic pressure (e.g., laparoscopy).[27]

When SPV and PPV values remain in an intermediate range (e.g., PPV 9% to 13%), then a positive response to a fluid bolus is less clear. Other commonly encountered conditions affecting the accuracy of SPV and PPV in predicting fluid responsiveness include low tidal volume ventilation, which lowers SPV and PPV and can produce false-negative values, and right heart failure, which can produce false-positive values.

Advancements in technology have allowed the estimation of stroke volume using noninvasive, proprietary pulse oximeter and arterial waveform devices (e.g., FloTrac, LidCO). These devices can estimate stroke volume and its changes after a fluid challenge to assess fluid responsiveness. The passive leg raise test can predict fluid responsiveness in critically ill patients; however, surgical conditions may preclude its use.[28] A detailed review of surrogate markers of stroke volume illustrates the complexities and clinical use of these measurements.[29,30]

Central venous pressure (CVP) measurement remains a controversial method of assessing volume status and predicting fluid responsiveness. CVP is a static surrogate marker for cardiac preload but can be affected by overall cardiac function, mechanical ventilation, patient positioning, and venous compliance. Although elevated CVP is likely a sign of cardiac and venous congestion and has been associated with increased risk of kidney injury and poor outcomes in the critically ill, overall predictive value of fluid responsiveness with CVP has been consistently poor.[31-33]

PERIOPERATIVE FLUID STRATEGIES FOR OPTIMAL VOLUME STATUS

Despite much research on strategies for perioperative fluid management that optimize intravascular volume status and minimize postsurgical morbidity, there remains no consensus on the ideal approach. Beginning in the 1960s, one approach to evaluating fluid deficit was derived from the pediatric literature and used the "4-2-1" rule to determine maintenance fluid requirements. Using this rule, total maintenance fluids are calculated based on a patient's weight (in kg) with the following equation: 4 mL/kg/hr for the first 10 kg + 2 mL/kg/hr for the second 10 kg + 1 mL/kg/hr for the remainder of the weight. For example, a 70-kg patient would require (4 mL/kg/hr × 10kg) + (2 mL/kg/hr × 10 kg) + (1 mL/kg/hr × 50 kg) = 110 mL/hr. In addition to maintenance fluid requirements, the clinician would calculate the fluid deficit from a patient's NPO (nothing by mouth) status, in addition to intraoperative blood loss and other insensible fluid losses. Using this method, it was not uncommon to find patients receiving >5 L of fluid replacement intraoperatively.[34]

Strategies for fluid management then shifted towards a target of "net-zero" weight balance after one seminal trial in patients undergoing elective colorectal surgery found increased postsurgical morbidity among patients who were randomized to a standard intraoperative and postoperative fluid regimen, compared with a restricted regimen with a goal of unchanged body weight.[35] A 2016 consensus statement from the Enhanced Recovery After Surgery (ERAS) Society provided moderate recommendations for keeping net-zero perioperative fluid balance.[36] Successful ERAS protocols reported decreased hospital length of stay and readmission rates, particularly for elective colorectal surgery, but the approach to intraoperative fluid management across institutions was nonuniform. For example, some institutions recommended keeping total fluid intake to less than 2 L; others recommended using fluid boluses of 250-mL increments in addition to a basal infusion rate (<10 mL/kg/hr) to achieve urine output of >0.5 mL/kg/hr; and yet others recommended fluid boluses based on surrogate markers of cardiac output, such as the Kuper protocol.[37-39] After some concern that intraoperative fluid restriction was associated with increased risk of AKI, a large international trial was conducted among patients undergoing major abdominal surgery with an increased risk of complications. In that study patients were randomized to a liberal intravenous fluid regimen (10 mL/kg fluid bolus on induction followed by 8 mL/kg/hr infusion intraoperatively, up to 100 kg) or a restrictive intravenous fluid regimen (fluid boluses of up to 5 mL/kg with 5 mL/kg/hr infusion intraoperatively). Although the rate of disability-free survival at 1 year was the same in both groups, in a secondary outcome, AKI was more common in the restrictive group (8.6%) compared with the liberal group (5%).[39,40]

Similar to other realms of perioperative and critical care, optimal fluid management is likely dependent on individual hemodynamic status, and any overarching strategies will likely harm some patients and benefit others. Indeed, the ERAS Society provides a strong recommendation for using advanced hemodynamic monitoring (i.e., arterial line monitoring and stroke volume monitoring) in high-risk patients undergoing major surgery with large intravascular fluid loss in order to practice a strategy of goal-directed fluid therapy (GDFT). In a GDFT-based strategy fluid therapy is titrated in response to advanced hemodynamic monitoring, which serves as a surrogate for optimizing stroke volume and cardiac output. Several studies, primarily of high-risk patients undergoing major abdominal surgery, have concluded that the use of GDFT algorithms has improved postoperative morbidity and decreased intensive care unit length of stay.[41,42] Importantly, many published strategies of GDFT have included the use of inotropic agents for persistently low cardiac output despite appropriate fluid challenges.

Box 24.1 Perioperative Fluid Management Considerations

- Use balanced crystalloid solutions instead of normal saline
- Avoid hydroxyethyl starch solutions because of potential nephrotoxicity
- If considering albumin administration, recall that potential benefit is unclear and cost is higher than crystalloids
- Avoid fluid overload, but consider that restrictive fluid practices are associated with increased risk of acute kidney injury
- Consider use of advanced hemodynamic monitoring to assess fluid responsiveness and guide fluid administration in high-risk patients undergoing major surgery

---

CONCLUSIONS

As technology improves to provide better monitoring of cardiac output and tissue perfusion, optimal strategies for fluid therapy will likely become more apparent. Box 24.1 lists general recommendations for perioperative fluid management.

ACKNOWLEDGMENT

The editors and publisher would like to thank Dr. Elizabeth A.M. Frost for contributing to this chapter in the previous edition of this work. It has served as the foundation for the current chapter.

REFERENCES

1. Miller R, Eriksson L, Fleisher L, Wiener-Kronish J, Cohen N, Young W Perioperative fluid and electrolyte therapy. Miller's Anesthesia. Saunders; 2014. 8th ed.
2. Weinbaum S, Tarbell JM, Damiano ER. The structure and function of the endothelial glycocalyx layer. *Annu Rev Biomed Eng.* 2007;9:121–167. doi:10.1146/annurev.bioeng.9.060906.151959.
3. Uchimido R, Schmidt EP, Shapiro NI. The glycocalyx: A novel diagnostic and therapeutic target in sepsis. *Crit Care.* 2019;23(1):16. doi:10.1186/s13054-018-2292-6.
4. Hippensteel JA, Uchimido R, Tyler PD, et al. Intravenous fluid resuscitation is associated with septic endothelial glycocalyx degradation. *Crit Care.* 2019;23(1):259. doi:10.1186/s13054-019-2534-2.
5. Legrand M, Alexander B, Joosten A Perioperative maintenance fluid therapy in patients undergoing thoracic surgery: More risks than benefits? Intensive Care Med. 03. 2020;46(3):552–553. doi:10.1007/s00134-020-05936-4.
6. Heming N, Moine P, Coscas R, Annane D Perioperative fluid management for major elective surgery. *Br J Surg.* 01 2020;107(2):e56-e62. doi:10.1002/bjs.11457.
7. O'Malley CM, Frumento RJ, Hardy MA, et al. A randomized, double-blind comparison of lactated Ringer's solution and 0.9% NaCl during renal transplantation. *Anesth Analg.* 2005;100(5):1518–1524. doi:10.1213/01.ANE.0000150939.28904.81. Maytable of contents.

8. Young JB, Utter GH, Schermer CR, et al. Saline versus Plasma-Lyte A in initial resuscitation of trauma patients: A randomized trial. *Ann Surg.* Feb 2014;259(2):255–262. doi:10.1097/SLA.0b013e318295feba.
9. Soussi S, Ferry A, Chaussard M, Legrand M. Chloride toxicity in critically ill patients: What's the evidence? *Anaesth Crit Care Pain Med.* 2017;36(2):125–130. doi:10.1016/j.accpm.2016.03.008.
10. Chaussard M, Dépret F, Saint-Aubin O, et al. Physiological response to fluid resuscitation with Ringer lactate versus Plasmalyte in critically ill burn patients. *J Appl Physiol.* 2020;128(3):709–714. doi:10.1152/japplphysiol.00859.2019 (1985).
11. Mehta BR, Fischer D, Ahmad M, Dubose TD. Effects of acetate and bicarbonate hemodialysis on cardiac function in chronic dialysis patients. *Kidney Int.* 1983;24(6):782–787. doi:10.1038/ki.1983.228.
12. Selby NM, Fluck RJ, Taal MW, McIntyre CW. Effects of acetate-free double-chamber hemodiafiltration and standard dialysis on systemic hemodynamics and troponin T levels. *ASAIO J.* 2006;52(1):62–69. doi:10.1097/01.mat.0000189725.93808.58 2006.
13. Bark BP, Persson J, Grände PO. Importance of the infusion rate for the plasma expanding effect of 5% albumin, 6% HES 130/0.4, 4% gelatin, and 0.9% NaCl in the septic rat. *Crit Care Med.* 2013;41(3):857–866. doi:10.1097/CCM.0b013e318274157e.
14. Myburgh JA, Finfer S, Bellomo R, et al. Hydroxyethyl starch or saline for fluid resuscitation in intensive care. *N Engl J Med.* 2012;367(20):1901–1911. doi:10.1056/NEJMoa1209759.
15. Caironi P, Tognoni G, Masson S, et al. Albumin replacement in patients with severe sepsis or septic shock. *N Engl J Med.* 2014;370(15):1412–1421. doi:10.1056/NEJMoa1305727.
16. Caraceni P, Tufoni M, Bonavita ME. Clinical use of albumin. *Blood Transfus.* 2013;11(Suppl 4):s18–s25. doi:10.2450/2013.005s.
17. Finfer S, Bellomo R, Boyce N, et al. A comparison of albumin and saline for fluid resuscitation in the intensive care unit. *N Engl J Med.* 2004;350(22):2247–2256. doi:10.1056/NEJMoa040232.
18. Westphal M, James MF, Kozek-Langenecker S, Stocker R, Guidet B, Van Aken H. Hydroxyethyl starches: Different products–different effects. *Anesthesiology.* 2009;111(1):187–202. doi:10.1097/ALN.0b013e3181a7ec82.
19. Perner A, Haase N, Guttormsen AB, et al. Hydroxyethyl starch 130/0.42 versus Ringer's acetate in severe sepsis. *N Engl J Med.* 2012;367(2):124–134. doi:10.1056/NEJMoa1204242.
20. Futier E, Garot M, Godet T, et al. Effect of hydroxyethyl starch vs saline for volume replacement therapy on death or postoperative complications among high-risk patients undergoing major abdominal surgery: The FLASH Randomized Clinical Trial. *JAMA.* 2020;323(3):225–236. doi:10.1001/jama.2019.20833.
21. Barron ME, Wilkes MM, Navickis RJ. A systematic review of the comparative safety of colloids. *Arch Surg.* 2004;139(5):552–563. doi:10.1001/archsurg.139.5.552.
22. Kapiotis S, Quehenberger P, Eichler HG, et al. Effect of hydroxyethyl starch on the activity of blood coagulation and fibrinolysis in healthy volunteers: Comparison with albumin. *Crit Care Med.* 1994;22(4):606–612. doi:10.1097/00003246-199404000-00016.
23. Falk JL, Rackow EC, Astiz ME, Weil MH. Effects of hetastarch and albumin on coagulation in patients with septic shock. *J Clin Pharmacol.* 1988;28(5):412–415. doi:10.1002/j.1552-4604.1988.tb05751.x.
24. Trumble ER, Muizelaar JP, Myseros JS, Choi SC, Warren BB. Coagulopathy with the use of hetastarch in the treatment of vasospasm. *J Neurosurg.* 1995;82(1):44–47. doi:10.3171/jns.1995.82.1.0044.

25. Wheeler AP, Bernard GR, Thompson BT, et al. Pulmonary-artery versus central venous catheter to guide treatment of acute lung injury. *N Engl J Med.* 2006;354(21):2213–2224. doi:10.1056/NEJMoa061895.

26. Marik PE, Cavallazzi R, Vasu T, Hirani A. Dynamic changes in arterial waveform derived variables and fluid responsiveness in mechanically ventilated patients: A systematic review of the literature. *Crit Care Med.* 2009;37(9):2642–2647. doi:10.1097/CCM.0b013e3181a590da.

27. Mathis MR, Schechtman SA, Engoren MC, et al. Arterial pressure variation in elective noncardiac surgery: Identifying reference distributions and modifying factors. *Anesthesiology.* 2017;126(2):249–259. doi:10.1097/ALN.0000000000001460.

28. Bentzer P, Griesdale DE, Boyd J, MacLean K, Sirounis D, Ayas NT. Will this hemodynamically unstable patient respond to a bolus of intravenous fluids? *JAMA.* 2016;316(12):1298–1309. doi:10.1001/jama.2016.12310.

29. Chaves RCF, Corrêa TD, Neto AS, et al. Assessment of fluid responsiveness in spontaneously breathing patients: A systematic review of literature. *Ann Intensive Care.* 2018;8(1):21. doi:10.1186/s13613-018-0365-y.

30. Perel A, Pizov R, Cotev S. Respiratory variations in the arterial pressure during mechanical ventilation reflect volume status and fluid responsiveness. *Intensive Care Med.* 2014;40(6):798–807. doi:10.1007/s00134-014-3285-9.

31. Eskesen TG, Wetterslev M, Perner A. Systematic review including re-analyses of 1148 individual data sets of central venous pressure as a predictor of fluid responsiveness. *Intensive Care Med.* 2016;42(3):324–332. doi:10.1007/s00134-015-4168-4.

32. Marik PE, Cavallazzi R. Does the central venous pressure predict fluid responsiveness? An updated meta-analysis and a plea for some common sense. *Crit Care Med.* 2013;41(7):1774–1781. doi:10.1097/CCM.0b013e31828a25fd.

33. Legrand M, Dupuis C, Simon C, et al. Association between systemic hemodynamics and septic acute kidney injury in critically ill patients: A retrospective observational study. *Crit Care.* 2013;17(6):R278. doi:10.1186/cc13133.

34. Holte K, Kehlet H. Fluid therapy and surgical outcomes in elective surgery: A need for reassessment in fast-track surgery. *J Am Coll Surg.* 2006;202(6):971–989. doi:10.1016/j.jamcollsurg.2006.01.003.

35. Brandstrup B, Tønnesen H, Beier-Holgersen R, et al. Effects of intravenous fluid restriction on postoperative complications: Comparison of two perioperative fluid regimens: A randomized assessor-blinded multicenter trial. *Ann Surg.* 2003;238(5):641–648. doi:10.1097/01.sla.0000094387.50865.23.

36. Feldheiser A, Aziz O, Baldini G, et al. Enhanced Recovery after Surgery (ERAS) for gastrointestinal surgery, part 2: Consensus statement for anaesthesia practice. *Acta Anaesthesiol Scand.* 2016;60(3):289–334. doi:10.1111/aas.12651.

37. Kuper M, Gold SJ, Callow C, et al. Intraoperative fluid management guided by oesophageal Doppler monitoring. *BMJ.* 2011;342:d3016. doi:10.1136/bmj.d3016.

38. Koerner CP, Lopez-Aguiar AG, Zaidi M, et al. Caution: Increased acute kidney injury in Enhanced Recovery after Surgery (ERAS) protocols. *Am Surg.* 2019;85(2):156–161.

39. Marcotte JH, Patel K, Desai R, et al. Acute kidney injury following implementation of an Enhanced Recovery after Surgery (ERAS) protocol in colorectal surgery. *Int J Colorectal Dis.* 2018;33(9):1259–1267. doi:10.1007/s00384-018-3084-9.

40. Myles PS, Bellomo R. Restrictive or liberal fluid therapy for major abdominal surgery. *N Engl J Med.* 2018;379(13):1283. doi:10.1056/NEJMc1810465.

41. Gan TJ, Soppitt A, Maroof M, et al. Goal-directed intraoperative fluid administration reduces length of hospital stay after major surgery. *Anesthesiology.* 2002;97(4):820–826. doi:10.1097/00000542-200210000-00012.

42. Benes J, Giglio M, Brienza N, Michard F. The effects of goal-directed fluid therapy based on dynamic parameters on post-surgical outcome: A meta-analysis of randomized controlled trials. *Crit Care.* 2014;18(5):584. doi:10.1186/s13054-014-0584-z.

43. Noritomi DT, Pereira AJ, Bugano DD, Rehder PS, Silva E. Impact of Plasma-Lyte pH 7.4 on acid-base status and hemodynamics in a model of controlled hemorrhagic shock. *Clinics (Sao Paulo).* 2011;66(11):1969–1974. doi:10.1590/s1807-59322011001100019.

25 BLOOD THERAPY

David Shimabukuro, Ronald D. Miller

The practice of transfusing blood has been around for centuries. The science of transfusion medicine started in the early twentieth century with the discoveries of human blood types and sodium citrate. Human blood typing is the pillar and foundation for safe blood transfusions, and citrate allowed for the storage of blood. The concept of collecting and storing blood (blood banking) was another major development, beginning in the 1930s. In the 1960s and 1970s transfusion practice focused on using whole blood in trauma (and war) for resuscitation and to stop bleeding. In the 1970s, 1980s, and 1990s transfusion was focused on the reduction in transmission of infections from a blood transfusion and moving toward blood component therapy instead of whole blood. In the 1990s and 2000s important topics in transfusion included when not to transfuse and what to transfuse. From the 2010s until now, the focus has been on patient blood management, which includes strategies to mitigate the need for transfusion and refining the precision of the indications for blood transfusions.

Red blood cell (RBC) transfusions given for specific clinical situations can decrease mortality rates. Conversely, severe complications can occur when multiple transfusions are given to a patient. For example, the term *lethal triad* describes hypothermia, acidosis, and coagulopathy and is an important negative indicator for trauma patient outcome in transfusion medicine. Similarly, the patient who requires high-volume transfusion (>10 units packed red blood cells [PRBCs] in 24 hours) experiences an increased mortality rate: a 10% increase for every 10 units of blood given. Thus if 50 units of blood are given, there is a 50% mortality rate.[1]

Despite the understanding that blood is a scarce resource and comes with possible complications, the practice of transfusing blood is quite commonplace. In 2019 in the United States alone over 10,000,000 units of blood products were transfused.[2] This underscores the importance of transfusion medicine and how the need for

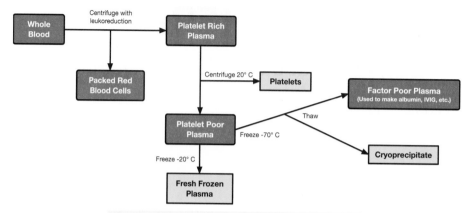

Fig. 25.1 Whole-blood processing by the blood center.

blood transfusions has helped this field evolve over the past 60 years.

The American Society of Anesthesiologists (ASA) Task Force on Perioperative Blood Management analyzed the literature and solicited opinions from experts and ASA members that were published as a practice guideline in 2015.[3] These guidelines will be periodically reviewed and updated in the future after review by the ASA Committee on Standards and Practice Parameters.

BLOOD BANKING ESSENTIALS

Whole-Blood Processing

Currently, the majority of the blood supply in the United States is in its component form (PRBCs, fresh frozen plasma [FFP], cryoprecipitate, platelets) because, in this way, it can be used in a more efficacious manner (individualized component therapy). Whole blood, if available, is likely to be autologous in nature. Soon after collection, whole blood is separated into PRBCs and platelet-rich plasma. The platelets are then separated from the plasma, and the plasma is then frozen. Depending on how the plasma is frozen, it can either be thawed for patient use or further processed to cryoprecipitate and, eventually, albumin (Fig. 25.1). All components are stored appropriately until ready for use or discarded if not used within the designated time frame (see later). Of course, this is an oversimplification of the process that is highly regulated and prescribed by the AABB (formerly known as the American Association of Blood Banks).

Ensuring Donor-Recipient Compatibility

In addition to separating blood into its components for individualized therapy, the blood bank is responsible for

Table 25.1 Blood Group Typing

Blood Group	Antigen on Erythrocyte	Plasma Antibodies
A	A	Anti-B
B	B	Anti-A
AB	AB	None
O	None	Anti-A, Anti-B
Rh	Rh	Anti-Rh; acquired after exposure

determining donor–recipient compatibility. These procedures will be discussed next.

Blood Type

Determining the blood type (A, B, O, Rh) of the recipient and donor is the first step in selecting blood for transfusion therapy. Routine typing of blood is performed to identify the major surface antigen(s) (A, B, Rh), or their absence, on the membranes of erythrocytes (Table 25.1). Naturally occurring antibodies (anti-A, anti-B) are formed whenever erythrocyte membranes lack surface A or B antigens, or both. These antibodies are capable of causing rapid intravascular destruction of erythrocytes whose membranes express the corresponding antigen(s). Therefore in blood type A erythrocytes express the A antigen and have anti-B antibodies; in blood type B erythrocytes express the B antigen and have anti-A antibodies. For blood type AB, both antigens are expressed, whereas in blood type O, no antigens are expressed. Rh factor can also be expressed on the erythrocyte cell surface. However, unlike the A and B naturally occurring antibodies, Rh antibodies are only produced after exposure and are not produced *de novo*.

Antibody Screen

In addition to determining a patient's blood type, an antibody screen is performed using the recipient's serum to identify the presence of antibodies against common minor RBC surface antigens. It is a simple agglutination process in which the recipient's serum is placed in wells with known common RBC surface antigens; the presence of agglutination indicates the likely presence of an antibody. The "type and screen" is typically used when the surgical procedure is unlikely to require transfusion of blood (e.g., many laparoscopic procedures) but is one in which there is still a chance that blood could be needed. Blood typing and screening permit more cost-efficient use of stored blood because the blood is available to more than one patient. The chance of a significant hemolytic reaction related to the use of typed and screened blood is approximately 1 in 70,000 units transfused.

Crossmatch

A crossmatch occurs when the donor's erythrocytes are incubated with the recipient's plasma. A crossmatch is always done before the transfusion of blood. This entire process usually takes around 45 to 60 minutes. Rapid agglutination (within 5–10 minutes) occurs if the crossmatch is incompatible secondary to a major blood typing (A, B, O, Rh) mismatch or in the presence of recipient antibodies against MN, P, and/or Lewis. In addition to major incompatibility, the crossmatch checks for minor incompatibility by assessing for the presence of antibodies against minor surface antigens (e.g., Kell, Kidd, Fya, Fyb). This minor agglutination reaction can take as long as 45 to 60 minutes to occur. The term *type-specific blood* refers to the fact that only the ABO-Rh type has been determined. Presently, crossmatching can be done electronically when specific criteria are met and, mainly, several concordant blood types are in the electronic medical record along with a current negative antibody screen. With electronic crossmatching, PRBC allocation of compatible units can be done in 5 to 10 minutes.

Massive Transfusion/Emergency Release Protocols

In certain clinical situations (e.g., aortic rupture) blood needs to be released from the blood bank on an emergent basis before a patient's blood type can be determined. Every hospital should be able to release blood rapidly via a massive transfusion and/or emergency release protocol. This usually involves a call to the blood bank stating the need to activate the massive transfusion/emergency release protocol that results in the immediate release of a prespecified number of units of uncrossmatched RBCs (type O-negative), prespecified number of units of FFP (type AB-negative), and prespecified number of platelet units.

Table 25.2	Blood Compatibility		
Component	**ABO/Rh**	**Screen**	**Crossmatch**
WB/PRBCs	Yes	Yes	Yes
FFP	Yes	Yes	No
Cryo	No	No	No
Platelets	No/Yes[a]	No/Yes[a]	No/Yes[a]

Cryo, Cryoprecipitate; *FFP,* fresh frozen plasma; *PRBCs,* packed red blood cells; *WB,* whole blood.
[a]On rare occasion, platelets can be typed and crossmatched to improve longevity after transfusion (e.g., for patients with thrombocytopenia who are refractory to random-donor platelets).

In an emergency situation that requires transfusion before full compatibility testing is completed (Table 25.2) the most desirable approach is to transfuse type-specific, partially crossmatched PRBCs. The donor erythrocytes are mixed with recipient plasma and observed for macroscopic agglutination. If the time required to complete this examination (typically <10 minutes) is not acceptable, the second option is to administer type-specific, noncrossmatched PRBCs, if available, or O-negative PRBCs (universal red blood cell donor, as it has no major surface antigens). O-negative whole blood is not selected because it may contain high titers of anti-A and anti-B hemolytic antibodies in the plasma component. For adult patients, with the exception of women of childbearing age, emergency administration of O-positive PRBCs is considered acceptable practice until the patient's blood type is determined. If the patient's blood type becomes known and available after 2 units of type O-negative PRBCs have been transfused, classic teaching was that subsequent transfusions should probably continue with O-negative PRBCs. However, it is not clear if this practice is necessary, and the generally recommended approach is to switch to type-specific blood when it becomes available.

The general approach to the administration of FFP during an emergency is similar to that of PRBCs. If type-specific plasma is not available, the plasma of AB-negative blood type donors can be given to all individuals, as it does not contain antibodies against the major surface antigens found on RBCs.

As platelets contain no RBCs and very little plasma, the blood type of the donor and recipient are irrelevant in the majority of emergency transfusions.

Of note, despite its relative unavailability, fresh whole blood is extremely effective in restoring normal coagulation after severe injury. The effectiveness of fresh whole blood depends on how long it has been stored and its temperature. In Vietnam in the late 1960s the military used type-specific blood that was maintained at room temperature and stored for no longer than 24 hours. They found it was extremely effective in preventing and treating trauma-induced coagulopathies.[4] Not surprisingly, more

Table 25.3 Blood Components

Component	Dose	Volume per Unit	Shelf Life	Storage	Response
PRBCs	1 unit	200–250 mL	21–42 days	1–6°C	1 g/dL increase
FFP	10–15 mL/kg	200–300 mL	Frozen: 1 year Thaw: 24 hours	Frozen: <−18°C Thaw: 1–10°C	30% of normal coagulation factors
Cryo	1 unit/5 kg	15–20 mL	Frozen: 1 year Thaw: 4 hours	Frozen: <−18°C Thaw: 1–10°C	100 mg/dL increase in fibrinogen
Platelets	4–6 pooled WB derivative or 1 apheresis unit	200–250 mL	5 days	20–24°C with gentle agitation	30–60×10^9/L increase

Cryo, Cryoprecipitate; *FFP,* fresh frozen plasma; *PRBCs,* packed red blood cells.

recently, the use of fresh whole blood by surgical teams in Afghanistan was associated with improved survival compared with component therapy without platelets.[5]

Blood Storage

PRBCs can be stored in a variety of solutions that contain phosphate, dextrose, and/or adenine at temperatures of 1 to 6°C. Accepted storage time (hemolysis <1% with 75% viability of transfused erythrocytes 24 hours after transfusion) is up to 42 days, depending on the donor and storage medium. Adenine increases erythrocyte survival by allowing the cells to resynthesize the adenosine triphosphate needed to fuel metabolic reactions. Changes that occur in RBCs during storage are affected by the length of storage and the type of preservative used. For many years, fresh PRBCs (<5 days of storage) had been recommended for critically ill patients in an effort to improve the delivery of oxygen (2,3-diphosphoglycerate [2,3-DPG] concentrations are higher in fresh blood), though nowadays, it is more determined by what is available in the hospital blood bank. In the past, administration of younger PRBCs (<14 days of storage) was thought to be associated with better outcomes (i.e., decreased mortality rate and fewer postoperative complications), especially with major surgery. However, a 2016 study concluded that the death rate among a general hospital population was not related to the duration of blood storage.[6] This was further validated by a large European study published a year later and by a Cochrane Database systematic review published in 2018.[7,8]

FFP and cryoprecipitate are stored at −20°C; platelets are kept at room temperature (20°C) and are continuously gently agitated to prevent clumping. Because platelets are kept at room temperature, they have a short shelf life of 5 days. On the other hand, although FFP and cryoprecipitate can be kept frozen for a year, once thawed, they have to be used within 24 hours and 4 hours, respectively.

BLOOD COMPONENTS (TABLE 25.3)

Packed Red Blood Cells

In the perioperative period PRBCs (200–250 mL volume with a hematocrit of 70%–80%) are used for the treatment of anemia associated with anticipated and/or actual surgical blood loss. The major goal is to increase the oxygen-carrying capacity of blood with a resultant increase in oxygen delivery to tissues and vital organs. Although PRBCs can increase intravascular fluid volume, nonblood products, such as crystalloids and colloids, can also achieve that endpoint. A single unit of PRBCs will increase adult hemoglobin concentrations approximately 1.0 to 1.5 g/dL. Theoretically, the use of hypotonic solutions with PRBCs may cause hemolysis, and the calcium present in lactated Ringer's solution may lead to clotting in the blood filter and/or transfusion line.

The decision to administer PRBCs should be based on measured blood loss and inadequate oxygen-carrying capacity. Acute blood loss in the range of 1500 to 2000 mL (approximately 30% of an adult patient's blood volume) may exceed the ability of crystalloids to replace blood volume without jeopardizing the oxygen-carrying capacity of the blood. Hypotension and tachycardia are likely, but these compensatory responses may be blunted by anesthesia or other drugs (e.g., β-adrenergic blocking drugs). Compensatory vasoconstriction may conceal the signs of acute blood loss until at least 10% of the blood volume is lost, and healthy patients may lose up to 20% of their blood volume before signs of hypovolemia occur. To ensure an adequate oxygen content in blood, PRBCs should be administered when blood loss is sufficiently large. Administration of whole blood, when available, decreases the incidence of hypofibrinogenemia and perhaps coagulopathies associated with the administration of multiple units of PRBCs. In the Vietnam conflict fresh whole blood (typed and crossmatched, but not cooled) was quite effective, especially with massive transfusion-associated coagulopathies. Forty years later in Iraq, military physicians administered fresh whole blood from prescreened "walking donors," which also can treat or prevent thrombocytopenia. In fact, warm fresh whole blood may be more efficacious than stored component therapy when treating critically ill patients requiring massive blood transfusions. Also, whole blood may be preferable to PRBCs when replacing blood losses that exceed 30% of the blood volume. Practically speaking, specific ratios of PRBC transfusions with FFP and platelets have been used in place of whole blood. For example, a ratio of 1.5 units PRBC with 1 unit of FFP (i.e., for every 1.5 units of PRBCs administered, 1 unit of FFP should be given). In addition, 1 unit of apheresis platelets (or 6 pooled random donor units) for 6 units of RBCs has been recommended in patients with large blood losses and trauma. Interestingly, despite its wide acceptance in massive resuscitation in trauma patients, these ratios have not been conclusively proven to improve mortality.[9,10]

With acute blood loss, interstitial fluid and extravascular protein are transferred to the intravascular space, which tends to maintain plasma volume. For this reason, when crystalloid solutions are used to replace blood loss, they should be given in amounts equal to about three times the amount of blood loss, not only to replenish intravascular fluid volume but also to replenish the fluid lost from interstitial spaces. Albumin is a solution that is useful for acute expansion of the intravascular fluid volume. In contrast to crystalloid solutions, albumin is more likely to remain in the intravascular space for a longer period (about 12 hours). These solutions avoid complications associated with blood-containing products but do not improve the oxygen-carrying capacity of the blood and in large volumes (>20 mL/kg) may cause coagulation defects from ongoing dilution (also see Chapter 24).

Fresh Frozen Plasma

FFP is the fluid portion obtained from a single unit of whole blood that is frozen within 6 hours of collection. All coagulation factors, except platelets, are present in FFP, which explains the use of this component for the treatment of hemorrhage from presumed coagulation factor deficiencies. FFP transfusions during surgery are probably not necessary unless the prothrombin time/international normalized ratio (PT/INR) or activated partial thromboplastin time (aPTT), or both, are at least 1.5 times longer than normal. More recently, FFP has been given in specific ratios with PRBCs in trauma patients regardless of laboratory values. Other indications for FFP are an urgent reversal of warfarin and management of heparin resistance (i.e., FFP contains antithrombin III).

Cryoprecipitate

Cryoprecipitate is the fraction of plasma that precipitates when FFP is thawed from −70°C. It contains factor VIII, fibrinogen, fibronectin, von Willebrand factor, and factor XIII. This component is useful for treating hemophilia A (it contains high concentrations of factor VIII in a small volume) or von Willebrand factor deficiency that is unresponsive to desmopressin. Cryoprecipitate can also be used to treat hypofibrinogenemia because it contains more fibrinogen than FFP.

Platelets

Administration of platelets allows specific treatment of thrombocytopenia without the infusion of unnecessary blood components. Platelets are derived from volunteer donors and can be pooled from platelet concentrates derived from whole blood donation (random-donor platelets) or from a single donor (apheresis platelets). During surgery, platelet transfusions are probably not required unless the platelet count is less than 50,000 to 100,000 cells/mm^3 (usually dictated by the type and location of surgery) as determined by laboratory analysis or in predetermined ratios with PRBC and FFP in trauma patients, as described previously.

PATIENT BLOOD MANAGEMENT AND THE DECISION TO TRANSFUSE RED BLOOD CELLS

The decision to transfuse should be based on a combination of factors: (1) patient blood management (PBM) and preoperative anemia; (2) monitoring of blood loss; (3) assessment of how much additional blood loss may occur; (4) monitoring for inadequate perfusion and oxygenation of vital organs; (5) quantitation of intravenous fluids given overall; and (6) monitoring for transfusion indicators, typically based on laboratory data. Several of these concepts will be discussed in more detail next.

Patient Blood Management

PBM has been a major part of our transfusion terminology for the past 10 to 15 years and is focused primarily on the perioperative period. The concept is based on three main pillars: (1) optimization of RBC mass, (2) reduction of blood loss and bleeding, and (3) optimization of the patient's physiologic tolerance toward anemia.[11] Supporting the pillars are techniques and agents used during the intraoperative period to reduce blood loss, such as controlled hypotension and antifibrinolytic agents. PBM also emphasizes the use of allogeneic blood components to be selective and optimal, keeping in mind that the ultimate goal is to transfuse only at the appropriate time and with the appropriate therapy.[12,13]

Although PBM includes intraoperative and postoperative phases of care, one of the more prioritized components of PBM has been the identification and management of preoperative anemia.[14] Studies have demonstrated that preoperative anemia is a risk factor for a poorer clinical outcome and is, logically, a predisposing factor for intraoperative blood transfusions. PBM emphasizes that proper preoperative preparation can reduce the number of blood transfusions used intraoperatively and should ideally be addressed (e.g., with iron and, possibly, recombinant human erythropoietin) before coming for surgery. A higher presurgical hemoglobin level not only decreases the need for intraoperative blood transfusions but the overall morbidity and mortality rates as well (also see Chapter 42).

Monitoring for Blood Loss

Visual estimation is the simplest technique for quantifying intraoperative blood loss. The estimate is based on a combination of visualization and gravimetric measurements of blood on sponges and drapes and in suction devices. Specifically, differences in weight between dry and blood-soaked gauze pads can routinely be determined. However, these methods for measuring blood loss are only modestly accurate. Regardless, it is done every day and in nearly every surgical case performed in the operating room.

Monitoring for Inadequate Perfusion and Oxygenation of Vital Organs

Standard monitors, such as the electrocardiogram and those measuring arterial blood pressure, heart rate, and oxygen saturation, are commonly used. Analysis of arterial blood gases, mixed venous oxygen saturation, and echocardiography may be useful in select patients. Tachycardia is an insensitive and nonspecific indicator of hypovolemia, especially in patients receiving a volatile anesthetic. Maintenance of arterial blood pressure with normal systolic pressure variation/pulse pressure variation and urine output suggests adequate intravascular blood volume. Urinary output usually decreases during moderate to severe hypovolemia and the resulting tissue hypoperfusion. Hyperlactatemia secondary to increased anaerobic metabolism can arise from tissue hypoxia from inadequate oxygen delivery. Arterial pH may decrease only when tissue hypoperfusion becomes severe.

Monitoring for Transfusion Indicators

The decision to transfuse is primarily based on laboratory data, the risk of anemia to a patient, and the patient's ability to compensate for decreased oxygen-carrying capacity, in addition to the inherent risks associated with transfusion. Given the lack of clear evidence in the published literature, many of the variables used to guide transfusion therapy, especially PRBCs, are based on clinical judgment and specialty society guidelines.

In the past 20 years terminology on blood transfusion policy has increased. A clinician may be using a *restrictive* blood policy, meaning "give blood only when absolutely necessary." This restrictive approach evolved many years ago when fear of transmitting hepatitis and human immunodeficiency virus (HIV) was widespread. However, transmission of such diseases is now rare. Blood transfusions given in response to proper indications should ideally decrease patient mortality.

In parallel with this terminology, a general standard of care has evolved that patients with hemoglobin values more than 10 g/dL rarely require a PRBC transfusion, whereas those with hemoglobin values less than 6 g/dL almost always require a PRBC transfusion, especially when anemia or surgical bleeding (or both) are acute and continuing. Determination of whether intermediate hemoglobin concentrations (6–10 g/dL) justify or require a transfusion should be based on the patient's risk for complications of inadequate oxygen delivery. Certain clinical situations may warrant transfusion of blood at a higher hemoglobin value than that in otherwise healthy patients. For example, a hemoglobin concentration of 7 g/dL may be an appropriate threshold for transfusion in a surgical patient with no risk factors for ischemia, whereas a transfusion threshold of 9 g/dL may be justified in a patient who is considered to be at risk for cardiac ischemia (e.g., history of coronary artery disease). Controlled studies to determine the hemoglobin concentration at which PRBC transfusion improves outcome in a surgical patient with acute blood loss are few, yet centering on hemoglobin values in a complex clinical situation must be done with caution.[13]

More recently, PBM has focused on the words *restrictive* and *liberal* for PRBC transfusions. PBM uses a hemoglobin value as an indicator for PRBC transfusion. A liberal policy would allow giving blood when hemoglobin levels were more than 10 g/dL. A restrictive policy allowed giving blood only when the hemoglobin levels were preferably 7 g/dL or lower. Analysis of the overall literature clearly favors the restrictive approach.[15,16] However, some groups have recommended a liberal approach to perioperative patients. According to a 2015 metaanalysis, "according to randomized published evidence, perioperative adult patients have an improved survival when receiving a liberal blood transfusion policy."[17] Of note, at the time of this publication, this is not a widely accepted practice.

Transfusion of PRBCs in patients with hemoglobin concentrations higher than 10 to 12 g/dL does not substantially increase oxygen delivery. Further decreases in the hemoglobin concentration can sometimes be offset by increases in cardiac output. The exact hemoglobin value at which cardiac output increases varies among individuals and is influenced by age, whether the anemia is acute or chronic, and sometimes by anesthesia. For example, the cardiovascular response to anemia in the elderly is decreased, as it is with general anesthesia. Yet the focus on hemoglobin as a transfusion indicator has existed for many years and still continues.[16,18] Furthermore, the availability of a noninvasive spectrophotometric monitor allows the continuous monitoring of hemoglobin levels. Whether this monitor can be used for transfusion decisions without a laboratory cooximeter determination is not clear. More than likely, this monitor will provide more opportunity for defining the relationship between hemoglobin levels and transfusion requirements.[19]

In conclusion, the decision to give a PRBC transfusion requires a carefully thought-out process that is based on objective clinical indications and a knowledge of transfusion medicine overall.[11,20]

COMPLICATIONS OF BLOOD THERAPY

Blood transfusions are extremely valuable in clinical medicine and have become increasingly safer, mainly because of more effective donor screening and pretransfusion blood testing. Complications of blood therapy, like an adverse effect of any therapy, must be considered when evaluating the risk-to-benefit ratio for treatment of individual patients with blood products.

The Food and Drug Administration (FDA) analyzes and publishes mortality and morbidity data related to outcomes from blood transfusions on an annual basis. The most recent publication is for fiscal year 2019 (Table 25.4). It lists the types of fatal reactions associated with blood transfusions from 2015 to 2019 on a cumulative basis and in 2019 alone. According to these data, fatal reactions are rare and have been similar in occurrence for each of the previous 5 years. The leading causes of a fatal outcome from blood transfusions are transfusion-related acute lung injury (TRALI), transfusion-associated circulatory overload (TACO), and hemolytic transfusion reactions.[3] Regardless, from the general public's perspective, the transmission of infectious diseases (i.e., HIV, hepatitis B and C viruses, West Nile virus, Zika) and hemolytic

transfusion reactions continue to be the most feared complications of transfusion therapy. Currently, the FDA continues to report that blood transfusions are safer now than at any time in history.

In addition to acquiring an infection from a blood transfusion, blood transfusions have been linked with other health care–associated infections.[21,22] The concept is that transfusions may cause a patient to be more susceptible to infections via immunomodulation. This is discussed in more detail next.

Transmission of Infectious Diseases (Table 25.5)

The incidence of infection from blood transfusions has markedly decreased over the past 30 to 40 years. For example, in 1980 the incidence of hepatitis was as high as 10%. Improved donor blood testing and screening have dramatically decreased the risk of transmission of hepatitis C and HIV to less than 1 in 2 million transfusions.[23] Although many factors account for the marked decrease in the incidence of transmission of infectious agents by blood transfusion, the most important one is improved testing of donor blood. Currently, hepatitis C, HIV, and West Nile virus are tested by nucleic acid technology. In 2002 more than 30 cases of transfusion-transmitted West Nile virus occurred. One year later, in 2003, with a nearly universal screening of donor blood by nucleic acid technology, the incidence was reduced to that of HIV. Other less commonly transmitted infectious agents include Chagas disease, hepatitis B, human T-cell lymphotropic virus, cytomegalovirus, malaria, and possibly variant Creutzfeldt–Jakob disease.

Because platelets are stored at room temperature, they deserve special attention. One of the leading causes of transfusion-related fatalities in the United States is

Table 25.4	Comparison of Transfusion-Related Fatalities in the United States Between 2015 and 2019[2]		
Cause	FY2015 Through FY2019 (# and % of total)		FY2019 (#)
TRALI	45	23%	13
TACO	65	34%	14
HTR (non-ABO)	26	14%	13
HTR (ABO)	13	7%	4
Microbial contamination	25	13%	2
Anaphylaxis	14	7%	2

HTR, Hemolytic transfusion reaction; *TACO*, transfusion-associated circulatory overload; *TRALI*, transfusion-related acute lung injury.

Table 25.5	Estimated Risk of Infection Transmitted by Blood Transfusion[23]
Infection	Risk
Hepatitis B	1 in 2 million
Hepatitis C	1 in 2 million
HIV	1 in 2 million
HTLV-I/II	1 in 3 million
West Nile virus	<1 in 3 million
Zika virus	<1 in 3 million
Trypanosoma cruzi	<1 in 3 million
Variant Creutzfeldt-Jakob	None
Bacteria (leading to sepsis event)	Platelets: 1 in 100,000
	PRBC: <1 in 1 million

HIV, Human immunodeficiency virus; *HTLV-I/II*, human T-cell lymphotropic virus type I or type II; *PRBC*, packed red blood cell.

bacterial contamination, which is most likely to occur in platelet concentrates. Platelet-related sepsis can be fatal, with overall transfusion-related sepsis events occurring as frequently as 1 in 100,000 transfusions. However, it is probably underrecognized because of the many other confounding variables present in hospitalized patients, and some estimate it to be as high as 1 in 2000. When donor platelets are cultured before infusion (and not released until the culture is negative after a minimum of 24 hours' incubation), the incidence of sepsis may be significantly reduced, but sepsis is still possible. The fact that platelets are stored at 20 to 24°C instead of 4°C probably accounts for the greater risk of bacterial growth than with other blood products. As a result, any patient in whom a fever develops within 6 hours of receiving platelet concentrates should be considered to possibly be manifesting platelet-induced sepsis, and empiric antibiotic therapy should be strongly considered.

Noninfectious Hazards of Transfusion

The causes of noninfectious serious hazards of transfusion are numerous and dominated by TRALI and transfusion-related immunomodulation (TRIM).

Transfusion-Related Acute Lung Injury

TRALI is among the top two leading causes of transfusion-related deaths. TRALI is acute lung injury that occurs within 6 hours after transfusion of a blood product, especially FFP. It can be further subdivided into type 1 or type 2 depending on the preexistence of acute respiratory distress syndrome (ARDS) in the preceding 12 hours.[24] It is characterized by dyspnea and arterial hypoxemia secondary to noncardiogenic pulmonary edema; it is a diagnosis of exclusion. Immediate actions to take when TRALI is suspected include (1) stopping the transfusion; (2) supporting the patient's vital signs, especially oxygenation; (3) obtaining a complete blood count and chest radiograph; and (4) notifying the blood bank of possible TRALI so that other associated units can be quarantined.

Because the diagnosis is difficult to make, follow-up actions are especially important, including sending a patient's blood specimen along with the empty bags of blood administered back to the blood bank. All transfusion forms and copies of anesthetic records (if not already present in the electronic medical record) will be required to be sent to the blood bank. Exclusion of multiparous female blood donors has decreased the incidence of TRALI.[25,26]

Transfusion-Related Immunomodulation

Blood transfusion, especially PRBCs, suppresses lymphocyte function likely via arginase, which, when combined with other effects produced by surgical trauma, may place patients at risk for postoperative infection.[27] Conversely, patients who receive blood transfusions may

have more extensive disease and a poorer prognosis independent of the administration of blood. As such, the role of blood transfusions in postoperative infections is difficult to ascertain.

Metabolic Abnormalities

Metabolic abnormalities that accompany the storage of blood include accumulation of hydrogen ions and potassium and decreased 2,3-DPG concentrations. The citrate present in the blood preservative as an anticoagulant may also affect the recipient.

Hydrogen Ions

The addition of most preservatives promptly increases the hydrogen ion content of stored blood. Continued metabolic function of erythrocytes results in additional production of hydrogen ions, with the pH of stored blood being as low as 6.7. Despite these changes, metabolic acidosis in recipients caused by the transfusion of blood products, even with rapid infusion of large volumes of stored blood, does not occur. If there is an acidosis, in all likelihood, it arises from tissue hypoxia and not from the blood product itself.

Potassium

The potassium content of stored blood increases progressively with the duration of storage, but even massive transfusions rarely increase plasma potassium concentrations. Failure of plasma potassium concentrations to increase most likely reflects the small amount of potassium actually present in 1 unit of stored blood. It is estimated that 1 unit of PRBCs contains 5 to 6 mEq of potassium. Despite this relatively low amount, caution should be exercised when transfusing a large volume in patients with impaired renal function.

2,3-Diphosphoglycerate

Storage of blood is associated with a progressive decrease in concentrations of 2,3-DPG in erythrocytes, which results in increased affinity of hemoglobin for oxygen (decreased P50 values). Conceivably, this increased affinity could make less oxygen available for tissues and jeopardize tissue oxygen delivery. There had been speculation that young blood (with higher levels of 2,3-DPG) should be used for critically ill patients to better increase tissue oxygen delivery and thereby improve mortality. However, despite a few observational studies and sound theoretical advantages, the routine use of young blood and the clinical significance of the 2,3-DPG oxygen affinity changes remain controversial.

Citrate

Citrate metabolism to bicarbonate may contribute to metabolic alkalosis, whereas binding of calcium by citrate could result in hypocalcemia. Indeed, metabolic alkalosis rather than metabolic acidosis can follow within hours of massive blood transfusions. Severe hypocalcemia as a result of citrate binding of calcium is rare because of mobilization of calcium stores from bone and the ability of the liver to rapidly metabolize citrate to bicarbonate. Therefore arbitrary administration of calcium in the absence of objective evidence of hypocalcemia (i.e., prolonged QT intervals on the electrocardiogram, measured decrease in plasma ionized calcium concentrations) is not indicated. Supplemental calcium may be needed when (1) the rate of blood infusion is more rapid than 50 mL/min, (2) hypothermia or liver disease interferes with the metabolism of citrate, or (3) the patient is a neonate. Patients undergoing liver transplantation are the most likely to experience citrate intoxication, and these patients may require calcium administration during a massive transfusion of stored blood.

Hypothermia

Administration of blood stored at 6°C or less can result in a decrease in the patient's body temperature. Passage of blood through specially designed warmers greatly decreases the likelihood of transfusion-related hypothermia. Unrecognized malfunction of these warmers, causing them to overheat, may result in hemolysis of the blood being transfused. Hypothermia has been shown to worsen coagulopathy and is a part of the lethal triad in trauma patients. It has also been associated with an increase in surgical site infections and poor wound healing.

Coagulopathy

The conclusion that excessive microvascular bleeding is occurring should be the combined judgment of both the surgical and anesthesia teams. Laboratory tests are only a supplement to clinically determined excessive microvascular bleeding. Blood loss should be determined by checking suction canisters, surgical sponges, and drains. A decision needs to be made regarding whether the blood loss is from inadequate surgical control of vascular bleeding or a coagulopathy. A platelet count, PT/INR, partial thromboplastin time (PTT), and fibrinogen level can confirm both the presence and type of coagulopathy. Platelet concentrates may be administered if the platelet count is less than 50,000 cells/mm^3. A qualitative platelet defect from antiplatelet drugs or cardiopulmonary bypass may require platelet concentrates to be given, even with a normal platelet count. Administration of FFP should be considered when the PT is longer than 1.5 times normal or the INR is more than 1.5. When laboratory tests are unavailable, if more than one blood volume (about 70 mL/kg) has been lost and excessive microvascular bleeding is present, FFP should be empirically transfused. The dose of FFP (10–15 mL/kg) should achieve at least 30% of most plasma factor concentrations. As indicated previously, specific ratios of FFP and platelets

with administration of RBCs seem to decrease coagulation problems in patients with trauma and massive blood loss. The previous description of transfusion practice is based on laboratory-derived coagulation values (e.g., platelet count), which takes some time. Use of point-of-care viscoelastic testing with rotational thromboelastography (ROTEM) or thromboelastography (TEG) has been successfully used in several clinical situations. However, most of the published studies on transfusion medicine and bleeding are based on standard laboratory tests (also see Chapter 23).

Cryoprecipitate should be considered if fibrinogen levels are less than 100 mg/dL. Also, a highly purified, lyophilized virus-inactivated fibrinogen concentrate from human plasma can be used to treat hypofibrinogenemia and is effective in some broader-based coagulopathies. Low blood fibrinogen levels are increasingly associated with coagulopathies and massive blood transfusions. Accordingly, fibrinogen administration is increasingly recognized as being important in treating patients with significant blood loss. In addition, desmopressin or a topical hemostatic agent (fibrin glue) may be used for excessive bleeding. Recombinant activated factor VII or vitamin K four-factor prothrombin complex concentrate may be considered as a "rescue" drug when standard transfusion therapy has failed to successfully treat a coagulopathy. These "last-resort" agents have the risk of inducing thromboembolic complications.

Transfusion Reactions

Although transfusion reactions are traditionally categorized as febrile, allergic, and hemolytic, anesthesia—especially general anesthesia—may mask the signs and symptoms of all types of transfusion reactions. Regardless, when transfusing blood, it is important to periodically check for signs and symptoms of bacterial contamination, TRALI, and hemolytic transfusion reactions, including urticaria, hypotension, tachycardia, increased peak airway pressure, hyperthermia, decreased urine output, hemoglobinuria, and microvascular bleeding.[28] Before instituting therapy for transfusion reactions, be sure to stop the blood transfusion first.

Febrile Reactions

Febrile reactions are the most common adverse non-hemolytic response to the transfusion of blood, and they accompany 0.5% to 1% of transfusions. The most likely explanation for febrile reactions is an interaction between recipient antibodies and antigens present on the leukocytes or platelets of the donor. The patient's temperature rarely increases to above 38°C, and the condition is treated by slowing the infusion and administering antipyretics. Severe febrile reactions accompanied by chills and shivering may require discontinuation of the blood transfusion. Today, most blood is leukoreduced at the time of separation into its components.

Allergic Reactions

Allergic reactions to properly typed and crossmatched blood are manifested as increases in body temperature, pruritus, and urticaria. Treatment often includes intravenous administration of antihistamines and, in severe cases, discontinuation of the blood transfusion. Examination of plasma and urine for free hemoglobin is useful to rule out hemolytic reactions.

Hemolytic Reactions

Hemolytic reactions occur when the wrong blood type is administered to a patient. The common factor in the production of intravascular hemolysis and the development of spontaneous hemorrhage is activation of the complement system. With the exception of hypotension, the immediate signs (lumbar and substernal pain, fever, chills, dyspnea, skin flushing) of hemolytic reactions are masked by general anesthesia. Even hypotension may be attributed to other causes in an anesthetized patient. The appearance of free hemoglobin in plasma or urine is presumptive evidence of a hemolytic reaction. Acute renal failure reflects precipitation of stromal and lipid contents of hemolyzed erythrocytes in distal renal tubules. Disseminated intravascular coagulation causing a coagulopathy is initiated by material released from hemolyzed erythrocytes.

The treatment of acute hemolytic reactions is immediate discontinuation of the incompatible blood transfusion, followed by maintenance of urine output by infusion of crystalloid solutions and administration of mannitol or furosemide. The use of sodium bicarbonate to alkalinize the urine and improve the solubility of hemoglobin degradation products in the renal tubules is of unproven value, as is the administration of corticosteroids.

AUTOLOGOUS BLOOD TRANSFUSIONS

Although this chapter has focused primarily on allogeneic blood transfusions, a few words should be said about autologous blood transfusions. There are three types of autologous blood: (1) predeposited (preoperative) autologous donation (PAD), (2) intraoperative and postoperative blood salvage, and (3) normovolemic hemodilution. The primary reason for the use of autologous blood is to decrease or eliminate infectious complications from allogeneic blood transfusions. In the 1980s both patient and physician fear escalated because of a legitimate concern regarding infectious diseases, especially hepatitis C and HIV. Today, given the recent advances in testing over the past 40 years, there has been a marked reduction in the rate of infectious disease transmission from allogeneic blood.

Predeposited Autologous Donation

Patients scheduled for elective surgery who may require transfusion of blood may choose to predeposit (predonate) blood for possible transfusion in the perioperative period and avoid the use of allogeneic blood. Patient donors must have a hemoglobin concentration of at least 11 g/dL. Most patients can donate 10.5 mL/kg of blood approximately every 5–7 days (maximum, 2–3 units), with the last unit collected 72 hours or more before surgery to permit restoration of plasma volume. Oral iron supplementation is highly recommended during this process. Treatment with recombinant erythropoietin is very expensive, but it increases the amount of blood that patients can predeposit by as much as 25%. PAD is not generally a cost-effective alternative to allogeneic blood.

Intraoperative Blood Salvage

Intraoperative blood salvage for reinfusion into the patient decreases the amount of allogeneic blood needed. Typically, semiautomated systems are used in which the RBCs are collected, washed, and then delivered to a reservoir for future administration either intraoperatively or postoperatively. The presence of infection or malignant disease at the operative site is considered a relative contraindication to blood salvage. Complications of intraoperative salvage include dilutional coagulopathy, reinfusion of anticoagulant (heparin, though it is theoretically removed during the washing process), and hemolysis. A documented quality assurance program, as recommended by the AABB, is required for those who use intraoperative salvage techniques.

Normovolemic Hemodilution

Normovolemic hemodilution consists of withdrawing a portion of the patient's blood volume early in the intraoperative period and concurrent infusion of crystalloids or colloids to maintain intravascular volume. The endpoint is a patient hematocrit of 27% to 33%, depending on the patient's cardiovascular and respiratory status. By initially hemodiluting the patient, fewer blood cells will be lost per milliliter of blood loss during surgery. At the conclusion of surgery, the patient's blood, with its enhanced oxygen-carrying capacity by virtue of a higher hematocrit and its greater clotting ability by virtue of platelets and other coagulation factors, is reinfused. Whether the use of this technique actually decreases allogeneic blood administration is questionable. The survival of recovered RBCs appears to be similar to that of transfused allogeneic cells.

CONCLUSIONS AND FUTURE DIRECTIONS

Transfusion of blood products has become increasingly safer as a result of the dramatically decreased incidence of infectious disease transmission. If given in accordance with proper indications, patient mortality rate is not increased because of receiving blood transfusions per se. As indicated previously, increasing emphasis is being placed on defining ratios of blood products that should be given (e.g., 1:1 PRBCs with FFP or platelets during major trauma). Alternatively, perhaps in the future, whole blood will be given more often. This would also mitigate the impact of lengthy blood storage times. Regardless, component therapy will always be around, at least until alternatives are developed and the ultimate impact of storage time on overall transfusion practice is refined. As for RBCs, other possibilities include hemoglobin-based oxygen carriers (HBOCs). For over 20 years, with all of their advantages (e.g., no typing and crossmatching), we hoped that one or more of these products would partially replace human blood transfusions. However, an FDA and National Institutes of Health (NIH) conference in 2008 indicated that HBOC products would not be available soon and, unfortunately, that prediction has been correct. Finally, consistent with the practice of medicine, well-designed protocols will increasingly be the foundation upon which transfusion practice is based.

REFERENCES

1. Johnson DJ, Scott AV, Barodka VM, Park S, Wasey JO, Ness PM, Gniadek T, Frank SM. Morbidity and mortality after high-dose transfusion. *Anesthesiology*. 2016;124(2):387–395. doi:10.1097/ALN.0000000000000945 FebPMID: 26569167.
2. FDA's Center for Biologics Evaluation and Research. Fatalities reported to FDA following blood collection and transfusion: Annual summary for fiscal year 2019. Accessed April 17, 2021. https://www.fda.gov/vaccines-blood-biologics/report-problem-center-biologics-evaluation-research/transfusiondonation-fatalities.
3. American Society of Anesthesiologists Task Force on Perioperative Blood Management. Practice guidelines for perioperative blood management: An updated report by the American Society of Anesthesiologists Task Force on Perioperative Blood Management. *Anesthesiology*. 2015;122(2):241–275. doi:10.1097/ALN.0000000000000463.
4. Miller R. Massive blood transfusions: The impact of Vietnam military data on modern civilian transfusion medicine. *Anesthesiology*. 2009;110(6):1412–1416. doi:10.1097/ALN.0b013e3181a1fd54.
5. Gurney J, Staudt A, Cap A, et al. Improved survival in critically injured combat casualties treated with fresh whole blood by forward surgical teams in Afghanistan. *Transfusion (Paris)*. 2020;60(Suppl 3):S180–S188. doi:10.1111/trf.15767.
6. Heddle N, Cook R, Arnold D, et al. Effect of short-term vs. long-term blood storage on mortality after transfusion. *N Engl J Med*. 2016;375(20):1937–1945. doi:10.1056/NEJMoa1609014.
7. Halmin M, Rostgaard K, Lee B, et al. Length of storage of red blood cells and patient survival after blood transfusion: A Binational cohort study. *Ann Intern Med*. 2017;166(4):248–256. doi:10.7326/M16-1415.
8. Shah A, Brunskill S, Desborough M, Doree C, Trivella M, Stanworth S. Transfusion of red blood cells stored for shorter versus longer duration for all conditions. *Cochrane Database Syst Rev*. 2018;12(12). doi:10.1002/14651858.CD010801.pub3.
9. McQuilten Z, Crighton G, Brunskill S, et al. Optimal dose, timing, and ratio of blood products in massive transfusion: Results from a systematic review. *Transfus Med Rev*. 2018;32(1):6–15. doi:10.1016/j.tmrv.2017.06.003.
10. Meneses E, Boneva D, McKenney M, Elkbuli A. Massive transfusion protocol in adult trauma population. *Am J Emerg Med*. 2020;38(12):2661–2666. doi:10.1016/j.ajem.2020.07.041.
11. Desai N, Schofield N, Richards T. Perioperative patient blood management to improve outcomes. *Anesth Analg*. 2018;127(5):1211–1220.
12. AABB. AABB Guide to Patient Blood Management and Blood Utilization. *AABB*. 2020.
13. Mueller M, van Remoortel H, Meybohm P, et al. Patient blood management: Recommendations from the 2018 Frankfurt Consensus Conference. *J Am Med Assoc*. 2019;321(10):983–997. doi:10.1001/jama.2019.0554.
14. Warner M, Shore-Lesserson L, Shander A, Patel S, Perelman S, Guinn N. Perioperative anemia: Prevention, diagnosis, and management throughout the spectrum of perioperative care. *Anesth Analg*. 2020;130(5):1364–1380. doi:10.1213/ANE.0000000000004727.
15. Zhang W, Zheng Y, Yu K, Gu J. Liberal transfusion versus restrictive transfusion and outcomes in critically ill adults: A meta-analysis. *Transfus Med Hemotherapy*. 2021;48(1):60–68. doi:10.1159/000506751.
16. Carson J, Stanworth S, Roubinian N, et al. Transfusion thresholds and other strategies for guiding allogeneic red blood cell transfusion. *Cochrane Database Syst Rev*. 2016;10(10). doi:10.1002/14651858.CD002042.pub4.
17. Fominskiy E, Putzu A, Monaco F, et al. Liberal transfusion strategy improves survival in perioperative but not critically ill patients. A meta-analysis of randomised trials. *Br J Anaesthesiol*. 2015;115(4):511–519. doi:10.1093/bja/aev317.
18. Vlaar A, Oczkowski S, de Bruin S, et al. Transfusion strategies in non-bleeding critically ill adults: A clinical practice guideline from the European Society of Intensive Care Medicine. *Intensive Care Med*. 2020;46(4):673–696. doi:10.1007/s00134-019-05884-8.
19. Miller R, Ward T, Shiboski S, Cohen N. A comparison of three methods of hemoglobin monitoring in patients undergoing spine surgery. *Anesth Analg*. 2011;112(4):858–863. doi:10.1213/ANE.0b013e31820eecd1.
20. Hare G, Cazorla-Bak M, Ku SM, et al. When to transfuse your acute care patient? A narrative review of the risk of anemia and red blood cell transfusion based on clinical trial outcomes. *Can J Anesth*. 2020;67(11):1576–1594. doi:10.1007/s12630-020-01763-9.
21. Rohde J, Dimcheff D, Blumberg N, et al. Healthcare-associated infection after red blood cell transfusion: A systematic review and meta-analysis. *J Am Med Assoc*. 2014;311(13):1317–1326. doi:10.1001/jama.2014.2726.
22. Lv Y, Xiang Q, Lin J, et al. There is no dose-response relationship between allogeneic blood transfusion and healthcare-associated infection: A retrospective cohort study. *Antimicrob Resist Infect Control*. 2021;10(1):1–10. doi:10.1186/s13756-021-00928-5.

23. Busch M, Bloch E, Kleinman S. Prevention of transfusion-transmitted infections. *Blood.* 2019;133(17):1854–1864. doi:10.1182/blood-2018-11-833996.

24. Vlaar A, Toy P, Fung M, et al. A consensus redefinition of transfusion-related acute lung injury. *Transfusion (Paris).* 2019;59(7):2465–2476. doi:10.1111/trf.15311

25. Middelburg R, van Stein D, Zupanska B, et al. Female donors and transfusion-related acute lung injury: A case-referent study from the International TRALI Unisex Research Group. *Transfusion (Paris).* 2010;50(11):2447–2454. doi:10.1111/j.1537-2995.2010.02715.x

26. Caram-Deelder C, Kreuger A, Evers D, et al. Association of blood transfusion from female donors with and without a history of pregnancy with mortality among male and female transfusion recipients. *J Am Med Assoc.* 2017;318(15):1471–1478. doi:10.1001/jama.2017.14825.

27. Remy K, Hall M, Cholette J, et al. Mechanisms of red blood cell transfusion-related immunomodulation. *Transfusion (Paris).* 2018;58(3):804–815. doi:10.1111/trf.14488

28. Strobel E. Hemolytic transfusion reactions. *Transfus Med Hemotherapy.* 2008;35(5):346–353. doi:10.1159/000154811.

SPECIAL ANESTHETIC CONSIDERATIONS

26 CARDIOVASCULAR DISEASE

Grace C. McCarthy, Annemarie Thompson

Cardiovascular disease is the leading cause of global death, with an estimated 17 million deaths per year; it is also the leading cause of death in the United States.[1,2] Many of the risk factors identified to predict perioperative mortality are cardiovascular in origin, including coronary artery disease (CAD), peripheral vascular disease, recent myocardial infarction (MI) (in the past 6 months), presence of congestive heart failure (CHF), and aortic stenosis.[3,4] Management of anesthesia for patients with cardiovascular disease requires an understanding of the pathophysiology of the disease process; appropriate preoperative testing; application of perioperative risk reduction strategies; and careful selection of anesthetic, analgesic, neuromuscular, and autonomic blocking drugs.

CORONARY ARTERY DISEASE

CAD (ischemic heart disease) occurs in approximately 40% of adult patients undergoing surgery annually in the United States.[1] The presence of CAD in patients who undergo anesthesia for noncardiac surgery may be associated with increased morbidity and mortality rates. Important components of the routine preoperative cardiac evaluation include history, assessment of cardiac risk factors, determination of the patient's exercise tolerance, cardiac symptoms, physical examination with specific attention to cardiac and respiratory findings, and review of the electrocardiogram (ECG)[5] (also see Chapter 13). Risk factors for CAD include family history of CAD (especially at age 50 or younger), physical inactivity, overweight or obesity, unhealthy eating, and tobacco use.

The most common anginal symptom in men is shortness of breath with exertion (e.g., stair climbing), whereas in women the most common symptom is fatigue. It is important to ask whether patients have chest pain or shortness of breath when walking up stairs because the ability to walk slowly on level ground requires only minimal exertion (approximately 2 metabolic equivalents

---

Box 26.1 Grading of Angina*

Grade I
Ordinary physical activity does not cause angina, such as walking and climbing stairs. Angina with strenuous or rapid or prolonged exertion at work or recreation.

Grade II
Slight limitation of ordinary activity. Angina occurs when walking or climbing stairs rapidly; walking uphill; walking or stair climbing after meals; or in cold, or in wind, or under emotional stress; or only during the few hours after awakening. Walking more than two blocks on level ground and climbing more than one flight of ordinary stairs at a normal pace and in normal conditions.

Grade III
Marked limitation of ordinary physical activity. Angina occurs when walking one or two blocks on the level and climbing one flight of stairs in normal conditions and at normal pace.

Grade IV
Inability to carry on any physical activity without discomfort; anginal syndrome may be present at rest.

---

*About 70% of ischemic episodes are not associated with angina pectoris, and as many as 15% of acute myocardial infarctions are silent. From Owlia M, Dodson JA, King JB, et al. Angina severity, mortality, and healthcare utilization among veterans with stable angina. J Am Heart Assoc. 2019;8(15):e012811.

[METs]); patients who are asymptomatic walking on flat ground will often report symptoms when walking up stairs (approximately 4 METs for one flight of stairs). Other potential signs of significant cardiac disease include (1) the inability to lie flat, (2) awakening from sleep with angina or shortness of breath, and (3) angina at rest or with minimal exertion. Limited exercise tolerance in the absence of significant pulmonary disease is the most striking evidence of decreased cardiac reserve. The ability to achieve a moderate level of activity (a metabolic equivalent of task score (METS) of 4 or more) without anginal symptoms predicts a low risk of perioperative complications.[6]

Assessment of functional capacity or cardiorespiratory fitness (METS) should help direct subsequent preoperative testing and treatment decisions. Ultimately, the history and physical examination with specific attention to signs and symptoms of new-onset angina, change in anginal pattern, worsening angina (Box 26.1), recent MI, heart failure, or aortic stenosis and the presence of appropriate medical therapy should determine whether patients are in the best medical condition possible before elective cardiac or noncardiac surgery[5] (see Chapter 13). Fig. 26.1 provides a suggested protocol for preoperative evaluation.

An increased heart rate is more likely than hypertension to produce signs of myocardial ischemia. Tachycardia increases myocardial oxygen requirements while at the same time decreases the duration of diastole, thereby decreasing left ventricular coronary blood flow (which occurs in diastole) and the delivery of oxygen to the left ventricle. Increased systolic and diastolic blood pressure, while increasing oxygen consumption, simultaneously increases

coronary perfusion despite the presence of atherosclerotic coronary arteries. Avoidance of tachycardia is important in the perioperative care of patients with significant CAD.

Prior Myocardial Infarction

For patients with prior MI, the incidence of myocardial reinfarction in the perioperative period is related to the time elapsed since the previous MI.[7-9] The incidence of perioperative myocardial reinfarction generally does not stabilize at 5% to 6% until 6 months after the MI. A common recommendation is to delay elective surgery, especially thoracic, upper abdominal, or other major procedures, for a period of 2 to 6 months after an MI. The exact duration of suggested delay is unclear. According to the 2014 American College of Cardiology/American Heart Association (ACC/AHA) guidelines for perioperative cardiac evaluation before noncardiac surgery, no fewer than 60 days should elapse between recent MI and noncardiac surgery. Though significant risk reduction occurs by 60 days post-MI, the risk of reinfarction remains elevated for up to 1 year after MI. After 6 months, the 5% to 6% incidence of myocardial reinfarction is about 50 times higher than the 0.13% incidence of perioperative MI in patients undergoing similar operations but in the absence of a prior MI.[10]

Most perioperative myocardial reinfarctions occur in the first 48 to 72 hours postoperatively. However, if ischemia is initiated by the stress of surgery, there can be an increased risk of MI for several months after surgery.[3]

The risk of noncardiac surgery for patients with prior MI is reduced in the setting of coronary artery revascularization by stenting (percutaneous coronary intervention [PCI]) or coronary artery bypass grafting.[9] Although PCI can mitigate the risk associated with preoperative MI, the ACC/AHA recommend against routine PCI outside of current clinical practice guidelines. Based on the need for dual antiplatelet therapy after PCI, elective noncardiac surgery should be delayed according to the following recommendations: 14 days after balloon angioplasty, 30 days after bare-metal stent placement, and 6 months after drug-eluting stent placement.[11] Coronary angiography is also not routinely recommended for preoperative evaluation.

Perioperative Risk Reduction Therapy/Medications

Knowledge of the pharmacology of the drugs often taken by patients with CAD and potential adverse interactions with anesthetics is an important preoperative consideration (also see Chapter 13). Continuation versus preoperative initiation of medications such as β-blockers and statins to reduce adverse outcomes remains controversial. Current recommendations include continuation of *existing* statin and β-blocker therapies, which has been demonstrated to be of benefit, whereas preoperative

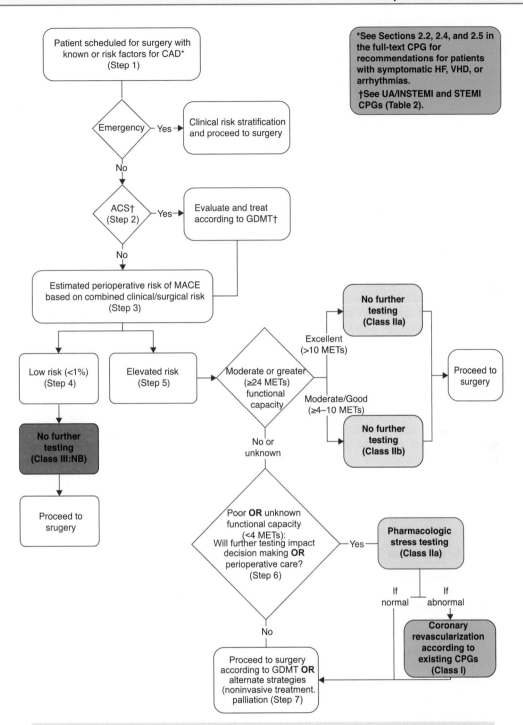

Fig. 26.1 Stepwise approach to perioperative cardiac assessment for coronary artery disease (CAD). *ACS,* Acute coronary syndrome; *CPG,* clinical practice guideline; *GDMT,* guideline-directed medical therapy; *HF,* heart failure; *MACE,* major adverse cardiac event; *MET,* metabolic equivalent; *NB,* no benefit; *STEMI,* ST-segment elevation myocardial infarction; *UA/NSTEMI,* unstable angina/non–ST-segment elevation myocardial infarction; *VHD,* valvular heart disease. (From Fleisher L, Fleischmann K, Auerbach AD, et al. 2014 ACC/AHA guideline on perioperative cardiovascular evaluation and management of patients undergoing noncardiac surgery. A report of the American College of Cardiology/American Heart Association Task Force on Practice Guidelines. J Am Coll Cardiol. 2014;64[22]:e77–e137.)

IV

Table 26.1 Area of Myocardial Ischemia as Reflected by the Electrocardiogram

Electrocardiogram Leads	Coronary Artery Responsible for Myocardial Ischemia	Area of Myocardium That May Be Involved
II, III, aVF	Right coronary artery	Right atrium Sinus node Atrioventricular node Right ventricle
V_3–V_5	Left anterior descending coronary artery	Anterolateral aspect of the left ventricle
I, aVL	Circumflex coronary artery	Lateral aspect of the left ventricle

introduction of these medical therapies should be decided based on risk estimation and clinical judgment.[5]

Despite the potential for adverse drug interactions, cardiac medications being taken preoperatively should, in general, be continued without interruption through the perioperative period. Holding angiotensin-converting enzyme (ACE) inhibitors and angiotensin receptor blockers (ARBs) perioperatively may be considered because continuation has been associated with an increased incidence of intraoperative hypotension.[12] In patients who do not require general anesthesia or who are undergoing low- to intermediate-risk procedures it is likely beneficial to continue all cardiac medications.

Patients with recently placed intracoronary stents receiving platelet inhibitors have a high risk of intracoronary thrombosis and death when the platelet inhibitors are discontinued for perioperative care. Guidelines provide recommendations for duration of antiplatelet therapy[11]; however, treatment should be individualized based on the patient's risk of stent thrombosis versus surgical bleeding (see Chapter 13).

Monitoring (Also See Chapter 20)

The intensity of monitoring in the perioperative period is influenced by the complexity of the operative procedure and the severity of the cardiovascular disease. The five-lead ECG serves as a noninvasive monitor of the balance between myocardial oxygen requirements and myocardial oxygen delivery in unconscious patients. When this balance is unfavorably altered, myocardial ischemia occurs, as evidenced on the ECG by at least a 1-mm downsloping of the ST segment from the baseline (Table 26.1). A precordial V_5 lead is a useful selection for detecting ST-segment changes characteristic of ischemia of the left ventricle during anesthesia, whereas lead II is the most sensitive for detection of arrhythmias. Intraarterial pressure monitoring can speed the identification and treatment of hemodynamic changes. Ventricular wall motion abnormalities observed by transesophageal echocardiogram (TEE) may be the most sensitive indicator of myocardial ischemia, but this monitor is expensive, invasive, and requires additional training; however, it is routinely used for detecting myocardial ischemia. As part of goal-directed therapy, continuous measurement of stroke volume variation (SVV) or pulse pressure variation (PPV) can predict fluid responsiveness and be used to optimize fluid administration, though there is controversy on whether there is any difference in outcomes[13] (also see Chapter 24).

Intraoperative monitoring of pulmonary artery pressures or use of TEE should be reserved for selected high-risk patients (e.g., cardiac surgery, recent MI, current heart failure, unstable angina).[1] Although few or no data support the use of pulmonary artery catheters,[14] in selected patients, a pulmonary artery catheter in combination with a TEE probe may be helpful for monitoring responses to intravenous fluid replacement and the therapeutic effects of drugs on left ventricular function and cardiac output. When compared with TEE, monitoring with a pulmonary artery catheter is not a highly sensitive approach for detecting myocardial ischemia. TEE allows assessment of regional wall motion, global ventricular function, valvular function, intravascular fluid volume, and associated ventricular filling.

Management of Anesthesia

Management of anesthesia in patients with CAD is based on a preoperative evaluation of left ventricular function (Table 26.2) and the maintenance of a favorable balance between myocardial oxygen requirements and myocardial oxygen delivery so as to prevent myocardial ischemia (Box 26.2). Any event associated with persistent tachycardia, systolic hypertension, diastolic hypotension, or arterial hypoxemia can adversely influence this delicate balance. Heart rate higher than 100 beats/min increases the risk of postoperative death in patients with risk for CAD; heart rates higher than 120 beats/min significantly increase the risk.

Maintaining heart rate and systemic arterial blood pressure within 20% of the awake values is commonly recommended. Monitoring with an intraarterial catheter greatly improves the ability to maintain stable systemic arterial blood pressures. Nevertheless, an estimated one-half of all new perioperative ischemic episodes are not preceded by or associated with significant changes in heart rate or systemic arterial blood pressure.[15] A single 1-minute episode of myocardial ischemia detected by a 1-mm ST-segment

Table 26.2 Evaluation of Left Ventricular Function

Assessment Feature	Good Function	Impaired Function
Previous myocardial infarction	No	Yes
Evidence of congestive heart failure	No	Yes
Ejection fraction	>0.55	<0.4
Left ventricular end-diastolic pressure	<12 mm Hg	>18 mm Hg
Cardiac index	>2.5 L/min/m²	<2 L/min/m²
Areas of ventricular dyskinesia	No	Yes

Box 26.2 Determinants of Myocardial Oxygen Requirements and Delivery

Myocardial Oxygen Requirements
- Heart rate
- Systolic blood pressure
- Myocardial contractility
- Ventricular volume

Myocardial Oxygen Delivery
- Coronary blood flow
- Oxygen content of arterial blood

elevation or depression increases the risk of cardiac events 10-fold and the risk for death 2-fold.[3,4] Tachycardia for 5 minutes above 120 beats/min in the postoperative period can increase the risk of death 10-fold. Prevention or treatment of tachycardia can reduce the risk of perioperative myocardial ischemia and associated death.

Preoperative anxiety can worsen myocardial ischemia because of increased catecholamine release and an increase in myocardial oxygen requirements secondary to an increase in heart rate and systemic blood pressure. Judicious preoperative use of a benzodiazepine or dexmedetomidine can be considered.

Choice and dose of induction and maintenance agents need to reflect the patient's underlying cardiac disease and function. In high-risk patients preinduction placement of an intraarterial catheter to monitor arterial blood pressure allows rapid pharmacologic manipulations and ability to achieve a more stable induction of anesthesia. Regardless of anesthetic choice, the main goals include avoidance of tachycardia and maintenance of hemodynamic stability.

Administration of opioids reduces the stimulation produced by tracheal intubation and attenuates the surgical stress response. β-Adrenergic blockers are effective in attenuating heart rate increases associated with tracheal intubation. Perioperative dexmedetomidine has been shown to reduce delirium after both cardiac surgery and noncardiac surgery.[16,17]

All volatile anesthetics induce ischemic preconditioning to varying degrees and may protect the myocardium from subsequent ischemia.[18] Regional myocardial ischemia associated with drug-induced vasodilation is known as *coronary artery steal*. The myth that isoflurane increases the risk of coronary steal has been debunked. There is no increased risk of coronary steal when hemodynamic variables are tightly controlled.[19,20] A large clinical trial in patients undergoing cardiac surgery failed to demonstrate a difference between halothane, enflurane, isoflurane, and narcotic-based anesthetics.[21]

Decreases in body temperature that occur intraoperatively may predispose to shivering on awakening, leading to abrupt increases in myocardial oxygen requirements. After high-risk surgery, intensive and continuous postoperative monitoring is useful for detecting myocardial ischemia, which is often asymptomatic. Most deaths after noncardiac surgery are linked to cardiovascular causes. MI after surgery independently raises the risk of 30-day mortality and stroke.[22] Perioperative monitoring of high-risk patients, including after surgery, is important to ensure the best recovery and patient outcomes.

VALVULAR HEART DISEASE

The most frequently encountered forms of valvular heart disease produce pressure overload (mitral stenosis, aortic stenosis) or volume overload (mitral regurgitation, aortic regurgitation).[23] The net effect of valvular heart disease is interference with forward flow of blood from the heart into the systemic circulation. TEE has revolutionized the evaluation and intraoperative management of valvular heart disease. Selection of anesthetic drugs for patients with valvular heart disease is often based on the likely effects of drug-induced changes in cardiac rhythm, heart rate, systemic arterial blood pressure, systemic vascular resistance (SVR), and pulmonary vascular resistance (PVR) relative to the maintenance of cardiac output in these patients. Monitoring intraarterial pressure is helpful in patients with clinically significant valvular heart disease.

Mitral Stenosis

Mitral stenosis is characterized by mechanical obstruction of left ventricular diastolic filling secondary to a progressive decrease in the orifice of the mitral valve. The obstruction produces an increase in left atrial and pulmonary venous pressure. Increased PVR is likely when the left atrial pressure is chronically higher than 25 mm Hg. Distention of the left atrium predisposes to atrial fibrillation, which can result in stasis of blood, the formation of thrombi, and systemic emboli. Chronic anticoagulation or antiplatelet therapy (or both) in patients with atrial fibrillation can reduce the risk of systemic embolic events. Mitral stenosis is commonly the result of the fusion of the mitral

IV

> **Box 26.3** Anesthetic Considerations in Patients With Mitral Stenosis
>
> - Avoid tachycardia and maintain sinus rhythm
> - Maintain systemic vascular resistance to maintain diastolic coronary perfusion
> - Arterial hypoxemia, hypoventilation, or hypercarbia may exacerbate pulmonary hypertension and precipitate right ventricular failure
> - Increased circulatory volume may lead to flash pulmonary edema and hypoxemia

> **Box 26.4** Anesthetic Considerations in the Patient With Mitral or Aortic Regurgitation
>
> - Maintain sinus rhythm with normal to slightly elevated heart rate (HR 80–100 bpm)
> - Maintain diastolic pressure; mild decrease in systemic vascular resistance will improve forward flow
> - Sudden increases in systemic vascular resistance may worsen mitral or aortic regurgitation

valve leaflets during the healing process of acute rheumatic carditis. Symptoms of mitral stenosis do not usually develop until about 20 years after the initial episode of rheumatic fever. A sudden increase in the demand for cardiac output as produced by pregnancy or sepsis, however, may unmask previously asymptomatic mitral stenosis.

Management of Anesthesia

Patients with mitral stenosis can be more susceptible than normal individuals to the ventilatory depressant effects of sedative drugs used for preoperative medication. If patients are given sedative drugs, supplemental oxygen may increase the margin of safety. Drugs used for induction and maintenance of anesthesia should cause minimal changes in heart rate and in SVR and PVR (Box 26.3). Furthermore, these drugs should not greatly decrease myocardial contractility. No one anesthetic has been proven to be superior. Intraoperative intravenous fluid therapy must be carefully titrated because these patients are susceptible to intravascular volume overload and to the development of left ventricular failure and pulmonary edema. Likewise, the head-down position may not be well tolerated because the pulmonary blood volume is already increased.

Monitoring intraarterial pressure and SVV or PPV is helpful to guide the adequacy of intravascular fluid replacement (also see Chapters 20 and 24). If central pressures are measured, an increase in right atrial pressure could also reflect pulmonary vasoconstriction, suggesting the need to check for causes, which may include nitrous oxide, desflurane, acidosis, hypoxia, increased mitral regurgitation, or light anesthesia.

Postoperatively, patients with mitral stenosis who undergo noncardiac surgery are at high risk for developing pulmonary edema and right-sided heart failure. Mechanical ventilation may be necessary, particularly after major thoracic or abdominal surgery. The shift from positive-pressure ventilation to spontaneous ventilation with weaning and extubation may lead to increased venous return and increased central venous pressures with worsening of heart failure.

Mitral Regurgitation

Mitral regurgitation is characterized by left atrial volume overload and decreased left ventricular forward stroke volume caused by the backflow of part of each stroke volume through the incompetent mitral valve back into the left atrium. This regurgitant flow is responsible for the characteristic V waves seen on the recording of the pulmonary artery occlusion pressure. Common causes of mitral regurgitation include mitral valve prolapse, ischemia leading to left ventricular dilation, and chronic hypertension. Mitral regurgitation secondary to rheumatic fever usually has a component of mitral stenosis. Isolated mitral regurgitation may be acute, reflecting papillary muscle dysfunction after an MI or rupture of chordae tendineae secondary to infective endocarditis.

Management of Anesthesia

Management of anesthesia in patients with mitral regurgitation should attempt to improve the forward left ventricular stroke volume. Cardiac output can be improved by mild increases in heart rate and mild decreases in SVR (Box 26.4). Preinduction placement of intraarterial pressure monitoring can speed the identification and treatment of hemodynamic changes in patients with clinically significant valvular disease.

A general anesthetic is the usual choice for patients with significant mitral regurgitation. Although decreases in SVR are theoretically beneficial, the rapid onset and uncontrolled nature of this response with a spinal anesthetic may detract from the use of this technique. Local or regional anesthesia may be used safely for surgery on peripheral body sites. Surgical stimulation can lead to undesirable increases in systemic arterial blood pressure and SVR. Intravascular fluid volume must be maintained to ensure adequate venous return and ejection of an optimal forward left ventricular stroke volume.

Aortic Stenosis

Aortic stenosis is characterized by increased left ventricular systolic pressure to maintain the forward stroke volume through a narrowed aortic valve. The magnitude of the pressure gradient across the valve serves as an estimate of the severity of valvular stenosis. Hemodynamically significant aortic stenosis is associated with mean systolic pressure gradients more than 40 mm Hg or valve areas less than 1.0 cm². The combination of symptoms (angina, heart failure, or syncope), signs (serious left ventricular dysfunction and progressive cardiomegaly), and a reduced valve area also indicate the diagnosis of critical aortic stenosis requiring surgical replacement. Increased intraventricular pressures are accompanied by compensatory increases in the thickness of the left ventricular wall, which leads to diastolic and systolic dysfunction. Angina pectoris occurs often in these patients in the absence of CAD, reflecting an increased myocardial oxygen demand associated with myocardial hypertrophy in combination with higher intraventricular pressures. There is a decrease in oxygen delivery secondary to the aortic valve pressure gradient in combination with an increase in oxygen requirements from the increase in left ventricular stroke work. Thus aortic stenosis results in an increase in left ventricular stroke work and oxygen requirements (increased demand) while reducing coronary blood flow (reduced supply).

Isolated nonrheumatic aortic stenosis usually results from progressive calcification and stenosis of a congenitally abnormal (usually bicuspid) valve. Aortic stenosis caused by rheumatic fever almost always occurs in association with mitral valve disease. Likewise, aortic stenosis is usually accompanied by some degree of aortic regurgitation. Regardless of the cause of aortic stenosis, the natural history of the disease includes a long latent period, often 30 years or more, before symptoms occur. Because aortic stenosis may be asymptomatic, it is important to listen for this cardiac murmur (systolic murmur in the second right intercostal space that may radiate to the right carotid) in patients scheduled for surgery. The incidence of sudden death is increased in patients with aortic stenosis.

Management of Anesthesia

With the advent of transcatheter aortic valve replacement (TAVR), the indications for aortic valve replacement (AVR) have changed, and many patients previously thought too high risk for surgical AVR (SAVR) are now considered candidates for TAVR. Patients with critical aortic stenosis or aortic stenosis with reduced ventricular function or symptoms of angina or heart failure should be evaluated for AVR before elective surgery.

Goals during management of anesthesia in patients with aortic stenosis are avoidance of arterial hypotension; maintenance of normal sinus rhythm; and avoidance of extreme and prolonged alterations in heart rate, SVR, and intravascular fluid volume (Box 26.5). The most important aspect of management for patients with aortic

---

Box 26.5 Anesthetic Considerations in Patients With Aortic Stenosis

- Maintain sinus rhythm with normal to slightly decreased heart rate (HR 60-90 bpm)
- Avoid hypotension; maintain systemic vascular resistance to maintain diastolic coronary perfusion
- Given underlying left ventricular hypertrophy, reduced intracavity volume, and associated diastolic dysfunction, fluid management may be challenging

---

stenosis is careful avoidance of hypotension. Preservation of normal sinus rhythm is critical because the left ventricle is dependent on properly timed atrial contractions to ensure optimal left ventricular filling and stroke volume. Marked increases in heart rate (more than 100 beats/min) decrease the time for left ventricular filling and ejection and decrease coronary blood flow while increasing myocardial oxygen consumption. Coronary blood flow to the left ventricle occurs during diastole, and changes in heart rate primarily affect diastolic time. Bradycardia (fewer than 50 beats/min) can lead to acute overdistention of the left ventricle. In severe aortic stenosis intraarterial pressure monitoring before induction of anesthesia can speed the identification and treatment of hemodynamic changes. Prophylactic infusions of vasoconstrictors such as phenylephrine started before induction may reduce hemodynamic changes.

Intravascular fluid volume should be maintained in order to maintain end-diastolic volume. This may be challenging in the setting of underlying left ventricular hypertrophy (LVH), reduced left ventricular filling, and diastolic dysfunction. A cardiac defibrillator should be promptly available when anesthesia is administered to patients with severe aortic stenosis because external cardiac compressions are unlikely to generate an adequate stroke volume across a severely stenosed aortic valve. Cardiopulmonary resuscitation (CPR) has a lower success rate in patients with aortic stenosis secondary to low coronary perfusion pressures as a result of the stenotic aortic valve (also see Chapter 45).

Aortic Regurgitation

Aortic regurgitation is characterized by decreased forward left ventricular stroke volume resulting from regurgitation of part of the ejected stroke volume back into the left ventricle through an incompetent aortic valve. A gradual onset of aortic regurgitation results in marked LVH and eventual dilation. Increased myocardial oxygen requirements secondary to LVH, plus a characteristic decrease in aortic diastolic pressure that decreases coronary blood flow, can manifest as angina pectoris in the absence of CAD. Coronary blood flow to the left ventricle occurs during diastole. In severe or acute aortic regurgitation with low diastolic pressures and elevated end-diastolic ventricular pressures coronary blood flow can be severely compromised. Acute aortic regurgitation is most often caused by infective endocarditis, trauma, or dissection of a thoracic aortic aneurysm. Chronic aortic regurgitation is usually the result of prior rheumatic fever. In contrast to aortic stenosis, the occurrence of sudden death in patients with aortic regurgitation is rare.

Management of Anesthesia

Management of anesthesia for noncardiac surgery in patients with aortic regurgitation is similar to the approach described for patients with mitral regurgitation (see Box 26.4). Preinduction intraarterial pressure monitoring can speed the identification and treatment of hemodynamic changes and should be used for patients with significant aortic regurgitation. Anesthetics with minimal effects on SVR or cardiac function should be selected.

DISTURBANCES OF CARDIAC CONDUCTION AND RHYTHM

The ECG is a valuable tool for diagnosing disturbances of cardiac conduction and rhythm (also see Chapter 20). Ambulatory ECG monitoring (Holter monitoring) is useful in documenting the occurrence of life-threatening cardiac dysrhythmias and assessing the efficacy of antidysrhythmic drug therapy. The incidence of intraoperative cardiac dysrhythmias depends on the definition (benign vs. life threatening), patient characteristics, and the type of surgery (frequent incidence during cardiothoracic surgery) (Table 26.3).

Heart Block

Disturbances of cardiac impulse conduction can be classified according to the site of the conduction block relative to the atrioventricular (AV) node. Heart block occurring above the AV node is usually benign and transient. Heart block occurring below the AV node tends to be progressive and permanent.

A theoretical concern in patients with bifascicular heart block is that perioperative events, such as alterations in systemic arterial blood pressure, arterial oxygenation, or electrolyte concentrations, might compromise conduction in the one remaining intact fascicle, leading to the acute onset intraoperatively of third-degree (complete) AV heart block. However, surgery performed during general or regional anesthesia does not predispose to the development of third-degree heart block in patients with coexisting bifascicular block. Therefore placement of a prophylactic artificial cardiac pacemaker is not required before anesthesia and surgery, but transcutaneous pacing should be available.

Cardiac Implantable Electronic Devices

The number of patients presenting for surgery with cardiac implantable electronic devices (CIEDs) is increasing. Permanent pacemakers are most commonly implanted for sinus node dysfunction and high-grade AV block. Biventricular pacemakers are specific types of pacing devices indicated for symptomatic patients with moderate to severe cardiac failure with left ventricular ejection fraction (EF) of <35% and a widened QRS interval. Biventricular pacing, often termed *chronic resynchronization therapy (CRT),* optimizes the timing of right and left ventricular contraction, which is otherwise uncoordinated,

with sole right ventricular pacing. Biventricular pacemakers (CRT) may be combined with an implantable cardioverter-defibrillator (ICD) (CRT-D).

Preoperative evaluation of the patient with a CIED includes determination of the type of device (pacemaker/ICD/CRT-D), reason for implantation, dependency on device, brand, model, and magnet mode settings. History should include symptoms suggesting device malfunction, such as dizziness, syncope, or signs of deteriorating cardiac function. A device under the skin may not be a pacemaker or ICD. Implanted devices include loop recorders, deep brain stimulators, intravenous pumps or ports, spinal stimulators, bladder stimulators, gastric stimulators, and vagal stimulators.

Electromagnetic interference (EMI) from monopolar electrosurgery may adversely affect the normal functioning of CIEDs. EMI is particularly important to consider in a patient who is pacemaker-dependent because oversensing may result in inappropriate inhibition of pacing and lead to hemodynamic compromise. For surgeries above the umbilicus, EMI of pacing cannot be reliably eliminated. For patients with true pacing dependency at high risk of EMI exposure during surgery, management requires either magnet placement (if the device is a pacemaker) or reprogramming (sole choice with an ICD, optional choice with a pacemaker). In the case of ICDs EMI may be falsely interpreted as a shockable rhythm with the risk of intraoperative shock delivery. Disabling the defibrillator function of an ICD before exposure to EMI is therefore advised.[24] The device should be reactivated after the surgical procedure and examined for proper function.

Selection of drugs or techniques for anesthesia is not influenced by the presence of CIEDs, as there is no evidence that the threshold and subsequent response of these devices is altered by drugs administered in the perioperative period. However, patients with CIEDs have a frequent incidence of coexisting cardiac disease and should be monitored carefully and anesthetized with care. Patients with ICDs frequently have poor ventricular function. Insertion of a pulmonary artery catheter will not disturb epicardial electrodes but might dislodge recently placed (less than 2 weeks) transvenous endocardial electrodes.

A suggested algorithm for perioperative management of transvenous pacemakers/ICDs is shown in Fig. 26.2.

HEART FAILURE

Heart failure is a syndrome caused by cardiac dysfunction (systolic, diastolic, or both) characterized by pulmonary and/or systemic venous congestion and/or inadequate peripheral oxygen delivery. The definitions and clinical data standards for heart failure were updated in 2021 (Table 26.4).[35] The term *guideline-directed management*

Table 26.3 Cardiac Conduction and Rhythm Abnormalities

Condition	Comments	Treatment	ECG Display
Third-degree (trifascicular, complete) AV block	Surgery and/ or anesthesia in patients with bifascicular block does not increase risk of developing third-degree heart block	Permanent pacemaker; temporary tx: emergency transvenous pacing or transesophageal pacing, IV isoproterenol	
Sick sinus syndrome	Malfunctioning sinus node resulting in sinus bradycardia, sinus arrest, brady-tachy syndrome	Permanent pacemaker; β-blockers for tachycardias	
Ventricular premature beats or premature ventricular complexes (PVCs)	Causes include myocardial ischemia, hypoxia, hypercarbia, hypokalemia, mechanical irritation of the ventricles	Identify underlying cause and correct; β-Blockers, calcium channel blockers, IV lidocaine (1–1.5 mg/kg)	
Ventricular tachycardia at least three wide QRS complexes (>120 ms) at a heart rate >120 beats/min	Causes include myocardial ischemia, hypoxia, electrolyte abnormalities, myocardial stimulation by surgeons	Stable: IV amiodarone, procainamide, lidocaine Unstable: synchronized cardioversion	
Wolff-Parkinson-White syndrome (preexcitation syndrome) PR <120 ms, wide QRS, delta wave	Often associated with paroxysmal atrial tachycardia. SVTs with 1:1 conduction may lead to hemodynamic collapse. Avoid events/drugs that increase sympathetic activity and predispose to tachydysrhythmias	Catheter ablation of accessory pathways; Stable: IV adenosine, procainamide, β-blockers Unstable: synchronized cardioversion	

Continued

Table 26.3	Cardiac Conduction and Rhythm Abnormalities—cont'd		
Condition	**Comments**	**Treatment**	**ECG Display**
Prolonged QT interval syndrome (>440 ms)	Associated with ventricular dysrhythmias, syncope, and sudden death. Avoid drugs that prolong the QT interval (i.e., droperidol)	β-blockers, left stellate ganglion block	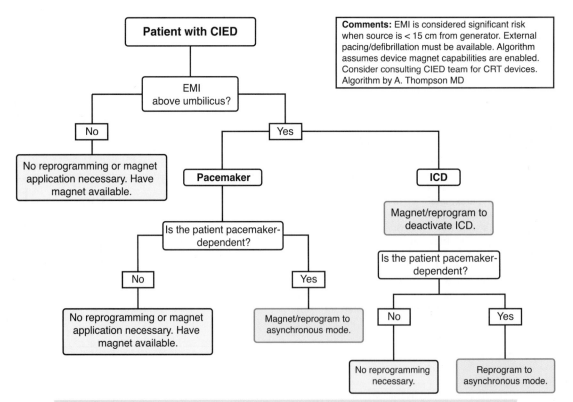

Figure A1 modified from Donald M, Kosowsky JM. Rosen's Emergency Medicine: Concepts and Clinical Practice. Yealy; December 31, 2017: 929–958.e2. © 2018. Fig. 69.15.

Figure A2 modified from Donald M, Kosowsky JM. Rosen's Emergency Medicine: Concepts and Clinical Practice. Yealy; December 31, 2017: 929–958.e2. © 2018. Fig. 69.11.

Figure A3 modified from Donald M, Kosowsky JM. Rosen's Emergency Medicine: Concepts and Clinical Practice. Yealy; December 31, 2017: 929–958.e2. © 2018. Fig. 69.16.

Figure A4 modified from Donald M, Kosowsky JM. Rosen's Emergency Medicine: Concepts and Clinical Practice. Yealy; December 31, 2017: 929–958.e2. © 2018. Fig. 69.36.

Figure A5 modified from Zimetbaum P. Goldman-Cecil Medicine. December 31, 2019: 331–343.e4. © 2020. Fig. 58.1.

Figure A6 modified from Perez M, Fonda H, Le V-V, Mitiku T, Ray J, Freeman JV, Ashley E, Froelicher VF. Current problems in cardiology. 2009. Nov 30; 34 (12): 586–662. © 2009. Fig. 3.

Fig. 26.2 Algorithm for perioperative management of CIEDs.

Table 26.4	Universal Definition and Classification of Heart Failure (HF)

Definition

HF is a clinical syndrome with current or prior symptoms and/or signs caused by structural and/or functional cardiac abnormalities and corroborated by at least one of the following:

- Elevated natriuretic peptide levels
- Objective evidence of cardiogenic pulmonary or systemic congestion

Classification by Stage

At Risk (Stage A)

Patients at risk for HF, but without current or prior symptoms or signs of HF and without structural cardiac changes or elevated biomarkers or heart disease

Pre-HF (Stage B)

Patients without current or prior symptoms or signs of HF with evidence of <u>one</u> of the following:

- Structural heart disease
- Abnormal cardiac function
- Elevated natriuretic peptide or cardiac troponin levels

HF (Stage C)

Patients with current or prior symptoms and/or signs of HF caused by a structural and/or functional cardiac abnormality

Advanced HF (Stage D)

Severe symptoms and/or signs of HF at rest, recurrent hospitalizations despite GDMT, refractory or intolerant to GDMT, requiring advanced therapies such as transplantation, mechanical circulatory support, or palliative care

Classification by EF

HF with reduced EF (HFrEF) – HF with LVEF < 40%

HF with mildly reduced EF (HFmrEF) – HF with LVEF 41-49%

HF with preserved EF (HFpEF) – HF with LVEF >50%

HF with improved EF (HFimpEF) – HF with baseline LVEF of <40%, a 10-point increase from baseline LVEF, and a second measurement of LVEF of >40%

From Bozkurt B, Coats AJS, Tsutsui H, et al. Universal definition and classification of heart failure: A report of the heart failure society of America, heart failure association of the European society of cardiology, Japanese heart failure society and writing committee of the universal definition of heart failure. J Card Fail. 2021;27:387–413

and therapy (GDMT) is used to encompass clinical evaluation, diagnostic testing, and pharmacologic and procedural treatments for heart failure. Pharmacologic treatment for stage C heart failure with reduced EF begins with an ACE inhibitor or ARB plus GDMT with a β-blocker (e.g., bisoprolol or carvedilol), with diuretics as needed.[2,26]

Elective surgery should not be performed in patients with untreated heart failure. The preoperative presence of heart failure is often associated with significant postoperative morbidity or mortality rates. Cardiology consultation is frequently helpful in patients with heart failure symptoms, as consideration of surgical or interventional revascularization and optimization of medical therapy can improve cardiac function. Preoperative initiation of β-blockers and vasodilator therapy with ACE inhibitors can improve ventricular function and reduce operative risk. These drugs should be started by physicians with expertise in treating heart failure, with drug doses increased slowly as tolerated over 3 to 6 months as the heart function recovers.

Management of Anesthesia

When surgery cannot be delayed, however, the drugs and techniques chosen to provide anesthesia must be selected with the goal of minimizing detrimental effects on cardiac output. Optimal cardiac output can be obtained when the impedance of the vasculature (preload and afterload) matches the impedance of the heart and can be achieved by careful preload and afterload management.

Positive-pressure ventilation of the lungs may be beneficial by decreasing pulmonary congestion, improving arterial oxygenation, and eliminating the work of breathing. Care must be taken on extubation of patients with heart failure, as the resumption of negative intrathoracic pressures with spontaneous ventilation can lead to increased filling pressures and worsening heart failure. Maintenance of arterial blood pressure with vasoconstrictors should precede increasing myocardial contractility with continuous intravenous infusions of inotropic drugs. The use of β-agonists in patients with heart failure may decrease the chance of survival and should be used only when necessary.

Regional anesthesia (also see Chapters 17 and 18) should be considered for patients with heart failure requiring peripheral or minor surgery. Anesthetics with minimal hemodynamic effects are optimal. If general anesthesia is required, additional monitoring (e.g., intraarterial pressure, central venous pressure, pulmonary artery pressure, TEE) may be required depending on the invasiveness of the surgical procedure and patient physiology.

HYPERTROPHIC CARDIOMYOPATHY

Hypertrophic cardiomyopathy (HCM) is characterized by left ventricular outflow tract obstruction (LVOTO) produced by asymmetric hypertrophy of the basal interventricular septum and systolic anterior motion (SAM) of the anterior mitral valve leaflet.[27,28] Associated LHV, in an attempt to overcome the obstruction, may be so massive that the volume of the left ventricular chamber is decreased, leading to smaller left ventricular end-diastolic volume, which can reduce stroke volume despite a normal EF. This disease is often hereditary and is an important

IV

Box 26.6 Management and Treatment of Left Ventricular Outflow Tract Obstruction (LVOTO) in Hypertrophic Cardiomyopathy

Decrease Myocardial Contractility and Heart Rate
- β-Adrenergic blockade

Increase Preload
- Increase intravascular fluid volume (fluids and head-down position)
- Increase diastolic filling time by decreasing heart rate

Increase Afterload
- α-Adrenergic stimulation (phenylephrine)
- Vasopressin

Arrhythmia Suppression/Treatment
- β-Adrenergic blockade
- Implantable cardiac defibrillator

Surgical Treatment of LVOTO
- Septal myectomy
- Septal ablation

---

cause of sudden cardiac death, especially in young adults. Though patients can remain asymptomatic for decades, common presenting symptoms include angina, dyspnea, exercise intolerance, dizziness, syncope, or sudden death. Treatment for patients with HCM includes β-blockers for heart rate control and arrhythmia suppression, ICDs to manage malignant arrhythmias, and surgical myectomy and septal ablation to decrease LVOTO (Box 26.6).

Management of Anesthesia

The goal during management of anesthesia for patients with HCM is to decrease the pressure gradient across the left ventricular outflow tract (see Box 26.6). This can be accomplished by decreasing heart rate and/or myocardial contractility, increasing preload (ventricular volume), and increasing afterload. Maintenance of sinus rhythm is also important because of increased dependence on atrial contraction for maintaining cardiac output in the setting of LVH and decreased left ventricular compliance.

Patient anxiety, intubation, surgical incision, and postoperative pain can lead to sympathetic stimulation. Anesthetic drugs and surgical blood loss can lead to changes in preload, afterload, and contractility. Increases in heart rate, rhythm disturbances, and decreases in afterload will exacerbate LVOTO and may cause hemodynamic deterioration. Increases in contractility and decreases in preload will also accentuate LVOTO, highlighting the dynamic component of HCM. Intraoperative hypotension is generally treated with intravenous fluids and vasoactive medications that do not increase heart rate or contractility such as phenylephrine or vasopressin. The Trendelenburg position will assist in increasing preload. Drugs with β-agonist activity are not likely to be used to treat hypotension because any increase in cardiac contractility or heart rate could increase

LVOTO. Vasodilators should be used with caution because decreases in SVR can also increase LVOTO. In the case of sudden onset of atrial fibrillation that is hemodynamically unstable direct current cardioversion may be necessary.[29]

PULMONARY HYPERTENSION

Pulmonary hypertension is defined as a mean pulmonary arterial pressure (mPAP) greater than 20 mm Hg at rest, measured during right heart catheterization.[30] Increased pulmonary pressure and resistance increase the afterload on the right heart, resulting in hypertrophy and dilation of the right ventricle. Initial adaptive remodeling of the right ventricle is followed by maladaptive hypertrophy and progressive right ventricular dysfunction and decreased cardiac output. Patients with pulmonary hypertension have a significantly increased risk of perioperative morbidity and mortality and should be treated with care. Patients with known or suspected pulmonary hypertension undergoing elective surgery should have a proper evaluation and optimization before surgery.

Management of Anesthesia

Goals during management of anesthesia in patients with pulmonary hypertension are to avoid events or drugs that could increase PVR and lead to right heart failure. Sympathetic stimulation caused by anxiety, stress, pain, and inflammation can increase PVR. Circumstances likely to exacerbate pulmonary hypertension include hypoxemia, hypercapnia, acidosis, hypothermia, hypervolemia, and insufficient anesthesia and analgesia. Using a regional anesthesia technique offers the advantage of maintaining spontaneous ventilation, and a continuous regional technique can be used for postoperative analgesia. Epidural anesthesia may be preferable over spinal because of the avoidance of an abrupt decrease in SVR leading to decreased coronary perfusion and worsening right heart failure. The main advantages of general anesthesia are control of oxygenation and ventilation and a secure airway during surgery. An intubated patient also allows for delivery of an inhaled pulmonary vasodilator (e.g., inhaled nitric oxide, inhaled milrinone, iloprost). All standard induction agents have no influence on PVR and therefore can be used. Volatile anesthetics are useful for relaxing vascular smooth muscle and attenuating airway responsiveness to stimuli produced by an endotracheal tube. All volatile anesthetics up to 1 MAC may be administered without causing an increase in PVR.[31] Nitrous oxide may increase PVR and should be avoided.[32]

For patients with severe pulmonary hypertension, intraarterial pressure monitoring is very helpful for hemodynamic management. Depending on the surgery, monitoring of pulmonary arterial or right atrial pressure (or both) may be helpful to detect any adverse effect on pulmonary vasculature. TEE monitoring can be very helpful in blood volume management and monitoring of right heart function. In patients with right heart dysfunction inotropic support with β-agonists can improve cardiac function. Therapy should be chosen based on the hemodynamic problem (volume, SVR, chronotropy, inotropy, and pulmonary hypertension). β-Agonists must be used carefully to avoid myocardial ischemia. In severe right ventricular failure combinations of β-agonists and phosphodiesterase inhibitors (amrinone or milrinone) can provide synergistic improvements in ventricular function and vasodilation (amrinone or milrinone), thus improving cardiac output.

CARDIAC TAMPONADE

Cardiac tamponade is characterized by (1) decreases in diastolic filling of the ventricles, (2) decreases in stroke volume, and (3) decreases in systemic arterial blood pressure caused by increased intrapericardial pressure from accumulation of fluid in the pericardial space (Box 26.7). Decreased stroke volume from inadequate ventricular filling results in activation of the sympathetic nervous system (tachycardia, vasoconstriction) as the cardiovascular system attempts to maintain the cardiac output. Cardiac output and systemic arterial blood pressure are maintained only as long as the pressure in the central veins exceeds the right ventricular end-diastolic pressure.

Although continuous intravenous infusions of catecholamines (epinephrine, norepinephrine, dopamine, dobutamine, or isoproterenol) and vasoconstrictors may be necessary to maintain cardiac output and arterial blood pressure, the primary therapy is pericardial drainage. A common sign of cardiac tamponade is hemodynamic collapse and cardiogenic shock unresponsive to fluids and inotropes. Systolic ventricular function is not the cause; rather, diastolic dysfunction from increased pericardial pressure is the primary problem. Once the pericardium is drained, venous return can enter the heart and hemodynamics will rapidly normalize.

Box 26.7 Manifestations of Cardiac Tamponade

- Increased pericardial pressure leading to decreased cardiac filling
- Hypotension
- Tachycardia
- Increased systemic vascular resistance
- Low cardiac output
- Equalization of left and right diastolic filling pressures
- Exaggeration of arterial blood pressure variation/pulsus paradoxus with respiration
- Fixed and reduced stroke volume (cardiac output and systemic arterial blood pressure dependent on heart rate)
- Failure to respond to volume and multiple inotropes with cardiogenic shock

---

Management of Anesthesia

Before the induction of general anesthesia in patients with significant cardiac tamponade, the patient should be positioned on the operating room table. Intraarterial monitoring is helpful if time permits. The chest and abdomen should be prepped and draped for surgery. Before anesthetic induction, the surgeons should be scrubbed, gowned, gloved, and at the operating room table, ready for incision. It is optimal if anesthetic induction, intubation, incision, and drainage of the pericardial tamponade can occur in extremely rapid succession. Institution of general anesthesia and positive-pressure ventilation of the lungs in the presence of cardiac tamponade can lead to immediate and profound hypotension or death, reflecting anesthetic-induced peripheral vasodilation, direct myocardial depression, and decreased venous return from positive-pressure ventilation. When percutaneous pericardiocentesis cannot be performed using local anesthesia, the induction and maintenance of general anesthesia are extremely dangerous but may be achieved while carefully maintaining spontaneous respiration. If possible, positive-pressure ventilation of the lungs should be avoided until drainage of the pericardial space is imminent.

ANEURYSMS OF THE AORTA

Aneurysms of the aorta most often involve the abdominal aorta but may involve any part of the thoracic or abdominal aorta. Most patients have hypertension, and many have associated atherosclerosis. A dissecting aneurysm denotes a tear in the intima of the aorta that allows blood to enter and penetrate between the walls of the vessel, producing a false lumen. Ultimately, the dissection may reenter the lumen through another tear in the intima or rupture through the adventitia.

Elective repair of an abdominal aneurysm is often recommended when the estimated diameter of the aneurysm is more than 5 cm. The incidence of spontaneous rupture increases dramatically when the size of the aneurysm exceeds this diameter. Extension of the abdominal aneurysm to include the renal arteries occurs in about 5% of patients.

Management of Anesthesia

All surgery patients with vascular disease should be considered for prophylactic β-blocker and statin therapy. Perioperative administration of β-blockers reduces the perioperative mortality rate 50% to 90%. β-blocking drugs should be started as soon as patients are identified as needing surgery.[5] Perioperative statin use may also be beneficial in reducing mortality.[33]

Anesthetic technique must take into account the surgical approach. Endovascular aneurysm repair is

IV

less invasive and may require only regional anesthesia, although in prolonged cases general anesthesia is preferred. Open procedures for aortic aneurysm surgery are major procedures and require general anesthesia. All patients undergoing anesthesia for resection of an abdominal aortic aneurysm should have monitoring of intraarterial pressures. Epidural catheter placement may be helpful for the management of postoperative pain. Continuous cardiac output monitoring with calculation of SVV or PPV can be used for goal-directed fluid therapy to guide volume replacement (also see Chapter 20).

CARDIOPULMONARY BYPASS

The introduction of cardiopulmonary bypass (CPB) ushered in the modern era of cardiac surgery, providing a bloodless and motionless field to allow detailed repair of the heart and great vessels while still supplying oxygenated blood to the organs. By providing extracorporeal replacement of lung function, oxygenation and ventilation, heart function, and perfusion of oxygenated blood to organs, CPB earns its ubiquitous nickname as the "heart–lung machine."

A schematic of a basic CPB circuit is shown in Fig. 26.3. The four basic components of a CPB circuit are a venous reservoir, pump, heat exchanger, and oxygenator. To access the circulatory system, there are typically two main cannulas: the venous cannula inserted in the right atrium or both the superior and inferior vena cavae, which drains blood from the right side of the heart to the CPB reservoir, and the arterial cannula inserted into the aorta, which returns oxygenated blood from the CPB circuit to the patient. There are many variations on this basic central cannulation strategy, but the main principles of venous blood drainage and oxygenated arterial blood return apply to all. There are additional components to a CPB circuit that aid in the management of blood loss (cardiotomy suckers), avoidance of

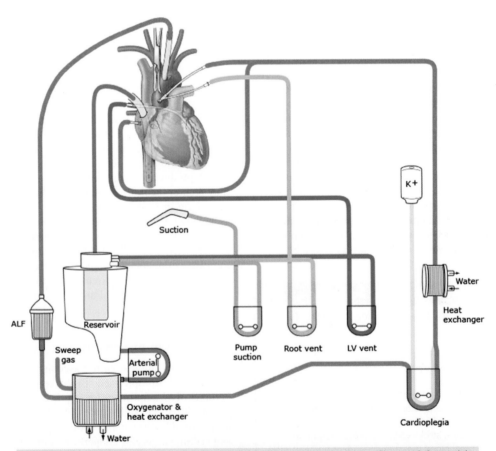

Fig. 26.3 Schematic Diagram of Cardiopulmonary Bypass Circuit. *ALF,* Arterial line filter; *LV,* left ventricle. (From https://www.uptodate.com/contents/management-of-cardiopulmonary-bypass#H3860522344 Graphic 93255, Version 5.0.)

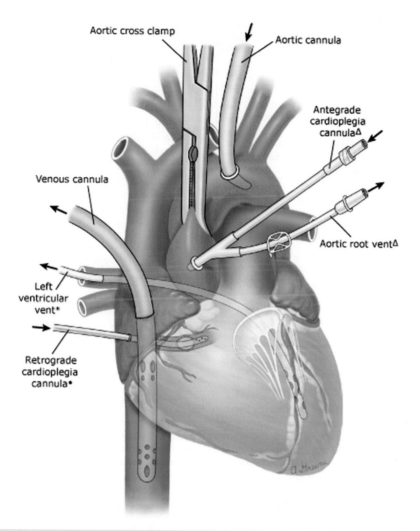

Aortic cross clamp

Aortic cannula

Antegrade
cardioplegia
cannula△

Venous cannula

Aortic root vent△

Left
ventricular
vent*

Retrograde
cardioplegia
cannula•

Fig. 26.4 Cardiopulmonary Bypass Cannulae Insertion Sites. * Left ventricular vent enters right upper pulmonary vein then passes into left ventricle through mitral valve. The arrows denote directional blood flow.
• Retrograde cardioplegia cannula enters right atrium and passes into coronary sinus.
△ Aortic root vent allows suction to be applied to the aortic root, thereby indirectly emptying the left ventricle. (From https://www.uptodate.com/contents/management-of-cardiopulmonary-bypass#H3860522344 Graphic 97188, Version 6.0.)

left ventricular distension (cardiac vent cannula), and maintenance of motionless surgical field and deairing (coronary sinus cannula and cardioplegia/root vent cannula). Cannula insertion sites are illustrated in Fig. 26.4.

The steps for initiation of CPB are described in Table 26.5. As CPB is initiated, venous blood enters the bypass circuit either by gravity, where drainage is determined by the height difference between the patient and the reservoir, or by vacuum-assisted drainage. Additional cannulae can be added as needed for cardioplegia and venting.

Blood gases are monitored during CPB. Oxygen delivery to the circuit is supplied by an oxygenator, and carbon dioxide elimination is determined by the gas flow rate. There are two blood gas management strategies: alpha stat and pH stat.[34] The best strategy has not been definitively determined, with each method having advantages and potential drawbacks. Their differences in measurement, advantages, and potential disadvantages are detailed in Box 26.8 (also see Chapter 22).

IV

Box 26.8 pH Stat Versus Alpha Stat Management During CPB

Alpha Stat

Description: arterial blood gas (ABG) is temperature uncorrected (i.e., ABG measured at 37°, regardless of body temperature)

Advantages: easier to implement; physiologic response to hypothermia is maintained; cerebral autoregulation is maintained

Disadvantages: can cause cerebral vasoconstriction because of alkalemia; leftward shift of oxyhemoglobin dissociation curve can reduce supply to vulnerable tissues

pH Stat

Description: ABG is temperature-corrected to the patient's temperature. CO_2 solubility is increased at lower temperatures, leading to a decline in Pco_2. To maintain normal pH, carbon dioxide is added to the circuit. Cerebral autoregulation is uncoupled.

Advantages: cerebrovascular vasodilatation and improved cerebral blood flow, particularly during deep hypothermic circulatory arrest; improved global and regional cooling.

Disadvantages: potential for increased embolic burden to cerebrovascular system.

Weaning from CPB refers to the gradual withdrawal of extracorporeal support. The heart and lungs will resume their native functions as CPB is discontinued. The actions involved with discontinuation of CPB are described in Table 26.6. Once separation of CPB is complete and the patient is determined not to require any additional repair, protamine is administered to neutralize the heparin given for CPB. Protamine should be given slowly over 10 to 15 minutes to avoid hypotension related to fast infusion, known as a *type I reaction*. There is also a type II and type III reaction associated with protamine, which causes anaphylaxis and pulmonary hypertensive crisis, respectively. Once protamine is given, an activated clotting time (ACT) is performed to confirm normalization of values.

ACKNOWLEDGMENTS

The authors, editors and publisher would like to thank Dr. Arthur Wallace for contributing to this chapter in previous editions of this work. It has served as a foundation for the current chapter.

Table 26.5	Steps for Initiation of Cardiopulmonary Bypass (CPB)
Heparinization	Blood in the CPB tubing and reservoir is prone to catastrophic clotting if the patient is not anticoagulated. The tubing and reservoir are non-endothelialized surfaces and represent a large surface area of foreign material that can activate native inflammatory responses as well as the coagulation cascade. An activated clotting time, or ACT, of 400-500 seconds is required for CPB to prevent clotting.
Arterial cannulation	Once the ACT is of sufficient duration, the aorta is cannulated.
Venous cannulation	This is typically performed after arterial cannulation when central venous cannulation (meaning the right atrium or vena cavae are cannulated). Manipulation of the right atrium can induce arrhythmias, cause mechanical obstruction of inflow to the right atrium, or tear the right atrium. With arterial cannulation having already been completed, volume can be administered if necessary through the arterial cannula to compensate for the hemodynamic effects of right atrial manipulation.

Table 26.6	Steps for Discontinuation of Cardiopulmonary Bypass
1. Rewarming	Although cooling can be rapid upon initiation of CPB, the same is not true for rewarming as rapid rewarming and hyperthermia have been associated with cerebral injury.
2. De-airing	Intracardiac air should be vented through a deairing cannula prior to separation from CPB to avoid air embolization to the heart, brain, and other organs. The anterior position of the right coronary artery in the supine patient makes it a frequent site of air embolism that can manifest as inferior ST elevations, ventricular dysfunction (particularly right ventricular dysfunction, but left ventricular dysfunction can also occur), and arrhythmias.
3. In addition, the following parameters should be addressed when discontinuation of CPB is imminent:	
a. Rate	Does the patient have a heart rate adequate to sustain cardiac output once CPB is discontinued? If the heart rate is too low, as in severe bradycardia or heart block, the patient will need an alternate method of pacing via epicardial wires.
b. Drips	CPB can induce an inflammatory response that results in significant vasoplegia. Additionally, myocardial dysfunction, either pre-existing or anticipated, can affect cardiac output after separation from CPB. Vasopressors and/or inotropes may be required to successfully separate from CPB.
c. Gas (anesthesia)	Are anesthetic gas flows restarted on the ventilator? Volatile agents are added to the CPB circuit during bypass, but a general anesthetic agent must be continued after CPB.
d. Oxygen	Ensure the oxygen flows are on. Initially an FiO2 =1 is often used until the post-CPB blood gas is collected.
e. Ventilation	Ensure the ventilator is on.

REFERENCES

1. Mangano DT, Goldman L. Preoperative assessment of patients with known or suspected coronary disease. *N Engl J Med*. 1995;333(26):1750–1756.
2. Virani SS, Alvaro A, Aparicio HJ, Benjamin Emelia J, Bittencourt Marcio S, Callaway Clifton W, Carson April P, et al. Heart Disease and Stroke Statistics-2021 update: A report from the American Heart Association. *Circulation*. 2021;143(8):e254–e743.
3. Mangano DT. Long-term cardiac prognosis following noncardiac surgery. *JAMA*. 1992. https://doi.org/10.1001/jama.1992.03490020081035.
4. Mangano DT, Browner WS, Hollenberg M, London MJ, Tubau JF. Association of perioperative myocardial ischemia with cardiac morbidity and mortality in men undergoing noncardiac surgery. *Surv Anesthesiol.*. 1991. https://doi.org/10.1097/00132586-199110000-00010.
5. Fleisher LA, Fleischmann KE, Auerbach AD, Barnason Susan A, Beckman Joshua A, Bozkurt Biykem, Davila-Roman Victor G, et al. 2014 ACC/AHA guideline on perioperative cardiovascular evaluation and management of patients undergoing noncardiac surgery: A report of the American College of Cardiology/American Heart Association Task Force on Practice Guidelines. *J Am Coll Cardiol*. 2014;64(22):e77–137.
6. Jetté M, Sidney K, Blümchen G. Metabolic equivalents (METS) in exercise testing, exercise prescription, and evaluation of functional capacity. *Clin Cardiol*. 1990;13(8):555–565.
7. Larsen K. Changing risk of perioperative myocardial infarction. *Perm J*. 2012. https://doi.org/10.7812/tpp/12-033.
8. Livhits M, Ko CY, Leonardi MJ, Zingmond DS, Gibbons MM, de Virgilio C. Risk of surgery following recent myocardial infarction. *Ann Surg*. 2011;253(5):857–864.
9. Livhits M, Gibbons MM, de Virgilio C, O'Connell JB, Leonardi Michael J, Ko Clifford Y, Zingmond David S. Coronary revascularization after myocardial infarction can reduce risks of noncardiac surgery. *J Am Coll Surg*. 2011;212(6):1018–1026.
10. Landesberg G, Beattie WS, Mosseri M, Jaffe AS, Alpert JS. Perioperative myocardial infarction. *Circulation*. 2009;119(22):2936–2944.
11. Levine GN, Bates ER, Bittl JA, Brindis Ralph G, Fihn Stephan D, Fleisher Lee A, Granger Christopher B, et al. 2016 ACC/AHA guideline focused update on duration of dual antiplatelet therapy in patients with coronary artery disease: A report of the American College of Cardiology/American Heart Association Task Force on Clinical Practice Guidelines: An update of the 2011 ACCF/AHA/SCAI guideline for percutaneous coronary intervention, 2011 ACCF/AHA guideline for coronary artery bypass graft surgery, 2012 ACC/AHA/ACP/AATS/PCNA/SCAI/STS guideline for the diagnosis and management of patients with stable ischemic heart disease, 2013 ACCF/AHA guideline for the management of ST-elevation myocardial infarction, 2014 AHA/ACC guideline for the management of patients with non–ST-elevation acute coronary syndromes, and 2014 ACC/AHA guideline on perioperative cardiovascular evaluation and management of patients undergoing noncardiac surgery. *Circulation*. 2016. https://doi.org/10.1161/cir.0000000000000404.
12. Hollmann C, Fernandes NL, Biccard BM. A systematic review of outcomes associated with withholding or continuing angiotensin-converting enzyme inhibitors and angiotensin receptor blockers before noncardiac surgery. *Anesth Analg*. 2018;127(3):678.
13. Meng L, Heerdt PM. Perioperative goal-directed haemodynamic therapy based on flow parameters: A concept in evolution. *Br J Anaesth*. 2016;117(suppl 3):iii3–iii17.
14. Bootsma IT, Boerma EC, Scheeren T WL, de Lange F. The contemporary pulmonary artery catheter. Part 2: Measurements, limitations, and clinical applications. *JoJ Clin Monit Comput*. 2021. https://doi.org/10.1007/s10877-021-00673-5.

IV

15. Slogoff S, Keats AS. Further observations on perioperative myocardial ischemia. *Anesthesiology.* 1986;65(5):539–542.

16. Wu M, Liang Y, Dai Z, Wang S. Perioperative dexmedetomidine reduces delirium after cardiac surgery: A meta-analysis of randomized controlled trials. *J Clin Anesth.* 2018;50(November):33–42.

17. Pan H, Liu C, Ma X, Xu Y, Zhang M, Wang Y. Perioperative dexmedetomidine reduces delirium in elderly patients after non-cardiac surgery: A systematic review and meta-analysis of randomized-controlled trials. *Can J Anesth.* 2019;66(12):1489–1500.

18. Lemoine S, Tritapepe L, Hanouz JL, Puddu PE. The mechanisms of cardioprotective effects of desflurane and sevoflurane at the time of reperfusion: Anaesthetic post-conditioning potentially translatable to humans? *Br J Anaesth.* 2016;116(4):456–475.

19. Leung JM, Goehner P, O'Kelly BF, Hollenberg Milton, Pineda Nito, Cason Brian A, Mangano Dennis T, Group Spi Research. Isoflurane anesthesia and myocardial ischemia: Comparative risk versus sufentanil anesthesia in patients undergoing coronary artery bypass graft surgery. *Anesthesiology.* 1991;74(5):838–847.

20. Hartman JC, Kampine JP, Schmeling WT, Warltier DC. Steal-prone coronary circulation in chronically instrumented dogs: Isoflurane versus adenosine. *Anesthesiology.* 1991;74(4):744–756.

21. Slogoff S, Keats AS. Randomized trial of primary anesthetic agents on outcome of coronary artery bypass operations. *Anesthesiology.* 1989;70(2):179–188.

22. Abbott TEF, Pearse RM, Andrew Archbold R, Ahmad Tahania, Niebrzegowska Edyta, Wragg Andrew, Rodseth Reitze N, Devereaux Philip J, Ackland Gareth L. A prospective international multicentre cohort study of intraoperative heart rate and systolic blood pressure and myocardial injury after noncardiac surgery: Results of the VISION Study. *Anesth Analg.* 2018;126(6):1936–1945.

23. Carabello BA, Crawford FA. Valvular Heart Disease. *NEJM.* 1997. https://doi.org/10.1056/nejm199707033370107.

24. Crossley GH, Poole JE, Rozner MA, Asirvatham Samuel J, Cheng Alan, Chung Mina K, Ferguson T Bruce, et al. The Heart Rhythm Society (HRS)/American Society of Anesthesiologists (ASA) Expert Consensus Statement on the perioperative management of patients with implantable defibrillators, pacemakers and arrhythmia monitors: Facilities and patient management: This document was developed as a joint project with the American Society of Anesthesiologists (ASA), and in collaboration with the American Heart Association (AHA), and the Society of Thoracic Surgeons (STS). *Heart Rhythm.* 2011;8(7):1114–1154.

25. Heart Failure Society of America. Section 2: Conceptualization and working definition of heart failure. *J Card Fail.* 2010;16(6):e34–e37. ISSN 1071-9164. https://doi.org/10.1016/j.cardfail.2010.05.011.

26. Yancy CW, Jessup M, Bozkurt B, Butler J, Jr Casey DE, Colvin MM, Drazner MH, Filippatos GS, Fonarow GC, Givertz MM, Hollenberg SM, Lindenfeld J, Masoudi FA, McBride PE, Peterson PN, Stevenson LW, 2017 Westlake C. ACC/AHA/HFSA focused update of the 2013 ACCF/AHA guideline for the management of heart failure: A report of the American College of Cardiology/American Heart Association Task Force on Clinical Practice Guidelines and the Heart Failure Society of America. *Circulation.* 2017 Aug 8;136(6):e137–e161. doi:10.1161/CIR.0000000000000509. Epub 2017 Apr 28. PMID: 28455343.

27. Marian AJ, Braunwald E. Hypertrophic cardiomyopathy: Genetics, pathogenesis, clinical manifestations, diagnosis, and therapy. *Circ Res.* 2017;121(7):749–770.

28. Hensley N, Dietrich J, Nyhan D, Mitter N, Yee M, Brady M. Hypertrophic cardiomyopathy: A review. *Anesth Analg.* 2015;120(3):554–569.

29. Poliac LC, Barron ME, Maron BJ. Perianesthetic management of hypertrophic cardiomyopathy. *Anesthesiology.* 2006. https://doi.org/10.1097/00000542-200609000-00040.

30. Simonneau G, Montani D, Celermajer DS, Denton Christopher P, Gatzoulis Michael A, Krowka Michael, Williams Paul G, Souza Rogerio. Haemodynamic definitions and updated clinical classification of pulmonary hypertension. *Eur Respir J..* 2019;53(1). https://doi.org/10.1183/13993003.01913-2018.

31. Pritts CD, Pearl RG. Anesthesia for patients with pulmonary hypertension. *Curr Opin Anaesthesiol.* 2010. https://doi.org/10.1097/aco.0b013e32833953fb.

32. Hilgenberg JC, McCammon RL, Stoelting RK. Pulmonary and systemic vascular responses to nitrous oxide in patients with mitral stenosis and pulmonary hypertension. *Anesth Analg.* 1980;59(5):323–326.

33. London MJ, Schwartz GG, Hur K, Henderson WG. Association of perioperative statin use with mortality and morbidity after major noncardiac surgery. *JAMA Internal Medicine.* 2017;177(2):231–242.

34. Pokela M, Sebastian D, Fausto B, Vilho Vainionpää, Salomäki Timo, Kiviluoma Kai, Rönkä Erkka, et al. pH-stat versus alpha-stat perfusion strategy during experimental hypothermic circulatory arrest: A microdialysis study. *Ann Thorac Surg.* 2003;76(4):1215–1226.

35. Bozkurt B, Coats AJ, Tsutsui H, et al. Universal Definition and Classification of Heart Failure: A report of the Heart Failure Society of America, Heart Failure Association of the European Society of Cardiology, Japanese Heart Failure Society and Writing Committee of the Universal Definition of Heart Failure. *J Card Fail.* 2021;27:387–413.

27 CHRONIC PULMONARY DISEASE

Andrew J. Deacon, Peter D. Slinger

INTRODUCTION

Chronic respiratory problems include obstructive and restrictive lung diseases, obstructive sleep apnea (OSA), and pulmonary hypertension. Obstructive lung diseases are commonly divided into reactive airway disorders (asthma) and chronic obstructive pulmonary disease (COPD). However, many patients have more than one type of lung disease. Using regional or local rather than general anesthesia is preferable for patients with chronic respiratory diseases.

History

Common symptoms elicited in all patients include cough, wheezing, shortness of breath, chest tightness, sputum production, and reduced exercise tolerance. Important components of the history are recent exacerbations, current and previous therapies (including hospital admissions), emergency room visits, and tobacco use.

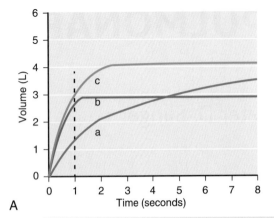

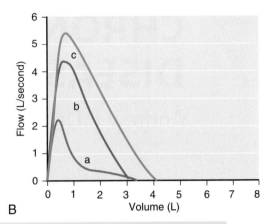

Fig. 27.1 Simple spirometry patterns in obstructive lung disease *(a)*, restrictive lung disease *(b)*, and normal patients *(c)*. (A) Volume–time curves. The exhaled volume during the first second of a maximal expiratory effort is the forced expiratory volume in 1 second (FEV$_1$). The maximal expired volume is the forced vital capacity (FVC). (B) Flow-volume curves. The maximal flow during a forced expiration is the peak expiratory flow (PEF). (From Patterson GA, Cooper JD, Deslauriers J, et al., eds. *Pearson's Thoracic and Esophageal Surgery.* 3rd ed. Philadelphia: Elsevier; 2008, used with permission.)

Physical Examination

Signs of chronic respiratory disease include tachypnea, cyanosis, use of accessory muscles of respiration, and clubbing of the fingers. Important examination findings are the presence of unequal breath sounds, wheezing, and rales during auscultation.

Laboratory Examination

Chest Imaging

A recent preoperative chest x-ray examination is not required for all patients but should be considered in any patient with a chronic respiratory disease or a patient with a recent change in respiratory symptoms or signs.

Spirometry

Simple spirometry (expired volume or flow vs. time), forced vital capacity (FVC), and forced expiratory volume in 1 second (FEV$_1$) (Fig. 27.1) are not required in all stable patients but should be ordered if there is any doubt about the severity of disease, such as a recent change in symptoms, if the patient is unable to give a clear history, or if any patient with chronic lung disease is having lung surgery. Full pulmonary function tests (plethysmography) (Fig. 27.2), including measurement of residual volume (RV), functional residual capacity (FRC), and measurement of the lung diffusing capacity for carbon monoxide (D$_{LCO}$) are only indicated if the diagnosis or severity of the lung disease is unclear from the simple spirometry procedure.

Gas Exchange

Oxygen saturation (pulse oximetry: Sp$_{O_2}$%) should be documented preoperatively in every patient with a chronic respiratory disease. Arterial blood gases are required preoperatively in patients with moderate or severe chronic respiratory disease who are at risk of requiring postoperative mechanical ventilation (major abdominal, thoracic, cardiac, spine, or neurosurgery) or if symptoms have become more intense.

ASTHMA

Clinical Presentation

Asthma is a common form of episodic recurrent lower airway obstruction that affects 3% to 5% of the population. Sixty-five percent of people with asthma become symptomatic before age 5 years.[1] Patients with childhood asthma often become quiescent with time but can have recurrences. Inflammation of the airways is a hallmark of asthma. Steroids (inhaled, oral, or both) are the most effective medications in controlling this inflammation. The inflamed airway is hyperresponsive to irritant stimuli with subsequent bronchospasm, small airway edema, and mucous secretions. Bronchospastic stimuli can include allergens, dust, cold air, instrumentation of the airways, and medications (nonsteroidal antiinflammatory drugs or histamine-releasing drugs). Patients with asthma are at risk for life-threatening bronchospasm during anesthesia, particularly during or recently after a respiratory tract infection. Elective surgery should therefore be delayed at least 6 weeks after a respiratory infection in these patients.

The severity of asthma, defined by the amount of treatment required to control symptoms, includes intermittent, mild persistent, moderate persistent, and severe persistent asthma[2,3] (Box 27.1). Most patients will be in steps 1 or 2 of this treatment protocol. Caution is

Lung volumes and capacities

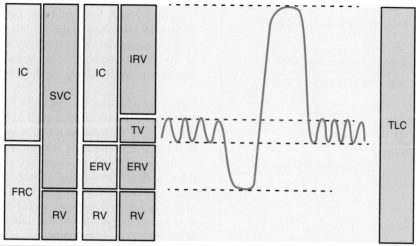

Fig. 27.2 Complete pulmonary function testing will provide data on lung volumes and capacities to differentiate obstructive from restrictive diseases. *ERV,* Expiratory reserve volume; *FRC,* functional residual capacity; *IC,* inspiratory capacity; *IRV,* inspiratory reserve volume; *RV,* residual volume; *SVC,* slow vital capacity; *TLC,* total lung capacity; *TV,* tidal volume. (Reprinted from Patterson AG, Cooper JD, Deslauriers J, et al., eds. *Pearson's Thoracic and Esophageal Surgery.* 3rd ed. Philadelphia: Elsevier; 2008. p. 1168, with permission.)

Box 27.1   Stepwise Therapy for the Treatment of Asthma

Step 1: Inhaled short-acting β_2-agonists (SABA) PRN (e.g., salbutamol [aka albuterol] 100–200 µg prn)
Step 2: Daily low-dose inhaled corticosteroids (ICS) and SABA PRN, or PRN concomitant with ICS and SABA (e.g., inhaled fluticasone 88 mcg twice daily)
Step 3: Daily and PRN combination low-dose ICS-formoterol*
Step 4: Daily and PRN combination medium-dose ICS-formoterol
Step 5: Daily medium-high dose ICS-LABA plus long-acting muscarinic antagonist† (LAMA) and PRN SABA
Step 6: Daily high-dose ICS-LABA plus oral systemic corticosteroids plus PRN SABA

prn, As needed.
*Formoterol is a long-acting inhaled β_2-agonist (LABA); there are several formulations of formoterol combined with an inhaled corticosteroid in a single inhaler.
†Long-acting muscarinic antagonists include tiotropium bromide and aclidinium bromide.
Stepwise approach for asthma management according to the National Asthma Education and Prevention Program Coordinating Committee. Step 1 is for patients with intermittent asthma only; the remaining steps are for patients with persistent asthma. Alternative management steps and additional treatment recommendations are available in Expert Panel Working Group of the National Heart, Lung, and Blood Institute (NHLBI) administered and coordinated National Asthma Education and Prevention Program Coordinating Committee (NAEPPCC), Cloutier MM, Baptist AP, Blake KV, et al. 2020 Focused updates to the asthma management guidelines: A report from the National Asthma Education and Prevention Program Coordinating Committee Expert Panel Working Group. J Allergy Clin Immunol. 2020;146(6):1217–1270.

required when anesthetizing patients after step 3. A history of severe or life-threatening exacerbations, requiring endotracheal intubation or admission to intensive care, is indicative of patients at increased risk of major pulmonary complications. Peak expiratory flow (PEF) rate is a simple and useful measurement of asthma severity. Many patients measure their own PEF to guide their therapy. PEF rates less than 50% of the predicted value (corrected for age, gender, and height) indicate severe asthma. A PEF increase of more than 15% after bronchodilator administration suggests inadequate treatment of asthma.

Suppression of the hypothalamic-pituitary-adrenal (HPA) axis may occur with corticosteroid therapy. Adrenal crisis may be precipitated by the stress of surgery. Short courses of oral prednisone used to treat asthma exacerbations can affect HPA function for up to 10 days, but dysfunction is unlikely to be prolonged. Large doses, prolonged therapy (>3 weeks), evening dosing, and continuous (as opposed to alternate day) dosing all increase suppression of the HPA axis and may take up to a year before returning to normal. Inhaled steroids are less likely to cause suppression of the HPA axis.

Management of Anesthesia

The adequacy of asthma control should be assessed during preoperative evaluation and symptoms uncharacteristic of asthma excluded (Table 27.1). Principles of perioperative management of patients with asthma are

IV

Table 27.1 Preoperative Assessment for Asthma	
History Suggestive of Inadequate Asthma Control	
Frequency of symptoms	
Use of β_2-agonist medications/relievers frequently	
Hospital attendances (e.g., emergency department, physician office visit)	
Hospital/intensive care unit (ICU) admissions	
Use of oral steroids/high-dose inhaled steroids	
Features Uncharacteristic of Asthma	**Differential Diagnosis**
Unremitting wheeze/stridor	Suggestive of fixed airway obstruction
Persisting wet cough/ productive cough	Suggestive of suppurative lung disease
Wheeze present from birth (rare with asthma)	Tracheomalacia/ bronchomalacia
A monophonic wheeze loudest over the glottis	Vocal cord dysfunction

Box 27.2 Principles of Perioperative Management of Asthma

- Usual inhalers per normal on day of surgery. Inhaled β_2-agonists before anesthesia.
- Avoid lower airway manipulation (e.g., endotracheal intubation) if possible. Use regional anesthesia or an LMA/mask for general anesthesia if possible.
- Avoid medications that release histamine (e.g., thiopental, morphine, atracurium).
- Use anesthetic drugs that promote bronchodilation (propofol, ketamine, sevoflurane).
- If instrumentation of the lower airway is necessary, it should be performed after attaining a deep level of general anesthesia to decrease airway reflexes.

LMA, Laryngeal mask airway.

outlined in Box 27.2. Volatile anesthetics, particularly sevoflurane,[4] reduce bronchomotor tone and produce a degree of bronchodilation (except desflurane) that may be helpful in patients with obstructive lung disease or bronchoconstriction.[5]

CHRONIC OBSTRUCTIVE PULMONARY DISEASE

Clinical Presentation

The pathologic hallmarks of COPD include inflammation of the small airways and destruction of lung parenchyma. The FEV_1/FVC ratio will be less than 70%, and the RV will be increased. The severity of COPD is assessed by the percent of FEV_1: stage I, more than 50% predicted (this category includes both mild and moderate COPD); stage II, 35% to 50%; and stage III, less than 35%.[6] Stage I patients should not have significant dyspnea, hypoxemia, or hypercarbia. Specific complications of COPD to be considered preoperatively are described next.

Carbon Dioxide Retention (Baseline $Paco_2$ >45 mm Hg)

Some patients with stage II or III COPD have an elevated $Paco_2$ at rest. Patients with CO_2 retention cannot be differentiated from patients without retention on the basis of history, physical examination, or spirometry. When these patients are given supplemental oxygen, their $Paco_2$ values increase because of an increase in alveolar dead space from a decrease in regional hypoxic pulmonary vasoconstriction and the Haldane effect.[7] However, supplemental oxygen must be administered to these patients to prevent the hypoxemia associated with the postoperative decrease in FRC. Increased CO_2 concentrations above baseline lead to respiratory acidosis, which causes cardiovascular changes (tachycardia, hypertension, and pulmonary vasoconstriction). $Paco_2$ levels more than 80 mm Hg can cause a decreased level of consciousness. The increase in $Paco_2$ in these patients postoperatively should be anticipated and monitored. To identify these patients preoperatively, patients with stage II or III COPD should have an analysis of arterial blood gas performed.

Right Ventricular Dysfunction

Right ventricular dysfunction occurs in up to 50% of patients with severe COPD. Chronic recurrent hypoxemia is the cause of right ventricular dysfunction and subsequent progression to cor pulmonale. Cor pulmonale occurs in 70% of adult COPD patients with an FEV_1 less than 0.6 L. Mortality risk in these patients is primarily related to chronic hypoxemia. Administration of oxygen is the only therapy that improves long-term survival and decreases right-sided heart strain associated with COPD. Patients who have a resting Pao_2 less than 55 mm Hg should receive supplemental oxygen to maintain Pao_2 at 60 to 65 mm Hg at home.

Bullae

Many patients with moderate or severe COPD develop cystic air spaces in the lung parenchyma known as *bullae.* These bullae will often be asymptomatic unless they occupy more than 50% of the hemithorax, in which case the patient will present with findings of restrictive respiratory disease in addition to their obstructive disease. A bulla is actually a localized loss of structural support tissue in the lung with elastic recoil of surrounding parenchyma. The pressure in a bulla is the mean pressure in the surrounding alveoli averaged over the respiratory cycle. Whenever positive-pressure ventilation is used, the pressure in a bulla will become positive in relation to the adjacent lung tissue and the bulla will expand, with the attendant risk of rupture, tension pneumothorax, and bronchopleural fistula. Positive-pressure ventilation can be used safely in patients with bullae, provided the airway pressures are low and adequate expertise and equipment are immediately available to insert a chest drain and obtain lung isolation if necessary. Nitrous oxide will diffuse into a bulla more quickly than the less soluble nitrogen can diffuse out and may lead to rupture of the bulla. The presence of bullae should be ascertained by examination of the chest imaging of any patient with COPD preoperatively.

Flow Limitation

Severe COPD patients are often flow limited, even during normal breathing. Flow limitation occurs when any increase in expiratory effort will not produce an increase in flow at that given lung volume. Flow limitation is present in normal patients only during a forced expiratory maneuver and in patients with COPD as a result of the loss of lung elastic recoil. During positive-pressure ventilation, this can lead to the development of an intrinsic positive end-expiratory pressure (auto-PEEP). Severely flow-limited patients are at risk of hemodynamic collapse during positive-pressure ventilation because of dynamic hyperinflation of the lungs leading to obstruction of pulmonary blood flow.

Perioperative Management

Four treatable complications of COPD must be actively sought and managed at the time of preoperative assessment: atelectasis, bronchospasm, respiratory tract infections, and congestive heart failure. Atelectasis impairs local lung lymphocyte and macrophage function, predisposing to infection. Wheezing may be a symptom of both airway obstruction and congestive heart failure. Patients with COPD should receive bronchodilator therapy as guided by their symptoms. If sympathomimetic and anticholinergic bronchodilators provide inadequate therapy, a trial of corticosteroid therapy should be instituted.

COPD patients have fewer postoperative pulmonary complications when intensive chest physiotherapy is initiated preoperatively. Even in patients with severe COPD, exercise tolerance can be improved with physiotherapy[8] of at least 1 month or more. Among COPD patients, those with excessive sputum benefit the most from chest physiotherapy. A comprehensive program of pulmonary rehabilitation involving physiotherapy, exercise, nutrition, and education has been shown consistently to improve functional capacity for patients with severe COPD. These programs typically have a duration of several months and are generally not an option in resections for malignancy.

INTERSTITIAL LUNG DISEASE

Interstitial lung disease (ILD) is a chronic restrictive pulmonary disease (i.e., FEV_1 <70% predicted, FEV_1/FVC ratio normal or increased, and RV decreased). Approximately 35% of ILD cases are attributable to an identifiable cause, such as exposure to inorganic dust, organic antigens, drugs, or radiation. The inciting agent in the remaining 65% of patients is unknown. In many of these patients, the lung is part of an autoimmune disorder.

Elastic recoil of the lungs increases as a consequence of inflammation and fibrosis of the alveolar walls, which results in decreased lung volumes. Early in the disease, patients adapt to smaller tidal volumes by increasing their respiratory rate. As the disease progresses, increased respiratory effort and energy are required to maintain sufficient tidal volumes to prevent alveolar hypoventilation. Uneven disease distribution throughout the lung can cause significant ventilation/perfusion mismatch and is the primary cause of hypoxemia in patients with ILD.

Controlled ventilation via an endotracheal tube is often the most reliable and safest approach to optimizing oxygenation and ventilation in patients with ILD when a general anesthetic is required. The goal of mechanical ventilation in patients with ILD is to maintain adequate ventilation and oxygenation while minimizing the risks of barotrauma and acute lung injury. Potential strategies to minimize airway pressures include the use of long durations of inspiration compared with the duration of expiration ratios (e.g., ratios of 1:1 to 1:1.5), small tidal volumes, and rapid respiratory rates. In contrast to obstructive lung disease PEEP can be used safely in ILD.

CYSTIC FIBROSIS

Cystic fibrosis is an autosomal recessive disorder that results in impaired transport of sodium, chloride, and water across epithelial tissue. This leads to exocrine gland malfunction with abnormally viscous secretions, which can cause obstruction of the respiratory tracts, pancreas, biliary system, intestines, and sweat glands. It presents as a mixed obstructive and restrictive lung disease. Inability to clear the thick purulent secretions enhances bacterial growth and leads to bronchiectasis as the disease advances.[9]

The early mortality of cystic fibrosis is primarily the result of pulmonary complications, including air-trapping, pneumothorax, massive hemoptysis, and respiratory failure. Effective sputum elimination is a key goal in the long-term management of cystic fibrosis. To optimize patients with cystic fibrosis for anesthesia, chest physiotherapy should be performed immediately before surgery. Endotracheal intubation with a large endotracheal tube is preferred, as it facilitates endobronchial toileting with a suction catheter, bronchoscopy, or both.

IV

Box 27.3 Clinical Signs and Symptoms Suggestive of Obstructive Sleep Apnea

1. Predisposing clinical characteristics:
   - Body mass index (BMI) ≥35 kg/m² (or 95th percentile for age and gender)
   - Neck circumference of ≥17 inches (men) or ≥16 inches (women)
   - Craniofacial abnormalities affecting the airway
   - Anatomic nasal obstruction
   - Tonsils touching or nearly touching in the midline
2. History of apparent airway obstruction during sleep (two or more of the following are present):
   - Frequent snoring
   - Observed pauses in breathing during sleep
   - Awakens from sleep with choking sensation
   - Frequent arousals from sleep
3. Somnolence:
   - Frequent somnolence or fatigue despite adequate "sleep"
   - Falls asleep easily in a nonstimulating environment despite "adequate sleep"

If a patient has signs or symptoms in two or more of the previous categories, there is a significant probability that he or she has obstructive sleep apnea (OSA). The severity of OSA can be determined using a sleep study. In the absence of a sleep study patients should be treated as though they have moderate sleep apnea unless one of the previous signs or symptoms is severely abnormal (i.e., markedly increased BMI), in which case they are classified as having severe sleep apnea.

Table 27.2 Determination of Severity of Obstructive Sleep Apnea on the Basis of a Sleep Study

Adult AHI	Pediatric AHI	OSA Severity	OSA Severity Score
6-20	1-5	Mild	1
21-40	6-10	Moderate	2
>40	>10	Severe	3

AHI, Apnea–hypopnea index; *OSA*, obstructive sleep apnea.

can lead to cognitive dysfunction manifesting as intellectual impairment and hypersomnolence.

The diagnosis of OSA can be based on clinical impression or a formal sleep study. OSA should be suspected when a patient with predisposing clinical risk factors reports heavy snoring and excessive daytime sleepiness, which are the cardinal features of OSA. OSA is characterized by frequent episodes of apnea or hypopnea during sleep. Apnea is defined as complete cessation of breathing for 10 seconds or more. Hypopnea is defined as more than 50% decrease in ventilation or oxygen desaturation of more than 3% to 4% for 10 seconds or more. It is definitively diagnosed by polysomnography in a sleep laboratory. The severity of OSA is measured by using the apnea–hypopnea index (AHI), which is the number of apneic or hypopneic episodes occurring per hour of sleep (Table 27.2).

OBSTRUCTIVE SLEEP APNEA (ALSO SEE CHAPTER 48)

Clinical Presentation

OSA affects approximately 4% of middle-aged men and 2% of middle-aged women.[10] Obesity is the most important physical characteristic associated with OSA, though OSA may be present in patients with a normal body mass index (BMI) and absent in the obese.

Patients with risk factors (male gender, middle age, BMI >28 kg/m², alcohol and sedative use) presenting for surgery should be screened for signs and symptoms of OSA (Box 27.3).

The pathophysiology of airflow obstruction is related primarily to upper airway pharyngeal collapse. Upper airway patency depends on the action of dilator muscles (i.e., tensor palatine, genioglossus muscle, and hyoid muscles). During sleep, laryngeal muscle tone is decreased, and apnea occurs when the upper airway collapses. Nonobese patients may develop OSA as a result of adenotonsillar hypertrophy or craniofacial abnormalities (retrognathia). Recurrent episodes of apnea or hypopnea lead to hypoxia, hypercapnia, increased sympathetic stimulation, and arousal from sleep. Patients may develop cardiopulmonary dysfunction manifesting as systemic or pulmonary hypertension and cor pulmonale. Nonrestoration of sleep

Treatment of Obstructive Sleep Apnea

Treatment should include correction of reversible exacerbating factors by means of weight reduction, avoidance of alcohol and sedatives, and nasal decongestants, if needed. Patients with mild OSA can achieve clinical improvement through lifestyle modification. For severe OSA, the three main therapeutic options are continuous positive airway pressure (CPAP), dental appliances, and upper airway surgery.

Preoperative Evaluation of Patients With Obstructive Sleep Apnea

The goals of the preoperative assessment are to identify anticipated difficulties in airway management (difficult facemask ventilation, endotracheal intubation, or both) and coexisting cardiovascular disease. Associated medical conditions should be treated, to the extent possible, before elective surgery. Patients with OSA may have perioperative issues in multiple organ systems, as described in Box 27.4.

Perioperative Management

Patients with OSA are sensitive to the respiratory depressant and sedative effects of benzodiazepines and opioids,

> **Box 27.4** Potential Organ System Involvement in Patients With OSA
>
> 1. *Airway:* Anticipated difficulties with airway management include difficult ventilation via a mask and difficult tracheal intubation.
> 2. *Respiratory system:* Patients with obesity will have evidence of restrictive lung disease on pulmonary function testing secondary to decreased chest wall compliance.
> 3. *Cardiovascular system:* Preoperative evaluation should be directed toward the detection of end-organ dysfunction resulting from chronic hypoxemia, hypercarbia, and polycythemia. Systemic hypertension, pulmonary hypertension, and signs of biventricular dysfunction (cor pulmonale and congestive heart failure) should be sought.
> 4. *Endocrine and gastrointestinal systems:* Fasting blood glucose levels should be sought to screen for type 2 diabetes. Symptoms of esophageal reflux should lead to aspiration prophylaxis before induction of anesthesia. Liver function tests may indicate fatty liver infiltration causing hepatic dysfunction in severe cases.

Table 27.3 Scoring Invasiveness of Surgery and Anesthesia

Surgery	Anesthesia	Invasive Score
Superficial or peripheral	Local infiltration or peripheral nerve block with no sedation	0
	Moderate sedation Spinal or epidural	1
	General anesthetic	2
Major or airway	General anesthetic	3

Table 27.4 Scoring of Opioid Requirement

Opioid Requirement	Score
None	0
Low-dose oral	1
High-dose oral	2
Parenteral or spinal/epidural	3

which can cause upper airway obstruction or apnea. These medications should be withheld preoperatively or used with caution in a monitored environment.

Intraoperative anesthetic concerns in patients with OSA relate to (1) airway management; (2) choice of anesthetic technique; (3) patient positioning; (4) monitoring, inaccurate noninvasive blood pressure measurements and significant underlying cardiorespiratory disease may warrant insertion of an arterial line for analysis of arterial blood gas monitoring and beat-to-beat blood pressure measurements; and (5) vascular access, difficult intravenous (IV) access secondary to excess adipose tissue may necessitate central line placement.

Upper airway abnormalities or increased airway adiposity in patients with OSA predisposes them as difficult to adequately ventilate with a bag and mask apparatus after induction of anesthesia. Oral and nasopharyngeal airways should be readily available. Excessive pharyngeal adipose tissue can make exposure of the glottic opening difficult during direct laryngoscopy and endotracheal intubation.

The intraoperative use of short-acting drugs (e.g., sevoflurane, desflurane, propofol) and multimodal nonopioid analgesia decreases the risk of postoperative respiratory depression. Nitrous oxide is best avoided in patients with coexisting pulmonary hypertension. Short- to intermediate-acting neuromuscular blocking drugs can be used for muscle relaxation if required.

The anesthesia provider should consider tracheal extubation with the patient in a semiupright position with an oral or nasopharyngeal airway in place to facilitate spontaneous ventilation. Supplemental oxygen and a small amount of PEEP may be provided via high-flow nasal cannula immediately after extubation. A two-person bag and mask ventilation may be required and possible reintubation of the trachea should acute airway obstruction develop. Administration of supplemental oxygen should be provided during transfer of the patient to the postanesthesia care unit (PACU). CPAP must be available for postoperative use in patients on CPAP or bilevel positive airway pressure (BiPAP) preoperatively.

Postoperative Management

Multimodal analgesia with nonsteroidal antiinflammatory drugs (NSAIDs), acetaminophen, and regional analgesia aims to minimize opiate analgesia and resultant respiratory depression. CPAP should be reinstituted postoperatively. Surveillance in a high-dependency unit such as the PACU, step-down unit, or intensive care unit (ICU) is prudent for patients with severe OSA.

Postoperative disposition of OSA is influenced by three factors:

1. Severity of the OSA (either by historical information or objective findings of a sleep study) (see Table 27.2)
2. Invasiveness of the surgical procedure and anesthesia (Table 27.3)
3. Predicted postoperative opioid use (Table 27.4)

A patient with increased perioperative risk of airway obstruction and resultant hypoxemia (perioperative OSA risk score greater than 4) should receive continuous oxygen saturation monitoring in either the ICU, a step-down unit, or telemetry unit (Box 27.5).

Box 27.5 Determination of Perioperative Obstructive Sleep Apnea Risk Score

OSA Severity Score (1–3)
+
Invasiveness of anesthesia or surgery (1–3)
   OR
Postoperative opioid requirement (1–3) (whichever is greater)
   If risk score = 4 → increased perioperative risk
   If risk score ≥5 → significantly increased perioperative risk

OSA, Obstructive sleep apnea.

Box 27.6 Management Principles for Pulmonary Hypertension Secondary to Lung Disease

- Avoid hypotensive and vasodilating anesthetic drugs whenever possible
- Ketamine does not exacerbate pulmonary hypertension
- Support mean blood pressure with vasopressors: norepinephrine, phenylephrine, vasopressin
- Use inhaled pulmonary vasodilators (nitric oxide, prostacyclin) in preference to intravenous vasodilators as needed
- Use thoracic epidural local anesthetics cautiously and with inotropes as needed
- Monitor cardiac output if possible

Obesity Hypoventilation Syndrome

Obesity hypoventilation syndrome (OHS) is defined by chronic daytime hypoxemia (Pao_2 <65 mm Hg) and hypoventilation ($Paco_2$ >45 mm Hg) in an obese patient without coexisting COPD. It results from an interaction of sleep-disordered breathing, decreased respiratory drive, and obesity-related respiratory impairment. Patients exhibit signs of central sleep apnea (apnea without respiratory efforts). This may culminate in the pickwickian syndrome characterized by obesity, daytime hypersomnolence, hypoxemia, and hypercarbia.

Preoperatively, obese patients should be screened for OHS with pulse oximetry. Patients with oxygen saturation less than 96% warrant analysis of arterial blood gases to assess carbon dioxide retention.

Ultimately, the information obtained from preoperative investigations allows the anesthesia provider to optimize the patient's clinical status before elective surgery and plan perioperative care, including arrangements for appropriate postoperative monitoring (i.e., step-down bed, ICU). Interventions may include treatment of coexisting conditions (systemic hypertension, cardiac dysrhythmias, congestive heart failure) and initiation of CPAP. A 2-week period of CPAP therapy is usually effective in correcting the abnormal ventilatory drive of patients with OHS.

PULMONARY HYPERTENSION

Pathophysiology

Patients with pulmonary hypertension (mean pulmonary artery pressure >25 mm Hg by catheterization or systolic pulmonary artery pressure >50 mm Hg on echocardiography)[11] may present for a variety of noncardiac surgical procedures.[12] Patients with pulmonary hypertension are at increased risk of respiratory complications and prolonged intubation after noncardiac surgery.[13]

Preoperative Evaluation

There are two commonly encountered types of pulmonary hypertension: pulmonary hypertension from left-sided heart disease and pulmonary hypertension from lung disease. Patients who present for noncardiac surgery are more likely to have pulmonary hypertension because of lung disease. Much of what has been learned about anesthesia for patients with pulmonary hypertension resulting from lung disease has come from clinical experience in pulmonary endarterectomies[14] and lung transplantation. Avoiding hypotension is the key to managing these patients (Box 27.6).

Management of Anesthesia

The increased right ventricular transmural and intracavitary pressures associated with pulmonary hypertension may restrict perfusion of the right coronary artery during systole, especially as pulmonary artery pressures approach systemic levels. The impact of pulmonary hypertension on right ventricular dysfunction has several anesthetic implications. The hemodynamic goals are similar to other conditions in which cardiac output is relatively fixed. Care should be taken to avoid physiologic states that will worsen pulmonary hypertension, such as hypoxemia, hypercarbia, acidosis, and hypothermia. Conditions that impair right ventricular filling, such as tachycardia and arrhythmias, are not well tolerated. Ideally, during anesthesia, right ventricular contractility and systemic vascular resistance are maintained or increased while pulmonary vascular resistance is decreased. Ketamine is a useful anesthetic in pulmonary hypertension caused by lung disease.[15] Inotropes and inodilators, such as dobutamine and milrinone, may improve hemodynamics in patients with pulmonary hypertension caused by left-sided heart disease. However, inodilators decrease systemic vascular tone and can cause tachycardia, potentially leading to a deterioration in the hemodynamics of patients with pulmonary hypertension caused by lung disease. Vasopressors such as phenylephrine, norepinephrine, and vasopressin are commonly used to maintain a systemic blood pressure greater than pulmonary pressures. Vasopressin can increase systemic blood pressure significantly without affecting pulmonary artery pressure in patients with pulmonary hypertension.[16] In patients with severe pulmonary hypertension selective

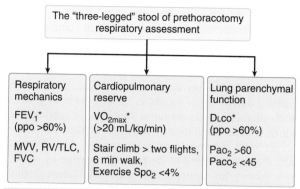

Fig. 27.3 The three-legged stool of prethoracotomy respiratory assessment. *Most valid test (see text). *D*lco, Lung diffusing capacity for carbon monoxide; *FEV₁*, forced expiratory volume in 1 second; *FVC*, forced vital capacity; *MVV*, maximum voluntary ventilation; *Paco₂*, partial pressure of carbon dioxide in mm Hg; *Pao₂*, partial pressure of oxygen (arterial) in mm Hg; *ppo*, predicted postoperative; *RV*, residual volume; *Spo₂*, pulse oximeter saturation; *TLC*, total lung capacity; *VO₂max*, maximal oxygen consumption. (Adapted from Slinger PD, ed. *Pearson's Thoracic and Esophageal Surgery.* New York: Springer; 2011, used with permission.)

inhaled pulmonary vasodilators, including nitric oxide (10 to 40 ppm)[17] or nebulized prostaglandins (prostacyclin 50 ng/kg/min),[18] should be considered.

Lumbar epidural analgesia and anesthesia have been used in obstetric patients with pulmonary hypertension,[19] and occasionally thoracic epidural analgesia is used in patients with pulmonary hypertension. Patients with pulmonary hypertension caused by lung disease seem to be extremely dependent on tonic cardiac sympathetic innervation for normal hemodynamic stability.[20] These patients will often require a low-dose infusion of inotropes or vasopressors during management with thoracic epidural local analgesia.

ANESTHESIA FOR LUNG RESECTION

Thoracic surgery is a relatively young specialty that has been significantly aided by the development of positive-pressure ventilation in the early 1950s, and advanced by the use of double-lumen endobronchial tubes (DLTs) and flexible bronchoscopes. These developments now enable a thoracic anesthesiologist to employ reliable lung isolation, allowing surgical access to the thorax and managing anesthesia during one-lung ventilation (OLV).

Preoperative Assessment for Pulmonary Resection

Preoperative assessment before pulmonary resection aims to identify patients at increased risk of perioperative morbidity and mortality in order to focus resources and

improve their outcome. Postoperative preservation of respiratory function is proportional to the amount of lung parenchyma preserved. The major causes of perioperative morbidity and mortality after thoracic surgery are respiratory complications. Major respiratory complications, such as atelectasis, pneumonia, and respiratory failure, occur in 15% to 20% of patients and account for much of the 3% to 4% mortality rate.[21] Objective measures of pulmonary function are required to guide anesthetic management and to transmit information easily between members of the health care team.

Objective Assessment of Pulmonary Function

Preoperative anesthetic assessment before lung resection continues to evolve as surgical techniques and perioperative care have expanded what is considered operable pathology. An "operable" patient is one who can tolerate the proposed resection with acceptable risk.

No single test of respiratory function is adequate for preoperative assessment. Before surgery, respiratory function should be assessed in three related but independent areas: respiratory mechanics, gas exchange, and cardiorespiratory interaction (Fig. 27.3). This "three-legged stool" approach can be used to plan intraoperative and postoperative management.

Respiratory Mechanics

Of all objective measures obtained via spirometry (e.g., FVC, FEV₁, ratio of FEV₁:FVC), the FEV₁ is most helpful. Spirometry measurements should be expressed as a percentage of predicted volume corrected for age, sex, and height (e.g., an FEV₁ of 74%). The predicted postoperative FEV₁ (ppoFEV₁%) is the most effective test for prediction of postthoracotomy respiratory complications.[22] It is calculated as follows (Eq. 1):

$$\text{ppoFEV}_1\% = \text{preoperative FEV}_1\%$$
$$\times (100 - \% \text{ of functional tissue removed}/100)$$

Counting the number of lung segments to be removed allows estimation of the percentage of functional lung tissue removed (Fig. 27.4). Patients with a ppoFEV₁ of more than 60% are at low risk of postoperative pulmonary complications, whereas those with a ppoFEV₁ of less than 30% are at high risk.[23]

Lung Parenchymal Function

Lung parenchymal function refers to the ability of the lung to exchange oxygen and carbon dioxide between the pulmonary vascular bed and the alveoli. The most useful indicator of lung parenchymal function is the Dlco obtained during lung function testing. The Dlco correlates with the total functioning surface area of the alveolar–capillary interface. The corrected Dlco can be used to calculate a predicted postresection (ppo) value using the same calculation as FEV₁ (see Eq. 1). Like FEV₁, a ppo Dlco greater than 60% correlates with a low risk of postoperative

IV

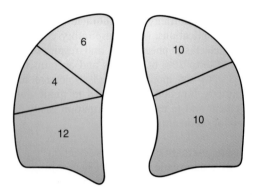

Lung segments
Total subsegments = 42

Example: Right lower lobectomy
postoperative FEV$_1$ decrease = 12/42 (29%)

Fig. 27.4 The number of subsegments of each lobe is used to calculate the predicted postoperative (ppo) pulmonary function. In this example after a right lower lobectomy, a patient with a preoperative FEV$_1$ 70% of normal would be expected to have a ppoFEV$_1$ of 70% × (100 − 29/100) = 50%. (From Slinger PD, ed. *Pearson's Thoracic and Esophageal Surgery.* New York: Springer; 2011, used with permission.)

pulmonary complications. Traditionally, analysis of arterial blood gas data, such as a partial pressure of oxygen (Pao$_2$) less than 60 mm Hg or a partial pressure of carbon dioxide (Paco$_2$) more than 45 mm Hg, has been used as an indicator of increased risk of respiratory failure.

Cardiopulmonary Interaction
The final step in assessment of respiratory function is the assessment of cardiopulmonary interaction. Formal laboratory exercise testing is the gold standard,[24] with the maximal oxygen consumption (V̇O$_{2max}$) being the most useful predictor of postthoracotomy outcome, and should be used for patients with a ppoFEV$_1$ or D$_{LCO}$ <60%. The risks of morbidity and mortality are low if the (V̇O$_{2max}$) is greater than 20 mL/kg/min, with less than 10 mL/kg/min considered very high risk.[23] Complete laboratory exercise testing is expensive and not available to all centers. Several alternatives, including the stair climb test (SCT), shuttle walk test (SWT), and the 6-minute walk test (6MWT), are valid surrogate tests for prethoracotomy assessment (outlined in Fig. 27.3).

Ventilation-Perfusion Scintigraphy
Prediction of postresection pulmonary function can be further refined by assessment of the preoperative contribution of the lung or lobe to be resected using ventilation-perfusion scintigraphy (V̇/Q̇ scan). If the lung to be resected is minimally functional, this will modify the ppoFEV$_1$.

Preoperative Cardiac Assessment
Cardiac complications are the second most common cause of perioperative morbidity and death in the thoracic surgical population. Intrathoracic surgery is considered a risk factor for major adverse cardiac events by the American College of Cardiology and American Heart Association.[25] Further, dysrhythmia occurs in 12% to 44% of patients after thoracic or esophageal surgery, the majority of which is atrial fibrillation.[26] The onset of atrial fibrillation occurs most commonly on postoperative days 2 and 3, with the risk reverting to the patient's baseline by week 6. Risk factors for postoperative atrial fibrillation include male sex, older age, magnitude of lung or esophagus resected, history of congestive cardiac failure, concomitant lung disease, and length of procedure. It may be reasonable to give high-risk patients (e.g., older patients undergoing pneumonectomy) prophylactic diltiazem or amiodarone to decrease the incidence of postoperative atrial fibrillation.[27]

Smoking Cessation

Pulmonary complications are reduced in patients undergoing lung resection who cease smoking perioperatively, with the benefits increasing proportionally to the length of cessation.[28] Patients should be encouraged to stop smoking at the preoperative assessment, as they may be more receptive to the message at this time. Nicotine replacement and behavioral management increase the rate of smoking cessation.

Assessment of the Patient With Lung Cancer

Patients undergoing lung resection for malignancy should be assessed for the four Ms: *m*ass effects, *m*etabolic abnormalities, *m*etastases, and *m*edications. These considerations are outlined in Box 27.7.

Box 27.7 Anesthetic Considerations in Patients With Lung Cancer (the Four Ms)	
Mass effects	Obstructive pneumonia, lung abscess, superior vena cava syndrome, tracheobronchial distortion, Pancoast syndrome, recurrent laryngeal nerve or phrenic nerve paresis, chest wall or mediastinal extension
Metabolic abnormalities	Lambert-Eaton syndrome, hypercalcemia, hyponatremia, Cushing syndrome
Metastases	Particularly to brain, bone, liver, adrenal gland
Medications	Chemotherapy drugs, pulmonary toxicity (bleomycin, mitomycin), cardiac toxicity (doxorubicin), renal toxicity (cisplatin)

Box 27.8 Indications for One-Lung Ventilation

- Allow OLV and therefore surgical exposure to the thorax and adjacent structures, such as for lung resection, mediastinal, cardiac, vascular, esophageal, and spinal surgery.
- Control ventilation, such as a patient with a bronchopleural fistula.
- Prevent contralateral lung soiling, such as pulmonary hemorrhage, bronchopleural fistula, and whole-lung lavage.
- Allow for differential patterns of ventilation in patients with unilateral lung injury.

Indications for Lung Isolation

Lung isolation techniques have several goals, as described in Box 27.8.

Options for Lung Isolation

There are several options to facilitate selective ventilation of one lung. These include a DLT (Fig. 27.5), a bronchial blocker (BB) placed through a single-lumen endotracheal tube (SLT) (see Fig. 27.12), and a single-lumen tube (standard endotracheal tube or endobronchial tube) placed directly into a bronchus. The advantages and disadvantages of each device are listed in Table 27.5.

Airway Anatomy

To place a device for lung isolation, the anesthesia provider must appreciate the bronchial anatomy (Fig. 27.6). Without this knowledge, it is easy to place a device incorrectly and is difficult to recognize and troubleshoot malposition.[29]

Salient aspects of the bronchial anatomy are highlighted in Box 27.9. For a more detailed description of bronchial anatomy, please see the online bronchoscopy simulator.[30]

Sizing a Double-Lumen Endobronchial Tube

There is no consensus as to the optimal method to size a DLT. An ideally sized DLT should have a bronchial external diameter 1 to 2 mm smaller than the bronchial diameter in order to fit the deflated bronchial cuff. Chest x-ray images may be used to assist DLT selection.[31] The authors' preference is a simplified method based on patient sex and height (Table 27.6). A further important step before placement is to check a chest x-ray, or ideally, a computed tomography (CT) chest coronal slice to exclude aberrant anatomy such as endoluminal obstruction, significant tracheal deviation, or aberrant right upper lobe take-off. DLTs have a larger external diameter than SLTs and should not be advanced against resistance (Fig. 27.7).

IV

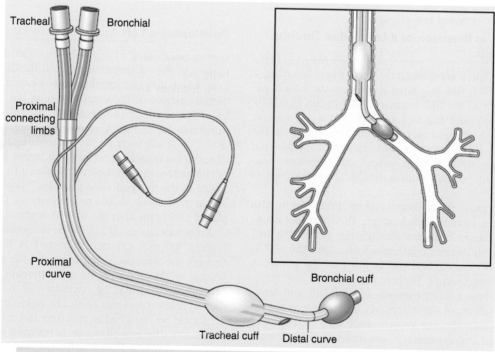

Fig. 27.5 Left-sided double-lumen endobronchial tube.

Table 27.5	Options for Lung Isolation	
Option	**Advantages**	**Disadvantages**
Double-lumen tube	• Easy to place successfully • Repositioning rarely required • Bronchoscopy to isolated lung • Suction to isolated lung • CPAP easily applied • Can alternate one-lung ventilation to either lung easily • Placement possible if bronchoscopy not available	• Size selection more difficult • Difficult to place in patients with difficult airways or abnormal tracheas • Not optimal for postoperative ventilation • Potential laryngeal and bronchial trauma
Bronchial blockers	• Size selection rarely an issue • Easily added to regular ETT • Allows ventilation during placement • Easier placement in patients with difficult airways and in children • Postoperative two-lung ventilation easy by withdrawing blocker • Selective lobar isolation possible • CPAP to isolated lung possible	• More time required to position • Repositioning required more often • Bronchoscope essential for positioning • Limited right-lung isolation because of RUL anatomy • Bronchoscopy to isolated lung impossible • Minimal suction to isolated lung • Difficult to alternate one-lung ventilation to either lung
Endobronchial tube	• Easier placement in patients with difficult airways • Short cuff designed for lung isolation	• Bronchoscopy necessary for placement • Does not allow for bronchoscopy, suctioning, or CPAP to isolated lung • Difficult one-lung ventilation to right lung
Endotracheal tube advanced into bronchus	• Easier placement in patients with difficult airways	• Bronchoscopy necessary for placement • Does not allow for bronchoscopy, suctioning, or CPAP to isolated lung • Cuff not designed for lung isolation • Extremely difficult one-lung ventilation to right lung

CPAP, Continuous positive airway pressure; *ETT*, endotracheal tube; *RUL*, right upper lobe of lung.

Methods of Insertion of a Left-Sided Double-Lumen Tube

Two techniques are commonly used when inserting a left-sided DLT. One is a blind technique: the endobronchial lumen of the DLT is passed through the glottis by laryngoscopy and the DLT is then turned 90 degrees counterclockwise and advanced until resistance is felt (Fig. 27.8). Blind insertion alone results in malposition in approximately 35% of cases, and therefore confirmation of position with a flexible bronchoscope is important.[32,33]

The alternative technique involves direct vision with the use of a flexible bronchoscope. The tip of the endobronchial lumen is passed through the glottis, the DLT is rotated 90 degrees counterclockwise, and the DLT is advanced so the tracheal cuff is just past the glottis. A flexible bronchoscope is then inserted into the endobronchial lumen to its opening, and the DLT and bronchoscope advanced simultaneously into the correct bronchus. Alternatively, the bronchoscope may be advanced through the endobronchial lumen and into the left main bronchus, with the DLT advanced over it.

Positioning a Left-Sided Double-Lumen Tube

Correct positioning of a DLT is important to avoid ventilation of the collapsed lung (i.e., if the DLT is too shallow), which may obscure the surgeon's field, and to avoid partial collapse of the ventilated lung (i.e., if the DLT is too deep), resulting in hypoxemia. Auscultation alone is unreliable for confirmation of DLT placement. It is still useful, as it will increase the anesthesia provider's index of suspicion regarding malposition before bronchoscopy, as troubleshooting an incorrectly placed DLT can be confusing to the inexperienced provider.[29] Both auscultation and bronchoscopy should be used when a DLT is initially placed and again after the patient is repositioned.

Bronchoscopy using a pediatric bronchoscope (approximately 4.0 mm external diameter) is first performed through the tracheal lumen to ensure the endobronchial portion of the DLT is in the left bronchus and the blue endobronchial cuff is approximately 5 to 10 mm below the tracheal carina (Fig. 27.9). The right upper lobe takeoff should be identified at this time to confirm anatomic landmarks. The bronchoscope is removed and reinserted into the bronchial lumen, ensuring both the left upper

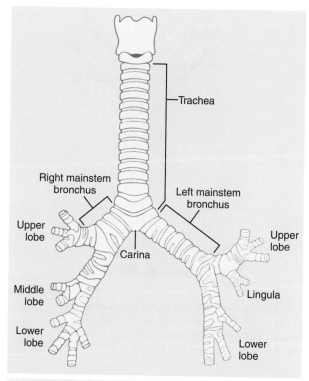

Fig. 27.6 Tracheobronchial anatomy. Right main bronchus is typically 1.5 to 2 cm. Left main bronchus is typically 4.5 to 5 cm.

Box 27.9 Bronchial Anatomy Relevant to Lung Isolation

- Carina: bifurcation is "sharp" with no further divisions seen in the left or right lumen
- Right main bronchus: typically 1.5–2 cm long
- Right upper lobe: the only trifurcation within the tracheobronchial tree, with a distinct appearance on fiberoptic bronchoscopy; aberrant take-off at or above carina in 1 in 250 patients
- Left main bronchus: typically 4.5–5 cm long
- Lower lobes: can be identified bilaterally as the longitudinal fibers of the trachealis muscle descend into them

---

Table 27.6	Selection of Double-Lumen Tube Size Based on Adult Patient's Sex and Height	
Sex	**Height (cm)**	**Size of Double-Lumen Tube (Fr)**
Female	>160 (63 in)	37
	<153–159	35
	<152 (60 in)	consider 32
Male	>170 (67 in)	41
	<160–169	39
	<159 (63 in)	consider 37

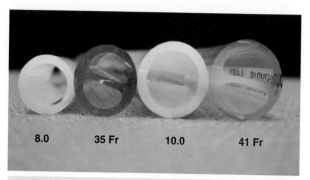

Fig. 27.7 Photograph of the cut cross sections of several single-lumen tubes and double-lumen tubes illustrating comparative size. (Courtesy Professor Jerome Klafta, Department of Anesthesia and Critical Care, University of Chicago.)

and lower lobes can be seen. Both lobes must be identified to ensure that distal migration of the endobronchial lumen has not led to insertion into the left lower lobe and occlusion of the left upper lobe.

Right-Sided Double-Lumen Tube Indications

Although a left-sided DLT is used most frequently for thoracic procedures, there are specific clinical situations in which the use of a right-sided DLT is indicated (Box 27.10). A right-sided DLT incorporates a modified cuff and slot in the endobronchial lumen that allows ventilation of the right upper lobe (Fig. 27.10). Tracheobronchial anatomy must be checked before insertion of the right-sided DLT (CT scan or bronchoscopy) to confirm normal positioning of the right upper lobe orifice.

Positioning a Bronchial Blocker

The unifying principle of a BB is that it is inserted within an SLT and advanced into the left or right main bronchus or, less commonly, into a lobe. The cuff of the BB is inflated to obstruct the lumen (Fig. 27.11), allowing lung isolation, and a small channel within the blocker is used to allow gas to escape, allowing lung deflation; to apply suction to the lung; to intermittently insufflate oxygen; and to apply PEEP. An adaptor attaches to the SLT, allowing insertion of a BB or flexible bronchoscope and attachment to the anesthetic circuit. The method of insertion of a BB depends on the blocker's design. Four commercially available BBs are shown in Fig. 27.12. The advantages and disadvantages of BBs compared with other methods of lung isolation are listed in Table 27.5.

Physiologic Considerations of One-Lung Ventilation in the Lateral Position

Initiation of OLV with an open chest in the lateral position exposes physiologic changes that improve

IV

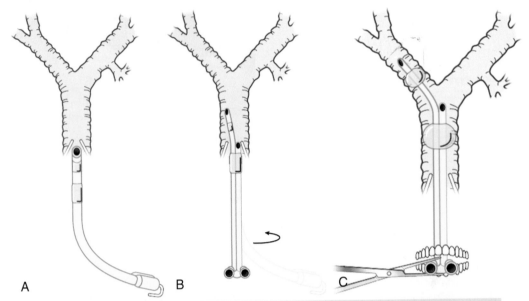

Fig. 27.8 Blind method for placement of a left-sided double-lumen tube. (A) The double-lumen tube is passed with laryngoscopy beyond the vocal cords. (B) The double-lumen tube is rotated 90 degrees counterclockwise. (C) The double-lumen tube is advanced to an appropriate depth (generally 27 to 29 cm marking at the level of the teeth). (From Campos JH. How to achieve successful lung separation. *SAJAA.* 2008;14:22–26.)

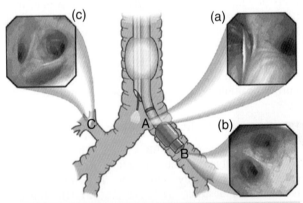

Fig. 27.9 Bronchoscopic examination of an optimally placed Mallinckrodt left-sided double-lumen tube. *(a)* The bronchoscope is passed through the tracheal lumen, and the edge of the endobronchial cuff is seen 5 mm below the tracheal carina. A white line marker is seen above the tracheal carina. *(b)* The bronchoscope is advanced through the endobronchial lumen, and a clear view of the left bronchial bifurcation (left upper and left lower bronchi) is seen. *(c)* A clear view of the right upper lobe bronchus and its three orifices confirms this is the right side. (From Campos JH. Update on tracheobronchial anatomy and flexible fiberoptic bronchoscopy in thoracic anesthesia. *Curr Opin Anaesthesiol.* 2009;22:4–10.)

> **Box 27.10** Indications for a Right-Sided Double-Lumen Tube
>
> Distorted anatomy of the entrance of the left main bronchus
> External or intraluminal tumor compression
> Descending thoracic aortic aneurysm
> Site of surgery involving the left main bronchus:
>   Left lung transplantation
>   Left-sided tracheobronchial disruption
>   Left-sided pneumonectomy[a]
>   Left-sided sleeve resection

[a]It is possible to manage a left pneumonectomy with a left-sided double-lumen tube (DLT) or bronchial blocker, but the DLT or blocker will have to be withdrawn before stapling the left main bronchus.

ventilation and perfusion matching compared with two-lung ventilation (TLV) with a closed chest. Perfusion to the nonventilated, nondependent lung is decreased from hypoxic pulmonary vasoconstriction and gravity, thereby favoring perfusion of the ventilated, dependent lung and decreasing shunt (Fig. 27.13). Changes in cardiac output can have varying effects, but typically shunt is lowest (and arterial Po_2 is greatest) at a "normal" cardiac output during OLV.[34,35]

Ventilation of the nondependent lung is stopped by virtue of lung isolation. The compliance of the ventilated, dependent lung decreases because of the cephalad shift of the diaphragm after induction of anesthesia and muscle relaxation, mediastinal shift after opening of the chest, and surgical pushing and manipulation of the mediastinum. This decrease in compliance and FRC can be improved with the application of PEEP. PEEP (5 to

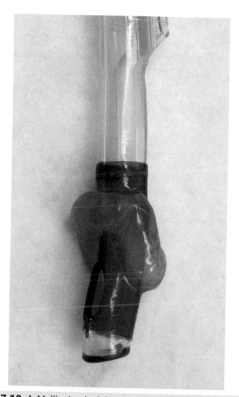

Fig. 27.10 A Mallinckrodt right-sided double-lumen tube. Note the modified cuff allowing right-lung isolation and slot in the endobronchial lumen allowing ventilation of the right upper lobe. (Courtesy Dr. Andrew Deacon, Department of Anesthesia, The Canberra Hospital, Australia.)

10 cm H_2O) to the ventilated, dependent lung also helps to reduce blood flow to the nonventilated, nondependent lung, as pulmonary vascular resistance is lowest at FRC (Fig. 27.14). Excessive PEEP may increase pulmonary vascular resistance, thereby increasing blood flow to the nonventilated, nondependent lung and worsening shunt.

Conduct of Anesthesia

Any anesthetic technique that provides safe and stable general anesthesia can be used for thoracic surgery. Although volatile anesthetics impair hypoxic pulmonary vasoconstriction, they do so only at a minimum alveolar concentration (MAC) greater than routine use, and there is no clear advantage of a propofol total intravenous anesthetic compared with a volatile anesthetic in terms of shunt fraction or hypoxemia.[36-38]

The majority of thoracic surgical procedures are of moderate duration (2 to 4 hours) and performed in the lateral position with an open hemithorax and OLV. Further, the surgeon is operating in close proximity to important structures, such as the heart and great vessels, and access to the patient is limited after lateral positioning. Thus the risk–benefit ratio for intraoperative monitoring and intravenous access favors being overly invasive at the outset.

Choice of monitoring should be guided by a knowledge of which complications are likely to occur (Table 27.7). An intraarterial catheter allows hemodynamic monitoring and analysis of arterial blood gases. It is the authors' practice to place an intraarterial catheter in all but the most simple

IV

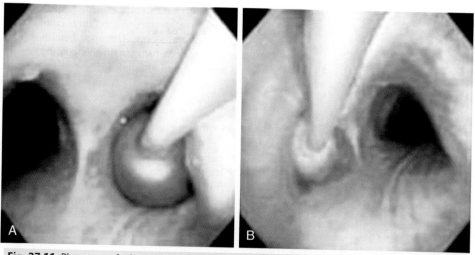

Fig. 27.11 Placement of a bronchial blocker. Correct positioning of a blocker in the right (A) and left (B) main bronchi as seen through a bronchoscope in the trachea just above the carina. (From Campos JH. How to achieve successful lung separation. *SAJAA.* 2008;14:22–26.)

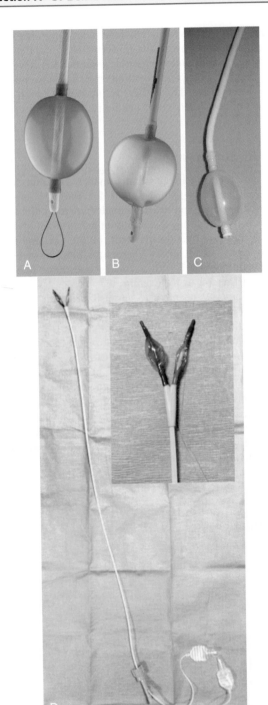

Fig. 27.12 Three commercially available endobronchial blockers. (A) The Arndt endobronchial blocker (Cook Critical Care, Bloomington, IN). (B) The Cohen Flexitip blocker (Cook Critical Care, Bloomington, IN). (C) The Fuji Uniblocker (Fuji Systems Corporation, Tokyo, Japan). (D) The Rusch EZ-Blocker (Contract Medical International GmbH, Dresden, Germany). (D from Piccioni F, Vecchi I, Spinelli E, et al. Extraluminal EZ-blocker placement for one-lung ventilation in pediatric thoracic surgery. *J Cardiothorac Vasc Anesth.* 2015;29[6]:e71–e73.)

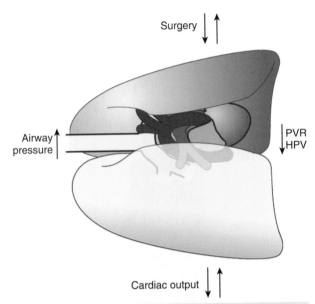

Fig. 27.13 Factors affecting the distribution of pulmonary blood flow during one-lung ventilation. Hypoxic pulmonary vasoconstriction *(HPV)* and the collapse of the nonventilated lung, which increases pulmonary vascular resistance *(PVR)*, tend to redistribute blood flow toward the ventilated lung. The airway pressure gradient between the ventilated and nonventilated thoraces tends to encourage blood flow to the nonventilated lung. Surgery and cardiac output can have variable effects, either increasing or decreasing the proportional flow to the ventilated lung.

thoracic case (e.g., wedge resection) being performed on a patient without comorbid disease. A central venous catheter allows vasoactive agents to be infused, assisting hemodynamic stability in a patient who is at risk of intraoperative hemorrhage or postoperative hypervolemia, such as for pneumonectomy, complex procedures, and redo-thoracotomy. The open hemithorax provides a large surface area for evaporative cooling; therefore devices to measure and maintain patient normothermia are required.

Another useful monitor during OLV is continuous spirometry. Available on most modern ventilators, this allows for continuous monitoring of inspiratory and expiratory volumes, pressures, and flows. Attention to the difference between the inspired and expired volumes during OLV may indicate an air leak and loss of lung isolation (>30 mL/breath). During TLV after lung resection, this difference correlates to an air leak through the lung parenchyma. The development of gas trapping in patients with obstructive lung disease is indicated by persistent end-expiratory flow.

Approach to Intravenous Fluid Management

The administration of the "right" amount of intravenous fluid to patients undergoing lung resection remains challenging. Patients undergoing lung resection are at risk

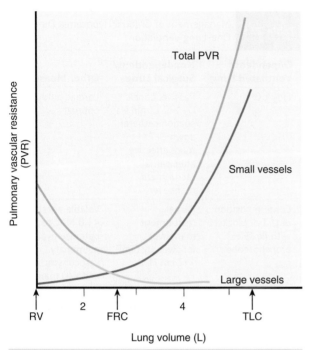

Fig. 27.14 The relationship between pulmonary vascular resistance *(PVR)* and lung volume. PVR is lowest at functional residual capacity *(FRC)* and increases as the lung volume decreases toward residual volume *(RV)*, caused primarily by an increase in the resistance of large pulmonary vessels. PVR also increases as lung volume increases above FRC toward total lung capacity *(TLC)* as a result of an increase in the resistance of small interalveolar vessels.

Table 27.7	Intraoperative Complications That Occur With Increased Frequency During Thoracotomy

Complication	Cause
Hypoxemia	Intrapulmonary shunt during one-lung ventilation
Sudden hypotension	Surgical compression of the heart or great vessels
Sudden changes in ventilating pressure or volume	Movement of endobronchial tube/blocker, air leak
Arrhythmia	Mechanical irritation of the heart
Bronchospasm	Direct airway stimulation, increased frequency of reactive airways disease
Hemorrhage	Surgical blood loss from great vessels or inflamed pleura
Hypothermia	Heat loss from open hemithorax

Box 27.11 Fluid Management for Pulmonary Resection Surgery

- 2–3 mL/kg/h until patient the patient can drink, then discontinue IV fluids.
- Total positive fluid balance should not exceed 20 mL/kg in the first 24-hour perioperative period.
- No fluid administration for third-space fluid losses during pulmonary resection.
- Urine output greater than 0.5 mL/kg/hr is unnecessary.
- If increased tissue perfusion is required postoperatively, it is advisable to use invasive monitoring and inotropes/vasopressors rather than cause fluid overload.

regimens should be avoided in favor of euvolemia,[40] that is, replacement of intravascular volume deficits and maintenance only with a balanced salt solution. Box 27.11 describes the authors' approach to fluid management.

Approach to One-Lung Ventilation

A suggested approach to lung-protective ventilation before and during OLV is outlined in Table 27.8.

Prediction of Intraoperative Hypoxia

There are many patient-, surgical-, and position-related factors that can be used to predict which patients are at risk of hypoxemia during OLV. These factors are outlined in Box 27.12.

Management of Hypoxia During One-Lung Ventilation

Less than 5% of patients develop hypoxia during OLV.[41] Although there is no consensus as to the lowest acceptable Spo_2 or Po_2 during OLV, an Spo_2 less than 94% typically indicates a problem. A stepwise plan for management of this complication is shown in Table 27.9. The most common cause of desaturation during OLV is DLT malposition (i.e., the DLT has advanced and is occluding the upper lobe)[41] and should therefore be investigated with a bronchoscope.

Conclusion of Surgery

A suggested plan for tracheal extubation at the conclusion of lung resection is outlined in Fig. 27.15. A prerequisite for extubation of the trachea is a patient who is alert, warm, and comfortable (AWaC).

Pain Management

Posterolateral thoracotomy is one of the most painful surgical incisions. Improvements in analgesic techniques over the last 30 years have contributed to a decrease

IV

of developing interstitial and alveolar edema, with the risk proportional to the extent of lung resected. Conversely, the incidence of acute kidney injury is higher with restrictive fluid regimens.[39] Very restrictive or liberal

Table 27.8	A Suggested Approach to One-Lung Ventilation

Parameter	Suggested Application	Explanation
Fio_2	Induction and early maintenance Fio_2 1.0 Decrease Fio_2 during OLV if tolerated	Aids absorption atelectasis in nondependent lung, speeding lung collapse
Tidal volume	TLV 6–8 mL/kg OLV 4–6 mL/kg[a]	Peak airway pressure <35 cm H_2O, Plateau airway pressure <25 cm H_2O
Recruitment maneuver	Before lung isolation During OLV as needed	Reverses atelectasis in ventilated lung, improving Po_2 during OLV[a]
Positive end-expiratory pressure	Routine PEEP 5–10 cm	No PEEP in patients with obstructive disease
Respiratory rate	Respiratory rate 12–16 breaths/min	May be higher if required
Pco_2	Permissive hypercapnia during OLV	Aim to keep pH ≥7.20
Mode	Volume or pressure controlled	Pressure control for patients at risk of lung injury, such as bullae, preexisting lung disease, pneumonectomy, lung transplantation

OLV, One-lung ventilation; PEEP, positive end-expiratory pressure; TLV, two-lung ventilation.
[a]Unzueta C, Tusman G, Suarez-Sipmann F, et al. Alveolar recruitment improves ventilation during thoracic surgery: A randomized controlled trial. Br J Anaesth. 2012;108:517–524.

Box 27.12	Factors That Correlate With an Increased Risk of Hypoxemia During One-Lung Ventilation

- Higher percentage of ventilation or perfusion to the operative lung on preoperative $\dot{V}/\dot{Q}$ scan
- Poor Pao_2 during two-lung ventilation, particularly in the lateral position intraoperatively
- Right-sided thoracotomy
- Normal preoperative spirometry (FEV_1 or FVC) or restrictive lung disease
- Supine position during one-lung ventilation

FEV_1, Forced expiratory volume in 1 second; FVC, functional residual capacity; Pao_2, partial pressure of oxygen (arterial); $\dot{V}/\dot{Q}$, ventilation/perfusion ratio.

Table 27.9	Management of Gradual Hypoxemia During One-Lung Ventilation

Dependent/ Ventilated Lung	Nondependent/ Surgical Lung	Other Measures
Fio_2 1.0	Passive, apneic O_2 1–2 L/min via suction catheter down DLT, more effective after partial recruitment maneuver	Cardiac output optimal
Confirm position of DLT or blocker with flexible bronchoscope	Partial recruitment maneuver followed by CPAP 1–2 cm H_2O	Volatile anesthetic <1.0 MAC to optimize hypoxic pulmonary vasoconstriction and V/Q matching
Recruitment maneuver (this will transiently make hypoxemia worse)	Intermittent positive-pressure ventilation	Venovenous ECMO
Apply PEEP 5–10 cm (except in patients with emphysematous pathology)	Flexible bronchoscopic lobar insufflation using O_2 connected to working channel	
	Selective lobar collapse using a bronchial blocker	
	Small tidal volume ventilation	
	Mechanical restriction of blood flow to the nonventilated lung (clamping pulmonary artery)	

CPAP, Continuous positive airway pressure; DLT, double-lumen tube; ECMO, extracorporeal membrane oxygenation; MAC, minimum alveolar concentration; OLV, one-lung ventilation; PEEP, positive end-expiratory pressure.
Note: Sudden and severe hypoxemia should be managed by informing the surgeon of the problem, reinflation of the isolated lung (provided it is safe to do so), and two-lung ventilation while attempting to identify and manage the cause. Methods of oxygenating the nondependent/surgical lung are listed from least intrusive to most intrusive to surgical access.

in postoperative mortality rate for these procedures.[42] No single analgesic technique can block the multiple sensory afferents that transmit nociceptive stimuli after thoracotomy (thoracic and cervical spinal nerves, vagus and phrenic nerves); therefore analgesia should

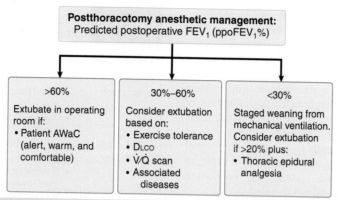

Fig. 27.15 Anesthetic management guided by preoperative assessment and the amount of functioning lung tissue removed during surgery. Dlco, Lung diffusing capacity for carbon monoxide; FEV$_1$, forced expiratory volume in 1 second; $\dot{V}/\dot{Q}$, ventilation/perfusion. (From Slinger PD, ed. *Pearson's Thoracic and Esophageal Surgery.* New York: Springer; 2011, used with permission.)

be multimodal. The optimal choice is based on patient factors (contraindications, preferences), surgical factors (type of incision), and system factors (available equipment, monitoring, nursing support, institutional familiarity with techniques). The ideal postthoracotomy analgesic technique includes opioid-sparing analgesics (e.g., acetaminophen, NSAIDs, opioids [systemic or neuraxial], and regional anesthesia).

MEDIASTINOSCOPY

Mediastinoscopy to stage lung cancer before resection has been largely superseded by endobronchial ultrasound-guided transbronchial needle aspiration (EBUS),[43] which may aid in the diagnosis of anterior and superior mediastinal masses and mediastinal lymphadenopathy.

The most common surgical approach is via a small (2 to 3 cm) midline, transverse incision superior to the suprasternal notch. Surgical access is limited, and there are many structures that may be compressed or transected, such as the trachea and bronchi, pleura, great vessels (particularly the innominate artery and vein), lymphatic vessels, phrenic and recurrent laryngeal nerves, and esophagus.

Any anesthetic technique can be used for mediastinoscopy. Although local anesthesia can be used for cooperative and motivated patients with relatively superficial lesions, general anesthesia with an SLT is typical. It is important the patient be still, as movement or coughing may result in surgical complications. An arterial line is typically unnecessary unless there are unusual patient or surgical factors. It is useful to monitor the pulse in the right hand (pulse oximeter, manual palpation by anesthesia provider's finger, arterial line), as compression of the innominate artery supplying blood to the right carotid artery may occur by the mediastinoscope. A noninvasive blood pressure cuff placed on the left arm confirms innominate compression.

> **Box 27.13** Anesthetic Management of Mediastinoscopy Hemorrhage
>
> 1. Stop surgery and pack the wound. There is a serious risk that the patient will approach the point of hemodynamic collapse if the surgery-anesthesia team does not realize soon enough that there is a problem.
> 2. Begin resuscitation and call for help, both anesthetic and surgical.
> 3. Obtain large-bore intravenous access in the lower limbs.
> 4. Place an arterial line (if not placed at induction).
> 5. Obtain crossmatched blood in the operating room.
> 6. Place a double-lumen tube or bronchial blocker if the surgeon thinks thoracotomy is a possibility.
> 7. Once the patient is stabilized and all preparations are made, the surgeon can reexplore the surgical incision.
> 8. Convert to sternotomy or thoracotomy if indicated.

Massive mediastinal hemorrhage is perhaps the most feared complication of mediastinoscopy and requires a median sternotomy or thoracotomy to control. A suggested approach to managing this complication is outlined in Box 27.13.

MEDIASTINAL MASSES

Patients with mediastinal masses, particularly anterior and superior masses, present unique problems for anesthesia care. Mediastinal masses may cause obstruction of major airways distal to an endotracheal tube and/or major vascular structures, such as the main pulmonary arteries, atria, and superior vena cava. Patients who are symptomatic or have significant compression of these vital structures visible on CT scans are likely to be at high risk of life-threatening respiratory or cardiovascular collapse. Anesthetic deaths occur mainly in children because of the more compressible cartilaginous airway, difficulty in obtaining a history of positional symptoms, and the requirement for general anesthesia for imaging in young children.

General anesthesia is potentially dangerous for a patient with a mediastinal mass for several reasons. General anesthesia leads to a decrease in lung volume with cephalad shift of the diaphragm and relaxation of bronchial smooth muscle, resulting in more compressibility of the airway by the overlying mass. Further, muscle relaxant–induced paralysis leads to a loss of the normal transpleural pressure gradient and a subsequent decrease in airway caliber. If possible, spontaneous ventilation should be maintained and paralysis avoided.

A suggested approach to the management of potential complications is outlined in Table 27.10. Flow-volume loops for assessment of severity of intrathoracic airway obstruction are unreliable and not recommended for decision making.[44,45]

If a patient is considered high risk for cardiovascular collapse, femorofemoral cardiopulmonary bypass should be initiated before induction of anesthesia, as there is insufficient time for this to be started after cardiovascular collapse.

Table 27.10 Management of Potentially Life-Threatening Complications of Mediastinal Masses

Complication	Options for Management
Airway obstruction	• Maintenance of spontaneous ventilation, avoidance of muscle relaxants • Awake fiber-optic intubation with single-lumen endotracheal or endobronchial tube placed distal to the obstruction • Patient repositioning: optimal position determined preinduction based on patient's symptoms • Rigid bronchoscopy and ventilation distal to the obstruction; experienced bronchoscopist and equipment in the room at induction
Cardiovascular collapse	• Lower limb intravenous (IV) access (large-bore IV with or without central line) • Patient repositioning • Elective cardiopulmonary bypass preinduction in extreme cases

REFERENCES

1. Fanta CH. Asthma. *N Engl J Med.* 2009;360:1002–1014.
2. McCracken JL, Veeranki SP, Ameredes BT, Calhoun WJ. Diagnosis and Management of Asthma in Adults: A Review. *JAMA.* 2017;318(3):279–290. https://doi.org/10.1001/jama.2017.8372.
3. Expert Panel Working Group of the National Heart, Lung, and Blood Institute (NHLBI) administered and coordinated National Asthma Education and Prevention Program Coordinating Committee (NAEPPCC), Cloutier MM, Baptist AP, Blake KV, Brooks EG, Bryant-Stephens T, DiMango E, Dixon AE, Elward KS, Hartert T, Krishnan JA, Lemanske Jr RF, Ouellette DR, Pace WD, Schatz M, Skolnik NS, Stout JW, Teach SJ, Umscheid CA, Walsh CG. 2020 Focused Updates to the Asthma Management Guidelines: A Report from the National Asthma Education and Prevention Program Coordinating Committee Expert Panel Working Group. *J Allergy Clin Immunol.* Dec. 2020;146(6):1217–1270. https://doi.org/10.1016/j.jaci.2020.10.003 .
4. Rooke GA, Choi JH, Bishop MJ. The effect of isoflurane, halothane, sevoflurane, and thiopental/nitrous oxide on respiratory system resistance after tracheal intubation. *Anesthesiology.* 1997;86:1294–1299.
5. Goff MJ, Arain SR, Ficke DJ, et al. Absence of bronchodilation during desflurane anesthesia: a comparison to sevoflurane and thiopental. *Anesthesiology.* 2000;93:404–408.
6. Rennard SI. Chronic obstructive pulmonary disease: definition, clinical manifestations, diagnosis, and staging. In: Stoller JK, ed. *UpToDate*: Waltham: UpToDate; 2015. Accessed July 29, 2015.
7. Wilson FA, Heunks L. Oxygen induced hypercapnia in COPD: myths and facts. *Crit Care.* 2012;16:323–328.
8. Morano M, Araujo A, Nascimento F, et al. Preoperative pulmonary rehabilitation versus chest physical therapy in patients undergoing lung cancer resection. *Arch Phys Med Rehab.* 2013;94:53–58.
9. Huffmayer J, Littlewood K, Nemergut E. Perioperative management of the adult with cystic fibrosis. *Anesth Analg.* 2009;109:1949–1961.
10. Olsen E, Chung F, Seet E. Surgical risk and the preoperative evaluation and management of adults with obstructive sleep apnea. In: Jones S, Collop N, eds. *UpToDate*: Waltham: UpToDate; 2014. (accessed July 29, 2015).
11. Galie N, Hoeper MM, Humbert H, et al. Guidelines for the diagnosis and treatment of pulmonary hypertension. *Eur Heart J.* 2009;30:2493–2537.
12. Pilkington SA, Taboada D, Martinez G. Pulmonary hypertension and its management in patients undergoing non-cardiac surgery. *Anaesthesia.* 2015;70:56–70.
13. Lai HC, Lai HC, Wang KY, et al. Severe pulmonary hypertension complicates postoperative outcome of non-cardiac surgery. *Br J Anaesth.* 2007;99(2):184–190.
14. Banks DA, Pretorius GV, Kerr KM, Manecke GR. Pulmonary endarterectomy: part II. Operation, anesthetic management, and postoperative care. *Semin Cardiothorac Vasc Anesth.* 2014;18(4):331–340.
15. Maxwell BG, Jackson E. Role of ketamine in the management of pulmonary hypertension and right ventricular failure. *J Cardiothorac Vasc Anesth.* 2012;26:e24.
16. Currigan DA, Hughes RJA, Wright CE, et al. Vasoconstrictor responses to vasopressor agents in human pulmonary and radial arteries. *Anesthesiology.* 2014;121:930–936.
17. Wauthy P, Abdel Kafi S, Mooi WJ, et al. Inhaled nitric oxide versus prostacyclin in chronic shunt-induced pulmonary hypertension. *J Thorac Cardiovasc Surg.* 2003;126(5):1434–1441.
18. Jerath A, Srinivas C, Vegas A, et al. The successful management of severe protamine-induced pulmonary hypertension using inhaled prostacyclin. *Anesth Analg.* 2010;110:365–369.
19. Bonnin M, Mercier FJ, Sitbon O, et al. Severe pulmonary hypertension during pregnancy: mode of delivery and anesthetic management of 15 consecutive

cases. *Anesthesiology.* 2006;102:1133–1137.

20. Missant C, Claus P, Rex S, Wouters PF. Differential effects of lumbar and thoracic epidural anesthesia on the haemodynamic response to acute right ventricular pressure overload. *Br J Anaesth.* 2009;104:143.

21. Brunelli A, Salati M, Rocco G, et al. European risk models for morbidity (EuroLung1) and mortality (EuroLung2) to predict outcome following anatomic lung resections: an analysis from the European Society of Thoracic Surgeons database. *European Journal of Cardio-Thoracic Surgery.* 2016;51:490–497.

22. Lim E, Baldwin D, Beckles M, et al. British Thoracic Society; Society for Cardiothoracic Surgery in Great Britain and Ireland. Guidelines on the radical management of patients with lung cancer. *Thorax.* 2010;65(suppl 3):iii1–iii27.

23. Brunelli A, Kim AW, Berger KI, et al. Physiologic evaluation of the patient with lung cancer being considered for resectional surgery: Diagnosis and management of lung cancer, 3rd ed: American College of Chest Physicians evidence-based clinical practice guidelines. *Chest.* 2013;143:e166S–e190S.

24. Weisman IM. Cardiopulmonary exercise testing in the preoperative assessment for lung resection surgery. *Semin Thorac Cardiovasc Surg.* 2001;13:116–125.

25. Fleisher LA, Fleishmann KE, Auerbach AD, et al. 2014 ACC/AHA guideline on perioperative cardiovascular evaluation and management of patients undergoing noncardiac surgery. *J Am Coll Cardiol.* 2014;64(22):e77–e137.

26. Fernando HC, Jaklitsch MT, Walsh GL, et al. The society of thoracic surgeons practice guideline on prophylaxis and management of atrial fibrillation associated with general thoracic surgery: executive summary. *Ann Thorac Surg.* 2011;92:1144–1152.

27. Frendl G, Sodickson AC, Chung MK, Waldo AL, Gersh BJ, Tisdale JE, Calkins H, Aranki S, Kaneko T, Cassivi S, Smith Jr SC, Darbar D, Wee JO, Waddell TK, Amar D, Adler D. American Association for Thoracic Surgery. 2014 AATS guidelines for the prevention and management of perioperative atrial fibrillation and flutter for thoracic surgical procedures. *J Thorac Cardiovasc Surg.* Sep. 2014;148(3):e153–e193. https://doi.org/10.1016/j.jtcvs.2014.06.036 Epub 2014 Jun 30. PMID: 25129609; PMCID: PMC4454633.

28. Pierre S, Rivera C, Le Maitre B, et al. Guidelines on smoking management during the perioperative period. *Anaesthesia Critical Care & Pain Medicine.* 2017;36:195–200.

29. Campos JH, Hallam EA, Van Natta T, et al. Devices for lung isolation used by anesthesiologists with limited thoracic experience: comparison of double-lumen endotracheal tube, Univent torque control blocker, and Arndt wire-guided endobronchial blocker. *Anesthesiology.* 2006;104(2):261–266.

30. Toronto General Hospital Department of Anesthesia. Perioperative Interactive Education. http://pie.med.utoronto.ca/VB/.

31. Brodsky JB, Macario A, Mark JB. Tracheal diameter predicts double-lumen tube size: a method for selecting left double lumen tubes. *Anesth Analg.* 1996;82:861–864.

32. Klein U, Karzai W, Bloos F, et al. Role of fiberoptic bronchoscopy in conjunction with the use of double-lumen tubes for thoracic anesthesia: a prospective study. *Anesthesiology.* 1998;88:346–350.

33. de Bellis M, Accardo R, Di Maio M, et al. Is flexible bronchoscopy necessary to confirm the position of double-lumen tubes before thoracic surgery? *Eur J Cardiothorac Surg.* 2011;40:912–918.

34. Slinger P, Scott WA. Arterial oxygenation during one-lung ventilation. A comparison of enflurane and isoflurane. *Anesthesiology.* 1995;82:940–946.

35. Russell WJ, James MF. The effects on arterial haemoglobin oxygenation saturation and on shunt of increasing cardiac output with dopamine or dobutamine during one-lung ventilation. *Anaesth Intensive Care.* 2004;32:644–648.

36. Beck DH, Doepfmer UR, Sinemus C, et al. Effects of sevoflurane and propofol on pulmonary shunt fraction during one lung ventilation for thoracic surgery. *Br J Anaesth.* 2001;86:38–43.

37. Pruszkowski O, Dalibon N, Moutafis M, et al. Effects of propofol vs sevoflurane on arterial oxygenation during one-lung ventilation. *Br J Anaesth.* 2007;98:539–544.

38. Von Dossow V, Welte M, Zaune U, et al. Thoracic epidural anesthesia combined with general anesthesia: the preferred anesthetic technique for thoracic surgery. *Anesth Analg.* 2001;92:848–854.

39. Myles PS, Bellomo R, Corcoran T, et al. Restrictive versus Liberal Fluid Therapy for Major Abdominal Surgery. *N Engl J Med.* 2018;378:2263–2274.

40. Batchelor TJP, Rasburn NJ, Abduelnour-Bertold E, et al. Guidelines for enhanced recovery after lung surgery: recommendations of the Enhanced Recover After Surgery (ERAS) Society and the European Society of Thoracic Surgeons (ESTS). *European Journal of Cardio-Thoracic Surgery.* 2019;55:91–115.

41. Brodsky JB, Lemmens JM. Left double-lumen tubes: clinical experience with 1,170 patients. *J Cardiothorac Vasc Anesth.* 2003;17:289–298.

42. Licker M, Widikker I, Robert J, et al. Operative mortality and respiratory complications after lung resection for cancer: impact of chronic obstructive pulmonary disease and time trends. *Ann Thorac Surg.* 2006;81:1830–1837.

43. Czarnecka A, Yasufuku K. Endobronchial ultrasound-guided transbronchial needle aspiration for staging patients with lung cancer with clinical N0 disease. *Ann Am Thorac Soc.* 2015;12(3):297–299.

44. Vander Els NJ, Sorhage F, Bach AM, et al. Abnormal flow volume loops in patients with intrathoracic Hodgkin's disease. *Chest.* 2000;117(5):1256–1261.

45. Hnatiuk OW, Corcoran PC, Sierra P. Spirometry in surgery for anterior mediastinal masses. *Chest.* 2001;120:1152–1156.

IV

28 RENAL, LIVER, AND BILIARY TRACT DISEASE

Anup Pamnani, Vinod Malhotra

RENAL DISEASE

Normal renal function is important for the excretion of anesthetics and medications, maintaining fluid and acid–base balance, and regulating hemoglobin levels in the perioperative period.

Renal disease is quite prevalent in patients presenting for surgery and is associated with an increased likelihood of poor postoperative outcomes. Even mild renal dysfunction is associated with a more likely risk of postoperative complications.[1]

Multiple preoperative risk factors have been identified that predict renal dysfunction in the postoperative period (Box 28.1).[2] Several perioperative clinical conditions are also associated with renal dysfunction and should be considered carefully in patients with preoperative risk factors. These include planned major surgery, critical illness, septic shock, exposure to nephrotoxic drugs, and radiocontrast.[3,4]

Renal Blood Flow

Although the kidneys represent only 0.5% of total body weight, their blood flow is equivalent to about 20% of cardiac output. Approximately two-thirds of renal blood flow is distributed to the renal cortex. Renal blood flow and the glomerular filtration rate (GFR) remain relatively constant at renal arterial blood pressures in the range of 80 to 180 mm Hg (Fig. 28.1). Being able to maintain renal blood flow at a constant rate independent of changes in perfusion pressure is known as *autoregulation*. It is achieved by adjustment of afferent arteriolar tone, which alters the resistance to blood flow. Autoregulation protects the glomerular capillaries from hypertension during acute hypertensive episodes and maintains GFR and renal tubule function during modest decreases in arterial blood pressure. When mean arterial blood pressure is outside the autoregulatory range, renal blood flow becomes pressure dependent. Autoregulation is reset by

Box 28.1 Risk Factors for Postoperative Acute Kidney Injury (AKI)

- GFR <60 m:/min/1.73 m^2
- Diabetes mellitus
- Age >50 years
- Male sex
- Heart failure
- Ascites
- Hypertension
- Emergency surgery
- Intraperitoneal surgery
- Increased number of chronic medications
- Use of ACE inhibitors or ARBs
- High ASA physical status score
- Albuminuria

ACE, Angiotensin-converting enzyme; *ARB*, angiotensin receptor blocker; *ASA*, American Society of Anesthesiologists; *GFR*, glomerular filtration rate.
Patients with chronic kidney disease and/or diabetes are at particularly high risk of AKI.
From Prowle JR, Forni LG, Bell M, et al. Postoperative acute kidney injury in adult non-cardiac surgery: Joint consensus report of the Acute Disease Quality Initiative and PeriOperative Quality Initiative. *Nat Rev Nephrol*. 2021;17(9):605-618.

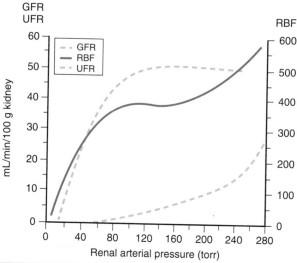

Fig. 28.1 Autoregulation of Renal Blood Flow (*RBF*) and the Glomerular Filtration Rate (*GFR*). The relationships between RBF, GFR, and urine flow rate (*UFR*) and mean renal arterial pressure in dogs are shown as renal arterial pressure is varied from 20 to 280 mm Hg. Autoregulation of RBF and GFR is observed between about 80 mm Hg and 180 mm Hg. (Redrawn from Hemmings HC. *Anesthetics, adjuvants and drugs and the kidney*. In Malhotra V, ed. *Anesthesia for Renal and Genitourinary Surgery*. New York: McGraw-Hill; 1996:18.)

chronic hypertension and can be significantly altered in the diabetic kidney.

Renal blood flow is also strongly influenced by the activity of the sympathetic nervous system and by release of renin and other hormones. Sympathetic nervous system stimulation can produce renal vasoconstriction and a marked decrease in renal blood flow even if systemic blood pressure is within the autoregulatory range.

Glomerular Filtration Rate

GFR reflects glomerular function and is a measure of the ability of the glomerular membrane to allow filtration. About 90% of the fluid filtered at the glomeruli is reabsorbed from renal tubules into peritubular capillaries and thus returned to the circulation (Fig. 28.2). Normal GFR is approximately 125 mL/min and is highly dependent on glomerular filtration pressure (GFP). GFP, in turn, is a function of renal artery pressure, afferent and efferent arteriolar tone, and glomerular oncotic pressure. Hydrostatic pressure within the glomerular capillaries is about 50 mm Hg. This pressure forces water and other low-molecular-weight substances such as electrolytes through the glomerular capillaries into the Bowman space. Plasma oncotic pressure is about 25 mm Hg at the afferent arteriole and with filtration increases to about 35 mm Hg at the efferent arteriole. Despite a relatively low net filtration pressure, the glomerular capillaries are able to filter plasma at a rate equivalent to about 125 mL/min. GFR is reduced by significantly decreased mean arterial pressure or renal blood flow. Afferent arteriolar constriction decreases GFR by decreasing glomerular flow. Conversely, afferent arteriolar dilation and mild efferent vasoconstriction increase GFP and GFR.

Humoral Mediators of Renal Function

Renin-Angiotensin-Aldosterone System
Renin is a proteolytic enzyme secreted by the juxtaglomerular apparatus of the kidneys in response to (1) sympathetic nervous system stimulation, (2) decreased renal perfusion pressure, and (3) decreases in the delivery of sodium to the distal convoluted renal tubules. Renin acts on angiotensinogen (a circulating globulin in plasma) to form angiotensin I. Angiotensin I is converted in the lungs by angiotensin-converting enzyme to angiotensin II. Angiotensin II, a potent vasoconstrictor, stimulates the release of aldosterone from the adrenal cortex. Angiotensin II selectively increases efferent renal arteriolar tone at low levels and causes afferent arteriolar constriction at higher levels. Aldosterone, in turn, stimulates reabsorption of sodium and water in the distal tubule and collecting ducts.

Prostaglandins
Prostaglandins are produced in the renal medulla via the enzymes phospholipase A$_2$ and cyclooxygenase and released in response to sympathetic nervous system stimulation, hypotension, and increased levels of angiotensin II. During periods of hemodynamic instability,

IV

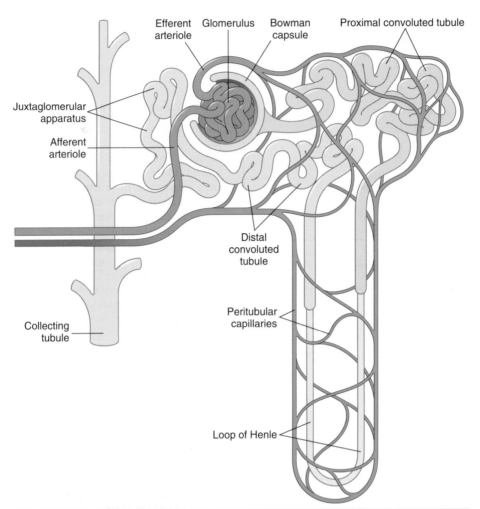

Fig. 28.2 Anatomy of a Nephron. The glomerulus is formed by the invaginated and blind end of the nephron known as the Bowman capsule. Hydrostatic pressure in these capillaries causes water and low-molecular-weight substances to filter through the glomerulus. Glomerular filtrate travels along the renal tubule (proximal convoluted tubule, loop of Henle, distal convoluted tubule), during which most of its water and various amounts of solutes are reabsorbed from the renal tubular lumen into peritubular capillaries. The remaining glomerular filtrate becomes urine.

prostaglandins act to modulate the effects of arginine vasopressin (AVP), the renin–angiotensin system, and norepinephrine by vasodilating juxtamedullary vessels and maintaining cortical blood flow.

Arginine Vasopressin

Previously known as *antidiuretic hormone,* AVP regulates osmolality and diuresis. Although secreted in the supraoptic and paraventricular nuclei in the hypothalamus, it exerts significant effects on the renal collecting system. AVP actions are concentrated on collecting duct V_2 receptors to increase membrane permeability and facilitate water reabsorption. The overall effect of AVP is to decrease serum osmolality and increase urine osmolality.

Atrial Natriuretic Peptide

Atrial natriuretic peptide (ANP) is secreted when stretch receptors in the atria of the heart and other organs are stimulated by increased intravascular volume. ANP acts by relaxing vascular smooth muscle to cause vasodilation, inhibiting the renin–angiotensin system, and stimulating diuresis and natriuresis. The net effect of ANP is to decrease systemic blood pressure and intravascular volume.

Drug Clearance

Excretion of drugs or their metabolites into urine depends on three mechanisms: (1) glomerular filtration, (2) active secretion by the renal tubules, and (3) passive reabsorption by the tubules. The glomerular filtration of small molecules characteristic of anesthetic drugs depends on the GFR and the fractional plasma protein binding. Drugs that are highly protein bound will be inefficiently filtered at the glomerulus. Nonionized acidic and basic compounds undergo passive reabsorption by back-diffusion in the proximal and distal renal tubules. However, the ionized forms of these weak acids and bases are trapped within renal tubules, accounting for increased renal elimination by either alkalinization or acidification of urine. Conjugation of drugs in the liver to water-soluble metabolites is another mechanism by which renal excretion of substances is achieved.

Renal Function Tests

Renal function can be evaluated preoperatively by using several laboratory tests (Table 28.1). These tests are not particularly sensitive measurements, and significant renal disease (more than a 50% decrease in renal function) can exist while laboratory values remain normal. Furthermore, the normal values established in healthy individuals may not be adjusted for age or be applicable during anesthesia. Trends are more useful for evaluating renal function than a single laboratory measurement.

Serum Creatinine

Serum creatinine concentration, which reflects the balance between creatinine production by muscle and its renal excretion, is often used as a marker of GFR. In contrast to blood urea nitrogen (BUN) concentration,

the serum creatinine level is not influenced by protein metabolism or the rate of fluid flow through renal tubules. It is, however, influenced by skeletal muscle mass. Furthermore, increases in serum creatinine are not typically noted until GFR has declined by at least 50%. Thus an increased creatinine level may serve as a late marker of renal injury. For example, elderly patients with known decreases in GFR frequently display normal serum creatinine concentrations because of decreased creatinine production as a consequence of the decrease in skeletal muscle mass. Indeed, mild increases in the serum creatinine concentration in elderly patients may suggest significant renal disease. Likewise, in patients with chronic renal failure serum creatinine concentrations may not accurately reflect the GFR because of (1) decreased creatinine production, (2) the presence of decreased skeletal muscle mass, or (3) nonrenal (gastrointestinal tract) excretion of creatinine. GFR can be estimated from serum creatinine by a variety of methods, including the following formula:

$$GFR = (140 - age) \times weight\,(in\,kg)/(serum\,creatinine \times 72)$$

Blood Urea Nitrogen

BUN concentrations, which are normally 10 to 20 mg/dL, vary with changes in GFR. The relationship between serum creatinine and BUN levels is particularly useful in diagnosing the cause of renal failure. Like serum creatinine, increases in BUN level are frequently a late sign of renal injury and are affected by dietary intake, coexisting illnesses, and intravascular fluid volume. For example, high-protein diets or gastrointestinal bleeding can increase the production of urea and thereby result in increased BUN concentrations (azotemia) despite a normal GFR. Other causes of increased BUN concentrations in the presence of normal GFR are increased catabolism during febrile illnesses and dehydration. Conversely, BUN concentrations can remain normal in the presence of low-protein diets despite decreases in GFR.

Increased BUN concentrations relative to serum creatinine in the presence of dehydration likely reflect increased urea absorption caused by decreased urinary flow through the renal tubules, which results in a BUN–creatinine ratio greater than 20. Although BUN concentration is susceptible to multiple extraneous influences, values more than 50 mg/dL inevitably reflect a decreased GFR.

Creatinine Clearance

Creatinine clearance (normal, 110–150 mL/min) is a measurement of the ability of the glomeruli to excrete creatinine into urine for a given serum creatinine concentration. Because clearance does not depend on corrections for age or the presence of a steady state, measurement of GFR is more reliable than the serum BUN or creatinine

Table 28.1	Tests Used for Evaluation of Renal Function	
Test	**Normal Value**	**Factors That Influence Interpretation**
Test of Glomerular Filtration		
Blood urea nitrogen	8–20 mg/dL	Dehydration Variable protein intake Gastrointestinal bleeding Catabolism
Serum creatinine	0.5–1.2 mg/dL	Age Skeletal muscle mass Catabolism
Creatinine clearance	120 mL/min	Accurate urine volume measurement
Tests of Tubular Function		
Urine specific gravity	1.003–1.030	All are affected by dehydration, solutes, filtrates, proteins, diuretics, dehydration, drugs, and extremes of age
Urine osmolality	350–500 mOsm	
Urine sodium	20–40 mEq	

values. The principal disadvantage of this test, however, is the need for timed urine collections. Typically, a 24-hour collection yields the most accurate results; however, a 2-hour collection may be acceptable. Creatinine clearance (CrCl) and, by proxy, GFR can be calculated from the formula

$$GFR = CrCl = Ucr \times V/Pcr$$

where Ucr is urine creatinine, Pcr is plasma creatinine drawn at the midpoint of the timed collection, and V is urinary flow rate.

Proteinuria

Small amounts of protein are normally filtered through glomerular capillaries and then reabsorbed in the proximal convoluted tubules. Proteinuria (excretion of more than 150 mg of protein per day) is more likely the result of abnormally high filtration rather than impaired reabsorption by the renal tubules. Intermittent proteinuria occasionally occurs in healthy individuals when standing and disappears when supine. Other nonrenal causes of proteinuria include exercise, fever, and congestive heart failure.

Urine Indices

Measurement of urine osmolality and urinary sodium and calculation of the fractional excretion of sodium can help differentiate between prerenal and renal tubular causes of azotemia.

Newer Tests of Renal Function

Several additional markers of renal function have recently been identified. Serum cystatin C, a ubiquitous protein that is exclusively excreted by glomerular filtration, is less influenced by variations in muscle mass and nutrition than creatinine. It may better predict risk of death and end-stage renal disease (ESRD) across diverse populations.[5]

Other biomarkers such as N-acetyl-β-D-glucosaminidase, kidney injury molecule-1, and interleukin-18 are promising in the early detection of kidney injury. These biomarkers may have a role in reducing morbidity and mortality rates associated with kidney injury in the perioperative setting.[6]

Pharmacology of Diuretics

Thiazide Diuretics

Thiazide diuretics (hydrochlorothiazide, chlorthalidone) are generally administered for the treatment of essential hypertension and for mobilization of the edema fluid that is associated with renal, hepatic, or cardiac dysfunction. Diuresis occurs as a result of the inhibition of reabsorption of sodium and chloride ions from the early distal renal tubules. Side effects associated with diuretic-induced hypokalemia may include (1) skeletal muscle

| Table 28.2 | Side Effects of Diuretics |

Diuretic Class	Hypokalemic, Hypochloremic Metabolic Alkalosis	Hyperkalemia	Hyperglycemia
Thiazide diuretics	Yes	No	Yes
Loop diuretics	Yes	No	Minimal
Osmotic diuretics	No	No	No
Aldosterone antagonists	No	Yes	No

weakness, (2) increased risk for digitalis toxicity, and (3) enhancement of nondepolarizing neuromuscular blocking drugs (Table 28.2).

Loop Diuretics

Loop diuretics (ethacrynic acid, furosemide, bumetanide) inhibit the reabsorption of sodium and chloride and augment the secretion of potassium, primarily in the loop of Henle. Intravenous administration of these drugs produces a diuretic response within minutes. Chronic administration of loop diuretics may result in hypochloremic, hypokalemic metabolic alkalosis, and, in rare instances, deafness.[7]

Osmotic Diuretics

The most frequently administered osmotic diuretic is the six-carbon sugar mannitol. Mannitol produces diuresis because it is filtered by the glomeruli and not reabsorbed within the renal tubules. This leads to increased osmolarity of the renal tubule fluid and associated excretion of water.

Mannitol increases fluid movement from intracellular spaces into extracellular spaces such that intravascular fluid volume expands acutely. This redistribution of fluid from intracellular to extracellular compartments decreases brain size and intracranial pressure (also see Chapter 30). Mannitol may further diminish intracranial pressure by decreasing the rate of cerebrospinal fluid formation.

Aldosterone Antagonists

Spironolactone blocks the renal tubular effects of aldosterone and offsets the loss of potassium from administration of thiazide diuretics. Ascites and peripheral edema secondary to cirrhosis of the liver is often treated with spironolactone. The most serious toxic effect of spironolactone is hyperkalemia. Serum potassium concentration should be monitored closely in patients taking spironolactone.

Dopamine and Fenoldopam

Dopamine dilates renal arterioles via its agonist action at the DA1 receptor, leading to increased renal blood flow and GFR. Treatment with low-dose dopamine (0.5–3 µg/kg/min) may increase urine output but yet not alter the course of renal failure. In addition, dose-dependent side effects of dopamine include tachydysrhythmias, pulmonary shunting, and tissue ischemia (gastrointestinal tract, digits).[8,9]

Fenoldopam, a dopamine analog, also possesses DA1 agonist activity but lacks the adrenergic activity of dopamine. It also increases renal blood flow and GFR, which may help the treatment of acute kidney injury (AKI). Several meta analyses (one in critically ill patients, the other two in cardiovascular surgery patients) had suggested that fenoldopam was associated with a significant reduction in postoperative AKI. However, a 2015 meta analysis of patients undergoing major surgery did not demonstrate an impact on renal replacement therapy use or improvement in hospital mortality.[10]

Pathophysiology of End-Stage Renal Disease

ESRD causes profound physiologic changes that affect several organs (Box 28.2 and Table 28.3).

Cardiovascular Disease

Cardiovascular disease is the predominant cause of death in patients with ESRD. Acute myocardial infarction, cardiac arrest of unknown cause, cardiac dysrhythmias, and cardiomyopathy account for more than 50% of deaths in patients receiving dialysis. Hypertension commonly exists in patients with ESRD. This systemic hypertension can be severe and refractory to antihypertensive therapy. Hypervolemia and excess activation of the renin–angiotensin–aldosterone system are the most common causes.

Additionally, the accumulation of uremic toxins and metabolic acids may contribute to poor myocardial performance. Yet the presence of ESRD with significantly depressed cardiac function does not necessarily contraindicate renal transplantation because cardiac ventricular function often improves after transplantation.

Uremia causes changes in lipid metabolism that lead to increased concentrations of serum triglycerides and reduced levels of protective high-density lipoproteins. Thus ESRD accelerates the progression of atherosclerosis. Pericardial disease and cardiac dysrhythmias can also be encountered in patients with ESRD. Pericardial effusions typically resolve when patients are adequately dialyzed.

Metabolic Disease

Many patients with ESRD also have diabetes mellitus. Kidney failure as a result of diabetes develops in nearly 30% to 40% of patients with ESRD and accounts for 30% of those on the waiting list for kidney transplantation. In fact, nephropathy develops in nearly 60% of insulin-dependent diabetic patients. Patients with ESRD and diabetes are more likely to develop cardiovascular disorders than patients with renal failure alone.[11]

Once patients are unable to excrete their dietary fluid and electrolyte loads, abnormalities in plasma electrolyte concentrations (sodium, potassium, calcium, magnesium, and phosphate) can develop. The most life-threatening electrolyte abnormality is hyperkalemia. The risk of hyperkalemia remains significant even in patients with ESRD undergoing maintenance hemodialysis; the incidence of hyperkalemia is lower in patients treated with continuous peritoneal dialysis.

Anemia and Abnormal Coagulation

Patients with renal failure generally display a normochromic, normocytic anemia because of decreased erythropoiesis and retained toxins that are secondary to renal failure. Treatment with recombinant erythropoietin can frequently increase hemoglobin concentrations. Symptoms of fatigue are reduced, and both cerebral function and cardiac function are improved. Occasionally, recombinant erythropoietin therapy may exacerbate preexisting essential hypertension. Patients with renal failure may also display uremia-induced defects in platelet function.

Differential Diagnosis and Management of Perioperative Oliguria

Prerenal Oliguria

Prerenal oliguria is characterized by the excretion of concentrated urine that contains minimal amounts of sodium (Table 28.4). Excretion of highly concentrated and sodium-poor urine confirms that renal tubular function is intact and reflects an attempt by the kidneys to

---

Box 28.2 Changes Characteristic of Chronic Renal Disease

- Anemia
- Decreased ejection fraction
- Decreased platelet adhesiveness
- Hyperkalemia
- Unpredictable intravascular fluid volume
- Metabolic acidosis
- Systemic hypertension
- Pericardial effusion
- Decreased sympathetic nervous system activity

Table 28.3 Stages of Chronic Renal Failure

Stage	Glomerular Filtration Rate (mL/min/1.73 m²)
1	>90
2	60–89
3	30–59
4	15–29
5	<15

IV

Table 28.4	Prerenal Oliguria Versus Acute Tubular Necrosis: Preoperative Differential Diagnosis	
Diagnostic Feature	Prerenal Oliguria	Acute Tubular Necrosis
Fractional excretion of sodium	<1%	>3%
Urine specific gravity	>1.015	1.01–1.015
Urine sodium (mEq/L)	<40	>40
Urine osmolality (mOsm/L)	>400	<400
Causes	Decreased renal blood flow (hypotension, hypovolemia, decreased cardiac output)	Renal ischemia, nephrotoxins, free hemoglobin or myoglobin

conserve sodium and restore intravascular fluid volume in response to decreased renal blood flow. The decreased renal blood flow most likely reflects an acute decrease in intravascular fluid volume or decreased cardiac output. Other causes of decreased renal blood flow are sepsis, liver failure, and congestive heart failure.[12]

The initial management of patients with perioperative oliguria is influenced by their risk for the development of acute renal failure. A brisk diuresis in response to an intravascular fluid challenge suggests that an acute decrease in intravascular fluid volume is the cause of the prerenal oliguria. When intravascular fluid replacement does not result in increased urine output, intrinsic renal disease or hemodynamic causes should be considered. Prompt recognition and treatment of prerenal oliguria is critical, as prolonged severe ischemia can lead to necrosis of renal tubules and convert reversible injury to true structural injury.

Administration of diuretics to maintain or stimulate urine flow in the perioperative period is controversial. One theory is that prevention of renal tubule urine stasis with diuretics can prevent prerenal oliguria from progressing to acute tubular necrosis. Nevertheless, urine output that is enhanced by the administration of a diuretic does not necessarily predict postoperative renal function. There is no evidence that drug-induced diuresis (dopamine, furosemide, mannitol) in the presence of reduced cardiac output or hypovolemia, or both, protects renal function. In fact, a 2013 meta analysis of clinical trials did not find reliable evidence that any interventions (e.g., diuretics, dopamine and its analogs, calcium channel blockers, angiotensin-converting enzyme inhibitors, specific hydration fluids, N-acetylcysteine, ANP, or erythropoietin) can reduce the risk of perioperative renal failure.[12]

Intrinsic Renal Disease

Acute tubular necrosis, glomerulonephritis, and acute interstitial nephritis are intrinsic renal causes of oliguria. In contrast to oliguria secondary to hypovolemia, the urine of patients with acute tubular necrosis is poorly concentrated and contains excessive amounts of sodium. Intrinsic renal disease is the most severe of the different forms of oliguria and is typically the hardest to reverse.

Postrenal Oliguria

An obstruction that is distal to the renal collecting system usually involves a mechanical problem such as a blood clot in the ureter, bladder, or urethra. Surgical ligation, renal calculi, and edema are other postrenal causes of low urine output. Another common postrenal cause is bladder catheter obstruction. Postrenal oliguria is frequently reversible once the source of the obstruction is removed.[13]

Postoperative Acute Kidney Injury

Postoperative AKI is a clinical syndrome that is usually multifactorial in cause. Risk factors are listed in Box 28.1. A 2021 consensus group recommended defining postoperative AKI as occurring when the Kidney Disease Improving Global Outcomes (KDIGO) criteria for AKI are met within 7 days of an operative intervention[2] (Box 28.3). The oliguria criteria are more commonly seen in the intraoperative and postoperative period than the serum creatinine criteria. Treatment of AKI should be targeted to underlying causes, as described earlier.

Management of Anesthesia in Patients With End-Stage Renal Disease

General anesthesia with tracheal intubation provides acceptable hemodynamics, excellent skeletal muscle relaxation, and a predictable depth of anesthesia in patients with ESRD who are undergoing major operations. Patients with advanced stages of comorbid conditions may require more extensive monitoring, such as continuous monitoring of systemic blood pressure and perhaps central venous pressure. Large variations in arterial blood pressure may occur, with hypotension being more likely than hypertension during maintenance of anesthesia. This is especially the case if the patient has recently been hemodialyzed in preparation for the surgical procedure. Those with the most severe comorbid conditions, such as symptomatic coronary artery disease or a history of congestive heart failure, may benefit from monitoring with a pulmonary artery catheter or transesophageal echocardiography (TEE).

The status of hemodialysis shunts or fistulas should be monitored and documented (e.g., presence of a palpable thrill) during positioning and intraoperatively to confirm

From Ilum JA, Lameire N; KDIGO AKI Guideline Work Group. Diagnosis, evaluation, and management of acute kidney injury: A KDIGO summary (Part 1). *Crit Care*. 2013;17(1):204.

Box 28.3 Kidney Disease Improving Global Outcomes (KDIGO) Criteria for AKI

AKI is defined as any of the following (not graded):
  Increase in SCr by ≥0.3 mg/dL (≥26.5 µmol/L) within 48 hours
  Increase in SCr to ≥1.5 times baseline, which is known or presumed to have occurred within the prior 7 days
  Urine volume <0.5 mL/kg/hr for 6 hours

continued patency. Peripheral lines and arterial blood pressure monitoring cuffs should not be placed in proximity to such implanted vascular access devices.

Normal saline (NS) is often given instead of lactated Ringer's solution for intravascular fluid resuscitation in patients with ESRD. The rationale is the hypothesized risk of hyperkalemia from potassium contained in lactated Ringer's solution. Yet this conclusion has not been proved to be likely. For example, two prospective randomized double-blind clinical trials comparing the two intraoperative fluid therapies in ESRD patients undergoing renal transplantation have shown more hyperkalemia and a greater degree of acidosis with NS than lactated Ringer's solution.[14,15]

Patients with uremia and other comorbid conditions (e.g., diabetes mellitus) are at an increased risk for aspiration of gastric contents during induction of anesthesia. The use of a rapid-sequence induction of anesthesia technique may be indicated in such patients. Succinylcholine is not contraindicated in patients with ESRD. The increase in serum potassium concentration after a large dose of succinylcholine is approximately 0.6 mEq/L for patients both with and without ESRD. This increase can be tolerated without imposing a significant cardiac risk, even if initial (i.e., preanesthetic) serum potassium concentration is more than 5 mEq/L.

Several strategies have achieved adequate heart rate and arterial blood pressure control during induction of anesthesia. Moderate to large doses of opioids, such as fentanyl, can blunt the response to laryngoscopy. However, systemic blood pressure is frequently more difficult to maintain after induction of anesthesia, and hypotension may require treatment with vasoconstrictors. The short-acting β-adrenergic blocker esmolol can blunt the hemodynamic response to tracheal intubation and is ideally suited for patients with an adequate ejection fraction.

Drugs or their metabolites that depend on renal elimination (pancuronium, vecuronium, morphine, meperidine) should be used cautiously or avoided. Cisatracurium is a good choice, as most of it is metabolized by spontaneous Hoffman degradation, which makes its duration of action independent of liver or kidney function. The elimination half-life of rocuronium is increased because of increased volume of distribution with no change in clearance. Mivacurium is metabolized by plasma cholinesterase, but its action may be prolonged by 10 to 15 minutes as a result of reduced cholinesterase activity in these patients (also see Chapter 11). Because morphine has long-acting renally excreted metabolites such as morphine-6-glucuronide, alternative opioid choices are preferred (e.g., fentanyl, sufentanil, alfentanil, remifentanil).

Appropriate choices of inhaled anesthetics include desflurane, isoflurane, and sevoflurane. The metabolism of sevoflurane to inorganic fluoride has been implicated in experimental studies of renal toxicity, although no controlled human studies are available to indicate either safety concerns or danger when using sevoflurane in the setting of ESRD.

LIVER DISEASE

The liver is responsible for the production of essential plasma proteins, the metabolism and detoxification of drugs and deleterious xenobiotics, the absorption of critical nutrients, and carbohydrate metabolism. Impaired liver function affects nearly every organ system in the body. Fig. 28.3 summarizes the end-organ implications of cirrhosis.

Hepatic Blood Flow

The liver is unique in that it receives a dual afferent blood supply that is equal to about 25% of cardiac output (Fig. 28.4). Approximately, 70% of hepatic blood flow is supplied by the portal vein, with the remainder supplied by the hepatic artery. Under normal conditions, each blood vessel contributes roughly 50% to the liver's oxygen supply. Portal vein flow is not regulated and is susceptible to systemic hypotension and decreases in cardiac output.

Intrinsic Determinants of Hepatic Blood Flow

Reduction in portal flow (up to a 50% reduction) is compensated for by modulating hepatic artery tone to maintain perfusion to the liver. This is primarily mediated via the hepatic arterial buffer response, which reciprocally varies hepatic arterial blood flow to changes in portal flow mediated by adenosine. The response is stimulated by low pH and O_2 content and increased P_{CO_2}. Volatile anesthetics and cirrhosis of the liver attenuate this reciprocal relationship and render the liver vulnerable to ischemia.

Extrinsic Determinants of Hepatic Blood Flow

Hepatic perfusion pressure (mean arterial or portal vein pressure minus hepatic vein pressure) and splanchnic

IV

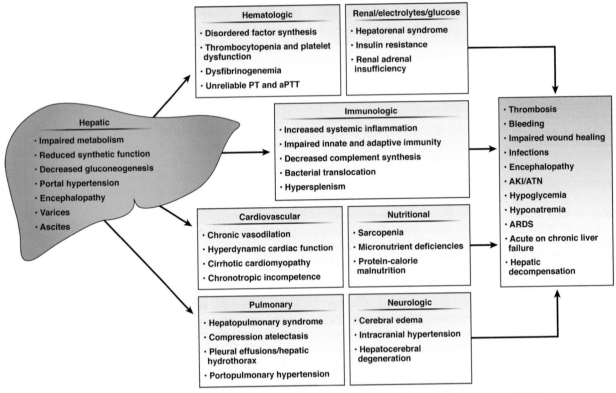

Fig. 28.3 Metabolic, Anatomic, and Physiologic Changes of Cirrhosis and Potential Consequences in the Surgical Patient. *AKI,* Acute kidney injury; *ARDS,* acute respiratory distress syndrome; *ATN,* acute tubular necrosis; *PT,* prothrombin time. (From Newman KL, Johnson KM, Cornia PB, et al. Perioperative evaluation and management of patients with cirrhosis: Risk assessment, surgical outcomes, and future directions. *Clin Gastroenterol Hepatol.* 2020;18[11]:2398-2414.e3, Fig. 1.)

vascular resistance determine hepatic blood flow. The splanchnic vessels receive vasomotor innervation from the sympathetic nervous system. Splanchnic nerve stimulation (pain, arterial hypoxemia, surgical stress) increases splanchnic vascular resistance and decreases hepatic blood flow.

Surgical stimulation and the proximity of the operative site to the liver are important determinants of the magnitude of the decrease in hepatic blood flow seen during general anesthesia. β-Adrenergic receptor blockers such as propranolol are associated with decreases in hepatic blood flow. Positive-pressure ventilation of the lungs, congestive heart failure, and administration of excessive intravascular fluid cause increased central venous pressure, resulting in increased hepatic venous pressure, which effectively decreases hepatic perfusion pressure and blood flow.

Glucose Homeostasis

The liver is the main organ for the storage and release of glucose. Hepatocytes extract glucose via an insulin-mediated mechanism, where it can be stored as glycogen. Glucagon-mediated catabolism of glycogen (glycogenolysis) releases glucose back into the systemic circulation for maintenance of euglycemia. Surgical stress, starvation, and sympathetic nervous system activation stimulate glycogen depolymerization to glucose. When glycogen stores are depleted, hepatic gluconeogenesis from substrates such as lactate, glycerol, and certain amino acids restores blood glucose levels.

Coagulation

Hepatocytes are responsible for the synthesis of the majority of procoagulant proteins in addition to regulators such as proteins C and S and antithrombin III. An important exception to this is factor VIII, which is partially produced in endothelial cells. Vitamin K, which is absorbed by bile secretion into the gastrointestinal tract, plays an important role in catalysis of some of the procoagulant proteins to produce factors II, VII, IX, and X. Laboratory studies such as prothrombin time (international normalized ratio [INR]), partial thromboplastin time (PTT), and fibrinogen

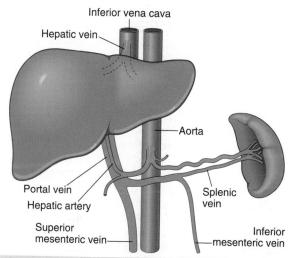

Fig. 28.4 Schematic Depiction of the Dual Afferent Blood Supply to the Liver Provided by the Portal Vein and Hepatic Artery. About 70% of hepatic blood flow is via the portal vein, with the remainder via the hepatic artery. Total hepatic blood flow is directly proportional to perfusion pressure across the liver and inversely related to splanchnic vascular resistance. Cirrhosis of the liver increases resistance to blood flow through the portal vein and decreases hepatic blood flow.

levels can be used to evaluate impaired coagulation and hepatic function. Impaired laboratory studies reflect significant hepatic dysfunction because most coagulation factors maintain function at up to 20% to 30% of their normal levels. In the intraoperative period point-of-care coagulation testing, such as rotational thromboelastometry (ROTEM), can be used to evaluate coagulation and guide therapy (also see Chapter 23).

Drug Metabolism

Hepatic drug metabolism is characterized by the conversion of lipid-soluble drugs to more water-soluble forms to facilitate renal excretion, transformation to pharmacologically less active substances, and excretion in bile.

Three major pathways are used to accomplish these goals. Phase 1 metabolism involves an increase in polarity of drugs via cytochrome P and mixed-function oxidases. Phase 2 metabolism involves conjugation of metabolites to water-soluble substrates. Phase 3 elimination relies on energy-dependent excretion of drugs into bile. Chronic liver disease may interfere with the metabolism of drugs because of the decreased number of enzyme-containing hepatocytes or the decreased hepatic blood flow that typically accompanies cirrhosis of the liver. Prolonged elimination half-times for morphine, alfentanil, diazepam, lidocaine, pancuronium, and vecuronium occur in patients with cirrhosis of the liver. Likewise, chronic drug therapy can inhibit hepatic enzymes and inhibit metabolism of anesthetic drugs, leading to higher circulating blood levels. Conversely, enzyme induction, particularly of cytochrome P isoforms, can also occur as a response to chronic therapy with drugs such as phenytoin, isoniazid, and rifampin or as a result of alcohol use disorder. Induction of hepatic enzymes can increase metabolism of administered anesthetic and therapeutic drugs, thereby reducing plasma levels.

Heme Metabolism

Although fetal erythrocyte production occurs exclusively in the liver, hepatic hematopoiesis accounts for only 20% of adult heme synthesis, with the remainder produced in the bone marrow. Heme synthesis occurs from glycine and succinyl coenzyme A (CoA) through a reaction catalyzed by aminolevulinic acid (ALA) synthase. ALA synthase is the rate-limiting step in the heme synthesis pathway and is regulated by feedback inhibition by its end product heme. Porphyrias are rare genetic diseases characterized by interruption of feedback inhibition of ALA synthase.

Heme degradation, primarily by the reticuloendothelial system, results in the formation of bilirubin as an end product. Formed bilirubin is then bound to plasma albumin for transport to the liver, where it is extracted and conjugated for secretion into canalicular bile. The majority of bilirubin excretion occurs in the gut, although a small portion is recirculated to the liver via the enterohepatic circulation. This accounts for the small amount of bilirubin conjugates present in blood. Conjugated bilirubin is water soluble, and about 10% is excreted in the urine.

Cholesterol and Lipid Metabolism

The liver stores dietary fat as triglycerides, cholesterol, and phospholipids and releases free fatty acids via triglyceride hydrolysis. In addition, the liver synthesizes free fatty acids from glucose, lipids, and protein. The liver also plays an important role in the regulation of cholesterol uptake, metabolism, and transport. Bile salts, the end product of cholesterol synthesis, serve as regulators of lipid metabolism. Elimination of cholesterol is achieved by biliary secretion and by excretion of bile acids.

Protein Metabolism

The liver plays a vital role in protein metabolism. Numerous biologically active proteins, including albumin, cytokines, hormones, and coagulation factors, are synthesized in the liver. In addition, nonessential amino acid synthesis can occur in hepatocytes when necessary. Protein degradation is another important function of the liver. The urea (Krebs) cycle is used by hepatocytes to convert the end products of amino acid degradation, such as ammonia and other nitrogenous waste products,

IV

507

to urea, which is readily excreted by the kidney. Severe hepatic dysfunction, such as that which occurs in end-stage liver disease (ESLD), leads to accumulation of ammonia in the serum resulting in hepatic encephalopathy (HE).

Pathophysiology of End-Stage Liver Disease

Cardiovascular Complications

Severe parenchymal disease that has advanced to the point of cirrhosis usually results in a hyperdynamic circulation. Hemodynamic measurements generally reveal normal to low systemic blood pressure, increased cardiac output, and decreased systemic vascular resistance. Decreased systemic vascular resistance occurs from vasodilation and abnormal anatomic and physiologic shunting. Physiologic shunting is the passage of blood from the arterial to the venous side of the circulation without effectively traversing a capillary bed. Abnormal blood vessels, such as those seen in the skin as spider angiomas, represent an anatomic shunt.[16,17]

Portal Hypertension

High resistance to blood flow through the liver, a hallmark of ESLD, causes an accumulation of blood in the vascular beds that are immediately upstream of the liver. Vessels draining the esophagus, stomach, spleen, and intestines dilate and hypertrophy, which leads to the development of splenomegaly and esophageal, gastric, and intraabdominal varices. Symptoms of portal hypertension include anorexia, nausea, ascites, esophageal varices, spider nevi, and HE. It is central to the pathogenesis of a variety of complications associated with ESLD, including massive variceal hemorrhage, increased susceptibility to infection, renal failure, and mental status changes.

Pulmonary Complications

ESLD is associated with hepatopulmonary syndrome and portopulmonary hypertension. Hepatopulmonary syndrome develops as a result of intrapulmonary arteriovenous communications that are not ventilated, impairment of hypoxic pulmonary vasoconstriction, atelectasis, and restrictive pulmonary disease secondary to ascites and pleural effusion. Arterial hypoxemia, secondary to the hepatopulmonary syndrome, may improve somewhat with supplemental oxygen in the early stages of the disease, but oxygen may not be effective with disease progression.

Portopulmonary hypertension is an increase in pulmonary arterial pressure in patients with portal hypertension. The cause is not well established. This syndrome occurs in less than 5% of patients, including the liver transplant population. Nevertheless, these patients are at increased risk for acute right-sided heart failure if physiologic conditions that increase pulmonary vascular resistance (acidosis, arterial hypoxemia, hypercapnia) occur during anesthesia. Hepatic hydrothorax, defined as pleural effusions occurring in the absence of cardiopulmonary disease, can also occur in up to 10% of cirrhotic patients. In some patients the pleural effusions from hepatic hydrothorax are large enough to impair oxygenation.

Hepatic Encephalopathy

Altered mental state is a frequent complication of both acute and chronic liver failure, with a clinically variable presentation ranging from minor changes in brain function to deep coma. The pathophysiology of HE is complex and not fully understood. When hepatic failure occurs, ammonia that is normally released by gut flora into the portal circulation accumulates and is shunted to the systemic circulation. The high level of systemic ammonia can lead to neuronal dysfunction and some of the clinical manifestations of HE. Other mechanisms are also implicated in the pathogenesis of this complex phenomenon, including alterations in the blood–brain barrier, γ-aminobutyric acid (GABA) receptor agonism, manganese toxicity, lactate, and dopamine metabolites.[18]

Therapy is primarily aimed at reducing ammonia levels. Lactulose reduces intestinal ammonia absorption via its laxative effect and a variety of mechanisms that alter the gut microbiome. Antibiotics like rifaximin and neomycin, which also alter gut microbial flora, are often used as ancillary therapies. L-Ornithine L-aspartate, probiotics, and branched-chain amino acids also have use in the management of this condition.

Impaired Drug Binding

When liver disease is so severe that albumin production is decreased, fewer sites are available for drug binding. This limited availability can increase levels of the unbound, pharmacologically active fraction of drugs, such as thiopental and alfentanil. Increased drug sensitivity as a result of decreased protein binding is most likely to be manifested when plasma albumin concentrations are lower than 2.5 g/dL.

Ascites

Ascites is a common complication of cirrhosis, affecting up to 50% of cirrhotic patients. The development of ascites is associated with significant morbidity and heralds the end stages of cirrhosis. Complications associated with ascites include marked abdominal distention (leading to atelectasis and restrictive pulmonary physiology), spontaneous bacterial peritonitis, and circulatory instability caused by compression of the inferior vena cava and right atrium. Although the exact mechanism of ascites is unclear, excess sodium retention by the kidney, decreased oncotic pressure because of hypoalbuminemia, and portal hypertension appear to play a central role. Initial therapy includes restriction of fluid administration, reduction of sodium intake, and administration of diuretics. In severe cases abdominal paracentesis can be effective at transiently reducing abdominal distention and restoring hemodynamic stability.[19,20] Some patients with refractory ascites are candidates for transjugular intrahepatic portosystemic shunt (TIPS), an interventional radiologic procedure to place a stent between a branch of the hepatic vein and portal vein (also see Chapter 38).

Renal Dysfunction and Hepatorenal Syndrome

Renal dysfunction can develop in a significant portion of patients with cirrhosis. A variety of etiologic factors, including diuretic therapy, reduced intravascular volume secondary to ascites or gastrointestinal hemorrhage, nephrotoxic drugs, and sepsis, can provoke acute renal failure and ultimately acute tubular necrosis in cirrhotic patients.

In the absence of obvious factors precipitating renal failure hepatorenal syndrome (HRS) can be diagnosed. HRS is a type of AKI, now called *HRS-AKI*, that is characterized by intense renal vasoconstriction.[21] Before the development of new criteria for AKI, patients with HRS were divided into two types. Type 1 HRS (now called HRS-AKI) typically presented as rapidly progressing prerenal failure and poor prognosis in the absence of therapeutic intervention. Conversely, type 2 HRS, with a more gradual increase in serum creatinine, now falls within the current definition of chronic kidney disease. The treatment of HRS-AKI includes 20% to 25% albumin administration, withdrawal of diuretics, vasoconstrictors (e.g., terlipressin, norepinephrine, or combined midodrine/octreotide), and reversal of precipitating factors.[21]

Effects of Anesthesia and Surgery on the Liver

Impact of Anesthetics on Hepatic Blood Flow

Inhaled anesthetics and regional anesthesia both typically decrease hepatic blood flow 20% to 30% in the absence of surgical stimulation. These changes reflect drug- or technique-induced effects on hepatic perfusion pressure or splanchnic vascular resistance, or both. For example, reduced hepatic blood flow from volatile anesthetics, in addition to regional anesthesia (T5 sensory level), is likely the result of decreased hepatic perfusion pressure. Autoregulation (increased hepatic artery blood flow offsetting decreases in portal vein blood flow) of hepatic blood flow may be best maintained with isoflurane. However, hepatic blood flow during the administration of desflurane and sevoflurane is maintained by a similar mechanism.

Volatile Anesthetic–Induced Hepatic Dysfunction

A rare but life-threatening form of hepatic dysfunction may reflect an immune-mediated hepatotoxicity caused by halothane. Two patterns of hepatic injury have occurred with use of halothane. A mild form occurs in up to 20% of patients and is associated with minimal sequelae. A rare fulminant form is associated with a fatality rate of 50% to 70%. Risk factors for development of this condition include prior exposure to halothane, age older than 40 years, obesity, and female sex. Isoflurane and desflurane are also capable of causing hepatic dysfunction, but the incidence of hepatitis after exposure to these volatile anesthetics is extremely rare, mainly because of the decreased magnitude of metabolism in comparison with halothane. Given its rare incidence and the disappearance of halothane in modern clinical practice, volatile anesthetic–induced hepatic dysfunction remains a diagnosis of exclusion in the patient presenting with hepatitis in the perioperative period.[22]

Management of Anesthesia in Patients With End-Stage Liver Disease

Preoperative Evaluation of Liver Disease

Preoperative liver function tests (Table 28.5) can be used to detect the presence of liver disease. Often, these tests are not very specific. Furthermore, the large reserve of the liver means that considerable hepatic damage can be present before liver function test results are altered. Indeed, cirrhosis of the liver may cause little alteration in liver function tests. Additional stressors, such as anesthesia and surgery, sometimes reveal underlying liver disease.

Historically, the Child-Turcotte-Pugh (CTP) score was used to classify liver dysfunction in patients with cirrhosis and portal hypertension (Table 28.6). In general, the risk of surgical mortality increases with increasing CTP class. Patients with CTP class C cirrhosis are not considered candidates for elective surgery. However, more contemporary studies have not demonstrated as strong of a correlation with mortality risk, most likely because

Table 28.5	Hepatic and Biliary Function Tests With Normal Values

Test	Normal Values[a]
Albumin	3.5–5.5 g/dL
Bilirubin	0.3–1.1 mg/dL
Unconjugated bilirubin (indirect reacting)	0.2–0.7 mg/dL
Conjugated bilirubin (direct reacting)	0.1–0.4 mg/dL
Aspartate aminotransferase (i.e., SGOT)	10–40 U/mL
Alanine aminotransferase (i.e., SGPT)	5–35 U/mL
Alkaline phosphatase	10–30 U/mL
Prothrombin time	12–14 s

[a]Normal values for each individual laboratory should be considered in interpreting liver function test results.
SGOT, Serum glutamic-oxaloacetic (acid) transaminase; *SGPT*, serum glutamate-pyruvate transaminase.

IV

Table 28.6 Child-Turcotte-Pugh (CTP) Score

Category	Description	Points
Encephalopathy	None	1
	Stage 1–2	2
	Stage 3–4	3
Ascites level	Absent	1
	Slight	2
	Moderate or severe	3
Serum albumin (g/dL)	>3.5	1
	2.8–3.5	2
	<2.8	3
Total bilirubin (mg/dL)	<2	1
	2–3	2
	>3	3
International normalized ratio (INR)	<1.7	1
	1.7–2.3	2
	>2.3	3

The CTP score is based on three laboratory tests and two physical findings in a patient with cirrhosis. The total number of points is used to assign the class.
CTP class A: 5–6 points
CTP class B: 7–9 points
CTP class C: 10–15 points
From Pugh RN, Murray-Lyon IM, Dawson JL, et al. Transection of the oesophagus for bleeding oesophageal varices. *Br J Surg.* 1973; 60(8):646–649.

Box 28.4 MELD Score and MELD-Na Formulas for Liver Disease

MELD score = (0.957 × $\log_e$ [serum creatinine (mg/dL)] + 0.378 × $\log_e$ [total serum bilirubin (mg/dL)] + 1.120 × $\log_e$ [INR]) × 10
–Minimum for all values is 1.
–Maximum value for creatinine is 4.
MELD-Na Score Formula
MELD-Na = MELD + 1.32 × (137 − Na) − [0.033 × MELD × (137 − Na)]
–Sodium values less than 125 mmol/L are set to 125, and values greater than 137 mmol/L are set to 137.

MELD, Model for End-Stage Liver Disease.

Intraoperative Management

Most major operations in patients with significant liver disease involve the use of general anesthesia. Regional techniques can be considered in selected patients who have normal coagulation values.

The magnitude of the operation determines the extent of invasive monitoring that is required. Major operations during which significant blood loss is likely require continuous monitoring of arterial blood pressure (arterial line) and filling pressure (central venous line). Patients with significant comorbid conditions (including cardiac diseases) undergoing procedures involving large anticipated blood loss may require placement of a pulmonary artery catheter or perioperative echocardiography.

Correction of severe coagulopathy before vascular line placement should be considered. Ultrasound guidance can reduce the risk of complications related to vascular access. Communication with the blood bank (also see Chapter 25) before surgery is crucial to ensure adequate availability of red blood cells, platelets, and clotting factors, including fresh frozen plasma and cryoprecipitate. For patients with esophageal varices, the risk of bleeding from insertion of a TEE probe may be increased.

Most patients have well-preserved cardiac function and no significant systemic or pulmonary hypertension. Induction of anesthesia can be achieved with an intravenous anesthetic such as propofol or etomidate, along with opioids and neuromuscular blocking drugs. Intravenous anesthetics have minimal impact on hepatic blood flow as long as arterial blood pressure is adequately maintained. Adequate anesthetic depth is necessary because sympathetic stimulation has an adverse effect on hepatic blood flow. A rapid-sequence or modified rapid-sequence induction of anesthesia is warranted if patients have significant ascites or delayed gastric emptying. Hypotension after induction of anesthesia occurs commonly because of the low systemic vascular resistance and relative hypovolemia. This can usually be treated with small doses of vasoconstrictors such as phenylephrine. Except for halothane, all volatile anesthetics are

surgery is avoided in patients with decompensated class C cirrhosis.[23]

The Model of End-Stage Liver Disease (MELD) score was initially developed in 2000 to predict 90-day mortality in patients who required TIPS procedures. The formula is complex but requires three laboratory tests: serum bilirubin, INR, and serum creatinine (Box 28.4). One advantage of the MELD score is its relative objectivity compared with the CTP score, which relied on physical examination for two of its components (ascites and encephalopathy). Preoperative MELD score correlates with postoperative mortality.[23] The Mayo Clinic created a risk calculator that incorporates MELD, age, and American Society of Anesthesiologists (ASA) physical status to provide a risk estimate for patients with cirrhosis undergoing major surgery.[24,25] Incorporation of serum sodium into the MELD score calculation (MELD-Na score) improves its accuracy in predicting mortality in patients listed for liver transplantation[26] (see Box 28.4). However, the MELD-Na score has not been evaluated as a postoperative surgical risk predictor. Postoperative mortality in patients with cirrhosis depends on factors related to the patient, surgical procedure, and anesthesia management (Fig. 28.5).

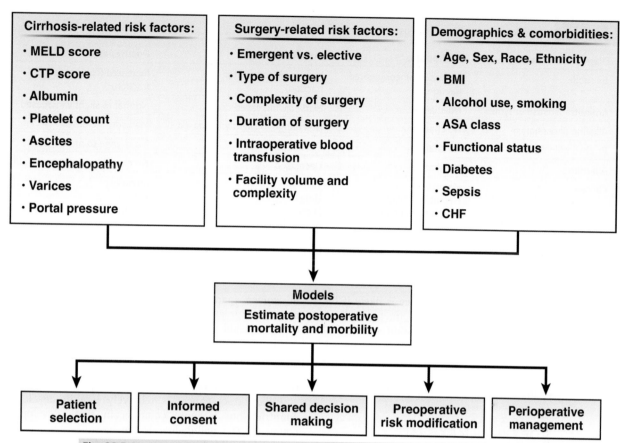

| Cirrhosis-related risk factors: | Surgery-related risk factors: | Demographics & comorbidities: |

Cirrhosis-related risk factors:

- MELD score
- CTP score
- Albumin
- Platelet count
- Ascites
- Encephalopathy
- Varices
- Portal pressure

Surgery-related risk factors:

- Emergent vs. elective
- Type of surgery
- Complexity of surgery
- Duration of surgery
- Intraoperative blood transfusion
- Facility volume and complexity

Demographics & comorbidities:

- Age, Sex, Race, Ethnicity
- BMI
- Alcohol use, smoking
- ASA class
- Functional status
- Diabetes
- Sepsis
- CHF

Models

Estimate postoperative mortality and morbidity

| Patient selection | Informed consent | Shared decision making | Preoperative risk modification | Perioperative management |

Fig. 28.5 Postoperative mortality in patients with cirrhosis depends on cirrhosis-related, surgery-related, and comorbidity-related factors. Currently, there are no comprehensive models to incorporate all of these factors. *ASA,* American Society of Anesthesiologists; *BMI,* body mass index; *CHF,* congestive heart failure; *CTP,* Child-Turcotte-Pugh; *MELD,* Model for End-Stage Liver Disease. (From Newman KL, Johnson KM, Cornia PB, et al. Perioperative evaluation and management of patients with cirrhosis: Risk assessment, surgical outcomes, and future directions. *Clin Gastroenterol Hepatol.* 2020;18[11]:2398–2414.e3, Fig. 2.)

suitable for patients with severe liver disease. No optimal anesthetic technique has been established for the maintenance of anesthesia.

Management of Coagulopathy

Traditionally, surgical blood loss and coagulopathy have been managed by administering blood products either by clinical judgment alone (if bleeding is rapid) or guided by conventional laboratory tests (e.g., PTT, INR, platelet count) (if bleeding is controlled) (also see Chapter 23). Standard laboratory testing, however, can be slow to yield results and does not provide information about the qualitative aspects of clot formation.

Advances in point-of-care coagulation technology, such as ROTEM and platelet function analysis, however, allow the clinician to rapidly diagnose and manage coagulopathy associated with ESLD in the perioperative setting. Additional information, unavailable through conventional laboratory tests, such as clot strength, platelet function, and hyperfibrinolysis, can be assessed rapidly at the bedside with these newer techniques.[27]

The use of factor concentrate therapies, such as prothrombin complex concentrate and fibrinogen concentrate may also play a significant role in blood product management in patients with ESLD. Hemostatic algorithms that use point-of-care coagulation testing and factor concentrate–based therapy are showing considerable promise in the management of patients with coagulopathy related to liver disease.[28]

Postoperative Jaundice

Halothane or other volatile anesthetics are often implicated as the cause of postoperative jaundice, but there are many other and probably more likely causes (Table 28.7).

Table 28.7 Classification and Causes of Postoperative Liver Dysfunction

Diagnostic Feature	Prehepatic	Intrahepatic	Posthepatic
Bilirubin	Increased (unconjugated fraction)	Increased (conjugated fraction)	Increased (conjugated fraction)
Aminotransferase enzymes	No change	Markedly increased	Normal to slightly increased
Alkaline phosphatase	No change	No change to slightly increased	Markedly increased
Prothrombin time	No change	Prolonged	No change to prolonged
Albumin	No change	Decreased	No change to decreased
Causes	Hemolysis Hematoma reabsorption Bilirubin overload from whole blood	Viruses Drugs Sepsis Arterial hypoxemia Congestive heart failure Cirrhosis	Stones Cancer Sepsis

A surgical cause of postoperative jaundice is likely if the operation involved the liver or biliary tract. Similarly, multiple blood transfusions and resorption of surgical hematoma can lead to jaundice in the perioperative period. Drugs, including antibiotics, and other metabolic or infectious causes, such as sepsis, must also be considered in the differential diagnosis of postoperative jaundice.

DISEASES OF THE BILIARY TRACT

The biliary tract refers to a system of organs and ducts that produce bile. The main functions of this system are to drain waste products from the liver and to aid in digestion.

Bile Metabolism and Secretion

Bile is an aqueous secretion that originates from hepatocytes and is modified distally by absorptive and secretory transport systems in the bile duct epithelium. It functions to excrete exogenous and endogenous substances, emulsify dietary fats to facilitate intestinal absorption, eliminate cholesterol, assist with immunoprotection in the intestine, and excrete hormones and pheromones.[29] Excess bile is stored in the gallbladder, a pouched organ, connected to the common bile duct via the cystic duct. In addition to acting as a reservoir, the gallbladder actively adjusts the ratio of biliary components during storage. A variety of pathologic and physiologic conditions can alter bile composition, secretion, and storage leading to gallstone formation.[30]

Pathophysiology of the Biliary Tract

The prevalence of gallstones is between 10% and 15% of the adult population. There is a higher prevalence in women (particularly during pregnancy), the obese, and those greater than 40 years of age. Dyslipidemia, diabetes, rapid weight loss, and dietary factors can also predispose to gallstone formation.[31] Gallstones typically present with steady right upper quadrant pain and intolerance to fatty foods. Presence of fever is usually indicative of acute cholecystitis or cholangitis.

Biliary tract cancer is relatively rare in developed countries but is more common in some developing countries. The gallbladder is the most common organ involved. Gallbladder cancer is characterized by delayed presentation of symptoms and difficulty with treatment. Chronic infection, environmental exposure to chemicals, and dietary and genetic factors have all been linked to the development of gallbladder cancer.[32] Treatment typically involves surgery and adjuvant therapies. Survival, particularly in advanced stages, can be low.

Gilbert syndrome, a benign disorder causing elevation in unconjugated bilirubin, is one of the most common causes of jaundice and may occasionally be mistaken for postoperative hepatobiliary dysfunction. Conversely, Dubin-Johnson and Rotor syndromes are congenital disorders leading to elevated conjugated bilirubin levels that can be exacerbated by surgery.

Management of Anesthesia for Biliary Tract Surgery

Anesthesia for cholecystectomy or exploration of the common bile duct, or both, should account for the effect of anesthetic drugs on intraluminal pressure in the biliary tract. Specifically, opioids can produce spasm of the choledochoduodenal sphincter, which increases common bile duct pressure. Such spasm may impair the passage of contrast medium into the duodenum and erroneously suggest the need for sphincteroplasty or the presence of common bile duct stones. However, opioids have been used in many instances without adverse effect, which emphasizes the fact that not all patients respond to opioids with choledochoduodenal sphincter spasm. Treatment of biliary spasm includes naloxone, glucagon, and nitroglycerin.

Laparoscopic Cholecystectomy

Anesthetic considerations for laparoscopic cholecystectomy are similar to those for other laparoscopic procedures. For example, insufflation of the abdominal cavity (pneumoperitoneum) with carbon dioxide introduced through a needle placed via a supraumbilical incision results in increased intraabdominal pressure that may interfere with ventilation of the lungs and venous return. During laparoscopic cholecystectomy, placement of the patient in the reverse Trendelenburg position favors movement of the abdominal contents away from the operative site and may facilitate mechanical ventilation of the lungs. This position, however, may further interfere with venous return.

Generous intravascular fluid replacement during laparoscopic cholecystectomy may facilitate recovery from this type of surgery.[33]

Monitoring end-tidal carbon dioxide concentrations during laparoscopic abdominal surgical procedures is useful because of the unpredictability of systemic absorption of the carbon dioxide used to create the pneumoperitoneum. Intraoperative decompression of the stomach with a nasogastric or orogastric tube may decrease the risk for visceral puncture at the time of needle insertion and may subsequently improve laparoscopic visualization. Administration of nitrous oxide during laparoscopic cholecystectomy has typically not been recommended because of the possibility that it could expand bowel gas volume, causing interference with surgical working conditions and the theoretical possibility that diffusion into the abdominal cavity could support combustion.[34] Loss of hemostasis or injury to the hepatic artery or liver may require prompt intervention via a conventional laparotomy incision.

REFERENCES

1. Mooney JF, Chow CK, Hillis GS. Perioperative renal function and surgical outcome. *Curr Opin Anesthesiol.* 2014;27:195–200.
2. Prowle JR, Forni LG, Bell M, et al. Postoperative acute kidney injury in adult noncardiac surgery: Joint consensus report of the Acute Disease Quality Initiative and PeriOperative Quality Initiative. *Nat Rev Nephrol.* 2021 Sep;17(9):605–618. doi:10.1038/s41581-021-00418-2 Epub 2021 May 11. PMID: 33976395; PMCID: PMC8367817.
3. Joannidis M, Druml W, Forni LG, et al. Prevention of acute kidney injury and protection of renal function in the intensive care unit: Update 2017. *Intensive Care Med.* 2017;43:730–749.
4. Hoste E, Clermont G, Kersten A, et al. RIFLE criteria for acute kidney injury are associated with hospital mortality in critically ill patients: A cohort analysis. *Crit Care.* 2006;10:R73.
5. Shlipak MG, Coresh J, Gansevoort RT. Cystatin C versus creatinine for kidney function-based risk. *N Engl J Med.* 2013;369:2457–2459.
6. Mårtensson J, Martling CR, Bell M. Novel biomarkers of acute kidney injury and failure: Clinical applicability. *Br J Anaesth.* 2012;109(6):843–850.
7. Sica DA. Diuretic use in renal disease. *Nat Rev Nephrol.* 2011;8:100–109.
8. ANZICS Clinical Trials Group. Low-dose dopamine in patients with early renal dysfunction: A placebo-controlled randomized trial. *Lancet.* 2000;356:2139–2143.
9. Friedrich JO, Adhikari N, Herridge MS, et al. Meta-analysis: Low dose dopamine increases urine output but does not prevent renal dysfunction or death. *Ann Intern Med.* 2005;142:510–524.
10. Gillies MA, Kakar V, Parker RJ, et al. Fenoldopam to prevent acute kidney injury after major surgery—A systematic review and meta-analysis. *Crit Care.* 2015;19:449.
11. Jones DR, Lee HT. Perioperative renal protection. *Best Pract Res Clin Anaesthesiol.* 2008;22:193–208.
12. Zacharias M, Mugawar M, Herbison GP, et al. Interventions for protecting renal function in the perioperative period. *Cochrane Database Syst Rev.* 2013;9:CD003590.
13. Sear JW. Kidney dysfunction in the postoperative period. *Br J Anaesth.* 2005;95:20–32.
14. O'Malley CM, Frumento RJ, Hardy MA, et al. A randomized, double-blind comparison of lactated Ringer's solution and 0.9% NaCl during renal transplantation. *Anesth Analg.* 2005;100:1518–1524.
15. Weinberg L, Harris L, Bellomo R, et al. Effects of intraoperative and early postoperative normal saline or Plasma-Lyte 148® on hyperkalaemia in deceased donor renal transplantation: A double-blind randomized trial. *Br J Anaesth.* 2017 Oct 1;119(4):606–615. doi:10.1093/bja/aex163 PMID: 29121282.
16. Kiamanesh D, Rumley J, Moitra VK. Monitoring and managing hepatic disease in anaesthesia. *Br J Anaesth.* 2013;111(suppl 1):i50–i61.
17. Moller S, Henriksen JH. Cardiovascular complications of cirrhosis. *Gut.* 2008;57:268–278.
18. Encephalopathy Wijdicks EFHepatic. *N Engl J Med.* 2016;375:1660–1670.
19. Gines P, Cardenas A, Arroyo V, et al. Management of cirrhosis and ascites. *N Engl J Med.* 2004;350:1646–1654.
20. Schuppan D, Afdhal NH. Liver cirrhosis. *Lancet.* 2008;371:838–851.
21. Simonetto DA, Gines P, Kamath PS. Hepatorenal syndrome: Pathophysiology, diagnosis, and management. *BMJ.* 2020 Sep 14;370:m2687. doi:10.1136/bmj.m2687 PMID: 32928750.
22. Hoetzel A, Ryan H, Schmidt R. Anesthetic considerations for the patient with liver disease. *Curr Opin Anaesthesiol.* 2012;25:340–347.
23. Northup PG, Friedman LS, Kamath PS. AGA clinical practice update on surgical risk assessment and perioperative management in cirrhosis: Expert review. *Clin Gastroenterol Hepatol.* 2019 Mar;17(4):595–606. doi:10.1016/j.cgh.2018.09.043 Epub 2018 Sep 28. PMID: 30273751.
24. Teh SH, Nagorney DM, Stevens SR, et al. Risk factors for mortality after surgery in patients with cirrhosis. *Gastroenterology.* 2007 Apr;132(4):1261–1269. doi:10.1053/j.gastro.2007.01.040 Epub 2007 Jan 25. PMID: 17408652.
25. Mayo Clinic. Postoperative mortality risk in patients with cirrhosis. https://www.mayoclinic.org/medical-professionals/transplant-medicine/calculators/postoperative-mortality-risk-in-patients-with-cirrhosis/itt-20434721. Accessed November 25, 2021.
26. Biggins SW, Kim RW, Terrault NA, et al. Evidence-based incorporation of serum sodium concentration Into MELD. *Gastroenterology.* 2006;130(6):1652–1660.

IV

27. Mallett SV. Clinical utility of viscoelastic tests of coagulation (TEG/ROTEM) in patients with liver disease and during liver transplantation. *Semin Thromb Hemost.* 2015;41(5):527–537.

28. Theusinger OM, Stein P, Levy JH. Point of care and factor concentrate-based coagulation algorithms. *Transfus Med Hemother.* 2015;42(2):115–121.

29. Boyer JL. Bile formation and secretion. *Compr Physiol.* 2013;3(3):1035–1078.

30. Dosch RA, Imagawa DK, Jutric Z. Bile metabolism and lithogenesis: An update. *Surg Clin North Am.* 2019;99(2):215–229 2019.

31. Stinton LM, Shaffer EA. Epidemiology of gallbladder disease: Cholelithiasis and cancer. *Gut Liver.* 2012;6(2):172–187.

32. Sharma A, Sharma KL, Gupta A, et al. Gallbladder cancer epidemiology, pathogenesis and molecular genetics: Recent Update. *World J Gastroenterol.* 2017;23(22):3978–3998.

33. Gerges FJ, Kanazi GE, Jabbour-Khoury SI. Anesthesia for laparoscopy: A review. *J Clin Anesth.* 2006;18:67–78.

34. Diemunsch PA, Torp KD, Van Dorsselaer T, Mutter D. Nitrous oxide fraction in the carbon dioxide pneumoperitoneum during laparoscopy under general inhaled anesthesia in pigs. *Anesth Analg.* 2000;90:k951–k953.

29 NUTRITIONAL, GASTROINTESTINAL, AND ENDOCRINE DISEASE

Sophia P. Poorsattar, Solmaz Poorsattar Manuel

NUTRITIONAL DISORDERS

Obesity

Obesity is a condition characterized by excessive accumulation and storage of adipose tissue. Obesity is most commonly quantified by body mass index (BMI), the ratio of a person's weight (in kilograms) to the square of their height (in meters). The Centers for Disease Control and Prevention and the World Health Organization provide definitions of obesity (Table 29.1).[1,2] Measuring the degree of obesity is of clinical relevance, because with increasing severity, there are adverse metabolic, biomechanical, and psychosocial health consequences. Although BMI is a simple and reproducible measure of obesity and its related metabolic risk, it does not account for sex- or ethnic-related differences, muscle mass, adipose tissue distribution, or frame size. Additional methods to quantitatively assess obesity include abdominal circumference, body fat percentage, and waist-to-hip ratio.

Obesity is a complex disease with its morbidity affecting every organ system in the body (Table 29.2). Associated conditions that are most likely to impact anesthesia care include pulmonary (obstructive sleep apnea, obesity hypoventilation syndrome, restrictive pulmonary physiology with impaired ventilation-perfusion matching, and reduced functional residual capacity with related rapid desaturation during apnea); cardiovascular (hypertension with related structural heart disease, pulmonary hypertension with cor pulmonale); and endocrine (insulin resistance and diabetes mellitus) disorders.[3]

Obesity is independently associated with various adverse outcomes in the perioperative setting, including greater hospital length of stay, greater estimated blood loss, longer operative times, increased surgical site infections, increased risk of renal failure, and prolonged assisted ventilation.[4] As a BMI calculation alone may not accurately predict metabolic health and comorbid

Table 29.1	CDC/WHO Obesity Definitions in Adults Over 20 Years Old

	BMI
Preferred BMI	18.5-24.9 kg/m²
Overweight	25.0-29.9 kg/m²
Class I obesity	30.0-34.9 kg/m²
Class II obesity	35.0-39.9 kg/m²
Class III obesity	≥40.0 kg/m²

Data from Refs. 1 and 2.
BMI, Body mass index; *CDC*, Centers for Disease Control and Prevention; *WHO*, World Health Organization.

Table 29.2	Medical Conditions Associated With Obesity[3,4]

Organ System	Associated Conditions
Central nervous system	Cognitive decline, dementia Depression
Respiratory system	Obstructive sleep apnea Obesity hypoventilation syndrome Restrictive lung disease
Cardiovascular system	Arrhythmias Systemic hypertension Coronary arterial disease Congestive heart failure Pulmonary hypertension Cor pulmonale Cerebrovascular disease Peripheral vascular disease Venous thromboembolism Hypercholesterolemia Hypertriglyceridemia Sudden cardiac death
Endocrine system	Metabolic syndrome Diabetes mellitus Cushing syndrome Hypothyroidism Infertility
Gastrointestinal system	Hiatal hernia Gastroesophageal reflux disease Nonalcoholic steatohepatitis Fatty infiltration of the liver Cholelithiasis
Musculoskeletal system	Degenerative joint disease Osteoarthritis Joint pain Inguinal hernia
Malignancy	Breast Gastric Pancreatic Liver, gallbladder Kidney Prostate Cervical, uterine, endometrial Colorectal
Other	Kidney failure Hypercoagulable syndromes Shorter life expectancy

conditions because of its previously mentioned limitations, a complete systems-based assessment is essential for determining a patient's perioperative risk (also see Chapter 13).

The combination of the metabolic risk factors associated with obesity is called *metabolic syndrome*. Metabolic syndrome is an important risk factor for the subsequent development of type 2 diabetes mellitus (T2DM) and/or cardiovascular disease, and its diagnosis is associated with a higher risk of morbidity after surgery.[5] There are six components to metabolic syndrome: abdominal obesity, atherogenic dyslipidemia, hypertension, insulin resistance, proinflammatory state, and prothrombotic state. Because the metabolic traits cooccur, a diagnosis of metabolic syndrome can be made in the presence of just three of the following five criteria: abdominal obesity, increased serum triglycerides, decreased high-density lipoproteins, hypertension, and increased fasting blood glucose levels.[4]

The development and maintenance of obesity are multifactorial and involve genetic, neuroendocrine, environmental, and psychosocial factors. The major therapeutic goals in these patients are to focus on weight reduction and increased physical activity and to pharmacologically treat the previously mentioned metabolic disturbances if they persist despite lifestyle modification.

Perioperative Considerations

Changes in anatomy and physiology related to obesity affect anesthetic planning and management. Preoperative assessment should focus on determining the presence and status of comorbid conditions. This assessment will allow for measures to be taken to minimize the risk of perioperative complications, including determining if certain additional testing is required, if the patient is scheduled at an appropriate surgical venue, and if adequate postoperative resources are available if needed.[6]

Standard preoperative fasting guidelines should be observed and the decision to use aspiration prophylaxis made on an individual basis for those patients who are high risk or symptomatic.[7] Careful consideration should be made regarding the use of sedative premedication to achieve anxiolysis, as patients with obesity may be more sensitive to the respiratory depressant effects. If used, these should be given in incremental doses and carefully titrated to effect.

Depending on the habitus of the patient, several logistical challenges may be encountered related to monitoring, procedures, and positioning. The amount and distribution of subcutaneous fat in the extremities may make obtaining peripheral intravenous access difficult and necessitate central venous access depending on the procedure. Similarly, the increased width or conical shape of the upper arms may make the use of a noninvasive blood pressure cuff inaccurate or unreliable and necessitate alternative cuff location (forearm or lower leg) or invasive arterial line access for blood pressure monitoring.[8] As operative room tables are often narrow, positioning may be a challenge (also see Chapter 19). Additional reinforcement or pressure point padding may be required to ensure adequate security and support, especially in the event that extreme angles of tilt are required for the procedure.

Before induction of anesthesia, an airway assessment should be made to determine risk factors for difficult mask ventilation or laryngeal intubation (also see Chapter 16). Securing an airway in patients with obesity may be challenging because of the redundancy of oropharyngeal tissue, increased neck circumference, reduced mobility of the cervical spine, or increased anterior-posterior chest dimension. Induction of anesthesia may also be complicated by rapid desaturation with apnea. A rapid decrease in blood oxygen saturation is multifactorial with causes including increased metabolic requirements (increased oxygen consumption and carbon dioxide production) and reduced functional residual capacity.[4,9] Ensuring adequate preoxygenation or providing apneic oxygenation allows for increased time to desaturation. Optimizing positioning by placing the patient in reverse Trendelenburg (back up or ramped position) will increase functional residual capacity by reducing atelectasis in dependent areas of the lung, improve ventilation-perfusion matching, and caudally displace chest tissue to allow for easier mask ventilation and view on laryngoscopy.[10]

No anesthetic type has proven superior in patients with obesity. However, in patients with elevated risk for respiratory or airway-related problems regional anesthesia should be considered if feasible. When general anesthesia is used, ventilatory management may be challenging and require additional pressure support or positive end-expiratory pressure to ensure adequate ventilation and avoid alveolar collapse. Choice of medications depends on patient-specific factors and comorbidities with consideration of altered drug metabolism and elimination with increased adipose tissue. As mentioned previously, anesthetic medications should be administered in incremental doses and titrated to effect to avoid oversedation or hypoventilation on emergence or postextubation. Ensuring adequate extubation criteria is important, as sedation or interim airway swelling and edema from the surgery or positioning may further complicate an already challenging intubation. As patients with obesity are at increased risk for postoperative pulmonary complications, including hypoxemia or hypercarbia from atelectasis, hypoventilation, or airway obstruction, additional

noninvasive ventilatory support in the recovery room may be required to ensure adequate ventilation and gas exchange.[11]

Bariatric Surgery

Adult bariatric surgery is a therapeutic option in patients with severe obesity who have failed conservative treatments, such as lifestyle modifications and medical management. Bariatric surgery results in significant sustained weight loss and a reduction in obesity-related comorbidities and cardiovascular events. The strategic approaches for surgically assisted weight loss fall into three categories: gastric restriction, intestinal malabsorption, or a combination of both.

Malabsorptive procedures include jejunoileal bypass or biliopancreatic diversion. These operations have the advantage of promoting significant weight loss by extensively bypassing the small intestine. Although these were the most commonly performed approaches when bariatric surgery was first created, they are now infrequently performed because of their related nutritional and metabolic complications.[12]

Restrictive procedures include gastric banding and sleeve gastrectomy. By creating a small gastric pouch and outlet, these procedures promote weight loss through several mechanisms, including appetite suppression and early satiety, reduced secretion of gastric hormones (i.e., ghrelin), and possibly vagal nerve compression. Whereas sleeve gastrectomies involve resection of the greater curvature of the stomach, banding procedures use adjustable or fixed bands to wrap the top portion of the stomach to the desired size. Gastric banding has fewer complications and lower morbidity and mortality, as it requires no cutting into gastrointestinal structures. Restrictive-based procedures take a longer time to achieve weight loss. However, the normal absorptive physiology of the small intestine is left intact, and nutritional deficiencies rarely occur.[12]

The most common combined bariatric procedure is the Roux-en-Y gastric bypass. This procedure involves creating a small gastric pouch, which is then connected to the jejunum. It is the most complex of the approaches and requires the longest operative time and hospital length of stay. Because of its combined gastric restriction and malabsorption approaches, it promotes the greatest weight loss and improvement in obesity-related comorbidities; however, these patients require lifelong nutritional surveillance and supplementation. As such, it is often reserved for patients with clinically severe obesity.

Bariatric surgeries are often performed laparoscopically because of the benefits of decreased pain, decreased complication rates, shorter recovery times, and outcome efficacy comparable to that of their open counterparts. In addition to the weight loss and high-resolution rate of comorbid conditions such as hypertension and diabetes, patients report improvement in their quality of life.

IV

Overall, perioperative mortality from bariatric surgeries ranges from 0.1% to 2.0%, with gastric banding having the lowest mortality and Roux-en-Y gastric bypass having the highest. Risk factors for mortality include male sex, older age, BMI ≥50.0 kg/m², diabetes mellitus, obstructive sleep apnea, and performance at a low-volume bariatric surgical center.[13]

Malnutrition

Malnourishment is an imbalance between energy expenditure and energy intake. This term may refer to excessive intake, such as occurs in individuals with obesity, or deficient intake, such as occurs in individuals with undernutrition.[14] For the purpose of this section, malnutrition will be used synonymously with undernutrition. In undernutrition, the supply of nutrients and energy to the body does not meet the demand necessary for cellular growth, maintenance, and function. Undernutrition can be divided into four subforms: wasting (low weight for height), shunting (low height for age), underweight (low weight for age), and micronutrient deficient. Malnourishment may occur as a result of a variety of pathologic and environmental causes and presents in a variety of forms. To account for this variation, the Global Leadership Initiative on Malnutrition developed a consensus on the diagnostic criteria for malnutrition that requires the combination of at least one phenotype and one etiologic criteria: nonvolitional weight loss, low BMI, or reduced muscle mass (phenotype criteria) or reduced food intake or absorption, or underlying inflammation resulting from acute disease/injury or chronic disease (etiologic criteria).[15]

Malnutrition is a complex metabolic disorder, involving inflammatory and neurohumoral mediators, which, when severe, affect every organ system in the body (Table 29.3).

Treatment is aimed at balancing nutritional intake with energy needs, taking into consideration the level of activity or stress of the patient. When it is evident that patients will not be able to meet their nutritional needs, nutritional supplementation may be indicated, either through enteral (oral or tube) feeding or parenteral (intravenous) feeding. When possible, enteral support is preferred over parenteral support because of its relative simplicity, safety, lower cost, and decreased rates of complications. Total parenteral nutrition (TPN) is required when the gastrointestinal tract is not functional. When used for brief periods, peripheral parenteral nutrition may be provided; however, when long-term or high caloric support is indicated, central venous access is required to allow for the infusion of hypertonic solutions at a lower volume. Numerous complications are associated with TPN, including metabolic and electrolyte derangements, renal dysfunction, liver dysfunction, altered coagulation, bacterial translocation from the gastrointestinal tract, and infection or sepsis.

Table 29.3 Body Systems Affected by Malnutrition

Organ System	Features
Central nervous system	Psychological disturbance, depression Depressed cognitive function Fatigue and generalized weakness
Cardiovascular system	Reduction in cardiac output Increased vagal tone Conduction abnormalities, arrhythmias Peripheral vasoconstriction
Respiratory system	Reduced respiratory muscle strength and function Decreased respiratory compliance Spontaneous pneumothorax
Gastrointestinal system	Gut atrophy, bacterial translocation, and impaired immune function Delayed gastric emptying, gastric dilatation
Musculoskeletal system	Reduced muscle mass and strength, myopathy Reduced bone mass, secondary fractures Impaired wound healing Impaired thermoregulation
Renal system	Reduced glomerular filtration rate Total body water proportionally higher Proteinuria, uremia
Electrolyte and metabolic	Hypokalemia Hypocalcemia Hypoglycemia Metabolic acidosis Increased cortisol
Pharmacologic	Delayed or reduced absorption of drugs Decreased protein binding from hypoalbuminemia Prolonged treatment with nondepolarizing muscle relaxants Lower dosing thresholds for toxicity

Modified from Edwards S. Anaesthetising the malnourished patient. *Update Anaesth.* 2016;31:31–37.

Perioperative Considerations

Malnutrition is associated with several complications in the perioperative period, including increased rates of infection, poor wound healing and anastomotic integrity, bacterial overgrowth in the gastrointestinal tract, increased time spent in the intensive care unit and hospital length of stay, and increased need for mechanical ventilation. It is also associated with increased mortality after organ transplant, major intraabdominal, or cardiothoracic surgeries. As such, it is important to identify patients who are malnourished and, when possible, intervene to improve their nutritional state in an effort to reduce complications and improve outcomes.

Assessing nutritional status preoperatively is complex; however, the combined use of a comprehensive history and physical examination and nutritional risk screening tool is a helpful approach. Certain laboratory testing may also help to identify malnourishment, including reduced serum protein markers, such as albumin, prealbumin, or transferrin. Of these, prealbumin may allow for the earliest detection of changes in nutritional status, given that its half-life is only 2 days; however, it should be measured in conjunction with C-reactive protein levels, as inflammation can raise the level of prealbumin and affect result interpretation. Reduced serum levels of cholesterol, zinc, iron, vitamin B_{12}, or folic acid may also indicate malnourishment. In the postoperative setting the adequacy of nutritional support may be assessed by the patient's overall clinical course and wound healing. Daily clinical assessment, trend in lean body mass, calorimetry, and laboratory results may also inform the patient's nutritional status.

Refeeding syndrome describes the metabolic disturbance that occurs after rapid nutritional repletion in a severely malnourished patient. Hypophosphatemia is the hallmark disturbance of the syndrome and occurs for several reasons. Initial glucose load from feeding leads to increased insulin levels, which in turn result in a rapid movement of extracellular phosphate, potassium, and magnesium into the intracellular compartment. Insulin also leads to the production of molecules that require phosphate, such as adenosine triphosphate and 2,3-diphosphoglycerate, which leads to further phosphate depletion. Hypophosphatemia in turn leads to tissue hypoxia, myocardial dysfunction, respiratory failure, hemolysis, rhabdomyolysis, and seizures. Refeeding syndrome can be avoided by having a cautious and carefully titrated approach to nutritional repletion.[16]

For severely malnourished patients, TPN or enteral feeding should be administered for 7 to 10 days before an electric surgery to improve outcomes. Nutritional replacement should be continued as long as possible before a surgical procedure. With TPN, consideration should be made regarding the presence of insulin in the infusion, as regular monitoring of the patient's glucose and electrolytes may be required. With enteral replacement, consideration should be made regarding the patient's risk of aspiration of gastric contents with the benefit of continued nutritional replacement to keep the patient at goal level.[16]

Intraoperative goals for anesthetic management rely on considering the various metabolic, physiologic, and pharmacologic changes in malnourished patients. General principles for management include preventing hypoglycemia, preventing hypothermia, treating and preventing dehydration, correcting electrolytes, identifying and treating infections, correcting micronutrient deficiencies, careful positioning and padding, and emotional support.

GASTROINTESTINAL DISORDERS

Inflammatory Bowel Disease

Inflammatory bowel disease (IBD) is a group of inflammatory disorders of the small intestine and colon. The two principal types are ulcerative colitis (UC) and Crohn disease (CD). UC primarily affects the colon and rectum and results in relapsing and remitting episodes of mucosal inflammation. CD may involve any portion of the gastrointestinal tract from the mouth to the perianal area and results in transmural inflammation, which may be complicated by fibrosis, stricture, fistula, or abscess formation. Although the two disorders have some distinct pathologic and clinical characteristics, there is substantial overlap, and differentiation of the two may be difficult.

The pathophysiology of IBD is complex and arises from interaction of both genetic and environmental factors, ultimately triggering an immunologic response and inflammation in the intestine. Known environmental risk factors include smoking, sedentary lifestyle, sleep deprivation, stress, appendectomy, antibiotics, oral contraceptives, and nonsteroidal antiinflammatory drugs (NSAIDs).[17] Diagnosis is often made based on the location and nature of the intestinal and extraintestinal manifestations coupled with findings on imaging and endoscopy. Fecal calprotectin may also suggest the diagnosis, but it is not specific for IBD.

Medical therapy for both types is aimed at alleviating the severity of symptoms and is not curative. In addition to medical therapy, up to 70% of patients may require surgical intervention. Although surgery cannot definitively cure CD, most cases of UC can be cured by proctocolectomy, although the patient's extraintestinal symptoms may persist.[18] In patients with advanced IBD of either type surgery may be indicated for various reasons, including disease complications (fistula, stricture, abscess, toxic megacolon, perforation), surgical complications (adhesions, bowel obstruction), intractable symptoms, or cancer prevention.

Perioperative Considerations

As the proportion of older patients with IBD is increasing, there is an increase in the complexity of comorbid conditions that require care in the perioperative setting. Increased perioperative morbidity of patients with IBD is seen in those who are malnourished, aged 60 to 80 years, on long-term immunosuppressive therapy, requiring emergent operation, and treated in low-volume centers. Type of surgical intervention is also related to perioperative morbidity, with increased risk in patients undergoing a total proctocolectomy with J pouch rather than ileostomy, a repair for fistulizing disease rather than strictureplasty or stoma revision, and an open rather than laparoscopic approach.[19]

IV

Before elective surgery, medical optimization should be performed to address possible nutritional deficiencies and associated coagulopathy, hypovolemia, and electrolyte or acid–base disturbance in order to reduce the associated morbidity. Because of the elevated risk for venous thromboembolic events in patients with IBD, perioperative pharmacologic prophylaxis is recommended. Perioperative medical management in patients with IBD varies depending on the type of IBD, the clinical circumstance of the patient, and the urgency of the surgery. The classes of medications used for patients with IBD include antidiarrheals, antiinflammatories, immunosuppressants, antibiotics, and other investigational drugs. Special consideration should be taken requiring the discontinuation and resumption of each type of immunosuppressive medication, as failure to hold or continue them may increase the risk of perioperative complications. Glucocorticoids should continue throughout the perioperative period with consideration for supplemental stress dosing before surgery.[19]

Although no specific type of anesthetic is preferred for patients with IBD, consideration should be taken regarding the interaction of common IBD drugs with anesthetic medications. Cyclosporine increases minimum alveolar concentration of volatile anesthetics. Azathioprine may partially antagonize the effect of nondepolarizing neuromuscular blocking agents, and cyclosporine and infliximab may enhance their potency.[19]

Gastroesophageal Reflux Disease

Gastroesophageal reflux disease (GERD) is a condition defined by the symptoms and complications associated with the reflux of gastric contents through the lower esophageal sphincter (LES) into the esophagus. Some degree of reflux is physiologic, but for patients with GERD, reflux is pathologic and leads to symptoms or mucosal injury. The classic symptoms of GERD are heartburn (burning retrosternal sensation) and regurgitation (perception of flow of refluxed gastric contents into the hypopharynx or mouth). The prevalence of heartburn and/or regurgitation symptoms is between 10% and 30% worldwide.[20] Other nonspecific manifestations of GERD include dysphagia, globus sensation, chest pain, laryngitis, hoarseness, cough, dental erosions, adult-onset asthma, and aspiration.

Several mechanisms contribute to the development of GERD, including the imbalance of symptom-eliciting factors and defensive factors. Symptom-eliciting factors include reflux events, acidity of refluxed contents, and esophageal hypersensitivity. Defensive factors include esophageal acid clearance and mucosal integrity.[21] Symptom severity is reflective of this imbalance in combination with impaired esophageal mobility, LES function, and/or gastric motility. Normally, the LES acts as an antireflux barrier at the level of the gastroesophageal junction (GEJ). The LES contributes to reflux prevention by maintaining a pressure higher than intraabdominal (or intragastric) pressure. Reflux occurs if the LES barrier becomes incompetent, such as with transient LES relaxations (i.e., belching), a hypotensive LES (reduced LES muscle tone and LES pressure), or an anatomic disruption of the LES. In patients with normal LES anatomy and function reflux can still occur if intraabdominal pressure exceeds LES pressure.

Several conditions are associated with the development of GERD, including hiatal hernia, obesity, pregnancy, obstructive sleep apnea, gastric hypersecretion, gastric outlet obstruction, gastric neuropathy, and increased intraabdominal pressure (Table 29.4).

Diagnosis is made based on a combination of symptom presentation, objective testing (endoscopy, ambulatory reflux monitoring), and response to empiric antisecretory therapy.[22] Conservative management with lifestyle modification and medications are the mainstay of treatment for GERD. Lifestyle interventions include

Table 29.4	Conditions Associated With GERD	
Condition	**Mechanism**	**Comments**
Hiatal hernia	Esophageal dysmotility, impaired emptying, cephalad displacement of LES into thoracic cavity, supradiaphragmatic postprandial acid pocket	Multifactorial
Obesity and weight gain	Increased intraabdominal pressure, LES dysfunction	Also increased incidence of hiatal hernia
Pregnancy	Hormonal factors (estrogen and progesterone-mediated reduction in LES tone), mechanical factors (gravid uterus causing increased intraabdominal pressure, delayed gastric emptying and decreased bowel transit)	Also see Chapter 33
Food and medications	LES dysfunction	Large meals, fatty foods, spicy foods, alcohol; medications may include aspirin/NSAIDs, anticholinergics, antidepressants

LES, Lower esophageal sphincter; *NSAID,* nonsteroidal antiinflammatory drug.

Table 29.5 Drug Therapies for GERD

Medication	Mechanism	Comments
Antacids	Neutralize gastric fluid acidity by providing base to react with hydrogen ions	Antacids can be particulate (e.g., TUMS) or nonparticulate (e.g., Bicitra).
Mucoprotective drugs (e.g., sucralfate)	Provide a mucosal barrier from stomach acids	
Prokinetic agents (e.g., metoclopramide)	Promote esophageal and gastric motility through the combined effect of increased muscarinic activity and dopamine and serotonin receptor antagonism	Metoclopramide may cause extrapyramidal side effects, such as tardive dyskinesia.
Histamine$_2$-receptor antagonists (e.g., famotidine)	Reduce the secretion of gastric acid	Histamine$_2$-receptor antagonists may cause adverse central nervous system effects, such as confusion, agitation, and psychosis, especially in the elderly.
Proton pump inhibitors (PPIs; e.g., pantoprazole)	Reduce the secretion of gastric acid	PPIs provide faster and more complete symptom relief and wound healing. Certain PPIs have drug–drug interactions, including inhibiting the metabolism and elimination of warfarin, digoxin, phenytoin, and benzodiazepines.

From Katz PO, Gerson LB, Vela MF. Guidelines for the diagnosis and management of gastroesophageal reflux disease. *Am J Gastroenterol.* 2013;108(3):308–329.

weight loss, head of bed elevation, and smoking cessation. Further, avoidance of late-night meals or foods that can potentially aggravate symptoms by lowering LES tone is recommended.

Drug therapies are aimed at relieving symptoms through several mechanisms (Table 29.5).[22]

Perioperative Considerations

Patients with GERD are at greater risk for aspiration. As such, anesthetic planning and management aim to minimize the chance for pulmonary aspiration of gastric contents and its associated morbidity. Depending on the volume, acidity, and composition of the gastric contents, aspiration may lead to airway obstruction, chemical injury and inflammation, pneumonia, acute respiratory distress syndrome, and/or respiratory failure. Risk factors for aspiration pneumonitis include gastric fluid pH less than 2.5, volume of aspirate more than 0.4 mL/kg, aspirate containing particulate matter, and pregnancy greater than 18 weeks' gestation. Premedication with antacids or histamine$_2$-receptor antagonists may help to reduce the extent of injury if aspiration occurs, and prokinetic agents may help to reduce the aspirate volume. Proton pump inhibitors (PPIs) should be continued leading up to surgery.

Rapid-sequence induction and intubation (RSII) is often the induction technique of choice in patients at risk of aspiration pneumonitis. The goal of RSII is to complete the sequence of events from awake with intact airway reflexes to endotracheal intubation with the cuff inflated within the shortest time interval allowable. It is during this interval that the complete loss of airway reflexes occur and pulmonary aspiration risk is the highest. If a difficult intubation is anticipated on preoperative airway evaluation, an awake intubation may be indicated over an RSII. With RSII, achieving adequate depth of anesthesia (with or without neuromuscular blockade) is essential to avoid coughing, straining, or active vomiting with airway manipulation. Positive-pressure ventilation is avoided between induction and intubation to decrease the risk of gastric insufflation. Thorough preoxygenation and apneic oxygenation are necessary to increase the time until hypoxemia develops with apnea. Positioning with the head of the bed elevated places the larynx above the LES and aids in reducing the risk of passive regurgitation and aspiration. Although the application of cricoid pressure during RSII is often used to reduce the incidence of aspiration of gastric contents, its use is controversial. Multiple studies of cricoid pressure during RSII provide inconclusive results regarding technique and efficacy, and some studies suggest potential harm with cricoid pressure.[23–25] Patients at risk for aspiration on induction and intubation are also at risk on emergence and extubation. Precautions to minimize aspiration during emergence include decompressing the stomach with an orogastric tube, elevating the head of the bed, and ensuring intact airway reflexes before extubation.

Surgical management of GERD is reserved for patients unable to tolerate medical therapy, for those with persistent symptoms necessitating long-term therapy, or for those who develop complications despite optimal medical therapy. Of the various endoscopic and surgical

IV

interventions available, the most common antireflux operation is the Nissen fundoplication. The operation is most often performed laparoscopically and consists of reducing the herniated stomach, repairing the diaphragmatic defect, and performing a gastric wrap around the stomach and LES to prevent the regurgitation of gastric contents. Although the Nissen fundoplication is the most effective and durable antireflux procedure, it also has the greatest potential for postoperative dysphagia, difficulty with vomiting, and gas bloating.

ENDOCRINE DISORDERS

Diabetes Mellitus

In the United States diabetes mellitus is the seventh leading cause of death among adults and has a prevalence of approximately 13%.[26] Diabetes is a disorder of impaired glucose, fat, and protein metabolism that results from an inadequate supply of insulin, an inadequate tissue response to insulin, or a combination of both. The hallmark of the disease is increased circulating levels of serum glucose that, when left untreated, lead to diffuse microvascular and macrovascular lesions progressing to end-organ dysfunction. Notably, diabetes is the leading cause of renal failure requiring dialysis in young and middle-aged adults and the leading cause of blindness among adults aged 20 to 74 years. Patients with diabetes have a twofold increase in risk of cardiac death or ischemic stroke compared with patients without diabetes. Diabetes is classified into four broad categories: type 1 diabetes mellitus (T1DM), type 2 diabetes mellitus, gestational diabetes mellitus (GDM), and diabetes resulting from other causes.[27] T1DM is characterized by the absence of insulin production caused by autoimmune destruction of pancreatic β-cells, whereas T2DM involves a progressive loss of insulin secretion in combination with insulin resistance. GDM is glucose intolerance with onset first recognized during pregnancy. Diabetes resulting from other causes includes various disease states that either damage the pancreas or lead to imbalances in hormones affecting the action of insulin.

The most prevalent forms of diabetes are T1DM and T2DM, with the former accounting for 5% to 10% of cases and the latter for the remaining 90% to 95% of cases.[27] Historical paradigms characterized T1DM as rapidly progressive with juvenile onset and dependent on insulin. In contrast, T2DM was characterized by a more insidious presentation with adult onset and noninsulin dependent. In reality, both T1DM and T2DM are heterogenous diseases with considerable variability in clinical presentation and disease progression. Many individuals with diabetes do not easily fit into a single class; therefore the label is less important than understanding the underlying pathogenesis of the hyperglycemia in order to effectively guide treatment.

> **Box 29.1** Diagnostic Criteria for Diabetes Mellitus
>
> 1. Glycated hemoglobin (HbA$_{1C}$) ≥6.5%,
> 2. Fasting plasma glucose ≥126 mg/dL (7.0 mmol/L) after 8 hours of no caloric intake
> 3. Two-hour plasma glucose ≥200 mg/dL (11.1 mmol/L) during an oral glucose tolerance test
> 4. A random plasma glucose ≥200 mg/dL (11.1 mmol/L) in a patient with classic symptoms of hyperglycemia or hyperglycemic crisis

Data from American Diabetes Association. 2. Classification and diagnosis of diabetes: Standards of medical care in diabetes—2020. *Diabetes Care.* 2020; 43(Suppl 1):S14-S31.

Several different techniques may confirm a diagnosis of diabetes (Box 29.1). Classic symptoms of hyperglycemia include polyuria, polydipsia, weight loss, and blurred vision. As a surrogate for end-organ complications, each diagnostic criterion reflects the glycemic threshold observed for the risk of developing retinopathy.

Monitoring of blood glucose control is best performed by measuring HbA$_{1C}$ levels. During hyperglycemia, glucose can permanently combine with hemoglobin in red blood cells and form HbA$_{1C}$. Because red blood cells have a 120-day life span, HbA$_{1C}$ levels reflect the average blood glucose levels over a 2- to 3-month period and provide an indication of how well diabetes has been controlled during this time. Although HbA$_{1C}$ level is a reliable marker of chronic glycemia, random or fasting serum blood glucose levels provide information regarding acute control.

The primary goal of treatment for all forms of diabetes is glucose control, with a reasonable target for an HbA$_{1C}$ <7%. Although treatment starts with education regarding dietary and lifestyle interventions, most patients require pharmacologic therapy. Various classes of medications aim to address hyperglycemia via increasing insulin availability (endogenously or exogenously), improving sensitivity to insulin, delaying the delivery and absorption of carbohydrates from the gastrointestinal tract, increasing urinary glucose excretion, or a combination of these approaches.

Because of its efficacy and favorable risk profile, metformin is the preferred initial noninsulin glucose-lowering agent for T2DM. Metformin is a biguanide that decreases hepatic glucose output and enhances tissue sensitivity to insulin. If this fails to adequately control glucose, additional therapeutics may be indicated. A newer class of oral medications for T2DM are the sodium-glucose cotransporter-2 (SGLT2) inhibitors, also called "gliflozins," which promote urinary glucose excretion as the means to reduce blood glucose levels.[28] In 2015 the US. Food and Drug Administration (FDA) issued a safety warning that these drugs may lead to diabetic ketoacidosis (DKA) with glucose levels lower

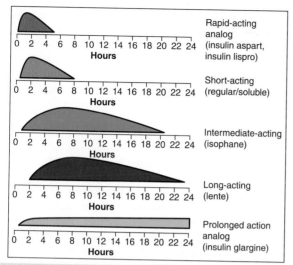

Fig. 29.1 Comparison of the onset and duration of different insulin preparations after subcutaneous administration. (From Chouhan R, Goswami S, Bajpai A. Recent advancements in oral delivery of insulin: From challenges to solutions. In Andronescu E, Grumezescu A, eds. *Nanostructures for Oral Medicine.* Elsevier; 2017:Figure 15.6.)

Table 29.6	Medical Conditions Associated With Diabetes	
Organ System	**Associated Conditions**	
Central nervous system	Retinopathy, vision loss Peripheral neuropathies Autonomic neuropathies Cerebrovascular disease, stroke Depression Cognitive impairment Disordered sleep	
Respiratory system	Inadequate ventilatory response to hypoxemia and hypercarbia	
Cardiovascular system	Hypertension Hyperlipidemia Orthostatic hypotension Cardiovascular instability Arrhythmias Accelerated atherosclerosis Congestive heart failure Coronary arterial disease, myocardial infarction Peripheral vascular disease, tissue ulceration	
Genitourinary system	Impotence Neurogenic bladder Renal failure	
Gastrointestinal system	Gastroparesis	
Musculoskeletal system	Decreased joint mobility Bone fractures	
Other	Delayed wound healing Increased susceptibility to infection Chronic pain Obesity Cancer	

than expected for DKA. This condition has been called "euglycemic DKA."

In patients with absolute or relative deficiencies in insulin, such as all patients with T1DM and many with advanced T2DM, insulin therapy is indicated. Insulin is categorized as rapid, intermediate, or long-acting (Fig. 29.1). With the goal of achieving a steady near-normoglycemic state, in the outpatient setting, insulin therapy is administered via continuous or intermittent subcutaneous injection with a combination of rapid and/or long-acting formulations tailored based on the anticipated glucose fluctuations of the individual patient.

Maintaining long-term near-normoglycemia is important for preventing and slowing the progression of the microvascular and macrovascular multiorgan diseases related to chronic systemic glucotoxicity (Table 29.6). Only a small fraction of patients with diabetes have no comorbidities. The most common comorbid diseases are retinopathy, nephropathy, autonomic neuropathy, cardiovascular disease, cerebrovascular disease, and obesity.

Perioperative Considerations

In the perioperative period the presence of many of the earlier-mentioned risk factors increases the incidence of adverse events. As such, before surgery, the evaluation and treatment of these diseases are essential in order to ensure optimization and subsequently avoid preventable morbidity and mortality. In addition to preexisting end-organ disease, extremes of glucose in the immediate perioperative period lead to injury. Hypoglycemia, when severe, can result in permanent brain damage. Hyperglycemia can result in decreased immune function, increased oxidative stress, endothelial dysfunction, increased inflammatory factors, procoagulant state, fluid shifts, and electrolyte fluxes.[29] This may subsequently result in poor wound healing, increased infections, delayed recovery, and further end-organ damage. Accordingly, an elevated HbA_{1c} or blood glucose preoperatively predicts worse perioperative outcome and may warrant postponement of a nonemergent surgery depending on the degree of elevation and associated conditions.[30]

The general goals of perioperative glucose control include the avoidance of hypoglycemia, the avoidance of hyperglycemia, and the prevention of acute, life-threatening consequences of both extremes, including ketoacidosis or nonketotic hyperosmolar syndrome. Preoperative diabetic medications should be adjusted to achieve these goals. Although most medication strategies

IV

are determined on a case-by-case basis, it is generally recommended to hold oral and/or noninsulin injectable hypoglycemic drugs the morning of surgery. Similarly, it is recommended to reduce the nighttime and/or morning dose of insulin by 20% to 50% in order to prevent hypoglycemia associated with preoperative fasting.[31] Intraoperatively, there is no consensus on a target glycemic range beyond avoidance of extremes in blood glucose. Adapted from studies mostly performed in the intensive care setting, such as the NICE-SUGAR trial, most society guidelines suggest maintaining glucose levels between 140 and 180 mg/dL (7.8 and 10 mmol/L) throughout surgery, as levels outside this range showed an increase in adverse events, including death.[30]

For patients with diabetes, blood glucose levels should be measured before and after surgery. The frequency of monitoring during the perioperative period depends on several factors, including if the patient has labile glycemic control, if they have received insulin of any type, and if they are critically ill. Additional perioperative factors that may contribute to glucose fluctuations include stress-induced neuroendocrine changes, decreased activity levels, altered nutritional intake, and glucocorticoid therapy. Because anesthesia may mask the signs and symptoms of hypoglycemia, glucose monitoring via point-of-care fingerstick or laboratory method may be necessary every hour. Medications to treat hypoglycemia, such as glucagon or dextrose, should be readily available. Laboratory monitoring to ensure physiologic electrolyte, acid–base, and fluid balance may be required as well.[30]

Additional perioperative planning depends on the end-organ complications of each patient. Preparation for anticipated difficult mask ventilation or intubation may be required in a patient with obesity or limited joint mobility. Aspiration precautions must be considered if there is concern for gastroparesis. Advanced cardiovascular monitoring may be indicated in patients with cardiac or cerebrovascular disease. The presence of renal insufficiency may alter drug and fluid management. Patients with existing neuropathies and arthropathies require careful positioning and pressure point padding (also see Chapter 19).

Thyroid Disease

The thyroid gland is situated in the anterior neck, wrapping around the front of the larynx and trachea. The secretion of thyroid hormones, triiodothyronine (T_3) and thyroxine (T_4), is regulated by thyroid-stimulating hormone (TSH), which is secreted from the anterior pituitary gland.

Thyroid hormones have many essential roles in the body, including regulation of metabolic rate, body temperature, gut motility and absorption, breakdown of glucose, breakdown of fats, cardiac inotropy and chronotropy,

respiratory rate, and oxygen consumption. Thyroid hormones are also essential for normal growth and brain development.

Thyroid disorders include hypothyroidism, hyperthyroidism, thyroid inflammation (thyroiditis), and thyroid enlargement (goiter), all of which may have implications for anesthetic management.[32]

Hypothyroidism

Hypothyroidism is characterized by deficient secretion of thyroid hormones. The most common causes are iodine deficiency and autoimmune (Hashimoto thyroiditis). Symptoms include unexpected weight gain, fatigue, constipation, heavy menstrual bleeding, hair loss, cold intolerance, bradycardia, and depression. Severe hypothyroidism can present with decreased mental status, hypoventilation, hypothermia, hypotension, congestive heart failure, hyponatremia, and hypoglycemia. Laboratory testing shows elevated TSH levels or reduced T_4 levels. Treatment of hypothyroidism includes thyroid hormone replacement. In severe presentations a stress dose steroid is often also given to mitigate complications from coexisting adrenal insufficiency.[32]

Perioperative Considerations

Patients should be clinically stable and medically euthyroid before elective surgeries. Prescribed medical therapy should be continued on the day of surgery. Coexisting conditions to screen for include adrenal insufficiency, hypoglycemia, anemia, and hyponatremia. If a goiter is present, preoperative evaluation and imaging should be done to assess risk factors for difficult intubation or hemodynamic collapse on induction, including dyspnea, dysphagia, voice change, assessment of airway or great blood vessel compression, tracheal deviation, tracheomalacia, or retrosternal extension.

If a symptomatic hypothyroid patient must undergo urgent or emergent surgery, extra caution is required. Hypothyroid patients may be hypersensitive to the respiratory depressant effects of premedications. In addition, because of reduced cardiac output and diminished baroreceptor reflexes, induction agents that preserve hemodynamic stability such as etomidate or ketamine should be considered. Mask ventilation and intubation may be more difficult in patients with a large goiter or enlarged tongue. Hypothyroid patients are also more susceptible to intraoperative hypothermia, slow drug metabolism, and delayed emergence from anesthesia.

Hyperthyroidism and Thyroid Storm

Hyperthyroidism is characterized by excess circulating thyroid hormone (T_3 or T_4). The most common causes are autoimmune (Graves disease), toxic multinodular goiter, and thyroiditis. Symptoms include weight loss, muscle weakness, insomnia, heat intolerance, diarrhea, tremor, tachyarrhythmias (e.g., new-onset atrial fibrillation), and anxiety. Goiters may be present in severe cases.

Laboratory testing shows elevated serum T_4 and T_3 with a reduced TSH level. Rapid management of symptoms can be achieved with β-blockers. Long-term management aimed at thyroid suppression may be achieved with medications (propylthiouracil, carbimazole, and methimazole), radioactive iodine destruction, or surgical removal.

Perioperative Considerations

Patients should be clinically stable, asymptomatic, and medically euthyroid (normal serum T_4 and T_3) before elective surgeries. Medical therapy, including β-blockers and thyroid suppression medications, should be continued on the day of surgery. Patients with goiters should be evaluated for potential airway compromise or mediastinal extension.

If a patient with uncontrolled hyperthyroidism must undergo urgent or emergent surgery, adrenergic overactivity and tachycardia can be controlled with short-acting β-blockers. Avoid sympathomimetic drugs such as ketamine and ephedrine. Relative hypovolemia in active hyperthyroidism has the potential to exacerbate hemodynamic changes. Exophthalmos is associated with an increased risk of corneal abrasion.

In addition, laryngoscopy, surgical stimulation, or tissue manipulation may precipitate a *thyroid storm,* which can present any time in the perioperative period. The presentation may include tachycardia, hemodynamic lability, fever, and diaphoresis. It can be distinguished from malignant hyperthermia by lack of rigidity or respiratory acidosis. Management includes supportive care, hydration, β-blockade, antithyroid medication, and removal of the precipitating cause.[33]

Thyroidectomy Postoperative Complications

Anesthesia providers should be aware of potential immediate postoperative complications after thyroid surgery. Recurrent laryngeal nerve (RLN) damage presents as hoarseness (unilateral) or stridor (bilateral). Transient hoarseness is also common and may result from glottic edema. Intraoperative real-time monitoring of RLN function assists in identification and protection and results in decreased incidence of injury. Some surgeons request placement of a neural integrity monitor (NIM) endotracheal tube, which incorporates electromyography (EMG) as part of the RLN identification process. Specifically, the surgeon uses a sterile probe that administers a small electrical current. If the RLN is stimulated, the vocal cords move, producing an EMG signal that is converted to an audible signal. Neuromuscular blockade must be avoided during this portion of the procedure.

Postoperative neck hematoma may also cause airway compromise and require bedside reopening of the surgical incision for hematoma management and urgent airway management. Risk of hematoma formation can be reduced by mitigating hypertension and coughing during emergence and extubation. Based on risk factors and comfort, consider deep extubation or administration of remifentanil, dexmedetomidine, or lidocaine at emergence. If there is stridor after extubation, immediate reintubation may be necessary.

Acute hypocalcemia resulting from unintentional removal of the parathyroid glands can present within 12 to 72 hours after surgery. Postoperative measurement of serum calcium with or without parathyroid hormone (PTH) aids in diagnosis. Preemptive calcium and vitamin D supplementation may be administered. Alternatively, PTH levels can be measured intraoperatively.[33]

Parathyroid Disease

Four parathyroid glands are typically located on the posterior side of the lateral lobes of the thyroid gland. The major function of the parathyroid glands is to produce and secrete PTH, which regulates the body's serum calcium and phosphate levels. In response to PTH, serum calcium levels are increased through increased bone resorption, reduced renal excretion, and increased gastrointestinal absorption. Parathyroid disorders include those that cause hyperparathyroidism and those that cause hypoparathyroidism.

Primary hyperparathyroidism results in excess levels of circulating PTH and serum calcium. Though the most common presentation is asymptomatic hypercalcemia, symptoms related to hypercalcemia may include bone pain (because of increased bone resorption), dehydration, and altered mental status. Primary hyperparathyroidism is most often managed by surgical removal of the abnormal parathyroid gland.[34,35]

Secondary hyperparathyroidism is most commonly the result of chronic kidney disease (CKD) or vitamin D deficiency. Patients with CKD have reduced urinary phosphate excretion. Phosphate retention induces hypocalcemia, which results in parathyroid hyperplasia with elevated PTH and low serum calcium or vitamin D. PTH-related peptide secreted by various types of malignant tumors is the most common cause of hypercalcemia in hospitalized patients.

Hypoparathyroidism is most commonly the result of postsurgical or autoimmune destruction of the parathyroid glands. Pseudohypoparathyroidism occurs when parathyroid glands appropriately produce PTH but target organs do not respond appropriately to the hormone. Symptoms of the hypocalcemia associated with these conditions include tetany (Chvostek sign or Trousseau sign), laryngospasm, stridor, altered mental status, paresthesias, seizures, and congestive heart failure. Hypoparathyroidism and pseudohypoparathyroidism are managed with calcium supplementation.

IV

Perioperative Considerations

Patients should have normalized serum calcium levels and be asymptomatic without electrocardiogram changes before elective surgery. In addition, their preoperative evaluation should rule out concurrent thyroid disease. During parathyroidectomy, intraoperative PTH testing can help determine when an overactive parathyroid gland has been removed. Blood samples can be drawn from a peripheral vein, arterial catheter, or by the surgeon from the internal jugular vein in the operative field. Postoperatively patients should be monitored for hematoma, vocal cord dysfunction, and symptomatic hypocalcemia.[35]

Adrenal Cortex Dysfunction

The adrenal glands, situated in the retroperitoneum above the kidneys within the renal fascia, are composed of an outer cortex and inner medulla. The adrenal cortex produces three main types of steroid hormones: mineralocorticoids, glucocorticoids, and androgens. The adrenal medulla contains chromaffin cells that produce the catecholamines epinephrine and norepinephrine.

Mineralocorticoids, such as aldosterone, help regulate blood pressure and electrolyte homeostasis. Glucocorticoids, such as cortisol, regulate metabolism and immune function. Both of these are essential hormones with major physiologic significance, and dysfunction in either of the systems has anesthetic implications.

Mineralocorticoid Excess

Hyperaldosteronism occurs when there are increased levels of aldosterone. In primary hyperaldosteronism there is hypersecretion of aldosterone by the adrenal cortex in the setting of a unilateral adenoma (Conn syndrome), bilateral hyperplasia, or adrenal gland carcinoma. Secondary hyperaldosteronism occurs in the setting of a disease state that stimulates aldosterone secretion through activation of the renin–angiotensin–aldosterone system, such as congestive heart failure, hepatic cirrhosis, nephrotic syndrome, and certain types of hypertension. Clinical manifestations of hyperaldosteronism are a result of increased tubular exchange of sodium for potassium and hydrogen ion, and include hypokalemic alkalosis, hypertension and fluid retention, skeletal muscle weakness, and fatigue.

Patients with primary aldosteronism have higher rates of stroke, myocardial infarction, and atrial fibrillation compared with patients with non–aldosterone-mediated hypertension.[36] Preoperative assessment may require cardiac imaging, including chest x-ray and echocardiography, to determine the extent and status of cardiovascular disease. Perioperative management in these patients focuses primarily on correcting intravascular volume and electrolyte status. Elevated blood pressure and hypokalemia may be addressed by administration of an aldosterone antagonist (e.g., spironolactone) or restricting sodium intake. Hypokalemia is associated with increased myocardial excitability and an increased risk of arrhythmias.[36] Careful potassium repletion may be required to restore intracellular and extracellular potassium balance.

Glucocorticoid Excess

Glucocorticoid excess may be related to hyperfunction of the adrenal cortex (primary disease), hypersecretion of adrenocorticotropic hormone (ACTH) by a pituitary adenoma (Cushing disease), production of ACTH-like substance by a nonpituitary tumor, or exogenous glucocorticoid administration. In each scenario cortisol excess produces Cushing syndrome, which is characterized by hypertension and fluid retention, impaired glucose metabolism, central obesity, hyperlipidemia, hypercoagulability, osteoporosis, altered mental status and emotional lability, and muscular weakness.

Perioperative planning must take the various systemic effects of Cushing syndrome into consideration. An assessment of cardiac risk factors should guide additional workup as necessary. Before surgery, hyperlipidemia and hypertension should be optimized. Similar to hyperaldosteronism, diuresis with spironolactone may help to mobilize excess intravascular fluid and restore electrolyte balance. Serum glucose should be monitored and corrected as necessary. Patients with bone density loss are at increased risk for fracture, and careful pressure point padding and positioning may be required. Patients receiving exogenous steroids may require supplemental steroid administration, as their adrenal glands may be unable to respond appropriately to the stress of surgery. Similarly, patients undergoing unilateral or bilateral adrenal resection will require glucocorticoid replacement therapy. In patients with significant skeletal muscle wasting consideration should be taken regarding the use of muscle relaxants.

Adrenal Insufficiency

Undersecretion of adrenal steroid hormones may result from either an inability of the adrenal glands to produce adequate amounts of hormones (primary adrenal insufficiency or Addison disease) or a deficiency in the production of ACTH (secondary adrenal insufficiency). Primary adrenal insufficiency is commonly caused by atrophy or destruction of the adrenal glands, whereas secondary adrenal insufficiency is often caused by pituitary dysfunction, traumatic brain injury, or long-term exogenous glucocorticoid use. Whereas primary adrenal insufficiency results in a combined deficiency of both mineralocorticoids and glucocorticoids, secondary adrenal insufficiency results primarily in an isolated deficiency of glucocorticoids with preserved mineralocorticoid production. It is uncommon for any type of adrenal insufficiency to result in an isolated deficiency of mineralocorticoids. Symptoms depend on the extent of adrenal function loss, whether mineralocorticoid function is preserved, and the degree of physiologic stress. Common features of any type of adrenal insufficiency include fatigue, weight loss, nonspecific abdominal complaints, myalgias, and arthralgias. Patients with primary adrenal insufficiency may also present with skin hyperpigmentation, salt craving, and postural hypotension.

Preoperative laboratory tests should include an electrolyte panel. Hyponatremia, hyperkalemia, or hypoglycemia should be appropriately addressed. Even asymptomatic adrenally insufficient patients may experience acute adrenal insufficiency, or *adrenal crisis,* during the perioperative period. During stress caused by illness or surgery, the secretion of cortisol by the adrenal cortex can transiently increase from a basal rate of approximately 10 mg/day up to 150 mg/day, depending on the stressor or magnitude of surgery. This relative lack of cortisol can lead to vasodilation and hypotension. Although the predominant manifestation is shock or hypotension unresponsive to typical vasopressors and fluid support, patients often have nonspecific symptoms such as acute abdominal pain, weakness, electrolyte disturbance, unexplained fever, confusion, or coma. Patients with primary adrenal insufficiency are at significantly higher risk for developing perioperative symptoms than those with a secondary deficiency. Maintenance steroid supplementation should not be missed, including on the day of surgery. An additional "stress dose" steroid should be administered to patients with primary adrenal insufficiency before any physiologically stressful procedure. For patients with secondary adrenal insufficiency from exogenous steroid administration, the administration of additional steroids beyond the baseline dose is an area of controversy.[37] One approach is to continue the preoperative steroid dose and administer a "rescue" steroid dose (e.g., hydrocortisone 50 to 100 mg) only if refractory hypotension develops. Another approach is to administer additional steroid based on the risk of hypothalamic–pituitary–adrenal axis (HPAA) suppression and the stress of surgery. For example, a patient with high risk of HPAA suppression (e.g., on prednisone at least 20 mg/day for >3 weeks) undergoing major surgery (e.g., cardiac surgery, esophagectomy, acute trauma) will receive hydrocortisone 100 mg IV before incision and 50 mg every 8 hours for 24 hours. A patient with low risk of HPAA suppression (e.g., on steroids <3 weeks or on prednisone less than 5 mg/day) would not receive stress-dose steroids unless refractory hypotension developed.[37]

Pheochromocytoma and Paraganglioma

Pheochromocytoma is a rare chromaffin cell tumor that occurs inside of the adrenal gland (adrenal medulla), and a paraganglioma is a chromaffin cell tumor that occurs outside of the adrenal gland. These neuroendocrine tumors, when hormonally active, can produce and release large amounts of catecholamines and metanephrines.

The signs and symptoms of hormonally active pheochromocytomas and paragangliomas are caused by sympathetic nervous system hyperactivity. The classic triad includes paroxysmal headaches (hypertension), tachycardia, and diaphoresis. Other common symptoms include heat intolerance, weight loss, chest discomfort, nausea and vomiting, orthostatic hypotension, constipation, anxiety, hyperglycemia, and hyperresponsiveness to noxious stimuli. Symptoms may be constant or paroxysmal. Severe catecholamine surges can cause hypertensive emergencies with end-organ damage.[38]

Pheochromocytoma multisystem crisis is a rare and extreme presentation with hemodynamic instability, hyperthermia (>40°C), neurologic manifestations, and multiorgan failure. This severe presentation may not respond to α-antagonism, and emergent surgery may be required. Another rare presentation is severe hemodynamic instability during induction of anesthesia, intubation, or surgical manipulation.[38,39]

The gold standard for diagnosing pheochromocytomas is elevated plasma fractionated metanephrines (metanephrine and normetanephrine) along with anatomic evidence of the tumor. Twenty-four-hour urinary metanephrines are used when plasma testing is unavailable. Anatomic imaging with contrast-enhanced computed tomography (CT) or T2-weighted magnetic resonance imaging (MRI) is used to localize the tumor and also gain information about size and relation to adjacent anatomic structures.[39,40]

Pheochromocytomas and paragangliomas are treated with surgical resection. Depending on size, location, and adjacent structure involvement, a minimally invasive (laparoscopic or robotic) or open technique may be chosen.[39]

Perioperative Considerations

Multidisciplinary teams should be involved in the preoperative evaluation and optimization of patients with pheochromocytomas and paragangliomas. The primary goals are to minimize catecholamine surges and evaluate for end-organ damage.

End-organ effects that may have implications for anesthetic management include the following: hypovolemia, aortic dissection, myocardial ischemia, toxic myocarditis, catecholamine-induced cardiomyopathy, hypertrophic or dilated cardiomyopathy, congestive heart failure, tachyarrhythmias, and acute stroke. Preoperative electrocardiogram and echocardiogram are indicated to evaluate cardiovascular function.[36,38] In addition, preoperative laboratory tests should include electrolytes, blood glucose, blood urea nitrogen, creatinine, and complete blood count.[36,38]

Perioperative catecholamine surges may be triggered by a variety of medications, noxious stimuli

IV

(including intubation), or intraoperative tumor manipulation. Therefore adequate preoperative adrenergic blockade is essential. The US Endocrine Society in conjunction with the European Society of Endocrinology recommends preoperative α-adrenoceptor blockade for 7 to 14 days before surgery to allow adequate time to normalize hemodynamic parameters.[40] Moderate symptoms can be managed with a selective, short-acting α$_1$ adrenoceptor antagonist (doxazosin, prazosin, terazosin). More significant clinical presentations are preferentially treated with a nonselective α$_1$ and α$_2$ adrenoceptor antagonist (phenoxybenzamine). Calcium channel blockers can also be used either in conjunction with α-blockade or when side effects are not tolerated.[36,38]

β-Adrenoceptor antagonists are also used to control heart rate after α-blockade has adequately normalized blood pressure.[41,42] Selective β$_1$ adrenoceptor antagonists (atenolol, metoprolol) are preferred. However, it is advised that β-antagonists should never be used alone or started before α-antagonists because blockade of vasodilatory peripheral β-adrenergic receptors with unopposed α-adrenergic stimulation can lead to uncontrolled hypertension.[38,40]

Relative hypovolemia caused by catecholamine excess activity makes individuals susceptible to intraoperative hypotension. Society guidelines recommend a high-sodium diet and adequate fluid intake before surgery.[40] In addition, preoperative intravascular volume resuscitation may be considered.[36]

Intraoperative management should begin with premedication as necessary to minimize anxiety. It is recommended to achieve an adequate depth of anesthesia before intubation and incision. Communication between anesthesia provider and surgeon, along with familiarity with the steps of the resection, help to anticipate and mitigate intraoperative hemodynamic variability. The first phase of the surgery, during which the tumor and its vascular supply are manipulated and isolated, is often the most turbulent. Hypertension can be treated with intravenous phentolamine, nitroprusside, nicardipine, clevidipine, labetalol, or esmolol. Magnesium has also emerged as an antihypertensive and antiarrhythmic medication with a favorable side effect profile. Tachyarrhythmias can be treated with esmolol, lidocaine, or amiodarone. After the tumor's efferent blood supply is clamped, hypotension necessitating vasopressor support is a common occurrence. Hypotension can be treated with volume resuscitation, phenylephrine, norepinephrine, vasopressin, and/or dopamine.[38]

General anesthesia with endotracheal intubation is the most common anesthetic approach. Continuous intraarterial blood pressure monitoring is appropriate for patients with hormonally active tumors, often placed before induction and intubation. Large-bore intravenous access for volume resuscitation in addition to a reliable line for vasoactive medications are recommended.[38] For open surgical procedures, epidural analgesia can help manage perioperative pain. When placing an epidural in patients with pheochromocytomas and paragangliomas, consider giving premedication to reduce anxiety, avoiding epinephrine in the test dose, and running low-concentration local anesthetic intraoperatively to avoid significant vasodilation and sympathectomy-induced hemodynamic lability.

Multiple common perioperative medications have the potential to trigger catecholamine surges. Anesthesia providers should attempt to avoid sympathomimetic medications (ketamine, ephedrine, meperidine), dopamine-blocking medications (metoclopramide, chlorpromazine, prochlorperazine, droperidol, haloperidol), proarrhythmics (halothane), and histamine-stimulating medications (morphine, atracurium).[38]

The most common postoperative concern is postresection hypotension caused by residual α-adrenoceptor antagonism after the removal of the catecholamine-secreting tumor. This is a particular issue with the use of phenoxybenzamine, which is an irreversible, long-acting α-adrenergic blocking agent. Postoperative hypertension is also common for 1 to 3 days after surgery. If the hypertension persists, this may be caused by incomplete resection, pain, or coexisting essential hypertension. Blood glucose fluctuations should be monitored, as hypoglycemia could develop after catecholamine suppression of insulin activity subsides. β-blockade and residual anesthesia may mask symptoms of hypoglycemia.[36] Other less common complications include adrenal insufficiency with bilateral adrenalectomies, acute kidney injury, volume overload, pulmonary complications, and thromboembolic events.[43]

Pituitary Gland Dysfunction

The pituitary gland, or hypophysis, is an endocrine gland that sits in the sella turcica of the sphenoid bone at the base of the brain. The anterior pituitary secretes hormones that regulate several physiologic processes, including human growth hormone (hGH), ACTH, TSH, gonadotropic hormones (luteinizing hormone [LH] and follicle-stimulating hormone [FSH]), and prolactin. The posterior pituitary secretes hormones produced in the hypothalamus, including vasopressin (antidiuretic hormone [ADH]) and oxytocin.

The pituitary gland disorders most impactful to anesthetic management include acromegaly, Cushing syndrome (described earlier), prolactinoma, panhypopituitarism, syndrome of inappropriate antidiuretic hormone secretion (SIADH), and diabetes insipidus (DI).

Acromegaly

Acromegaly is characterized by excess growth hormone in adults (after growth plates have closed). Presenting signs and symptoms include enlarged hands and feet, enlarged facial features, deepening of the voice, head-aches, obstructive sleep apnea, hypertension, and glucose intolerance. These patients also have increased inci-dence of left ventricular hypertrophy, heart failure, and arrhythmias. Acromegaly is most commonly caused by a pituitary adenoma; transsphenoidal surgical resection is the preferred treatment.

Preoperative evaluation of patients with acromegaly should include a careful cardiac evaluation with electrocar-diogram. Blood sugar should be monitored perioperatively and treated as appropriate. An airway management plan should take into account potentially increased difficulty in mask ventilation and/or endotracheal intubation caused by upper airway changes common in acromegaly: macroglos-sia, enlarged epiglottis, enlarged mandible, subglottic nar-rowing, and enlarged nasal turbinates. For patients with obstructive sleep apnea, it should be noted that postopera-tive noninvasive positive-pressure ventilation is relatively contraindicated after transsphenoidal surgery.

Prolactinoma

A prolactinoma is a hyper-prolactin-secreting tumor of the pituitary gland. Prolactinomas are the most common type of functional pituitary tumor and are classified as either microprolactinoma (<10 mm) or macroprolacti-noma (>10 mm). Hyperprolactinemia causes galactor-rhea, amenorrhea, hypogonadism, and gynecomastia. Tumors with mass effect cause headaches, visual field changes, and cranial nerve palsies. Medical management with dopamine agonists (bromocriptine, cabergoline) help reduce tumor size and normalize prolactin levels. Unfortunately, they both have significant side effects. Transsphenoidal surgical resection is suggested if medical therapy is not tolerated or fails.

Hypopituitarism

Hypopituitarism describes decreased secretion of one or more of the hormones secreted by the pituitary gland. With any pituitary dysfunction, all other pituitary hor-mone levels should be checked and replaced with exog-enous hormone supplements as appropriate.

Syndrome of Inappropriate Antidiuretic Hormone Secretion

SIADH is characterized by excessive secretion of ADH, which results in water retention, volume overload, serum hyponatremia and hypoosmolarity, and urine hyperna-tremia (urine sodium > 30 mEq/L) and hyperosmolarity (urine osmolality > 100 mOsm/kg H_2O). Perioperative man-agement of SIADH depends on severity and acuity of the hyponatremia and whether symptoms are present. Plasma sodium levels should be closely followed. Asymptomatic and mild hyponatremia can be treated with salt intake and fluid restriction. Symptomatic and moderate hyponatremia can be treated with furosemide and normal saline infu-sion. For patients with severe symptoms of hyponatremia (confusion, seizures, coma), 3% hypertonic saline should be used cautiously. A risk of over-rapid correction of serum sodium levels is osmotic demyelination syndrome.

Central Diabetes Insipidus

Central DI is characterized by decreased ADH production resulting in polyuria, hypernatremia, hypokalemia, and dehydration. Perioperatively, it is important to moni-tor urine output and serum electrolytes and attempt to maintain euvolemia. Administration of preoperative vas-opressin analogue (desmopressin) or intraoperative vaso-pressin helps prevent significant intraoperative fluid loss.

Neuroendocrine Tumors

Neuroendocrine tumors are neoplasms that arise from cells of the neuroendocrine system. The majority of these tumors are nonfunctional; however, some functional tumors are capable of hormone overproduction. Surgical resection is the treatment of choice for localized pancre-atic neuroendocrine tumors, and surgical debulking may be of benefit in metastatic disease.[44]

Functional neuroendocrine tumors with implications for anesthetic management include insulinomas, gas-trinomas, VIPomas, and carcinoid tumors. Insulinomas secrete excess insulin, causing hypoglycemia that can worsen with preoperative fasting. Hyperglycemia may occur after insulinoma resection. Close blood glucose monitoring and treatment are required perioperatively. Gastrinomas secrete excess gastrin causing peptic ulcer disease, diarrhea, and esophageal reflux. Perioperative care includes treatment with H2 antagonists and PPIs, rapid-sequence intubation, and rehydration. VIPomas secrete excess vasoactive intestinal peptide (VIP) caus-ing watery diarrhea, flushing, hypotension, dehydration, hypokalemia, achlorhydria, and metabolic acidosis. Fluid deficits should be corrected preoperatively and a soma-tostatin analogue (octreotide) started.[45]

Carcinoid Tumor

Carcinoid tumors are neuroendocrine tumors that secrete excess vasoactive hormones, notably serotonin, brady-kinins, prostaglandins, tachykinins, substance P, and/or histamine. Carcinoid tumors primarily occur in the gas-trointestinal tract, most commonly in the midgut (ileum and appendix). Vasoactive substances released by tumors isolated to the gastrointestinal tract are largely metabo-lized by the liver, preventing significant systemic effects. However, when vasoactive substances do not go through hepatic degradation in the setting of metastatic spread, the symptoms of carcinoid syndrome are seen.

Carcinoid syndrome presents as flushing, tachycardia, hypotension, lacrimation, peripheral edema, abdominal pain, diarrhea, dehydration, electrolyte abnormalities, bronchoconstriction, and right-sided valvular heart dis-ease. In the short term, somatostatin analogs (octreotide)

IV

can ameliorate symptoms of carcinoid syndrome by blocking the production and release of vasoactive mediators; however, with time, patients often become refractory to somatostatin analogs. Surgical resection is the most effective treatment.

Preoperative evaluation of patients with carcinoid tumor should determine the severity and impact of symptoms. Cardiac evaluation should include electrocardiogram and echocardiography. Fluid and electrolyte abnormalities should be corrected.

The primary goal of intraoperative management of patients with carcinoid tumor is to minimize vasoactive substance release. Octreotide should be started preoperatively, continued intraoperatively, and tapered off postoperatively. Other common premedications include benzodiazepines (anxiolysis), antihistamines, and ondansetron (antiserotonin).

Intraoperative management aims to minimize anxiety, noxious stimuli, hypercapnia, and hypothermia, all of which may stimulate vasoactive substance release. Hypotension can be treated with fluid bolus, octreotide, phenylephrine, and/or vasopressin. Sympathomimetic agents (e.g., epinephrine) and histamine-stimulating medications can theoretically stimulate the release of vasoactive substances from the tumor and exacerbate hemodynamic instability. Intraoperative hypertension can be treated with octreotide or β-adrenergic blockade.[46]

REFERENCES

1. Centers for Disease Control and Prevention (CDC). Prevalence of overweight, obesity, and extreme obesity among adults: United States, 2017–2018. February 2020. https://www.cdc.gov/nchs/products/databriefs/db360.htm. Accessed October 13, 2020.
2. World Health Organization (WHO). Obesity and overweight fact sheet. 2020. https://www.who.int/news-room/fact-sheets/detail/obesity-and-overweight. Accessed October 13, 2020.
3. Adams JP, Murphy PG. Obesity in anaesthesia and intensive care. *Br J Anaesth.* 2000;85:91–108.
4. Lang LH, Parekh K, Tsui BYK, Maze M. Perioperative management of the obese surgical patient. *Br Med Bull.* 2017;124(1):135–155.
5. Glance LG, Wissler R, Mukamel DB, et al. Perioperative outcomes among patients with the modified metabolic syndrome who are undergoing noncardiac surgery. *Anesthesiology.* 2010;113:859.
6. Joshi GP, Ahmad S, Riad W, et al. Selection of obese patients undergoing ambulatory surgery: A systematic review of the literature. *Anesth Analg.* 2013;117:1082.
7. American Society of Anesthesiologists Committee. Practice guidelines for preoperative fasting and the use of pharmacologic agents to reduce the risk of pulmonary aspiration: Application to healthy patients undergoing elective procedures: An updated report by the American Society of Anesthesiologists Committee on Standards and Practice Parameters. *Anesthesiology.* 2011;114:495.
8. Eley VA, Christensen R, Guy L, Dodd B. Perioperative blood pressure monitoring in patients with obesity. *Anesth Analg.* 2019;128:484.
9. Jensen MD, Ryan DH, Apovian CM, et al. 2013 AHA/ACC/TOS guideline for the management of overweight and obesity in adults: A report of the American College of Cardiology/American Heart Association Task Force on Practice Guidelines and the Obesity Society. *Circulation.* 2014;129(25 suppl 2):S102–S138.
10. De Jong A, Molinari N, Pouzeratte Y, et al. Difficult intubation in obese patients: incidence, risk factors, and complications in the operating theatre and in intensive care units. *Br J Anaesth.* 2015;114:297–306.
11. Hodgson LE, Murphy PB, Hart N. Respiratory management of the obese patient undergoing surgery. *J Thorac Dis.* 2015;7:943–952.
12. Baker MT. The history and evolution of bariatric surgical procedures. *Surg Clin North Am.* 2011;91:1181–1201.
13. Wolfe BM, Kvach E, Eckel RH. Treatment of obesity: Weight loss and bariatric surgery. *Circ Res.* 2016;118(11):1844–1855.
14. World Health Organization. What is malnutrition? 2016. www.who.int/features/qa/malnutrition/en (Accessed on October 22, 2020).
15. Jensen GL, Cederholm T, Correia MITD, et al. GLIM criteria for the diagnosis of malnutrition: A consensus report from the Global Clinical Nutrition Community. *JPEN J Parenter Enteral Nutr.* 2019;43:32.
16. Edwards S. Anaesthetising the malnourished patient. *Update Anaesth.* 2016;31:31–37.
17. Ananthakrishnan AN. Epidemiology and risk factors for IBD. *Nat Rev Gastroenterol Hepatol.* 2015;12(4):205–217.
18. Nickerson, et al. Perioperative considerations in Crohn disease and ulcerative colitis. *Clin Colon Rectal Surg.* 2016;29:80–84.
19. Kumar A, Auron M, Aneja A, Mohr F, Jain A, Shen B. Inflammatory bowel disease: Perioperative pharmacological considerations. *Mayo Clin Proc.* 2011;86(8):748–757.
20. El-Serag HB, Sweet S, Winchester CC, Dent J. Update on the epidemiology of gastro-oesophageal reflux disease: A systematic review. *Gut.* 2014;63(6):871–880.
21. Boeckxstaens G, El-Serag HB, Smout AJ, Kahrilas PJ. Symptomatic reflux disease: The present, the past and the future. *Gut.* 2014;63:1185.
22. Katz PO, Gerson LB, Vela MF. Guidelines for the diagnosis and management of gastroesophageal reflux disease. *Am J Gastroenterol.* 2013;108(3):308–329.
23. Zdravkovic M, Rice MJ, Brull SJ. The clinical use of cricoid pressure: First, do no harm. *Anesth Analg.* 2019.
24. Algie CM, Mahar RK, Tan HB, et al. Effectiveness and risks of cricoid pressure during rapid sequence induction for endotracheal intubation. *Cochrane Database Syst Rev.* 2015: CD011656.
25. Birenbaum A, Hajage D, Roche S, et al. Effect of cricoid pressure compared with a sham procedure in the rapid sequence induction of anesthesia: The IRIS randomized clinical trial. *JAMA Surg.* 2019;154:9.
26. Center for Disease Control. National Diabetes Statistics Report, 2020. *Estimates of diabetes and its burden in the United States.* www.cdc.gov/diabetes/pdfs/data/statistics/national-diabetes-statistics-report.pdf Accessed on December 10, 2020.
27. American Diabetes Association 2. Classification and diagnosis of diabetes: *Standards of Medical Care in Diabetes* 2020. Jan;43(Supplement 1):S14–S31.
28. Peacock SC, Lovshin JA, Cherney DZI. Perioperative considerations for the use of sodium-glucose cotransporter-2

inhibitors in patients with type 2 diabetes. *Anesth Analg.* 2018 Feb;126(2):699–704. doi:10.1213/ANE.0000000000002377. PMID: 28786838.

29. Akhtar S, Barash PG, Inzucchi SE. Scientific principles and clinical implications of perioperative glucose regulation and control. *Anesth Analg.* 2010;110(2):478–497.

30. Sudhakaran S, Surani SR. Guidelines for perioperative management of the diabetic patient. *Surg Res Pract.* 2015;2015:284063.

31. Alexanian SM, McDonnell ME, Akhtar S. Creating a perioperative glycemic control program. *Anesthesiol Res Pract.* 2011;2011:465974.

32. Bacuzzi A, Dionigi G, Del Bosco A, Cantone G, Sansone T, Di Losa E, Cuffari S. Anaesthesia for thyroid surgery: Perioperative management. *Int J Surg.* 2008;6(Suppl 1):S82–S85.

33. Patel KN, Yip L, Lubitz CC, Grubbs EG, Miller BS, Shen W, Angelos P, Chen H, Doherty GM, Fahey TJ 3rd, Kebebew E, Livolsi VA, Perrier ND, Sipos JA, Sosa JA, Steward D, Tufano RP, McHenry CR, Carty SE. The American Association of Endocrine Surgeons guidelines for the definitive surgical management of thyroid disease in adults. *Ann Surg.* 2020 Mar;271(3):e21–e93 .

34. Bilezikian JP, Bandeira L, Khan A, Cusano NE. Hyperparathyroidism. *Lancet.* 2018 Jan 13; 391(10116):168–178.

35. Wilhelm SM, Wang TS, Ruan DT, et al. The American Association of Endocrine Surgeons guidelines for definitive management of primary hyperparathyroidism. *JAMA Surg.* 2016;151(10):959–968.

36. Phitayakorn R, McHenry CR. Perioperative considerations in patients with adrenal tumors. *J Surg Oncol.* 2012;106(5):604–610.

37. Liu MM, Reidy AB, Saatee S, Collard CD. Perioperative steroid management: Approaches based on current evidence. *Anesthesiology.* 2017 Jul;127(1):166–172. doi:10.1097/ALN.0000000000001659 PMID: 28452806.

38. Naranjo J, Dodd S, Martin YN. Perioperative management of pheochromocytoma. *J Cardiothorac Vasc Anesth.* 2017 Aug;31(4):1427–1439.

39. Newell KA, Prinz RA, Pickleman J, et al. Pheochromocytoma multisystem crisis: A surgical emergency. *Arch Surg.* 1988;123(8):956–959.

40. Lenders JW, Duh QY, Eisenhofer G, et al. Pheochromocytoma and paraglioma: An Endocrine Society clinical practice guideline. *J Clin Endocrinol Metab.* 2014;99:1915–1942.

41. Weingarten TN, Welch TL, Moore TL, et al. Preoperative levels of catecholamines and metanephrines and intraoperative hemodynamics of patients undergoing pheochromocytoma and paraganglioma resection. *Urology.* 2017;100:131–138.

42. Neumann HPH, Young WF Jr, Eng C. Pheochromocytoma and paraglioma. *N Engl J Med.* 2019;381(6):552–565.

43. Tischler AS, de Krijger RR, Gill AJ, et al. Phaechromocytoma: In: *WHO Classification of Tumours of Endocrine Organs.* 4th ed. Lyon, France: International Agency for Research on Cancer; 2017:183–190.

44. Scott AT, Howe JR. Evaluation and management of neuroendocrine tumors of the pancreas. *Surg Clin North Am.* 2019 Aug;99(4):793–814 .

45. Singh S, Dey C, Kennecke H, Kocha W, Maroun J, Metrakos P, Mukhtar T, Pasieka J, Rayson D, Rowsell C, Sideris L, Wong R, Law C. Consensus recommendations for the diagnosis and management of pancreatic neuroendocrine tumors: Guidelines from a Canadian national expert group. *Ann Surg Oncol.* 2015 Aug;22(8):2685–2699 .

46. Kunz PL, Reidy-Lagunes D, Anthony LB, Bertino EM, Brendtro K, Chan JA, Chen H, Jensen RT, Kim MK, Klimstra DS, Kulke MH, Liu EH, Metz DC, Phan AT, Sippel RS, Strosberg JR, Yao JC; North American Neuroendocrine Tumor Society. Consensus guidelines for the management and treatment of neuroendocrine tumors. *Pancreas.* 2013 May;42(4):557–577 .

IV

30 CENTRAL NERVOUS SYSTEM DISEASE

Lingzhong Meng, and Alana Flexman

The central nervous system (CNS) deserves special consideration in the perioperative setting for several reasons. First, anesthesia care is often required for patients undergoing treatment for CNS diseases, such as intracranial tumors or aneurysms, carotid disease, or diseases of the spine. Second, anesthesia providers commonly encounter patients with concurrent CNS diseases (e.g., Parkinson disease or prior stroke) who present for nonneurologic procedures. Third, neurocognitive dysfunction or other neurologic complications, such as stroke and delirium, can occur after surgery. Finally, the CNS is highly vulnerable to ischemia, as it is metabolically active with little oxygen reserve and is therefore sensitive to hypoxia even for very brief periods. The latter is especially important in vulnerable patients with altered cerebrovascular pathophysiology leading to poor regulatory reserve of cerebral blood flow (CBF). This chapter discusses the relevant knowledge base and clinical care needed when taking care of patients with CNS diseases or who are at risk for neurocognitive complications in the perioperative setting.

NEUROANATOMY

Supratentorial and Infratentorial Compartments

Conceptually, the cranium is divided into supratentorial and infratentorial compartments. The supratentorial compartment contains the cerebral hemispheres and diencephalon (thalamus and hypothalamus), and the brainstem (midbrain, pons, and medulla) and cerebellum make up the infratentorial compartment. For intracranial surgery, the location of the lesion has important implications for operative position and anesthetic management. For example, antiepileptic medications are commonly

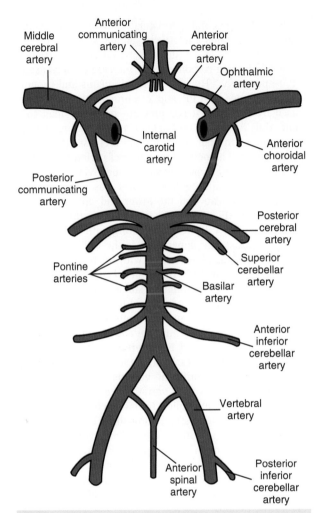

Fig. 30.1 Anatomy of the circle of Willis.

Middle cerebral artery

Anterior communicating artery

Anterior cerebral artery

Ophthalmic artery

Internal carotid artery

Anterior choroidal artery

Posterior communicating artery

Posterior cerebral artery

Pontine arteries

Superior cerebellar artery

Basilar artery

Anterior inferior cerebellar artery

Vertebral artery

Anterior spinal artery

Posterior inferior cerebellar artery

approximately 50% or more of the population has an abnormal circulation, implying that collateralization may not be complete. The clinical significance of an abnormal circle of Willis may depend on the pattern of the abnormality and coexisting cerebrovascular diseases. Anesthesia providers should carefully maintain adequate cerebral perfusion pressure (CPP) in anesthetized surgical patients with hemodynamically significant obstructive cerebrovascular lesions (e.g., carotid stenosis) or abnormal collateral circulation. Unfortunately, this information is not available in most patients; therefore consistently avoiding relative hypotension in the perioperative period is a reasonable approach.

Cranial Nerves

There are 12 pairs of intracranial nerves, each with a unique distribution and sensorimotor and autonomic function. Some neurosurgical procedures can potentially jeopardize specific intracranial nerves during surgery. For example, resection of acoustic neuroma can injure or sacrifice the vestibulocochlear nerve. Intracranial nerves can be monitored intraoperatively to facilitate timely detection of reversible injury and theoretically prevent permanent deficit. If intraoperative neuromonitoring is used, the anesthesiology and neurophysiologic monitoring teams need to be in close communication to ensure that appropriate equipment is available and a compatible anesthesia technique is chosen to facilitate monitoring, with the goal of maintaining a stable anesthetic depth that avoids overly suppressing neurophysiologic function. Anesthetic technique should be tailored to the intraoperative neuromonitoring used. For example, volatile anesthetic agents are typically minimized during somatosensory and motor evoked potential monitoring, and neuromuscular blocking agents should be avoided when motor evoked potentials are used. Glossopharyngeal nerve and hypoglossal nerve monitoring require placement of monitoring needles inside of the mouth, and caution should be taken until all needles are removed. Vagus nerve monitoring requires the placement of a special endotracheal tube with electrodes. If motor evoked potentials are used, a bite block must be placed to avoid trauma to the tongue and oropharynx, because masseter and temporalis muscle contraction commonly occur during stimulation.

Blood–Brain Barrier

The anatomic and functional integrity of the blood–brain barrier has important clinical implications. The blood–brain barrier is composed of capillary endothelial cells with tight junctions that prevent free passage of electrolytes, macromolecules, or proteins. In contrast, lipid-soluble substances (carbon dioxide, oxygen, anesthetic agents) cross the blood–brain barrier easily. The

considered during supratentorial, rather than infratentorial, brain tumor resection. In addition, intracranial lesions may be classified as either intraaxial or extraaxial, defined as within or outside the brain parenchyma, respectively. The location of intraaxial mass lesions is particularly relevant, as some lesions may compromise eloquent areas such as the language centers and motor cortex of the brain. In this case functional preservation during surgery becomes a critical focus.

Cerebral Vasculature

The arterial blood supply to the brain is through the left and right internal carotid arteries (anterior circulation) and the vertebrobasilar system (posterior circulation). Anastomoses between these vessels form the circle of Willis (Fig. 30.1) and create a collateral blood supply to protect against focal ischemia. However, this ring should not be assumed to be complete in all patients;

IV

blood–brain barrier may be disrupted in the event of hypertensive crisis, trauma, infection, arterial hypoxemia, severe hypercapnia, tumors, and sustained seizure activity. Osmotic therapy (e.g., mannitol) for brain edema, intracranial hypertension, or intraprocedural brain relaxation relies on an intact blood–brain barrier in order to move the free water from the brain parenchyma to the intravascular space.

NEUROPHYSIOLOGY

Regulation of Cerebral Blood Flow

Normal CBF is approximately 50 mL/100 g/min and represents 12% to 15% of total cardiac output. The brain, representing 2% of the body weight, receives a disproportionately large share of cardiac output because of its high metabolic rate and inability to store energy. As preservation of oxygen delivery is critical, the brain is equipped with robust regulatory mechanisms to regulate blood flow. Physiologic measures that regulate CBF include the following: (1) cerebral metabolic rate via neurovascular coupling, (2) CPP via cerebral autoregulation, (3) arterial blood carbon dioxide and oxygen partial pressure ($Paco_2$ and Pao_2, respectively) via cerebrovascular reactivity, (4) sympathetic nervous activity, (5) cardiac output, and (6) anesthetic agents directly. Different regulatory mechanisms may exert distinctive and sometimes opposing effects on CBF; however, these effects are integrated at the level of cerebral resistance arteries/arterioles to determine the CBF.[1,2]

Cerebral Metabolic Rate and Neurovascular Coupling

Cerebral metabolic rate of oxygen ($CMRO_2$) is often used as an index of the cerebral metabolic activity. $CMRO_2$ and CBF are closely related—an increase or decrease in $CMRO_2$ results in a proportional increase or decrease in CBF, respectively. This mechanism is known as *neurovascular coupling* or *cerebral metabolism-flow coupling*. In the perioperative setting $CMRO_2$ can be reduced by hypothermia and most intravenous anesthetic drugs, which produces a coupled reduction in CBF in healthy brains (CBF decreases 7% for every 1°C decrease in body temperature below 37°C).[3] In contrast, $CMRO_2$ and therefore CBF may be dramatically increased by seizure activity.

Cerebral Perfusion Pressure and Cerebral Autoregulation

CPP is the difference between mean arterial pressure (MAP) and intracranial pressure (ICP) or central venous pressure, whichever is greater. How CPP affects CBF is determined by cerebral autoregulation, which is a mechanism that maintains a relatively stable CBF in the face of a fluctuating CPP as a result of cerebral vasoconstriction or vasodilation in response to an increase or decrease in CPP, respectively.[1] That is, the simultaneous and proportionate changes in CPP and cerebrovascular resistance caused by cerebrovascular pressure reactivity lead to a stable CBF. However, as static cerebral autoregulation takes minutes to take effect, a rapid increase or decrease in MAP may be associated with a brief period of cerebral hyperperfusion or hypoperfusion, respectively.[4]

The cerebral autoregulation curve has three portions that are the plateau and the lower and upper limits of autoregulation (Fig. 30.2). The lower limit is the CPP level below which the CBF decreases along with a decreasing CPP. In contrast, the upper limit is the CPP level above which the CBF increases along with an increasing CPP. The plateau is the CPP range between the lower and upper limits where CBF remains stable (approximately 50 mL/100 g/min in awake adults and lower in anesthetized adults). The frequently quoted limits of autoregulation are a lower limit of 60 mm Hg and an upper limit of 150 mm Hg. However, it is important to recognize that although these numbers may apply to young and healthy humans, there is significant variation, and they may not apply in patients with various medical and surgical comorbidities.[5] For example, chronic uncontrolled hypertension or sympathetic stimulation shifts the autoregulatory curve to the right, and these patients require a higher minimum CPP to maintain adequate CBF. Autoregulatory curves are an individualized phenomenon; perioperative blood pressure or CPP management should incorporate individual variation and factors to avoid jeopardizing cerebral perfusion.

Cerebral autoregulation may be impaired in various circumstances. It can be abolished after traumatic brain injury and intracranial surgery. As a result, CBF becomes pressure passive, implying that it no longer remains stable across the autoregulatory CPP range and instead changes along with changes in CPP. Severe hypercapnia, often as a result of hypoventilation, can also impair cerebral autoregulation. Inhaled anesthetic agents are potent cerebral vasodilators and impair autoregulation to varying degrees depending on the dose used. In contrast, intravenous anesthetic agents do not typically disrupt this regulatory mechanism. In circumstances where cerebral autoregulation is impaired it is important to carefully control CPP because changes in CPP lead directly to changes in CBF, leading to either inadequate or overzealous perfusion of the brain.

Cerebrovascular $Paco_2$ and Pao_2 Reactivity

Both $Paco_2$ and Pao_2 are powerful modulators of CBF, reflecting a robust cerebrovascular $Paco_2$ and Pao_2 reactivity. Changes in $Paco_2$ produce corresponding and

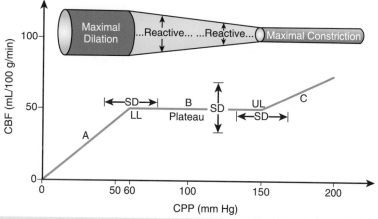

Fig. 30.2 Cerebral autoregulation describes the relationship between cerebral blood flow (CBF) and cerebral perfusion pressure (CPP). The three key elements of an autoregulation curve are the lower limit (*LL*), the upper limit (*UL*), and the plateau. *CBF* remains stable in the CPP range between the lower and upper limits and is pressure passive beyond this range. The frequently quoted numbers are the lower limit = 60 mm Hg, the upper limit = 150 mm Hg, and the plateau = 50 mL/100 g/min. However, these numbers may not be representative of all patients, and these parameters may vary, as indicated by the standard deviation (*SD*) in this illustration, especially in the context of poorly controlled hypertension. The cerebrovascular reactivity is also illustrated. (Figure 1 of Reference 1)[1]

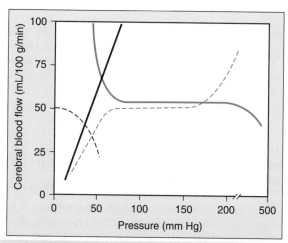

Fig. 30.3 Schematic depiction of the impact of intracranial pressure (*dashed black line*), Pao_2 (*solid red line*), $Paco_2$ (*solid black line*), and cerebral perfusion pressure (mean arterial pressure minus intracranial pressure or central venous pressure, whichever is greater) (*dashed red line*) on cerebral blood flow.

same directional changes in CBF between a $Paco_2$ of 20 and 80 mm Hg (Fig. 30.3). CBF increases or decreases approximately 1 mL/100 g/min, or 2%, for every 1 mm Hg increase or decrease in $Paco_2$ from 40 mm Hg. Such changes in CBF reflect the effect of carbon dioxide–mediated alterations in perivascular pH that lead to cerebral arteriole dilation or constriction. The $Paco_2$-related change in CBF only lasts for about 6 to 8 hours because

of the compensatory change in bicarbonate (HCO_3^-) concentration. Both extreme hyperventilation and hypoventilation should be avoided, as they lead to cerebral hypoperfusion and hyperperfusion, respectively. There is evidence to suggest that prolonged and aggressive hyperventilation after traumatic brain injury is associated with poorer neurologic outcome.[6] In contrast, decreases in Pao_2 below a threshold value of about 50 mm Hg result in an exponential increase in CBF (see Fig. 30.3), likely a compensatory mechanism to maintain cerebral oxygen delivery. Cerebral oxygen delivery equals arterial blood oxygen content times CBF. Therefore if arterial blood oxygen content decreases because of acute anemia or hemoglobin desaturation, CBF can increase to maintain cerebral oxygen delivery.

Effects of Anesthetic Agents on CBF (Also See Chapters 7 and 8)

Intravenously administered anesthetic agents such as propofol and thiopental cause simultaneous reduction of $CMRO_2$ and CBF. The effect of intravenous anesthetics on CBF is attributed to neurovascular coupling; that is, the decrease in $CMRO_2$ leads to a corresponding decrease in CBF. The reported effects of ketamine on cerebrovascular physiology and ICP have varied, which likely reflects different research study conditions.[7] When ketamine is given on its own without control of ventilation, $Paco_2$, CBF, and ICP all increase, whereas when given in the presence of another sedative/anesthetic drug in patients

IV

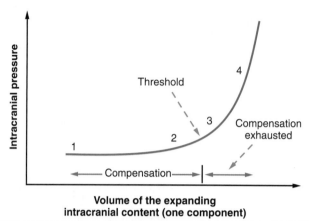

Fig. 30.4 Illustration of the effect of an expanding intracranial component on intracranial pressure (ICP). As the volume of an intracranial component increases from point 1 to point 2 on the curve, ICP remains relatively stable because of the compensatory mechanisms, including the translocation of cerebrospinal fluid from the intracranial space into the spinal subarachnoid space. Between points 1 and 2, the volumetric sum of all intracranial components remains relatively constant. Patients with intracranial tumors who are between point 1 and point 2 on the curve are unlikely to manifest clinical symptoms of increased ICP. The compensation ability is exhausted on the rising portion of the curve (point 3) when a small volumetric increase of the expanding intracranial component leads to a noticeable increase of ICP. Clinical signs and symptoms attributable to increased ICP are likely at this stage. Additional increases in intracranial volume at this point, as produced by increased CBF secondary to hypercapnia or inhaled anesthesia, can precipitate abrupt further increases in ICP (point 4).

whose ventilation is controlled, these effects were not observed. Because of this controversy, however, ketamine is often avoided in patients with known intracranial disease or increased ICP.

Benzodiazepines and opioids decrease $CMRO_2$ and CBF, analogous to propofol and thiopental, although to a lesser extent. However, if these medications result in respiratory depression and elevation of $Paco_2$, the opposite effect may occur. Opioids should be used with caution in patients with intracranial disease because of their depressant effects on consciousness and ventilation with associated increases in $Paco_2$, and therefore ICP.

Alpha-2 agonists (e.g., clonidine and dexmedetomidine) are unique sedatives in that they do not cause significant respiratory depression. They reduce arterial blood pressure, CPP, and CBF with minimal effects on ICP. Alpha-2 agonists can be used intraoperatively to reduce the dose of other anesthetic agents and blunt hemodynamic responses, or postoperatively as sedatives and to attenuate postoperative hypertension and tachycardia.

In contrast to intravenous anesthetics, volatile anesthetic agents are potent cerebral vasodilators. At low doses, this vasodilation is balanced by a reduction in CBF induced via flow metabolism coupling and a reduction in $CMRO_2$. However, when administered during normocapnia at concentrations higher than 0.5 minimum alveolar concentration (MAC), desflurane, sevoflurane, and isoflurane induce dose-dependent vasodilation and

increases in CBF even though $CMRO_2$ is decreased. Therefore volatile anesthetic agents produce divergent changes in $CMRO_2$ and CBF that are distinct from intravenous anesthetic agents, particularly at high doses. When used in isolation, nitrous oxide increases CBF and possibly $CMRO_2$; however, these effects appear to be attenuated by the coadministration of other anesthetic agents.

INTRACRANIAL PRESSURE AND BRAIN RELAXATION

ICP and brain relaxation are related but distinct. ICP is the pressure measured inside of the cranium with the cranium closed/intact. Brain relaxation is the volumetric relationship between the brain and intracranial space and the tactile feeling of the firmness of the brain by the surgeon with the cranium opened.[8] When the cranium is opened, the ICP equals the atmospheric pressure (i.e., zero); however, the brain may or may not be regarded as relaxed. Nonetheless, the management strategies for ICP and brain relaxation are similar.

Determinants of ICP and the Compensation for an Elevated ICP

The intracranial compartment normally contains three components: (1) brain matter, (2) cerebrospinal fluid (CSF), and (3) blood. Increases in any of these components

Box 30.1 Methods to Decrease Intracranial Pressure

Cerebral Blood Volume Reduction
Decrease Cerebral Blood Flow
  Intravenous anesthetic drugs are preferred
  Decrease $CMRO_2$ (propofol, barbiturates)
  Employ hyperventilation
  Avoid cerebral vasodilators
  Avoid extreme hypertension

Increase Venous Outflow
  Elevate head
  Avoid constriction at the neck
  Avoid PEEP and excessive airway pressure

Cerebrospinal Fluid Reduction
External ventricular drain
Lumbar drain
Head elevation (translocation of intracranial cerebrospinal fluid)
Acetazolamide (Diamox)

Cerebral Edema Reduction
Osmotic therapy (mannitol, hypertonic saline)
Furosemide (Lasix)
Prevention of ischemia and secondary edema
Dexamethasone to reduce peritumoral vasogenic edema

Resection of Space-Occupying Lesions

Decompressive Craniectomy

$CMRO_2$, Cerebral metabolic rate of oxygen; *PEEP*, positive end-expiratory pressure.

or the addition of a pathologic lesion (e.g., tumor) can result in an elevated ICP, normally defined as a sustained increase of ICP greater than 15 mm Hg. Marked increases in ICP can decrease CPP, and therefore CBF, to the point of causing cerebral ischemia. However, several compensatory physiologic mechanisms can help to reduce ICP, including compensatory reduction of other intracranial components such as translocation of CSF from the intracranial space to the extracranial space. When these compensatory mechanisms are exhausted, ICP starts to rise and cerebral blood vessels are eventually compressed (Fig. 30.4). It is important to differentiate CBF from cerebral blood volume (CBV) because the former is a dynamic concept representing flow, whereas the latter is a static concept representing the intracranial blood volume. These two terms are related but not interchangeable. The treatment of intracranial hypertension is primarily via the reduction of various intracranial components, including CBV (Box 30.1). Theoretically, the reduction of CBV should not compromise CBF; otherwise, the brain will experience hypoperfusion or ischemia.

Effect of Anesthetic Agents on ICP

Most intravenous anesthetic drugs reduce CBF because of the reduction of $CMRO_2$ (neurovascular coupling), and this reduction is associated with a decrease in ICP caused

by the simultaneous decrease in CBV. However, in this case the decrease in CBF is appropriate and induced by a simultaneous decrease in $CMRO_2$. These drugs should be considered in patients whose ICP is abnormally elevated. In patients refractory to initial treatment of intracranial hypertension a deep level of anesthesia such as propofol-induced burst suppression or barbiturate coma can be considered as alternative options. However, this must be done carefully, as large doses of propofol or thiopental may adversely affect blood pressure and cardiac output and compromise cerebral perfusion.

An increased frequency of excitatory peaks on the electroencephalogram (EEG) of patients receiving etomidate, as compared with thiopental, suggests etomidate should be administered with caution to patients with a history of epilepsy, because seizures increase $CMRO_2$, CBF, and ICP as a consequence.[9] Opioids and benzodiazepines reduce ICP through reductions in $CMRO_2$ and CBF, although this benefit will be offset if respiratory depression and increases in $Paco_2$ occur. The effect of ketamine is controversial, as discussed earlier.

Volatile anesthetic agents are cerebral vasodilators and produce dose-dependent increases in ICP that parallel the increases in CBF and CBV, although the clinical importance of this increase is unclear. Hyperventilation to decrease $Paco_2$ to <35 mm Hg attenuates the tendency for volatile anesthetic agents to increase ICP. In patients undergoing craniotomy for supratentorial tumors with evidence of a midline shift, neither isoflurane nor desflurane significantly affected lumbar CSF pressure when moderate hypocapnia ($Paco_2$ of 30 mm Hg) was maintained.[10] Although there are no data on the impact of anesthesia type on meaningful clinical outcomes, intravenous agents can be considered in patients with exhausted ICP-compensating mechanisms, as evidenced by elevated ICP, abnormal mental status, or imaging studies.

Neuromuscular blocking drugs do not directly affect ICP unless they induce release of histamine or hypotension. Histamine can cause cerebral vasodilation, leading to an increase in ICP. Succinylcholine may increase ICP through increases in CBF, although this phenomenon is inconsistently reported in the literature because of differences in study design and patient neurologic status.[11]

NEUROPROTECTION

Many anesthetic agents have been proposed as neuroprotectants given their potential to reduce cerebral metabolic rate and excitotoxicity during periods of oxygen deprivation. Animal studies support the ability of many anesthetic agents, including volatile anesthetic agents, barbiturates, propofol, and xenon, to provide neuroprotection, although convincing human data are lacking.[12] Hypothermia has been investigated extensively as a method of cerebral protection during acute injury. Although numerous animal studies have supported temperature reduction to reduce ischemic injury, several large prospective, randomized trials of hypothermia in aneurysm surgery and traumatic brain injury have failed to reproduce a consistent clinical benefit to date.[3] Cooling of patients with return of spontaneous circulation after cardiac arrest has been shown to improve neurologic outcome in a randomized controlled trial,[13] although a more recent trial contradicted these findings.[14] In contrast, hyperthermia worsens ischemic injury and should be avoided in patients vulnerable to cerebral ischemia.

NEUROPHYSIOLOGIC MONITORING

Neurophysiologic monitoring is employed during various neurologic surgeries with increasing frequency because of minimal risk to patients and the potential to reduce intraprocedural neurologic injuries. An understanding of the effects of anesthetic agents on various monitoring modalities, including the EEG, somatosensory and motor evoked potentials, and intracranial nerve monitoring, is critical in neuroanesthesia. The monitoring techniques can use a transcranial, direct cortical or subcortical approach. Different monitoring modalities often require different anesthetic regimens to preserve the quality of monitoring. Generally speaking, narcotics have a minimal impact, whereas intravenous and volatile anesthetics cause a dose-dependent suppression of monitoring signals. Anesthesia providers should facilitate neurophysiologic monitoring, avoiding major fluctuations in anesthetic level during monitoring. The impact of anesthetics on evoked potentials is discussed further in Chapter 20. Of note, electrocorticography (ECoG) is sometimes used during neurologic surgery to identify epileptic foci or activity. ECoG is sensitive to anesthetic agents that change the seizure threshold (e.g., benzodiazepines, propofol, and volatile anesthetic agents) and requires close communication and collaboration with the neurophysiologic monitoring team.

ANESTHESIA FOR NEUROSURGERY

Preoperative Assessment

Patients presenting for neurosurgical procedures can have a wide range of symptoms. Patients with intracranial mass lesions may present with seizures, altered level of consciousness, headaches, cranial nerve abnormalities, and motor or sensory deficits. Aneurysms and arteriovenous malformations (AVMs) can present with a severe ("thunderclap") headache, if ruptured, and focal deficits or visual impairment from compression of the optic

Box 30.2 Preoperative Evidence of Increased Intracranial Pressure
Positional headache
Nausea and vomiting
Hypertension and bradycardia
Altered level of consciousness
Altered patterns of breathing
Papilledema

chiasm when unruptured. Some neurosurgical patients are asymptomatic, having discovered their intracranial pathology incidentally through imaging.

Evidence of increased ICP should be elicited during the preoperative visit. Clinical signs may be consistent with, but do not reliably indicate, the level of ICP (Box 30.2). Imaging may reveal midline shift, encroachment of expanding brain on cerebral ventricles, cerebral edema, hydrocephalus, or any combination of these signs. In symptomatic patients preoperative medications that cause sedation or depression of ventilation are usually avoided. Drug-induced depression of ventilation can lead to increased $Paco_2$ and subsequent increases in CBF and ICP. In alert patients small doses of benzodiazepines may provide a useful degree of anxiolysis but should be used judiciously, if at all.

Patient medications related to CNS disease include antiepileptic drugs (e.g., levetiracetam), drugs used to reduce peritumor edema (e.g., dexamethasone), and drugs used to reduce brain free water (e.g., mannitol, hypertonic saline). Other medications may include antihypertensive drugs, drugs used for blood glucose control, drugs for chronic pain, and anticoagulants. Abnormal laboratory results should be investigated and corrected if clinically indicated. Coagulation profile, including platelet count and international normalized ratio (INR), and studies such as echocardiography and brain magnetic resonance imaging (MRI)/computed tomography (CT)/angiogram should be reviewed. The side of the brain lesion, left versus right, should be specifically noted.

Monitoring

In addition to standard monitors, continuous monitoring of arterial blood pressure via an intraarterial catheter is recommended for intracranial procedures. The advantages of invasive blood pressure monitoring include the ability to continuously assess CPP and intravascular volume using systolic pressure variation and pulse pressure variation (also see Chapter 20). In addition, these catheters allow for arterial blood gas sampling and accurate determination of $Paco_2$. Central venous catheters are not routinely used, although they can be considered in patients with difficult peripheral venous access or where there is a potential for massive transfusion. Measurement of the exhaled carbon dioxide concentration (capnography) is used to adjust mechanical ventilation or assess spontaneous breathing if the patient is awake or sedated. The electrocardiogram (ECG) allows prompt detection of cardiac dysrhythmias caused by surgical stimulation or traction on the brainstem, intracranial nerves, or dura. Neuromuscular blockade is monitored with a peripheral nerve stimulator. Because of the length of these surgical procedures and the use of diuretics, a bladder catheter is often necessary and helps to guide fluid therapy. A continuous monitor of ICP is helpful but rarely used after the bone flap is removed and the dura is opened. Two types of ICP monitors are inserted by neurosurgeons. The intraventricular catheter or external ventricular device (EVD) permits direct measurement of ICP and drainage of CSF. The subarachnoid or subdural bolt is placed through a burr hole and can be inserted quickly in an emergency setting, but it does not allow for CSF drainage.

Induction of Anesthesia

The goal of induction of anesthesia is to achieve a sufficient level of anesthesia to blunt the stimulation of direct laryngoscopy and tracheal intubation without compromising systemic hemodynamics and cerebral perfusion. Propofol produces reliable and prompt onset of unconsciousness and is unlikely to adversely increase ICP. Etomidate is rarely used in neurosurgical patients. However, the dose of a drug being chosen in a particular patient is a clinical decision that depends on the patient's age, physical condition, and comorbidities. Hemodynamic support with sympathomimetic drugs, such as phenylephrine and ephedrine, may be necessary, and such drugs should be readily available, particularly in cases where CPP is already compromised. A nondepolarizing neuromuscular blocking drug or succinylcholine is used to facilitate tracheal intubation, mechanical ventilation of the lungs, and patient positioning on the operating table. Increases in ICP may occur after the administration of succinylcholine, but the extent of the increase is usually short-lived and clinically inconsequential.[11] The patient's trachea is intubated after the confirmation of skeletal muscle paralysis so that coughing and acute increases in ICP are avoided. Injection of additional intravenous anesthetics before initiating direct laryngoscopy may attenuate the increase in systemic blood pressure and ICP.

Positioning (Also See Chapter 19)

During intracranial procedures, the head of the operating table is frequently turned 90 to 180 degrees away from the anesthesia workstation. Anesthesia providers typically have limited access to the patient's head, and the endotracheal tube should be safely secured before draping. The eyelids are closed and covered by transparent and waterproof film dressing to avoid abrasion and chemical injury to the eyes from prep solutions. A soft bite block should be placed and secured to prevent injury from biting secondary to motor monitoring or seizures.

Resection of supratentorial tumors and intracranial vascular lesions is typically accomplished with the patient in supine, semilateral, or lateral position. Resection of posterior fossa/infratentorial tumors frequently requires placement of the patient in a prone or sitting position. The sitting position facilitates surgical exposure of posterior fossa tumors, but because of the high risk of venous air embolism (>25% incidence), the prone position is frequently used instead. Other risks associated with the sitting position include upper airway edema as a result of venous obstruction from excessive cervical flexion and quadriplegia from spinal cord compression and ischemia, especially in the presence of preexisting cervical stenosis. An alternative approach is the "park bench position," in which the patient is placed in a lateral position but rolled slightly forward with the head further rotated to "look" at the floor. This position allows the surgeon full access to the posterior fossa and minimizes the risk for venous air embolism.

Extreme rotation, flexion and extension of the head and neck should be avoided, especially in patients with cervical spine diseases or elderly patients with arthritis or osteoporosis. Twisting, stretching, and compression of the neck vascular structures should also be avoided. A chest roll is frequently used in patients positioned lateral or in the park bench position, but not semilateral position. Pressure points should be adequately padded to avoid compression injury. The body weight should be borne by multiple points, not a single point, in a fashion of even distribution. Slight flexion of elbows and knees is recommended. Mechanisms to prevent patients from slipping should be instituted if the operating table is tilted during surgery. The patient's tolerance and ease of airway instrumentation, when needed, should also be taken into consideration during positioning for any procedure that is to be done under monitored anesthesia care such as deep brain stimulator placement or awake craniotomy.

A special consideration during neurologic surgery is the application of a head frame using pins. Caution must be exercised to avoid bucking or movement during the placement and removal of the head frame and while the patient is fixed in the frame to avoid injury to the patient. Additional doses of propofol and/or opioids are frequently administered immediately before head frame placement to blunt the hemodynamic fluctuation. A bolus of remifentanil (1 to 2 mcg/kg) is a commonly used and effective medication for this purpose.

Maintenance of Anesthesia

The goal of anesthetic care during neurosurgical procedures is to provide appropriate levels of unconsciousness and analgesia; facilitate brain relaxation while

IV

maintaining optimal cerebral perfusion; facilitate neurophysiologic monitoring; and enable a smooth and prompt emergence without confusion, agitation, nausea, and shivering.[15] Deep levels of anesthesia may adversely affect the quality of neurophysiologic monitoring and prolong emergence. Targeting a lighter plane of anesthesia facilitates neurophysiologic monitoring and enables a quicker emergence, although it may risk patient movement if used without muscle paralysis.

Anesthesia is often maintained using a combination of propofol and remifentanil infusion, with or without a low-dose volatile anesthetic agent (MAC 0.3–0.4). Some practitioners add dexmedetomidine infusion. The use of nitrous oxide and ketamine infusion during neurosurgical procedures is controversial. Volatile anesthetic agents must be used carefully because of their ability to increase ICP. The choice of anesthetic agents should also take into account the neurophysiologic monitoring being used because certain agents (e.g., volatile anesthetic agents and nitrous oxide) may adversely affect the quality of monitoring. High doses of propofol may affect EEG monitoring. Collaboration with the neuromonitoring team is essential to facilitate appropriate monitoring and communication if any issues arise during the procedure.

Direct-acting vasodilating drugs (hydralazine, nitroprusside, nitroglycerin, calcium channel blockers) may increase CBF and ICP despite causing simultaneous decreases in systemic blood pressure; therefore use of these drugs, particularly before the dura is open, is not encouraged. On the contrary, sympathomimetic drugs such as phenylephrine or norepinephrine are often infused to maintain arterial blood pressure and an ideal CPP.

Inadequate depth of anesthesia can result in patient movement, coughing, or reacting to the presence of the tracheal tube during intracranial procedures. These responses can lead to complications such as increases in ICP, surgical bleeding, and brain swelling. Because deep levels of anesthesia may impede neurophysiologic monitoring, the depth of anesthesia should be carefully titrated. Muscle paralysis provides insurance against movement or coughing but is not possible in cases with motor monitoring. In these cases anesthesia providers can consider the use of an opioid infusion (e.g., remifentanil or fentanyl) with a propofol infusion, with the possible addition of a low-dose volatile agent.

ICP Reduction and Brain Relaxation

As discussed earlier, ICP reduction and brain relaxation are related but distinct concepts. Osmotic agents such as mannitol (0.25–1 g/kg IV) or 3% hypertonic saline are frequently administered to reduce cerebral water content and decrease ICP before craniectomy and improve brain relaxation after craniectomy.[16] The onset of action is 5 to 10 minutes, maximum effects are seen in 20 to 30 minutes, and the effects last for about 2 to 4 hours. However, if administered rapidly, mannitol can also cause peripheral vasodilation (hypotension) and short-term intravascular volume expansion, which could result in increased ICP and volume overload. Mannitol is a relatively well-tolerated drug.[16] Furosemide (0.3–0.5 mg/kg IV) is sometimes used in combination with mannitol to decrease brain water and ICP and is thought to be synergistic with mannitol in decreasing ICP. However, hypovolemia secondary to diuresis may adversely affect cardiac output and tissue perfusion. Intravascular volume replacement should take into account losses resulting from diuresis. Hyperventilation is an effective strategy to reduce ICP and improve brain relaxation, with immediate onset. Intravenous agents may be preferred over volatile agents when ICP reduction and brain relaxation are critical, although there are no clinical outcome data to support one anesthetic technique over another. The patient's position is also important, as placing the patient in a head-up position will decrease ICP. Finally, any constriction around the neck should be avoided, as it may impair venous drainage.

Ventilation Adjustment

After tracheal intubation, ventilation of the lungs is controlled at a rate and tidal volume sufficient to maintain Pa_{CO_2} between 30 and 35 mm Hg. There is no evidence of additional therapeutic benefit when Pa_{CO_2} is decreased below this range. It remains unclear whether a smaller tidal volume is lung protective during neurologic procedures. Use of high levels of positive end-expiratory pressure (PEEP) is not encouraged because of impairment of cerebral venous drainage and potential for increased ICP, but this can usually be counteracted by raising the head 10 to 15 cm above the level of the chest. Recruitment maneuvers or large increases in intrathoracic pressure can increase ICP and reduce blood pressure and should be avoided. Hypoventilation is detrimental, as hypercapnia causes cerebral vasodilation, increased CBF and ICP, and impaired cerebral autoregulation.[1] Overall, the current consensus is to maintain eucapnia during intracranial surgery and use relative hyperventilation only as a temporizing measure.

Fluid Management

Maintaining euvolemia is recommended. Dextrose solutions are not recommended because they are rapidly distributed throughout body water, and if blood glucose concentrations decrease more rapidly than brain glucose concentrations, water crosses the blood–brain barrier and cerebral edema results. Furthermore, hyperglycemia augments ischemic neuronal cell damage by promoting neuronal lactate production, which worsens cellular injury. Therefore crystalloid solutions such as normal saline, PlasmaLyte, and lactated Ringer solution are recommended. Colloids such as 5% albumin are also an acceptable replacement fluid but have not been shown to improve outcomes compared with crystalloids and may be detrimental in patients with traumatic brain injury.[17] Goal-directed fluid therapy shows promise but requires further study in brain-injured patients.

Blood Product Administration and Anticoagulant Management

The transfusion trigger for red blood cells remains controversial in patients undergoing neurosurgical procedures. The decision to transfuse is based on the patient's age, baseline hemoglobin, ongoing blood loss during surgery, comorbidities, and signs of organ dysfunction. Currently available evidence suggests that a hemoglobin of less than 9 to 10 g/dL is associated with worse outcomes in neurologically impaired patients, although the role of transfusion remains to be determined. Ultimately, the decision to transfuse should be individualized. Coagulopathy and thrombocytopenia are associated with a higher risk of perioperative bleeding and should be corrected, particularly given the risk of intracranial hematoma. Anticoagulants, including aspirin, are typically stopped before surgery; however, specific practice varies, as there is no consensus for patients undergoing neurosurgery.

Emergence From Anesthesia and Postoperative Care

On awakening from anesthesia, coughing or straining by the patient should be avoided, given the risk of inducing an intracranial hemorrhage or cerebral edema. Remifentanil can be used to facilitate a smooth emergence, particularly if a low-dose infusion is continued through emergence. A prior intravenous bolus of lidocaine, opioid, or both may help decrease the likelihood of coughing during tracheal extubation. After extubation, early and frequent neurologic assessments are important to identify neurologic injury or ischemia or intracranial hematoma. Delayed return of consciousness or neurologic deterioration in the postoperative period should be immediately assessed with consideration for further urgent imaging (e.g., CT or MRI). Intracranial hemorrhage, stroke, and tension pneumocephalus should be ruled out as early as possible. The postoperative sympathetic stress response (hypertension, tachycardia) should be attenuated using labetalol, nicardipine, or opioids to avoid precipitating intracranial hematoma. Drugs that reduce MAP without cerebral vasodilation are preferred.

Venous Air Embolism

Neurosurgical procedures are considered at higher risk of venous air embolism for several reasons. These procedures often require significant elevation of the head, which elevates the operative site above the level of the heart and increases the risk for venous air embolism.[18] In addition, the venous sinuses in the cut edge of bone or dura may not collapse when transected, which can allow air to enter the venous system. Once air is entrained, it enters the pulmonary circulation and becomes trapped in small vessels and acutely increases dead space. Massive air embolism may cause air to be trapped in the right ventricle and subsequently cause acute right ventricular failure. Microvascular bubbles may also cause reflex bronchoconstriction and activate the release of endothelial mediators causing pulmonary edema. Death is usually the result of cardiovascular collapse and arterial hypoxemia. Air may reach the coronary and cerebral circulations (paradoxical air embolism) by crossing a patent foramen ovale, which is present in 20% to 30% of adults, and result in myocardial infarction or stroke. Furthermore, transpulmonary passage of venous air is possible even in the absence of a patent foramen ovale.

Transesophageal echocardiography is the most sensitive method to detect air embolism, but it is invasive and may be impractical during intracranial surgery. A precordial Doppler ultrasound transducer placed over the right heart (over the second or third intercostal space to the right or left of the sternum to maximize audible signals from the right atrium) is the next most sensitive, detecting amounts of air as small as 0.25 mL.[19] This monitor represents a practical noninvasive indicator of the presence of intracardiac air. A sudden decrease in end-tidal concentrations of carbon dioxide reflects increased dead space secondary to continued ventilation of nonperfused alveoli. An increased end-tidal nitrogen concentration may reflect nitrogen from venous air embolism if the inspired oxygen fraction is 100%, but end-tidal nitrogen is rarely monitored. Aspiration of air through a correctly positioned central venous catheter can also be used to diagnose air embolism. A right atrial catheter with the tip positioned at the junction of the superior vena cava and the right atrium may allow rapid aspiration of air. During controlled ventilation of the lungs, sudden attempts (gasps) by patients to initiate spontaneous breaths may be an early indication of venous air embolism. Hypotension, tachycardia, cardiac dysrhythmias, hypoxemia, and a "mill wheel" murmur are late signs of air embolism. A pulmonary artery catheter may show an abrupt increase in pulmonary artery pressure. In awake patients additional signs of venous air embolism include chest pain, coughing, and anxiety.

Once recognized, the management includes avoiding further entrainment of air and supportive care. The surgeon should be notified immediately whenever venous air embolism is suspected in order to minimize further air entry into the circulation. Venous air embolism is treated by (1) irrigation of the operative site with fluid, in addition to the application of occlusive material to bone edges (e.g., bone wax) to occlude potential sites of air entry; (2) placement of the patient in a head-down position; (3) gentle compression of the internal jugular veins and intravenous fluids to increase venous pressure; (4) ensuring 100% inspired oxygen fraction; and (5) hemodynamic support. If nitrous oxide is being administered, it should be promptly discontinued to avoid the risk of increasing the size of air bubbles. Despite the logic of applying PEEP to decrease entrainment of air, the efficacy of this maneuver has not been confirmed. Furthermore, PEEP could reverse the pressure gradient between the left and right atria and predispose to passage of air across a patent foramen ovale.

COMMON CLINICAL CASES

Intracranial Mass Lesions (Box 30.3)

The pathology of an intracranial mass lesion may be a primary brain tumor or a metastatic tumor. The signs and symptoms are diverse and often nonspecific. The clinical manifestations may or may not reflect increases in ICP. The initial diagnosis is usually made by MRI. Abrupt increases in ICP should be avoided when caring for patients with a large intracranial mass lesion. The patient's position during surgery is determined by the location of the tumor and surgical approach. Dexamethasone is commonly used to reduce peritumor edema, particularly after tumor resection. Patients with supratentorial tumors will sometimes receive an intraoperative dose of antiepileptics. Strategies to increase brain relaxation are frequently required with large tumors, particularly if there is significant preoperative peritumor edema or midline shift. Awake craniotomy with intraoperative mapping may be indicated for lesions residing in close proximity to eloquent areas of the brain.[20]

Sitting-position craniotomy for posterior fossa tumor resection has several additional considerations, although this approach is rarely used. A patent foramen ovale can be excluded using preoperative echocardiography. As the neck is flexed, there is a risk of tongue edema and airway compromise. CPP should be accurately measured by ensuring the transducer of the arterial line is positioned no lower than the external ear canal level, and hypotension should be minimized. Given the high risk of venous air embolism, a properly positioned central venous catheter and precordial Doppler are recommended. Adequate hydration is warranted to compensate for the blood pooling in the lower body. Posterior fossa operations have the potential of stimulating or injuring vital brainstem respiratory and circulatory centers and can result in intraoperative arrhythmias, hemodynamic instability, and postoperative respiratory insufficiency. The cranial nerves can also be stimulated or affected, which can lead to intraoperative dysrhythmias and postoperative impairment of protective airway reflexes. Postoperatively, the

---

Box 30.3 Management of Anesthesia for Patients With Intracranial Masses

Preoperative
- Avoid sedatives and opioids if ICP is elevated.
- Standard anxiolytics can be given if ICP is not elevated.

Monitors

Supratentorial Masses
- Standard ASA monitors, arterial line, temperature, and Foley catheter are used.

Infratentorial Masses—Depending on Positioning
- Prone or park bench position: Standard ASA monitors, arterial line, temperature, and Foley catheter are adequate.
- Sitting position (associated with increased frequency of VAE): Standard monitors plus central venous catheter, precordial Doppler, or TEE are required.

Induction
- Adequate anesthesia and skeletal muscle paralysis are obtained before direct laryngoscopy/tracheal intubation to avoid increasing ICP while maintaining CPP.

Maintenance
- Maintain adequate CPP.
- Assure adequate brain relaxation.
- Opioid (e.g., remifentanil infusion) plus propofol infusion and/or low MAC volatile anesthetic.
- Avoid intraoperative muscle relaxant if motor function is tested/mapped.
- Mannitol (0.25–1 g/kg IV) for brain relaxation.
- Maintain euvolemia.
- Eucapnia if normal ICP; temporary hyperventilation for a tight brain only.

Postoperative
- Avoid coughing, straining, and systemic hypertension during tracheal extubation.
- Rapid awakening allows early neurologic assessment.

ASA, American Society of Anesthesiologists; *CPP,* cerebral perfusion pressure; *ICP,* intracranial pressure; *MAC,* mean alveolar concentration; *TEE,* transesophageal echocardiography; *VAE,* venous air embolism.

---

decision to extubate is based on the patient's ability to protect their airway and the risk of ventilatory failure.

Intracranial Aneurysms (Box 30.4)

Intracranial aneurysms occur in 2% to 4% of the population. The risk of rupture (subarachnoid hemorrhage) in these individuals is 1% to 2% per year. Although many aneurysms are found incidentally, many present for the first time after rupture. Subarachnoid hemorrhage leads to a sudden onset of severe headache, nausea, vomiting, focal neurologic signs, and/or altered consciousness. Subarachnoid hemorrhage can result in major complications, including death, rebleeding, vasospasm, acute hydrocephalus, and delayed cerebral ischemia. Aneurysmal subarachnoid hemorrhage is a common

---

Box 30.4 Anesthetic Management of Patients With Intracranial Aneurysms

Preoperative
- Neurologic evaluation is performed to look for evidence of increased intracranial pressure and vasospasm.
- Electrocardiogram changes are often present.
- HHH therapy when vasospasm present is becoming controversial.
- Nimodipine therapy is considered standard care.

Induction
- Avoid increases in systemic blood pressure.
- Maintain cerebral perfusion pressure to avoid ischemia.

Maintenance
- Opioid (e.g., remifentanil infusion) plus propofol infusion and/or low MAC volatile anesthetic
- Mannitol (0.25-1 g/kg IV) for brain relaxation
- Maintain normal to increased systemic blood pressure to avoid ischemia during surgical retraction and temporary clipping.
- Maintain euvolemia.
- Maintain eucapnia; avoid unnecessary hyperventilation.
- EEG burst suppression can be considered.
- Avoid hyperthermia.

Postoperative
- Maintain normal to increased systemic blood pressure
- Early awakening is recommended to facilitate neurologic assessment
- HHH therapy should be used with caution in patients with vasospasm

HHH, Hypervolemia, hypertension, hemodilution.

cause of intracranial hemorrhage that requires treatment in interventional radiology suites or operating rooms. Short- to medium-term outcomes are similar in patients treated surgically versus endovascular insertion of platinum coils, although the long-term benefits of one technique over the other continue to be debated.[21] Some patients are unsuitable candidates for endovascular coiling because of the anatomy and location of their aneurysms; in these cases surgical clipping is required.

Early treatment is advocated to reduce the rebleeding risk, but surgery may be associated with greater technical difficulty because of a swollen inflamed brain. Cerebral vasospasm is generally manifested clinically 3 to 5 days after subarachnoid hemorrhage and is the foremost cause of morbidity and mortality. Transcranial Doppler and cerebral angiography can detect cerebral vasospasm before clinical symptoms (worsening headache, neurologic deterioration, loss of consciousness) occur. So-called "triple H" therapy (hypervolemia, hypertension, hemodilution) was used in the past to treat vasospasm, but its use has been questioned because of the lack of convincing evidence of benefit.[22] Nimodipine decreases the morbidity and mortality from vasospasm and is one of the few medical treatments for vasospasm with proven beneficial

effects.[23] Other treatment modalities include selective intraarterial injection of vasodilators and balloon dilation (angioplasty) of the affected arterial segments in the interventional neuroradiology suite (also see Chapter 38).

Other complications of subarachnoid hemorrhage include seizures (10%), acute and chronic hydrocephalus, and intracerebral hematoma. Changes on the ECG (T-wave inversions, U waves, ST depressions, prolonged QT, and rarely Q waves) and mild elevation of cardiac enzymes are frequent but do not usually correlate with significant myocardial dysfunction or poor outcome. Hyponatremia is commonly seen after subarachnoid hemorrhage. Significant electrolyte, acid–base abnormalities, or hemodynamic derangements should be corrected if present, and a cardiac workup should ensue if Q waves are seen on ECG.

The anesthetic care for intracranial aneurysm clipping is designed to (1) prevent sudden increases in systemic arterial blood pressure, which would increase the aneurysm's transmural pressure and could result in rupture or rebleeding, and (2) facilitate surgical exposure and access to the aneurysm. Induction and maintenance of anesthesia must be designed to minimize the hypertensive responses evoked by noxious stimulation, such as direct laryngoscopy and placing the patient's head in immobilizing pins. Conversely, CPP must be maintained to prevent ischemia during surgical retraction or temporary vessel occlusion or as a result of vasospasm.

Hemodynamic control is important during dissection of the aneurysm to prevent intraoperative rupture. Temporary occlusive clips applied to the major feeding artery of the aneurysm can create regional arterial hypotension and cerebral ischemia. It is judicious to maintain a normal or even increased systemic arterial blood pressure to facilitate perfusion through collateral circulations. In addition to maintaining collateral cerebral circulations via systemic relative hypertension, drugs such as propofol or thiopental may be administered, via either boluses or high-rate infusion to the point of burst suppression on electroencephalography monitoring, in the hope that they can provide some protection from cerebral ischemia. Occasionally, hypothermic circulatory arrest may be used for very large complex aneurysms. Unfortunately, convincing evidence supporting the benefits of these maneuvers is lacking.

The patient's trachea is generally extubated at the completion of surgery unless there is significant neurologic impairment or other intraoperative complications. Measures to prevent vasospasm and seizures while maintaining adequate CPP should be continued during care of these patients postoperatively.

Arteriovenous Malformations

The incidence of AVMs in the general population and annual rate of rupture are similar to aneurysms, at 2%

IV

to 4% and 2%, respectively. Up to 10% of patients diagnosed with an AVM have an associated aneurysm.[24] Risk of hemorrhage is related to the anatomic features of AVM, including size and characteristics of the feeding arteries. These patients may be treated in several ways: expectantly, open resection, endovascular embolization, or with stereotactic radiosurgery (gamma knife). Preoperative embolization is frequently employed to reduce blood loss and facilitate surgical resection.

Anesthesia for resection or embolization of AVMs is similar to that of aneurysms with a few distinct considerations. Because of their flow characteristics (low-pressure, high-flow shunts), AVMs are unlikely to rupture during acute systemic hypertension, such as during laryngoscopy. Despite this, hypertension should still be avoided during induction, given the high rate of associated aneurysms. Finally, anesthesia for intracranial AVM resection must include preparation for massive, persistent blood loss and postoperative cerebral swelling.

Carotid Disease (Box 30.5)

In the United States stroke is the fifth leading cause of death and a significant cause of disability. A significant proportion of strokes is the result of atherosclerotic stenosis of the carotid artery. Despite the technical advancement and increasing adoption of carotid artery stenting (CAS), carotid endarterectomy (CEA) remains the "gold standard" in treating symptomatic carotid disease.[25] Although the perioperative risk of stroke and death (approximately 4%–7%) must be taken into account, CEA may be beneficial in asymptomatic patients as well.[26] Data suggest that early CEA (<30 days after symptom onset) is optimal given the presence of unstable atherosclerotic plaque.[27]

Preoperative assessment of patients undergoing CEA should focus on assessment of perioperative risk of cardiac ischemia, as these patients typically have atherosclerotic cardiovascular disease. Either general or regional anesthesia (deep and superficial cervical plexus block) may be used for this procedure. Although an awake patient may provide a more accurate intraoperative assessment of the patient's neurologic status and more stable hemodynamic profile, it requires a cooperative and motionless patient. Current evidence suggests that outcomes are similar whether CEA is performed with regional or general anesthesia.[28]

Goals of anesthesia for CEA include (1) prevention of cerebral ischemia through maintenance of adequate CPP and (2) prevention of myocardial ischemia through avoidance of acute peaks in blood pressure and heart rate. Invasive hemodynamic monitoring with a peripheral arterial catheter is indicated to ensure adequate CPP. This is especially important during intraoperative clamping of the carotid artery. The anesthesia provider should ensure that the MAP is maintained above the patient's baseline

---

Box 30.5 Management of Anesthesia for Patients With Carotid Stenosis

Preoperative
- Neurologic examination is indicated to look for preoperative deficits.
- Screen for associated CAD.
- Anxiolytics may be useful.

Monitors
- Standard ASA monitors, arterial line, and Foley catheter are used.
- Cerebral ischemia monitoring depends on institutional and individual practitioner's preference.

Induction
- Avoid increases in mean arterial pressure or heart rate if CAD is suspected.
- Maintain adequate CPP.

Maintenance
- Maintain adequate CPP (baseline to 20 % above) during carotid clamping.
- Opioid (e.g., remifentanil infusion) plus propofol infusion and/or low MAC volatile anesthetic
- Close intraoperative monitoring for cerebral ischemia during carotid clamping by keeping the patient awake or based on various monitoring modalities

Postoperative
- Avoid coughing, straining, and systemic hypertension during tracheal extubation.
- Rapid awakening allows early neurologic assessment.
- Monitor for hyperperfusion syndrome and airway compromise.

ASA, American Society of Anesthesiologists; *CAD*, coronary artery disease; *CPP*, cerebral perfusion pressure.

---

pressure (within 20%) to ensure adequate collateral flow through the circle of Willis. Hypocarbia should be avoided, given the risk of cerebral vasoconstriction and ischemia. Many methods have been employed to detect intraoperative cerebral ischemia and need for shunting during clamping, including EEG, evoked potentials, transcranial Doppler, cerebral oximetry, and stump pressure, although none have been shown to definitively improve outcome.

Postoperative complications include cardiovascular ischemia and neurologic deficits secondary to intraoperative emboli. Hypertension should be avoided because it may lead to two complications: neck hematoma with airway compromise and/or hyperperfusion syndrome. Cerebral hyperperfusion syndrome, although rare, can cause symptoms ranging from severe headache and eye and facial pain to focal neurologic deficits, seizures, and loss of consciousness.[29] The mechanism most commonly cited is impairment of cerebral autoregulation. Management includes maintaining postprocedure blood pressure lower than 140/90, or possibly lower based on patient and procedure characteristics.

REFERENCES

1. Meng L, Gelb AW. Regulation of cerebral autoregulation by carbon dioxide. *Anesthesiology.* 2015;122(1):196–205.

2. Meng L, Hou W, Chui J, Han R, Gelb AW. Cardiac output and cerebral blood flow: The integrated regulation of brain perfusion in adult humans. *Anesthesiology.* 2015;123(5):1198–1208.

3. Polderman KH. Mechanisms of action, physiological effects, and complications of hypothermia. *Crit Care Med.* 2009;37(7 Suppl):S186–S202.

4. Dagal A, Lam AM. Cerebral autoregulation and anesthesia. *Curr Opin Anaesthesiol.* 2009;22(5):547–552.

5. Meng L, Wang Y, Zhang L, McDonagh DL. Heterogeneity and variability in pressure autoregulation of organ blood flow: Lessons learned over 100+ years. *Crit Care Med.* 2019;47(3):436–448.

6. Guidelines for the management of severe traumatic brain injury. *J Neurotrauma.* 2007;24(Suppl 1):S1–S106.

7. Albanèse J, Arnaud S, Rey M, Thomachot L, Alliez B, Martin C. Ketamine decreases intracranial pressure and electroencephalographic activity in traumatic brain injury patients during propofol sedation. *Anesthesiology.* 1997;87(6):1328–1334.

8. Li J, Gelb AW, Flexman AM, Ji F, Meng L. Definition, evaluation, and management of brain relaxation during craniotomy. *Br J Anaesth.* 2016;116(6):759–769.

9. Reddy RV, Moorthy SS, Dierdorf SF, Deitch RD, Link L. Excitatory effects and electroencephalographic correlation of etomidate, thiopental, methohexital, and propofol. *Anesth Analg.* 1993;77(5):1008–1011.

10. Muzzi DA, Losasso TJ, Dietz NM, Faust RJ, Cucchiara RF, Milde LN. The effect of desflurane and isoflurane on cerebrospinal fluid pressure in humans with supratentorial mass lesions. *Anesthesiology.* 1992;76(5):720–724.

11. Kovarik WD, Mayberg TS, Lam AM, Mathisen TL, Winn HR. Succinylcholine does not change intracranial pressure, cerebral blood flow velocity, or the electroencephalogram in patients with neurologic injury. *Anesthesia & Analgesia.* 1994;78(3):469–473.

12. Meng L. General anesthetic agents are not neuroprotective and may be neurotoxic. *J Neurosurg Anesthesiol.* 2019;31(4):362–364.

13. Bernard SA, Gray TW, Buist MD, et al. Treatment of comatose survivors of out-of-hospital cardiac arrest with induced hypothermia. *N Engl J Med.* 2002;346(8):557–563.

14. Nielsen N, Wetterslev J, Cronberg T, et al. Targeted temperature management at 33°C versus 36°C after cardiac arrest. *N Engl J Med.* 2013;369(23):2197–2206.

15. Flexman AM, Wang T, Meng L. Neuroanesthesia and outcomes: Evidence, opinions, and speculations on clinically relevant topics. *Curr Opin Anesthesiol.* 2019;32(5):539–545.

16. Zhang W, Neal J, Lin L, et al. Mannitol in critical care and surgery over 50+ years: A systematic review of randomized controlled trials and complications with meta-analysis. *J Neurosurg Anesthesiol.* 2019;31(3):273–284.

17. Myburgh J, Cooper DJ, Finfer S, et al. Saline or albumin for fluid resuscitation in patients with traumatic brain injury. *N Engl J Med.* 2007;357(9):874–884.

18. Muth CM, Shank ES. Gas embolism. *N Engl J Med.* 2000;342(7):476–482.

19. Schubert A, Deogaonkar A, Drummond JC. Precordial Doppler probe placement for optimal detection of venous air embolism during craniotomy. *Anesth Analg.* 2006;102(5):1543–1547.

20. Meng L, McDonagh DL, Berger MS, Gelb AW. Anesthesia for awake craniotomy: A how-to guide for the occasional practitioner. *Can J Anaesth.* 2017;64(5):517–529.

21. Thomas AJ, Ogilvy CS. ISAT: Equipoise in treatment of ruptured cerebral aneurysms? *Lancet.* 2015;385(9969):666–668.

22. Dankbaar JW, Slooter AJ, Rinkel GJ, Schaaf IC. Effect of different components of triple-H therapy on cerebral perfusion in patients with aneurysmal subarachnoid haemorrhage: A systematic review. *Crit Care.* 2010;14(1):R23.

23. Wang J, McDonagh DL, Meng L. Calcium channel blockers in acute care: The links and missing links between hemodynamic effects and outcome evidence. *Am J Cardiovasc Drugs.* 2021;21(1):35–49.

24. Ogilvy CS, Stieg PE, Awad I, et al. Recommendations for the management of intracranial arteriovenous malformations: A statement for healthcare professionals from a special writing group of the Stroke Council, American Stroke Association. *Circulation.* 2001;103(21):2644–2657.

25. Kolkert JL, Meerwaldt R, Geelkerken RH, Zeebregts CJ. Endarterectomy or carotid artery stenting: The quest continues part two. *Am J Surg.* 2015;209(2):403–412.

26. Raman G, Moorthy D, Hadar N, et al. Management strategies for asymptomatic carotid stenosis: A systematic review and meta-analysis. *Ann Intern Med.* 2013;158(9):676–685.

27. Rerkasem K, Rothwell PM. Systematic review of the operative risks of carotid endarterectomy for recently symptomatic stenosis in relation to the timing of surgery. *Stroke.* 2009;40(10):e564–e572.

28. Lewis SC, Warlow CP, Bodenham AR, et al. General anaesthesia versus local anaesthesia for carotid surgery (GALA): A multicentre, randomised controlled trial. *Lancet.* 2008;372(9656):2132–2142.

29. Lin YH, Liu HM. Update on cerebral hyperperfusion syndrome. *J Neurointerv Surg.* 2020;12(8):788–793. doi:10.1136/neurintsurg-2019-015621 AugEpub 2020 May 15. PMID: 32414892; PMCID: PMC7402457.

IV

31 OPHTHALMOLOGY AND OTOLARYNGOLOGY

Steven Gayer, Howard D. Palte

Surgical procedures of the head and neck present unique anesthetic challenges. Operative field isolation places the anesthesia provider at a distance from the airway and hampers access to the patient. The region's extensive parasympathetic innervations predispose patients to intraoperative bradycardia and asystole. Ophthalmic and otolaryngologic procedures require smooth induction and emergence from anesthesia. Coughing and bucking increase venous and intraocular pressure (IOP), which may negatively affect surgical outcome.

OPHTHALMOLOGY

More than 2 million cataract operations are completed nationally each year. Most eye procedures are considered low risk for perioperative complications; however, ophthalmic patients are often at greater risk during surgery because typically they include the elderly (also see Chapter 35), who frequently have multiple concomitant medical issues, or pediatric patients (also see Chapter 34), who may be premature or have associated syndromes.[1] Additionally, most operations are conducted on an ambulatory basis (also see Chapter 37), emphasizing the importance of preoperative evaluation (also see Chapter 13).

Most ophthalmologic procedures are performed via monitored anesthesia care (MAC) and some form of regional or topical eye anesthetic.[2] Aside from intraoperative analgesia and akinesia, advantages of ophthalmic regional blocks include suppression of the oculocardiac reflex (OCR) and provision of postoperative pain management. An understanding of regional block techniques and management of their complications is requisite. General anesthesia is reserved for operations of prolonged duration; more invasive orbital procedures; and patients unable to remain relatively still such as neonates, infants, and children.

Anesthetic drugs and maneuvers may affect ocular dynamics and surgical outcomes, and ophthalmic medications can cause adverse anesthesia reactions or may significantly affect systemic physiology. Appreciation of factors affecting IOP and vigilance vis-à-vis the OCR are critical.

Intraocular Pressure

Adequate pressure within the eye serves to maintain refracting surfaces, corneal contour, and functionally correct vision. IOP is primarily derived from a balance between aqueous humor production and drainage. Aqueous humor is actively secreted from the posterior chamber's ciliary body and flows through the pupil into the anterior chamber, where it is admixed with aqueous humor passively produced by blood vessels on the iris's forward surface. After washing over the avascular lens and corneal endothelium, aqueous humor filters through the spongy trabecular meshwork into the canal of Schlemm tubules at the base of the cornea. From there, it exits the eye into episcleral veins and ultimately to the superior vena cava and right atrium. Therefore any obstruction of venous return from the eye to the right side of the heart can increase IOP. Lesser factors that influence IOP include force transmitted to the globe by contraction of the orbicularis oculi or extraocular muscles in addition to hardening of the lens, vitreous, and sclera that can occur with aging.

IOP ranges between 10 and 22 mm Hg in the intact normal eye. Typically, there is a 2 to 5 mm Hg diurnal variation. Small transient changes occur with each cardiac contraction and with eyelid closure, mydriasis, and postural changes. These changes are normal and have no bearing on the intact eye. A sustained increase in IOP during anesthesia, however, has the potential to produce acute glaucoma, retinal ischemia, hemorrhage, and permanent visual loss.

Factors That Influence Intraocular Pressure

Venous congestion resulting from obstruction at any point from the episcleral veins to the right atrium may cause a substantive increase of IOP. Before induction of anesthesia, Trendelenburg positioning or presence of a tight cervical collar can increase intraocular blood volume, dilate orbital vessels, and inhibit aqueous drainage. Straining, retching, or coughing during induction of anesthesia will markedly increase venous pressure and can readily precipitate an increase in IOP of 40 mm Hg or more. Should this occur while the globe is open during surgery, such as during corneal transplant, loss of vitreous, hemorrhage, and expulsion of eye contents may lead to permanent damage to the eye or even blindness. Arterial hypertension can transiently increase IOP but has much less impact than perturbations of venous drainage. External compression on the globe by a tightly applied facemask, laryngoscopy, and tracheal intubation also elevate IOP, but placement of a supraglottic airway has minimal impact. Hypoxemia and hypoventilation can increase IOP. Hyperventilation and hypothermia have the opposite effect.

Anesthetic Drugs and Intraocular Pressure

Inhaled and most intravenous anesthetics produce dose-related reductions in IOP. Although the exact mechanisms are not known, IOP is probably reduced by a combination of central nervous system depression, diminished aqueous humor production, enhanced aqueous outflow, and relaxation of extraocular muscles. There is controversy surrounding the effect of ketamine on IOP. Although ketamine may not increase IOP, it does cause rotatory nystagmus and blepharospasm, making it a less-than-ideal anesthetic for eye surgery.

In the absence of alveolar hypoventilation, nondepolarizing neuromuscular blocking drugs decrease IOP via relaxation of the extraocular muscles. In contrast, succinylcholine produces an increase of about 9 mm Hg in 1 to 4 minutes after intravenous administration, with a subsequent diminution to baseline within 7 minutes. The increase in IOP is probably the result of several mechanisms, including tonic contraction of extraocular muscles, relaxation of orbital smooth muscle, choroidal vascular dilation, and aqueous outflow-impeding cycloplegia. Many clinicians avoid using succinylcholine with eye surgery patients; however, pretreatment with a small dose of a nondepolarizing neuromuscular blocking drug, lidocaine, β-blocker, or acetazolamide may attenuate the increase in IOP associated with induction of anesthesia with succinylcholine, direct laryngoscopy, and endotracheal intubation.

Ophthalmic Medications

Systemic absorption of topical ophthalmic drugs from either the conjunctiva or via drainage through the nasolacrimal duct onto the nasal mucosa can produce untoward side effects. These drops include acetylcholine, anticholinesterases, cyclopentolate, epinephrine, phenylephrine, and timolol (Table 31.1). Phospholine iodide (echothiophate) is a miosis-inducing anticholinesterase that profoundly interferes with metabolism of succinylcholine. Prolonged paralysis after a single dose of succinylcholine may ensue. Phenylephrine drops are available in concentrations of 2.5% and 10%. Systemic absorption via the nasolacrimal duct of 10% phenylephrine drops can induce transient malignant hypertension. Parenteral administration of a long-acting antihypertensive drug may result in untoward hypotension after resolution of the short-acting phenylephrine. Some systemic ophthalmic drugs, such as glycerol, mannitol, and acetazolamide, may also produce untoward side effects.

Oculocardiac Reflex

The OCR is a sudden profound decrease in heart rate in response to traction on the extraocular muscles or

Table 31.1	Drugs Administered to Ophthalmic Surgery Patients		
Ophthalmic Indication	**Drug**	**Mechanism of Action**	**Systemic Effect**
Miosis	Acetylcholine	Cholinergic agonist	Bronchospasm, bradycardia, hypotension
Glaucoma (increased intraocular pressure)	Acetazolamide	Carbonic anhydrase inhibitor	Diuresis, hypokalemic metabolic acidosis
	Echothiophate	Irreversible cholinesterase inhibitor	Prolongation of succinylcholine's effects
			Reduction in plasma cholinesterase activity up to 3–7 weeks after discontinuation
			Bradycardia, bronchospasm
	Timolol	β-Adrenergic antagonist	Atropine-resistant bradycardia, bronchospasm, exacerbation of congestive heart failure; possible exacerbation of myasthenia gravis
Mydriasis, ophthalmic capillary decongestion	Atropine	Anticholinergic	Central anticholinergic syndrome (*mad as a hatter*, delirium, agitation; *hot as a hare*, fever; *red as a beet*, flushing; *dry as a bone*, xerostomia, anhidrosis)
			Blurred vision (cycloplegia, photophobia)
	Cyclopentolate	Anticholinergic	Disorientation, psychosis, convulsions, dysarthria
	Epinephrine	α-, β-Adrenergic agonist	Hypertension, tachycardia, cardiac dysrhythmias; epinephrine paradoxically leads to decreased intraocular pressure and can also be used for glaucoma
	Phenylephrine	α-Adrenergic agonist, direct-acting vasopressor	Hypertension (1 drop, or 0.05 mL, of a 10% solution contains 5 mg of phenylephrine)
	Scopolamine	Anticholinergic	Central anticholinergic syndrome (see atropine earlier)

external pressure on the globe. There is a wide range of reported incidence, varying from approximately 15% to 80%. This reflex occurs more commonly in young patients. The reflex arc has a trigeminal nerve afferent limb that generates an efferent vagal response that may precipitate a variety of dysrhythmias, including junctional or sinus bradycardia, atrioventricular block, ventricular bigeminy, multifocal premature ventricular contractions, ventricular tachycardia, and asystole.

The OCR is most often encountered during strabismus surgery but can occur during any type of ophthalmic surgery. OCR may also occur while performing an ophthalmic regional anesthetic nerve block. Hypercarbia, hypoxemia, and light planes of anesthetic depth augment the incidence and severity of OCR.

Prompt removal of the instigating surgical stimulus frequently results in rapid recovery. Unrelenting tension may induce cardiac arrest, so heart rate must be continuously monitored during eye regional block and surgery. At the first sign of dysrhythmia, surgery must stop and all pressure on the eye or traction on eye muscles discontinued. The ventilatory status and depth of anesthesia should be reassessed. The reflex may extinguish itself after a few minutes; it also can be abated by administration of a parasympatholytic drug such as atropine or glycopyrrolate. The OCR can also be eradicated by an anesthetic eye block, thereby abolishing its afferent arc. Paradoxically, initial placement of a regional block can induce the OCR.

The prophylactic use of intramuscular anticholinergics for adult ophthalmic surgery patients is not recommended, as the tachycardia after atropine or glycopyrrolate may have significant consequences for geriatric patients with coexisting cardiac disease (also see Chapter 26). In children (also see Chapter 34) who are more dependent on heart rate to maintain cardiac output, prophylactic intravenous administration of atropine (0.01 to 0.02 mg/kg) or glycopyrrolate may be prudent just before commencing eye surgery.

Preoperative Assessment

Patients having eye surgery are often at the extremes of age, —ranging from premature babies with retinopathy to the elderly. Hence, special age-related considerations such as altered pharmacokinetics and pharmacodynamics apply (also see Chapter 35). The elderly, pediatric patients with various syndromes, and premature infants frequently have multiple comorbid conditions. Preoperative evaluation is vital, but routine laboratory testing is not appropriate. For cataract surgery, in particular, routine testing is associated with a significant increase in health care spending.[3] Physician assessment and judgment determine the need for indicated laboratory testing.[4] Cessation of antiplatelet/anticoagulant drugs before eye surgery is controversial.[5] The risk of intraocular bleeding versus the risk of perioperative stroke, myocardial ischemia, and deep venous thrombosis must be assessed.[6]

One of the most important preoperative assessments is the likelihood of patient movement during surgery. Inability to remain supine and relatively still during intraocular surgery with MAC may result in eye injury and have devastating long-term visual consequences.[7]

Anesthetic Options

Anesthetic options for most ophthalmic procedures include general anesthesia, retrobulbar (intraconal) block, peribulbar (extraconal) anesthesia, sub-Tenon block, and topical analgesia (Box 31.1). Often, there is minimal exposure to regional anesthetic eye block techniques during anesthesia training, creating a reluctance to perform such blocks. Professional societies dedicated to teaching safe ophthalmic regional anesthesia can provide valuable instruction.[8] Site of surgery errors is more common for eye procedures than all other surgeries (except dental and digital). Of prime importance is confirmation of the correct side of surgery (i.e., right eye versus left eye) immediately before anesthesia and surgery.

Needle-Based Ophthalmic Regional Anesthesia

The anatomic foundation of needle-based eye blocks rests upon the concept of the orbital cone. This structure consists of the four ocular rectus muscles extending from their origin at the apex of the orbit to the globe anteriorly. These muscles and their surrounding connective tissue form a compartment behind the globe akin to the brachial plexus sheath in the axilla.

A retrobulbar block is performed by inserting a steeply angled needle from the inferotemporal orbital rim into this muscle cone such that the tip of the needle is behind (retro) the globe (bulbar).[9] A more descriptive term is

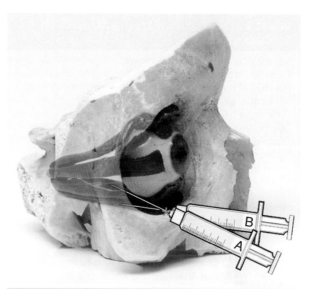

Fig. 31.1 Needle-Based Regional Anesthesia for Ophthalmic Surgery. (A) An intraconal (retrobulbar) block is placed deeper and is more steeply angled. (B) An extraconal (peribulbar) block is shallower and minimally angled. Asterisk indicates needle entry point. A portion of the lateral orbital rim is removed. (Model courtesy of Dr. Roy Hamilton.)

intraconal block (Fig. 31.1).[10] Injection of a small volume of local anesthetic into this compartment will produce rapid onset of akinesia and analgesia.

The boundary separating the intraconal from extraconal space is porous, and thus local anesthetics injected outside the muscle cone diffuse inward. A peribulbar block can be achieved by directing a minimally angled needle to a shallow depth such that the tip remains outside the cone (see Fig. 31.1). This extraconal block is theoretically safer because the needle is not directed toward the apex of the orbit; hence, the needle tip is ultimately situated farther from key intraorbital structures. This distance minimizes the potential for optic nerve trauma, optic nerve sheath injection, orbital epidural, and brainstem anesthesia. Complications of needle-based eye blocks are listed in Box 31.2. Because extraconal block local anesthetics are injected at a farther distance from the nerves, larger volumes and more time for diffusion of the local anesthetic are needed. Thus intraconal versus extraconal anesthesia is somewhat analogous to subarachnoid versus epidural anesthesia in terms of volume, onset, and density of block.

Altered physiologic status after an ophthalmic anesthetic block has important implications. Differential diagnosis includes oversedation, brainstem anesthesia, and intravascular injection of local anesthetic (Table 31.2). Abrupt onset of seizure activity is characteristic of intravascular injection. Convulsions are typically of brief and limited duration. A small dose of induction agent (e.g., propofol) or benzodiazepine may be beneficial. Brainstem

Box 31.1 Goals for Anesthesia Management of Ophthalmic Surgery
Safety
Analgesia
Akinesia (when indicated)
Control of intraocular pressure
Avoidance of the oculocardiac reflex
Awareness of possible drug interactions
Awakening without coughing, nausea, or vomiting

IV

Box 31.2 Complications of Regional Anesthesia for Ophthalmic Surgery

Superficial or retrobulbar hemorrhage
Elicitation of the oculocardiac reflex
Puncture of the globe
Intraocular injection
Optic nerve trauma
Seizures (intravenous injection of local anesthetic solution)
Brainstem anesthesia (spread of local anesthetic to the
    brainstem causing delayed-onset loss of consciousness,
    respiratory depression, paralysis of the contralateral
    extraocular muscles)
Central retinal artery occlusion
Blindness

Table 31.2 Differential Diagnosis of Altered Physiologic Status After Regional Anesthesia for Ophthalmic Surgery

Alteration	Oversedation	Brainstem Anesthesia	Intravascular Injection
Loss of consciousness	±	+	+
Apnea	±	+	±
Cardiac instability	±	+	±
Seizure activity	Ø	Ø	+
Contralateral mydriasis	Ø	±	Ø
Contralateral eye block	Ø	±	Ø

+, Likely; ±, may or may not be present; Ø, not present.

anesthesia may have a gradual latency of onset and persist for 10 to 40 minutes or longer. Patients must be continuously monitored after anesthetic eye blocks for signs of oversedation, brainstem anesthesia, and intravascular absorption of local anesthetics.

Branches of the facial nerve that innervate the eyelid's orbicularis oculi muscle are blocked by the larger volume of local anesthetic used with extraconal injection. This prevents eyelid squeezing and is a distinct advantage during corneal transplantation. An intraconal block requires a separate facial nerve injection to limit blepharospasm.

Cannula-Based Ophthalmic Regional Anesthesia

Ophthalmic anesthesia can also be achieved by instilling local anesthetics through a cannula into the space between the globe's rigid sclera and sub-Tenon capsule (Fig. 31.2).[11] The capsule consists of fascia that envelops the eye, providing a smooth friction-free interface in which to rotate.

Anteriorly, it originates near the limbal margin, where it is fused to the conjunctiva. As the capsule extends posteriorly, it surrounds the eye, with portions reflected onto the extraocular muscles. Local anesthetics injected into the sub-Tenon space block ciliary nerves that penetrate the capsule and the optic nerve posteriorly.

A cannula is introduced into the episcleral (or sub-Tenon) space through a dissection accomplished with blunt scissors. Alternatively, the dissection can be created with a blunt conjunctival probe or by using a blunt-tipped, side-ported rigid cannula.[12]

Topical Ophthalmic Regional Anesthesia

Topical anesthesia is typically achieved using local anesthetic lidocaine gel. The gel acts as a barrier to antiseptic, so 5% betadine drops are instilled before application of gel. Local anesthetic drops are placed to minimize the astringency of the betadine. Intraoperatively, the surgeon can inject preservative-free local anesthetic into the anterior chamber to supplement anesthesia.

Anesthesia Management of Specific Ophthalmic Procedures

Retina Surgery

The globe's posterior inner wall is lined by the retina, sensory tissue that converts incoming light into neural output and, ultimately, vision. The densely packed macula near its center provides fine detailed vision. Perfusion comes from the choroid layer situated between the sclera and the retina. The retina may break or detach from the choroid, leading to ischemia and compromised vision. Patients with diabetic retinopathy or extreme myopia are at particular risk. Surgical options include combinations of scleral buckle, vitrectomy, laser, cryotherapy, and injection of intravitreal gas.

Preoperative evaluation of patients with diabetes and coexisting comorbid conditions (also see Chapter 13) is important, and appropriate changes should be made to ensure that these patients are in optimal medical condition for surgery. Sudden death during retina surgery can occur because of venous air embolism introduced into the choroid blood flow during the air/fluid exchange portion of vitrectomy.[13] Retina surgery is often prolonged and associated with more extensive manipulation of the eye, therefore requiring general anesthesia or dense regional anesthetic block with MAC. Perfluorocarbons such as sulfur hexafluoride (SF6) and C3F8 are inert, relatively insoluble gases that are injected to internally tamponade the retina onto the choroid. Resorption can take 10 to 28 days depending on which drug is selected. As nitrous oxide is over 100-fold more diffusible than SF6, it can expand the size of the gas bubble, increase IOP, and potentially cause retinal ischemia and permanent loss of vision.[14] Nitrous oxide should be discontinued 20 minutes before gas injection or omitted altogether.

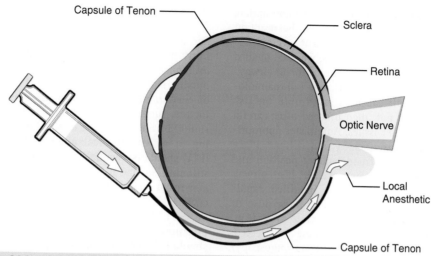

Fig. 31.2 Sub-Tenon Block. Local anesthetic is infused via a cannula into the potential space between the capsule of Tenon and the sclera, ultimately arriving at the optic nerve.

Glaucoma

Glaucoma is commonly characterized as a sustained increase in IOP that leads to diminished perfusion of the optic nerve and eventual loss of vision. Various forms of glaucoma exist, each presenting with differing degrees of IOP variation. Terminology can be confusing, resulting in several classifications: acquired versus congenital, high IOP versus normal pressure, acute versus chronic, and open versus narrow or closed angle. Angle-closure (acute) glaucoma occurs when the angle between the iris and cornea narrows and obstructs outflow. Open-angle (chronic) glaucoma results from sclerosis of the trabecular meshwork and impaired aqueous drainage. Outflow is improved with constriction of the pupil by miotic drugs. Administration of atropine drops into the eye produce mydriasis and are contraindicated. Intravenous atropine, on the other hand, is minimally absorbed by the eye and should be used when indicated during anesthesia. Infantile glaucoma may readily progress to blindness, making early surgery more urgent. Congenital glaucoma is often a component of many syndromes, several of which have important anesthesia implications.

Many adult glaucoma procedures can be managed with regional anesthesia and MAC. General anesthesia is requisite for pediatric glaucoma cases. Anesthesia implications include (1) avoiding mydriasis by continuing all miotic drops; (2) understanding the interactions of antiglaucoma medications and anesthetics (see Table 31.1); and (3) preventing increases in IOP associated with induction, maintenance, and emergence from anesthesia.

Strabismus Surgery

Strabismus surgery is performed to correct misalignment of extraocular muscles and realign the visual axis. Most patients are pediatric (also see Chapter 34). Special considerations include (1) frequent incidence of intraoperative OCR, (2) potential increased risk for malignant hyperthermia, and (3) marked prevalence of postoperative nausea and vomiting (PONV).

Nausea and Vomiting

The incidence of PONV after strabismus surgery varies widely but has been quoted as high as 85%. PONV is the most common reason for pediatric inpatient admission after outpatient surgery and is probably a vagal-mediated response to surgical manipulation of extraocular muscles. Multimodal antiemetics with differing mechanisms of action may be more effective than individual medications for those patients at most risk of PONV after eye surgery.

Malignant Hyperthermia

Strabismus is a neuromuscular disorder that can be associated with other myopathies. The frequency of masseter muscle spasm after succinylcholine is fourfold greater than baseline. Suspect malignant hyperthermia if hypertension, tachycardia, hypercarbia, and increasing temperature occur (also see Chapter 7).

Traumatic Eye Injuries

Eye injury occurs from penetrating or blunt trauma. The anesthesia plan must balance specific risks. Increased IOP resulting from a tightly applied facemask, laryngoscopy, and endotracheal intubation, or because of coughing or bucking, can cause extrusion of globe contents and jeopardize vision. Additionally, in emergency situations, the patient may be nonfasting and at risk of aspiration of gastric contents upon induction of general anesthesia. Control of the airway can be achieved with a rapid-sequence induction of anesthesia, including succinylcholine; however, succinylcholine can also cause a transient increase in

IOP.[15] Awake endotracheal intubation may be appropriate for patients with difficult airways; however, the resultant increases in IOP can be disastrous. The risks of succinylcholine or awake intubation on IOP must be weighed against the dangers imposed by a full stomach or difficult airway.

The anesthesia provider should ask the ophthalmologist if the operative repair can be delayed until the risk of aspiration is lower. If not, then proceed after careful evaluation to rule out other issues. Administer appropriate drugs to decrease gastric acidity and volume. Place the patient in slight reverse Trendelenburg position and avoid any maneuvers that may increase IOP. If no airway problems are anticipated, consider a modified rapid-sequence induction of anesthesia with a large dose of a nondepolarizing neuromuscular blocking drug (e.g., rocuronium 1.2 mg/kg). If succinylcholine is selected, the IOP and systemic hypertension after laryngoscopy/intubation can be moderated by intravenous lidocaine, opioids, or a small pretreatment dose of nondepolarizing neuromuscular blocker before induction of anesthesia. Regional anesthesia may be an option for select injuries and patients at greater risk from general anesthesia.[16]

Postoperative Eye Issues

Corneal Abrasion

The most common cause of postoperative eye pain after general anesthesia is corneal abrasion. It manifests with conjunctivitis, tearing, and foreign body sensation. Damage may be mechanically incurred by dangling ID tags, the anesthesia mask, drapes, and other objects. During general anesthesia, abrasion may also occur because of the loss of the blink reflex, the drying effects of exposure to air, and diminished tear production. Preventive measures include gently taping the eyelids shut during mask ventilation, endotracheal intubation, and thereafter. Ointments may cause allergic reaction or blurred postemergence vision. Protective goggles may be best. Antibiotic ointment and patching the eye usually result in healing of corneal abrasions within a day or two.

Acute Glaucoma

Acute glaucoma can be very painful. Presence of a mydriatic pupil may be diagnostic. This is an urgent matter calling for consult with an ophthalmologist. Intravenous mannitol or acetazolamide can decrease IOP and relieve pain.

Postoperative Visual Loss

Painless loss of vision after surgery may be the result of ischemic optic neuropathy (ION) or brain injury (also see Chapter 19). Both are rare events. Risk is more frequent with spine surgery in the prone position and cardiac surgery.[17] Consultation with an ophthalmologist is mandatory, as early funduscopic examination may aid in diagnosis.

OTOLARYNGOLOGY

Ear, nose, and throat (ENT) surgery can make the airway fairly inaccessible and is commonly referred to as *field avoidance*. Preoperative planning with the surgeon and nursing staff is essential.[18] There is a distinct possibility of encountering a difficult airway because of anatomic factors, surgical issues, or underlying disease. Attention should be directed to the establishment and firm anchoring of an endotracheal airway. The endotracheal tube (ETT) should be manually supported during patient repositioning, such as turning of the head, because movement can result in endobronchial intubation, tube occlusion, cuff leaks, disconnections, or even frank dislodgement of the ETT and inadvertent extubation. Before surgical preparation or placement of drapes, the neck position should be reassessed and susceptible pressure points padded. During surgery, the airway may be compromised by often undetected bleeding, edema, or surgical manipulation. The use of posterior pharyngeal packs can minimize the risk of aspiration of gastric contents. Operating room personnel should be alerted to their placement, and there must be confirmation of the complete removal of all packs before extubation of the trachea.

Special Considerations for Head and Neck Surgery

The Difficult Airway (Also See Chapter 16)

Preoperative assessment of patients undergoing head and neck surgery may generate airway concerns; management should be discussed with the surgeon before entering the operating room. In anticipation, supplementary equipment should be readied and expert assistance immediately available. Modified techniques for securing the airway include video laryngoscopy, fiber-optic bronchoscopy, or even performance of a tracheostomy under local anesthesia. Importantly, tracheal retention sutures should be performed during tracheostomy in order to facilitate airway recapture when patency is compromised. Intratracheal procedures may result in significant edema and acute obstruction. In the acute postoperative phase some patients may remain intubated, whereas others may require treatment with humidified oxygen or nebulized bronchodilators.

Laryngospasm

The laryngeal reflex producing laryngospasm is mediated by vagal stimulation of the superior laryngeal nerve. Abrupt intense, prolonged closure of the larynx compromising gas exchange may occur secondary to instrumentation of the endolarynx, presence of blood or foreign body, and inadequate depth of anesthesia. In complete airway obstruction the anesthesia provider may be unable to ventilate despite an adequate mask fit. The resultant hypercarbia, hypoxia, and acidosis elicit an autonomic sympathetic response manifesting as hypertension and tachycardia. However, temporal reduction in brainstem firing to the superior laryngeal nerve eventually causes relaxation of the vocal cords. In small children even brief laryngospasm is perilous because hypoxemia develops rapidly as a result of their reduced functional residual capacity and high cardiac output (also see Chapter 34). Prompt recognition and intervention are essential. Treatment modalities include the administration of 100% oxygen via positive-pressure facemask ventilation, placement of an oral or nasal airway, and deepening of anesthesia with intravenously administered anesthetics. Small doses of succinylcholine (0.25 to 0.5 mg/kg) and tracheal intubation may be necessary in refractory cases. The likelihood of encountering laryngospasm may be reduced with the use of intravenous or topical lidocaine spray before laryngoscopy and endotracheal intubation.

Upper Respiratory Infections

Patients, especially children, scheduled for elective ENT surgery may present with an unresolved upper respiratory infection (URI) predisposing to airway hyperreactivity. These children are at enhanced risk of intraoperative breath-holding, hypoxemia, and postoperative croup.[19] Postponing surgery for uncomplicated pediatric URI is controversial and may not be required for brief non-airway ENT procedures such as myringotomy and tube placement (also see Chapter 34).

Epistaxis

Patients with massive epistaxis are often anxious, hypovolemic, and hypertensive. Rehydration and reassurance are essential. These patients are considered at high risk for regurgitation and aspiration of gastric contents because large amounts of blood are swallowed. A large-bore peripheral intravenous cannula with generous rehydration is vital because blood loss is occult, and hypotension or further hemorrhage may occur after induction of anesthesia.

Obstructive Sleep Apnea (Also See Chapter 48)

Obstructive sleep apnea (OSA) is characterized by upper airway obstruction and disordered breathing patterns during sleep. Symptoms include snoring, headache, sleep disturbance, daytime somnolence, and personality changes. Polysomnography (sleep study) establishes the diagnosis and severity of the disorder but is not routinely performed. Pediatric patients may have behavior and growth disturbances in addition to poor school performance. Patients with OSA are often obese with short, thick necks and large tongues. These factors contribute to difficult airway management during mask ventilation, direct laryngoscopy, tracheal intubation, and extubation.[20]

In addition, patients with OSA are exquisitely sensitive to the side effects of hypnotics (sedation) and narcotics (respiratory depression) resulting in prolonged recovery

times. High-flow (70 L/min) nasal oxygen has been used during induction of anesthesia to decrease the risk of hypoxemia during laryngoscopy.[21]

Airway Fires

Airway fires are a direct patient hazard and source of medical litigation. Three elements are needed to produce a fire in the operating room: (1) heat or a source of ignition (laser or electrosurgical unit); (2) fuel (paper drapes, ETT, or gauze swabs); and (3) oxidizer (O_2, air, or N_2O).

The danger of an airway fire is not limited to general anesthesia. It may also occur during face and neck procedures conducted under MAC because electrocautery is used in close proximity to an open source of oxygen, such as nasal cannula.[22]

Anesthesia Management of Specific Otolaryngology Procedures

Ear Surgery

There are several points to consider for anesthesia and ear surgery, discussed in the following sections.

Nitrous Oxide

Nitrous oxide is more soluble than nitrogen in blood and diffuses into air-filled cavities faster than nitrogen. The resultant increase in middle ear pressure may be problematic because of potential for dislodgement of eardrum grafts. Furthermore, acute discontinuation of high concentrations of nitrous oxide markedly decreases pressure in the middle-ear cavity, producing serous otitis. Nitrous oxide should be avoided or used in moderate concentration (<50%) and discontinued at least 15 minutes before application of an eardrum graft.

Facial Nerve Monitoring

The surgeon may elect to use a facial nerve monitor to avoid inadvertent injury to the facial nerve branches during surgery. The administration of long-acting neuromuscular blocking agents will hinder detection of facial nerve activity by the monitor. Therefore use of nondepolarizing neuromuscular blocking drugs should be limited to induction; succinylcholine is a viable alternative. Also, a neuromuscular monitor can be used to confirm a response to train-of-four stimulation of a peripheral nerve and absence of full paralysis before surgical dissection in the middle ear (also see Chapter 11).

Epinephrine

Epinephrine is frequently injected during ear microsurgery to decrease bleeding and improve surgical field visualization. Systemic uptake may precipitate tachydysrhythmias. Hence, epinephrine concentration should be limited to a 1:200,000 solution.[23] Other means to control bleeding include moderate reverse Trendelenburg (head-up) positioning to decrease venous congestion and the use

IV

of volatile anesthetics to decrease systolic arterial blood pressures within an acceptable range. The use of vasoactive drugs and controlled hypotension is controversial.

Emergence

Head and neck manipulation during the application of bandages at the conclusion of surgery produces movement of the ETT and airway irritation. Coughing and bucking increase venous pressure, which can lead to graft disruption or acute bleeding. In the patient with an uncomplicated airway extubation of the trachea at a deep plane of anesthesia may be beneficial.

Postoperative Nausea and Vomiting (Also See Chapter 39)

As a result of manipulation of the vestibular apparatus, PONV is common after middle ear surgery. Factors exacerbating PONV include anesthetic technique (use of nitrous oxide and narcotics), inadequate rehydration, and postoperative movement. The number and dosing of prophylactic agents to prevent PONV are guided by a graded risk analysis.[24] Prophylactic interventions may include use of one or more antiemetics, including corticosteroid, 5-HT3-receptor antagonist, neurokinin-1 receptor antagonist, scopolamine patch, low-dose propofol, and gastric decompression. Scopolamine may cause confusion and probably should not be used in elderly patients.

Myringotomy and Tube Insertion

Myringotomy and tube insertion are performed for children with disorders of the middle ear who have a history of repeated ear infections with unsatisfactory response to antibiotic therapy. There may be residual middle ear inflammation and upper airway irritability. An inhalation induction and maintenance via spontaneous respiration with a facemask is preferred for this brief procedure. Also, premedication may not be necessary because residual sedation may delay a rapid recovery.

Tonsillectomy and Adenoidectomy

Most patients undergoing this procedure are young and healthy. Common surgical perioperative issues include airway obstruction, bleeding, cardiac arrhythmias, and croup (postextubation airway edema). Patients frequently have upper airway obstruction that only becomes apparent during sleep (OSA). In general, a comprehensive history and physical examination are sufficient, but symptoms of sleep-disordered breathing, obesity, or a bleeding diathesis warrants further investigation. Sedative premedication is best avoided in children with OSA, obesity, intermittent airway obstruction, or significant tonsillar hypertrophy.

In young children inhalational induction of anesthesia is preferred because preoperative establishment of an intravenous line may be difficult or traumatic. Intravenous access is secured once the child is anesthetized. Loss of pharyngeal muscle tone upon induction of anesthesia

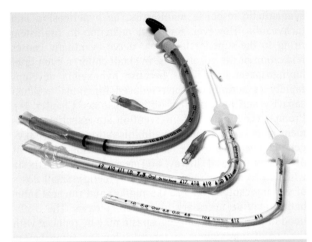

Fig. 31.3 Armored and cuffed preformed curved oral endotracheal tubes.

may cause airway obstruction and require assistance with positive airway pressure. Placement of a cuffed preformed curved oral ETT optimizes field visualization and decreases the likelihood of accidental extubation of the trachea (Fig. 31.3). An air leak at 20 cm H_2O peak airway pressure reduces the probability of tissue edema, a critical factor for pediatric patients who have narrower airway diameters than adults. A precordial stethoscope is useful to monitor breath sounds because ETT dislodgement can occur with movement of the head or mouth gag. The supraglottic area is occasionally packed with gauze to protect against aspiration. Before extubation of the trachea, the pack must be removed and the stomach should be decompressed. Tracheal extubation can be safely performed when the child is fully awake and responsive. However, some anesthesia providers opt for tracheal extubation under deep anesthesia in order to minimize cough and laryngospasm.

Intravenous dexamethasone may decrease edema and postoperative pain in addition to PONV. Postoperative airway obstruction may occur for a variety of reasons, including secretions or blood on the vocal cords or a retained pharyngeal pack. Notably, airway obstruction and respiratory efforts against a closed glottis may result in marked negative intrathoracic pressure and pulmonary edema. This pressure is transmitted to interstitial tissue and promotes the flow of fluid from the pulmonary circulation into the alveoli. Young children (younger than 4 years old) are susceptible to airway obstruction as late as 24 hours postoperatively and may benefit from prolonged postoperative monitoring.

Tonsillar Bleeding After Tonsillectomy and Adenoidectomy

The family expectation is that children undergoing tonsillectomy will have an uneventful and uncomplicated procedure and anesthesia. However, serious complications can occur. Hemorrhage after tonsillectomy normally occurs within a few hours of surgery and presents with expectoration of red blood, repeated swallowing, tachycardia, and PONV.[25] In fact, occult (swallowed) blood loss is underestimated. Intravenous rehydration is critical before surgery. A rapid-sequence induction is mandated because these patients are considered to have a stomach full of blood. The rapid-sequence induction prerequisites include preoxygenation, application of cricoid pressure (Sellick maneuver), administration of hypnotic and neuromuscular blocking drugs in rapid succession, and availability of a working suction catheter.

Epiglottitis

Acute epiglottitis is an infectious disease caused by *Haemophilus influenzae* type B, most often affecting children between 2 and 7 years of age with a history of sudden onset of fever and dysphagia.[26] Symptomatic progression from pharyngitis to airway obstruction and respiratory failure can be rapid (within hours). The child appears agitated, drools, and leans forward keeping the head in an extended position. Progression to exhaustion may result from labored breathing against a compromised airway.

Direct visualization of the glottis should not be attempted because stimulation of the patient and struggling may result in complete airway obstruction. Anesthesia commences only when all emergency airway equipment is immediately available and a surgeon adept at rigid bronchoscopy and tracheostomy is at the bedside. An inhaled induction of anesthesia maintaining spontaneous ventilation is preferred. Atropine may be given to avoid bradycardia and to dry secretions. The edematous airway necessitates use of a small ETT. Because the degree of airway narrowing is unpredictable, a range of ETT sizes should be available. In the event of any difficulty the surgeon should intervene and secure the airway with a rigid bronchoscope or establish a surgical airway.

Foreign Body in Airway

Tracheal aspiration of a foreign body is an emergency, especially in the pediatric population (also see Chapter 34). Clinical manifestations include sudden dyspnea, dry cough, hoarseness, and wheezing. Mutual cooperation between the anesthesia provider and surgeon is vital to avoid inadvertent distal displacement of the foreign body and complete airway obstruction.

Removal of the foreign body is achieved either via direct laryngoscopy or rigid bronchoscopy, without application of positive airway pressure.[27] The surgeon should be present and ready to perform emergency cricothyrotomy or tracheostomy in the event of complete airway occlusion. Total intravenous anesthesia maintaining spontaneous respiration avoids exposing operating room personnel to volatile anesthetics. Postoperatively, the patient should breathe humidified oxygen and remain under close observation for airway edema.

Nasal and Sinus Surgery

Nasal surgery is performed for either cosmetic or functional purposes. Common surgical operations include polypectomy, septoplasty, functional endoscopic sinus surgery, and rhinoplasty. Patients undergoing nasal surgery often have significant nasal passage obstruction that may hinder ventilation via facemask. Furthermore, nasal polyps are associated with allergy and asthma. The rich vascular supply can result in substantial intraoperative blood loss that may go undetected as blood trickles backward into the pharynx. Many nasal procedures can be performed with regional anesthesia and sedation.

The anterior ethmoidal and sphenopalatine branches of the trigeminal nerve provide sensory innervation to the nasal septum and lateral walls. Topical anesthesia is achieved by packing the nose with local anesthetic-soaked pledgets. Previously, the advantages of using cocaine included production of topical anesthesia, vasoconstriction of vascular tissue, and shrinking of the mucosa. Because of cocaine's disadvantages, including altered sensorium and deleterious cardiovascular effects, it has been largely replaced by a "pseudococaine" mixture of local anesthetic and vasoconstrictor.[28]

Anesthesia can be supplemented with submucosal local anesthetic infiltration. When general anesthesia is chosen, the airway should be secured with a cuffed ETT. A posterior pharyngeal pack can prevent aspiration of gastric contents and decrease PONV caused by swallowed blood. Extubation of the trachea should be performed only on return of protective airway reflexes.

Cochlear Implant Surgery

Cochlear implant is the treatment of choice for bilateral sensorineural hearing loss. The majority of these procedures are performed under general anesthesia with endotracheal intubation. In select cases the procedure may be conducted with MAC.[29]

Endoscopic Surgery

Endoscopy includes esophagoscopy, bronchoscopy, laryngoscopy, and microlaryngoscopy (with or without laser surgery). Airway evaluation is performed for a variety of pathologic conditions, ranging from foreign body, gastroesophageal reflux, and papillomatosis to tumors or tracheal stenosis. The compromised airway requires careful preoperative assessment. Airway issues should be discussed with the surgeon, and preoperative investigations such as analysis of arterial blood gases, flow-volume loops, radiographic studies, or magnetic resonance imaging may be warranted.

A proactive airway management plan is necessary. Consideration must be given to an awake fiber-optic endotracheal intubation if doubts exist about the efficacy of successful mask ventilation and direct laryngoscopy. Sedative premedication should be cautiously considered in the presence of upper airway obstruction.

IV

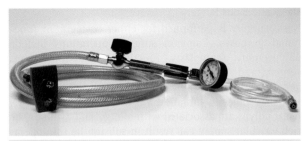

Fig. 31.4 Sanders injector apparatus uses high-flow oxygen insufflations through a small-gauge catheter placed in the trachea.

Administration of an anticholinergic drug will diminish secretions and facilitate airway visualization. Stridor and inspiratory retractions are definitive signs of airway obstruction.

Several techniques can be employed to provide oxygenation and ventilation during endoscopy. The trachea can be intubated with a small-diameter pediatric ETT, but these tubes are frequently too short for use in adults and offer high resistance to flow. Because an ETT impairs visualization of the posterior commissure, a technique using high-flow oxygen insufflations through a small-gauge catheter placed in the trachea is useful (Fig. 31.4).[30] Another alternative is a manual jet ventilator, which attaches to a side port of the laryngoscope or bronchoscope. The oxygen source is connected to "wall" pressure (30 to 50 psi), but can be regulated to the lowest pressure that produces chest rise (typically 15 to 20 psi). Oxygen flow is delivered during inspiration and concomitantly entrains air into the trachea via the Venturi effect. This technique carries a risk of pneumothorax and pneumomediastinum from rupture of alveolar blebs.

An adequate degree of masseter relaxation is required for introduction of a suspension laryngoscope by the endoscopist. A succinylcholine infusion can be administered but may produce a phase II neuromuscular block (also see Chapter 11).

Laser Surgery

Laser (light amplification by stimulated emission of radiation) surgery affords precision in targeting lesions, provides hemostasis, causes minimal tissue edema, and promotes rapid healing. Its physical properties depend on the medium used to create the beam. Laser is used in the treatment of vocal cord papillomas, laryngeal webs, and resection of subglottic occlusive tissue. The use of a small-diameter ETT is necessary for maximum exposure.[31] Laser energy can cause retinal damage and can produce a laser plume of toxic fumes with potential to transmit disease. An efficient smoke evacuator and special masks are necessary because small particles are readily inhaled. The patient's eyes should be taped, and operating room personnel must wear protective eyeglasses.

The greatest danger during laser surgery is ETT fire, so suitable precautions should be taken (Box 31.3). Flexible

stainless steel laser-resistant tubes are available for the specific type of laser employed (Fig. 31.5). To dissipate heat and detect cuff rupture, the tube cuff should be filled with saline and an indicator dye. Although polyvinylchloride tubes are flammable, they may be modified with a metallic tape wrap. Nonetheless, they retain risk for ignition and can reflect the laser beam onto nontargeted tissue. The tissue adjacent to the surgical field should be protected with moist packing. Postoperatively, patients should be monitored for laryngeal edema.

Neck Dissection Surgery

Neck dissection may be complete, modified, or functional. Anatomically, the structures principally involved are (1) the sternocleidomastoid muscle, (2) cranial nerve XI, and (3) internal and external jugular veins and carotid artery. Frequently, neck dissection is performed for removal of a tumor and may also involve partial or total glossectomy. Patients with such tumors may have a history of tobacco and alcohol use disorder. Pulmonary disease is likely and is an indication for a preoperative pulmonary evaluation.

Box 31.3 Operating Room Precautions for Laser Surgery

Preoperative Period
1. Arrange surgical drapes to avoid accumulation of combustible gases (O_2, N_2O).
2. Allow time for flammable skin preparations to dry.
3. Moisten gauze and sponges in vicinity of laser beam.

Intraoperative Period
1. Alert surgeon and OR personnel about ignition risk.
2. Assign specific roles to each OR member in case of fire.
3. Use appropriate laser-resistant ETT.
4. Reduce inspired O_2 to minimal values (monitor Spo_2).
5. Replace N_2O with air.
6. Wait a few minutes after steps 3 to 5 before activating laser.

ETT, Endotracheal tube; *OR*, operating room; *Spo$_2$*, oxygen saturation measured by pulse oximetry.

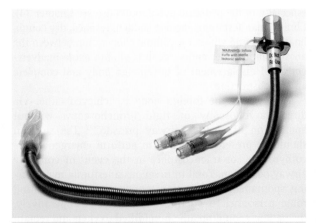

Fig. 31.5 Laser endotracheal tube—stainless steel.

In many cases the neck dissection may be bilateral, and a tracheostomy may be performed to maintain a patent airway. Upper airway management may be difficult in these patients, especially if there is a history of radiation treatment of the larynx and pharynx or if a mass is present in the oral cavity. Neuromuscular blocking drugs are ideally avoided. Traction or pressure on the carotid sinus can provoke prolongation of the QT interval, bradydysrhythmias, and even asystole. Treatment consists of early detection, cessation of surgical stimulus, and administration of atropine. The carotid sinus reflex can be blocked with local anesthetic infiltration. During dissection, open veins carry a risk of venous air embolism.

Postoperative Complications

In the postoperative period the anesthesia provider should be aware of potential nerve injuries. Damage to the recurrent laryngeal nerve can cause vocal cord dysfunction and, when bilateral, results in airway obstruction. The phrenic nerve also traverses through the operative field, and injury to it can result in paralysis of the ipsilateral hemidiaphragm. Pneumothorax can also occur in the postoperative period. Excessive coughing or agitation may cause bleeding and airway compromise. The patient should be closely monitored in the postoperative phase when a tracheostomy is not performed.

Thyroid and Parathyroid Surgery

Thyroid storm may be encountered in a patient who has inadequately controlled hyperthyroidism. It manifests with signs of massive catecholamine release, including tachycardia, hypertension, and diaphoresis. Intraoperative anesthesia considerations again focus on airway management. Surgical manipulation of the head and neck can occlude a standard ETT, so an armored ETT may be beneficial (see Fig. 31.3). Airway obstruction after thyroid or parathyroid surgery can be caused by bleeding from the operative site compressing the trachea. Emergency measures include prompt incision and opening of the wound to release the accumulated hematoma. Surgical trauma to one or both recurrent laryngeal nerves can manifest as postextubation hoarseness or stridor. Some surgeons use electromyography (EMG) to monitor recurrent laryngeal nerve integrity, using a special ETT and EMG monitor. Parathyroid injury or removal may cause hypocalcemia with clinical signs of tetany, cardiac dysrhythmias, and laryngospasm (also see Chapter 29).

Parotid Surgery

The parotid gland may be excised in toto, or surgery may be limited to the superficial portion of the gland. Because the parotid is traversed by the facial nerve, nerve function can be monitored with a facial nerve monitor in order to circumvent surgical trauma.[32] The facial nerve may need to be sacrificed during radical parotidectomy and then reconstructed with a graft from the contralateral greater auricular nerve (branch of the superficial cervical plexus). Nasotracheal intubation is appropriate if a mandibular resection is planned.

Facial Trauma

Facial fractures are characterized by the LeFort classification of maxilla fractures (Fig. 31.6).[33] Orotracheal intubation is necessary when intranasal damage is a possibility. In orthognathic surgery LeFort fractures are created for cosmetic repair.

IV

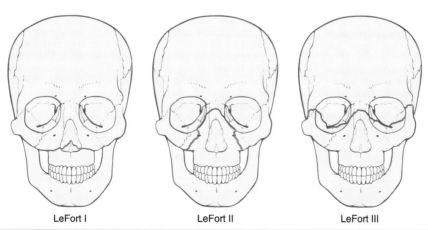

LeFort I   LeFort II   LeFort III

Fig. 31.6 Facial Injuries and the LeFort Fracture Classification. A LeFort I fracture extends across the lower portion of the maxilla but does not continue up into the medial canthal region. A LeFort II fracture also extends across the maxilla, but at a more cephalad level, and it continues upward to the medial canthal region. A LeFort III fracture is a high-level transverse fracture above the malar bone and through the orbits. It is characterized by complete separation of the maxilla from the craniofacial skeleton. (From Myer CM. Trauma of the larynx and craniofacial structures: Airway implications. *Paediatr Anaesth.* 2004;14:103–106, used with permission.)

REFERENCES

1. Gayer S, Zuleta J. Perioperative management of the elderly undergoing eye surgery. *Clin Geriatr Med.* 2008;24(4):687–700.
2. Vann MA, Ogunnaike BO, Joshi GP. Sedation and anesthesia care for ophthalmologic surgery during local/regional anesthesia. *Anesthesiology.* 2007;107(3):502–508.
3. Chen CL, Lin GA, Bardach NS, et al. Preoperative medical testing in Medicare patients undergoing cataract surgery. *N Engl J Med.* 2015;372(16):1530–1538.
4. Schein OD, Katz J, Bass EB, et al. The value of routine preoperative medical testing before cataract surgery. Study of Medical Testing for Cataract Surgery. *N Engl J Med.* 2000;342:168–175.
5. Katz J, Feldman MA, Bass EB, et al. Risks and benefits of anticoagulant and antiplatelet medication use before cataract surgery. *Ophthalmology.* 2003;110(9):1784–1788.
6. McClellan AJ, Flynn Jr HW, Gayer S. The use of perioperative antithrombotic agents in posterior segment ocular surgery. *Am J Ophthalmol.* 2014;158(5):858–859.
7. Bhananker SM, Posner FW, Cheney KL, et al. Injury and liability associated with monitored anesthesia care. A closed claims analysis. *Anesthesiology.* 2006;104(2):228–234.
8. Ophthalmic Anesthesia Society. www.eyeanesthesia.org.
9. Fanning GL. Orbital regional anesthesia. *Ophthalmol Clin North Am.* 2006;19(2):221–232.
10. Gayer S. Ophthalmic anesthesia: More than meets the eye. *ASA Refresher Courses in Anesthesiology.* 2006;34(5):55–63.
11. Kumar CM, Dodds C. Sub-Tenon's anesthesia. *Ophthalmol Clin North Am.* 2006;19(2):209–219.
12. Gayer S, Palte H. "A novel technique for minimally invasive sub-Tenon's anesthesia". *Reg Anesth Pain Med.* 2019;44(1):131–132.
13. Gayer S, Palte HD, Albini TA, Flynn HW Jr, Martinez-Ruiz R, Salas N, McClellan AJ, Relhan N, Parel JM. In-vivo porcine model of venous air embolism during pars plana vitrectomy. *Am J Ophthalmol.* 2016;171(11):139–144.
14. Wolf GL, Capuano C, Hartung J. Nitrous oxide increases intraocular pressure after intravitreal sulfur hexafluoride injection. *Anesthesiology.* 1983;59:547–548.
15. Vachon CA, Warner DO, Bacon DR. Succinylcholine and the open globe. Tracing the teaching. *Anesthesiology.* 2003;99:220–223.
16. Gayer S. Rethinking anesthesia strategies for patients with traumatic eye injuries: Alternatives to general anesthesia. *Curr Anaesth Crit Care.* 2006;17:191–196.
17. Shen Y, Drum M, Roth S. The prevalence of perioperative visual loss in the United States: A 10 year study from 1996 to 2005 of spinal, orthopedic, cardiac, and general surgery. *Anesth Analg.* 2009;109(5):1534–1545.
18. Satloff RT, Brown AC. Special equipment in the operating room for otolaryngology—Head and neck surgery. *Otolaryngol Clin North Am.* 1981;14:669–686.
19. Tait AR, Malviya S, Voepel-Lewis T, et al. Risk factors for perioperative adverse respiratory events in children with upper respiratory tract infections. *Anesthesiology.* 2001;95:299–306.
20. Gross JB, Bachenberg KL, Benumof JL, et al. Practice guidelines for the perioperative management of patients with obstructive sleep apnea: A report by the American Society of Anesthesiologists (ASA) Task Force on Perioperative Management of patients with obstructive sleep apnea. *Anesthesiology.* 2006;104(5):1081–1093.
21. Renda T, Corrado A, Iskandar G, et al. High-flow nasal oxygen therapy in intensive care and anaesthesia. *BJA.* 2018;120(1):18–27.
22. Caplan RA, Barker SJ, Connis RT, et al. American Society of Anesthesiologists Task Force on Operating Room Fires Practice advisory for the prevention and management of operating room fires. *Anesthesiology.* 2008;108(5):786–801.
23. Dunlevy TM, O'Malley TP, Postma GN. Optimal concentration of epinephrine for vasoconstriction in neck surgery. *Laryngoscope.* 1996;106:1412–1414.
24. Apfel CC, Laara E, Koivuranta M, et al. A simplified risk score for predicting postoperative nausea and vomiting: Conclusions from cross-validations between two centers. *Anesthesiology.* 1999;91:693–700.
25. Randall DA, Hoffer ME. Complications of tonsillectomy and adenoidectomy. *Otolaryngol Head Neck Surg.* 1998;118:61–68.
26. Tanner K, Fitzsimmons G, Carrol ED, et al. *Haemophilus influenzae* type b epiglottitis as a cause of acute upper airways obstruction in children. *BMJ.* 2002;325:1099–1100.
27. Lam HC, Woo JK, van Hasselt CA. Management of ingested foreign bodies: A retrospective review of 5240 patients. *J Laryngol Otol.* 2001;115:954–957.
28. Lange RA, Cigarroa RG, Yancy Jr CW, et al. Cocaine-induced coronary-artery vasoconstriction. *N Engl J Med.* 1989;321:1557–1562.
29. Hamerschmidt R, Morero A, Wiemes G, et al. Cochlear implant surgery with local anesthesia and sedation: comparison with General Anesthesia. *Otol Neurol.* 2012;34:75–78.
30. Rajagopalan R, Smith F, Ramachandran PR. Anaesthesia for microlaryngoscopy and definitive surgery. *Can Anaesth Soc J.* 1972;19:83–86.
31. Rampil IJ. Anesthetic considerations for laser surgery. *Anesth Analg.* 1992;74:424–435.
32. Terrell JE, Kileny PR, Yian C, et al. Clinical outcome of continuous facial nerve monitoring during primary parotidectomy. *Arch Otolaryngol Head Neck Surg.* 1997;123:1081–1087.
33. Myer CM. Trauma of the larynx and craniofacial structures, airway implications. *Paediatr Anaesth.* 2004;14:103–106.

32 ORTHOPEDIC SURGERY

David Furgiuele, Mitchell H. Marshall,
Andrew D. Rosenberg

RHEUMATOLOGIC DISORDERS

Patients with rheumatoid arthritis (RA) and other rheumatologic disorders, such as ankylosing spondylitis, present for orthopedic surgery related to their disease state. Knowledge of these diseases and their underlying medical issues is essential for optimal anesthetic and perioperative management.

Rheumatoid Arthritis

RA is a chronic inflammatory disease that initially destroys joints and adjacent connective tissue and then progresses to a systemic disease affecting major organ systems (Fig. 32.1). Implicated predisposing causes include genetic (over 100 gene loci have been identified), environmental, bacterial, viral, and hormonal factors.[1–5] The role of T cells, autoimmunity, and inflammatory mediators are important in the progression of RA and may serve as sites for potential new treatments.[2–5]

Systemic manifestations of RA are widespread. They may include pulmonary involvement with interstitial fibrosis and cysts with honeycombing, gastritis and ulcers from aspirin and other analgesics, neuropathy, muscle wasting, vasculitis, and anemia. Ultimately, the anatomy of the airway is damaged and altered in patients with RA.[2–5]

Airway and Cervical Spine Changes
The patient must be carefully evaluated for both complexity and risks of endotracheal intubation. For example, the airway may be difficult to visualize when attempting intubation. Furthermore, the performance of maneuvers to intubate the trachea may result in an increased risk of cervical spine injury. Many airway abnormalities may occur in patients with RA. Normal mouth opening may be decreased as a result of temporomandibular arthritis. This difficulty may be compounded by the presence of a hypoplastic mandible, which may fuse early in patients

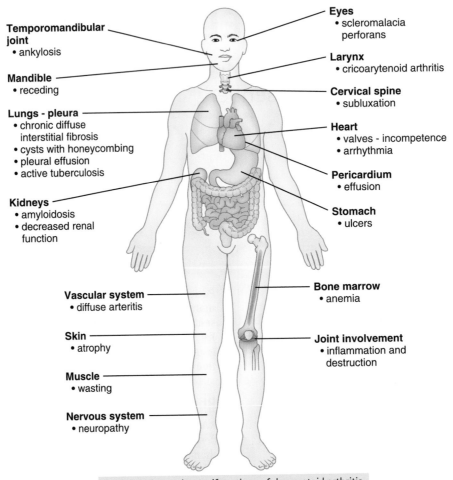

Fig. 32.1 Systemic manifestations of rheumatoid arthritis.

with juvenile RA. This results in the noticeable overbite in some patients with RA.[2-5]

As with other joints, the cricoarytenoid joint may be affected. Cricoarytenoid arthritis may result in shortness of breath and snoring. Patients with RA have been misdiagnosed as having sleep apnea as a result of this condition.[6] Patients with cricoarytenoid arthritis may present with stridor during inspiration, which may occur in the postanesthesia care unit (PACU) after surgery while recovering from anesthesia. Acute subluxation of the cricoarytenoid joint as a result of tracheal intubation can cause stridor as well and is not responsive to administration of racemic epinephrine.[3]

The cervical spine is abnormal in as many as 80% of patients with RA. Subluxation and unrestricted motion of the cervical spine can lead to impingement of the spinal cord and its injury.[7] Three anatomic areas of the cervical spine may become involved, resulting in atlantoaxial subluxation, subaxial subluxation, or superior migration of the odontoid (Fig. 32.2).

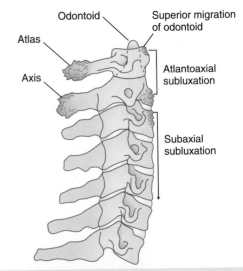

Fig. 32.2 Sites of potential involvement of rheumatoid arthritis in the cervical spine.

Atlantoaxial Subluxation

Atlantoaxial subluxation is the abnormal movement of the C1 cervical vertebra (the atlas) on C2 (the axis). Normally, the transverse axial ligament (TAL) holds the odontoid process, also referred to as the *dens,* which is the superior projection of the vertebra of C2, in place directly behind the anterior arch of C1 (Fig. 32.3A). With an intact TAL, as the cervical spine is flexed and extended, the odontoid moves with the cervical arch of C1 and the movement between the two is minimal. With destruction of the TAL by RA, movement of the dens is no longer restricted. As the neck is flexed and extended, the C1 vertebra can sublux on the C2 vertebra as the dens and C1 cervical spine no longer move together (see Fig. 32.3B). This can result in impingement of the spinal cord, placing it at risk for damage. Subluxation of C1 on C2, referred to as *atlantoaxial subluxation,* can be quantified by a measurement made between the back of the anterior arch of C1 and the front of the dens or odontoid. This distance is referred to as the *atlas-dens interval* (ADI). Flexion and extension radiographs of the cervical spine are obtained in order to determine the distance between the atlas and dens and the degree of subluxation (Fig. 32.4). If the ADI is 4 mm or more, atlantoaxial instability is present, the amount of subluxation is considered significant, and the patient is considered to be at risk for spinal cord injury. Because the ring of the cervical arch is an enclosed space, as the ADI increases, the safe area

for the cord (SAC), that area left within the arch of C1, decreases and motion can lead to impingement of the cord. In a situation in which the TAL is disrupted, extension of the head minimizes the ADI and increases the SAC, whereas flexion increases the ADI (Fig. 32.5) and decreases the SAC, making flexion a position of greater risk. However, as RA affects more than just the TAL, all neck movements in patients with RA have to be evaluated carefully because extension of the neck can also lead to problems. Although uncommon, asymptomatic patients can have ADI measurements as high as 8 mm to 10 mm. These asymptomatic patients are able to compensate for their cervical spine instability with use of local musculature while awake, but this is not possible when anesthetized. Therefore neck motion should be minimized after administration of sedation or general anesthesia in patients with atlantoaxial subluxation.[2–5,7–10]

Subaxial Subluxation

Subluxation of 15% or more of one cervical vertebra on another below the level of the axis (C2) is referred to as *subaxial subluxation.* This can result in significant spinal cord impingement and neurologic symptoms. The C5–C6 level is the most common area for subaxial subluxation.[9,10] As a result, neck motion can increase impingement and result in spinal cord injury. Therefore minimal motion of the cervical spine is recommended in patients with this condition.

Superior Migration of the Odontoid

Inflammation and bone destruction can result in cervical spine collapse in patients with RA. Not all areas of the cervical spine are equally affected in any given patient. For example, if the odontoid is spared, cervical spine collapse may actually result in an intact odontoid process projecting up through the foramen magnum and into the skull. The odontoid can impinge on the brainstem, and patients may suffer neurologic symptoms, including quadriparesis or paralysis (Fig. 32.6). This pathologic anatomic condition is referred to as *superior migration of the odontoid.* The odontoid needs to be removed in order to decompress the spinal cord and brainstem. A complicated operative procedure, a transoral odontoidectomy, may accomplish this and involves an incision in the posterior pharyngeal wall, followed by removal of the arch of C1 and then removal of the odontoid, or pannus, or both, which is causing the neurologic symptoms. With completion of the transoral portion of the procedure, the cervical spine is very unstable, necessitating a posterior spinal fusion.

The Trachea in Rheumatoid Arthritis

Although the cervical spine is affected by RA and may collapse from bone destruction, the trachea is usually spared. This results in the trachea twisting in a characteristic manner as the cervical spine collapses, only serving

IV

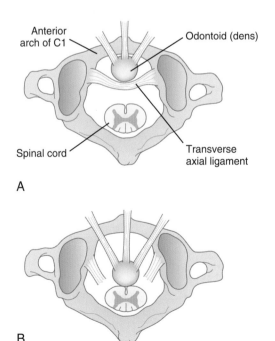

Fig. 32.3 (A) Cross-sectional view demonstrating intact transverse axial ligament (*TAL*) holding the odontoid in place against the anterior arch of C1 vertebra. (B) Rupture of TAL may result in spinal cord impingement.

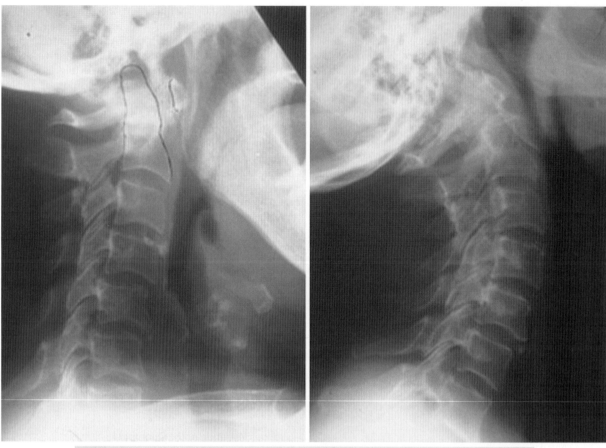

Fig. 32.4 Radiographs of cervical spine in flexion and extension. Note significant atlantoaxial instability with flexion in the left panel where the odontoid and arch of C1 are outlined. Note contrast in the right panel where in extension the odontoid and arch of C1 are in close proximity.

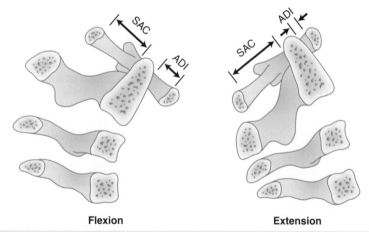

Flexion   **Extension**

Fig. 32.5 Flexion and extension views demonstrating how flexion increases the atlas-dens interval (*ADI*) and decreases the safe area for the spinal cord (*SAC*). In extension the ADI is decreased and the SAC is increased.

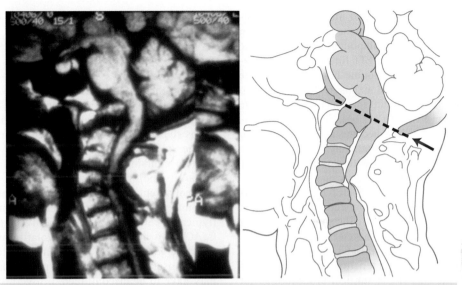

Fig. 32.6 Magnetic resonance image (*MRI*) and reconstruction demonstrating superior migration of the odontoid through the foramen magnum and impingement on medulla and pons. Also note subaxial subluxation. (MRI courtesy of Malcolm Dobrow, MD.)

to increase the difficulty of intubating these patients.[9] Tracheal intubation aids such as a fiber-optic bronchoscope, Glidescope, Airtraq, or intubating laryngeal mask airway (LMA) should be available for assistance in intubating these patients should it be needed (also see Chapter 16).

Ankylosing Spondylitis

Ankylosing spondylitis is an inflammatory rheumatologic disorder in which repetitive minute bone fractures followed by healing result in the characteristic bamboo spine, disease of the sacroiliac joint, fusion of the posterior elements of the spinal column, and fixed neck flexion that are characteristic in this patient population. There is an association between ankylosing spondylitis and HLA-B27, although most HLA-B27–positive patients are not affected with the disease. Patients also develop thoracic and costochondral involvement, which may result in a rapid shallow breathing pattern.[3,11] The cervical spine becomes rigid, and direct laryngoscopy and airway manipulation should be performed only after careful assessment. A tracheal intubation assist device can help secure the airway. Return of the neck to the neutral position via cervical spine surgery involves removal of all the bony elements of the posterior portion of the spine followed by extension of the head back into a neutral position. This is a very complicated and dangerous procedure, especially at the time when the neck is extended back to the neutral position, which relies on spinal cord monitoring to assess neurologic function as the spine is manipulated.

SPINE SURGERY

Posterior spinal fusion, scoliosis correction, and combined anteroposterior spine procedures may be long, complex operations associated with significant blood loss, marked fluid shifts, and major hemodynamic alterations. These factors necessitate adequate patient preparation for the perioperative period, including a detailed preoperative evaluation (also see Chapter 13), anticipation regarding perioperative intravenous fluid administration, and appropriate monitoring requirements. Some patients have underlying neuromuscular disorders that could influence the timing of tracheal extubation. Preoperative pulmonary function testing will facilitate clinical decisions in this patient population. Appropriate size and number of intravenous catheters, in addition to hemodynamic and neurologic monitoring needs, should be determined. In addition, the blood bank needs to be advised that significant blood loss can occur, requiring rapid administration of blood and blood products (also see Chapter 25).

Anterior spine surgery may be performed via abdominal or thoracic approaches. Thoracic surgery may involve open thoracotomy or thoracoscopic techniques. Preoperative discussion with the surgeon is crucial to determine the surgical approach, as there may be a need to provide lung isolation and one-lung ventilation. High thoracic and thoracoscopic procedures frequently require one-lung ventilation to ensure adequate visualization (also see Chapter 27). This can be accomplished with the use of a double-lumen or a bronchial blocker tube.

IV

If the procedure is a combined anteroposterior procedure, a double-lumen endotracheal tube (ETT) can be used for the anterior component, with the tube exchanged for a single-lumen ETT for the posterior portion of the surgery. Although double-lumen ETTs provide value in facilitating surgical exposure, they can also create risks, such as difficult intraoperative exchange of the double-lumen ETT to a single-lumen ETT. Reintubation of the trachea can become difficult, owing to airway edema, and may be traumatic. Alternatively, a bronchial blocker can be used with a single-lumen ETT (Fig. 32.7).[4,12]

Advantages of the bronchial blocker include avoiding the need to change the tube between different stages of the procedure or at the end of the surgery. Deflating the cuff and withdrawing the catheter back into its casing and recapping the proximal end return the ETT to its single-lumen tube characteristics. If extubation of the trachea at the end of the surgical procedure is not indicated, the ETT does not have to be changed at the end of the operation, thereby avoiding the possibility of changing an ETT in the presence of potentially significant airway edema or difficult endotracheal intubation. The PACU or intensive care unit staff needs to be properly educated as to the various ports of the bronchial blocker.[3,4,12]

Some surgeons are using CO_2 insufflation as the sole means of moving the lung away from the surgical field, even in high thoracic spine surgical procedures. This allows for the use of a single-lumen ETT for the entire procedure, bypassing the need for either a double-lumen tube or a bronchial blocker.

Anesthetic Technique

The anesthetic technique is geared to provide anesthesia and analgesia for the procedure while avoiding drugs that may interfere with acquisition of the waveforms required for perioperative neurologic evaluation of the spine. Nitrous oxide/oxygen or air/oxygen are used in combination with opioids and an infusion of propofol and/or dexmedetomidine. If somatosensory evoked potentials (SSEPs) alone are being monitored, an inhaled anesthetic, equivalent to a small percentage (typically <50%) of 1 minimum alveolar concentration (MAC), can be administered. Volatile anesthetics may interfere with signal acquisition in patients monitored with transcranial motor evoked potentials (TCMEPs) and may have to be discontinued, if used at all, if adequate signals cannot be obtained. Although neuromuscular blockade may be used to facilitate tracheal intubation, paralysis should not be maintained if TCMEPs are being continuously monitored. If the patient is having pedicle screws placed, then the neuromuscular blockade needs to be terminated before the electromyograms (EMGs) are obtained so that testing can be properly performed. A small dose of ketamine, either as a bolus or continuous infusion, can be given in the perioperative period as an additional pain relief modality to provide analgesia for major surgery, including spine surgery (also see Chapter 8).[13,14]

Awareness

Intraoperative awareness is a concern for patients and physicians alike. Patients undergoing spine surgery may be at increased risk for intraoperative awareness as a result of the requirement that the anesthetic techniques administered to them be modified to allow for adequate intraoperative neurophysiologic monitoring waveforms to assess spinal cord function. Therefore the use of brain function monitoring in these patients may help avoid intraoperative awareness. However, this is not a standard, and as noted in the Practice Advisory for Intraoperative Awareness and Brain Function Monitoring,[15] a decision should be made on a case-by-case basis by the individual practitioner for selected patients (e.g., if light anesthesia is being administered). There was a consensus in the advisory that brain function monitoring is not routinely indicated for patients undergoing general anesthesia as the "general applicability of these monitors in the prevention of intraoperative awareness had not been established." In fact, a large randomized trial of processed EEG versus end-tidal anesthetic monitoring demonstrated that awareness is not decreased with use of brain function monitoring.[16] The need for brain monitoring is still not clear.

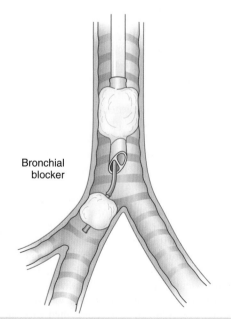

Bronchial blocker

Fig. 32.7 Depiction of how a bronchial blocker is placed to isolate the lung for one-lung ventilation.

Blood Conservation During Spine Surgery

Methods to decrease blood loss in spine surgery patients include predonation, hemodilution, wound infiltration with a dilute epinephrine solution, hypotensive anesthetic techniques, use of cell salvage devices, positioning to diminish venous pressure, careful surgical hemostasis, and administration of antifibrinolytics (also see Chapter 23). Medications that have been employed to decrease blood loss during spine surgery include the antifibrinolytics aprotinin, tranexamic acid (TXA), and ε-aminocaproic acid. Aprotinin, a serine protease inhibitor, effectively decreases blood loss in cardiac patients and has also been demonstrated to be efficacious in patients undergoing spine surgery.[17-19] The synthetic lysine analogs TXA and ε-aminocaproic acid have also been employed in patients undergoing orthopedic joint replacement surgery.[19] TXA can be administered by an initial bolus injection of 50 mg/kg over 30 minutes followed by a continuous infusion of 10 mg/kg/hr, although other regimens may be used. TXA may alternatively be given topically or intraarticularly in appropriate patients.

A metaanalysis of the use of antifibrinolytics in orthopedic patients demonstrated that although both aprotinin and TXA are effective in decreasing blood loss, the data were not sufficient to demonstrate efficacy with ε-aminocaproic acid.[18] However, the negative side effects of aprotinin in cardiac patients include (1) increased risk of myocardial infarction (MI) or heart failure by approximately 55%, nearly double the risk of stroke; (2) increased long-term risk of mortality; and (3) a more frequent death rate in patients receiving aprotinin as demonstrated in a study over a 5-year period comparing aprotinin with lysine analogs in high-risk cardiac surgery. The study was terminated early and resulted in relabeling and ultimately withdrawing aprotinin from the market.[20-22]

Positioning

Spine surgery is often performed with the patient in the prone position (also see Chapter 19). Careful positioning is crucial to avoid patient injury. Movement to the prone position should be performed in a carefully coordinated manner with the surgical team. The neck should not be hyperextended or hyperflexed but placed in the neutral position and the ETT positioned so that it is not kinked. Contact areas are padded, and the face and eyes are protected. Prolonged prone positioning has resulted in pressure ulcers on the face, especially the chin and forehead, and other areas. When possible, periodic repositioning of the head during prolonged procedures may minimize the risk of such injuries. Direct pressure on the eye can result in visual loss. Pressure and stretch on nerves are avoided by proper padding and avoiding any extension over 90 degrees. The abdomen needs to be hanging free to avoid increased venous pressure and thereby increased venous bleeding. The prone position alters pulmonary dynamics, so pulmonary function must be reassessed in this position.

Intraoperative Spinal Cord Monitoring

Monitoring spinal cord function is an important component of major surgical procedures involving distraction and rotation of the spine, such as with major anteroposterior spinal fusions and scoliosis surgery (also see Chapter 20). Spinal cord monitoring is employed in order to detect and hopefully reverse in a timely manner any adverse effects noted during the operative period. Spinal cord monitoring may include use of SSEPs, motor evoked potentials (MEPs) including TCMEPs, EMGs, or a wake-up test. The anesthetic technique must be adjusted appropriately when spinal cord monitoring is employed. Some anesthetics interfere with acquisition of the waveforms that are obtained intraoperatively and used to analyze spinal cord integrity.

SSEPs are sensory evoked potential waves generated in the cerebral cortex that result from sensory stimuli caused by repetitive peripheral nerve stimulation in the extremities that propagate up through the dorsum or sensory portion of the spinal cord and into the brain. These waveforms are then detected via electrodes placed over the scalp. Specific areas on the scalp coincide with the brain's sensory areas for the upper and lower extremities, and proper signal acquisition obtained over these sites indicates an intact sensory or dorsal portion of the spinal cord. The SSEP waveform generated from multiple repetitive stimulations is analyzed for its latency and amplitude (Fig. 32.8). An increase in latency of more than 10% or a decrease in amplitude of 60% or more, in addition to an inability to obtain a proper waveform or signal, may be indicative of spinal cord dysfunction or disruption. Many factors can alter waveforms unrelated to surgery. They should be properly detected and eliminated. Surgically unrelated causes may include hypotension, hypothermia, high concentrations of volatile anesthetics, benzodiazepines, hypercarbia or hypocarbia, and anemia. Only a small concentration of volatile anesthetic (typically 1% to 2% desflurane) should be employed when SSEP monitoring is used. Midazolam and other benzodiazepines are avoided because they may interfere with obtaining a waveform. Some anesthesia providers avoid nitrous oxide and use a combination of air in oxygen.[3-5,13,14]

Surgically related conditions resulting in loss of SSEPs include direct injury or trauma to the cord or impairment of blood supply. Distraction, rotation, excessive bleeding, and severing or clamping of arterial blood supply can result in ischemia to the cord and neurologic injury. Unlike direct injury, which is demonstrated immediately by changes in SSEPs, ischemia may take time, up to half an hour or longer, to manifest itself. Some areas of the spinal cord are more vulnerable and therefore more

IV

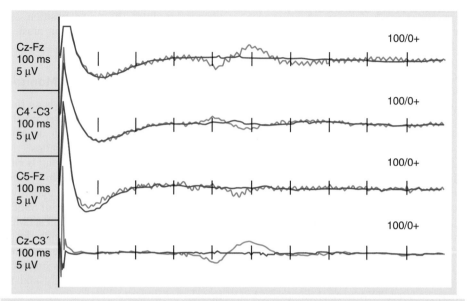

Fig. 32.8 Somatosensory evoked potentials (*SSEPs*) of tibial nerve demonstrating loss of SSEP waveform. Note how the newly acquired waveforms (*purple*) are flattened when compared with baseline tracings (*red*) as amplitudes of tracings are decreased and latency increased. Tracings returned to normal after retraction of the cauda equina was released. (Courtesy of Department of Neurophysiology, NYU Hospital for Joint Diseases.)

prone to ischemia, as their blood supply is dependent on watershed blood flow. Surgical intervention as a result of either direct contact or stretching may impair blood supply and thus render the cord ischemic.[23] Once a significant change in SSEPs or other monitor is noted, specific maneuvers should be used such as releasing the rotation and distraction of the spine if it has occurred. In addition, as a result of distraction, there may be insufficient blood supply to the spine, and therefore, the mean arterial blood pressure should be increased in an effort to restore adequate blood flow. All variables such as hemoglobin, temperature, CO_2, and arterial blood pressure should be considered. Once these are all evaluated, a wake-up test (see following discussion) may be necessary if the waveforms do not improve.

Transcranial Motor Evoked Potentials

As SSEP monitoring only helps determine adequate status of the dorsal or sensory portion of the spinal cord, a method to monitor the motor or ventral aspect of the spinal cord became necessary.[24] Initially this was provided via neurogenic MEPs, but these waveforms could be obtained only while the surgical incision was open and the spinous processes available for insertion of electrodes. Thus some vulnerable operative periods remained unmonitored. TCMEPs allow for monitoring the patient's motor pathways throughout the entire procedure. Stimulation over the motor cortex of the brain generates a waveform, which is propagated down the

motor pathways and detected distally in the arm or leg. This stimulation results in a characteristic waveform (Fig. 32.9). Loss of the wave may be indicative of neurologic injury (see Fig. 32.9). As with SSEP waveforms, loss of the tracings requires the following steps: an evaluation to determine the cause, attention to physiologic variables, intervention to increase arterial blood pressure, and possibly a wake-up test as well.[25]

To generate TCMEPs, the patient cannot have a residual neuromuscular blockade (also see Chapter 11). Importantly, it should be understood that the electric current causing the stimulus over the motor cortex also stimulates muscles directly in the area of the electrodes placed in the scalp—the masseter muscle and muscles of mastication. This muscle contraction may result in a strong bite, which can potentially injure the tongue, lip, and ETT. Instances of significant tongue lacerations and damage to ETTs can occur and potentially develop into emergency situations, especially with the patient in the prone position.[26] The tongue should not protrude through the teeth. Placing a bite block made of tongue depressors and gauze in the back of the mouth along the teeth line bilaterally will help prevent injury. In the prone (face-down) position, any motion may allow for the tongue to slip and fall between the teeth, rendering it vulnerable to laceration. Each stimulus is associated with a masseter muscle contraction, so the patient is at risk as long as waveforms are being generated.[25,26]

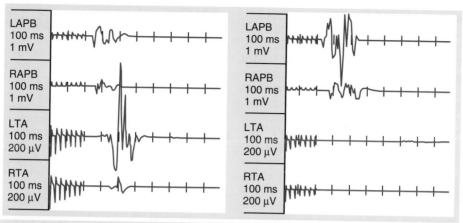

Fig. 32.9 Normal transcranial motor evoked potentials (*left*) and loss of waveform (*right lower two panels*) indicating possible neurologic issue with motor component of the spinal cord. (Courtesy of Department of Neurophysiology, NYU Hospital for Joint Diseases.)

Electromyograms

After pedicle screw placement, the surgeon may request EMGs to determine if the screw is in close proximity to a nerve root, as this can result in neurologic deficits. An electric current is sent through the screw, and EMGs are measured distally. If a low milliampere (mA) current can stimulate the nerve root, then the screw is too close to the nerve root. Therefore in general, a current greater than 7 mA is sent to generate a response to know that screws are not too close to nerve roots. For accurate muscle EMGs, residual neuromuscular blockade must be terminated or reversed.

Wake-Up Test

The wake-up test was traditionally used to assess spinal cord integrity in many scoliosis cases. Development of sophisticated spinal cord monitoring is now standard in many hospitals, and the wake-up test is generally reserved for those situations in which monitoring is unobtainable or a significant intraoperative change in spinal cord monitoring waveforms is noted. During the wake-up test, the anesthetic is discontinued and the patient is asked to move the extremities. Potential complications of this approach include increased bleeding, venous air embolism, and even inadvertent extubation of the trachea in the prone position with the wound exposed. The wake-up test is performed as follows: Turn off all inhaled anesthetics; reverse any neuromuscular blocking drug-induced paralysis; and stop infusions such as dexmedetomidine, propofol, or ketamine. If spontaneous respirations do not begin, inject naloxone 0.04 mg at a time to reverse any residual narcotic effect. The patient's head should be held to reduce the risk of self-extubation of the trachea. Before assessing lower extremity function, confirm upper extremity function. This can be accomplished by having the patient squeeze an observer's hand. Patient compliance denotes adequate recovery from general anesthesia. Then, while someone is observing the feet, ask the patient to wiggle his or her toes. A rapid-acting anesthetic such as propofol should be ready to be administered as soon as the assessment is complete, so the patient can rapidly be reanesthetized. If the wake-up test is not successful in demonstrating adequate motor movement, further surgical intervention may be warranted and the patient may require transport to the radiology suite for additional imaging studies.[3,5,27]

Conclusion of the Case

At the conclusion of the operation, the patient is placed in the supine position. All lines and tubes are secured so that intravenous line, arterial line, and airway access are not lost at this crucial time. Carefully reassess the patient for hemodynamic status, intravascular volume status, hematocrit, blood loss, degree of fluid and blood replacement, temperature, and the potential for airway edema. Premature extubation of the trachea must be avoided. Also facial edema, respiratory effort, the amount of pain medication, and the presence of splinting and pain should be evaluated before extubating the trachea. After the decision is made to extubate the trachea or not, the patient may be properly transported to the PACU. Supplemental oxygen should be used in the PACU. Electrolytes, hemoglobin, and clotting studies should be ordered as indicated.

Postoperative pain management (also see Chapter 40) may prove complicated after spine surgery, as some patients may be taking significant amounts of pain medications, particularly opioids, before surgery. For these patients and for narcotic-naïve patients, a perioperative pain management plan can be developed and incorporated in the patient's care plan. In fact, the pain management pathway should consider using preoperative oral pain

IV

medications, intraoperative infusion of pain medications, and postoperative medications to supply a multimodal pain regimen with the goal of maximizing pain relief while considering methods to decrease narcotic-related respiratory depression. Applying individual consideration to a standard pain pathway, preoperative pain medications may include acetaminophen, gabapentin, or other antiinflammatory pain medications. Patient-controlled analgesia (PCA) may be effective postoperatively, with the dose tailored to the patient's needs. Some centers use ketamine as an analgesic adjunct, either intraoperatively or postoperatively. The use of nonsteroidal antiinflammatory drugs (NSAIDs), such as ketorolac, needs careful consideration, as they will interfere with bone formation and therefore should be avoided in patients who have just undergone spinal fusion.[28] NSAIDs can be considered on an individual basis when bone healing is not a factor, with cautionary consideration of cardiac-related issues resulting from their administration. Other oral medications are helpful in the perioperative period and may be considered for administration preoperatively and postoperatively. These drugs may include acetaminophen, anticonvulsants (e.g., gabapentin and pregabalin), antispasmodics that work at the spinal cord level (e.g., baclofen, tizanidine), antiinflammatory medications, and opioids. Intravenous acetaminophen is an excellent addition to the pain management regimen in patients who are nil per os, or nothing by mouth (NPO).

Vision Loss

Postoperative visual loss (POVL) is a rare but potentially devastating complication occurring in patients undergoing spine surgery (also see Chapters 19 and 31).[29-36] Although its cause is unclear, patients having prolonged spine surgery (>6 hours) in the prone position who have large blood loss (>1 L) are particularly at risk.[29] Yet patients with small blood loss and short procedures also have had visual loss. Perioperative factors such as anemia, hypotension, prolonged surgery, blood loss, increased venous pressure from positioning in the prone position, edema, a compartment syndrome within the orbit, and resistance to blood flow such as direct pressure on the eye, in addition to systemic diseases such as diabetes, hypertension, and vascular disease have all been considered possible etiologic factors.[29-36]

Ischemic optic neuropathy (ION) is a major cause of POVL. Variations in blood supply to the optic nerve may play a role in the development of ION, including reliance on a watershed blood supply to critical areas of the optic nerve. The head-down position allows edema to develop in the orbit, and this increase in venous pressure may affect arterial blood flow. Ocular perfusion pressure (OPP), or the blood pressure supplying blood flow to the optic nerve, is a function of the mean arterial pressure (MAP) and intraocular pressure (IOP) such that

> **Box 32.1** Summary of the ASA Practice Advisory
>
> - There is a subset of patients who undergo spine procedures in the prone position and are at increased risk for perioperative visual loss. Patients who may be at increased risk are those having long procedures or substantial blood loss or both.
> - Consider informing high-risk patients that there is a small, unpredictable risk of perioperative visual loss.
> - The use of deliberate hypotensive techniques during spine surgery is not associated with perioperative visual loss.
> - In patients who have substantial blood loss, colloids should be administered in addition to crystalloids to maintain intravascular volume.
> - There is no apparent transfusion "trigger" that would eliminate the risk of perioperative visual loss related to anemia.
> - When positioning high-risk patients, the head should be level with or higher than the heart when possible. In addition, when possible, the head should be maintained in a neutral forward position (e.g., without significant neck flexion, extension, lateral flexion, or rotation).
> - Staged spine procedures should be considered in high-risk patients.

From American Society of Anesthesiologists Task Force on Perioperative Visual Loss. Practice advisory for perioperative visual loss associated with spine surgery: An updated report by the American Society of Anesthesiologists Task Force on Perioperative Visual Loss. *Anesthesiology*. 2012;116(2):274–285. *ASA*, American Society of Anesthesiologists.

OPP = MAP – IOP. Increases in IOP or decreases in MAP can have a negative impact on OPP.[12] Increases in IOP can decrease OPP and lead to ischemia, and the prone position is associated with increases in IOP.[31]

A visual loss registry has been established by the American Society of Anesthesiologists (ASA) to facilitate establishing the cause of POVL.[30] An ASA Practice Advisory points to ION as the most likely cause of POVL (Box 32.1).[29-36] In a published report of 93 cases reported in the POVL registry, 83 resulted from ION, with the remainder attributed to central retinal artery occlusion (CRAO). CRAO may be embolic in nature or the result of direct pressure on the eyeball and tends to be unilateral. Most patients in the registry were healthy and placed in the prone position for spine surgery. Blood loss more than 1 L and procedures of 6 hours or longer were present in 96% of cases. Fifty-five of the POVL cases were bilateral, with 47 having total visual loss. The registry publication reveals that blood loss in patients with POVL varied widely with a mean of 2 L but ranged from 0.1 to 25 L.[30,34,35] The advisory and registry publications promote a preoperative discussion with the patient, and some suggest staged spine procedures for prolonged surgeries.[30,34,35]

A study comparing 80 patients who suffered ION reported in the registry publication with matched control subjects revealed more insight concerning risk. An increased incidence of ION was noted in patients with the following risk factors: males, obese patients, patients who underwent surgery on a Wilson frame, longer anesthesia time, cases with larger blood loss, and those who received a smaller percentage of colloid.[37]

SURGERY IN THE SITTING POSITION

Shoulder surgery is frequently performed with patients in the sitting, or "beach chair," position, with the head and upper torso elevated 30 to 90 degrees from the supine position (also see Chapter 19). Anesthesia in this position is associated with rare but significant and devastating neurologic complications, including stroke, ischemic brain injury, and vegetative states.[38,39] The cause is a decrease in cerebral perfusion pressure resulting in insufficient blood supply to the brain. This is caused by the arterial blood pressure gradient that develops between the heart and brain in this position. For each centimeter of head elevation above the level of the heart, there is a decrease in arterial blood pressure of 0.77 mm Hg. Therefore arterial blood pressure measured at the level of the heart is not the blood and perfusion pressure at the brain. Measurements obtained at the level of the heart must be recalculated. A 20-cm height differential is not uncommon, which calculates to approximately a 15 to 16 mm Hg gradient. A convenient point for measuring height difference between the heart and brain is the external auditory meatus, which is at the same level as the circle of Willis (COW). Even so, there is still a significant amount of brain tissue above this level. If arterial blood pressure decreases, or the surgeon's request for significant hypotensive anesthesia is followed, cerebral hypotension, and therefore a significantly diminished cerebral perfusion pressure, may occur at the level of the COW and the brain. Therefore significant hypotension should be avoided in these patients, especially those elderly, hypertensive patients whose autoregulatory curve is undoubtedly compromised.

FRACTURED HIP

Hip fractures occur frequently in elderly patients, who often also suffer from multiple preexisting medical conditions or comorbid conditions. Factors predisposing to fracture include medical comorbid conditions, osteoporosis, lower limb dysfunction, visual impairment, increasing age, Parkinson disease, previous fracture, stroke, female gender, dementia, institutionalized patients, excess alcohol or caffeine consumption, cold climate, and use of psychotropic medications.[40] Mortality rates can range up to 14% to 36% in the first year after fracture.[40] Medical status affects morbidity and mortality risks. One example is the number of preexisting comorbid conditions from which the patient suffers. A prospective cohort study of over 2000 patients over the age of 60 years with an acute hip fracture reported that the presence of three or more comorbid conditions was the strongest preoperative risk factor.[41] The most common postoperative complications were chest infection and heart failure; each was associated with greater risk of death.

Generally, when significant comorbid conditions that need correction exist, patients benefit from delay in surgery while their medical status is improved. Mortality rate in high-risk patients was decreased from 29% to 3% in one study when time was taken to correct physiologic abnormalities.[42] In a 2005 prospective study of 2660 patients who underwent surgical treatment for hip fracture the overall mortality rate was 9% at 30 days, 19% at 90 days, and 30% at 12 months. Healthy patients did well as long as surgery was performed within 4 days.[43] Patients with comorbid conditions had a nearly 2.5 times increased mortality rate at 30 days as compared with healthy patients. Also, patients admitted to the hospital immediately after fracture did better than those admitted more than a day later.[43] A metaanalysis of over 200,000 elderly patients with hip fracture noted that operative delay beyond 48 hours after admission was associated with increased mortality rate and suggested that undue delay may be harmful to patients, especially young or low-risk patients.[44]

Preoperative evaluation (also see Chapter 13) is especially important. The diagnosis of a recent MI illustrates how these evaluations have changed. Previously, surgery was delayed up to 6 months after an MI, but now, the tendency is to risk-stratify patients based on the severity of their MI to determine wait time until surgery.[45] The recent MI needs to be evaluated on a risk–benefit ratio comparing the risk of surgery after a recent MI with the negative side effects of keeping a patient bed bound with its attendant risks of pneumonia, pulmonary embolism, pain, loss of ability to walk, and decubitus ulcers. Factors to consider are the extent of the MI, additional myocardium that may be at risk, presence of postinfarction angina, and presence of congestive heart failure (CHF). Although ongoing angina or the presence of CHF may preclude early surgery, a small subendocardial MI with minimal increase in cardiac enzymes and normal echocardiogram and stress test would allow consideration for an earlier intervention. A fractured hip usually prevents the patient from undergoing a normal exercise stress test. Therefore if indicated, a pharmacologic stress test may be needed.

Anesthetic Technique

A long-standing issue is whether one anesthetic technique, general or regional, is associated with better outcomes in patients undergoing hip fracture repair. In general, the data accumulated over many years

IV

and many different studies have not documented a clear advantage of one technique over another.[3,5,46,47] Therefore choice of spinal or general anesthesia should be made on a case-by-case basis taking the patient's specific medical issues into consideration. The pros and cons of both spinal and general anesthesia must be considered when choosing the technique for a given patient (also see Chapter 14). General anesthesia, although easy to administer, does not provide any thromboembolic protection for the patient that may be provided by a regional technique.[3,5] In what may prove to be a clearer elucidation of whether anesthetic technique (neuraxial or general anesthesia) affects outcome in hip fracture patients, a 2012 retrospective study involving over 18,000 hip fracture patients revealed that use of regional anesthesia resulted in lower mortality rates and fewer pulmonary complications in patients with intertrochanteric hip fractures but not in those patients suffering femoral neck fractures.[48] In 2021, a multi-center, pragmatic, randomized study compared spinal anesthesia with general anesthesia in 1,600 older (age 50 and above) hip fracture patients (Regional vs General Anesthesia for Promoting Independence After Hip Fracture, or REGAIN). Spinal anesthesia was not found to be superior to general anesthesia with respect to survival and recovery of ambulation at 60 days. Furthermore, there was no significant difference in the incidence of postoperative delirium between groups.[49]

The anesthesia provider should consider the type of fracture when preparing for surgery. Intertrochanteric fractures are associated with larger blood losses and longer operations, because a plate and screw are inserted, than intracapsular fractures that may be repaired with cannulated screws or a hemiarthroplasty depending on the viability of the femoral head.

Advantages of regional anesthesia, such as provided by a spinal anesthetic, include the following: (1) it avoids endotracheal intubation and airway manipulation and the medications that need to be administered to accomplish this, (2) it decreases the total amount of systemic medication the patient receives throughout the procedure, and (3) it may play a role in decreasing the risk of thromboembolism. The vasodilatory effect of the spinal anesthetic may help the patient with CHF. However, intravascular fluid still should be given cautiously because CHF may worsen as the intravascular vasodilatory effect of the spinal recedes.[3,5]

Preoperatively, intravascular volume status is a concern, as fractures can result in significant blood loss, and a spinal anesthetic in the presence of hypovolemia can result in profound hypotension. An additional concern is the amount of time the patient must lie on the fracture table, especially in the elderly, as even small amounts of sedation can result in significant respiratory depression.

Peripheral nerve blocks, including lumbar plexus, femoral, and lateral femoral cutaneous nerve (LFCN) blocks, may also be used in selected situations. Lumbar plexus block can be performed with the nerve stimulator technique or the use of ultrasound guidance.[50] Fracture repair requiring only cannulated pins may be performed with combined femoral and LFCN blocks. The femoral nerve block provides analgesia in the region of the hip, and the LFCN block will anesthetize the region of cannulated pin insertion located on the lateral aspect of the thigh. An LFCN block is performed by administering a fan of local anesthetic in a cephalad direction from a point 1 cm medial and inferior to the anterior superior iliac spine. The LFCN is a sensory nerve and therefore not amenable to location with a nerve stimulator. Alternatively, the nerve can be blocked using ultrasound guidance.

Intraoperative considerations for patients undergoing fractured hip repair include proper positioning and padding on the fracture table, maintaining adequate intravascular volume status as blood is lost, and adequately maintaining body temperature. Observation for hemodynamic alterations and other unanticipated responses in the elderly patient is especially important as the procedure progresses.

At the conclusion of the surgery, reassess hemodynamic status, ensuring that the patient has received adequate blood and fluid replacement. Determine if the dose of narcotic the patient received is going to have a prolonged effect, thereby resulting in respiratory depression once the patient is extubated. Check for hypothermia and anemia, and evaluate the patient's end-tidal CO_2, as the elderly can be slow to awaken and can easily hypoventilate as a result of the opioids they received. Once the trachea is extubated, administer supplemental oxygen. The dose and frequency of pain medication should be determined cautiously, as increased circulation time and the cumulative effect of administered opioids may become evident when not expected.

TOTAL JOINT REPLACEMENT

Total hip, knee, and shoulder replacements are frequently performed in patients suffering from osteoarthritis, rheumatologic disorders, and trauma. Operations may include replacement of an entire joint, partial joint replacement, replacement of individual components, or resurfacing procedures. Major concerns include the patient's age, concurrent medical conditions, blood loss, proper positioning and padding, hemodynamic variations during the procedure, the response to methylmethacrylate cement (MMC), and the risk of fat and pulmonary emboli.

Tranexamic Acid in Orthopedics

TXA use in total joint arthroplasty, as in spine surgery, has gained wide acceptance, as a number of studies have shown its efficacy in decreasing blood loss in these procedures. TXA is an antifibrinolytic that prevents clot breakdown by binding to plasminogen and inhibiting fibrinolysis. In 2018 the American Society of Regional Anesthesia and Pain Medicine, along with the American Association of Hip and Knee Surgeons and the American Academy of Orthopaedic Surgeons, published a consensus statement on the use of TXA in total joint arthroplasty. The intent was to establish evidence-based guidelines for TXA administration in total hip and knee arthroplasty to improve treatment and reduce practice variation. Major guideline recommendations include the following: (1) that either IV, topical, or oral administration of TXA is effective at reducing perioperative blood loss; (2) multiple doses of TXA do not have any significant benefit over a single dose in reducing blood loss and need for transfusion; (3) TXA administration before incision is more effective than if given after incision; and (4) TXA administration does not increase the risk of venous thromboembolism in patients without a history of venous thromboembolic events.[51] A 2021 systematic review of 216 studies suggested that intravenous TXA, irrespective of dosing, does not increase the risk of venous thromboembolic events.[52]

As the use of TXA has increased, there have been multiple case reports of inadvertent intrathecal administration of TXA, resulting in significant morbidity and mortality. A 2019 review article identified 21 reports of intrathecal TXA administration. In 20 cases there were significant neurologic and cardiac complications requiring prolonged intensive care treatment, leading to 10 deaths.[53] A 2021 case report was published of a patient undergoing a total knee arthroplasty who received intrathecal TXA instead of local anesthetic, which resulted in myoclonic seizures and hypertension.[54] Treatments employed in these reports included administration of anticonvulsants, general anesthesia, cerebrospinal fluid (CSF) lavage, and intensive hemodynamic and neurologic monitoring.

In September 2020 the National Alert Network published an advisory that highlighted the dangers of the use of TXA in orthopedics. There were three cases in which a medication error occurred and TXA was injected into the intrathecal space. This was felt to be the result of the vials having a similar appearance to commonly used local anesthetics (Fig. 32.10). When TXA is administered via the spinal route, it acts as a neurotoxin with a mortality rate as high as 50%.[55] The U.S. Food and Drug Administration (FDA) issued its own alert to health care providers in December 2020. It noted that injection of TXA into the spinal space could cause disastrous effects, including seizures, arrhythmias, permanent neurologic injury, and death.[56]

IV

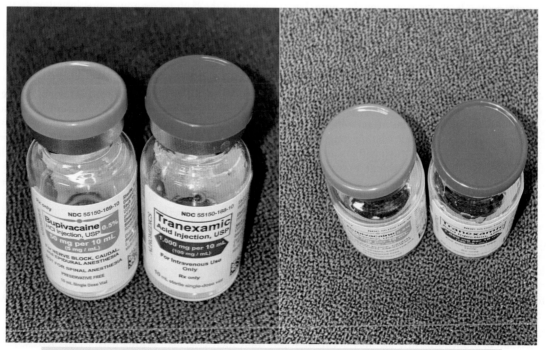

Fig. 32.10 Comparison of bupivacaine and tranexamic acid vials, illustrating similarities between them.

Institutions should rapidly establish protocols with safety measures to prevent these avoidable occurrences. Risk-reduction measures include having the pharmacy provide nonvial preparations of TXA, two-person verification of medications to be injected into the intrathecal space, and having TXA made available for intravenous injection only after spinal anesthesia has been completed.

Total Hip Replacement

Total hip replacements (THRs) are performed with patients traditionally in either the supine or lateral decubitus position. A relatively new approach, the anterior approach to the hip, is frequently performed with the patient in the supine position on a special operating room table. Using this technique, selected patients are candidates for same-day hip replacement. In the supine position, the arm that is on the same side as the hip needs to be flexed away from the side. In the lateral position, an axillary roll is placed just caudal to the axilla to protect the axillary artery and brachial plexus from compression (also see Chapter 19). Patients having procedures in the lateral position also have a lateral positioner placed to stabilize their pelvis. The positioner can push abdominal contents cephalad and interfere with respiratory function.

A THR may have MMC used to secure the prosthesis. Younger patients tend to receive noncemented joint replacements. The use of MMC is associated with cardiopulmonary side effects such as hypoxia, bronchoconstriction, hypotension, cardiovascular collapse, and even death. The cause for the systemic reaction to MMC may result from the liquid MMC monomer itself, which is used in producing the cement for cementing the prosthesis, or may be the result of air, fat, or bone marrow elements being forced into circulation. The higher the liquid content of the liquid monomer in the mix with the polymer MMC at the time of insertion, which occurs from not adequately mixing or not waiting long enough for mixing to occur, the more frequently side effects are noted.[3,4,57] High-risk patients include those who are hypovolemic at the time of cementing, those who are hypertensive, and those with significant preexisting cardiac disease.[3,42]

Transesophageal echocardiographic evaluation of cardiac structure and function during reaming and cementing does indicate that MMC and fat emboli flow centrally to the heart from the surgical site.[57] If a patient has a patent foramen ovale, these emboli can theoretically cross the patent foramen into the left ventricle and then move into the arterial circulation. If the patient has a probe-patent foramen ovale, an increase in pulmonary pressures as a result of bronchoconstriction may occur. MMC, for example, can increase right atrial pressure and shunt blood flow directly across the probe-patent foramen

ovale. Many patients may have a decreased Pao_2 during the reaming and cementing process intraoperatively. An increase in the Fio_2 of 1.0 may be necessary.

At the conclusion of surgery, the patient is transferred to the PACU. Supplemental oxygen is administered, and a hemoglobin count should be considered. Further testing is based upon the patient's underlying medical condition. A postoperative pain management plan should be considered preoperatively (also see Chapter 40). Pain pathways are used at some medical centers that include preoperative oral medications. More comprehensive protocols to optimize management for same-day procedures are also being used. They may include recommendations for intravascular fluid management, dosing of spinal anesthetics, and medications to promote bladder contractility. For inpatients, postoperative pain management may include epidural infusion with epidural PCA, intravenous PCA, oral medications, or peripheral nerve block including lumbar plexus block. The postoperative pain management the patient receives may be influenced by the thromboembolism prophylaxis administered.

Total Knee Replacements and Tourniquets

Total knee replacements (TKRs) are frequently performed with a tourniquet in place to provide a bloodless surgical field. The tourniquet should be carefully placed on the upper thigh over appropriate padding. The leg may be wrapped with an Esmarch elastic bandage to help exsanguinate the limb before tourniquet inflation. In the lower extremity, the tourniquet is inflated to approximately 100 mm Hg above the systolic blood pressure, as this will prevent arterial blood from entering the exsanguinated limb.[3,4,58]

As tourniquets render the limb ischemic, there is a limit to inflation time before the ischemia can result in permanent limb damage. The safe upper limit of ischemia time is about 2 hours. The surgeon should be informed of tourniquet inflation time at 1 hour and then as the tourniquet approaches the 2-hour limit so it can be deflated in a timely manner. If the total tourniquet time exceeds the 2-hour limit, the tourniquet should be deflated at 2 hours for a period of at least 15 to 20 minutes before it is reinflated. This will allow for the "wash-out" of acidic metabolites from the ischemic limb as the limb is reperfused with oxygenated blood. Recirculation of the ischemic limb with release of the tourniquet is noted by a decrease in arterial blood pressure and an increase in end-tidal CO_2 as the acid products recirculate.[3] The hypotension usually responds to intravascular fluid administration and vasopressors if necessary.[3,58]

Pain is noted as the duration of tourniquet inflation time increases, manifesting itself as an increase in arterial blood pressure and heart rate. Overaggressively treating the increase in arterial blood pressure with opioids and other medications can result in hypotension after the tourniquet is released. Animal models have determined the pain to occur as a result of C-fiber firing. A regional block proximal to the tourniquet can prevent C-fibers from firing.[3,58,59]

Complications noted with tourniquet use include nerve damage, vessel damage (especially in patients with atherosclerosis), pulmonary embolism, and skin damage. Skin injury may be the result of the antiseptic prep solution if it is allowed to seep under the tourniquet and tourniquet padding at the time of skin prep, causing a chemical burn. Additional concerns at the time of tourniquet deflation are pulmonary embolism and a decrease in core temperature as the isolated extremity is reperfused.[3,45,46]

After deflating the tourniquet, the surgical field should be observed for evidence of bleeding. Occasionally the tourniquet is deflated at the tourniquet control box but there is no bleeding because the tubing to the tourniquet is kinked. This is a significant complication, as the tourniquet is effectively still inflated and the patient is then at risk for prolonged tourniquet inflation time, limb ischemia, and complications. One method to help ensure tourniquet deflation is to disconnect the tubing from the tourniquet box and observe the incision for bleeding, which is an indicator of tourniquet deflation.

TKRs are frequently performed under regional anesthesia with intravenous sedation. As a tourniquet is used during the operation, in the operating room blood loss is usually not significant. However, if much blood loss occurs into drains in the PACU, hypotension may result. Some surgeons do not deflate the tourniquet until the wound is closed and the dressing is on the patient. In this situation blood loss is usually less but there is a risk of postoperative bleeding.[60]

Debate exists as to whether bilateral TKRs should be performed in one setting. Many patients have undergone bilateral TKRs in one day or during one hospital admission.[60-64] If bilateral TKRs are scheduled, they should be performed after careful patient selection. Many institutions have guidelines delineating those patients felt to be acceptable candidates for bilateral procedures based on comorbid conditions and ASA physical status. Intraoperatively, the anesthesia provider should be aware that drainage from the first total joint will be occurring into the wound drainage system, which may be hidden from view. If bleeding is significant, hypotension can occur for what might be unrecognized reasons.

TKR patients have more postoperative pain than patients receiving THR. A postoperative pain management plan should be delineated to address anticipated pain. This plan may include oral and intravenous pain medications and nerve blocks. Preoperative oral pain medications such as acetaminophen, gabapentin, or NSAIDs (with cardiovascular risk considered) are employed by some as part of a total knee pain pathway. With early ambulation becoming popular, even as early as in the PACU, there is a need to provide adequate pain relief for mobilization. Peripheral nerve blocks, such as a femoral or an adductor canal block, can supply such pain relief.[65] The adductor canal block potentially spares motor components of the femoral nerve, preserving motor strength in the femoral nerve distribution. It is not clear that use of femoral or adductor canal blocks results in a more frequent incidence of falls.[66] Postoperative pain relief may also include PCA, continuous infusions through catheters, individual nerve blocks of the lower extremities, and intravenous or oral medications. The use of intravenous dexamethasone administered at the time of a peripheral nerve block prolongs the block's duration, which may be useful in this setting.[67] In lieu of peripheral nerve blocks, some surgeons are using "off-label" periarticular infiltrations of liposomal bupivacaine at the end of surgery to achieve extended postoperative analgesia. One randomized trial comparing intraarticular liposomal bupivacaine to single-shot femoral nerve blockade after TKR reported similar inpatient pain control.[68]

Deep Venous Thrombosis and Thromboembolism Prophylaxis

The need for, and technique of, perioperative deep venous thrombosis (DVT) prophylaxis varies by surgeon and institution. Thromboembolism management should be coordinated with the anesthesia providers. Options for DVT prophylaxis include warfarin, low-molecular-weight heparin (LMWH), sequential compression boots, and aspirin. Although guidelines do exist as to which medications to use, the choice of DVT thromboprophylaxis is still variable. The surgeon's choice and timing of DVT prophylaxis will influence the choice of technique: general, spinal, combined spinal and epidural, epidural, peripheral block, or nerve block and catheter. At issue is concern that catheter manipulation while a patient is anticoagulated will result in bleeding, and if the catheter is in the epidural space, its removal can potentially result in epidural bleeding, epidural hematoma formation, and paralysis. Once an epidural hematoma develops, the catheter must be removed expeditiously before irreversible paralysis occurs. Although epidural hematomas classically present with severe pain and onset of numbness and weakness, in patients receiving epidural infusions of local anesthetics, these classic symptoms may be masked.

LMWH was used for postoperative anticoagulation in Europe without significant problems. However, after introduction of the LMWH enoxaparin in the United States, the incidence of epidural hematomas increased. Several factors may have contributed, including twice-daily LMWH (compared with once daily in Europe), performance of neuraxial anesthesia or removal of epidural catheters while the anticoagulation effect of LMWH was

IV

still present, use of multiple medications with anticoagulation properties simultaneously, or the lack of attention to dosing schedule. This prompted a 1998 warning from the FDA noting "reports of epidural or spinal hematomas with concurrent use of low molecular weight heparin and spinal/epidural anesthesia or spinal puncture." Consensus statements from the American Society of Regional Anesthesia and Pain Medicine (ASRA) addressed the issue in an evidence-based guideline, currently in its fourth edition, published in 2018.[69] The FDA issued an updated drug safety communication in 2013 that recommended waiting at least 12 hours before neuraxial needle placement in a patient who received a prophylactic dose of enoxaparin and waiting 4 hours (increased from the previous 2-hour waiting period) before dosing enoxaparin after an epidural catheter is removed.[70] Patients receiving warfarin should have their catheter removed only when the international normalized ratio (INR) is less than 1.5. Other anticoagulants and antiplatelet medications should be avoided when LMWH is being used and an epidural catheter is in place.[69]

When given alone, aspirin and NSAIDs do not appear to increase the risk of spinal hematoma in patients undergoing neuraxial anesthesia. However, several potent antiplatelet drugs place a patient at an increased risk for a neuraxial hematoma if a spinal or epidural anesthetic is performed while their effects are present. The medications listed in Box 32.2 should be withheld for the recommended period, or a nonneuraxial technique should be used instead.[69] These guidelines will likely undergo revision as new medications are added and as additional experience is considered (also see Chapter 23).

Box 32.2 Discontinuation of Antiplatelet Agents Before Neuraxial Blockade

Medication	Time Interval*
Ticlopidine	10 days
Clopidogrel	5–7 days
Prasugrel	7–10 days
Ticagrelor	5–7 days

From Horlocker T, Vandermeulen, E, Kopp S, et al. Regional anesthesia in the patient receiving antithrombotic or thrombolytic therapy: American Society of Regional Anesthesia and Pain Medicine Evidence-Based Guidelines (Fourth Edition). Reg Anesth Pain Med. 2018;43(3):286.
*Time interval between medication discontinuation and neuraxial blockade.

REFERENCES

1. Okada Y, Wu D, Trynka G, et al. Genetics of rheumatoid arthritis contributes to biology and drug discovery. *Nature.* 2014;506(7488):376–381.
2. Klippel JH, Crofford LJ, Stone JH, Weyland CM, eds. Rheumatoid arthritis. Epidemiology, pathology and pathogenesis. *Primer on the Rheumatic Diseases.* 12th ed. Atlanta: Arthritis Foundation; 2001:209–232.
3. Bernstein RL, Rosenberg AD. *Manual of Orthopedic Anesthesia and Related Pain Syndromes.* New York: Churchill Livingstone; 1993.
4. Rosenberg AD. Current issues in the anesthetic treatment of the patient for orthopedic surgery. *ASA Refresher Courses in Anesthesiology.* 2004;32:169–178.
5. Rosenberg AD. Anesthesia for major orthopedic surgery. *ASA Refresher Courses in Anesthesiology.* 1997;25:131–144.
6. Bienenstock H, Ehrlich GE, Freyberg RH. Rheumatoid arthritis of the cricoarytenoid joint: A clinicopathological study. *Arthritis Rheum.* 1963;6:48–63.
7. Skues MA, Welchew EA. Anaesthesia and rheumatoid arthritis. *Anaesthesia.* 1993;48:989–997.
8. Steel HH. Anatomical and mechanical considerations of the atlantoaxial articulations. *J Bone Joint Surg Am.* 1968;50:1481–1490.
9. Keenan MA, Stiles CM, Kaufman RL. Acquired laryngeal deviation associated with cervical spine disease in erosive polyarticular arthritis. Use of the fiberoptic bronchoscope in rheumatic disease. *Anesthesiology.* 1983;58:441–449.
10. Macarthur A, Kleiman S. Rheumatoid cervical joint disease—a challenge to the anesthetist. *Can J Anaesth.* 1993;40(2):154–159.
11. Klippel JH, Crofford LJ, Stone JH, Weyland CM, eds. Seronegative spondyloarthropathies, ankylosing spondylitis. Primer on the Rheumatic Diseases. 12th ed. Atlanta, GA: Arthritis Foundation; 2001:250–254.
12. Rosenberg AD. Annual Meeting 58th Refresher Course Lectures and Basic Science Review RCL American Society of Anesthesiology. *Anesthesiology.* 2007;119.
13. Zakine J, Samarcq D, Lorne E, et al. Postoperative ketamine administration decreases morphine consumption in major abdominal surgery: A prospective, randomized, double-blind, controlled study. *Anesth Analg.* 2008;106(6):1856–1861.
14. Subramaniam K, Subramaniam B, Steinbrook RA. Ketamine as adjuvant analgesic to opioids: A quantitative and qualitative systematic review. *Anesth Analg.* 2004;99:482–495.
15. American Society of Anesthesiologists Task Force on Intraoperative Awareness. Practice advisory for intraoperative awareness and brain function monitoring: A report by the American Society of Anesthesiologists Task Force on Intraoperative Awareness. *Anesthesiology.* 2006;104:847–864.
16. Avidan MS, Zhang L, Burnside BA, et al. Anesthesia awareness and the bispectral index. *N Engl J Med.* 2008;358:1097–1108.
17. Urban MK, Jules-Elysee K, Urquhart B, et al. The efficacy of antifibrinolytics in the reduction of blood loss during complex adult reconstructive spine surgery. *Spine (Phila Pa 1976).* 2001;26:1152–1156.
18. Zufferey P, Merquiol F, Laporte S, et al. Do antifibrinolytics reduce allogeneic blood in orthopedic surgery? *Anesthesiology.* 2006;105(5):1034–1046.
19. Neilipovitz DT, Murto K, Hall L, et al. A randomized trial of tranexamic acid to reduce blood transfusion for scoliosis surgery. *Anesth Analg.* 2001;93:82–87.
20. Mangano DT, Tudor IC, Dietzel C, et al. The risk associated with aprotinin in cardiac surgery. *N Engl J Med.* 2006;354:353–365.
21. Mangano DT, Miao Y, Vuylsteke A, et al. Mortality associated with aprotinin during 5 years following coronary bypass graft surgery. *JAMA.* 2007;297:471–479.
22. Fergusson DA, Hebert PC, Mazer CD, et al. A comparison of aprotinin and lysine analogues in high-risk cardiac surgery. *N Engl J Med.* 2008;358:2319–2331.
23. Pasternak BM, Boyd DP, Ellis FH. Spinal cord injury after procedures on the aorta. *Surg Gynecol Obstet.* 1972;135:29–34.

24. Owen JH, Laschinger J, Bridwell K, et al. Sensitivity and specificity of somatosensory and neurogenic motor evoked potentials in animals and humans. *Spine (Phila Pa 1976)*. 1988;13(10):1111–1118.

25. Hilibrand AS, Schwartz DM, Sethuraman V, et al. Comparison of transcranial electric motor and somatosensory evoked potential monitoring during cervical spine surgery. *J Bone Joint Surg Am*. 2004;86:1248–1253.

26. MacDonald D. Intraoperative motor evoked potential monitoring: overview and update. *J Clin Monit Comput*. 2006;20(5):347–377.

27. Vauzelle C, Stagnara P, Jouvinroux P. Functional monitoring of spinal cord activity during spinal surgery. *Clin Orthop Relat Res*. 1973;93:173–178.

28. Glassman SD, Rose SM, Dimar JR, et al. The effect of postoperative nonsteroidal antiinflammatory drug administration on spinal fusion. *Spine (Phila Pa 1976)*. 1998;23:834–838.

29. Williams EL. Postoperative blindness. *Anesthiol Clin North Am*. 2002;20:605–622.

30. Lee L, Roth S, Posner K, et al. The American Society of Anesthesiologists Postoperative Visual Loss Registry: Analysis of 93 spine surgery cases with postoperative visual loss. *Anesthesiology*. 2006;105(4):652–659.

31. Cheng MA, Todorov A, Tempelhoff R, et al. The effect of prone positioning on intraocular pressure in anesthetized patients. *Anesthesiology*. 2001;95:1351–1355.

32. Lee L, Lam A. Unilateral blindness after position lumbar spine surgery. *Anesthesiology*. 2001;95:793–795.

33. Roth S, Barach P. Postoperative visual loss: Still no answers—yet. *Anesthesiology*. 2001;95:575–577.

34. Warner MA. Postoperative visual loss: Experts, data and practice. *Anesthesiology*. 2006;105:641–642.

35. American Society of Anesthesiologists Task Force on Perioperative Visual Loss. Practice advisory for perioperative visual loss associated with spine surgery: An updated report by the American Society of Anesthesiologists Task Force on Perioperative Visual Loss. *Anesthesiology*. 2012;116(2):274–285.

36. Roth S. Perioperative visual loss: What do we know, what can we do? *Br J Anaesth*. 2009;103(suppl):i31–i40.

37. The Postoperative Visual Loss Study Group. Risk factors associated with ischemic optic neuropathy after spine surgery. *Anesthesiology*. 2012;116(1):15–24.

38. Pohl A, Cullen DJ. Cerebral ischemia during shoulder surgery in the upright position: A case series. *J Clin Anesth*. 2005;17:463–469.

39. Cullen DJ, Kirby RB. Beach chair position may decrease cerebral perfusion pressure. Catastrophic outcomes have occurred. *APSF Newsl*. 2007;22(2):25.

40. Zuckerman J. Hip fracture. *N Engl J Med*. 1996;334:1519–1525.

41. Roche JJ, Wenn RT, Sahota O, et al. Effect of comorbidities and postoperative complications on mortality after hip fracture in elderly people: Prospective observational cohort study. *BMJ*. 2005;331(7529):1374.

42. Schultz RJ, Whitfield GF, LaMura JJ, et al. The role of physiologic monitoring in patients with fractures of the hip. *J Trauma*. 1985;25:309–316.

43. Moran CG, Wenn RT, Sikand M, et al. Early mortality after hip fracture: Is delay before surgery important? *J Bone Joint Surg Am*. 2005;87:483–489.

44. Shiga T, Wajimaa Z, Ohe Y. Is operative delay associated with increased mortality of hip fracture patients? Systematic review, meta-analysis, and meta-regression. *Can J Anaesth*. 2008;55:146–154.

45. Shah KB, Kleinman BS, Sami H, et al. Reevaluation of perioperative myocardial infarction in patients with prior myocardial infarction undergoing noncardiac operations. *Anesth Analg*. 1990;71:231–235.

46. Valentin N, Lomholt B, Jensen JS, et al. Spinal or general anaesthesia for surgery of the fractured hip? A prospective study of mortality in 578 patients. *Br J Anaesth*. 1986;58:284–291.

47. Davis FM, Woolner DF, Frampton C, et al. Prospective multi-centre trial of mortality following general or spinal anesthesia for hip fracture surgery in the elderly. *Br J Anaesth*. 1987;59:1080–1088.

48. Neuman MD, Silber JH, Elkassabany NM, et al. Comparative effectiveness of regional versus general anesthesia for hip fracture surgery in adults. *Anesthesiology*. 2012;117:72–92.

49. Neuman Mark D, Feng Rui, Carson Jeffrey L, et al., REGAIN Investigators. Spinal Anesthesia or General Anesthesia for Hip Surgery in Older Adults. *N Engl J Med*. 2021;385(22):2025–2035. doi:10.1056/NEJMoa2113514. 34623788.

50. Touray ST, de Leeuw MA, Zuurmond WW, Perez RS. Psoas compartment block for lower extremity surgery: A meta-analysis. *Br J Anaesth*. 2008 Dec;101(6):750–760. doi:10.1093/bja/aen298 Epub 2008 Oct 22. PMID: 18945717.

51. Fillingham YA, Ramkumar DB, Jevsevar DS, et al. Tranexamic acid in total joint arthroplasty: The endorsed clinical practice guides of the American Association of Hip and Knee Surgeons, American Society of Regional Anesthesia and Pain Medicine, American Academy of Orthopaedic Surgeons, Hip Society, and Knee Society. *Reg Anesth Pain Med*. 2019;44(1):7–11.

52. Taeuber I, Weibel S, Herrmann E, et al. Association of intravenous tranexamic acid with thromboembolic events and mortality: A systematic review, meta-analysis, and meta-regression. *JAMA Surg*. 2021:e210884.

53. Patel S, Robertson B, McConachie I. Catastrophic drug errors involving tranexamic acid administered during spinal anaesthesia. *Anaesthesia*. 2019;74(7):904–914.

54. Al-Taei MH, AlAzzawi M, Albustani S, Alsaoudi G, Costanzo E. Incorrect route for injection: Inadvertent tranexamic acid intrathecal injection. *Cureus*. 2021;13(2):e13055.

55. Dangerous Wrong-Route Errors with Tranexamic Acid. Institute for Safe Medication Practices. Sept. 9, 2020. www.ismp.org/alerts/dangerous-wrong-route-errors-tranexamic-acid. Accessed April 8, 2021.

56. FDA Alerts Healthcare Professionals About the Risk of Medication Errors with Tranexamic Acid Injection Resulting in Inadvertent Intrathecal (Spinal) Injection. Food and Drug Administration. Dec. 3, 2020. www.fda.gov/drugs/drug-safety-and-availability/fda-alerts-healthcare-professionals-about-risk-medication-errors-tranexamic-acid-injection-resulting. Accessed April 8, 2021.

57. Donaldson AJ, Thompson HE, Harper NJ, Kenny NW. Bone cement implantation syndrome. *Br J Anaesth*. 2009;102(1):12–22.

58. Odinsson A, Finsen V. Tourniquet use and its complications in Norway. *J Bone Joint Surg*. 2006;88:1090–1092.

59. Chabel C, Russell LC, Lee R. Tourniquet-induced limb ischemia: A neurophysiologic animal model. *Anesthesiology*. 1990;72:1038–1044.

60. Rama KR, Apsingi S, Poovali S, et al. Timing of tourniquet release in knee arthroplasty. Meta-analysis of randomized, controlled trials. *J Bone Joint Surg Am*. 2007;89:699–705.

61. Memtsoudis SG, Ma Y, Gonzalez Della Valle A, et al. Perioperative outcomes after unilateral and bilateral total knee arthroplasty. *Anesthesiology*. 2009;111:1206–1216.

62. Chan WC, Musonda P, Cooper AS, et al. One-stage versus two-stage bilateral unicompartmental knee replacement: A comparison of immediate post-operative complications. *J Bone Joint Surg*. 2009;91:1305–1309.

63. Ritter MA, Harty LD, Davis KE, et al. Simultaneous bilateral, staged bilateral, and unilateral total knee arthroplasty: A survival analysis. *J Bone Joint Surg Am*. 2003;85:1532–1537.

64. Restrepo C, Parvizi J, Dietrich T, et al. Safety of simultaneous bilateral total knee arthroplasty. A meta-analysis. *J Bone Joint Surg Am*. 2007;89:1220–1226.

IV

65. Kim DH, Lin Y, Goytizolo EA, et al. Adductor canal block versus femoral nerve block for total knee arthroplasy. *Anesthesiology.* 2014;120:540–555.

66. Memtsoudis AG, Danninger T, Rasul R, et al. Inpatient falls after total knee arthroplasty. The role of anesthesia type and peripheral nerve blocks. *Anesthesiology.* 2014;120:551–563.

67. Abdallah FW, Johnson J, Chan V, et al. Intravenous dexamethasone and perineural dexamethasone similarly prolong the duration of analgesia after supraclavicular block: A randomized, triple arm, double blind, placebo-controlled trial. *Reg Anesth Pain Med.* 2015;40(2):125–132.

68. Surdam JW, Licini DJ, Baynes NT, Arce BR. The use of exparel (liposomal bupivacaine) to manage postoperative pain in unilateral total knee replacement. *J Arthroplasty.* 2015;30(2):325–329.

69. Horlocker TT, Vandermeulen E, Kopp SL, Gogarten W, Leffert LR, Benzon HT. Regional Anesthesia in the Patient Receiving Antithrombotic or Thrombolytic Therapy: American Society of Regional Anesthesia and Pain Medicine Evidence-Based Guidelines (Fourth Edition). *Reg Anesth Pain Med.* 2018 Apr;43(3):263–309. Erratum in: *Reg Anesth Pain Med.* 2018 Jul;43(5):566. Vandermeulen, Erik [corrected to Vandermeulen, Erik]. PMID: 29561531. doi:10.1097/AAP.0000000000000763.

70. Food and Drug Administration. FDA Drug Safety Communication: Updated recommendations to decrease risk of spinal column bleeding and paralysis in patients on low molecular weight heparins. Nov. 6:2013 http://www.fda.gov/Drugs/DrugSafety/ucm373595.htm.

Chapter

33 OBSTETRICS

Christine M. Warrick, Mark D. Rollins

Providing peripartum analgesia and anesthesia requires an understanding of the physiologic changes that occur during pregnancy and labor and the effects of anesthetic care on the mother, fetus, and neonate. It also demands an understanding of the course of labor and delivery; knowledge of high-risk maternal conditions; ability to provide a variety of analgesic and anesthetic techniques; and preparation for potential obstetric emergencies and complications requiring immediate intervention, such as fetal distress and maternal hemorrhage.

PHYSIOLOGIC CHANGES IN PREGNANT WOMEN

During pregnancy, labor, and delivery, women undergo significant changes in anatomy and physiology as a result of (1) altered hormonal activity; (2) biochemical changes associated with increasing metabolic demands of a growing fetus, placenta, and uterus; and (3) mechanical displacement by an enlarging uterus.[1,2]

Cardiovascular System Changes

Changes in the cardiovascular system during pregnancy can be summarized as (1) an increase in intravascular fluid volume, (2) an increase in cardiac output, (3) a decrease in systemic vascular resistance, and (4) the presence of supine aortocaval compression (Table 33.1).

Intravascular Fluid and Hematology

Maternal intravascular fluid volume begins to increase in the first trimester. At term, the plasma volume has increased about 50% above the nonpregnant state, whereas the erythrocyte volume has increased only about 25%. This disproportionate increase in plasma volume accounts for the relative anemia of pregnancy. The hemoglobin decreases but normally remains at 11 g/dL or greater. This expanded intravascular fluid volume of 1000 to 1500 mL at term offsets the 300 to 500 mL blood loss that accompanies vaginal delivery and the average 800 to 1000 mL blood loss from cesarean delivery. After delivery, the contracted uterus auto-transfuses about 500 mL of blood.

The total plasma protein concentration is decreased as a result of the dilutional effect of the increased intravascular fluid volume, and colloid osmotic pressure is reduced from about 27 mm Hg down to 22 mm Hg by term. Pregnancy is a hypercoagulable state with increases in factors I, VII, VIII, IX, X, and XII and von Willebrand factor and decreases in factors XI and XIII, antithrombin III, and protein S. This results in an approximately 20% decrease in prothrombin time (PT) and partial thromboplastin time (PTT). Platelet count may remain normal or decrease 10% by term, and leukocytosis is common.

Table 33.1	Changes in the Cardiovascular and Pulmonary Systems During Pregnancy
System Parameter	**Value at Term Compared With Nonpregnant Value**
Cardiovascular System	
Intravascular fluid volume	Increased 35%–45%
Plasma volume	Increased 45%–55%
Erythrocyte volume	Increased 20%–30%
Cardiac output	Increased 40%–50%
Stroke volume	Increased 25%–30%
Heart rate	Increased 15%–25%
Peripheral circulation	
Systemic vascular resistance	Decreased 20%
Pulmonary vascular resistance	Decreased 35%
Central venous pressure	No change
Pulmonary capillary wedge pressure	No change
Femoral venous pressure	Increased 15%–50%
Pulmonary System	
Minute ventilation	Increased 45%–50%
Tidal volume	Increased 40%–45%
Breathing frequency	Increased 0%–15%
Lung volumes	
Expiratory reserve volume	Decreased 20%–25%
Residual volume	Decreased 15%–20%
Functional residual capacity	Decreased 20%
Vital capacity	No change
Total lung capacity	Decreased 0%–5%
Arterial blood gases and pH	
Pao_2	Normal or slightly increased
$Paco_2$	Decreased 10 mm Hg
pH	No change or minimal alkalosis
Oxygen consumption	Increased 20%

Data from Refs. 1 and 2.

Cardiac Output

Cardiac output increases by about 35% by the end of the first trimester and increases 40% to 50% above baseline by the third trimester. This augmentation of cardiac output is the result of increases in both stroke volume (25% to 30%) and heart rate (15% to 25%). The onset of labor is associated with further increases in cardiac output, with increases above prelabor values by 10% to 25% during the first stage and 40% in the second stage. The largest increase occurs immediately after delivery, when cardiac output is increased by as much as 80% above prelabor values. This presents a unique postpartum risk for patients with cardiac disease, such as fixed valvular stenosis or cardiomyopathy. Cardiac output decreases within the first hours after delivery and reaches prelabor values about 48 hours postpartum. By 2 weeks postpartum, it has decreased substantially toward pre-pregnant values.

Systemic Vascular Resistance

Although cardiac output and plasma volume increase, systemic blood pressure decreases in an uncomplicated pregnancy secondary to a 20% reduction in systemic vascular resistance. Systolic, mean, and diastolic blood pressure may all decrease 5% to 20% by 20 weeks' gestation and increase slightly towards pre-pregnant values as the pregnancy progresses. There is no change in central venous pressure during pregnancy despite the increased plasma volume because venous capacitance increases.

Aortocaval Compression

When supine, the gravid uterus can compress the aorta and vena cava. Compression of the vena cava can decrease preload, cardiac output, and systemic blood pressure (Fig. 33.1). In the supine position, some vena caval compression can occur near the beginning of the second trimester. By term, full occlusion when supine is typical, with venous return of blood from the lower extremities through the epidural, azygos, and vertebral veins. In addition, significant aortoiliac artery compression occurs in 15% to 20% of pregnant women. Nearly 15% of pregnant women at term experience significant hypotension in the supine position. Diaphoresis, nausea, vomiting, and changes in cerebration often accompany the hypotension. This constellation of symptoms is termed *supine hypotension syndrome*. Vena cava compression decreases cardiac output 10% to 20% and may also contribute to lower extremity venous stasis and thereby result in ankle edema, varices, and increased risk of venous thrombosis.

Echocardiography Changes

There are significant changes in echocardiography during pregnancy.[3] The heart is displaced anteriorly and leftward. Right-sided chambers increase in size by 20% and left-sided chambers increase in size by 10% with an associated left ventricular (LV) eccentric hypertrophy. The right ventricular systolic pressure remains unchanged despite increases in intravascular volume. Mitral, tricuspid, and pulmonic valve annuli diameters increase. Tricuspid and pulmonic valve regurgitation is common, and about one in four women have mitral regurgitation. In addition, small insignificant pericardial effusions may be present.

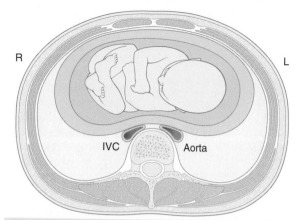

R   L

IVC   Aorta

Fig. 33.1 Schematic diagram showing compression of the inferior vena cava (IVC) and abdominal aorta by the gravid uterus in the supine position.

Compensatory Responses and Anesthetic Implications

Many pregnant women do not experience significant arterial hypotension when supine because they compensate for the reduction in preload with increases in systemic vascular resistance. This compensation is impaired by regional anesthetic techniques. Consequently, supine positioning is avoided during neuraxial anesthetic administration in the second and third trimesters. Significant lateral tilt (30 degrees) is frequently required to reduce hypotension and preserve fetal circulation by effectively displacing the gravid uterus off the inferior vena cava (Fig. 33.2).[4] Left uterine displacement can be accomplished by placing the patient in a left lateral position or by elevation of the right hip with a wedge or table tilt.

The gravid uterus can also compress the lower abdominal aorta. Such compression leads to arterial hypotension in the lower extremities, but decreases in systemic blood pressure measured in the arms may not reflect this decrease. The significance of aortocaval compression is the associated decrease in uterine and placental blood flow. Even with a healthy uteroplacental unit, prolonged maternal hypotension (more than a 25% decrease for an average patient) for longer than 10 to 15 minutes can significantly decrease uterine blood flow (UBF) and lead to progressive fetal acidosis.

The increased venous pressure distal to the level of vena caval compression diverts blood return from the lower half of the body via the paravertebral venous plexuses to the azygos vein. Flow from the azygos vein enters the superior vena cava and returns to the heart. Dilation of the epidural veins with pregnancy may increase the rate of unintentional intravascular placement of an epidural catheter and accidental intravascular injection of the local anesthetic solution. A "test dose" is therefore employed before dosing an epidural catheter in

IV

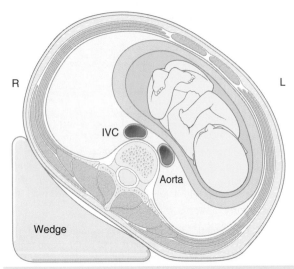

Fig. 33.2 Schematic diagram depicting left uterine displacement by elevation of the right hip with a wedge. This position deflects the gravid uterus off of the inferior vena cava (IVC) and aorta.

order to decrease the likelihood of an unintended intravascular placement before initiating neuraxial blockade. This technique is described in the section "Neuraxial Dosing and Delivery Techniques."

Pulmonary System Changes

The most significant changes in the pulmonary system during pregnancy include alterations in (1) the upper airway, (2) minute ventilation, (3) arterial oxygenation, and (4) lung volumes (see Table 33.1).

Upper Airway

During pregnancy there is significant capillary engorgement of the mucosal lining of the upper respiratory tract and increased tissue edema and friability. Additional care is needed during suctioning and placement of airways (e.g., avoid nasal instrumentation if possible) to prevent tissue bleeding with instrumentation. Mask ventilation, laryngoscopy, and intubation are all more challenging. A smaller cuffed tracheal tube (6.0 to 6.5 mm internal diameter) is typically selected because the vocal cords and arytenoids are often edematous. The presence of preeclampsia, upper respiratory tract infections, and active pushing with associated increased venous pressure further exacerbate airway tissue edema, making both ventilation and intubation more problematic. In addition, the weight gain associated with pregnancy, particularly in women of short stature or with coexisting obesity, can result in difficulty placing the laryngoscope because of a shorter neck and increased breast tissue.

Minute Ventilation and Oxygenation

Minute ventilation increases about 50% above pre-pregnant levels during the first trimester and is maintained for the remainder of the pregnancy. This increased minute ventilation is achieved primarily by a greater tidal volume, with small increases in the respiratory rate (see Table 33.1). Elevated circulating levels of progesterone and increased CO_2 production are presumed to be the stimulus for the increased minute ventilation. Resting maternal $Paco_2$ decreases from 40 mm Hg to approximately 30 mm Hg during the first trimester as a reflection of the increased minute ventilation. Arterial pH, however, remains only mildly alkalotic (7.42 to 7.44) because of increased renal excretion of bicarbonate ions (HCO_3^- is approximately 20 to 21 mEq/L).

Early in gestation, maternal Pao_2 while breathing room air is normally above 100 mm Hg because of the presence of hyperventilation and the associated decrease in alveolar CO_2. Later, Pao_2 will decrease towards pre-pregnancy values, likely reflecting airway closure and intrapulmonary shunt. Maternal hemoglobin (Hgb) is right-shifted, with the oxygen partial pressure associated with 50% Hgb saturation (P_{50}) increasing from 27 mm Hg up to approximately 30 mm Hg. This right-shift combined with the left-shifted fetal Hgb (a P_{50} of approximately 18 mm Hg) facilitates oxygen delivery across the placenta.

At term, maternal oxygen consumption is increased by 20%. The added work of labor results in further increases in both minute ventilation and oxygen consumption. During labor, oxygen consumption increases above prelabor rates by 40% during the first stage and 75% during the second stage.

Lung Volumes

The expiratory reserve volume (ERV) and residual lung volume (RV) do not begin to change until about the third month of pregnancy (see Table 33.1). With enlargement of the uterus, the diaphragm is forced cephalad, which is primarily responsible for the 20% decrease in functional residual capacity (FRC) present by term. This change is created by approximately equal decreases in the ERV and RV. As a result, FRC can be less than closing capacity for many small airways and may give rise to atelectasis in the supine position. Vital capacity is not significantly changed with pregnancy. The combination of increased minute ventilation and decreased FRC results in a greater rate at which changes in the alveolar concentration of inhaled anesthetics can be achieved. Respiratory measures of forced expiratory volume in 1 second (FEV_1), FEV_1/FVC (forced vital capacity), and closing capacity do not change significantly with pregnancy.

Anesthetic Implications

During induction of general anesthesia in a pregnant patient, Pao_2 decreases much more rapidly than in a nonpregnant patient because of decreased oxygen reserve (decreased FRC) and increased oxygen uptake (increased metabolic rate). For these reasons, the administration of supplemental oxygen, or "preoxygenation," before general anesthesia is critical for patient safety. The pregnant patient should breathe oxygen for 3 minutes before any anticipated period of apnea (such as induction) or take four maximal breaths over the 30 seconds just before induction if emergent general anesthesia is needed. In addition, the increased airway edema makes both ventilation and intubation more difficult and further increases the potential for complications and morbidity. Optimal positioning should be obtained and backup airway equipment readily available before induction of general anesthesia. See "Anesthesia for Cesarean Delivery."

Gastrointestinal Changes

Gastrointestinal changes during pregnancy make women beyond 20 weeks' gestation vulnerable to aspiration of gastric contents and the development of pneumonitis. Displacement of the stomach and pylorus cephalad by the enlarged uterus repositions the intraabdominal portion of the esophagus into the thorax and decreases the competence of the lower esophageal sphincter. Higher progesterone and estrogen levels of pregnancy further reduce esophageal sphincter tone. During vaginal delivery, gastric pressure is increased by both the gravid uterus and the lithotomy position. Gastrin, which is secreted by the placenta, stimulates gastric hydrogen ion secretion such that the pH of gastric fluid is predictably low in pregnant women. For these reasons, gastric fluid reflux into the esophagus with subsequent esophagitis (heartburn) is common and increases with the pregnancy gestational age. In addition, gastric emptying is delayed with the onset of labor or administration of opioids, further increasing the risk of aspiration.

Anesthetic Implications

Regardless of the time interval since the ingestion of food, women in labor are treated as having a full stomach and an increased risk for pulmonary aspiration. This includes the routine use of nonparticulate antacids, rapid-sequence induction, cricoid pressure, and cuffed intubation as part of the general anesthesia induction sequence in a pregnant woman after approximately 20 weeks gestational age. Pain, anxiety, and opioids administered during labor can further slow gastric emptying beyond an already prolonged transit time. Epidural analgesia using local anesthetics with low-dose fentanyl does not delay gastric emptying, but administering epidural boluses of fentanyl does.[5] The low pH of aspirated gastric fluid is important in the production and severity of acid pneumonitis and is the basis for the administration of antacids to pregnant women before induction of anesthesia. Current American Society of Anesthesiologists (ASA) guidelines[6] recommend the "timely administration of oral nonparticulate antacids, IV H2-receptor antagonists, and/or metoclopramide for aspiration prophylaxis" before the induction of anesthesia in pregnant women. Nonparticulate antacids such as sodium citrate (30 mL) work rapidly. Metoclopramide can significantly decrease gastric volume in as little as 15 minutes, although gastric hypomotility associated with prior opioid administration reduces the effectiveness of metoclopramide.[7] H2-receptor antagonists increase gastric fluid pH in pregnant women approximately 1 hour after administration without producing adverse effects. There is some evidence that antacids plus H2 antagonists are better than antacids alone in decreasing gastric acidity.[8] The physiologic effects of pregnancy on gastric function return to normal approximately 24 hours after delivery.[1]

Nervous System Changes

Volatile anesthetic requirements (minimum alveolar concentration [MAC]) decrease up to 40% during pregnancy in animal studies[9] and 28% in humans[10] within the first trimester of pregnancy. However, an electroencephalographic study suggests that anesthetic effects of sevoflurane are similar in pregnant and nonpregnant women.[11] Consequently, the degree of anesthetic reduction and mechanism remains uncertain, but progesterone activity may be partially responsible. A clinical implication of this decreased MAC is that alveolar anesthetic concentrations that would not routinely produce unconsciousness may approximate anesthetizing concentrations in pregnant women. Judicious administration of agents that depress the central nervous system (CNS) is required to prevent unintended impairment of upper airway reflexes and increased risk of pulmonary aspiration that is already elevated secondary to gastrointestinal changes detailed previously. Notably, rates of intraoperative awareness under general anesthesia are increased for cesarean delivery, and reducing standard anesthetic levels in stable pregnant patients is not advised.

Pregnant patients are more sensitive to the local anesthetics used during neuraxial blockade. There is a decrease in local anesthetic dose needed for epidural or spinal anesthesia in pregnant women at term. The observation of decreased neuraxial local anesthetic doses as early as the first trimester suggests a role for biochemical changes causing increased nerve sensitivity. Although this increased sensitivity is likely based on hormonal changes, there may be some role for mechanical changes as well. Engorgement of epidural veins as intraabdominal pressure increases with progressive enlargement of the uterus results in a decrease in both the size of the epidural space and volume of cerebrospinal fluid (CSF) in the subarachnoid space. The decreased volume of

IV

these spaces facilitates the spread of local anesthetics. However, CSF pressure itself does not increase with pregnancy.

Renal Changes

Renal blood flow and the glomerular filtration rate are increased about 50% to 60% by the third month of pregnancy and do not return to pre-pregnant levels until 3 months postpartum. Therefore, the normal upper limits of blood urea nitrogen and serum creatinine concentrations in pregnant women are only 50% of those in nonpregnant women. There is decreased tubular resorption of both protein and glucose, and excretion of these in the urine is common. A 24-hour urine collection of less than 300 mg protein or 10 grams glucose is considered the upper limit of normal in pregnancy.

Hepatic Changes

Liver blood flow does not change significantly with pregnancy. Plasma protein concentrations are reduced during pregnancy, and decreased serum albumin levels can result in elevated free blood levels of highly protein-bound drugs. Slightly elevated liver function tests are common in the third trimester. Plasma cholinesterase (pseudocholinesterase) activity is decreased about 25% to 30% from the tenth week of gestation up to 6 weeks postpartum. This decreased activity is unlikely to be associated with significant prolongation of the neuromuscular blockade of succinylcholine, but return of muscle strength should always be verified. In addition, incomplete gallbladder emptying and changes in bile composition increase the risk of gallbladder disease during pregnancy. Even without underlying pathology, alkaline phosphate levels double during pregnancy from placental production.

PHYSIOLOGY OF THE UTEROPLACENTAL CIRCULATION

The placenta is the interface of maternal and fetal tissue for the purpose of physiologic exchange. Maternal blood is delivered to the uterus and placenta by two uterine arteries. On the fetal side, nutrient-rich and waste-free blood is returned from the placenta to the fetus through a single umbilical vein, and fetal blood returns to interface with the maternal circulation via two umbilical arteries.

Uterine Blood Flow

UBF increases throughout gestation from about 100 mL/min before pregnancy to 700 mL/min (about 10% of cardiac output) at term gestation. About 80% of UBF perfuses the intervillous space (placenta) and 20% supports the myometrium. The uterine vasculature has limited autoregulation and remains essentially maximally dilated under normal pregnancy conditions. UBF can decrease from any cause of reduced uterine perfusion pressure such as systemic hypotension secondary to hypovolemia, aortocaval compression, or decreased systemic resistance from either general or neuraxial anesthesia. UBF can also decrease with increased uterine venous pressure. This can result from vena caval compression (supine position), prolonged or frequent uterine contractions, significant abdominal musculature contraction (Valsalva maneuver during pushing), or extreme hypocapnia ($Paco_2$ <20 mm Hg) associated with hyperventilation secondary to labor pain.

Epidural or spinal anesthesia does not significantly alter UBF as long as maternal hypotension is avoided. Although certain types and higher doses of vasopressors can increase uterine artery resistance and decrease UBF, phenylephrine, ephedrine, and norepinephrine can all be used safely to treat hypotension in standard clinical doses, See "Hypotension" section below.

Placental Exchange

Transfer of oxygen from the mother to the fetus is dependent on a variety of factors, including the ratio of maternal UBF to fetal umbilical blood flow, the oxygen partial pressure gradient, the respective hemoglobin concentrations and affinities, the placental diffusing capacity, and the acid–base status of the fetal and maternal blood (Bohr effect). The fetal oxyhemoglobin dissociation curve is left-shifted (greater oxygen affinity), whereas the maternal hemoglobin binding curve is right-shifted (decreased oxygen affinity), resulting in facilitated oxygen transfer to the fetus. The fetal Pao_2 is normally 20 to 40 mm Hg,[12] but can reach 60 mm Hg if the mother is breathing 100% oxygen.[13] This is because the placental exchange to the fetus from the mother represents more of a venous rather than arterial blood. CO_2 readily crosses the placenta and is not limited by diffusion, but rather flow.

Placental exchange of most drugs and other substances less than 1000 Daltons occurs principally by diffusion from the maternal circulation to the fetus and vice versa. Diffusion of a substance across the placenta to the fetus depends on maternal-to-fetal concentration gradients, maternal protein binding, molecular weight, lipid solubility, and the degree of ionization of that substance. Minimizing the maternal blood concentration of a drug is the most important method of limiting the amount that ultimately reaches the fetus.

The high molecular weight and poor lipid solubility of nondepolarizing neuromuscular blocking drugs result in limited ability of these drugs to cross the placenta. Succinylcholine has a low molecular weight but is highly ionized and therefore does not readily cross the placenta. Thus, during administration of a typical general anesthetic for cesarean delivery, the fetus/neonate is not paralyzed. Additionally, heparin, insulin, and glycopyrrolate have significantly limited placental transfer. Placental transfer of benzodiazepines, volatile anesthetics, local anesthetics, and opioids is facilitated by the relatively low molecular weights of these substances. In general, drugs that readily cross the blood–brain barrier also cross the placenta.

Fetal Uptake

Fetal uptake of a substance that crosses the placenta is affected by the lower pH (0.1 unit) of fetal blood compared with maternal. The lower fetal pH means that weakly basic drugs (e.g., local anesthetics) that cross the placenta in the nonionized form will become ionized in the fetal circulation. Because an ionized drug cannot readily cross the placenta and return to the maternal circulation, this drug will accumulate in the fetal blood against a concentration gradient. Therefore, in an acidotic fetus, higher concentrations of local anesthetic can accumulate (ion trapping), especially during periods of fetal distress. Increased concentrations of local anesthetics in the fetus can result in decreased neonatal neuromuscular tone. If direct maternal intravascular local anesthetic injection occurs, significant fetal toxicity can result in bradycardia, ventricular arrhythmia, acidosis, and severe cardiac depression. Placental transfer and fetal uptake of specific analgesic and anesthetic agents are detailed in the upcoming sections on "Methods of Labor Analgesia" and "Anesthesia for Cesarean Delivery."

Characteristics of the Fetal Circulation

The fetal circulation helps protect vital fetal organs from exposure to high concentrations of drugs initially present in umbilical venous blood. For example, about 75% of umbilical venous blood initially passes through the fetal liver such that significant portions of drugs are metabolized before reaching the fetal arterial circulation for delivery to the heart and brain. Despite decreased liver enzyme activity in comparison with adults, fetal/neonatal enzyme systems are adequately developed to metabolize most drugs. Moreover, drugs in the portion of umbilical venous blood that enter the inferior vena cava via the ductus venosus will be diluted by drug-free blood returning from the lower extremities and pelvic viscera of the fetus. These circulatory characteristics decrease the fetal plasma drug concentrations compared with maternal after an intravenous drug bolus.[14]

STAGES OF LABOR

The anesthesia provider may be consulted at any time to aid in a safe delivery. The labor course, mode of delivery,

and maternal comorbidities should all be considered in determining which analgesic or anesthetic technique is most appropriate. Understanding the stages of labor and common labor patterns is important to appreciate when labor is not progressing and obstetric intervention may be required. Progression of labor is reliably unpredictable. Retrospective reviews of the maternal labor course have led to a change of definitions for what constitutes normal labor progress.[15] Ideally, this change will decrease cesarean deliveries in the first stage of labor (active-stage arrest).

The course of labor is divided into three stages. The *first stage* begins with maternal perception of uterine contractions (latent phase) and continues with significant acceleration of cervical dilation (active phase), until the cervix is fully dilated. The latent phase can persist for hours to days. The active phase begins when the rate of cervical dilation increases (usually after 5 to 6 cm dilation). The *second stage* of labor begins with full cervical dilation and ends with neonatal birth. This stage is referred to as the "pushing and expulsion" stage. Once the neonate is born, the *third stage* begins and is completed when the placenta is delivered. Concern for abnormal labor and obstetric interventions may be indicated if progression through the stages of labor is halted or delayed.

If dilation slows or stops in the active phase of labor despite pharmacologic interventions, this is considered active-phase arrest and cesarean delivery will likely be considered by the obstetrician. Arrest of descent occurs during the second stage of labor, when the neonate cannot be born vaginally. The mode of delivery in this case depends on the location of the neonatal head when arrest of descent occurs. If the neonate is low enough in the pelvis, the obstetrician can perform an instrumented vaginal delivery (also known as an *operative vaginal delivery*) via vacuum or forceps. If the neonate remains too high in the pelvis, then the woman will likely need to undergo a cesarean delivery. Additionally, the fetal condition can dictate a change in delivery mode based on the fetal heart rate tracing.

ANATOMY OF LABOR PAIN

Uterine contractions, cervical dilation, and perineal distention cause pain during labor and delivery. Afferent somatic and visceral sensory fibers from the uterus and cervix travel to the spinal cord with sympathetic nerve fibers (Fig. 33.3). Most painful stimuli in the first stage of labor are the result of afferent nerve impulses from the lower uterine segment and cervix, with visceral pain arising from the uterine body. Nerve fibers from the uterus and cervix course with the hypogastric nerves and sympathetic chain to the dorsal root ganglia of levels T10–L1. In the second stage of labor, additional somatic pain is

IV

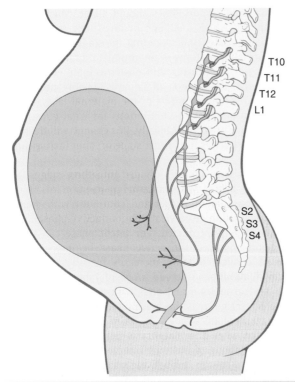

Fig. 33.3 Schematic Diagram of Pain Pathways During Pregnancy. Visceral pain during the first stage of labor is caused by uterine contraction and cervical dilation. Afferent sensory fibers from the uterus and cervix travel with sympathetic nerve fibers and enter the spinal cord at T10–L1. Somatic afferents from the vagina and perineum travel via the pudendal nerve to levels S2–S4.

transmitted from afferent nerves innervating the vagina and perineum and results from distension, ischemia, and tissue injury of these areas as the fetus descends into the pelvis and delivers. These afferent impulses travel primarily via the pudendal nerve to dorsal root ganglia of levels S2–S4. Neuraxial analgesic techniques must block levels T10–L1 to provide pain relief during the first stage of labor and also include S2–S4 for efficacy during the second stage of labor.

The mother, fetus, and labor course can all be affected by the physiologic effects of labor pain. Pain stimulates the sympathetic nervous system, elevates plasma catecholamine levels, creates reflex maternal tachycardia and hypertension, and can decrease UBF. In addition, changes in uterine activity can occur with the rapid decrease in plasma epinephrine concentrations associated with the onset of neuraxial analgesia. Variations in epinephrine levels can result in a range of uterine effects, including a transient period of uterine hyperstimulation (tachysystole), a period of uterine quiescence, or conversion of a dysfunctional uterine activity pattern to a more

regular pattern. There is variation in the severity of pain reported by women during labor and delivery. However, the intensity of pain during labor increases with cervical dilation. In the absence of medical contraindications to labor pain relief options, maternal request is a sufficient indication for treatment of pain during labor.[16]

METHODS OF LABOR ANALGESIA

Nonpharmacologic Techniques

There are many nonpharmacologic techniques for labor analgesia. Three theoretical models describe how these techniques work by their effects on endogenous labor pain pathways.[17] Hydrotherapy, massage, position changes, and transcutaneous electrical nerve stimulation (TENS) inhibit pain fiber transmission by providing tactile stimulation to an area of pain (gate control model). Acupuncture/acupressure, sterile water injections, and TENS cause pain at sites remote from labor pain, which stimulates the endorphin system, leading to decreased overall pain (diffuse noxious inhibitory control model). The CNS control model focuses on attention divergence from labor pain using Lamaze, meditation, hypnosis, relaxation, expectation management, and music. Though data for analgesic benefit with these techniques are limited and modest, acupuncture, acupressure, TENS, relaxation, and massage techniques offer some element of patient control and increased patient satisfaction.[18] Hypnosis and intradermal water injection techniques show no significant analgesic benefit beyond control populations. Nonetheless, perceived patient autonomy and patient control appear to substantially contribute to a woman's satisfaction with labor and delivery in comparison with analgesic efficacy. Additionally, a meta-analysis reviewing the effectiveness of a support individual (e.g., doula, family member) noted that women with a support individual used fewer pharmacologic analgesia methods, had a decreased length of labor, were more likely to have a vaginal birth, and were less likely to have negative feelings about childbirth.[19]

Systemic Medications

Systemic analgesics can be beneficial for women in the early stages of spontaneous or induced labor. However, use of these medications is typically limited by both dose and timing.[20] These limits are dictated by the potential for maternal sedation, respiratory compromise, loss of airway protection, and proximity to time of delivery because of concern for adverse neonatal effects. Whereas systemic opioid analgesics are commonly used for labor, use of sedatives, anxiolytics, and dissociative agents is rare.

Opioids (also see Chapter 9)

All opioids readily cross the placental barrier and can cause neonatal effects, including decreased fetal heart rate variability and neonatal dose-related respiratory depression. Additionally, maternal side effects are common and include nausea, vomiting, pruritus, and delayed gastric emptying.

Fentanyl has a short duration of action and no active metabolites, which makes it a preferable analgesic for labor. When administered in small intravenous (IV) bolus doses of 50 to 100 mcg per hour, there are no significant differences in neonatal Apgar scores and respiratory effort compared with newborns of mothers not receiving fentanyl.[21]

Meperidine has a longer duration of action (maternal half-life 2 to 3 hours) and is metabolized to an active metabolite (normeperidine). Meperidine can be administered IV (12.5 to 25 mg) or intramuscularly (IM) (25 to 50 mg). The fetal and neonatal half-life of meperidine is prolonged (13 to 23 hours) and highly variable. Increased levels of neonatal normeperidine have been associated with decreased Apgar scores, increased time to sustained respiration, lower fetal oxygen saturation levels, abnormal neurobehavior, and difficulty initiating breastfeeding.[17,22] Despite these undesirable side effects, it remains a commonly used labor analgesic worldwide, likely because of cost, ease of administration, and availability.

Morphine, like meperidine, also has an active metabolite (morphine-6-glucuronide) and a longer duration of action. Notably, morphine causes profound maternal sedation, has a prolonged half-life in neonates, and is no longer commonly used. It remains occasionally administered IM in combination with promethazine to provide latent labor analgesia (for 2.5 to 6 hours) and rest. This technique is termed *morphine sleep* and based on a prospective cohort study does not affect maternal or neonatal outcomes.[23]

Remifentanil has a rapid onset and fast elimination by plasma and tissue esterases with significant tissue metabolism.[17] The primary benefit of remifentanil over other opioid labor analgesics is the minimization of neonatal side effects because of its rapid metabolism. Although remifentanil patient-controlled analgesia (PCA) does not provide superior pain relief compared with epidural labor analgesia,[24] remifentanil provides better pain relief with improved patient satisfaction compared with other opioids and does not appear to adversely affect neonatal outcomes.[25] A retrospective comparison of remifentanil and fentanyl PCA for labor analgesia found more transient maternal desaturation with remifentanil, but fentanyl resulted in greater need for assisted neonatal ventilation and supplemental oxygen.[26] Because of maternal safety concerns (specifically related to respiratory effects), remifentanil use in labor is typically reserved for women with contraindications to neuraxial techniques. When remifentanil is used for labor analgesia, continuous pulse oximetry, end-tidal CO_2 monitoring, oxygen supplementation, and 1:1 nursing are recommended.[27]

Nitrous Oxide (also see Chapter 7)

Use of inhaled nitrous oxide (N_2O) for labor analgesia began in the 1880s, with increased use in the 1930s after invention of a portable device for administration. Although many countries have high utilization rates (>50%), it is only over the past decade that it has been widely available in the United States as an option for labor analgesia. The mechanisms of N_2O are not well understood, and there are few high-quality studies examining its efficacy, optimization, and potential adverse impacts.[28] N_2O is an *N*-methyl-d-aspartate (NMDA) antagonist, but may also modulate pain perception via alpha-2 receptors in the spinal cord dorsal horn and release endogenous opioids in the brain. N_2O possesses many desirable qualities for labor analgesia, including rapid onset, rapid elimination, and no effect on uterine contractility. It can be used in all stages of labor, with no studies to suggest a detrimental effect of N_2O on the fetus or neonate.[29] Although the Food and Drug Administration (FDA) issued a 2016 communication[30] warning against lengthy or repeated use of 11 anesthetic agents in children less than 3 and pregnant women during the third trimester, N_2O was not included. Side effects are well tolerated, most commonly nausea, dysphoria, and dizziness. Although N_2O provides less analgesic effect than epidural analgesia, it offers a safe and satisfactory analgesic option for many women that allows mobility and control of analgesic administration during labor.[31] It is self-administered in a fixed mixture of 50% N_2O with 50% oxygen via facemask. Out of concern for maternal respiratory depression and loss of airway reflexes with deeper levels of sedation, coadministration of systemic opioids or other sedating medications is not recommended.[29] Emissions of this greenhouse gas are significantly reduced in the labor setting with use of the demand valve, and occupational exposure risk is negligible when N_2O is administered with proper scavenging equipment (also see Chapter 49).

Neuraxial (Regional) Analgesia

In the United States, neuraxial analgesia (e.g., epidural, spinal, dural puncture epidural [DPE], combined spinal epidural [CSE]) is the most widely used method for labor analgesia. Neuraxial analgesia typically involves the administration of local anesthetics in combination with opioid analgesics into the epidural and/or intrathecal space. Adjuvant drugs such as epinephrine[32] and clonidine[33] have been shown to decrease the dose of local anesthetics or opioids required for analgesia. The FDA has issued a "black box" warning regarding increased risk of hypotension and bradycardia with neuraxial clonidine in obstetrics, and caution should be used.

Local Anesthetics

Local anesthetics are discussed in detail in Chapter 10. Bupivacaine and ropivacaine are the most commonly used local anesthetics for labor analgesia, and both are extremely safe when appropriately dosed for epidural or intrathecal administration. An accidental, large intravascular dose of any local anesthetic can result in significant maternal morbidity (seizures, loss of consciousness, severe arrhythmias, and cardiovascular collapse) or mortality and the potential for fetal accumulation (ion trapping); see previous section "Physiology of the Uteroplacental Circulation." Immediate recognition and treatment are essential, see "Systemic Toxicity and Excessive Blockade." Optimal local anesthetic concentration, dosing, and delivery techniques are discussed within "Neuraxial Dosing and Delivery Techniques."

Neuraxial Opioids

The neuraxial opioids fentanyl and sufentanil are commonly used in obstetric anesthesia in combination with local anesthetics to improve the quality of labor analgesia and allow a reduction in local anesthetic concentration. Although administration of opioids alone in the epidural space can provide moderate analgesia, the doses required are associated with significant maternal side effects (nausea, sedation, pruritus), and the analgesia is inferior compared with dilute solutions of local anesthetic alone. Coadministration of neuraxial opioids with local anesthetics improves the quality of analgesia and has local anesthetic-sparing effects. The addition of neuraxial opioids is associated with dose-related maternal side effects, including pruritus, sedation, and nausea. In addition, administration of intrathecal opioids can result in fetal bradycardia independent of hypotension.[20] The mechanism for fetal bradycardia is unclear but may result from uterine hyperactivity after the rapid onset of analgesia.

NEURAXIAL TECHNIQUES

The most effective form of labor pain relief with the highest rate of maternal satisfaction is neuraxial analgesia.[34] Excellent analgesia is achieved with a labor epidural, without sedating side effects, and the mother remains able to actively participate during labor. All of these factors can increase maternal satisfaction with the labor experience. However, a negative experience with the childbirth process can result when there is poor communication about neuraxial labor analgesia, provision of neuraxial pain relief is delayed, or analgesia is inadequate.[35]

Preoperative Assessment

Before initiation of any neuraxial blockade, anesthesia providers should assess the woman's pregnancy and health history; perform a focused physical examination; discuss risks, benefits, and alternatives; and obtain consent. Routine laboratory tests are not required in otherwise healthy women.[6] Resuscitation equipment and drugs must be immediately available to manage serious complications secondary to initiation of epidural or spinal blocks (see "Contraindications and Complications of Neuraxial Anesthesia" section below). During initiation of neuraxial blockade, the mother and fetus must be closely monitored (maternal vital signs and fetal heart rate monitoring).[36] Current recommendations allow otherwise healthy laboring women to have modest amounts of clear liquids regardless of whether a labor epidural is in place. In complicated labors (e.g., by morbid obesity, difficult airway, concerning fetal status), the anesthesia provider might consider restricting oral intake.[6]

Timing and Placement of Epidural

Regardless of cervical dilation, maternal request for relief of labor pain is sufficient justification for epidural placement according to current ASA and American College of Obstetricians and Gynecologists (ACOG) guidelines.[6,16] In the past, there were concerns that early epidural placement might adversely affect labor progress. However, randomized controlled clinical trials (RCTs) comparing women receiving either systemic opioids or neuraxial analgesia in early labor (both spontaneous and induced) demonstrated no difference in rates of cesarean delivery.[37,38] A Cochrane review based on studies up to 2017 comparing use of labor epidural with either no epidural or systemic opioid labor analgesia also noted no difference in rates of cesarean delivery, but a modest increase in the length of the second stage (about 15 minutes) and an increased rate of instrumented vaginal delivery in women using neuraxial labor analgesia.[39] However, a secondary analysis of trials conducted after 2005 found there was no longer an association between use of a labor epidural and need for instrumented vaginal delivery. A 2015 clinical trial found no difference between epidurals dosed with fentanyl alone vs. local anesthetic, suggesting a prolonged second stage is not a result of decreased pushing effort secondary to local anesthetic effects.[40] This increase in the second stage is not harmful to the infant or mother. As long as the fetal status remains reassuring and there is ongoing progress towards delivery, the duration of the second stage does not dictate intervention.[41]

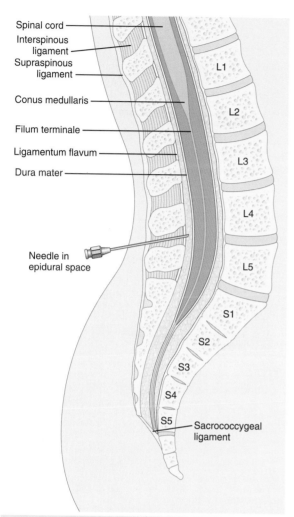

Spinal cord

Interspinous ligament

Supraspinous ligament

Conus medullaris

Filum terminale

Ligamentum flavum

Dura mater

L1

L2

L3

L4

L5

Needle in epidural space

S1

S2

S3

S4

S5 — Sacrococcygeal ligament

Fig. 33.4 Schematic diagram of lumbosacral anatomy showing needle placement for epidural block.

(e.g., chlorhexidine) for skin preparation, allowing for adequate drying time; (3) sterile draping of the patient; (4) aseptic techniques during equipment preparation (e.g., ultrasound) and placement of needles and catheters; and (5) use of sterile occlusive dressings at the catheter insertion site.[42] The needle is typically inserted between the L3 and L4 spinous processes. The needle traverses the skin and subcutaneous tissues, supraspinous ligament, interspinous ligament, the ligamentum flavum, and then reaches the epidural space (Fig. 33.5). The tip of the Tuohy needle should not penetrate the dura, which forms the boundary between the intrathecal or subarachnoid space and the epidural space. The epidural space is found using a tactile technique called *loss of resistance*. To perform this technique, an air- or saline-filled syringe is attached to the Tuohy needle, and tactile resistance is noted with pressure on the plunger of the syringe as the needle is advanced towards the epidural space. Resistance dramatically decreases when the tip of the needle is advanced through the ligamentum flavum (dense resistance) into the epidural space (no resistance). Average depth of the epidural space is about 5 cm from the skin. Once properly positioned, a catheter is inserted through the needle. The needle is removed and the epidural catheter is secured with 4 to 5 cm remaining in the epidural space for use with intermittent or continuous injection. To minimize unintended catheter migration, the catheter should be secured with a sterile dressing only after the patient has returned to a neutral upright or lateral position. Local anesthetics and/or opioids (discussed earlier) are administered via the epidural catheter to achieve and maintain analgesia throughout the labor and delivery course. The epidural catheter can also be used for instrumented vaginal or cesarean delivery and opioid (e.g., morphine) administration for postoperative analgesia when appropriate.

Epidural Technique (also see Chapter 17)

Epidurals provide continuous pain relief during labor via a catheter-based technique. Placement involves insertion of a specialized needle (Tuohy) between vertebral spinous processes in the back and into the epidural space (Fig. 33.4). To prevent unintentional dural puncture ("wet tap"), the Tuohy needle has a slightly curved blunt tip. Placement can occur with the patient in the sitting or lateral position, depending on the anesthesia provider's experience and the position that provides optimal exposure to anatomic landmarks. Aseptic techniques should always be used during neuraxial placement per ASA task force recommendations. These recommendations include (1) removal of jewelry (e.g., rings and watches), handwashing/use of hand sanitizer before donning sterile gloves, and wearing of caps, masks, and sterile gloves; (2) use of individual packets of antiseptic

Combined Spinal Epidural and Dural Puncture Epidural Techniques

The CSE and DPE techniques follow the epidural technique noted earlier, but after the loss of resistance a spinal needle (≤25 gauge, pencil-point) is inserted into the epidural needle, using a needle-through-needle technique. For a DPE, once CSF is visualized in the spinal needle hub, the spinal needle is removed and the epidural catheter is placed as described with the epidural technique. Compared with an epidural, the benefit of the DPE may be fewer one-sided blocks, less sacral sparing, and slightly faster onset of analgesia, with less hypotension and pruritis than a CSE.[20,43] The benefits of the DPE require use of a 25-gauge or larger spinal needle. For the CSE, an intrathecal dose of local anesthetic and/or opioid is administered through the spinal needle before removal. The benefit of the CSE is the quick onset (about 2 minutes) of analgesia, along with better sacral

IV

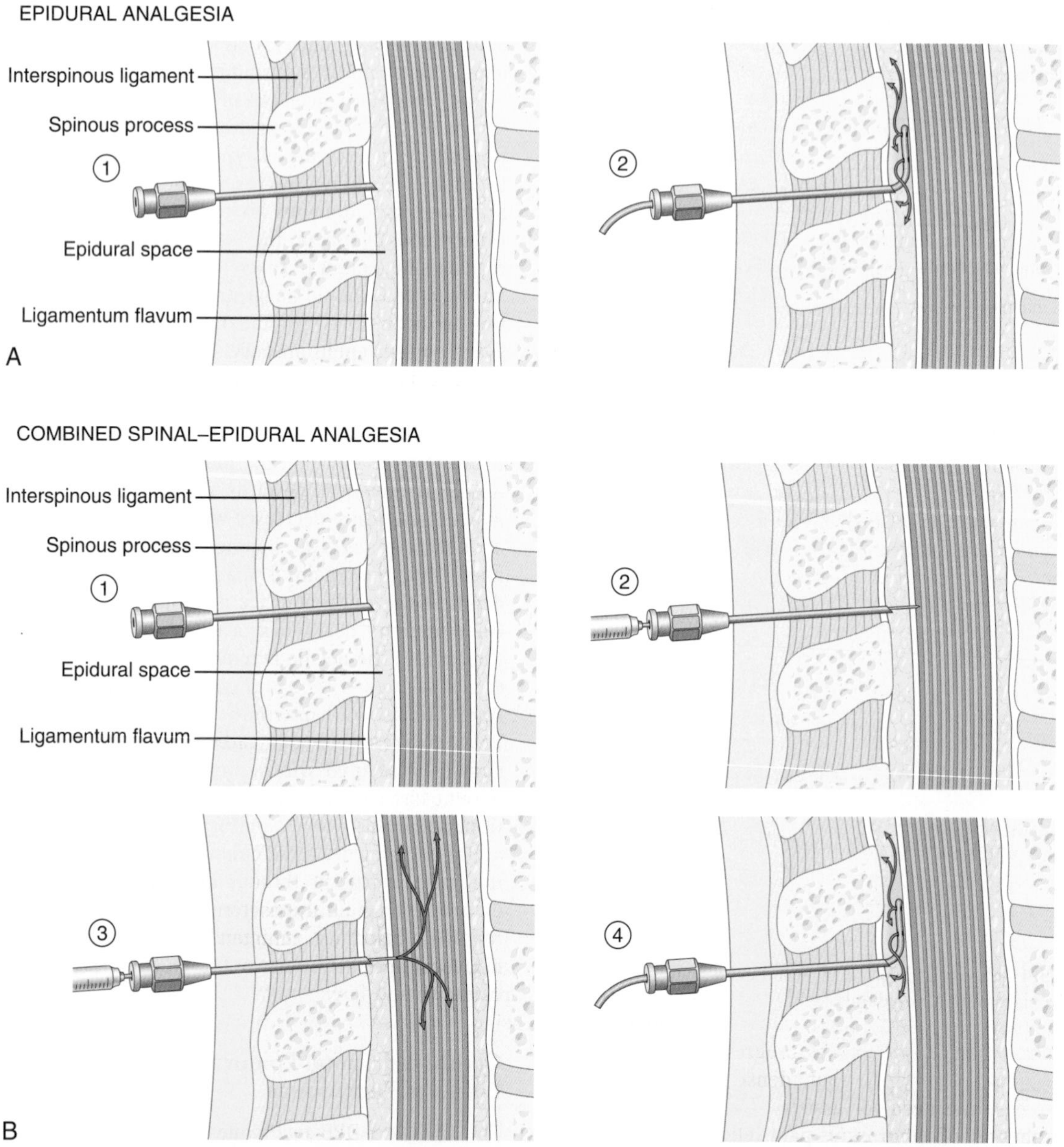

EPIDURAL ANALGESIA

COMBINED SPINAL–EPIDURAL ANALGESIA

Fig. 33.5 Technique of Epidural and Combined Spinal-Epidural Analgesia. (A) Epidural catheter placement for labor analgesia. (1) The desired epidural space L2–L4 is identified. After infiltration with local anesthetic, a Tuohy needle is seated in the intervertebral ligaments. A syringe is connected to the epidural needle for confirmation of degree of resistance using constant or periodic pressure on the plunger. As the needle tip is passed from the high resistance of the ligaments to the low resistance in the epidural space, a sudden loss of resistance is recognized by the anesthesia provider and advancement is stopped. (2) An epidural catheter is advanced through the needle into the space. Analgesic medications are administered through the catheter after a "test dose." (B) Combined spinal-epidural analgesia. (1) After Tuohy needle placement into the epidural space, (2) a spinal needle (24–26 gauge) is introduced through the epidural needle into the subarachnoid space. (3) Proper placement is confirmed by free flow of the cerebrospinal fluid. A bolus of local anesthetic and/or opioid is given through the spinal needle. (4) After spinal needle removal, an epidural catheter is advanced through the Tuohy into the epidural space. The epidural catheter can be used for continuation of labor analgesia. (Adapted from Eltzschig HK, Lieberman ES, Camann WR. Regional anesthesia and analgesia for labor and delivery. *N Engl J Med.* 2003;348:319–332.)

spread, fewer one-sided blocks, and fewer catheter failures compared with a plain epidural.[20] However, with a CSE compared with DPE or epidural, there appears to be increased opioid-based pruritus, increased risk of uterine tachysystole, and greater incidence of fetal bradycardia after block placement. Although there is not an increased risk of headache with a CSE technique compared with an epidural, use of a 25-gauge spinal needle required for optimal DPE efficacy requires further study regarding possible minimally increased risk of headache.[20,44]

Neuraxial Dosing and Delivery Techniques

An epidural catheter allows infusion of local anesthetic with or without opioid drugs. In addition, anesthesia providers can bolus the catheter with either the same or a more concentrated solution of local anesthetic. Programmable infusion pumps allow a patient-controlled epidural analgesia (PCEA) method of delivering the chosen anesthetic mixture with or without a background infusion. Compared with a continuous infusion alone, a PCEA method of delivery allows for a decrease in medical personnel, decreased motor block, improved patient satisfaction, and lower local anesthetic consumption.[6,45] Adding a background infusion to PCEA further improves labor analgesia, reduces the need for clinician boluses, and does not increase maternal or neonatal adverse events. Programmed intermittent epidural bolus (PIEB) is a more recent method of administering automated fixed epidural boluses at scheduled intervals. PIEB can be used alone or with a PCEA technique. A 2018 Cochrane systematic review suggests that compared with a continuous infusion technique, PIEB may reduce local anesthetic usage, improve maternal satisfaction, and decrease the need for rescue boluses.[46] Using PIEB with PCEA allows a basal analgesia with the ability for the patient to tailor additional analgesia depending on her own preferences, which may change as the labor progresses.

Because of concerns that dense motor blockade may increase the need for assisted vaginal delivery, the concentrations of labor epidural local anesthetics have decreased as practice has evolved. Typical maintenance infusion concentrations for epidural bupivacaine (0.04% to 0.125%) or ropivacaine (0.0625% to 0.2%) are both effective. Opioids such as fentanyl (2 mcg/mL) or sufentanil (0.2 mcg/mL) may be added to the infusion mixture to augment analgesia and decrease local anesthetic requirements, but increase the side effects of pruritus, nausea, and sedation in a dose-dependent fashion. Opioids can also be bolused through the epidural catheter with typical doses of fentanyl 50 to 100 mcg or sufentanil 5 to 10 mcg to improve analgesia. Dilute concentrations of epinephrine (1:300,000 to 1:800,000) can also be added to the epidural mixture to augment analgesia. If using a dilute solution (0.0625% bupivacaine with 2 mcg/ml fentanyl) with PIEB volumes of 10 mL, higher bolus rates of flow (500 mL/hr) and intervals of 40 to 45 minutes between each PIEB may improve efficacy of the labor analgesia.[47,48]

For CSEs the initial intrathecal dose can include an opioid, a local anesthetic, or a combination of the two. Typical intrathecal doses for opioids are fentanyl (10 to 20 mcg) or sufentanil (1.5 to 5 mcg), and local anesthetic doses include bupivacaine (1.25 to 3.5 mg) and ropivacaine (2 to 5 mg). Use of opioids alone is associated with increased rates of severe pruritus,[49] and higher-dose intrathecal opioids (e.g., sufentanil 7.5 mcg) are associated with increased risk of fetal bradycardia even in the absence of hypotension.[50] When combined with 2.5 mg intrathecal bupivacaine, 15 mcg of fentanyl appears to be an optimal dose, with increasing amounts not improving analgesic efficacy but potentially increasing undesired side effects.[51]

Before initiation of an epidural catheter, a *test dose* should be performed to evaluate the possibility of unintended IV or intrathecal catheter placement. Commonly, 3 mL of 1.5% lidocaine containing 1:200,000 epinephrine is used. Increases in heart rate and blood pressure >20% above baseline (intravascular placement) or rapid analgesia and lower extremity motor block (intrathecal placement) note epidural catheter misplacement. Maternal vital signs should be obtained before placement of neuraxial analgesia (heart rate, pulse oximetry, and blood pressure). Whenever bolusing the epidural catheter, aspirate the catheter first to help confirm it has not migrated into the intrathecal or intravascular space. Administer the anesthetic mixture incrementally while monitoring maternal vitals (blood pressure and pulse oximetry) and fetal heart rate (FHR). Unintended complications can occur when a catheter is initially bolused (e.g., unintended intrathecal administration, local anesthetic systemic toxicity). Consequently, the patient should be under direct observation by an anesthesia provider, labor nurse, or midwife for at least 20 minutes after initial administration of neuraxial medication, with maternal heart rate and pulse oximetry monitoring, and blood pressure measured at least every 5 minutes.[36]

Instrumented vaginal delivery may become necessary for arrest of descent and/or fetal indications. Use of forceps often requires a denser block with perineal anesthesia. Supplementation with 5 to 10 mL of an epidural local anesthetic (e.g., 2% lidocaine or 3% 2-chloroprocaine) may be needed.

Spinal Labor Analgesia

Placement of spinal medications provides rapid analgesia when delivery is imminent in the advanced second stage. It is also useful for instrumented (forceps/vacuum) delivery, management of retained placenta, or repair of high-degree perineal lacerations. A 25- to 27-gauge "pencil point" spinal needle is selected to reduce the risk of postdural puncture headache. Intrathecal medications

IV

are commonly administered in doses similar to those used in the spinal portion of a CSE (e.g., 2.5 mg bupivacaine with 15 mcg fentanyl) to provide analgesic onset within minutes. This type of labor analgesia lasts about 60 to 90 minutes and is significantly less than that needed for cesarean delivery. To optimize anesthesia for perineal laceration repair, hyperbaric local anesthetic can be administered followed by leaving the patient in the sitting position for 5 minutes to achieve a dense sensory block in the perineal region ("saddle block").

CONTRAINDICATIONS OF NEURAXIAL ANESTHESIA

Certain conditions contraindicate neuraxial procedures. These include (1) patient refusal, (2) infection at the needle insertion site, (3) significant coagulopathy, (4) hypovolemic shock, (5) increased intracranial pressure from mass lesion, and (6) inadequate resources or provider expertise.[52] Other conditions such as systemic infection, neurologic disease, and mild coagulopathies are relative contraindications that should be evaluated on a case-by-case basis using current guidelines. Human immunodeficiency virus (HIV) and hepatitis infection are not contraindications to neuraxial technique in pregnant women. For women with thrombocytopenia or receiving thromboprophylaxis, recent guidelines provide guidance on placement of neuraxial anesthesia[53-55] (also see Chapter 23).

COMPLICATIONS OF NEURAXIAL ANESTHESIA

The rates of inadequate neuraxial labor analgesia requiring catheter replacement are approximately 7% to 12% for epidurals and 3% to 7% for CSEs based on two retrospective studies.[56,57] The rate of accidental dural puncture during epidural catheter placement is approximately 1% to 2%, and about half of these will result in a severe headache, which is typically managed with analgesics, hydration, rest, caffeine, or blood patch if necessary. Other potential side effects from neuraxial blockade include pruritus, nausea, shivering, urinary retention, motor weakness, low back soreness, and a prolonged block. More serious complications of meningitis, epidural hematoma, and nerve or spinal cord injury are extremely rare. A multicenter database analysis of 257,000 obstetric patients examined rates of serious neurologic events.[58] The rate of epidural abscess or meningitis was 1:63,000, epidural hematoma was 1:251,000, and high neuraxial block 1:4,300. A 2006 meta-analysis of 1.37 million women receiving labor epidurals noted rates of deep epidural infections 1:145,000, epidural hematoma 1:168,000, and persistent neurologic injury remaining greater than 1 year at 1:240,000.[59] Discussion

of informed consent is essential before labor analgesia, and a patient's recall of neuraxial risks does not appear to be reduced in the presence of labor pain.[60]

Systemic Toxicity and Excessive Blockade (also see Chapter 10)

Infrequent but occasionally life-threatening complications can result from administration of neuraxial anesthesia. The most serious complications are from accidental IV or intrathecal injections of local anesthetics. An unintended bolus of IV local anesthetic causes dose-dependent consequences ranging from minor side effects (e.g., tinnitus, perioral tingling, mild blood pressure and heart rate changes) to major complications (seizures, loss of consciousness, severe arrhythmias, cardiovascular collapse). The severity depends on the dose, type of local anesthetic, and preexisting condition of the woman. Bupivacaine has more affinity for sodium channels than lidocaine and dissociates more slowly. In addition, its high protein affinity makes cardiac resuscitation more difficult and prolonged. Measures that minimize the likelihood of accidental intravascular injection include careful aspiration of the catheter before injection, test dosing, and incremental administration of therapeutic doses. Successful resuscitation and support of the mother will reestablish UBF. This will provide adequate fetal oxygenation and allow time for excretion of local anesthetic from the fetus. The neonate has an extremely limited ability to metabolize local anesthetics and may have prolonged convulsions if emergent delivery is required.

A high spinal (total spinal) can result from an unrecognized epidural catheter placed subdurally, migration of the catheter during its use, or an overdose of local anesthetic in the epidural space (i.e., high epidural). Both high spinals and high epidurals can result in severe maternal hypotension, bradycardia, loss of consciousness, and blockade of the motor nerves to the respiratory muscles.

Treatment

Treatment of complications resulting from both intravascular injection and high spinal are directed at restoring maternal and fetal oxygenation, ventilation, and circulation. Intubation, vasopressors, fluids, and advanced cardiac life support (ACLS) algorithms are often required. ACLS guidelines for pregnancy include use of manual left uterine displacement to relieve aortocaval compression, avoidance of lower extremity vessels for drug delivery, and no modifications to pharmacologic or defibrillation protocols except removal of fetal and uterine monitors before shock[61] (also see Chapter 45). If a local anesthetic overdose occurs, consider use of a 20% IV lipid emulsion to bind the drug and decrease toxicity.[62] For cardiac arrest with unsuccessful resuscitation where the fundal height is at or above the level of the umbilicus (approximately 20 weeks' gestation), the fetus should be emergently delivered if the mother is not resuscitated within 5 minutes of the arrest.[61] This guideline for emergent cesarean delivery increases the chances of survival for both the mother and neonate. In addition, the use of checklists and simulation can improve performance during rare but critical events.

Hypotension

Hypotension (decrease in systolic blood pressure >20%) secondary to decreased systemic vascular resistance is the most common complication of neuraxial blockade for labor analgesia, with rates of approximately 14%.[63] Prophylactic measures include left uterine displacement and hydration. Although a standard for timing, amount, and hydration fluid remain controversial, all agree dehydration should be avoided. Prehydration with up to 1 L IV crystalloid does not appear to significantly decrease rates of hypotension from low-dose labor epidurals.[64] Treatment of hypotension consists of further uterine displacement, IV fluids, and vasopressor administration. Either phenylephrine or ephedrine can be used to treat hypotension (see "Anesthesia for Cesarean Delivery"). If treated promptly, transient maternal hypotension does not lead to fetal depression or neonatal morbidity.

Increased Core Temperature

A rise in core maternal body temperature and fever are associated with labor epidural analgesia. Although it was originally believed that all laboring women who had epidural analgesia gradually increased their core temperature, more current studies suggest that only about 20% of women who receive epidural labor analgesia develop a fever, and the remaining 80% have no increase in core body temperature.[65] Although the etiology of the maternal temperature rise remains uncertain, an association with noninfectious inflammation mediated by proinflammatory cytokines is supported most consistently in the literature. This rise in maternal temperature is not associated with a change in white blood cell count or an infectious process and is not reduced with prophylactic antibiotics, so treatment is not necessary.[66] In addition, the fever associated with epidural labor analgesia does not increase the incidence of neonatal sepsis and need not affect neonatal septic workup. Although some studies note no effect on fetal well-being, other studies suggest maternal temperatures greater than 38°C are associated with adverse neonatal outcomes, including seizures, hypotonia, and need for a period of assisted ventilation.[66,67]

ANESTHESIA FOR CESAREAN DELIVERY

The majority of cesarean deliveries are performed with neuraxial anesthesia. Use of regional anesthesia (1) avoids the risks of maternal aspiration and difficult airway associated with general anesthesia, (2) allows less anesthetic exposure to the neonate, (3) has the benefit of an awake mother, and (4) allows placement of neuraxial opioids to decrease postoperative pain. Sometimes the severity of the fetal condition and emergent nature of the situation (e.g., fetal bradycardia or uterine rupture) necessitate the use of general anesthesia for its rapidity and reliability. Other times, general anesthesia is required when regional anesthesia is contraindicated (e.g., coagulopathy or severe hemorrhage). In addition to its rapid and dependable onset, benefits of general anesthesia over regional include a secure airway, controlled ventilation, and potential for less hemodynamic instability. Current ASA guidelines[6] recommend the "timely administration of oral nonparticulate antacids, IV H2-receptor antagonists, and/or metoclopramide for aspiration prophylaxis" before the induction of anesthesia in pregnant women. In emergent situations, an oral nonparticulate antacid may be most appropriate.

Spinal Anesthesia

For a pregnant woman without an epidural catheter, spinal anesthesia is the most common regional anesthetic technique used for cesarean delivery. The block is rapid in onset, does not carry the risk of systemic drug toxicity because of the smaller dose, and is more reliable in providing surgical anesthesia from the midthoracic level to the sacrum compared with epidural anesthesia. The incidence of postdural puncture headache has become low (<5%) with the introduction of smaller diameter (≤25 gauge), noncutting, "pencil-point" spinal needles. Maternal hypotension is more likely and more profound with spinal anesthesia than with epidural anesthesia. Untreated maternal hypotension can result in fetal bradycardia and acidosis. A consensus statement regarding hypotension after spinal anesthesia for cesarean delivery recommends prophylactic infusion of an alpha agonist (i.e., phenylephrine initiated at 25 to 50 mcg/min), rapid crystalloid infusion with initiation of spinal anesthesia (co-loading), and left uterine displacement to reduce the incidence and severity of hypotension.[68] The recommendation is to maintain systolic blood pressure above 80% of baseline. Because maternal heart rate correlates significantly with cardiac output, ephedrine and/or glycopyrrolate should also be considered in cases of low maternal heart rate.[68] Administration of prophylactic norepinephrine has been demonstrated to have improved maternal heart rate and cardiac output compared with phenylephrine.[69] However, phenylephrine is currently recommended because of the amount of supporting data. Spinal anesthesia can be safely used for patients with preeclampsia. A typical spinal anesthetic could consist of bupivacaine (10 to 15 mg), with fentanyl (15 mcg) and preservative-free morphine (150 mcg) added to augment the spinal and decrease

IV

postoperative pain. A large variety of other combinations of local anesthetic and opioid doses are also used. A hyperbaric solution of local anesthetic is often used to facilitate anatomic and gravitational control of the block distribution. The medication will flow with the spinal curvature to a block position near T4. The duration of a single-shot spinal anesthetic is variable, but normally provides adequate surgical anesthesia for ≥90 minutes.

A continuous spinal anesthetic technique with intrathecal catheter placement is a rarely used alternative, sometimes chosen in cases of accidental dural puncture during attempted epidural catheter placement. This allows the advantage of a titratable, reliable, dense anesthetic, but carries the risks of high spinal if the intrathecal catheter is mistaken for an epidural catheter or the provider is unfamiliar with the technique. The rates of rare complications such as meningitis or neurologic impairment from local anesthetic toxicity with use of a spinal catheter may be somewhat higher than the other neuraxial techniques but remain unknown. Some data suggest that leaving the spinal catheter in place for 24 hours after delivery decreases the risk of postdural puncture headache.[70]

Epidural Anesthesia

Epidural anesthesia is an excellent choice for cesarean delivery when an indwelling, functioning epidural catheter has been placed for labor analgesia. It allows titration to the desired level of anesthesia and ability to extend the block time if needed. It is also ideal for patients who cannot tolerate the sudden onset of sympathectomy, such as some patients with severe cardiac disease. Some disadvantages include a slower onset compared with spinal anesthesia and a greater risk of maternal systemic drug toxicity. The volume and concentration of local anesthetic drugs used for surgical anesthesia are larger than those used for labor analgesia; however, the technique of catheter placement, test dosing, and potential complications are similar. A standard dosing regimen for epidural anesthesia for cesarean delivery could include approximately 15 to 20 mL of 2% lidocaine or 3% 2-chloroprocaine in divided doses. For urgent cesarean deliveries, 3% 2-chloroprocaine is often selected because it has the most rapid onset of any epidural local anesthetics. Compared with lidocaine, 2-chloroprocaine diminishes both the efficacy and duration of epidural morphine administered for postoperative analgesia.[71] Addition of epinephrine (1:200,000) or fentanyl (50 to 100 mcg) can enhance the intensity and duration of the block and increase the systemic toxicity threshold. Typically, the anesthesia provider attempts to provide sensory anesthesia to the T4 level. Epidural block failure rates for cesarean delivery after use of a labor epidural range between 1.7% and 19.8%.[72] Predictors of failure to convert a labor epidural to surgical anesthesia for cesarean delivery include neuraxial block placement by a nonspecialist obstetric anesthesiologist (odds ratio [OR] 4.6), an increased number of manual boluses during labor (OR 4.4), and the urgency of a cesarean delivery (OR 2.5).[73] In some cases conversion to general endotracheal anesthesia may be required. Epidural morphine (e.g., 2 mg) is typically administered near the end of the procedure to decrease postoperative pain for up to 24 hours.

Combined Spinal Epidural Anesthesia

In selected circumstances, use of a CSE technique offers the advantage of a spinal anesthetic with rapid, reliable onset of a dense block and the ability to administer additional local anesthetic through the epidural catheter. This allows titration of the block level or extension of the block duration if the surgical procedure lasts for a longer period.

General Anesthesia

General anesthesia is used in obstetric practice for cesarean delivery, typically when neuraxial anesthesia is contraindicated or for emergencies because of its rapid and predictable action. Based on data from 1997 to 2002, the relative risk of general anesthesia is 1.7 times that of neuraxial anesthesia.[74] Although the mortality associated with general anesthesia can be caused by intubation failure or induction problems, a large portion of this mortality is the result of airway obstruction and/or hypoventilation occurring on extubation, in the postanesthesia care unit, or in the postpartum ward.[74] Appropriate airway examination, preparation, and familiarity with techniques and an algorithm for the difficult airway are critical for providing a safe anesthetic (Fig. 33.6), in addition to appropriate postoperative monitoring. A multiinstitutional database of adverse obstetric anesthesia events indicates that current rates of failed intubation are approximately 1:533, although none of the 10 failed obstetric intubations resulted in maternal mortality.[58] The sequence of events for inducing general anesthesia for cesarean delivery are detailed in Box 33.1.

After administration of a nonparticulate antacid, preoxygenation, and confirmation of surgical readiness, a rapid-sequence induction is typically performed and a cuffed endotracheal tube placed. Surgical incision is made after confirmation of tracheal intubation and adequate ventilation. Anesthesia is maintained by administration of a combination of a halogenated agent and benzodiazepines, opioid analgesics, propofol, nitrous oxide, and additional muscle relaxant if needed. During typical general anesthesia for cesarean delivery, opioids and benzodiazepines are administered after the baby is delivered to avoid placental transfer of these agents to

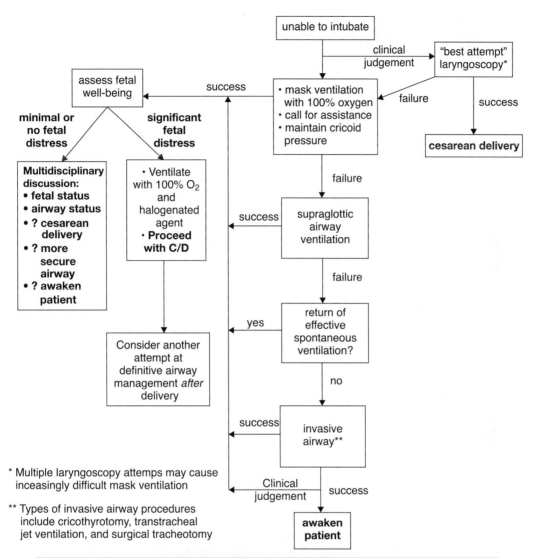

Fig. 33.6 Algorithm for Difficult Airway Management With Failed Intubation in Obstetrics. *C/D,* cesarean delivery. (Adapted from Hughes S, Levinson G, Rosen M. *Shnider and Levinson's Anesthesia for Obstetrics,* 4th ed. Lippincott, Williams & Wilkins Philadelphia, PA 2002.)

IV

the neonate. Before delivery of the baby, the primary anesthetic for the incision and delivery is the induction agent, as there is typically little time for significant uptake and distribution of the inhaled agents into either the mother or fetus. If intubation attempts fail, the cesarean delivery may proceed if the anesthesia provider can reliably ventilate the mother with either facemask or laryngeal mask airway[6] (see Fig. 33.6). Halogenated agents are often partially or completely replaced with other anesthetic agents (e.g., total intravenous anesthesia [TIVA] with propofol and opioids) after delivery to further reduce the risk of uterine atony.

Induction Drugs (also see Chapter 8)

A number of different drugs are used by anesthesia providers to rapidly induce general anesthesia. *Propofol* is a highly lipid-soluble drug with a rapid onset of action that renders the patient unconscious within approximately 30 seconds. Propofol is associated with decreased systemic arterial pressure after induction, especially when opioids are coadministered. Because it is preservative-free and lipid-based, propofol supports rapid microbial growth at room temperature and must be drawn up only hours before use. Propofol administration has no significant effect on neonatal behavior scores with induction doses

---

Box 33.1 General Anesthesia for Cesarean Section: A Suggested Technique

- Administer a nonparticulate oral antacid (sodium citrate) before induction of anesthesia
- Place standard monitors and maintain left uterine displacement
- Start an infusion of crystalloid solution through a large-bore intravenous catheter
- Preoxygenate for 3 minutes or four maximal breaths over 30 seconds
- After confirming surgeon is ready and patient prepped, an assistant should apply cricoid pressure and maintain it until the position of the endotracheal tube is verified*
- Administer induction agent and neuromuscular blocking agent in rapid sequence, wait 30 to 60 seconds, and then initiate direct laryngoscopy for tracheal intubation
- After confirming endotracheal tube placement, communicate to surgeon to begin incision
- Administer oxygen in air and a volatile anesthetic
- After delivery, anesthesia may be maintained by administering a combination of a halogenated agent and benzodiazepines, opioid analgesics, propofol, nitrous oxide and additional muscle relaxant as needed
- Extubate the trachea when the patient is fully awake and strong

*Not all agree that cricoid pressure is efficacious or required in every patient.

---

of 2.5 mg/kg, but larger doses (9 mg/kg) are associated with newborn depression.

Etomidate also has a rapid onset of action because of its high lipid solubility. Its rapid hydrolysis results in a relatively short duration of action. At typical induction doses (0.3 mg/kg), etomidate has minimal effects on the maternal cardiovascular system, making it an appropriate choice for patients with hemodynamic compromise. However, etomidate is painful on injection, can cause involuntary muscle tremors, has higher rates of nausea and vomiting (compared with propofol, which has antiemetic properties), and can increase the risk of seizures in patients with decreased thresholds. It also decreases neonatal cortisol production (typically <6 hours in duration), with uncertain clinical significance.

Ketamine produces a rapid onset of anesthesia, but unlike propofol, ketamine's sympathomimetic characteristics increase maternal arterial pressure, heart rate, and cardiac output through central stimulation of the sympathetic nervous system, making it also appropriate for patients with hemodynamic compromise. Doses greater than those typical for induction of general anesthesia (1 to 1.5 mg/kg) can lower seizure threshold and increase uterine tone, which reduces uterine arterial perfusion. In low doses (0.25 mg/kg), ketamine is a profound analgesic, but has been associated with undesirable psychomimetic side effects (bad dreams), which can be lessened by coadministration of benzodiazepines. Both ketamine and etomidate are considered appropriate for induction of anesthesia in a pregnant woman who is actively hemorrhaging, has uncertain blood volume, and is at risk for profound hypotension.

Neuromuscular Blocking Drugs and Reversal Agents (also see Chapter 11)

Succinylcholine (1 to 1.5 mg/kg IV) remains the neuromuscular blocking drug of choice for obstetric anesthesia because of its rapid onset (30 to 45 seconds) and short duration of action. Because it is highly ionized and poorly lipid soluble, only small amounts cross the placenta. It is normally hydrolyzed in maternal blood by the enzyme pseudocholinesterase and does not generally interfere with fetal neuromuscular activity. Although pseudocholinesterase activity is decreased in pregnancy, neuromuscular blockade by succinylcholine is not significantly prolonged. If large doses are administered (2 to 3 mg/kg), succinylcholine levels become detectable in umbilical cord blood; however, extremely high doses (10 mg/kg) are needed for the transfer to result in neonatal neuromuscular blockade. If the hydrolytic enzyme is present either in low concentration or in a genetically determined atypical form, prolonged maternal paralysis can occur, and the return of neuromuscular strength should always be verified before extubation or before additional nondepolarizing muscle relaxants are administered.

Rocuronium is an acceptable alternative to succinylcholine. It provides adequate intubating conditions in approximately 90 seconds at doses of 0.6 mg/kg and under 60 seconds at doses of 1.2 mg/kg. Unlike succinylcholine, it has a much longer duration of action, decreasing maternal safety in the event the anesthesia provider is unable to intubate or ventilate the patient. However, with a large intravenous dose of *sugammadex* (16 mg/kg), neuromuscular block with rocuronium can be rapidly reversed, and sugammadex is effective and safe to use at the conclusion of a cesarean delivery (typically 2 to 4 mg/kg).[75] The Society for Obstetric Anesthesia and Perinatology currently recommends avoidance in pregnant woman undergoing nonobstetric surgery, as sugammadex reduces unbound progesterone in pharmacologic studies and could theoretically affect the length of pregnancy.[76] Consequently, a standard reversal option is coadministration of *neostigmine* and *glycopyrrolate*. Glycopyrrolate is poorly transferred across the placenta, whereas neostigmine is more capable of crossing. Although this combination is frequently administered to pregnant women undergoing nonobstetric surgery for neuromuscular blockade reversal without adverse effect, there have been case reports of profound fetal bradycardia when glycopyrrolate and neostigmine were coadministered.[77] Consequently, it has been suggested that neostigmine be administered with atropine (which crosses the placenta) to pregnant women who require reversal of neuromuscular blockade. If administered after cesarean delivery, placental transfer is irrelevant.

Uterine smooth muscle is not affected by neuromuscular blockade. Under normal circumstances, nondepolarizing neuromuscular blockers do not cross the placenta in amounts significant enough to cause neonatal muscle weakness. However, when large doses are administered over long periods, neonatal neuromuscular blockade can occur. A paralyzed neonate will have normal cardiovascular function but no spontaneous ventilatory movements or reflex responses, and skeletal muscle flaccidity is present. Treatment consists of respiratory support until the neonate excretes the drug, which may take up to 48 hours. Antagonism of nondepolarizing neuromuscular blocking drugs with cholinesterase inhibitors may be attempted, but adequate respiratory support is the mainstay of treatment.

Maintenance of Anesthesia

Maintenance of anesthesia for cesarean delivery often includes the inhalation of a low concentration (<0.75 MAC) of halogenated anesthetic in addition to other agents (e.g., propofol), with opioids administered after the baby is delivered to avoid the concern of placental transfer to the neonate. Placental transfer of volatile anesthetics is rapid because they are nonionized, highly lipid-soluble substances of low molecular weight. Fetal concentrations depend on the concentration and duration of anesthetic administered to the mother. In 2016 the FDA published a warning that "repeated or lengthy use of general anesthetic and sedation drugs during surgeries or procedures in children younger than three years or in pregnant women during the third trimester may affect the development of children's brains."[30] This warning comes from concern that administration of drugs that bind to gamma-aminobutyric acid (GABA) or NMDA receptors could result in long-term effects on children's learning and behavior. No specific anesthetic agent (e.g., halogenated anesthetics, propofol, ketamine) is known to be safer than another, and there is no association known between use of general anesthesia for urgent cesarean delivery and neurocognitive disability later in life[78] (also see Chapter 12).

The impact of general anesthesia on neonatal outcome, especially in the presence of fetal distress, has been studied for many years. A depressed fetus is likely to be associated with a depressed neonate, and general anesthesia is selected because it is the most rapidly acting and reliable anesthetic technique to allow cesarean delivery. A Cochrane review of 16 studies comparing neuraxial blockade with general anesthesia in otherwise uncomplicated cesarean deliveries found that "no significant difference was seen in terms of neonatal Apgar scores of 6 or less and of 4 or less at one and five minutes and need for neonatal resuscitation."[79] The authors concluded that there was no evidence to show that neuraxial anesthesia

was superior to general anesthesia for neonatal outcome. The induction to delivery interval is not as important to neonatal outcome as the interval from uterine incision to delivery, when UBF may be compromised and fetal asphyxia may occur. A prolonged time from induction to delivery may result in a lightly anesthetized neonate but not an asphyxiated neonate. If excessive concentrations of volatile anesthetics are administered for extended periods, neonatal effects of these drugs, as evidenced by flaccidity, respiratory depression, and decreased tone, may be anticipated. Importantly, if neonatal depression is caused by the transfer of anesthetic drugs, the infant is merely anesthetized and should respond to simple treatment measures such as assisted ventilation of the lungs until the anesthetic is eliminated. Rapid improvement of the infant should be expected. If this does not occur, other causes of neonatal depression should be investigated. For these reasons, it is critical that clinicians experienced with neonatal ventilation are present at cesarean deliveries under general anesthesia. A discussion of the operative and anesthetic plan by the neonatologist, obstetrician, and anesthesia provider is crucial for optimizing the outcome of neonates in these situations.

ABNORMAL PRESENTATIONS AND MULTIPLE BIRTHS

Multiple Gestations

Around 3% of live births in the United States are from multiple gestation pregnancy, with 97% of these being twins. Multiple gestation pregnancies carry increased risks of preterm labor, hypertensive disorders of pregnancy, gestational diabetes, hyperemesis gravidarum, anemia, preterm premature rupture of membranes, intrauterine growth restriction, and intrauterine fetal demise. Approximately 50% of twin pregnancies result in preterm birth with threefold greater perinatal mortality than singleton pregnancies.[80] The cesarean delivery rate for multiple gestation pregnancies is approximately 75%. Compared with planned vaginal delivery, a planned cesarean delivery does not decrease the risk of fetal or neonatal death.[81] In most twin pregnancies, both fetuses are in the vertex (head down) position, although vaginal delivery can still be attempted when the second twin is breech. A discussion with the obstetrician and planning for a possible "breech extraction" is beneficial for all attempted twin vaginal deliveries regardless of positioning of each fetus. Additionally, an emergent cesarean delivery may be required if the second twin changes position after the first twin is delivered or if the second twin develops fetal bradycardia. Epidural placement should be strongly considered for women with twin gestation attempting vaginal delivery. Presence of an epidural catheter can facilitate delivery and extraction

IV

of the second twin. When the second twin is breech, epidural analgesia allows optimal analgesia and relaxation of the perineum during delivery of the head or if instrumented vaginal delivery is required to deliver the second twin. Administration of agents that provide rapid uterine relaxation (e.g., IV nitroglycerin) may be required to improve delivery conditions for the second twin and reduce the risk of head entrapment. Administration of a small volume of a more concentrated local anesthetic near delivery can optimize analgesia and potentially allow for rapid transition to neuraxial anesthesia for cesarean delivery in the event of head entrapment and/or fetal bradycardia.

Abnormal Presentations

Breech Presentation

Singleton breech presentation at term is uncommon (3% to 4%). However, the majority of women with breech presentation have a planned cesarean delivery. Although breech vaginal delivery is possible, few centers in the United States offer singleton vaginal breech delivery. In addition, current evidence demonstrates possible short-term benefits in neonatal and maternal morbidity from a planned cesarean delivery of a breech term fetus, although long-term benefits remain uncertain.[82] As a result, obstetric guidelines are flexible with regard to vaginal breech delivery recommendations depending on patient desires and the obstetrician's level of experience. Women should undergo pelvimetry, an ultrasound to determine fetal weight, and counseling by the obstetrician to review the risks of the procedure. Women attempting vaginal breech delivery should be encouraged to have an epidural placed during labor, as the anesthetic management and risks are similar to breech extraction of the second twin discussed earlier.

External cephalic version (ECV) is a procedure that involves rotating the fetus into a cephalic position via external palpation and pressure of the fetal parts. Ultrasound and fetal heart rate monitoring can help assess fetal distress during ECV. ECV has been shown to decrease the cesarean delivery rate.[82] Terbutaline is a tocolytic that facilitates uterine relaxation and nearly doubles success rates for ECV.[83] In a meta-analysis of 18 RCTs, ECV under neuraxial anesthesia had significantly higher odds of decreased pain, improved satisfaction, and successful fetal version compared with control (OR = 2.59).[84] Although neuraxial anesthesia is more likely to cause hypotension, the rates of nonreassuring fetal response and emergent cesarean delivery are not increased. Risks of ECV include placental abruption, fetal bradycardia, and rupture of membranes. Although these risks are low, ECV should be performed in a facility where cesarean delivery can occur and an anesthesia provider is immediately available in case an urgent or emergent cesarean delivery is needed.

Shoulder Dystocia

A shoulder dystocia is an obstetric emergency that occurs in up to 3% of vaginal deliveries. Diagnosis is made when expulsion of the infant after delivery of the fetal head is obstructed by the fetal shoulders within the maternal pelvis. Risk factors include macrosomia, maternal diabetes, history of dystocia, and instrumented delivery. The risks of postpartum hemorrhage (PPH) and fourth-degree laceration are increased for deliveries complicated by shoulder dystocia. Upon diagnosis of shoulder dystocia, the obstetrician performs a set of maneuvers to deliver the infant. Cases of shoulder dystocia occurring for 7 minutes or longer have a significant increased risk of neonatal brain injury. The final maneuver (Zavanelli maneuver) in a failed delivery because of shoulder dystocia requires pushing the fetal head back into the pelvis and proceeding with emergent cesarean delivery. Fetal injuries and sequelae of shoulder dystocia are brachial plexus injury (Erb palsy), neurologic injury from asphyxia, and fractured clavicle or humerus. These neurologic injuries typically improve over time with roughly less than 10% resulting in permanent Erb palsy. The average perinatal mortality rate is estimated at 0.4% to 0.5% for deliveries complicated by shoulder dystocia.[85]

HYPERTENSIVE DISORDERS OF PREGNANCY

The clinical spectrum of hypertensive diseases during pregnancy has a significant impact on maternal and neonatal mortality and morbidity. Hypertensive disorders in pregnancy are classified into four types: (1) preeclampsia-eclampsia, (2) chronic hypertension, (3) chronic hypertension with superimposed preeclampsia, and (4) gestational hypertension. *Gestational hypertension* is new-onset elevated blood pressure occurring after 20 weeks' gestation, most often near term and with the etiology unclear but with the need for increased surveillance during pregnancy. If the elevated blood pressure persists through 12 weeks postpartum, the woman is considered to have *chronic hypertension. Chronic hypertension* is elevated blood pressures predating pregnancy or occurring before 20 weeks' gestation. These women are at higher risk for developing superimposed preeclampsia.

Preeclampsia

Preeclampsia is a pregnancy-specific progressive disorder with multiorgan system involvement that affects 3% to 5% of all pregnancies.[86] The greatest risk factors for developing preeclampsia include a history of preeclampsia and chronic hypertension. Other risk factors include nulliparity, multigestation pregnancy, pregestational diabetes, systemic lupus erythematosus or antiphospholipid antibody syndrome, renal disease, body mass index greater than 30 kg/m^2, maternal age <17 or >35 years, and use of assisted reproductive therapy. Diagnostic criteria are detailed in Boxes 33.2 and 33.3, which define preeclampsia into two distinct categories: (1) preeclampsia and (2) preeclampsia with severe features. A subcategory of severe preeclampsia is *HELLP syndrome*, which is a constellation of *h*emolysis, *e*levated *l*iver enzymes, and *l*ow *p*latelet count. *Eclamptic seizures* develop in less than 2% of patients with preeclampsia and less than

4% of patients with preeclampsia and severe features.[87] Eclamptic seizures may take place before, during, or after labor and delivery. Although symptoms of headache and visual disturbances frequently occur before eclampsia, one in five patients with eclampsia report no symptoms before the seizure.[88] Interestingly, many women (20% to 38%) do not have typical signs of preeclampsia (hypertension or proteinuria) before the seizure episode.[87] Several mechanisms have been proposed in the development of preeclampsia, including chronic ischemia of the uteroplacental unit, maternal immune reactions, genetic factors, increased trophoblast apoptosis, and angiogenic factor imbalances.[87] Pathophysiology may include failure of spiral artery remodeling, which creates decreased placental perfusion, and subsequent placental hypoxia and oxidative stress.[86] Ultimately this damages placental villi and increases maternal angiogenic protein levels.

Definitive treatment of preeclampsia is with delivery. The timing of delivery versus expectant management is based on disease severity and gestational age.[87] In patients with stable preeclampsia without severe features, the pregnancy is typically monitored until 37 weeks' gestation. Delivery is recommended if severe features develop after 34 weeks' gestation. Before 34 weeks' gestation, expectant management may be considered with stable maternal and fetal condition, including controlled maternal blood pressure. Administration of corticosteroids is recommended to assist with fetal lung maturity if delivery before 34 weeks' gestation is anticipated. It is critical for the anesthesia provider to be aware of these patients and their clinical course, as they can rapidly deteriorate and require urgent or emergent delivery. Hypertensive disorders of pregnancy are associated with long-term biologic changes that confer a significantly increased future risk of cardiovascular disease, including stroke and hypertension later in life.[87,89]

Intrapartum Management

Invasive monitoring is not typically required, and central venous access may increase risk without clear benefit. However, in cases of preeclampsia with severe hypertension refractory to primary antihypertensive therapies, an invasive pressure line and/or central venous catheter may be beneficial. Judicious volume expansion before initiation of neuraxial blockade is generally supported, as patients with preeclampsia have low plasma oncotic pressure yet are prone to fluid overload, with potential for pulmonary complications.

Magnesium

Administration of magnesium sulfate to patients with preeclampsia decreases eclampsia rates by more than half and reduces the risk of placental abruption.[90] The risk of eclamptic seizures in patients with severe features is fourfold greater than in patients without severe features. Guidelines recommend magnesium sulfate for prevention of seizures in women with gestational hypertension with

IV

severe features and preeclampsia with severe features or eclampsia.[87] However, these guidelines do not recommend routine magnesium prophylaxis for patients with gestational hypertension or preeclampsia *without* severe features.[87,91] Magnesium can significantly increase the efficacy and duration of both depolarizing and non-depolarizing muscle relaxants. Magnesium sulfate also increases uterine and smooth muscle relaxation.

Magnesium sulfate is typically administered via a 4- to 6-gram IV loading dose over 20 to 30 minutes, followed by a continuous infusion of 1 g/hr until 12 to 24 hours after delivery. For women who require cesarean delivery before the onset of labor, the magnesium infusion should ideally begin before surgery and continue during surgery and for 24 hours after delivery.[87] For women who deliver vaginally, the infusion should also continue for 24 hours after delivery. The therapeutic range is 6 to 8 mg/dL for seizure prophylaxis. Magnesium toxicity can be evaluated by deep tendon reflexes, respiratory assessment, and neurologic status. At magnesium levels of 10 mg/dL, loss of deep tendon reflexes occurs; electrocardiogram (ECG) findings include prolonged P-R interval and widened QRS. Respiratory arrest occurs at magnesium levels of 15 to 20 mg/dL, with asystole occurring at levels greater than 20 to 25 mg/dL. Although half of the dietary intake of magnesium is absorbed in the intestine, regulation of serum magnesium is managed primarily by the kidney. Patients with oliguria and worsening renal function can rapidly develop magnesium toxicity. In addition to monitoring for signs of toxicity, determination of magnesium levels in patients with renal dysfunction should be considered.[87] If toxicity develops, IV calcium chloride (500 mg) or calcium gluconate (1 g) (which act as magnesium antagonists) should be administered, in addition to IV furosemide to promote urinary excretion of magnesium.

Antihypertensives

Current guidelines recommend expeditiously treating severe hypertension for prevention of heart failure or myocardial ischemia, renal injury, and/or intracerebral hemorrhage/ischemia.[92] Antihypertensive treatment should be started expeditiously for patients with *acute severe hypertension* (systolic blood pressure ≥160 mm Hg or diastolic blood pressure ≥110 mm Hg). First-line agents include IV labetalol or hydralazine and oral nifedipine. If blood pressure remains unresponsive, infusions of rapid-acting vasoactive medications (e.g., nicardipine) with placement of invasive arterial monitoring may be necessary.[87] Maternal blood pressure and fetal heart rate must be monitored closely during initiation of antihypertensive therapy. The therapeutic blood pressure goal is only 10% to 20% below the severe thresholds described earlier (i.e., goal blood pressure approximately 130/85) in order to maintain appropriate uteroplacental perfusion and prevent fetal compromise.

Neuraxial Analgesia Considerations

The ACOG considers neuraxial analgesia the preferred analgesic method for labor or cesarean delivery in patients with preeclampsia.[87] However, care to maintain appropriate maternal blood pressure and cardiac output is needed to prevent a reduction in uteroplacental perfusion pressure (see "Complications of Neuraxial Anesthesia"). Neuraxial analgesia offers the advantage of avoiding general anesthesia for urgent or emergent cesarean delivery in the setting of increased airway edema and risk for stroke with sympathetic response to direct laryngoscopy. For women with preeclampsia, a thorough evaluation of the patient's current status should be performed, including hemoglobin and platelet levels, before placement of any neuraxial block, given the potential for thrombocytopenia. A 2021 consensus statement from the Society for Obstetric Anesthesia and Perinatology addressed the use of neuraxial procedures in obstetric patients with thrombocytopenia. The statement concluded that the risk of epidural hematoma from neuraxial anesthesia with a platelet count ≥70 × 10⁹/L is likely to be very low, assuming no additional contraindications to neuraxial anesthesia exist.[53] Additionally, this consensus statement recommends evaluating a coagulation panel in the setting of preeclampsia and a platelet count less than 100×10^9/L. Regardless, the decision to place a neuraxial block should be based on a frank discussion with the patient of risk versus benefit, in addition to other anesthetic and analgesic alternatives. If an epidural is placed in a patient with thrombocytopenia, caution should be taken before epidural catheter removal, as platelet levels often decrease further after delivery. Bleeding time has no demonstrated value in this clinical context.

The anesthesia provider must be prepared for urgent delivery, given the potential for placental insufficiency with preeclampsia. Exaggerated upper airway edema is frequent in patients with preeclampsia, which increases the risk of difficult intubation if an emergent general anesthetic is required. Tracheal intubation may produce further hypertension during laryngoscopy; a small dose of nitroglycerine (2.0 mcg/kg) or esmolol (1.5 mg/kg) can attenuate this response when administered with propofol for induction.[93] If there is concern for a difficult airway, appropriate alternatives such as video laryngoscopy with the initial intubation attempt should be considered (also see Chapter 16). Postpartum uterine atony is common with magnesium sulfate infusion and is accentuated if inhaled anesthetic is used for maintenance of general anesthesia. Pitocin and prostaglandins are safe for uterine atony, but methylergonovine (Methergine) is contraindicated, as it can precipitate hypertensive crisis.

HEMORRHAGE IN PREGNANT WOMEN

Hemorrhage in pregnant women remains a significant cause of maternal mortality. Placenta previa, abruptio placentae, and uterine rupture are the major causes of bleeding and uncontrolled hemorrhage during the third trimester and labor. PPH occurs in approximately 3% of deliveries in the United States and is most commonly the result of uterine atony. Common problems identified with obstetric hemorrhages leading to significant morbidity and mortality include (1) poor quantification of blood loss, (2) unrecognized associated risk factors for hemorrhage, (3) delayed initiation of treatment, and (4) inadequate readiness and resources including insufficient transfusion of appropriate blood products in a massive hemorrhage situation.[94]

Placenta Previa

Placenta previa results from an abnormal uterine implantation of the placenta in front of the presenting fetus. The incidence is approximately 1 in 200 pregnancies. Risk factors include advanced age, multiparity, assisted reproductive techniques, prior hysterotomy, and prior placenta previa. Historically, the classic presentation of placenta previa is painless vaginal bleeding that occurs preterm in the third trimester. Most previas are now diagnosed antenatally by ultrasonography. A trial of labor is acceptable if the placental edge is farther than 2 cm from the internal os, but cesarean delivery is required if the placenta is within 1 cm of the cervical os.[95] For patients whose placentas lie between 1 and 2 cm from the cervical os or who have a shortened cervix or thickened placental edge, the optimal management remains uncertain, and delivery management is individualized based on current circumstances.[95] Neuraxial anesthesia is an appropriate choice if there is no active bleeding or hypovolemia. The use of two large-bore IV lines with fluid warmers and availability of invasive monitoring is suggested with cesarean delivery, given the increased risk of placenta accreta with known previa (see "Placenta Accreta Spectrum" below).

Massive Hemorrhage

For emergency situations with active hemorrhage, general anesthesia may be required. Ketamine (1 to 1.5 mg/kg IV) or etomidate (0.3 mg/kg) are useful drugs for induction of anesthesia. If a massive hemorrhage occurs, activation of a massive transfusion protocol with availability of fresh frozen plasma, platelets, and fibrinogen in addition to packed red blood cells may be needed for transfusion in ratios similar to a trauma resuscitation, as a dilutional coagulopathy can result in such a situation[96] (also see Chapter 43). In these cases of uncontrolled rapid hemorrhage, point-of-care testing can significantly assist in determining appropriate transfusion components. However, there may be situations of massive hemorrhage when there is not time to wait for the return of laboratory studies, and transfusion of appropriate blood products should be based on clinical judgement, with adjustments as laboratory information

becomes available. Use of tranexamic acid (1 to 2 g) in PPH reduces the risk of death from exsanguination, with the most treatment benefit if it is administered within 3 hours of delivery.[97] Neonates delivered from pregnant women in hemorrhagic shock are likely to be acidotic and hypovolemic and may need resuscitation. If hemorrhage is not controlled with standard measures, the obstetric team can consider (1) uterine artery ligation, (2) B-Lynch sutures, (3) an intrauterine balloon or vaccum device, (4) use of arterial embolization by interventional radiology (if the patient is stable for transport), or (5) hysterectomy.

Abruptio Placentae

Placental abruption is separation of the placenta after 20 weeks of gestation but before delivery. The incidence is approximately 0.4 to 1 in 100 pregnancies. Risk factors include advanced age, hypertension, trauma, smoking, cocaine use, chorioamnionitis, premature rupture of membranes, previa, and history of prior abruption. Placental abruption is associated with a greater risk of perinatal mortality; maternal mortality; and maternal morbidity, including hemorrhage, coagulopathy, thromboembolism, and acute kidney injury.[98] When the separation involves only the placental margin, the escaping blood can appear as vaginal bleeding often associated with uterine tenderness. Alternatively, large volumes of blood loss (>2 L) can remain entirely concealed in the uterus. Chronic bleeding and clotting between the uterus and placenta can cause maternal disseminated intravascular coagulopathy (DIC). Ultrasound is specific if abruption is noted, but has poor sensitivity, and a normal examination does not exclude abruption. Definitive treatment of abruptio placentae is to deliver the pregnancy. The anesthetic plan is based on both the delivery urgency and the abruption severity. Epidural analgesia can be used for labor and vaginal delivery if there are no signs of maternal hypovolemia, active bleeding, clotting abnormalities, or fetal distress. However, severe blood loss necessitates emergency cesarean delivery and the use of a general anesthetic similar to that described for massive hemorrhage. It is predictable that neonates born under these circumstances will be acidotic and hypovolemic.

Uterine Rupture

Uterine rupture is poorly defined and includes cases ranging from scar dehiscence to those with catastrophic uterine wall rupture. In addition to prior uterine scar, uterine rupture is associated with rapid spontaneous delivery, motor vehicle trauma, trauma from instrumented vaginal delivery, large or malpositioned fetus, and excessive oxytocin stimulation. After a single prior cesarean delivery with a low transverse incision, a trial of labor after cesarean (TOLAC) is associated with a ≤1% incidence of uterine rupture.[99] Spontaneous rupture of an

IV

unscarred uterus is far more rare. The clinical presentation is variable with no finding being 100% sensitive. Signs and symptoms may include fetal bradycardia, persistent abdominal pain, vaginal bleeding, cessation of contractions, loss of station, maternal hypotension, and breakthrough pain with epidural analgesia.[100] Persistent abdominal pain is not always a diagnostic finding but has a high correlation, and an abnormal FHR pattern is often the first and most common sign associated with uterine rupture. Neuraxial labor analgesia may be used as part of TOLAC and should not be expected to mask signs and symptoms of uterine rupture. Immediate evaluation, aggressive resuscitation, and general anesthesia for emergent cesarean delivery are normally required for management. Often uterine repair by the obstetrician can occur after an emergent cesarean delivery if a minor scar dehiscence is present, but hysterectomy is needed for most cases of uterine wall rupture of an unscarred uterus. When vaginal birth is planned after a previous cesarean delivery, it is recommended that "TOLAC be attempted in facilities that can provide cesarean delivery for situations that are immediate threats to the life of the woman or fetus"[99] should a uterine rupture occur. Appropriate staffing considerations include obstetric, anesthesia, pediatric, and nursing personnel.

Retained Placenta

Retained placenta, which occurs in about 2% to 3% of all vaginal deliveries, usually necessitates manual exploration of the uterus. If epidural analgesia was not used for vaginal delivery, manual removal of the placenta may be initially attempted with analgesia provided by IV administration of opioids. If uterine relaxation is necessary for placenta removal, boluses of IV nitroglycerin (200 mcg) are normally effective but have not been shown to reduce the need for manual uterine extraction. Additionally, relocation to the operating room and placement of neuraxial analgesia may be beneficial for thorough evaluation. Rarely, induction of general anesthesia with tracheal intubation and administration of a volatile anesthetic to provide uterine relaxation and anesthesia will be necessary. An effort to obtain accurate blood loss is critical in determining an appropriate anesthetic and resuscitation plan, as retained placenta is significantly associated with an increased risk of PPH and need for transfusion.

Uterine Atony

Uterine atony is a common cause of PPH and can occur immediately after delivery or several hours later. Risk factors for postpartum uterine atony include retained products, long labor, high parity, macrosomia, polyhydramnios, excessive oxytocin augmentation, and chorioamnionitis. Active management of the third stage using oxytocin administration, uterine massage, and umbilical cord traction are recommended to reduce PPH risk without increasing the risk of retained placenta.[101] The amount of oxytocin used to prevent PPH is highly variable and includes continuous infusions of 20 to 40 IU diluted in up to 1 L of crystalloid administered after delivery as a "wide open" IV infusion in addition to protocols using algorithms that bolus 3 IU at a time in an effort to reduce the overall oxytocin dose required to prevent PPH. No differences in the uterine tone, maternal hemodynamics, side effects, or blood loss were observed between these different methods of oxytocin dosing.[102] Whereas a dilute solution of oxytocin typically exerts minimal cardiovascular effects, rapid IV injection of even 3 to 5 IU is associated with tachycardia, vasodilation, and hypotension and should be administered over 30 seconds or more.[102]

Periodic communication between anesthesia providers and the obstetric team is key in reducing PPH by progressing rapidly to additional types of uterotonics if oxytocin is not effective. Methylergonovine (0.2 mg IM) is an ergot derivative administered to improve uterine tone. Because of the significant vasoconstriction, it is relatively contraindicated in patients with preeclampsia and patients with pulmonary hypertension or ischemic cardiac disease. The prostaglandin $F_{2\alpha}$ (0.25 mg IM) is another uterotonic used to treat refractory atony. It is associated with nausea, tachycardia, pulmonary hypertension, desaturation, and bronchospasm. It should be avoided in patients with asthma and pulmonary hypertension. Prostaglandin E_1 or misoprostol (600 mcg oral/sublingual/rectal) can also be effective in treating atony. It has no significant cardiac effects, but may cause hyperthermia. If PPH is not controlled with these initial methods, more invasive techniques and blood product transfusion will be urgently needed, as described earlier in "Massive Hemorrhage."

Placenta Accreta Spectrum

Placenta accreta spectrum (PAS) refers to the range of pathologic adherence and growth of the placenta into the uterine wall. Placental implantation beyond the endometrium gives rise to (1) *placenta accreta vera,* which is implantation and adherence onto the myometrium; (2) *placenta increta,* which is implantation into the myometrium; and (3) *placenta percreta,* which is penetration through the full thickness of the myometrium (Fig. 33.7). With placenta percreta, implantations may occur onto bowel, bladder, ovaries, or other pelvic organs and vessels. PAS can produce a markedly adherent placenta that cannot be removed without tearing the myometrium and producing a life-threatening severe hemorrhage.

The incidence of PAS is between 0.8 and 3.1 per 1000 pregnancies, and it is the most common cause of peripartum hysterectomy in the United States.[103] Ultrasonography diagnosis of placenta accreta has a positive predictive value of only 68% and a diagnostic sensitivity of 55%, with a negative predictive value of 98% and

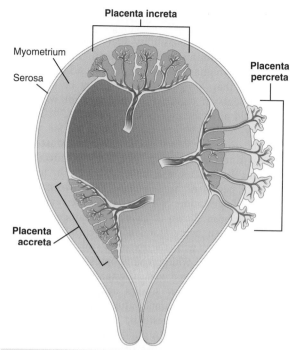

Fig. 33.7 Classification of Placenta Accreta Spectrum Based on the Degree of Penetration of Myometrium. (From Kamani AAS, Gambling DR, Chritlaw J, et al. Anesthetic management of patients with placenta accreta. *Can J Anaesth.* 1987;34:613-617, with permission.)

specificity of 88%.[104] Consequently, anesthetic management should not be exclusively guided by antepartum ultrasound results. These abnormal placental implantations occur more frequently in association with placenta previa. In patients with placenta previa and no previous cesarean delivery, the incidence of accreta is approximately 3%. However, the risk of PAS associated with placenta previa increases with the number of previous cesarean deliveries. With one previous uterine incision, the incidence of placenta accreta has been reported to be 11%; with two previous uterine incisions, the rate is 40%; and with three or more prior uterine incisions, the incidence rises to above 60%.[105]

In patients with PAS, massive and rapid intraoperative blood loss is common, with reported median blood loss ranging from 2000 to 5000 mL, and in some, substantially more. Coagulopathies develop in approximately 20% of these patients, and a significant portion require hysterectomies. Placenta accreta is not reliably diagnosed until the uterus is open. The anesthesia provider must keep this possibility in mind and be prepared to treat sudden massive blood loss. Choice of anesthesia technique (neuraxial, general, or neuraxial with conversion to general) may often be individualized and determined by patient comorbidities, degree and certainty of PAS, specific patient preferences, resource availability,

and provider familiarity and preference.[106] For patients with a preoperative diagnosis of PAS or high suspicion, preparations for massive hemorrhage are needed as noted earlier (e.g., large-bore IV access, invasive monitoring, blood products readily available). Use of intraoperative cell salvage and tranexamic acid administration should be considered for intraoperative management of PAS.[106]

AMNIOTIC FLUID EMBOLISM

The incidence of amniotic fluid embolism (AFE) is currently estimated between 1 and 6 cases per 100,000 deliveries.[58,107] Clinical features of AFE include the sudden onset of maternal hypotension, respiratory distress, altered mental status, DIC, cardiopulmonary arrest, and absence of fever.[108] AFE typically occurs during labor or within 30 minutes of delivery of the placenta. In rare instances, AFE may occur during the first or second trimester of pregnancy, at the time of pregnancy termination, or amniocentesis.[109] The exact cause and pathogenesis of AFE remain uncertain, but it is believed to be a type of hypersensitivity reaction with activation of proinflammatory mediators to some component of the amniotic fluid.

The diagnosis of AFE remains a clinical diagnosis of exclusion. Although aspirating amniotic fluid debris such as fetal squamous cells from the maternal pulmonary circulation was once considered diagnostic, it is now well established that fetal cells are present in the circulation of all pregnant women. There is no specific diagnostic laboratory or postmortem finding to either confirm or refute the diagnosis of AFE.[109,110] Conditions that mimic AFE include venous air embolism, pulmonary thromboembolism, acute hemorrhage (i.e., uterine rupture, atony, abruption, accreta), peripartum cardiomyopathy, sepsis, anaphylaxis, local anesthetic toxicity, high spinal, and aspiration of gastric contents. AFE should be considered in the differential diagnosis of any sudden cardiorespiratory collapse of a laboring or recently delivered patient, while working to rule out other pathologies. Point-of-care echocardiography is a valuable aid in both diagnosis and management of any patient having acute cardiovascular collapse (also see Chapter 21). Patients with AFE can have echocardiography findings of right ventricular failure, including a D-shaped septum, acute pulmonary hypertension, and right ventricular systolic dysfunction.[111]

Treatment of AFE is supportive and directed toward cardiopulmonary resuscitation with multidisciplinary care, inotropic support, determination of clotting status, possible transfusion, and correction of hypoxemia or postpartum uterine atony. Rapid onset of coagulopathy may occur, resulting in life-threatening hemorrhage. Tracheal intubation and mechanical ventilation are almost always required.[109,110]

IV

ANESTHESIA FOR NONOBSTETRIC SURGERY DURING PREGNANCY

The overall incidence of nonobstetric surgery during pregnancy is 1% to 2%, with trauma, appendicitis, cholecystitis, and malignancy being the most frequent indications.[112] In addition to management of hemodynamics and ventilation, taking into account the physiologic changes of pregnancy, anesthesia management objectives for pregnant women undergoing nonobstetric surgery include prevention of intrauterine fetal hypoxia and acidosis. Early in pregnancy, concerns include risk for spontaneous abortion with surgical procedures; later in pregnancy, concerns include premature labor associated with surgery. Elective procedures should always be delayed until after pregnancy. If surgery is required, the second trimester is often preferred. Regardless of trimester, a pregnant woman should never be denied an indicated surgical procedure or have that surgery delayed because this can adversely affect the health of the pregnant woman and fetus.[113] A retrospective cohort study of women who had nonobstetric general surgery during pregnancy and a matched cohort of women who were not pregnant noted that there were more emergency operations in the pregnant patient group, but found no difference in rates of mortality or morbidity.[114] Laparoscopic surgery is considered as safe as open approaches during any trimester, and the indications for its use are the same as nonpregnant patients. Most investigations comparing laparoscopic with open techniques note no significant difference in fetal or maternal outcomes. If a laparoscopic technique is used, in addition to considerations discussed later, low pneumoperitoneum pressures (10 to 15 mm Hg) should be used if feasible.

For operations during pregnancy, the anesthesia provider should (1) determine an anesthetic plan that optimizes the maternal and fetal condition; (2) consult an obstetrician and perinatologist in order to optimize plans for unexpected events; (3) determine a plan for fetal monitoring, if appropriate; and (4) discuss a plan in the event of a cesarean delivery or maternal arrest. When nonobstetric surgery is planned, the "surgery should be done at an institution with neonatal and pediatric services; an obstetric care provider with cesarean delivery privileges should be readily available; and a qualified individual should be readily available to interpret fetal heart rate patterns."[113] There is no evidence that a regional anesthetic technique is better than using general anesthesia for nonobstetric surgery during pregnancy, and there is some retrospective evidence that use of regional techniques for abdominal surgery may result in higher rates of preterm labor compared with general anesthesia.[115] Regional techniques should only be chosen over general anesthesia when typically used for a given surgery.

Avoidance of Teratogenic Drugs

There is always the possibility that anesthesia will be unknowingly administered to women with an early undiagnosed pregnancy. For this reason, ASA guidelines recommend that "pregnancy testing may be offered to female patients of childbearing age and for whom the result would alter the patient's management."[116] Routine pregnancy testing before elective surgery for women of childbearing age remains controversial. Most drugs, including anesthetics, have been demonstrated to be teratogenic in at least one animal species. In humans, the critical period of organogenesis is between 15 and 56 days of gestation. No currently used anesthetic agents have been shown to have any teratogenic effects in humans when using standard concentrations at any gestational age,[113] with the exception of cocaine. Neurodegeneration and widespread apoptosis after exposure to anesthetics has been clearly established in developing animals, and a few studies demonstrate cognitive impairment in adult animals after neonatal anesthetic exposure. No specific anesthetic agent is known to be safer than another. The FDA published a warning in 2016 that "repeated or lengthy use of general anesthetic and sedation drugs during surgeries or procedures in children younger than three years or in pregnant women during the third trimester may affect the development of children's brains."[117] This warning is based on concern that anesthetic or sedative drugs that bind to GABA or NMDA receptors could result in long-term effects on children's learning and behavior. Despite this warning, "there is no evidence that in utero human exposure to anesthetic or sedative drugs has any effect on the developing fetal brain"[113] (also see Chapter 12).

Avoidance of Intrauterine Fetal Hypoxia and Acidosis

Avoidance of decreased UBF and oxygenation is critical to fetal well-being, as both hypercapnia and hypocapnia result in reduced UBF and fetal acidosis. The development of intrauterine fetal hypoxia and acidosis is minimized by avoiding maternal hypotension with left uterine displacement after mid-gestation and by preventing arterial hypoxemia and excessive changes in $Paco_2$. High maternal inspired concentrations of oxygen do not increase the risk for in utero retrolental fibroplasia (retinopathy) because the oxygen consumption of the placenta plus the distribution of maternal and fetal blood flow in the placenta prevent fetal Pao_2 from exceeding 60 mm Hg, even if maternal Pao_2 exceeds 500 mm Hg.[13]

FHR monitoring via Doppler is possible at 16 to 18 weeks gestational age, but the utility of FHR variability as a marker of well-being is not established until 25 to 27 weeks of gestation. If the fetus is considered previable, preprocedure and postprocedure FHR assessment is generally considered sufficient. Regardless of fetal viability, ACOG and ASA state that the "decision to use fetal monitoring should be individualized and, if used, should be based on gestational age, type of surgery, and facilities available."[113] The greatest value of fetal monitoring is that by displaying fetal compromise, it allows further optimization of the maternal and fetal condition. Currently there is no evidence for the efficacy of FHR monitoring. In addition, interpretation is difficult because placement and signal acquisition may be challenging, a trained person is needed for FHR interpretation, and most anesthetics reduce FHR variability.

Prevention of Preterm Labor

The underlying pathology requiring surgery, and not the anesthetic technique, has been associated with an increased risk for preterm delivery. Intraabdominal procedures have a greater risk than minor peripheral procedures. After successful completion of surgery, both the FHR and maternal uterine activity should be monitored. Preterm labor can be treated with tocolytics (e.g., nifedipine or indomethacin) in consult with an obstetrician. Although magnesium sulfate does not demonstrate efficacy as a tocolytic, in situations where there is concern for preterm delivery, administration of magnesium sulfate can reduce the risk of cerebral palsy.[118] In addition, maternal corticosteroid administration is recommended for concern of significantly preterm delivery to decrease neonatal respiratory morbidity.[118] Postoperative analgesics can alter the perception of contractions, stressing the need for external monitoring.

Management of Anesthesia

Before proceeding, a plan for fetal monitoring, potential maternal arrest, and implications of an urgent cesarean delivery should be discussed with the surgeon, an obstetrician, and a perinatologist. When appropriate, neuraxial anesthetic techniques should be considered, given appropriate provider experience and circumstance, as they limit fetal drug exposure and maternal risks associated with general anesthesia. When a general anesthetic is chosen, aspiration prophylaxis and left uterine displacement should be used. Induction technique should be similar to that for cesarean delivery with general anesthesia previously discussed. Eucarbia should be maintained (30 mm Hg $ETco_2$), in addition to adequate uterine perfusion with fluids and appropriate vasopressor use such as phenylephrine. Regardless of the anesthetic technique selected, inspired oxygen concentration should be 50% or greater. Postoperative issues to address include deep venous thrombosis prophylaxis, FHR and uterine activity monitoring for at least 24 hours, and postoperative analgesia plan.

DIAGNOSIS AND MANAGEMENT OF FETAL DISTRESS

Overview

Intrapartum fetal monitoring evolved with the goal to identify fetal hypoxia during labor and allow clinicians to intervene before acidosis and long-term fetal damage occur. The fetal brain responds to peripheral and central stimuli via chemoreceptors, baroreceptors, and direct effects of metabolic changes within the CNS, which ultimately affect FHR. FHR monitoring was developed as a basic, nonspecific method of tracking fetal oxygenation and distress. Excellent external FHR monitors are available, but it is often necessary to apply an internal fetal scalp electrode to obtain accurate continuous FHR monitoring.

Key Evaluation Components

The assessment of FHR interpretation involves evaluation of (1) uterine contractions, (2) baseline FHR, (3) baseline FHR variability, (4) presence of accelerations, (5) periodic or episodic decelerations, and (6) changes or trends of FHR patterns over time.[119]

Uterine Contractions

Uterine contractions can be monitored externally or internally. External monitors only convey contraction frequency, but internal monitoring allows for both frequency and measurement of intrauterine pressure (in Montevideo units). Uterine activity and definitions are detailed in Box 33.4. Uterine contractions can decrease placental perfusion and oxygen delivery via constriction of the spiral arteries. If a tonic contraction or period of tachysystole occurs during labor, treatment with

---

Box 33.4 Uterine Activity Terminology

- Normal: ≤5 contractions in 10 minutes, averaged over a 30-minute window
- Tachysystole: >5 contractions in 10 minutes, averaged over a 30-minute window
- Characteristics of uterine contractions: tachysystole should be always qualified as to presence or absence of associated FHR decelerations.
  - Tachysystole applies to either spontaneous or stimulated labor. The clinical response to tachysystole may differ depending on whether contractions are spontaneous or stimulated.
  - Hyperstimulation and hypercontractility are not defined and should be abandoned.

Data from Macones GA, Hankins GD, Spong CY, et al. The 2008 National Institute of Child Health and Human Development workshop report on electronic fetal monitoring: Update on definitions, interpretation, and research guidelines. *J Obstet Gynecol Neonatal Nurs.* 2008;37(5):510–515.
FHR, Fetal heart rate.

IV

subcutaneous terbutaline or IV nitroglycerin can briefly relax the uterus and restore fetal perfusion.

Baseline FHR

Baseline FHR is determined by approximating the mean FHR rounded to increments of 5 bpm during a 10-minute window, excluding accelerations, decelerations, and periods of marked FHR variability (change >25 bpm). Normal baseline FHR ranges from 110 to 160 bpm; fetal bradycardia is defined as FHR <110 bpm; and fetal tachycardia is defined as FHR >160 bpm.

Variability

Baseline variability is also determined by examining fluctuations that are irregular in amplitude and frequency during a 10-minute window, excluding accelerations and decelerations. Variability is classified as follows: *absent FHR variability:* amplitude range undetectable; *minimal FHR variability:* amplitude range greater than undetectable and ≤5 bpm; *moderate FHR variability:* amplitude range 6 to 25 bpm; and *marked FHR variability:* amplitude range >25 bpm.

Accelerations

An acceleration is an abrupt increase in FHR defined as an increase from the acceleration onset to the peak in >30 seconds. In addition, the peak must be ≥15 bpm and last ≥15 seconds from the onset to return. Before 32 weeks of gestation, accelerations are defined as having a peak ≥10 bpm and a duration of ≥10 seconds.

Decelerations

Decelerations are classified as *variable* or *late* based on specific criteria (Fig. 33.8). A prolonged deceleration is present when there is a visually apparent decrease in the FHR from the baseline that is ≥15 bpm, lasting ≥2 minutes.

Late decelerations are a result of uteroplacental insufficiency causing relative fetal brain hypoxia during a contraction. The change results in sympathetic response and increased peripheral vascular resistance, elevating the fetal blood pressure, which is detected by the fetal baroreceptors and results in a decrease in the FHR. This response is termed a "reflex" late deceleration. A second type of late deceleration is caused by myocardial depression in the presence of worsening hypoxia. A moderate drop in FHR indicates some uteroplacental insufficiency; however, a more severe drop in FHR can indicate near total insufficiency. Although many texts associate *early deceleration* with head compression, this remains controversial, as early deceleration may reflect vagal activity from mild hypoxia that mirrors the uterine contraction.[120] Early decelerations are typically <20 bpm below baseline and though considered benign, might evolve into a more typical late deceleration. *Variable decelerations* are generally synonymous with umbilical cord compression. An ominous *sinusoidal* FHR pattern is defined as having a smooth sine wave–like pattern with a cycle frequency of 3 to 5/min that persists for ≥20 minutes and can be associated with placental abruption.[119]

Minimal to undetectable FHR variability in the presence of decelerations is associated with fetal acidemia. Severe decelerations (<70 bpm for >60 sec) are associated with fetal acidemia and are extremely ominous with the absence of variability.[121]

The FHR tracing is a nonspecific assessment of fetal acidosis and should be interpreted over time in relation to the clinical context and fetal and maternal factors. A normal fetus will experience episodes of hypoxia during labor and tolerate these periods without long-term neurologic sequelae.

FHR Categories

A three-tiered FHR classification system is currently used for a more general fetal assessment (Box 33.5).[122] An FHR classification may move between categories throughout the labor course. A *category I* FHR tracing is considered normal and predicts a normal fetal acid–base state at the time of assessment; no specific intervention is necessary. To qualify as category 1, all of the following criteria must be present: (1) baseline FHR of 110 to 160 bpm, (2) moderate baseline FHR variability, (3) no late or variable decelerations, (4) early decelerations may be present or absent, and (5) accelerations may be present or absent.

A *category II* FHR tracing is considered indeterminate and includes all tracings not in categories I or III. Examples include fetal tachycardia, prolonged decelerations more than 2 minutes but less than 10 minutes, and recurrent late decelerations with moderate baseline variability. Category II tracings require continued monitoring and reevaluation in light of the entire clinical scenario.

A *category III* FHR tracing is associated with an abnormal fetal acid–base status. Category III tracings include either (1) a sinusoidal FHR pattern or (2) absent FHR variability with recurrent late decelerations, recurrent variable decelerations, or bradycardia. These tracings require prompt patient evaluation and efforts to improve the fetal condition, such as intrauterine resuscitation with change in maternal position, treatment of hypotension, use of supplemental oxygen, and treatment of tachysystole if present. If the FHR tracing does not improve despite these interventions, expeditious delivery should proceed.

EVALUATION OF THE NEONATE AND NEONATAL RESUSCITATION

The transition from fetal to neonatal life involves an adjustment from a fluid- to an air-filled environment with major physiologic changes in the pulmonary and circulatory systems. Antepartum and intrapartum

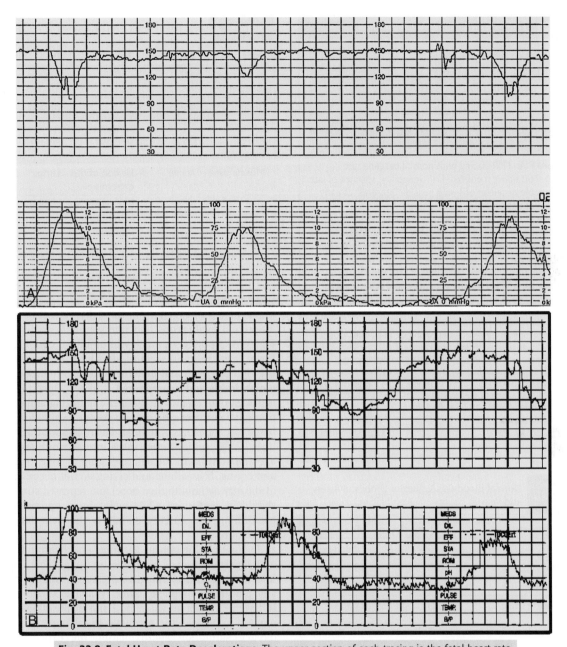

Fig. 33.8 Fetal Heart Rate Decelerations. The upper section of each tracing is the fetal heart rate. The lower section displays uterine activity. (A) Variable deceleration with minimal variability. (B) Late deceleration with minimal variability.

events can predict how safe and successful the transition to neonate will be. Umbilical cord gases are frequently sent at delivery as a measure of fetal assessment. Umbilical artery values reflect fetal well-being, and umbilical vein values are a reflection of maternal status and uteroplacental perfusion. Typical values are shown in Table 33.2.

Assessment of neonates immediately after birth is important to promptly identify depressed infants who require active resuscitation. The Apgar scoring system provides a simplified method for rapid neonatal assessment at 1, 5, and 10 minutes after delivery. Five parameters are assessed and assigned a numerical value (0, 1, or 2) to identify neonates who need resuscitation (Table 33.3). It has not been surpassed as a method of facilitating recognition and guiding resuscitation management of a newborn at birth. Approximately 10% of newborns need some assistance to begin breathing, and less than 1% require advanced cardiopulmonary resuscitation that includes chest compressions and

Box 33.5 FHR Tracing Criteria for Decelerations

Category	Color	Description
I	Green	No acidemia
IIa	Blue	No central fetal acidemia (adequate oxygen)
IIb	Yellow	No central fetal acidemia, but FHR pattern suggests intermittent reductions in O_2 which may result in fetal O_2 debt
IIc	Orange	Fetus potentially on verge of decompensation
III	Red	Evidence of actual or impending damaging fetal asphyxia

Category I. An FHR tracing with normal baseline rate (110–160 bpm), moderate FHR variability, absence of late or variable decelerations, and possible presence of early decelerations.

Category II. Everything not included in categories I and III. Most authorities believe that the middle category (category II) needs to be subdivided into three further subcategories, based on the severity of the periodic changes (IIb) and then reduction of FHR variability (IIc).

Category III. An FHR tracing with absent FHR variability, recurrent decelerations or bradycardia, or a sinusoidal pattern.

Data from Macones GA, Hankins GD, Spong CY, et al. The 2008 National Institute of Child Health and Human Development workshop report on electronic fetal monitoring: Update on definitions, interpretation, and research guidelines. *J Obstet Gynecol Neonatal Nurs.* 2008;37(5):510–515 and Parer JT, Ikeda T. A framework for standardized management of intrapartum fetal heart rate patterns. *Am J Obstet Gynecol.* 2007;197(1):26.e1-e6.

FHR, Fetal heart rate.

Table 33.2 Normal Blood Gas Values of Umbilical Artery and Vein

Measurement	Mean Artery	Mean Vein
pH	7.27	7.34
Pco_2 (mm Hg)	50	40
Po_2 (mm Hg)	20	30
Bicarbonate (mEq/L)	23	21
Base excess (mEq/L)	−3.6	−2.6

Data derived from Thorp JA, Rushing RS. Umbilical cord blood gas analysis. *Obstet Gynecol Clin North Am.* 1999;26(4):695–709.

Table 33.3 Evaluation of a Neonate Using the Apgar Score

Criterion	2	1	0
Heart rate (beats/min)	>100	<100	Absent
Breathing	Irregular, crying	Slow	Absent
Reflex irritability	Cry	Grimace	No response
Muscle tone	Active	Flexion of the extremities	Limp
Color	Pink	Body pink, extremities cyanotic	Cyanotic

For each of the five criteria, the value of 0, 1, or 2 is added to calculate a total score.

Cardiopulmonary Resuscitation

Management of neonates in the delivery room falls into 30-second evaluations and interventions, as detailed in Fig. 33.9. At delivery, a delay in umbilical cord clamping for at least 30 to 60 seconds after birth is recommended for vigorous term and preterm infants to increase hemoglobin levels and improve iron stores.[124] Once the infant is placed under a radiant warmer and drying and stimulation have occurred, the first 30-second evaluation begins based on the 2020 American Heart Association guidelines.[123] The initial survey takes into account gestational age and starts with the determination of tone, breathing, and crying. If breathing and crying do not occur, clearing of the airway (mouth then nose) and repeated stimulation should be performed while maintaining optimal airway positioning and euthermia–this is the next 30-second evaluation.

Evaluation for apnea, gasping, and heart rate occur with determination of the 1-minute Apgar score; possible interventions include positive pressure ventilation (PPV) and placement of pulse oximetry and ECG monitoring. Initiate PPV with air (21% Fio_2) and titrate supplemental oxygen to achieve the preductal (right upper extremity) oxygen saturation approximating the expected value after birth for healthy infants (see Fig. 33.9). In the event of heart rate <100, PPV efficacy should be evaluated by checking for chest movement, optimizing PPV delivery, and considering the need for intubation or laryngeal mask airway placement. If the heart rate drops below 60, then chest compressions, intubation, and ventilation with 100% oxygen should commence with ECG monitoring and preparation for umbilical vein cannulation. Infants greater than 36 weeks' gestation assessed to have moderate to severe hypoxic ischemic encephalopathy should be enrolled in a therapeutic hypothermia protocol.

If meconium is present, an individual skilled in tracheal intubation should be present at the time of birth.

administration of resuscitation medications.[123] Most newborns (Apgar ≥8) require little treatment other than suctioning of the nose and mouth, tactile stimulation to promote breathing, and avoiding hypothermia. The neonate's skin should be wiped dry and the baby placed on a radiantly heated bed, covered with warm blankets, or placed in skin-to-skin contact with the mother. Apgar scores of 10 are rare because the acrocyanosis persists in a normal newborn well past 5 minutes of life.

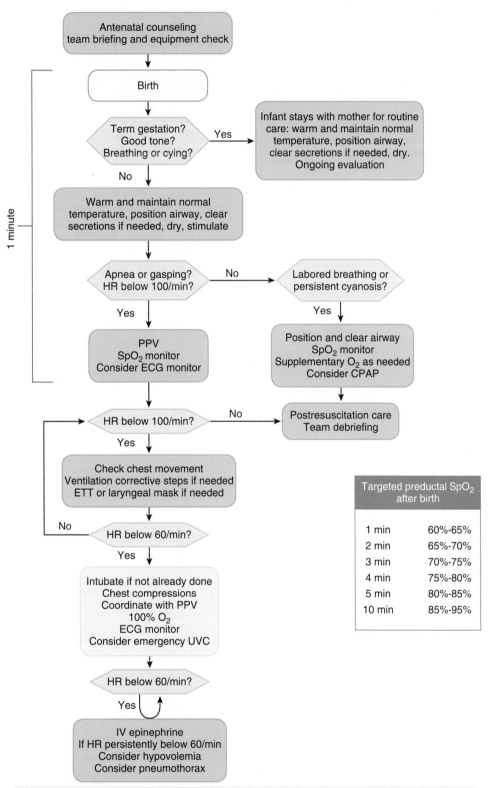

Fig. 33.9 NRP Resuscitation Flow Diagram. (Based on figure from Neonatal resuscitation: 2020 American Heart Association Guidelines update for cardiopulmonary resuscitation and emergency cardiovascular care. *Circulation*. 2020;142:S524–S550.)

IV

No significant interventions are needed if the infant is vigorous with good respiratory effort and muscle tone after delivery. However, if poor muscle tone and inadequate breathing efforts are present, resuscitation should commence with PPV if the infant is not breathing or the heart rate is less than 100/min.[123] Routine intubation for tracheal suction in this setting is no longer suggested. Instead, emphasis is made on initiating ventilation within the first minute of life in a nonbreathing or ineffectively breathing infant by clearing the airway and use of PPV.

Epinephrine

Epinephrine is indicated in the event the heart rate continues to stay below 60 despite PPV. The dose is 0.01 to 0.03 mg/kg IV administered rapidly. The dose may be repeated every 3 to 5 minutes, if necessary.

Hypovolemia

Although cardiac arrest secondary to hypovolemia is rare, the following conditions may lead to hypovolemia in the neonate: placental abruption, placenta previa, or vasa previa. Volume expansion should be instituted in a newborn who appears to have suffered blood loss or if shock has not responded to the resuscitation measures discussed previously. Blood or isotonic crystalloid (preferably normal saline) in 10 mL/kg aliquots may be administered in the delivery room.

Glucose

Hypoglycemia should be suspected after deliveries in which the newborn experienced severe asphyxia, intrauterine growth restriction, or maternal diabetes. During the resuscitation, a heelstick can determine the blood glucose level.

REFERENCES

1. Kacmar RM, Gaiser R. *Physiologic changes of pregnancy.* In: Chestnut DH, Wong CA, Tsen LC, Ngan Kee WD, Beilin Y, Mhyre JM, Bateman BT, eds. *Chestnut's Obstetric Anesthesia: Principles and Practice.* 6th ed. Philadelphia: Elsevier; 2020:13–37.
2. Page SM, Rollins MD. Physiology and pharmacology of obstetric anesthesia. In: Hemmings HC, Egan TD, eds. *Pharmacology and Physiology for Anesthesia, Foundations and Clinical Application.* 2nd ed. Philadelphia: Elsevier; 2019:732–751.
3. Afari HA, Davis EF, Sarma AA. Echocardiography for the Pregnant Heart. *Curr Treat Options Cardiovasc Med.* 2021;23:55.
4. Higuchi H, Takagi S, Zhang K, et al. Effect of lateral tilt angle on the volume of the abdominal aorta and inferior vena cava in pregnant and nonpregnant women determined by magnetic resonance imaging. *Anesthesiology.* 2015;122:286–293.
5. Porter JS, Bonello E, Reynolds F. The influence of epidural administration of fentanyl infusion on gastric emptying in labour. *Anaesthesia.* 1997;52:1151–1156.
6. Practice Guidelines for Obstetric Anesthesia: An Updated Report by the American Society of Anesthesiologists Task Force on Obstetric Anesthesia and the Society for Obstetric Anesthesia and Perinatology. *Anesthesiology.* 2016;124:270–300.
7. Hey VM, Ostick DG, Mazumder JK, et al. Pethidine, metoclopramide and the gastro-oesophageal sphincter. A study in healthy volunteers. *Anaesthesia.* 1981;36:173–176.
8. Paranjothy S, Griffiths JD, Broughton HK, et al. Interventions at caesarean section for reducing the risk of aspiration pneumonitis. *Cochrane Database Syst Rev.* 2014:CD004943.
9. Palahniuk RJ, Shnider SM. Eger EI, 2nd: Pregnancy decreases the requirement for inhaled anesthetic agents. *Anesthesiology.* 1974;41:82–83.
10. Gin T, Chan MT. Decreased minimum alveolar concentration of isoflurane in pregnant humans. *Anesthesiology.* 1994;81:829–832.
11. Ueyama H, Hagihira S, Takashina M, et al. Pregnancy does not enhance volatile anesthetic sensitivity on the brain: an electroencephalographic analysis study. *Anesthesiology.* 2010;113:577–584.
12. Morton SU, Brodsky D. Fetal Physiology and the Transition to Extrauterine Life. *Clin Perinatol.* 2016;43:395–407.
13. Haydon ML, Gorenberg DM, Nageotte MP, et al. The effect of maternal oxygen administration on fetal pulse oximetry during labor in fetuses with nonreassuring fetal heart rate patterns. *Am J Obstet Gynecol.* 2006;195:735–738.
14. Sanchez-Alcaraz A, Quintana MB, Laguarda M. Placental transfer and neonatal effects of propofol in caesarean section. *J Clin Pharm Ther.* 1998;23:19–23.
15. Caughey AB. Evidence-Based Labor and Delivery Management: Can We Safely Reduce the Cesarean Rate? *Obstet Gynecol Clin North Am.* 2017;44:523–533.
16. ACOG Practice Bulletin No. 209. Obstetric Analgesia and Anesthesia. *Obstet Gynecol.* 2019;133:e208–e225.
17. Markley JC, Rollins MD. Non-Neuraxial Labor Analgesia: Options. *Clin Obstet Gynecol.* 2017;60:350–364.
18. Arendt KW, Tessmer-Tuck JA. Nonpharmacologic labor analgesia. *Clin Perinatol.* 2013;40:351–371.
19. Bohren MA, Hofmeyr GJ, Sakala C, et al. Continuous support for women during childbirth. *Cochrane Database Syst Rev.* 2017;7:Cd003766.
20. Nanji JA, Carvalho B. Pain management during labor and vaginal birth. *Best Pract Res Clin Obstet Gynaecol.* 2020;67:100–112.
21. Rayburn W, Rathke A, Leuschen MP, et al. Fentanyl citrate analgesia during labor. *Am J Obstet Gynecol.* 1989;161:202–206.
22. Nissen E, Widstrom AM, Lilja G, et al. Effects of routinely given pethidine during labour on infants' developing breastfeeding behaviour. Effects of dose-delivery time interval and various concentrations of pethidine/norpethidine in cord plasma. *Acta Paediatr.* 1997;86:201–208.
23. Maykin MM, Ukoha EP, Tilp V, et al. Impact of therapeutic rest in early labor on perinatal outcomes: a prospective study. *Am J Obstet Gynecol MFM.* 2021;3:100325.
24. Freeman LM, Bloemenkamp KW, Franssen MT, et al. Patient controlled analgesia with remifentanil versus epidural analgesia in labour: randomised multicentre equivalence trial. *BMJ.* 2015;350:h846.

25. Weibel S, Jelting Y, Afshari A, et al. Patient-controlled analgesia with remifentanil versus alternative parenteral methods for pain management in labour. *Cochrane Database Syst Rev.* 2017;4:Cd011989.

26. Marwah R, Hassan S, Carvalho JC, et al. Remifentanil versus fentanyl for intravenous patient-controlled labour analgesia: an observational study. *Can J Anaesth.* 2012;59:246–254.

27. Van de Velde M, Carvalho B. Remifentanil for labor analgesia: an evidence-based narrative review. *Int J Obstet Anesth.* 2016;25:66–74.

28. Likis FE, Andrews JC, Collins MR, et al. Nitrous oxide for the management of labor pain: a systematic review. *Anesth Analg.* 2014;118:153–167.

29. Rollins MD, Arendt KW, Carabello BA, et al. Nitrous Oxide. American Society of Anesthesiologists (ASA) Guidelines. (Available at: https://www.asahq.org/about-asa/governance-and-committees/asa-committees/committee-on-obstetric-anesthesia/nitrous-oxide) 2020 - Accessed April 27, 2021.

30. American Society of Anesthesiologists. ASA Response to the FDA Med Watch Warning - December 16, 2016. (Available at: https://www.asahq.org/advocacy-and-asapac/fda-and-washington-alerts/washington-alerts/2016/12/asa-response-to-the-fda-med-watch) 2016 - Accessed April 27, 2021.

31. Richardson MG, Lopez BM, Baysinger CL, et al. Nitrous Oxide During Labor: Maternal Satisfaction Does Not Depend Exclusively on Analgesic Effectiveness. *Anesth Analg.* 2017;124:548–553.

32. Polley LS, Columb MO, Naughton NN, et al. Effect of epidural epinephrine on the minimum local analgesic concentration of epidural bupivacaine in labor. *Anesthesiology.* 2002;96:1123–1128.

33. Lee A, Landau R, Lavin T, et al. Comparative efficacy of epidural clonidine versus epidural fentanyl for treating breakthrough pain during labor: a randomized double-blind clinical trial. *Int J Obstet Anesth.* 2020;42:26–33.

34. Jones L, Othman M, Dowswell T, et al. Pain management for women in labour: an overview of systematic reviews. *Cochrane Database Syst Rev.* 2012;2012:Cd009234.

35. Attanasio L, Kozhimannil KB, Jou J, et al. Women's Experiences with Neuraxial Labor Analgesia in the Listening to Mothers II Survey: A Content Analysis of Open-Ended Responses. *Anesth Analg.* 2015;121:974–980.

36. American Society of Anesthesiologists Guidelines for Neuraxial Anesthesia in Obstetrics. (Available at: http://www.asahq.org/~/media/sites/asahq/files/public/resources/standards-guidelines/guidelines-for-neuraxial-anesthesia-in-obstetrics.pdf) 2021. Accessed - July 30, April 27, 2021.

37. Sng BL, Leong WL, Zeng Y, et al. Early versus late initiation of epidural analgesia for labour. *Cochrane Database Syst Rev.* 2014;10:CD007238.

38. Wong CA, Scavone BM, Peaceman AM, et al. The risk of cesarean delivery with neuraxial analgesia given early versus late in labor. *N Engl J Med.* 2005;352:655–665.

39. Anim-Somuah M, Smyth RM, Cyna AM, et al. Epidural versus non-epidural or no analgesia for pain management in labour. *Cochrane Database Syst Rev.* 2018;5:CD000331.

40. Craig MG, Grant EN, Tao W, et al. A randomized control trial of bupivacaine and fentanyl versus fentanyl-only for epidural analgesia during the second stage of labor. *Anesthesiology.* 2015;122:172–177.

41. American College of O, Gynecologists, Society for Maternal-Fetal M. Safe prevention of the primary cesarean delivery. *Am J Obstet Gynecol.* 2014;210:179–193.

42. Practice Advisory for the Prevention. Diagnosis, and Management of Infectious Complications Associated with Neuraxial Techniques: An Updated Report by the American Society of Anesthesiologists Task Force on Infectious Complications Associated with Neuraxial Techniques and the American Society of Regional Anesthesia and Pain Medicine. *Anesthesiology.* 2017;126:585–601.

43. Chau A, Bibbo C, Huang CC, et al. Dural Puncture Epidural Technique Improves Labor Analgesia Quality With Fewer Side Effects Compared With Epidural and Combined Spinal Epidural Techniques: A Randomized Clinical Trial. *Anesth Analg.* 2017;124:560–569.

44. Bradbury CL, Singh SI, Badder SR, et al. Prevention of post-dural puncture headache in parturients: a systematic review and meta-analysis. *Acta Anaesthesiol Scand.* 2013;57:417–430.

45. Heesen M, Bohmer J, Klohr S, et al. The effect of adding a background infusion to patient-controlled epidural labor analgesia on labor, maternal, and neonatal outcomes: a systematic review and meta-analysis. *Anesth Analg.* 2015;121:149–158.

46. Sng BL, Zeng Y, de Souza NNA, et al. Automated mandatory bolus versus basal infusion for maintenance of epidural analgesia in labour. *Cochrane Database Syst Rev.* 2018;5:CD011344.

47. Delgado C, Ciliberto C, Bollag L, et al. Continuous epidural infusion versus programmed intermittent epidural bolus for labor analgesia: optimal configuration of parameters to reduce physician-administered top-ups. *Curr Med Res Opin.* 2018;34:649–656.

48. Epsztein Kanczuk M, Barrett NM, Arzola C, et al. Programmed Intermittent Epidural Bolus for Labor Analgesia During First Stage of Labor: A Biased-Coin Up-and-Down Sequential Allocation Trial to Determine the Optimum Interval Time Between Boluses of a Fixed Volume of 10 mL of Bupivacaine 0.0625% With Fentanyl 2 µg/mL. *Anesth Analg.* 2017;124:537–541.

49. Asokumar B, Newman LM, McCarthy RJ, et al. Intrathecal bupivacaine reduces pruritus and prolongs duration of fentanyl analgesia during labor: a prospective, randomized controlled trial. *Anesth Analg.* 1998;87:1309–1315.

50. Van de Velde M. Neuraxial analgesia and fetal bradycardia. *Curr Opin Anaesthesiol.* 2005;18:253–256.

51. Wong CA, Scavone BM, Slavenas JP, et al. Efficacy and side effect profile of varying doses of intrathecal fentanyl added to bupivacaine for labor analgesia. *Int J Obstet Anesth.* 2021;13:19–24.

52. Neal JM, Barrington MJ, Brull R, et al. The Second ASRA Practice Advisory on Neurologic Complications Associated With Regional Anesthesia and Pain Medicine: Executive Summary 2015. *Reg Anesth Pain Med.* 2015;40:401–430.

53. Bauer ME, Arendt K, Beilin Y, et al. The Society for Obstetric Anesthesia and Perinatology Interdisciplinary Consensus Statement on Neuraxial Procedures in Obstetric Patients With Thrombocytopenia. *Anesth Analg.* 2021;132:1531–1544.

54. Horlocker TT, Vandermeulen E, Kopp SL, et al. Regional Anesthesia in the Patient Receiving Antithrombotic or Thrombolytic Therapy: American Society of Regional Anesthesia and Pain Medicine Evidence-Based Guidelines (Fourth Edition). *Reg Anesth Pain Med.* 2018;43:263–309.

55. Leffert L, Butwick A, Carvalho B, et al. The Society for Obstetric Anesthesia and Perinatology Consensus Statement on the Anesthetic Management of Pregnant and Postpartum Women Receiving Thromboprophylaxis or Higher Dose Anticoagulants. *Anesth Analg.* 2018;126:928–944.

56. Pan PH, Bogard TD, Owen MD. Incidence and characteristics of failures in obstetric neuraxial analgesia and anesthesia: a retrospective analysis of 19,259 deliveries. *Int J Obstet Anesth.* 2004;13:227–233.

57. Booth JM, Pan JC, Ross VH, et al. Combined Spinal Epidural Technique for Labor Analgesia Does Not Delay Recognition of Epidural Catheter Failures: A Single-center Retrospective Cohort Survival Analysis. *Anesthesiology.* 2016;125:516–524.

IV

58. D'Angelo R, Smiley RM, Riley ET, et al. Serious complications related to obstetric anesthesia: the serious complication repository project of the Society for Obstetric Anesthesia and Perinatology. *Anesthesiology.* 2014;120:1505–1512.
59. Ruppen W, Derry S, McQuay H, et al. Incidence of epidural hematoma, infection, and neurologic injury in obstetric patients with epidural analgesia/anesthesia. *Anesthesiology.* 2006;105:394–399.
60. Burkle CM, Olsen DA, Sviggum HP, et al. Parturient recall of neuraxial analgesia risks: Impact of labor pain vs no labor pain. *J Clin Anesth.* 2017;36:158–163.
61. Panchal AR, Bartos JA, Cabañas JG, et al. Part 3: Adult Basic and Advanced Life Support: 2020 American Heart Association Guidelines for Cardiopulmonary Resuscitation and Emergency Cardiovascular Care. *Circulation.* 2020;142:S366–s468.
62. Neal JM, Neal EJ, Weinberg GL. American Society of Regional Anesthesia and Pain Medicine Local Anesthetic Systemic Toxicity checklist: 2020 version. *Reg Anesth Pain Med.* 2021;46:81–82.
63. Simmons SW, Taghizadeh N, Dennis AT, et al. Combined spinal-epidural versus epidural analgesia in labour. *Cochrane Database Syst Rev.* 2012;10:CD003401.
64. Hofmeyr G, Cyna A, Middleton P. Prophylactic intravenous preloading for regional analgesia in labour. *Cochrane Database Syst Rev.* 2004:CD000175.
65. Arendt KW, Segal BS. The association between epidural labor analgesia and maternal fever. *Clin Perinatol.* 2013;40:385–398.
66. Sharpe EE, Arendt KW. Epidural Labor Analgesia and Maternal Fever. *Clin Obstet Gynecol.* 2017;60:365–374.
67. Greenwell EA, Wyshak G, Ringer SA, et al. Intrapartum temperature elevation, epidural use, and adverse outcome in term infants. *Pediatrics.* 2012;129:e447–e454.
68. Kinsella SM, Carvalho B, Dyer RA, et al. International consensus statement on the management of hypotension with vasopressors during caesarean section under spinal anaesthesia. *Anaesthesia.* 2018;73:71–92.
69. Ngan Kee WD, Lee SW, Ng FF, et al. Randomized double-blinded comparison of norepinephrine and phenylephrine for maintenance of blood pressure during spinal anesthesia for cesarean delivery. *Anesthesiology.* 2015;122:736–745.
70. Orbach-Zinger S, Jadon A, Lucas DN, et al. Intrathecal catheter use after accidental dural puncture in obstetric patients: literature review and clinical management recommendations. *Anaesthesia.* 2021;76:1111–1121.
71. Toledo P, McCarthy RJ, Ebarvia MJ, et al. The interaction between epidural 2-chloroprocaine and morphine: a randomized controlled trial of the effect of drug administration timing on the efficacy of morphine analgesia. *Anesth Analg.* 2009;109:168–173.
72. Carvalho B. Failed epidural top-up for cesarean delivery for failure to progress in labor: the case against single-shot spinal anesthesia. *Int J Obstet Anesth.* 2012;21:357–359.
73. Mankowitz SK, Gonzalez Fiol A, Smiley R. Failure to Extend Epidural Labor Analgesia for Cesarean Delivery Anesthesia: A Focused Review. *Anesth Analg.* 2016;123:1174–1180.
74. Abir G, Mhyre J. Maternal mortality and the role of the obstetric anesthesiologist. *Best Pract Res Clin Anaesthesiol.* 2017;31:91–105.
75. Richardson MG, Raymond BL. Sugammadex Administration in Pregnant Women and in Women of Reproductive Potential: A Narrative Review. *Anesth Analg.* 2020;130:1628–1637.
76. Society for Obstetric Anesthesia and Perinatology Statement on Sugammadex during pregnancy and lactation Ad Hoc task force: Willett, Butwick, Togioka, Bensadigh, Hofer, Zakowski April 22, 2019,
77. Clark RB, Brown MA, Lattin DL. Neostigmine, atropine, and glycopyrrolate: does neostigmine cross the placenta? *Anesthesiology.* 1996;84:450–452.
78. De Tina A, Palanisamy A. General Anesthesia During the Third Trimester: Any Link to Neurocognitive Outcomes? *Anesthesiol Clin.* 2017;35:69–80.
79. Afolabi BB, Lesi FE. Regional versus general anaesthesia for caesarean section. *Cochrane Database Syst Rev.* 2012;10:CD004350.
80. Murray SR, Stock SJ, Cowan S, et al. Spontaneous preterm birth prevention in multiple pregnancy. *Obstet Gynaecol.* 2018;20:57–63.
81. Melka S, Miller J, Fox NS. Labor and Delivery of Twin Pregnancies. *Obstet Gynecol Clin North Am.* 2017;44:645–654.
82. ACOG Committee Opinion No. 745. Mode of Term Singleton Breech Delivery. *Obstet Gynecol.* 2018;132:e60–e63.
83. External Cephalic Version. ACOG Practice Bulletin, Number 221. *Obstet Gynecol.* 2020;135:e203–e212.
84. Hao Q, Hu Y, Zhang L, et al. A Systematic Review and Meta-analysis of Clinical Trials of Neuraxial, Intravenous, and Inhalational Anesthesia for External Cephalic Version. *Anesth Analg.* 2020;131:1800–1811.
85. Dajani NK, Magann EF. Complications of shoulder dystocia. *Semin Perinatol.* 2014;38:201–204.
86. Chappell LC, Cluver CA, Kingdom J, et al. Pre-eclampsia. *Lancet.* 2021;398:341–354.
87. Gestational Hypertension and Preeclampsia: ACOG Practice Bulletin, Number 222. *Obstet Gynecol.* 2020;135:e237–e260.
88. Cooray SD, Edmonds SM, Tong S, et al. Characterization of symptoms immediately preceding eclampsia. *Obstet Gynecol.* 2011;118:995–999.
89. Grandi SM, Vallee-Pouliot K, Reynier P, et al. Hypertensive Disorders in Pregnancy and the Risk of Subsequent Cardiovascular Disease. *Paediatr Perinat Epidemiol.* 2017;31:412–421.
90. Duley L, Gulmezoglu AM, Henderson-Smart DJ, et al. Magnesium sulphate and other anticonvulsants for women with pre-eclampsia. *Cochrane Database Syst Rev.* 2010:CD000025.
91. Brown MA, Magee LA, Kenny LC, et al. The hypertensive disorders of pregnancy: ISSHP classification, diagnosis & management recommendations for international practice. *Pregnancy Hypertens.* 2018;13:291–310.
92. Committee Opinion No. 692. Emergent Therapy for Acute-Onset, Severe Hypertension During Pregnancy and the Postpartum Period. *Obstet Gynecol.* 2017;129:e90–e95.
93. Pant M, Fong R, Scavone B. Prevention of peri-induction hypertension in preeclamptic patients: a focused review. *Anesth Analg.* 2014;119:1350–1356.
94. Scavone BM, Main EK. The National Partnership for Maternal Safety: a call to action for anesthesiologists. *Anesth Analg.* 2015;121:14–16.
95. Vahanian SA, Vintzileos AM. Placental implantation abnormalities: a modern approach. *Curr Opin Obstet Gynecol.* 2016;28:477–484.
96. Salmanian B, Clark SL, Hui SR, et al. Massive Transfusion Protocols in Obstetric Hemorrhage: Theory versus Reality. *Am J Perinatol.* 2021.
97. Effect of early tranexamic acid administration on mortality, hysterectomy, and other morbidities in women with post-partum haemorrhage (WOMAN): an international, randomised, double-blind, placebo-controlled trial. *Lancet.* 2017;389:2105–2116.
98. Downes KL, Grantz KL, Shenassa ED. Maternal, Labor, Delivery, and Perinatal Outcomes Associated with Placental Abruption: A Systematic Review. *Am J Perinatol.* 2017;34:935–957.
99. ACOG Practice Bulletin No. 205. Vaginal Birth After Cesarean Delivery. *Obstet Gynecol.* 2019;133:e110–e127.
100. Guiliano M, Closset E, Therby D, et al. Signs, symptoms and complications of complete and partial uterine ruptures during pregnancy and delivery. *Eur J Obstet Gynecol Reprod Biol.* 2014;179:130–134.

101. Practice Bulletin No. 183. Postpartum Hemorrhage. *Obstet Gynecol.* 2017;130:e168–e186.

102. Kovacheva VP, Soens MA, Tsen LC. A Randomized, Double-blinded Trial of a "Rule of Threes" Algorithm versus Continuous Infusion of Oxytocin during Elective Cesarean Delivery. *Anesthesiology.* 2015;123:92–100.

103. Einerson BD, Weiniger CF. Placenta accreta spectrum disorder: updates on anesthetic and surgical management strategies. *Int J Obstet Anesth.* 2021;46:102975.

104. Silver RM, Barbour KD. Placenta accreta spectrum: accreta, increta, and percreta. *Obstet Gynecol Clin North Am.* 2015;42:381–402.

105. Silver RM, Landon MB, Rouse DJ, et al. Maternal morbidity associated with multiple repeat cesarean deliveries. *Obstet Gynecol.* 2006;107:1226–1232.

106. Warrick CM, Rollins MD. Peripartum Anesthesia Considerations for Placenta Accreta. *Clin Obstet Gynecol.* 2018;61:808–827.

107. Ito F, Akasaka J, Koike N, et al. Incidence, diagnosis and pathophysiology of amniotic fluid embolism. *J Obstet Gynaecol.* 2014;34:580–584.

108. Clark SL, Romero R, Dildy GA, et al. Proposed diagnostic criteria for the case definition of amniotic fluid embolism in research studies. *Am J Obstet Gynecol.* 2016;215:408–412.

109. Society for Maternal-Fetal Medicine. Electronic address psoPacheco LD, Saade G, et al. Amniotic fluid embolism: diagnosis and management. *Am J Obstet Gynecol.* 2016;215:B16–B24.

110. Clark SL. A Biomarker for Amniotic Fluid Embolism: The Search Continues. *Bjog.* 2021.

111. Simard C, Yang S, Koolian M, et al. The role of echocardiography in amniotic fluid embolism: a case series and review of the literature. *Can J Anaesth.* 2021.

112. Vasco Ramirez M, Valencia GC. Anesthesia for Nonobstetric Surgery in Pregnancy. *Clin Obstet Gynecol.* 2020;63:351–363.

113. ACOG Committee Opinion No. 775. Nonobstetric Surgery During Pregnancy. *Obstet Gynecol.* 2019;133:e285–e286.

114. Moore HB, Juarez-Colunga E, Bronsert M, et al. Effect of Pregnancy on Adverse Outcomes After General Surgery. *JAMA Surg.* 2015;150:637–643.

115. Hong JY. Adnexal mass surgery and anesthesia during pregnancy: a 10-year retrospective review. *Int J Obstet Anesth.* 2006;15:212–216.

116. American Society of Anesthesiologists Quality Management and Departmental Administration Committee. Pregnancy Testing Prior to Anesthesia and Surgery. (Available at: Pregnancy-Testing-Prior-to-anesthesia-and-surgery.pdf) 2016. Accessed - July 30, 2021

117. Andropoulos DB, Greene MF. Anesthesia and Developing Brains - Implications of the FDA Warning. *N Engl J Med.* 2017;376:905–907.

118. Tsakiridis I, Mamopoulos A, Athanasiadis A, et al. Antenatal Corticosteroids and Magnesium Sulfate for Improved Preterm Neonatal Outcomes: A Review of Guidelines. *Obstet Gynecol Surv.* 2020;75:298–307.

119. Macones GA, Hankins GD, Spong CY, et al. The 2008 National Institute of Child Health and Human Development workshop report on electronic fetal monitoring: update on definitions, interpretation, and research guidelines. *J Obstet Gynecol Neonatal Nurs.* 2008;37:510–515.

120. Lear CA, Galinsky R, Wassink G, et al. The myths and physiology surrounding intrapartum decelerations: the critical role of the peripheral chemoreflex. *J Physiol.* 2016;594:4711–4725.

121. Parer JT, King T, Flanders S, et al. Fetal acidemia and electronic fetal heart rate patterns: is there evidence of an association? *J Matern Fetal Neonatal Med.* 2006;19:289–294.

122. ACOG Practice Bulletin No. 106. Intrapartum fetal heart rate monitoring: nomenclature, interpretation, and general management principles. *Obstet Gynecol.* 2009;114:192–202.

123. Aziz K, Lee CHC, Escobedo MB, et al. Part 5: Neonatal Resuscitation 2020 American Heart Association Guidelines for Cardiopulmonary Resuscitation and Emergency Cardiovascular Care. *Pediatrics.* 2021;147.

124. Delayed Umbilical Cord Clamping After Birth: ACOG Committee Opinion Summary, Number 814. *Obstet Gynecol.* 2020;136:1238–1239.

IV

34 PEDIATRICS

Erin A. Gottlieb, Dean B. Andropoulos

Providing anesthetic care for infants and children poses unique challenges because of the profound differences in physiology, pharmacokinetics and pharmacodynamics of anesthetic drugs, and wide variety of procedures that these patients undergo, which are often very different from the adult population. The developmental physiology, pharmacology, fluid and transfusion therapy, and airway management in pediatric anesthesia will be defined. Anesthetic considerations and techniques in pediatric patients, especially in neonates, who are the most unique group of pediatric patients, will be reviewed. The new field of fetal surgery will be addressed, and the growing areas of anesthesia in remote locations for pediatric patients and anesthetic neurotoxicity in the developing brain will be discussed briefly. In the final section the most common types of congenital heart disease (CHD) and their pathophysiology will be reviewed.

DEVELOPMENTAL PHYSIOLOGY

Respiratory System

Lung Development

Lung development begins in the fourth week of gestation, but extrauterine survival becomes possible only when terminal air sacs begin to form and the capillary network surrounding them is sufficient for pulmonary gas exchange around the 26th week. Alveolar formation begins by the 36th postconceptual week, but most alveoli form postnatally. Type II pneumocytes begin producing surfactant around the 24th week of gestation, and production of this mixture of phospholipids and surfactant proteins is critical for reducing surface tension and facilitating the inflation of alveoli.

Chest Wall and Respiratory Muscles

The ribs extend from the vertebral column horizontally in infants compared with a caudad angle in adults. This configuration renders the accessory muscles of respiration ineffective in infants. The ribcage also tends to move inward during inspiration because of the high cartilage content in the ribs of neonates and infants. This paradoxical chest wall movement occurs commonly under general anesthesia and is the result of decreased tone of the intercostal muscles and upper airway obstruction. The diaphragm increases its work to maintain tidal volume, which can lead to fatigue.

The mature diaphragm has a low content of type I (slow twitch, high oxidative capacity) muscle fibers. Before 37 weeks' postconceptual age, less than 10% of the diaphragmatic fibers are type I. A term infant has approximately 25% type I fibers, and an adult has approximately 50%. This means that the diaphragm is more likely to become fatigued in premature and term infants, leading to earlier respiratory failure.

Chest wall compliance decreases throughout childhood and adolescence owing to the ossification of the ribs and development of thoracic muscle mass. The elastic recoil pressure of the lung increases throughout this time from an increase in pulmonary elastic fibers.

Respiratory Variables

There are some major differences in static lung volumes and respiratory variables among children of different ages and adults (also see Chapter 5). Table 34.1 illustrates the major differences in these and other variables between infants and adults. Total lung capacity (TLC) is much larger per kilogram in adults compared with infants. This is largely because of the relative efficiency and strength of adult muscles of inspiration and effort.

Functional residual capacity (FRC) is similar on a per kilogram basis among age groups. However, the mechanical reasons for this similarity differ. The FRC in adults is defined as the volume at which passive elastic forces of the chest wall are balanced by the recoil of the lung. This is the volume at end exhalation. In infants both the elastic recoil of the chest and the recoil pressure of the lung are very low. This would predict an FRC of about 10% of TLC. However, the FRC is about 40% of TLC owing to a prolongation of the expiratory time constant by a process known as *laryngeal braking*.

In an apneic infant the lung volume is smaller than the FRC. Thus an apneic infant has a disproportionately smaller store of intrapulmonary oxygen than an adult, and hypoxemia will develop rapidly if the airway is poorly maintained.

In infants the closing capacity (CC) is larger than the FRC, so during exhalation, small airways start to collapse and trap air. In adults the CC is smaller than the FRC.

Factors Affecting Respiration

In both infants and adults Pao_2, $Paco_2$, and pH control ventilation. An increase in $Paco_2$ increases minute ventilation by increasing respiratory rate and tidal volume. This response to hypercapnia is not enhanced by hypoxemia. In fact, hypoxia may depress the hypercapnic ventilatory response.

High inspired oxygen concentrations depress newborn respiratory drive, and low inspired oxygen concentrations stimulate it. However, continued hypoxia will eventually lead to respiratory depression. Hypoglycemia, anemia, and hypothermia also decrease respiratory drive.

Metabolic demand drives minute ventilation. As oxygen consumption increases, alveolar minute ventilation increases. Although tidal volume also increases, the increase in respiratory rate is the predominant variable that increases minute ventilation in infants.

Breathing Patterns

Normal newborn breathing is periodic. There are pauses of less than 10 seconds and periods of increased respiratory activity. Periodic breathing is different from apnea, a ventilatory pause associated with desaturation and bradycardia. Apnea is associated with prematurity and is treated with respiratory stimulants (e.g., caffeine) and with tactile stimulation such as stroking or rocking. Postoperative apnea in former premature infants is an important consideration in the planning of outpatient surgery.

Cardiovascular System

Fetal Circulation

The fetal circulation is characterized by (1) increased pulmonary vascular resistance (PVR) with very little pulmonary blood flow, (2) decreased systemic vascular resistance (SVR) with the placenta as the major low-resistance vascular bed, and (3) right-to-left blood flow through the ductus arteriosus and foramen ovale (Fig. 34.1). At birth, three events change the circulation into its postnatal configuration. First, alveolar oxygen concentration increases, and alveolar carbon dioxide concentration decreases with the expansion of the lungs. This results in a decrease in PVR. Second, the low-resistance placental bed is removed from the circulation when the umbilical cord is clamped. This results in an increase in SVR. The decrease in PVR leads to an increase in pulmonary blood flow and therefore an increase in blood return to the left

IV

Table 34.1 Age-Dependent Respiratory Variables

Variable	Units	Neonate	6 mo	12 mo	3 yr	5 yr	9 yr	12 yr	Adult
Approx. weight	kg	3	7	10	15	19	30	50	70
Respiratory rate	breaths/min	50 ± 10	30 ± 5	24 ± 6	24 ± 6	23 ± 5	20 ± 5	18 ± 5	12 ± 3
Tidal volume	mL	21	45	78	112	170	230	480	575
	mL/kg	6-8	6-8	6-8	6-8	7-8	7-8	7-8	6-7
Minute ventilation	mL/min	1050	1350	1780	2460	4000		6200	6400
	mL/kg/min	350	193	178	164	210		124	91
Alveolar ventilation	mL/min	665		1245	1760	1800		3000	3100
	mL/kg/min	222	125	117	95	60	44		
Dead space/tidal volume ratio		0.3	0.3	0.3	0.3	0.3	0.3	0.3	0.3
Oxygen consumption	mL/kg/min	6-8							3-4
Vital capacity	mL	120			870	1160		3100	4000
	mL/kg	40			58	61		62	57
Functional residual capacity	mL	80			490	680		1970	3000
	mL/kg	27			33	36		39	43
Total lung capacity	mL	160			1100	1500		4000	6000
	mL/kg	53			73	79		80	86
Closing volume as percentage of vital capacity	%					20		8	4
Number of alveoli	Saccules × 10^6	30	112	129	257	280			300
Specific compliance	CL/FRC:mL/cm H$_2$O/L	0.04	0.038			0.06			0.05
Specific conductance of small airways	mL/s/cm H$_2$O/g	0.02		3.1	1.7	1.2		8.2	13.4
Hematocrit	%	55 ± 7	37 ± 3	35 ± 2.5	40 ± 3	40 ± 2	40 ± 2	42 ± 2	43-48
Arterial pH	pH units	7.30-7.40		7.35-7.45					7.35-7.45
Paco$_2$	mm Hg	30-35		30-40					30-40
Pao$_2$	mm Hg	60-90		80-100					80-100

Modified and reproduced with permission from O'Rourke PP, Crone RK. The respiratory system. In Gregory GA, ed. *Gregory's Pediatric Anesthesia*. 2nd ed. New York: Churchill Livingstone: 1989:63-91.

side of the heart. The increase in left atrial pressure functionally closes the foramen ovale.

The three fetal channels that close after birth are the ductus arteriosus, ductus venosus, and foramen ovale. The ductus arteriosus is functionally closed in 98% of neonates at 4 days of life. It constricts because of an increase in arterial oxygen tension and a decrease in prostaglandins released from the placenta. Later, the constricted duct becomes fibrotic, becoming the ligamentum arteriosum. The ductus venosus closes with the clamping of the umbilical vein. The portal pressure decreases, and the ductus venosus closes. Via the ductus venosus, an umbilical venous catheter enters the inferior vena cava and becomes a true central venous catheter. The foramen ovale is patent in many infants and is probe patent in 30% of adults.

If pulmonary artery vasoconstriction occurs in the first few days of life as a result of hypoxemia, acidosis, or pulmonary hypertension, blood can shunt right to left through the previously functionally closed foramen ovale or the ductus arteriosus, resulting in profound hypoxemia and acidosis. This is termed *persistent fetal circulation* and can be life threatening. Treatment is directed toward decreasing PVR.

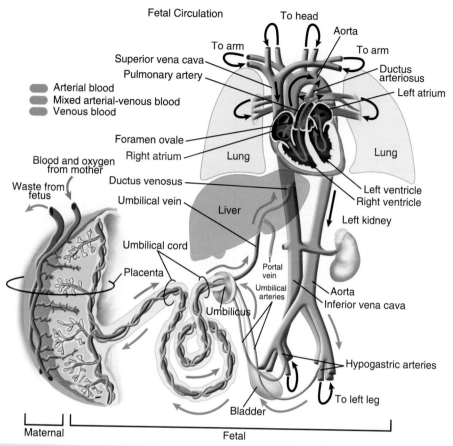

Fig. 34.1 Course of the fetal circulation in late gestation. Note the selective blood flow patterns across the foramen ovale and the ductus arteriosus. (From Greeley WJ, Cripe CC, Nathan AT. Anesthesia for pediatric cardiac surgery. In Miller RD, ed. *Miller's Anesthesia*, Vol 2, 8th ed. Philadelphia: Saunders; 2015:2799–2853.)

Neonatal Myocardium

The neonatal myocardium is characterized by poorly organized myocytes that contain fewer contractile elements than the adult myocardium, in which the myocytes are well organized in a parallel arrangement. The sarcoplasmic reticulum in the neonatal heart is immature with disorganized T-tubules. The neonatal myocardium depends heavily on the concentration of free ionized calcium for contractility. Transfusion of blood products to neonates may cause hypocalcemia and depressed cardiac function, which can be treated with calcium administration (also see Chapter 25).

Although the stroke volume of neonates is usually fixed and the cardiac output usually increases by increasing heart rate only, the neonate can increase stroke volume up to a point according to the Frank-Starling relationship if the afterload is kept low.[1]

Autonomic Innervation of the Heart

The parasympathetic nervous system predominates early in life, while the sympathetic nervous system is still developing. This imbalance is clinically relevant and can be seen as marked bradycardia or even asystole during laryngoscopy, orogastric tube placement, or tracheal suctioning in the neonate or infant. Many anesthesia providers will pretreat with an anticholinergic—atropine or glycopyrrolate—before airway instrumentation.

Newborn Cardiovascular Assessment

The newborn cardiovascular examination should focus on the hemodynamics, including heart rate and arterial blood pressure (in all extremities) and oxygen saturation measurements. Other parts of the examination include capillary refill, peripheral pulses, respiratory status, and the possible presence of a murmur or third or fourth heart sound on auscultation. Urine output trends should be assessed. Analysis of arterial, venous, or capillary blood gases should be performed if acidosis is suspected. If performed, results of a chest radiograph, electrocardiogram, or echocardiogram should be reviewed. Normal cardiovascular variables are displayed in Table 34.2.

IV

Table 34.2	Normal Heart Rate and Systolic Blood Pressure as Functions of Age	
	Normal Range	
Age Group	**Heart Rate (beats/min)**	**Systolic Blood Pressure[a] (mm Hg)**
Neonate (<30 days)	120–160	60–75
1–6 mo	110–140	65–85
6–12 mo	100–140	70–90
1–2 yr	90–130	75–95
3–5 yr	80–120	80–100
6–8 yr	75–115	85–105
9–12 yr	70–110	90–115
13–16 yr	60–110	95–120
>16 yr	60–100	100–125

[a]As measured using an oscillometric blood pressure device.

Renal System

Postnatally, the kidneys replace the placenta in maintaining metabolic homeostasis. The glomerular filtration rate (GFR) is 15% to 30% of adult values at birth and increases to 50% at 5 to 10 days of life. Adult values are reached by 1 year of age. The low GFR affects the neonate's ability to excrete sodium, water loads, and some drugs. Tubular function develops after 34 weeks of gestation. The tubules are immature and have a reduced threshold at which bicarbonate is no longer completely reabsorbed by the kidney. This is associated with the inability of young infants to respond to an acid load and the slightly reduced values of pH (7.37) and plasma bicarbonate (22 mEq/L). Infants also have decreased concentrating ability and a low level of production and excretion of urea. Blood urea nitrogen (BUN) remains normal because less urea is being produced. Creatinine immediately postnatally equals the maternal value and decreases in the first 48 hours to levels of 0.5 mEq/L or less if renal function is normal.

Hematologic System

The blood volume in the newborn ranges from 82 to 93 mL/kg for the term newborn to 90 to 105 mL/kg for the preterm newborn. After the first year of life, blood volume declines to approximately 70 to 80 mL/kg. The normal newborn hemoglobin is 14 to 20 g/dL. Fetal hemoglobin (HbF) makes up 70% to 80% of the hemoglobin at birth. HbF has a higher affinity for oxygen than does adult hemoglobin. The higher affinity of HbF for oxygen shifts the oxyhemoglobin dissociation curve to the left. The P_{50} of HbF is 18 to 20 mm Hg, and the P_{50} of adult hemoglobin is 27 mm Hg. The difference in

P_{50} between the two types of hemoglobin facilitates the uptake of oxygen by the fetus at the placental interface.

The physiologic nadir in hemoglobin occurs at 9 to 12 weeks of life and is 10 to 11 g/dL in the term infant. The decreased hemoglobin values do not affect oxygen delivery because of a shift in the oxyhemoglobin dissociation curve to the right. The rightward shift is caused by an increase in 2,3-diphosphoglycerate (2,3-DPG) and the replacement of HbF by adult hemoglobin, which facilitates the unloading of oxygen in the tissues. The hemoglobin concentration stabilizes at 11.5 to 12 g/dL until 2 years of age, after which it increases gradually to adult values during puberty.

At birth, the vitamin K–dependent coagulation factors (II, VII, IX, X) are present at 20% to 60% of adult levels. This may lead to a prolonged prothrombin time. It can take several weeks for these factors to reach normal values owing to synthesis in an immature liver. Prophylactic intramuscular (IM) vitamin K is given to all newborns. In addition, maternal ingestion of some drugs, including anticonvulsants and warfarin, can cause vitamin K deficiency in the newborn.

PHARMACOLOGIC DIFFERENCES

Pharmacokinetics

Protein binding of drugs is different between infants and adults. Some of this difference is because of a lower concentration of serum protein/albumin in younger children. There is also a lower affinity of protein-bound drugs for serum proteins in neonates compared with adults. With decreased protein binding, the concentration of free drug is increased, resulting in an increase in drug effect. The effect of decreased protein binding is most apparent in highly protein-bound drugs such as phenytoin, bupivacaine, barbiturates, and diazepam (also see Chapter 4).

The difference in body composition also has an effect on pharmacokinetics. Preterm and term neonates have a larger percentage of total body water compared with older children and adults. This is reflected in an increase in the volume of distribution (Vd). A larger initial dose of drug is needed to reach the same therapeutic serum level and pharmacologic effect when the Vd is increased. In neonates larger initial doses are required for digoxin, succinylcholine, and antibiotics. Fentanyl is an important example of a commonly used anesthetic in neonates that requires larger initial doses. Also, neonates and infants may be more sensitive to the effects of certain drugs and need lower serum blood levels to achieve the same effects. Medications should be given slowly and titrated to predetermined effects.

There is also a decreased percentage of fat and muscle in small infants compared with older children and adults. Drugs that rely on redistribution to these tissues for the termination of clinical effects may last longer in small infants. Thiopental and propofol, for example, depend on redistribution for awakening after a single dose.

Hepatic Metabolism

Hepatic metabolism of drugs changes lipid-soluble, pharmacologically active drugs into usually inactive, nonlipid-soluble drugs for excretion. The activity of most hepatic enzymes is reduced in neonates, as is blood flow to the liver. This can result in a longer duration of effect of some pharmacologic drugs. Again, fentanyl is an important example. Hepatic metabolism of drugs approximates 50% of adult values at birth in a full-term neonate, rapidly increases during the first month of life to near-adult values, and is fully mature by 1 or 2 years of age.

Renal Excretion

Neonatal kidneys become more efficient with age. Owing to immature glomerular and tubular function, drugs that depend on the kidney for excretion such as aminoglycosides have prolonged elimination half-times in neonates. Glomerular and tubular function is nearly mature at 20 postnatal weeks and is fully mature at 2 years.

Pharmacology of Inhaled Anesthetics

F_A/F_I is the ratio of concentration of alveolar (F_A) to inspired (F_I) anesthetic. At the beginning of an inhaled induction of anesthesia, F_A is zero and F_I is large. As the F_A/F_I increases toward 1, induction of anesthesia occurs. The F_A/F_I ratio increases more rapidly in neonates compared with adults, which means that anesthesia can be induced more rapidly than in adults.[2] There is a larger alveolar ventilation to FRC ratio (V_A/FRC) in neonates compared with adults and thus a more rapid increase in F_A/F_I. The ratio is 5:1 in neonates and 1.5:1 in adults (also see Chapter 7).

Infants and small children may have an increased cardiac output during an inhaled induction via a mask because of preoperative anxiety. Increased cardiac output is associated with increased pulmonary blood flow and higher uptake of anesthetic from the lungs, which decreases F_A and slows the increase in F_A/F_I. Therefore as a result of uptake, the rate of anesthetic induction would slow down. However, the increased cardiac output also increases anesthetic delivery to the vessel-rich group (VRG), and the partial pressure of anesthetic in the VRG equilibrates with F_A. The partial pressure of anesthetic in the venous blood approaches the partial pressure in the alveoli and speeds the increase in F_A/F_I.

In neonates there are also reduced tissue/blood solubility and reduced blood/gas solubility. Blood solubility of the higher-solubility inhaled anesthetics (e.g., isoflurane)

is 18% lower in neonates. Therefore there is less uptake from the alveoli, and the increase in F_A/F_I is more rapid. The blood solubility of the less soluble inhaled anesthetics, such as sevoflurane and desflurane, does not differ between infants and adults, and F_A/F_I does not increase as rapidly. The reduced tissue solubility of isoflurane also contributes to a more rapid increase in F_A/F_I in neonates compared with adults.

Effect of Shunt on Inhaled Induction of Anesthesia

Left-to-right shunts are mostly intracardiac (ventricular or atrial septal defects) and are associated with increased pulmonary blood flow. These have no real effect on the rate at which induction of anesthesia occurs. Right-to-left shunts involve a portion of the systemic venous return that bypasses gas exchange in the lungs and is circulated systemically. Right-to-left shunts can be either intracardiac (tetralogy of Fallot [TOF]) or intrapulmonary (endobronchial intubation, atelectasis). Right-to-left shunts slow the rise in F_A/F_I and delay induction of anesthesia. This is more pronounced with less soluble anesthetics such as sevoflurane and desflurane.

Minimum Alveolar Concentration

Minimum alveolar concentration (MAC) varies with age. The MAC of inhaled anesthetic drugs is highest in infants 1 to 6 months old. The MAC is 30% less in full-term neonates for isoflurane and desflurane. Sevoflurane MAC at term is the same as at age 1 month.[2] The presence and degree of prematurity decrease MAC. This may be because of the immaturity of the central nervous system or neurohumoral factors. Cerebral palsy and developmental delay also reduce the MAC by 25%[3] (also see Chapter 7).

FLUIDS AND ELECTROLYTES

Intraoperative Fluid Administration

Intravenous (IV) fluid given to children in the operating room serves one of four purposes: replacement of a deficit, maintenance fluids, balancing ongoing losses, and treatment of hypovolemia (also see Chapter 24). Although hypotonic solutions such as 0.2% normal saline with added dextrose and potassium are often used outside the operating room for maintenance fluid administration, generally, non–glucose-containing isotonic solutions are given in the operating room in order to avoid hyponatremia and serum potassium concentration abnormalities. Lactated Ringer solution and Plasma-Lyte A are the most commonly used isotonic solutions in pediatric patients. Administration of 5% albumin is the most common colloid used in pediatric patients, but disagreement exists as to the efficacy of this therapy versus isotonic crystalloid administration.

IV

Replacement of Preoperative Fluid Deficits

The preoperative deficit is the number of hours that a patient has had no oral intake or has been *nil per os* (NPO) multiplied by the hourly maintenance fluid requirement of the patient (Table 34.3). Generally, 50% of the deficit is replaced in the first hour of anesthesia, and the remaining 50% is replaced during the following 2 hours.[4]

Patients presenting for emergency surgery may have larger fluid deficits from vomiting, fever, third-space fluid loss, or blood loss that needs to be taken into account. The use of warmed fluids should be considered to avoid hypothermia with administration of large amounts of intravascular volume replacement.

Maintenance Fluids

The hourly maintenance rate should be calculated using the "4-2-1 rule" and should be administered in the form of isotonic solution throughout the case.

Ongoing Fluid Losses

Ongoing losses can be characterized as whole blood loss, third-space loss, and evaporation. When blood or colloid is used to replace blood loss, a ratio of 1:1 is used. When crystalloid is used to replace blood loss, a ratio of 3:1 is used. Third-space and evaporative losses vary with the invasiveness of the procedure, from noninvasive such as a strabismus repair to very invasive such as an exploratory laparotomy for necrotizing enterocolitis (NEC) (see Table 34.3). Third-space losses can be replaced with isotonic crystalloid.

Treatment of Hypovolemia

Intravascular volume can be monitored in pediatric patients by assessing the hemodynamic variables for the age group. Tachycardia and decreased arterial blood pressure suggest hypovolemia. Monitoring of urine output or central venous pressure can provide other information about intravascular volume status. If hypovolemia is suspected, a 10 to 20 mL/kg bolus of crystalloid or colloid can be given.

Glucose Administration

Glucose-containing solutions should not be used routinely in pediatric patients intraoperatively.[4] They should not be used to replace intravascular fluid deficits, third-space losses, or blood loss. In children older than 1 year of age the stress and catecholamine release associated with surgery usually prevent hypoglycemia. Glucose is commonly given to patients who are younger than 1 year of age or less than 10 kg. Pediatric patients at greater risk for developing hypoglycemia include premature and term neonates and any patient who is critically ill or who has hepatic dysfunction. Patients receiving total parenteral nutrition with high dextrose concentrations preoperatively can either be continued on a reduced rate of the same infusion or can be converted to a 5% or 10% dextrose-containing infusion to maintain the administration of glucose. An infusion pump should be used for high-concentration dextrose solutions to avoid bolus administration. Blood glucose concentration should be monitored closely in patients with risk of glucose instability.

TRANSFUSION THERAPY

Maximum Allowable Blood Loss

Before anesthesia, the maximum allowable blood loss (MABL) should be calculated for a given case and to prepare for possible transfusion of red blood cells (also

---

Table 34.3 Fluid Replacement in Children

Basis for Replacement	Fluid Requirements	
	Hourly	**24 Hr**
Maintenance		
Weight (kg)		
<10	4 mL/kg	100 mL/kg
11–20	40 mL + 2 mL/kg >10 kg	1000 mL + 50 mL/kg >10 kg
>20	60 mL + 1 mL/kg >20 kg	1500 mL + 20 mL/kg >20 kg
Replacement of Ongoing Losses[a]		
Type of surgery		
Noninvasive (e.g., inguinal hernia repair, clubfoot repair)	0–2 mL/kg/hr	
Mildly invasive (e.g., ureteral reimplantation)	2–4 mL/kg/hr	
Moderately invasive (e.g., elective bowel reanastomosis)	4–8 mL/kg/hr	
Significantly invasive (e.g., bowel resection for necrotizing enterocolitis)	≥10 mL/kg/hr	

[a]Replacement for ongoing losses with crystalloid must always be integrated with the patient's current cardiorespiratory status, status as evaluated during the surgical procedure, estimated blood loss with plans for blood product replacement, and baseline medical problems.

see Chapter 25). The estimated blood volume (EBV) is dependent on the age of the child and hematocrit (Hct):

$$MABL = EBV \times (Patient\ Hct - minimum\ acceptable\ Hct)/patient\ Hct$$

Initial treatment for blood loss is to maintain intravascular volume by administering crystalloid or colloid solution. When the Hct reaches the threshold, red blood cells should be transfused. The minimum acceptable Hct depends on patient age and comorbid conditions. For example, a higher Hct (e.g., 30%–45%) is desired in patients with cyanotic CHD, those with significant pulmonary disease, and infants with apnea/bradycardia or tachypnea/tachycardia.

Transfusion of Blood Products

Packed Red Blood Cells
Transfusion of 10 to 15 mL/kg of packed red blood cells (PRBCs) should increase the hemoglobin concentration by 2 to 3 g/dL. The estimated volume of transfusion of PRBCs should be predicted in advance in order to split units of cells in the blood bank into 10 to 15 mL/kg aliquots. This reduces the waste of a residual unit when only 60 mL, for example, is required for transfusion. It also allows the blood bank to reserve the remaining unit for later administration to the same patient, reducing multiple donor exposure for the patient.

Special processing of PRBCs, including leukocyte reduction and irradiation, is warranted in some settings, including young infants less than 4 months of age and immunosuppressed or transplant patients. Leukocyte reduction is achieved by removing white blood cells by filtration to a maximum concentration of 5×10^6 leukocytes per PRBC unit. White blood cells are responsible for febrile, nonhemolytic transfusion reactions; human leukocyte antigen (HLA) allosensitization; and transmission of cytomegalovirus.

Irradiation of blood products is necessary to reduce the risk of transfusion-associated graft-versus-host disease, a potentially fatal condition in which transfused lymphocytes engraft and proliferate in the bone marrow of the recipient. Irradiated blood should be given to immunocompromised children and to children with normal immunity who share an HLA haplotype with the donor. For this reason, all directed donor blood from family members is irradiated.

Platelets
Platelet concentrates are either derived from whole blood or collected by apheresis. They are suspended in plasma, which contains coagulation factors. Administration of 5 to 10 mL/kg of platelet concentrate should increase the platelet count by 50,000/dL to 100,000/dL. Indications for platelet transfusion are dependent on platelet number, function, and the presence or absence of bleeding.

Platelets are a cellular component of blood and may require irradiation using the same criteria noted earlier for PRBCs.

Fresh Frozen Plasma
Fresh frozen plasma (FFP) is administered to correct coagulopathy caused by insufficient coagulation factors. It contains all coagulation factors and regulatory proteins. Administration of 10 to 15 mL/kg will increase factor levels by 15% to 20%. Prothrombin complex concentrates are derived from human plasma and contain vitamin K–dependent coagulation factors. The use of these agents has been described as a substitute for FFP for emergent reversal of anticoagulation and for the treatment of coagulopathy after cardiopulmonary bypass surgery.[5-7]

Cryoprecipitate and Fibrinogen Concentrate
Cryoprecipitate and fibrinogen concentrate are sources of fibrinogen for replacement. Cryoprecipitate is primarily used as a source of fibrinogen, factor VIII, factor XIII, and von Willebrand factor. It is ideal for administration to infants because of high levels of these factors in a small volume. Administration of 1 unit (10–20 mL) for every 5 kg to a maximum of 4 units is usually adequate for correcting coagulopathy caused by insufficient fibrinogen. Fibrinogen concentrate is a plasma-derived source of fibrinogen. It is increasingly being used for fibrinogen replacement in pediatric cardiac surgery and other complex pediatric surgeries, including craniosynostosis and scoliosis repair. Viscoelastic testing, rotational thromboelastometry (ROTEM), or thromboelastography (TEG) is often used to guide replacement[8-10] (also see Chapter 23).

Antifibrinolytics

Antifibrinolytics include aprotinin, a serine protease inhibitor, and tranexamic acid and ε-aminocaproic acid, lysine analogs. These drugs can decrease bleeding and the transfusion requirements during pediatric cardiac, spine, and cranial reconstructive surgery. Aprotinin is not currently available for use owing to concerns about adverse effects in adults.

Recombinant Factor VIIa

Recombinant factor VIIa is indicated for the treatment and prevention of bleeding in patients with factor VII deficiency and hemophiliacs with inhibitors to factors VIII and IX. Over the last 10 years, there have been multiple reports of off-label use of the drug in nonhemophiliac pediatric patients in a variety of situations, including postcardiopulmonary bypass bleeding and trauma with a reduction in transfusion of blood products and normalization of coagulation studies. Concerns remain about the potential for thromboembolic complications.[11]

IV

PEDIATRIC AIRWAY

Airway Assessment

There is no valid airway assessment in children that is similar to the Mallampati classification in adults. Children are often uncooperative with examination. Care should be taken to inspect for micrognathia, midface hypoplasia, limited mouth opening or cervical mobility, and other craniofacial anomalies that can predict difficult laryngoscopy. The patient and parents should be questioned about the presence of loose teeth or orthodontic appliances that may be dislodged or broken during airway manipulation (also see Chapter 16).

Airway Management Techniques

Airway management techniques in children are similar to those in adult patients, although the anatomy differs. Infants and young children have larger craniums, and thus it is unnecessary to place a pillow under the occiput to achieve the "sniffing position" for airway management. The tongue is often relatively large in young infants and can more easily obstruct the airway. The cricoid ring is the narrowest part of the airway of the infant and young child instead of the laryngeal aperture at the vocal cords, as in adults. However, recent magnetic resonance imaging (MRI) and bronchoscopic data indicate that the pediatric airway is cylindrical, and the narrowest part is the glottis, as in adults.[12] The larynx is positioned relatively higher, at C4 in the neonate rather than C6 as in the adult. The epiglottis is omega-shaped and soft in the infant rather than U-shaped and stiff in the adult. Management of the airway using a facemask is more common in children. An appropriately sized mask should be selected, and care should be taken to optimally position the patient to avoid airway obstruction. If obstruction is encountered, continuous positive airway pressure of 5 to 10 cm H_2O or an oral airway can be introduced to restore airway patency.

Supraglottic airway (SGA) devices are also made in pediatric sizes and can be used for routine cases or as part of a difficult airway algorithm. SGA devices allow the patient to breathe spontaneously with no upper airway obstruction and without instrumentation of the trachea. They can also be used safely with pressure control mechanical ventilation in children. A 2014 metaanalysis found that the use of the laryngeal mask during pediatric anesthesia was associated with a decreased incidence of respiratory complications, including desaturation, laryngospasm, cough, and breath-holding, compared with tracheal intubation.[13] In a 2017 randomized controlled trial of SGA versus endotracheal tube in infants undergoing elective procedures there were fewer perioperative adverse respiratory events with the SGA as well.[14]

Endotracheal tubes are used for a large percentage of anesthetics in children. Historically, uncuffed tubes were the standard of care in children younger than 8 years of age because of concerns about subglottic stenosis and postextubation stridor. However, with the introduction of endotracheal tubes with high-volume/low-pressure cuffs, some studies suggest that there is no increased risk of airway edema with cuffed tubes and that the use of cuffed tubes may decrease the number of laryngoscopies and intubations caused by inappropriate tube size. As a result of innovation in material and design, cuffs are now very thin and do not enlarge the outer diameter of the tube, and downsizing the inner diameter tube size to compensate for the bulk of the cuff is no longer recommended.[15] A comparison of classic sizing for uncuffed and cuffed tubes and the new recommendations for cuffed tubes is displayed in Table 34.4. The Microcuff endotracheal tube differs from the conventional endotracheal tube in that it has a thinner polyurethane cuff that is positioned closer to the tip of the tube. With this design change, the Murphy eye was eliminated. There are some situations where this tube is advantageous, such as a distal tracheoesophageal fistula located very close to the carina, where ventilation with a conventional endotracheal tube may result in a loss of tidal volume through the fistula.[16] The lack of Murphy eye can also lead to an increased inability to ventilate when the tip becomes occluded with blood or secretions or when the tube is inappropriately deep (on the carina or in the mainstem bronchus). This can lead to barotrauma from an inability to exhale or the need for an emergent tube exchange.[17,18]

Table 34.4 Oral Endotracheal Tube (ETT) Size for Age

Age Group	Uncuffed ETT Size (ID mm)	Cuffed ETT Size (ID mm)
Preterm	2.5–3.0	NA
Term	3.0–3.5	3.0–3.5
1–6 mo	3.5	3.5
7–12 mo	4.0	3.5–4.0
1–2 yr	4.5	4.0–4.5
3–4 yr	4.5–5.0	4.5
5–6 yr	5.0–5.5	4.5–5.0
7–8 yr	NA	5.0–5.5
9–10 yr	NA	5.5–6.0
11–12 yr	NA	6.0–6.5
13–14 yr	NA	6.5–7.0
14+ yr	NA	7.0–7.5

Depth of insertion:
Multiplying the ID of the ETT by 3 yields the proper depth of insertion to the lips in centimeters. *Example:* 4.0 mm ETT × 3 = 12 cm for depth of insertion.

ID, Inner diameter.

Difficult Pediatric Airway

The difficult airway in children can be challenging because of a lack of patient cooperation in most age groups, which makes awake endotracheal intubation virtually impossible. Most techniques are performed under deep sedation or general anesthesia. A difficult airway should be anticipated in patients with craniofacial abnormalities or syndromes including Pierre Robin, Treacher Collins, and Goldenhar syndromes. A plan for management of the airway and equipment should be prepared.

Anesthesia can be induced intravenously or via inhalation. Adequacy of ventilation via a mask should be determined. At this point, the airway can be visualized or managed with a variety of airway adjuncts, including the optical stylet, videolaryngoscope, flexible fiber-optic bronchoscope, and the SGA, all of which are made in one or more pediatric sizes.[19] The SGA can be used as the primary airway management for the case or as a backup plan if tracheal intubation is required, either by temporarily securing the airway or as a conduit through which an endotracheal tube can be placed.[20] Maintaining oxygenation, either during periods of apnea or during intubation attempts in infants, can be accomplished using high-flow nasal cannula, modified nasopharyngeal airway, or modified nasal Ring-Adair-Elwyn (RAE) endotracheal tube.[21]

Prenatally diagnosed difficult airways (e.g., large cystic hygroma) are occasionally delivered as an *ex utero* intrapartum therapy (EXIT) procedure during which the fetus is partially delivered via cesarean section and the airway is secured while oxygenation is achieved via placental exchange (see later discussion).

ANESTHETIC CONSIDERATIONS

Preoperative Evaluation and Preparation

The preoperative evaluation of a pediatric patient differs from that of an adult for many reasons (also see Chapter 13). The age and weight of the child are extremely important, as equipment such as laryngoscopes, endotracheal tubes, masks, and IV fluid setups are based on the age and size of the child. Drugs are commonly dosed based on weight, and accuracy is critical to avoid underdosage and overdosage. A history of prematurity is important, including the gestational age at which the patient was delivered and any sequelae of prematurity such as cerebral palsy, chronic lung disease, and apnea and bradycardia. If the child has a genetic or dysmorphic syndrome, distinguishing features should be reviewed for potential impact on the anesthetic, including craniofacial or cervical spine abnormalities, that may lead to a difficult endotracheal intubation. Previous anesthetic history should be reviewed. A history of sleep-disordered breathing (obstructive sleep apnea), heralded by obstructed breathing or loud snoring during sleep, may be associated with difficult facemask ventilation and higher sensitivity to opioid-induced respiratory depression.

The family should be questioned about risk factors for malignant hyperthermia (MH), including family history of MH, patient history of MH, and congenital myopathies such as central core disease or King-Denborough syndrome. The parents should also be questioned about the presence of muscular dystrophies. Although possibly not associated with true MH, exposure to succinylcholine and inhaled anesthetics can result in hyperkalemia and rhabdomyolysis in patients with muscular dystrophy, and a nontriggering anesthetic (e.g., propofol) should be used.

A review of systems should be performed, and any pertinent positive findings should be explored. The patient and parent should be questioned about the presence or recent history of congestion, cough, fever, vomiting, or diarrhea, which may affect the decision to proceed with an elective procedure. Vital signs, including heart rate, respiratory rate, temperature, and arterial blood pressure, should be measured. Use of a pulse oximeter can be used to screen for occult cardiac or pulmonary disease.

Physical examination should include a general assessment of the patient's growth and development. The airway should be examined as thoroughly as possible with attention to craniofacial abnormalities, presence of micrognathia, and tonsillar size. The heart and lungs should be auscultated to evaluate for murmurs and wheezing or decreased breath sounds. The patient should be examined for any signs of infectious process, including rhinorrhea, tonsillar exudate, fever, and cough. Extremities should be examined for potential sites for IV access.

Preoperative Laboratory Testing

Routine preoperative laboratory testing for healthy children undergoing outpatient surgery is not indicated except in the case of urine pregnancy testing (UPT) (see later discussion). However, preoperative testing may be indicated in children with organ system dysfunction. For example, BUN, creatinine, and potassium levels should be tested preoperatively in patients with renal disease. Hemoglobin should be measured in former premature infants at risk for anemia having procedures associated with significant blood loss. Radiologic examination is not routinely performed. However, if recent radiographs, computed tomography (CT) scans, or MRIs are available, they should be reviewed. If echocardiogram results or subspecialist notes are available, they should also be reviewed.

Preoperative UPT of pediatric patients is a controversial topic. Adolescent females are unlikely to admit that they are sexually active or if there is a chance that they might be pregnant. Parents are reluctant to believe that their child might be pregnant. Asking the parent and child about the possibility of pregnancy can be uncomfortable for all parties. For these reasons, most hospitals

IV

have a policy on preoperative UPT and will test all female patients beginning at menarche or at an arbitrary age (e.g., 10 years old). Occasionally, a UPT will be positive, and there must be a process for verification. There must also be a process for revealing the results to the patient and parents and for counseling, based on local institutional considerations and individual state law.[22]

Recent Upper Respiratory Tract Infection

The presence or recent history of upper respiratory tract infection (URI) is another controversial topic. Whereas cancellations for URI were quite common in the past, the present view is that the risks associated with anesthetizing a child with URI are manageable with little morbidity. Still, there is a slightly increased risk of airway hyperreactivity with associated bronchospasm, laryngospasm, and postoperative arterial desaturation caused by atelectasis. Parents should be questioned about the presence of a URI. The patient should be examined for nasal congestion, cough, wheezing, and fever, and if a decision is made to proceed with the anesthetic, care should be taken to minimize risk of an adverse respiratory event.[23] Signs of lower respiratory tract infection (productive cough, fever, rales, wheezing, rhonchi, diminished or absent breath sounds) require cancellation of elective surgery. Practical considerations usually result in minor surgery being performed in the face of URI, especially ear, nose, and throat (ENT) procedures when URI is frequent, and the surgery will often decrease the frequency of these infections. Elective major surgery (i.e., intraabdominal, intrathoracic, cardiac) is usually postponed for 2 to 6 weeks.

Preoperative Fasting Guidelines

It is difficult for both the parents and the patient to keep a child NPO for an extended period, and fasting can lead to significant perioperative distress for the child and family. However, adherence to fasting guidelines minimizes the risk of aspiration of gastric contents. In the absence of bowel obstruction, gastroesophageal reflux, or other conditions leading to delayed gastric emptying NPO guidelines in children are as follows: Solid foods are allowed until 6 to 8 hours before anesthesia; milk, fortified breast milk, and infant formula until 6 hours before; unfortified breast milk until 4 hours before; and clear liquids until 2 hours before anesthesia.[24] Forethought in scheduling and giving preoperative instructions about NPO times can minimize the time without oral intake, and children who are scheduled later in the day are often able to ingest clear liquids until 2 hours before the beginning of the anesthetic. The American Society of Anesthesiologists guidelines currently reflect a fasting time of 2 hours for clear fluids. However, multiple global pediatric anesthesia societies (Europe, Australia, New Zealand) endorse a more liberal fasting time for clear fluids of 1 hour before an elective procedure. The 1-hour fasting time for clear liquids is being adopted at some large children's hospitals in the United States.[25,26]

Premedication

Both parental and patient anxiety can lead to significant perioperative stress and dissatisfaction. Attempts should be made to allay anxiety during the preoperative interview. If it appears that the family and child are significantly anxious, premedication may be required to calm and sedate the child. This may, in turn, improve parental anxiety.

The most widely used premedication in North America is midazolam. It can be administered via oral, intranasal, rectal, and IM routes. Midazolam 0.5 to 0.75 mg/kg provides adequate anxiolysis and sedation approximately 20 minutes after oral administration. Rarely, a child will experience a paradoxical reaction to midazolam characterized by agitation. Diazepam and lorazepam are most often used in older children and also produce sedation and amnesia.

Ketamine, a phencyclidine derivative, can also be used as an oral, nasal, rectal, or IM premedication. It produces sedation, amnesia, and analgesia, but it is also associated with excessive salivation, nystagmus, postoperative nausea and vomiting (PONV), and hallucinations. It does not depress airway reflexes, and airway tone is preserved. IM ketamine may be administered to agitated or developmentally delayed children who refuse to breathe via a mask or accept drugs for premedication.

The α_2-agonist clonidine, given orally, provides preoperative sedation that is similar to that produced by benzodiazepines. It acts centrally and peripherally to decrease arterial blood pressure. Anesthetic requirements are decreased so that a lower concentration of volatile anesthetic is required to produce the same effect. Clonidine does not cause airway obstruction and reduces requirements for postoperative pain medication. Clonidine has a longer onset of effect than most other drugs used for premedication and must be given at least 1 hour before the anesthetic. This reduces clonidine's utility in most busy, rapid-case-turnover settings.

Dexmedetomidine, another α_2-agonist, is becoming increasingly popular as a premedication. Though its onset is slightly longer than that of midazolam, it produces satisfactory sedation for parental separation and acceptance of breathing via a mask when given intranasally at a dose of 1 to 2 µg/kg. It also reduces the requirement for rescue analgesia and the incidence of postoperative agitation, delirium, and shivering.[27]

Parental presence at induction of anesthesia (PPIA) is another technique used to allay both patient and parental anxiety. The parent accompanies the child to either the operating room or an induction room for the induction of anesthesia. It can be comforting for both the parent and child. However, occasionally PPIA increases parental anxiety and can lead to increased patient anxiety and physiologic changes in the parent, including syncope. The temperament of both the child and the parent should be considered before the suggestion of PPIA.[28] A recent Cochrane review of nonpharmacologic interventions for assisting anesthetic induction in children concluded that PPIA is not useful. Other nonpharmacologic techniques, including low-sensory stimulation environment, hand-held video games, and behavioral intervention, are more likely to reduce anxiety and improve patient cooperation during induction of anesthesia.[29]

Perioperative Considerations

Thermoregulation and Heat Loss
Because of a larger surface area to weight ratio, small infants tend to lose heat more rapidly by both radiation and convection than adults when placed in a cold environment. Small infants are unable to shiver and rely on nonshivering thermogenesis by metabolizing brown fat for heat production. Heat loss can also be limited by thermoregulatory vasoconstriction. The warming of the operating room environment and the use of radiant warmers, warmed IV fluids, airway humidification, and forced air warming can help to preserve normothermia in children.

Perioperative hyperthermia may be caused by infection, inflammatory states, or overzealous warming. Hyperthermia is a late sign in MH; the first signs are usually tachycardia, hypercarbia, and acidosis.

Monitoring (Also See Chapter 20)
Standard American Society of Anesthesiologists monitors include electrocardiography (ECG), blood pressure monitoring, pulse oximetry, and capnography, and they should be used in every pediatric anesthetic. A nerve stimulator is recommended for monitoring neuromuscular blockade. The continuous auscultation of breath sounds via esophageal or precordial stethoscope is also recommended, but some surveys demonstrate that this monitor is being used less in favor of other monitors.[30] The monitoring of temperature is mandatory to detect MH or, more commonly, hypothermia.

Invasive arterial blood pressure and central venous pressure monitoring are indicated for invasive surgery and for patients with significant cardiopulmonary comorbid conditions. Monitoring cerebral oxygenation via near-infrared spectroscopy (NIRS) can be helpful during cardiac surgery and other cases in which cerebral perfusion may be compromised. Monitoring of processed electroencephalogram is also available for children to estimate and trend anesthetic depth, although there is some controversy over the reliability of this modality in children.[31]

Routes of Induction of Anesthesia
General anesthesia can be induced via inhalation or through the administration of IV or IM drugs in children.

An inhaled induction of anesthesia with sevoflurane in oxygen with or without nitrous oxide is a common method used in children because it does not require IV access. The child is taken to the operating or induction room, monitors are placed, and a facemask is applied. The concentration of inhaled anesthetic should be increased slowly in a cooperative child. As induction progresses, the child will usually pass through stage 2, the excitement phase. During this phase, coughing, vomiting, involuntary movement, and laryngospasm are possible. Attention should be devoted to the adequacy of the mask airway and the extent of obstruction. After the patient has passed through stage 2, an IV catheter can be placed. If laryngospasm occurs before placement of the peripheral IV catheter, treatment with continuous positive airway pressure or IM succinylcholine may be required.

IV induction is selected in children who already have IV access, who request an IV induction, or for whom an IV induction is indicated (full stomach, persistent gastroesophageal reflux disease, significant potential for cardiopulmonary compromise). In some medical centers a peripheral IV catheter is placed in all children presenting for surgery. The most common induction anesthetic in children is propofol 2 to 3 mg/kg. Neuromuscular blockade, usually rocuronium 0.6 to 1.2 mg/kg or vecuronium 0.08 to 0.1 mg/kg, is often used to facilitate tracheal intubation, particularly in older children. Intubation of the trachea without muscle relaxation, facilitated by a bolus of propofol 1 to 1.5 mg/kg after induction of anesthesia with sevoflurane, is a common approach in infants and young children without significant cardiopulmonary disease.

IM induction of anesthesia is used most commonly in developmentally delayed or severely uncooperative children and can be achieved with IM administration of ketamine (5 mg/kg). IM atropine or glycopyrrolate can be administered with the ketamine to decrease excess salivation. An IM ketamine induction may also be used in children with burns, poor peripheral veins, and a difficult airway because of extensive scarring for whom an inhaled induction of anesthesia may result in loss of both airway tone and the ability to ventilate the lungs via a mask.

Maintenance of Anesthesia
Anesthesia is maintained with inhaled anesthetic or IV administration of drugs or a combination of the two. Muscle relaxant can be used to facilitate operative exposure. However, neuromuscular blockade is probably used less frequently in children than in adults (also see Chapter 11).

Emergence
In pediatric anesthetic practice the decision to extubate the trachea while deeply anesthetized, or after emergence, must be made on a case-by-case basis. In

IV

some circumstances children are allowed to regain their airway reflexes and are extubated "awake." However, extubation during deep anesthesia and emergence without an endotracheal tube in place is a common practice in pediatric anesthesia. Advantages to waiting to extubate the trachea until the patient is awake include the ability to protect against aspiration of stomach contents or blood/secretions from the airway, and the relative safety of passing through stage 2 with an endotracheal tube in place. Advantages of extubation during deep anesthesia include no coughing or straining against suture lines or incisions and removal of the endotracheal tube before it leads to airway reactivity, both of which lead to a smoother emergence. The child then emerges in the operating room or in the recovery room, and meticulous attention is needed to ensure that laryngospasm or airway obstruction does not go undetected during or after transfer to the postanesthesia care unit (PACU).

Pain Management (Also See Chapter 40)

Analgesic drugs used for pain control in children include acetaminophen, nonsteroidal antiinflammatory drugs (NSAIDs), and opioids, and they can be administered by an oral, IM, or IV route. The most common opioids used in pediatric anesthesia are fentanyl and morphine. Side effects include sedation, respiratory depression, pruritus, and nausea/vomiting.

IV acetaminophen is now available and is a useful addition to systemic opioids in perioperative pain management. It is critical that perioperative acetaminophen administration is communicated between all providers and parents and documented on the medical record to prevent duplicate dosing and hepatotoxicity.

NSAIDs, including ketorolac, can be associated with platelet dysfunction, gastrointestinal bleeding, and renal dysfunction. Therefore patient comorbid conditions should be considered such as renal impairment and risk of bleeding (tonsillectomy, cardiac surgery) before administration of NSAIDs for pain control. Advantages of acetaminophen and NSAIDs include lack of excessive sedation and respiratory depression, which are common side effects of opioids.

Regional Anesthesia (Also See Chapters 17 and 18)

Regional anesthesia for intraoperative and postoperative pain control provides excellent analgesia with minimal side effects and decreases the requirement for opioid and nonopioid pain relievers. The single-shot caudal injection with local anesthetic is most commonly used for surgery at or below the level of the umbilicus. Alternatively, a catheter can be advanced into the caudal epidural space for delivery of an infusion of local anesthetic, which can be continued into the postoperative period. In children younger than 5 years of age the catheter can usually be advanced to any spinal level and deliver local anesthetic

to the associated dermatomes. In addition, the epidural space can be accessed relatively easily from the lumbar or thoracic level with subsequent placement of a catheter.

Other commonly performed regional blocks include brachial plexus, ilioinguinal nerve, femoral nerve, lateral femoral cutaneous nerve, sciatic and popliteal nerve, ankle, and penile blocks. These blocks are performed using landmark technique supplemented by ultrasound guidance; a peripheral nerve stimulator is also occasionally used by some anesthesia providers. When performing regional blocks in children, the child is commonly receiving a general anesthetic and is therefore unable to communicate the elicitation of a paresthesia or extreme pain on injection, which indicates a possible perineural injection. For this reason, guidance with ultrasound is widely assumed to increase the safety of peripheral nerve blocks in children.[32]

Spinal anesthesia has also been used as the sole anesthetic or in combination with a general anesthetic for a variety of cases. The technique gained popularity as an alternative to general anesthesia in former preterm infants having inguinal hernia repair who were at high risk for perioperative apnea. This technique has been expanded to infants undergoing longer urologic surgeries (e.g., hypospadias repair) for longer than 60 minutes.[33] Spinal anesthesia has also been used in older infants and children with and without increased risk for a general anesthetic.[34]

The Postanesthesia Care Unit (Also See Chapter 39)

Airway Monitoring

The PACU is a critical phase of the perioperative experience where a number of problems may be encountered. Many patients are transferred deeply anesthetized without an endotracheal tube from the operating room and will emerge from general anesthesia in the PACU. Transport from the operating room to the PACU must be carefully monitored to detect hypoventilation or airway obstruction; many institutions require supplemental oxygen administration and even pulse oximetry during transport. As the patient regains airway reflexes, there is an increased risk for airway obstruction. The airway must be monitored closely for signs of obstruction, laryngospasm, and hypoxemia, and a self-inflating or Jackson–Rees–style ventilating circuit and mask must be available to provide oxygen, continuous positive airway pressure, and ventilation. In addition, succinylcholine should be available to facilitate emergent reintubation or management of laryngospasm. The airway should also be monitored for stridor/postintubation croup caused by swelling. Treatment with dexamethasone, humidified oxygen, or nebulized racemic epinephrine may be warranted. Patients should also be monitored closely for apnea and hypoventilation in the recovery area.

Postoperative Nausea and Vomiting

PONV is ranked by parents as the most unwanted side effect of anesthesia. A recent study identified four risk factors that predict PONV in children: age 3 years and older, strabismus surgery, duration of surgery, and previous history of postoperative vomiting in the patient or in a parent or sibling. Risk reduction can be achieved with interventions or strategies including liberal fluid administration, the use of total IV anesthesia, the opiate-sparing effects of regional anesthesia/analgesia, and the use of IV acetaminophen or the alpha-$_2$ agonist dexmedetomidine or clonidine.[35] Two-drug pharmacologic prophylaxis with ondansetron and dexamethasone has an expected relative risk reduction for PONV of approximately 80%.[36] Aprepitant, an oral neurokinin-1 receptor antagonist, shows promise as a prophylactic antiemetic in pediatric patients. This may be helpful in patients who are at high risk of PONV but have a contraindication or relative contraindication to ondansetron (e.g., long QT) or corticosteroids (diabetes mellitus).[37] As administration of aprepitant and the IV NK-1 receptor antagonist fosaprepitant are associated with decreased efficacy of oral contraceptives, appropriate counseling of patients receiving the drug should be performed.[38]

Emergence Agitation and Delirium

Emergence agitation (EA) and emergence delirium (ED) are characterized by inconsolability, restlessness, nonpurposeful movements, incoherence, lack of eye contact, and decreased awareness of surroundings. EA/ED is frequently encountered in the PACU and can be troublesome to families, recovery room caregivers, and anesthesia care providers. Contributors to the development of EA/ED may include volatile anesthesia, type of surgery, the age of the patient, parental and/or patient anxiety, preexisting patient behavior, and the quality of interaction between the patient/family and health care staff. Unfortunately, EA/ED can be associated with postoperative maladaptive behavior lasting days to weeks.[39] The Pediatric Anesthesia Emergence Delirium (PAED) scale was developed to assist in the diagnosis of ED, as pain can be difficult to distinguish from EA/ED. Though many drugs, including propofol, fentanyl, clonidine, and dexmedetomidine, may decrease the incidence of ED, only low-dose ketamine and nalbuphine decrease the incidence without prolonging emergence.

Pain Control

The adequacy of pain control must be assessed frequently for pediatric patients of all ages from neonates to adolescents. Patients are recovering from a wide spectrum of procedures with differing amounts of associated pain. The children may be preverbal, nonverbal, or developmentally delayed and unable to communicate their pain level. There are several scales for assessing pain in children, including the FLACC (face, legs, activity, cry, consolability) and Wong–Baker Faces Pain Scale, along with evaluating vital signs. However, pain can be confused with anxiety, ED, and anger in children. Opioids can be titrated to effectively treat moderate to severe postoperative pain. NSAIDs or acetaminophen can also be administered, and if an epidural catheter is in place, it can be assessed for functionality and redosed.

Discharge Criteria

PACUs are often structured in two stages. Patients are transferred from the operating room directly to the first stage of recovery, where the airway is assessed continuously and acute postoperative pain and PONV are treated. After patients are awake with a stable airway and pain under control, they may be moved to a second stage to complete recovery. The modified Aldrete scoring system is the most frequently used scoring system to determine discharge readiness. In the outpatient setting patients may go directly from the operating room to second-stage recovery, known as *fast tracking.*

Behavioral Recovery

Children can develop maladaptive behavioral changes after surgery, including sleep and eating disturbances, separation anxiety, new-onset enuresis, and other behavioral issues. Parental anxiety, parental presence at induction, parental presence in the PACU, and the use of premedication have been shown to influence the incidence of these behavioral changes. Most of these behavioral changes do not persist beyond 3 days postoperatively. However, avoidance of negative behavior changes is associated with higher patient/parent satisfaction and a better overall perioperative experience.[28]

MEDICAL AND SURGICAL DISEASES AFFECTING THE NEONATE

Necrotizing Enterocolitis

NEC is a common surgical emergency in the neonate. This condition is primarily seen in premature infants, with over 90% of affected patients born before 36 weeks of gestation. The incidence of NEC among premature and low-birth-weight infants is 3% to 7% and is inversely proportional to gestational age. From 20% to 40% of infants with NEC will require surgery, with a surgical mortality rate of 23% to 36%.[40]

The pathophysiology of NEC involves intestinal mucosal ischemic injury secondary to reduced mesenteric blood flow, often in conjunction with a patent ductus arteriosus (PDA), with its resultant "steal" of blood flow away from the systemic circulation. Bacterial infection is also an important component, and signs of abdominal sepsis are prominent. Ischemia, infection, and inflammation may result in full-thickness necrosis of small

IV

intestine, particularly in the ileocolic region, with resultant intestinal perforation.

Clinical Manifestations

The patient presenting for surgery for NEC is most often a preterm infant, with other complications of prematurity such as respiratory distress syndrome, PDA, a history of birth asphyxia, or other cardiorespiratory instability. Clinical signs include abdominal distention; bloody stools; dilated intestinal loops and pneumatosis intestinalis on abdominal radiograph; temperature instability; and signs of sepsis, including thrombocytopenia, hemodynamic instability, and disseminated intravascular coagulopathy (DIC). Intestinal perforation is evident on abdominal radiography and is a surgical emergency; these patients are often critically ill or unstable with hypotension, DIC, metabolic acidosis, and worsening respiratory status.

Medical and Surgical Treatment

Initial treatment of NEC without intestinal perforation or other signs of extensive bowel necrosis is usually medical, with broad-spectrum antibiotics, gastric decompression, serial abdominal examination and radiographs, and careful monitoring for signs of cardiorespiratory decompensation. Originally, surgery for NEC with perforation was by laparotomy, resection of necrotic intestine, and creation of ostomies. This necessitated later reconstructive surgery and often resulted in resection of extensive lengths of small intestine, resulting in short-gut syndrome. In more recent years primary peritoneal drainage, whereby a small incision is made and a surgical drain is left in place, has gained popularity for smaller, sicker infants, who may then have definitive surgery later when their medical condition has improved. Some patients may not require further treatment at all, and survival using this more conservative approach is comparable in many series.[40]

Management of Anesthesia

Surgery for NEC is most often emergent, and preoperative preparation should focus on assessment and correction of fluid and electrolyte abnormalities, hemodynamic and respiratory instability, providing broad-spectrum antibiotics, and correcting coagulation abnormalities. Surgery for NEC can be performed at the bedside in the neonatal intensive care unit (NICU), necessitating a mobile surgical and anesthesia team and equipment. Most patients are already tracheally intubated. Monitoring often includes a peripheral arterial catheter; umbilical artery catheters are often removed because of concern over further mesenteric ischemia. Central venous access is often desirable, but attempts to secure invasive monitors should not delay emergent surgery.

Anesthesia with synthetic opioids such as fentanyl is the regimen best tolerated in the critically unstable neonate. Doses are titrated, starting at 2 to 5 µg/kg, but additional doses are added to provide 20 to 50 µg/kg fentanyl if tolerated. Volatile anesthetics are often not tolerated owing to vasodilatory effects, and small doses of benzodiazepines such as midazolam 0.05 to 0.1 mg/kg or ketamine 0.5 mg/kg may be added. Muscle relaxation with rocuronium, vecuronium, or another nondepolarizing neuromuscular blocking drug is necessary. Because of large fluid losses from exposed intestine undergoing resection, IV fluid requirements are often very large, at 10 to 20 mL/kg/hr, and 5% albumin, PRBCs, FFP, and platelets are often infused in the face of DIC and significant blood loss. Inotropic support in the form of dopamine 5 to 10 µg/kg/min or epinephrine 0.03 to 0.05 µg/kg/min is often needed and should be instituted early, rather than infusing excessive amounts of IV fluid to maintain blood pressure in unstable patients. Calcium chloride or gluconate bolus is often necessary to maintain normal ionized calcium levels to preserve myocardial contractility and vascular tone, particularly with infusion of significant volumes of citrated blood products. Frequent analysis of arterial blood gases to measure acid–base status and oxygenation, in addition to serum electrolytes, glucose, ionized calcium, and lactate, is often desirable to direct therapy. Mechanical ventilation is adjusted to maintain Pao_2 50 to 70 mm Hg and Spo_2 90% to 95% in the premature infant; however, in the extremely ill patient it is preferable to maintain somewhat higher oxygen tensions to allow for a margin of safety. Hemoglobin should be maintained at 10 to 15 g/dL to preserve oxygen-carrying capacity. Temperature management is critical, and these surgeries are often performed on the patient's overhead warming bed. The operating room temperature must be 85°F to 90°F (29–32°C) or higher, and forced air warming and warmed blood products must be used in an effort to maintain core temperature at 96.8°F (36°C) or higher. Postoperatively, mechanical ventilation, inotropic and fluid support, and antibiotics are continued, and a full report of the operation and anesthetic is given to the NICU team.

Abdominal Wall Defects: Gastroschisis and Omphalocele

Gastroschisis is an abdominal wall defect whereby the intestines protrude, usually to the right of the umbilical cord, without a covering sac, with the umbilical cord not part of the defect (Fig. 34.2).[41] These infants most often do not have associated congenital or chromosomal anomalies. An omphalocele is a midline defect with the intestines covered by a peritoneal sac and the umbilical cord incorporated into the defect (Fig. 34.3). These neonates frequently have other associated anomalies, including CHD.

Medical and Surgical Treatment

These diagnoses may be made prenatally, and presurgical management includes covering the exposed bowel

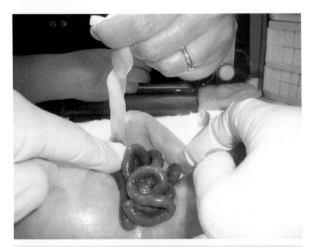

Fig. 34.2 Gastroschisis. Note position to the right of the umbilical cord, which is not included in the defect. It is also not covered with a peritoneal sac. (From Marven S, Owen A. Contemporary postnatal surgical management strategies for congenital abdominal wall defects. *Semin Pediatr Surg.* 2008;17:224, used with permission.)

with plastic or other synthetic material, attention to fluid replacement, and prevention of volvulus and bowel ischemia. Nasogastric decompression is important to minimize fluid and air accumulation. The size of the defects varies greatly; formerly even large defects were candidates for primary surgical reduction of the viscera and fascial closure, as this was thought to prevent later intestinal complications. However, with excessive increases in intraabdominal pressure, an abdominal compartment syndrome can arise, resulting in intestinal ischemia and renal failure. In addition, the sudden increase in intraabdominal pressure may lead to increased ventilatory requirements, often necessitating days of sedation, muscle relaxation, and careful monitoring of ventilatory and hemodynamic status. Now a staged approach is often used, which involves containing the viscera in a Silastic silo with its edges sutured to the peritoneum around the defect. Then, using gravity, compression of the bowel, traction, and expansion of the abdominal cavity, the viscera are gradually reduced into the peritoneal cavity over a period of days to weeks. Surgical closure of the peritoneum and skin is undertaken at the end of this period. Some small to moderate-sized defects can be managed with a similar staged reduction strategy, with the peritoneum and skin defects healing by secondary intention.

Management of Anesthesia

Because of the modern staged approach, the challenges of providing anesthesia for a one-stage reduction and closure are rarely encountered. Still, the initial surgery is often to suture the Silastic silo and partially reduce the viscera. Preoperative preparation includes maintaining

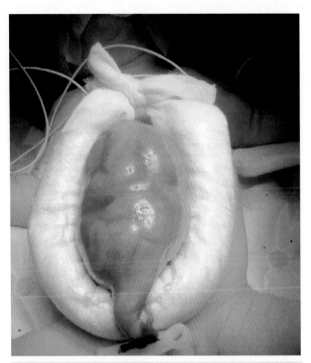

Fig. 34.3 A giant omphalocele supported with dressing collar. Note the midline position, covering with peritoneal sac, and inclusion of the umbilical cord. (From Marven S, Owen A. Contemporary postnatal surgical management strategies for congenital abdominal wall defects. *Semin Pediatr Surg.* 2008;17:223, used with permission.)

adequate fluid replacement to account for losses from the exposed viscera. These infants may be premature but are often full term and have a stable cardiorespiratory status. The general considerations noted earlier for NEC surgery concerning temperature management and fluid replacement apply to surgery for abdominal wall defects. Induction of anesthesia and tracheal intubation can be accomplished with a variety of drugs, with precautions to prevent aspiration of gastric contents. The umbilical vessels are not available, so secure large-bore venous access should be obtained, and possibly arterial catheter monitoring for patients with very large defects or unstable cardiorespiratory status. IV fluid replacement of 10 to 20 mL/kg/hr is important, along with administration of 5% or 10% dextrose at maintenance rates. Anesthesia can be maintained with volatile anesthetics, benzodiazepines, and opioids, with the dose depending on plans for tracheal extubation at the end of the procedure. If the primary procedure is silo placement without primary reduction, the tracheas of full-term infants can often be extubated at the end of the procedure, and subsequent reductions can be done at the bedside with small-dose sedation. The final fascial and skin closure will require a full general anesthetic. If a full reduction and closure of a major defect is planned, arterial and central venous

IV

pressure monitoring are important, along with bladder catheterization and careful management of cardiorespiratory status. This often requires significant increases in positive end-expiratory pressure, additional fluid administration, and inotropic support, in addition to prolonged postoperative ventilation, sedation, and muscle relaxation.

Tracheoesophageal Fistula

Tracheoesophageal fistula (TEF) is seen in five different anatomic configurations (Fig. 34.4), with the most common being type C, with esophageal atresia and a distal TEF. Diagnosis is made when the neonate experiences choking and cyanosis when attempting oral feeds. The chest and abdominal radiograph reveal an inability to pass an orogastric tube, which lodges in the blind esophageal pouch, and the presence of gas-filled intestines from the distal TEF. Infants with TEF often have other anomalies, and many have VACTERL association (*v*ertebral defects, imperforate *a*nus, *c*ardiac defects, *t*racheoesophageal fistula, *r*enal anomalies, *l*imb anomalies). A thorough evaluation for these additional defects, especially cardiac, should be undertaken in these infants. The severity of illness can be mild (e.g., feeding difficulties in a full-term neonate with no respiratory distress), but some patients are critically ill. Severe respiratory failure can result from continuous aspiration of gastric contents via the distal TEF, exacerbated by respiratory distress syndrome and massive abdominal distention from filling of the stomach with gas from the TEF. Patients at more frequent risk of perioperative morbidity and mortality include those with complex CHD, weight less than 2 kg, poor pulmonary

compliance, large pericarinal fistulas, and those scheduled for thoracoscopic repair.[42]

Surgical Approaches

Earlier approaches were usually staged, often first performing a gastrostomy under local anesthesia to decompress the stomach and allow some recovery of pulmonary function. Then, a right thoracotomy would be performed to ligate the TEF and possibly to reconstruct the esophageal atresia. Other approaches included a cervical esophagostomy to drain the upper esophageal pouch and prevent aspiration. In recent years the staged approach has largely been abandoned. In the current era a one-stage ligation of the TEF with primary esophageal repair, without a gastrostomy, is the preferred strategy in about 80% to 90% of patients.[43] Critically ill premature infants may still require gastrostomy before thoracotomy and TEF ligation, and if the gap between esophageal segments is too long, gastrostomy followed by esophageal dilation and stretching may be required after the initial thoracotomy. Outcomes of neonatal TEF surgery vary; the critically ill premature infant or neonate with multiple anomalies has a higher mortality and morbidity rate; the full-term neonate without other problems has an operative survival rate approaching 100%.

Anesthetic Management

The critically ill neonate with high ventilation pressures and gastric distention will emergently undergo anesthesia for right thoracotomy and ligation of the TEF. These infants may present in extremis owing to a large TEF, with most of the tidal volume being lost through the TEF, severely compromising ventilation. Manual ventilation, inotropic support, sodium bicarbonate, and vasoactive bolus drugs

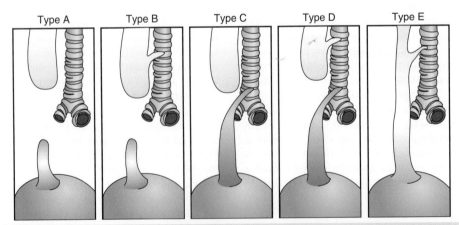

Fig. 34.4 Classification of tracheoesophageal anomalies in descending order of incidence. Type A (8%) is esophageal atresia without a tracheoesophageal fistula. Type B (1%) is esophageal atresia with a proximal tracheoesophageal fistula. Type C (86%) is esophageal atresia with a distal tracheoesophageal fistula. Type D (1%) is esophageal atresia with both proximal and distal tracheoesophageal fistulas. Type E (4%) is an H-type fistula without esophageal atresia. (From Gross RE. Artesia of the esophagus. In *The Surgery of Infancy and Childhood*. Philadelphia: Saunders; 1953:75–102.)

such as epinephrine and atropine may be needed until the TEF is ligated and the stomach decompressed. More commonly the trachea is intubated and there are varying degrees of difficulty with ventilation. After the patient is transported carefully to the operating room, anesthesia is carefully induced with the administration of IV or inhaled anesthetics and muscle relaxants. The patient is then positioned for right thoracotomy. An arterial catheter is essential for monitoring of arterial blood pressure and gas exchange. Very careful attention is paid to adequacy of ventilation during the entire case, as the endotracheal tube may migrate into the TEF and compromise ventilation. End-tidal CO_2, careful observation of lung inflation and chest movement, and a precordial stethoscope in the left axillary area are important monitors. Periods of difficult ventilation and hypoxemia during lung retraction and TEF ligation should be expected. Normally, after the TEF is ligated, ventilation improves dramatically.

In the patient whose trachea is not intubated awake tracheal intubation was classically considered to be the best technique, but in the modern era this is rarely practiced. Instead, either IV or inhaled induction of anesthesia, with muscle relaxation, can be achieved after suctioning the upper esophageal pouch and administration of oxygen. Then, an endotracheal tube is passed into the distal trachea, and gentle positive-pressure ventilation is accomplished with careful assessment of effectiveness of ventilation. Endotracheal tube migration into the TEF should be suspected with ventilation difficulties. Bronchoscopy is performed in some centers to assess the size and position of the TEF before surgery and to properly position the endotracheal tube; only in the presence of a large TEF (>3 mm) located near the carina is there likely to be difficulty with ventilation.[44] After ligation of the TEF, the esophagus is usually repaired primarily. Some centers are performing TEF repair via the video-assisted thoracoscopy approach, which itself can cause difficulty with ventilation secondary to the CO_2 insufflation. Although it is possible to extubate the trachea in the operating room in a vigorous full-term infant without complications, a more prudent approach is to leave the trachea intubated to allow adequate analgesic administration in the NICU. If the patient requires reintubation, the subsequent airway manipulation could disrupt the esophageal repair. A nasogastric tube is placed by the surgeon in the operating room for early gastric decompression and feeding.

Congenital Diaphragmatic Hernia

Congenital diaphragmatic hernia (CDH) is a defect in the diaphragm evident early in gestation, which results in the herniation of the intestines, spleen, and sometimes stomach or liver, into the thorax. Most commonly this is on the left side through the foramen of Bochdalek and results in severe restriction of lung development (Fig. 34.5). This lesion is often diagnosed prenatally;

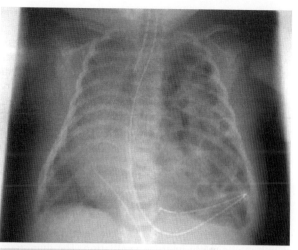

Fig. 34.5 Left-sided congenital diaphragmatic hernia. Note bowel loops filling the left hemithorax and nasogastric tube in the stomach, which is also herniated through the defect. The heart is shifted to the right side of the chest. (From de Buys Roessingh AS, Dinh-Xuan A. Congenital diaphragmatic hernia: Current status and review of the literature. *Eur J Pediatr.* 2009;168:398, used with permission.)

the neonate with significant defects presents with respiratory failure, requiring mechanical ventilation. These neonates present with a scaphoid abdomen, bowel sounds in the chest, respiratory distress, and cyanosis of varying degrees. Pulmonary hypertension from lung hypoplasia and immediate postnatal elevation in PVR cause right-to-left shunting through patent foramen ovale and ductus arteriosus, often resulting in severe cyanosis from persistent fetal circulation. In these cases surgical treatment, which consists of an abdominal or thoracoabdominal incision to reduce the viscera into the abdominal cavity and repair the diaphragm either primarily or with a synthetic mesh material, must be delayed while therapy is instituted to stabilize the medical condition of the infant. Laparoscopic repair has also been described. High-frequency oscillatory ventilation (HFOV) to improve gas exchange in hypoplastic lungs, inhaled nitric oxide (iNO) to treat the pulmonary hypertension, or extracorporeal membrane oxygenation (ECMO) to stabilize the cardiorespiratory status in the most severely affected neonates may be necessary. Surgical repair is then undertaken several days later, sometimes while on ECMO, which results in reduction of the abdominal viscera but does not solve the problem of lung hypoplasia and pulmonary hypertension, which may require days or weeks of support until they improve sufficiently.[45]

Management of Anesthesia

These infants are often critically ill. Transport to the operating room is achieved carefully. HFOV may need to

IV

be transitioned to conventional ventilation, as surgery with HFOV may not be possible. iNO should be continued throughout the operating room course. Anesthesia is often provided with high-dose synthetic opioids such as fentanyl 25 to 50 µg/kg or more to provide analgesia and blunt the pulmonary hypertensive response to painful stimuli. Volatile anesthetics are often not tolerated, so small doses of benzodiazepines or ketamine can provide amnesia. Monitoring of arterial and central venous pressures is essential, and inotropic support with dopamine or epinephrine is often necessary. Frequent arterial blood gases are analyzed, and changes in ventilation are made to maximize oxygenation, reduce $PaCO_2$, and increase pH to lower pulmonary artery pressures. After left thoracoabdominal incision at the costal margin, the abdominal contents are reduced out of the thorax, which may acutely improve ventilation. The diaphragm is reconstructed with a synthetic mesh material. Manual ventilation or ventilation with an intensive care unit (ICU) ventilator may be necessary throughout the case, as many standard anesthesia machine ventilators are often not capable of delivering the high inspired gas flows and small tidal volumes necessary to ventilate such patients. The patient is transported back to the NICU, where HFOV may need to be reinstated and iNO should be continued.

The most severely ill neonates with CDH receive ECMO support, and surgery may be done while on ECMO, which is problematic because of bleeding secondary to heparinization. Adequate blood products, including PRBCs, platelets, and FFP, must be available if the repair is done on ECMO. Anesthesia is provided with high-dose opioids, benzodiazepines, or ketamine.

Patent Ductus Arteriosus

The PDA is most often seen in the premature neonate and can result in pulmonary overcirculation and pulmonary edema, reduced ventilatory compliance, and ventilator dependence worsened by concurrent respiratory distress syndrome or pneumonia. The PDA may prevent weaning from the ventilator and result in secondary complications such as feeding intolerance or NEC. Clinical presentation includes persistent pulmonary edema, bounding pulses, and wide pulse pressure from diastolic runoff from the aorta to the pulmonary artery through the PDA. Sometimes, the large left-to-right shunt from the PDA causes cardiac failure and hypotension requiring inotropic support. Diagnosis is made with transthoracic echocardiography. Attempts at medical closure with indomethacin, ibuprofen, or acetaminophen may be successful, though some of these pharmacologic agents may adversely affect renal and platelet function. This should be considered in the preoperative evaluation of a neonate with PDA who has failed medical therapy and requires surgical intervention.[46]

Management of Anesthesia

The patient is often a small premature neonate weighing 500 to 1000 g who is ventilator dependent and may be hemodynamically unstable. Surgery may be done at the bedside in the NICU in some medical centers. Transport to the operating room must be done carefully with continuous monitoring. Anesthesia is normally provided with synthetic opioids such as fentanyl 25 to 50 µg/kg, muscle relaxation with a nondepolarizing drug, and small doses of benzodiazepines or ketamine, as volatile anesthetics are usually not tolerated. Arterial monitoring is useful for frequent assessment of hemodynamics and arterial blood gases. A left thoracotomy is done, and the PDA is approached via a retropleural dissection. Careful monitoring of ventilation with visual inspection, capnography, and a precordial or esophageal stethoscope is performed, as ventilation is easily compromised. Because of the risk of worsening retinopathy of prematurity (ROP), target PaO_2 is normally 50 to 80 mm Hg and SpO_2 90% to 95%, so high inspired FiO_2 is avoided unless absolutely necessary. The PDA is often larger than the descending thoracic aorta; monitoring with a pulse oximeter and blood pressure cuff on the lower extremity is important to ensure that the surgeon identifies and ligates the correct structure. The PDA can be ligated with sutures or surgical clips. PRBCs must be immediately available in case there is bleeding from damage to the paper-thin PDA. Maintenance of normothermia and provision of glucose is critically important during PDA ligation in the premature infant. Most infants will remain mechanically ventilated for some period after PDA ligation. In recent years, very small PDA occlusion devices have become available for transcatheter occlusion in premature infants in the cardiac catheterization laboratory. This approach has a low incidence of complications and has become the preferred method in many centers.[47]

In contrast to the premature infant with otherwise normal cardiac anatomy in whom the PDA must be closed, infants with CHD may be dependent on the PDA to provide pulmonary blood flow in the case of pulmonary atresia or stenosis, or systemic blood flow in the case of hypoplasia of left-sided cardiac structures such as severe coarctation of the aorta or hypoplastic left-sided heart syndrome. Prostaglandin E_1 is infused in these patients at 0.01 to 0.05 µg/kg/min and must be maintained until a stable source of pulmonary blood flow is established via surgical or transcatheter intervention.

Retinopathy of Prematurity

ROP is a vasoproliferative disease affecting premature or low-birth-weight infants. Five stages of ROP exist, and in stages 4 and 5, retinal detachment occurs, which can result in permanent visual loss.[48] The pathophysiology is complex, with the more premature infants at higher risk, but one of the main causes is excessive oxygen tensions in the vessels of the retina, accompanied by wide swings in oxygen tension such as those seen in cardiopulmonary instability with ventilated premature infants with respiratory distress syndrome, PDA, sepsis, apnea/bradycardia, and other problems associated with prematurity. Thus SpO_2 is maintained at 88% to 93% in many premature infants, with resulting oxygen tensions of 50 to 70 mm Hg targeted. Excessive oxygen tensions, as may be seen with general endotracheal anesthesia, are to be avoided, even if short-lived. The challenge for the anesthesia provider caring for such infants is to manage oxygenation with these restrictions in mind.

Premature infants hospitalized in the NICU receive regular retinal examinations, and if high-risk type I or greater ROP is diagnosed, urgent surgical therapy is undertaken within 24 to 72 hours to maximize visual outcomes. This often results in the urgent scheduling of treatment during evening and weekend hours. Retinal ablative therapy with indirect laser photocoagulation of proliferating vessels in one or both eyes is the treatment of choice. Cryotherapy may also be used, and at more severe stages, a vitrectomy may be required.

Management of Anesthesia

Because of the urgent or emergent nature of ROP surgery, the patient may not have feeding withheld. If the patient is still ventilated, any anesthetic technique, usually in conjunction with muscle relaxation, may be used. If the patient is not ventilated, any technique for induction, followed by muscle relaxation and endotracheal intubation, may be used. As these cases may last several hours, especially with extensive disease in both eyes, attention must be paid to patient temperature and provision of glucose during the surgery. Because of the often prolonged nature of the anesthetic, the risk of postanesthetic apnea in the premature infant, and the eye discomfort necessitating analgesia after the procedure, mechanical ventilation should be controlled after ROP surgery for 12 to 24 hours. Regardless of airway management after surgery, the patient must be carefully monitored in the NICU setting for postanesthetic problems.

Myelomeningocele

Myelomeningocele is a developmental defect of the neural tube, resulting in an open neural placode covered only by a thin membrane and cerebrospinal fluid. The defect is often diagnosed prenatally, varies in size, and may be located in the thoracolumbar or lumbosacral spine areas. The most common presentation is a lumbosacral myelomeningocele in a full-term infant. Preoperatively, it is critical not to allow the sac covering the spinal defect to rupture, which will increase the risk of meningitis. These infants are nursed prone, with a moist gauze covering the defect. Surgery is scheduled emergently and consists of dissection of nerve roots and covering the defect with

fascia and skin. In addition, over 75% of infants have hydrocephalus, and many have Arnold-Chiari malformation of the spinal cord and brainstem; these patients will require a ventriculoperitoneal shunt, usually done after the initial repair. Long-term outcome depends on early repair to prevent infection and the level of spinal cord dysfunction.[49]

Management of Anesthesia

Great care must be taken to prevent rupture of the sac covering the myelomeningocele during transport and positioning for induction of anesthesia and surgery. The infant cannot lie directly supine for this reason. Anesthetic induction and endotracheal intubation can be performed with the infant in the left lateral decubitus position. An alternative approach is to carefully place the infant supine in a doughnut-shaped padded foam bolster so that the myelomeningocele defect is in the center but not touching the operating room bed. After confirmation of endotracheal tube position, the infant is positioned prone for surgery. Any technique can be used for induction and maintenance of anesthesia, but the surgeon usually performs the repair under the microscope and requests that no muscle relaxant be used during the repair portion of the surgery so that motor function can be assessed. In addition, as patients with myelomeningocele repair at birth are at highest risk for developing latex allergy, all surgical gloves and all other materials in contact with the patient must be latex free. After surgery, the trachea can be extubated, using the same positioning techniques as for intubation. The patient then is turned prone and is kept in this position in which the infant will be nursed for several days. Myelomeningocele is now often repaired *in utero*, using open or fetoscopic techniques (see later).[50]

Pyloric Stenosis

Pyloric stenosis is hypertrophy of the pyloric muscle leading to a gastric outlet obstruction. A typical presentation is a young infant between 2 and 8 weeks of age with persistent projectile vomiting. This results in weight loss, dehydration, and electrolyte imbalance consisting of a hypochloremic, hypokalemic metabolic alkalosis from loss of hydrogen and chloride ions from stomach contents. These infants may develop severe dehydration, lethargy, poor skin turgor, sunken eyes and fontanel, poor urine output, and plasma chloride concentrations as low as 65 to 70 mEq/dL. Historically, these patients presented late with marked malnutrition.[51] Diagnosis is by clinical history; there is a 5:1 male predominance, and average age at presentation is 5 to 6 weeks. An olive-shaped and -sized mass may be palpable in the epigastrium; definitive diagnosis is made by ultrasound. Repair of pyloric stenosis is *not* a surgical emergency. The patient must be rehydrated, starting with a bolus of 10 to 20 mL/kg of normal saline or lactated

Ringer solution, followed by greater-than-maintenance-rate IV fluids (usually 5% dextrose in half-normal saline with potassium chloride). The fluid and electrolyte status is followed carefully and laboratory values rechecked periodically. When the patient has been rehydrated to a normal vascular volume and normal or near-normal electrolytes, the patient is ready for surgery. Some groups use a chloride value of >100 mEq/L and adequate urine output to determine readiness for surgery.[52] This preparation may require 12 to 72 hours, depending on the severity at presentation.[53] The degree of preoperative metabolic alkalosis also correlates with the duration of postoperative emesis, time to goal feeds, and length of stay.[54]

Management of Anesthesia

After adequate rehydration, the patient is brought to the operating room, and gastric contents are evacuated with a large-bore orogastric suction catheter before induction of anesthesia to reduce the risk of aspiration. Although awake tracheal intubation was the preferred technique in the past, this is rarely practiced in the modern era. After preoxygenation, the patient is administered an IV induction dose of propofol 2 to 2.5 mg/kg. Cricoid pressure is applied, and paralysis is achieved with succinylcholine 1 to 2 mg/kg (after pretreatment with atropine) or, preferably, a nondepolarizing muscle relaxant such as rocuronium. A modified rapid-sequence technique, with rapid small tidal volume via mask ventilation through cricoid pressure, may be used to prevent arterial desaturation in a young infant whose oxygen consumption is two to three times that of the adult. Inhalation induction may also be employed, though not as commonly in the United States.[55] After successful confirmation of tracheal intubation, maintenance of anesthesia proceeds with a volatile anesthetic. Opioids are often avoided because of the risk of postanesthetic apnea in pyloric stenosis. Instead, postoperative analgesia is provided by local anesthetic infiltration of the incision by the surgeon, in addition to acetaminophen or ketorolac. Supplemental regional anesthesia/analgesia, most commonly via a caudal approach, may also be employed.[55] Surgery proceeds either via small open epigastric incision or via laparoscopy with CO_2 insufflation of the abdomen. After conclusion of the surgery, a nasogastric tube may be left in place. The trachea is extubated after reversal of nondepolarizing muscle relaxant and full return of airway reflexes, in addition to a regular breathing pattern without pauses or apnea. Because of the metabolic alkalosis seen in many pyloric stenosis patients, cerebrospinal fluid pH may be increased, causing a reduction in respiratory drive, which is not corrected for 12 to 48 hours. This, in conjunction with respiratory drive that may not be fully mature until 44 weeks' postconceptual age, may place even full-term infants undergoing pyloromyotomy at risk for postanesthetic apnea. These patients should be monitored for 12 to 24 hours after anesthesia for this complication.[56]

CONGENITAL HEART DISEASE

CHD is present in approximately 1 in 100 live births and is the most common indication for surgery or invasive catheter treatment in the first year of life.[57] This section will describe the basic classification of CHD and the fundamental pathophysiology of the most common lesions. Preanesthetic evaluation and preparation are similar to that described earlier; in addition, an ECG, chest radiograph, and echocardiogram are available for cardiac surgery and most noncardiac procedures. Cardiac catheterization, CT, and MRI are also frequently employed to assist in preoperative planning. An important consideration is whether the patient has had previous corrective or palliative cardiac surgery and whether there are residual defects. Detailed anesthetic management of CHD is beyond the scope of this chapter and is available in a number of reference textbooks.[58,59]

Left-to-Right Shunts

Left-to-right shunts arise from a communication between the left and right chambers of the heart or between the great vessels—the aorta and pulmonary artery. Ventricular septal defect (VSD) (Figs. 34.6 and 34.7), atrial septal defect (ASD) (Fig. 34.8), and PDA (Fig. 34.9) are the three most common CHD lesions and together comprise approximately 50% of all lesions.[57] The pathophysiology of these lesions depends on the degree of left-to-right shunting, which in turn derives from a number of factors (Fig. 34.10), including the size and position of the defect, pressure gradient between chambers, relative pulmonary and systemic vascular resistance, and relative compliance of right versus left ventricle. Increased flow across the defect results in increased pulmonary blood flow and return to the left atrium and left ventricle. Significant shunting (i.e., greater than a pulmonary to systemic blood flow ratio of 2:1) may result in pulmonary venous congestion and interstitial pulmonary edema, which results in increased work of breathing manifested by tachypnea, intercostal retractions, and poor feeding in infants with congestive heart failure. Flow and pressure in the pulmonary artery are increased with large left-to-right shunts, which can result in permanent remodeling of the pulmonary vasculature if the defect is not closed. The resulting fixed pulmonary hypertension causes right ventricular (RV) hypertrophy, and pressure in the RV can exceed left ventricular (LV) pressure, resulting in reversal of the shunt to a right-to-left shunt. The patient then becomes cyanotic and can progress to Eisenmenger syndrome, a condition of long-standing irreversible cyanosis. Eisenmenger syndrome is very rare in the modern era because of the early correction of left-to-right shunting defects. Surgical or catheter repair of these defects is undertaken at any time in life, ranging from infancy to adulthood, depending on the size of the defect and severity of symptoms.

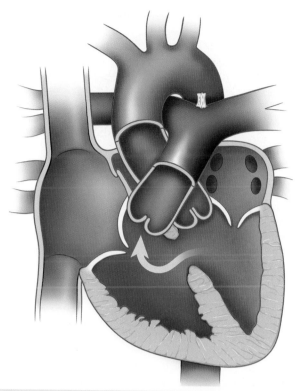

Fig. 34.6 Ventricular septal defect (VSD). Left-to-right shunt between left and right ventricles can result in pulmonary overcirculation and congestive heart failure. (Reproduced with permission from Cabrera AG, Bastrero P, Qureshi AM, et al. Ventricular septal defect. In Mery CR, Bastrero P, Hall SR, et al. [eds.] *Texas Children's Hospital Handbook of Congenital Heart Disease.* Houston: Texas Children's Hospital; 2020:97.)

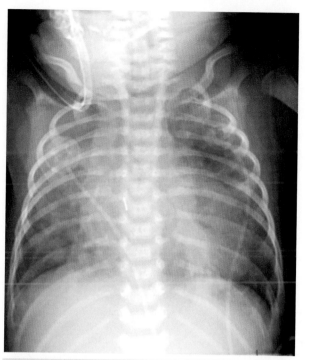

Fig. 34.7 Chest radiograph in an infant with large VSD demonstrating cardiomegaly and pulmonary edema. (Reproduced with permission from Cabrera AG, Bastrero P, Qureshi AM, et al. Ventricular septal defect. In Mery CR, Bastrero P, Hall SR, et al. [eds.] *Texas Children's Hospital Handbook of Congenital Heart Disease.* Houston: Texas Children's Hospital: 2020:99.)

IV

Right-to-Left Shunts

Right-to-left shunting lesions result from obstruction of outflow from the right ventricle and shunting across a VSD because of higher pressure in the right ventricle compared with the left ventricle. The degree of resulting cyanosis depends on the degree of obstruction in the right ventricle and the size of the VSD. In addition, SVR will also affect the amount of shunting. The most common right-to-left shunt lesion is TOF, about 6% of CHD patients,[57] consisting of RV outflow tract obstruction at the pulmonary subvalvar and valvar location, and large VSD with overriding aorta. The two additional components of the tetralogy are RV hypertrophy and right-sided aortic arch (in 25% of patients) (Figs. 34.11 and 34.12).

Obstructive Lesions

Obstructive lesions can be seen at multiple locations in the heart and great vessels; the most common is valvar pulmonic stenosis, with a prevalence of about 13% of

CHD. Coarctation of the aorta, usually near where the ductus arteriosus inserts, is observed in about 7% of CHD (Fig. 34.13) and valvar aortic stenosis in 5%.[57] Left-sided obstruction (i.e., to LV outflow) is less well tolerated; LV hypertrophy can occur and if untreated can result in coronary ischemia, ventricular arrhythmias, and death. Pulmonary valvar stenosis is usually well tolerated unless severe; the right ventricle can exhibit hypertrophy, but coronary ischemia usually does not result. Left- and right-sided obstructive lesions are amenable to surgical or catheter correction; timing will depend on symptoms and severity of pathophysiology and can range from the newborn period to adulthood.

Transposition of the Great Arteries

Dextro-transposition of the great arteries (d-TGA) occurs when the aorta arises from the right ventricle and the pulmonary artery from the left ventricle (Fig. 34.14). D-TGA comprises approximately 4% of CHD lesions.[57] This results in the systemic venous return being ejected from the aorta without being oxygenated in the lungs, resulting in profound cyanosis (Fig. 34.15). Survival at birth depends on mixing of oxygenated blood from the

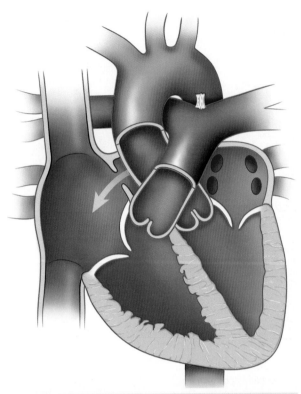

Fig. 34.8 Atrial septal defect. Note left-to-right shunting; because of the lower pressures in the atria, the degree of shunting tends to be much less than in moderate and large VSD, and symptomatology is less severe; small ASDs are often not diagnosed until later in childhood or even adulthood. (Reproduced with permission from Kailin J, Liou A, Adachi I. Atrial septal defect. In Mery CR, Bastrero P, Hall SR, et al. [eds.] *Texas Children's Hospital Handbook of Congenital Heart Disease*. Houston: Texas Children's Hospital; 2020:68.)

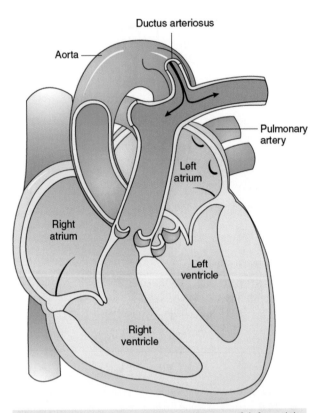

Fig. 34.9 Patent Ductus Arteriosus. Degree of left-to-right shunting from the high-pressure aorta to the pulmonary artery is influenced by the diameter, length, and tortuosity of the PDA. (Reproduced with permission from Andropoulos DB, Gottlieb EA. Congenital heart disease. In Fleischer LA [ed.] *Anesthesia and Uncommon Diseases*. 6th ed. Philadelphia: Elsevier; 2012:92.)

left side of the heart to the right side of the heart, at the ventricular, atrial, or PDA levels. Approximately 15% to 20% of neonates with d-TGA have a VSD and tend to have less cyanosis; if there is no VSD, the neonate is maintained on prostaglandin-E$_1$ to keep the ductus arteriosus patent. Many of these patients undergo a balloon atrial septostomy, a catheter-based procedure to create a large ASD to allow more mixing and better systemic oxygenation, which promotes physiologic stability before surgery. Surgery consists of the neonatal arterial switch operation performed in the first weeks of life. Surgery for d-TGA is a common neonatal procedure, comprising about 10% of neonatal cardiac surgeries.

Single-Ventricle Lesions

A functional single ventricle results from severe obstruction or atresia of structures on the left or right side of

the heart, that is, aortic or mitral stenosis or atresia resulting in hypoplastic left heart syndrome (HLHS) (Fig. 34.16) or tricuspid atresia resulting in hypoplastic right heart syndrome. Together, these conditions have a prevalence of approximately 4% of CHD,[57] but the patients undergo a disproportionate number of surgeries and catheter procedures as neonates and infants. In HLHS systemic blood flow depends on flow through the right ventricle, out the pulmonary artery, through a large PDA, and into the aorta. Aortic flow to the brachiocephalic vessels and the coronary arteries is retrograde because of no or very limited antegrade flow across the aortic valve. Complete mixing of the systemic and pulmonary circulations results, and as PVR declines over the first days of life, blood flow is preferentially directed toward the lungs, resulting in severe overcirculation, steal of flow from the systemic circulation, low systemic cardiac output, lactic acidosis and shock, and death if not treated (Fig. 34.17). The PDA is maintained with PGE$_1$, and staged palliative surgery is undertaken

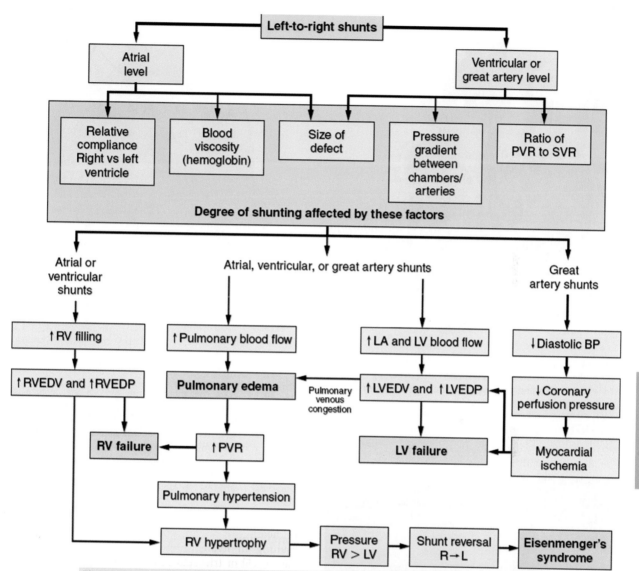

Fig. 34.10 Pathophysiology of left-to-right shunting lesions. The flow diagram depicts factors that affect left-to-right shunting at the atrial, ventricular, and great artery level and the pathophysiology produced by these shunts. A large shunt will result in LV failure, RV failure, and pulmonary edema. Increased pulmonary blood flow and pulmonary artery pressures lead to pulmonary hypertension and eventually Eisenmenger syndrome. These final common outcomes are highlighted in bold lettering. See text for detailed discussion. *BP*, Blood pressure; *LA*, left atrium; *LV*, left ventricle; *LVEDP*, left ventricular end-diastolic pressure; *LVEDV*, left ventricular end-diastolic volume; *PVR*, pulmonary vascular resistance; *RV*, right ventricle; *RVEDP*, right ventricular end-diastolic pressure; *RVEDV*, right ventricular end-diastolic volume; *SVR*, systemic vascular resistance. (Reproduced with permission from Andropoulos DB, Gottlieb EA. Congenital heart disease. In Fleischer LA [ed.] *Anesthesia and Uncommon Diseases*. 6th ed. Philadelphia: Elsevier; 2012:91.)

in the neonatal period to reconstruct the aortic arch and provide systemic flow through a neo-aortic valve (anatomic pulmonary valve) and a more stable and controllable source of pulmonary blood flow with a shunt or right ventricle to pulmonary artery conduit. Stage I palliation for HLHS is a common neonatal surgery, comprising about 10% of operations in this age group. Hypoplastic right heart also results in circulatory mixing but is usually much better tolerated because of the presence of a systemic left ventricle; neonatal surgical or catheter procedures to increase or decrease pulmonary blood flow may be necessary.

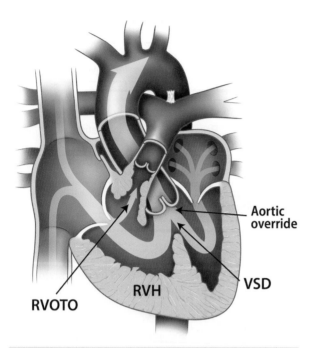

Fig. 34.11 Tetralogy of Fallot. Note large VSD and obstruction to RV outflow at the subvalvar and valvar level, resulting in right-to-left shunting and cyanosis. (Reproduced with permission from Cabrera AG, Bastrero P, Hall SR, et al. Tetralogy of Fallot. In Mery CR, Bastrero P, Hall SR, et al. [eds.] *Texas Children's Hospital Handbook of Congenital Heart Disease*. Houston: Texas Children's Hospital; 2020:113.)

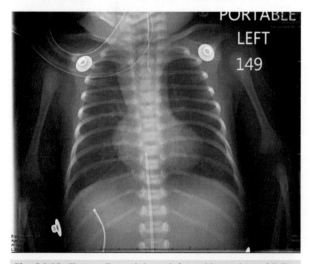

Fig. 34.12 Chest radiograph in an infant with tetralogy of Fallot. Note decreased vascular markings in lung fields from decreased pulmonary blood flow and "boot-shaped" heart from hypoplastic main pulmonary artery. (Reproduced with permission from Cabrera AG, Bastrero P, Hall SR, et al. Tetralogy of Fallot. In Mery CR, Bastrero P, Hall SR, et al. [eds.] *Texas Children's Hospital Handbook of Congenital Heart Disease*. Houston: Texas Children's Hospital; 2020:114.)

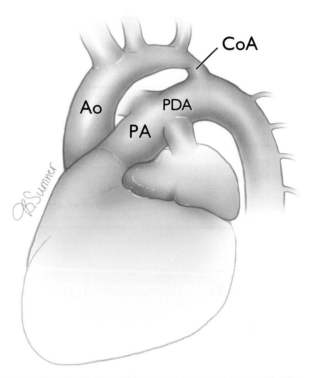

Fig. 34.13 Severe coarctation of the aorta in the neonate. A large patent ductus arteriosus (*PDA*) supplies blood flow to the aorta distal to the coarctation. *Ao*, Aorta; *CoA*, coarctation; *PA*, pulmonary artery; *PDA*, patent ductus arteriosus. (Reproduced with permission from Lopez KN, Tume SC, Hall SR, et al. Aortic coarctation and interrupted aortic arch. In Mery CR, Bastrero P, Hall SR, et al. [eds.] *Texas Children's Hospital Handbook of Congenital Heart Disease*. Houston: Texas Children's Hospital; 2020:209.)

Conclusion

The increased longevity in all forms of CHD that has resulted from the myriad of advances in surgical and medical therapy over the past 70+ years has resulted in a significant population of survivors of CHD numbering over 2.4 million children and adults in the United States.[57] The anesthesia provider is increasingly likely to provide care for these patients in the course of everyday practice.

SPECIAL ANESTHETIC CONSIDERATIONS

Anesthesia for the Former Premature Infant

Many former premature infants present for surgery, either during their initial hospitalization or later as outpatients. The most common procedures include inguinal herniorrhaphy, circumcision, eye examination, and strabismus surgery. Although many infants

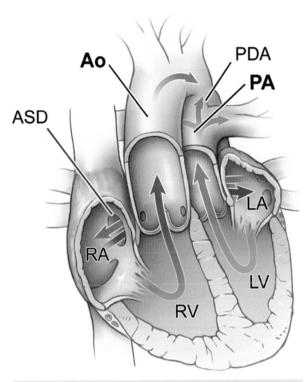

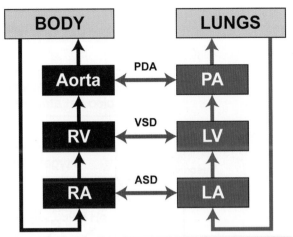

Fig. 34.15 Physiology in d-TGA. Oxygenated blood recirculates through the lungs; deoxygenated systemic venous blood recirculates through the body; survival depends on mixing of oxygenated blood into the systemic circulation by a communication at one or more levels. (Reproduced with permission from Cabrera AG, Checchia PA, Andropoulos DB, et al. Transposition of the great arteries. In Mery CR, Bastrero P, Hall SR, et al. [eds.] *Texas Children's Hospital Handbook of Congenital Heart Disease*. Houston: Texas Children's Hospital; 2020:120.)

IV

Fig. 34.14 d-transposition of the great arteries. Note the pulmonary artery (*PA*) arises from the left ventricle (*LV*), and the aorta (*Ao*) arises from the right ventricle (*RV*). There is an atrial septal defect (*ASD*) in this example. (Reproduced with permission from Cabrera AG, Checchia PA, Andropoulos DB, et al. Transposition of the great arteries. In Mery CR, Bastrero P, Hall SR, et al. [eds.] *Texas Children's Hospital Handbook of Congenital Heart Disease*. Houston: Texas Children's Hospital; 2020:120.)

have recovered well without sequelae, many have chronic conditions such as bronchopulmonary dysplasia (need for supplemental oxygen beyond 30 days of life after a diagnosis of respiratory distress syndrome), apnea and bradycardia, anemia, hydrocephalus from intraventricular hemorrhage, visual disturbances, and developmental delay. The infant's postconceptual age is important; an infant born at 28 weeks' gestation who presents at 12 weeks for surgery is now 40 weeks' postconceptual age and is equivalent in many respects to only a full-term infant, not an infant at 3 months of age. The major risk in this regard is postanesthetic apnea, which in some cases is fatal. The risk of postanesthetic apnea increases with increasing prematurity at birth and younger age at the time of the anesthetic.[60] Although the time at which the risk of apnea is eliminated is not clear, 50 weeks' postconceptual age or less is commonly used as the cutoff point for admitting former premature infants for 24 hours of apnea monitoring after receiving an anesthetic.

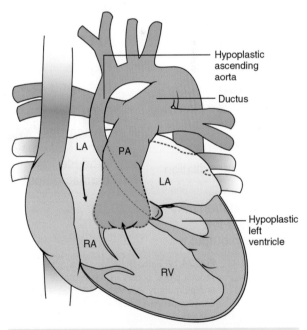

Fig. 34.16 Hypoplastic left heart syndrome. Mitral and aortic atresia are present in this example. Blood flows from the left atrium (*LA*) to the right atrium (*RA*), the right ventricle (*RV*), to the pulmonary artery (*PA*). Systemic blood flow is provided by the large ductus arteriosus into the aorta. Complete mixing of the pulmonary and systemic circulations occurs. (Reproduced with permission from Andropoulos DB, Gottlieb EA. Congenital heart disease. In Fleischer LA [ed.] *Anesthesia and Uncommon Diseases*, 6th ed. Philadelphia: Elsevier; 2012:120.)

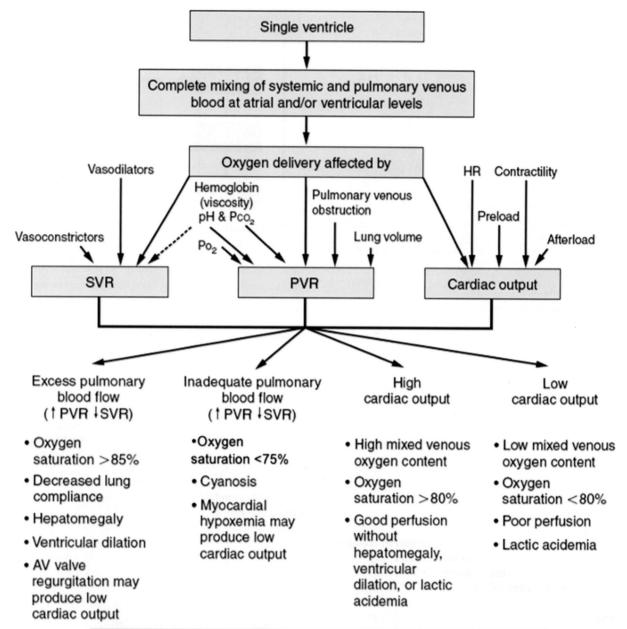

Fig. 34.17 Pathophysiology of single-ventricle lesions. Complete mixing of systemic and pulmonary venous blood occurs in the ventricle. Optimal oxygen delivery involves a balance between systemic and pulmonary vascular resistance. (Reproduced with permission from Andropoulos DB, Gottlieb EA. Congenital heart disease. In Fleischer LA [ed.] *Anesthesia and Uncommon Diseases*, 6th ed. Philadelphia: Elsevier; 2012:122.)

Anesthesia for Remote Locations

Anesthesia and sedation for diagnostic and therapeutic procedures are increasing for children in locations remote from the operating room, and the clinical complexity of the patients requiring care is also increasing (also see Chapter 38). These procedures include MRI and CT scans, interventional radiology procedures, bone marrow aspirations, gastrointestinal endoscopy, auditory brainstem evoked response testing, and cardiac catheterization. Techniques vary widely and include moderate or deep sedation, general anesthesia with IV drugs, volatile anesthetics with facemask or

SGA, or full general endotracheal anesthesia. Frequently used anesthetics include propofol, ketamine, barbiturates, benzodiazepines, and opioids. The central alpha-2 agonist dexmedetomidine is increasingly being used for nonpainful diagnostic studies such as MRI.[61] The same standards for preoperative evaluation, monitoring, and recovery must be maintained for anesthesia in remote locations to ensure safety in this environment.[62]

Ex Utero Intrapartum Therapy Procedure and Fetal Surgery

The EXIT procedure was first performed in 1989. The purpose is to secure the neonatal airway while the fetus is still being oxygenated via the placenta. The mother is placed under general anesthesia, a hysterotomy is made, and the fetus is partially delivered. This strategy can be used to oxygenate the fetus while the airway is secured by direct laryngoscopy, rigid bronchoscopy, or tracheostomy while on placental bypass. Indications include large neck masses, congenital airway obstruction, and previous tracheal occlusion for CDH. The EXIT procedure has also been used for patients with fetal anomalies in whom neonatal resuscitation may be difficult, including large thoracic masses, CDH, unilateral pulmonary agenesis, and some complex cardiac lesions. Maintenance of placental bypass provides time to establish IV access and an airway, give resuscitative drugs, and cannulate for ECMO when necessary in a controlled manner.[63]

Fetal interventions have been performed as open midgestational (hysterotomy-based) procedures involving exteriorization and replacement of the fetus and as minimally invasive procedures assisted by fetoscopy, ultrasound, and echocardiography. An open approach has been used to treat myelomeningocele, congenital cystic adenomatoid malformation, and sacrococcygeal teratoma with varied success. Minimally invasive approaches have been taken to treat CDH, bladder outlet obstruction, HLHS, and twin–twin transfusion syndrome, among others.

Open midgestational procedures and EXIT procedures are usually performed with maternal general anesthesia, and minimally invasive procedures can be performed with maternal local, sedation, regional, general, or combined regional and general techniques. General anesthesia with inhaled anesthetic provides anesthesia to both the mother and the fetus, and a high concentration volatile anesthetic (2 MAC) can be used to provide uterine relaxation. Anesthetic and resuscitative drugs can then be given directly to the fetus via an IM, IV, intracardiac, or intraamniotic route. For minimally invasive procedures, it is important to discuss the need for fetal immobility preoperatively. For some fetal cardiac procedures,

general anesthesia is required for the mother, and fentanyl, vecuronium, and atropine must be delivered directly to the fetus for safety reasons.

A preoperative plan should be made for intrauterine fetal resuscitation in advance. Maternal interventions, including left lateral positioning, oxygen delivery, and blood pressure augmentation with volume or vasopressor administration, can facilitate fetal resuscitation. Atropine, epinephrine, calcium gluconate, sodium bicarbonate, and PRBCs can be delivered to the fetus, and cardiac compressions and drainage of pericardial effusions can be carried out.[64,65]

Anesthetic Neurotoxicity and Neuroprotection in the Developing Brain

Neonatal rodent models of prolonged anesthesia with γ-aminobutyric acid agonists (isoflurane, midazolam, propofol) or *N*-methyl-D-aspartate antagonists (ketamine) produce accelerated apoptosis, or programmed cell death, of neurons in the developing brain.[66] These data raised concern that commonly used anesthetic drugs could be having similar effects in the developing human brain, generating intense interest and a number of new research avenues to determine if this effect applies to human neonates and infants. Criticism of the animal studies includes the fact that most were conducted in the absence of a surgical stimulus and that the exposure periods were quite prolonged compared with the corresponding exposure of a human infant during anesthesia and surgery. Other animal models have demonstrated that anesthetics such as ketamine and desflurane are neuroprotective in animal models that include surgery or painful stimuli. Recently completed studies investigating the effects of anesthetic exposure early in life include (1) the GAS study examining neurocognitive performance after either a general or spinal anesthetic during infancy[67]; (2) the PANDA (Pediatric Anesthesia & Neurodevelopment Assessment) study comparing neurocognitive performance in sibling cohorts in which one sibling had an anesthetic exposure before 3 years of age[68]; and (3) the MASK study comparing neurocognitive performance in children exposed to anesthesia before 3 years of age with those without an exposure.[69] These studies have reported no effect on pure cognitive neurodevelopmental testing (e.g., intelligence quotient) after brief single or multiple exposures to general anesthesia. A small effect on behavioral problems and executive function was reported after a single exposure and a small effect on fine motor and reading performance and behavioral problems after multiple exposures. Data are lacking on the effect of prolonged exposures over about 3 hours. Currently there is insufficient evidence to change the current approach to anesthesia in the infant (also see Chapter 12).

IV

REFERENCES

1. Andropoulos DB. Physiology and molecular biology of the developing circulation. In: Andropoulos DB, ed. *Anesthesia for Congenital Heart Disease*. 3rd ed. Oxford, UK: Wiley Blackwell; 2015: 84–105.

2. Lerman J. Inhalation agents in pediatric anaesthesia–An update. *Curr Opin Anaesthesiol*. 2007;20:221–226.

3. Frei FJ, Haemmerle MH, Brunner R, Kern C. Minimum alveolar concentration for halothane in children with cerebral palsy and severe mental retardation. *Anesthesia*. 1997;52:1056–1060.

4. Bailey AG, McNaull PP, Jooste E, et al. Perioperative crystalloid and colloid fluid management in children: Where are we and how did we get here?. *Anesth Analg*. 2010;110:375–390.

5. Navaratnam M, Ng A, Williams GD, et al. Perioperative management of pediatric en-bloc combined heart-liver transplants: A case series review. *Pediatr Anesth*. 2016;26:976–986.

6. Adams CB, Vollman KE, Leventhal EL, et al. Emergent pediatric anticoagulation reversal using a 4-factor prothrombin complex concentrate. *Am J Emerg Med*. 2016;34 1182.e1–1182.e2.

7. Jooste EH, Machovec KA, Einhorn LM, et al. 3-Factor prothrombin complex concentrates in infants with refractory bleeding after cardiac surgery. *J Cardiothorac Vasc Anesth*. 2016;30: 1627–1631.

8. Haas T, Spielmann N, Dillier C, et al. Higher fibrinogen concentrations for reduction of transfusion requirements during major paediatric surgery: A prospective randomized trial. *Br J Anaesth*. 2015;115:234–243.

9. Galas FR, de Almeida JP, Fukushima JT, et al. Hemostatic effects of fibrinogen concentrate compared with cryoprecipitate after cardiac surgery: A randomized pilot trial. *J Thorac Cardiovasc Surg*. 2014;148:1647–1655.

10. Romlin B, Wahlander H, Berggren H, et al. Intraoperative thromboelastometry is associated with reduced transfusion prevalence in pediatric cardiac surgery. *Anesth Analg*. 2011;112:30–36.

11. Alten JA, Benner K, Green K, et al. Pediatric off-label use of recombinant factor VIIa. *Pediatrics*. 2009;123:1066–1072.

12. Dalal PG, Murray D, Messner AH, et al. Pediatric laryngeal dimensions: An age-based analysis. *Anesth Analg*. 2009;108:1475–1479.

13. Luce V, Harkouk H, Brasher C, et al. Supraglottic airway devices vs tracheal intubation in children: A quantitative meta-analysis of respiratory complications. *Paediatr Anaesth*. 2014;24: 1088–1098.

14. Drake-Brockman TFE, Ramgolam A, Zhang G, et al. The effect of endotracheal tubes versus laryngeal mask airways on perioperative respiratory adverse events in infants: A randomized controlled trial. *Lancet*. 2017;389:701–708.

15. Salgo B, Schmitz A, Henze G, et al. Evaluation of a new recommendation for improved cuffed tracheal tube size selection in infants and small children. *Acta Anaesthesiol Scand*. 2006;50:557–561.

16. Gupta A, Gupta N. Ineffective ventilation in a neonate with a large pre-carinal tracheoesophageal fistula and bilateral pneumonitis–Microcuff endotracheal tube to our rescue!. *J Neonatal Surg*. 2017;6:14.

17. Lam H, Kitzman J, Matthews R, Young L, Austin TM. Symptomatic endotracheal tube obstruction in infants intubated with Microcuff® endotracheal tubes. *Pediatr Anesth*. 2016;26:767–775.

18. Matsuoka W, Ide K, Matsudo T, et al. The occurrence and risk factors of inappropriately deep tip position of Microcuff pediatric endotracheal tube during PICU stay: A retrospective cohort pilot study. *Pediatr Crit Care Med*. 2019;20:e510–e515.

19. Fiadjoe J, Stricker P. Pediatric difficult airway management: current devices and techniques. *Anesthesiol Clin*. 2009;27:185–195.

20. Jagannathan N, Sequera-Ramos L, Sohn L, et al. Elective use of supraglottic airway devices for primary airway management in children with difficult airways. *Br J Anaesth*. 2014;112:742–748.

21. Hsu G, Fiadjoe JE. The pediatric difficult airway: Updates and innovations. *Anesthesiol Clin*. 2020;38:459–475.

22. Wheeler M, Coté CJ. Preoperative pregnancy testing in a tertiary care children's hospital: A medico-legal conundrum. *J Clin Anesth*. 1999;11:56–63.

23. Tait AR, Malviya S. Anesthesia for the child with an upper respiratory tract infection: Still a dilemma?. *Anesth Analg*. 2005;100:59–65.

24. Practice guidelines for preoperative fasting and the use of pharmacologic agents to reduce the risk of pulmonary aspiration. Application to healthy patients undergoing elective procedures: a report by the American Society of Anesthesiologists Task Force on Preoperative Fasting. *Anesthesiology*. 1999;90(3):896–905.

25. Thomas M, Morrison C, Newton R, Schindler E. Consensus statement for clear fluids fasting for elective pediatric general anesthesia. *Pediatr Anesth*. 2018;28:411–414.

26. Isserman R, Elliott E, Subramanyam R, Kraus B, et al. Quality improvement project to reduce pediatric clear liquid fasting times prior to anesthesia. *Pediatr Anesth*. 2019;29:698–704.

27. Sun Y, Lu Y, Huang Y, et al. Is dexmedetomidine superior to midazolam as a premedication in children? A meta-analysis of randomized controlled trials. *Paediatr Anaesth*. 2014;24:863–874.

28. Sadhasivam S, Cohen LL, Szabova A, et al. Real-time assessment of perioperative behaviors and prediction of perioperative outcomes. *Anesth Analg*. 2009;108:822–826.

29. Mayande A, Cyna AM, Yip P, et al. Non-pharmacological interventions for assisting the induction of anaesthesia in children (review). *Cochrane Database Syst Rev*. 2015;7:CD006447.

30. Watson A, Visram A. Survey of the use of oesophageal and precordial stethoscopes in current paediatric anaesthetic practice. *Paediatr Anaesth*. 2001;11:437–442.

31. Davidson AJ. Monitoring the anaesthetic depth in children–An update. *Curr Opin Anaesthesiol*. 2007;20:236–243.

32. Pinto N, Sawardekar A, Suresh S. Regional anesthesia: Options for the pediatric patient. *Anesthesiol Clin*. 2020;38:559–575.

33. Trifa M, Tumin D, Whitaker EE, Bhalla T, Jayanthi VR, Tobias JD. Spinal anesthesia for surgery longer than 60 min in infants: Experience from the first 2 years of a spinal anesthesia program. *J Anesth*. 2018;32:637–640.

34. Tobias JD. Spinal anaesthesia in infants and children. *Paediatr Anaesth*. 2000;10:5–16.

35. Gan TJ, Belani KG, Bergese S, et al. Fourth Consensus Guidelines for the Management of Postoperative Nausea and Vomiting. *Anesth Analg*. 2020;131:411–448.

36. Engelman E, Salengros JC, Barvais L. How much does pharmacologic prophylaxis reduce postoperative vomiting in children? Calculation of prophylaxis effectiveness and expected incidence of vomiting under treatment using Bayesian meta-analysis. *Anesthesiology*. 2008;109:1023–1035.

37. Kanaparthi A, Kukura S, Slenkovich N, et al. Perioperative administration of Emend® (aprepitant) at a tertiary care children's hospital: A 12-month survey. *Clin Pharmacol*. 2019;11:155–160.

38. Bailard N, Rebello E. Aprepitant and fosaprepitant decrease the effectiveness of hormonal contraceptives. *Br J Clin Pharmacol*. 2018;84:602–603.

39. Mason KP. Paediatric emergence delirium: A comprehensive review and interpretation of the literature. *Br J Anaesthesia*. 2017;118:335–343.

40. Henry MC, Moss RL. Neonatal necrotizing enterocolitis. *Semin Pediatr Surg*. 2008;17:98–109.

41. Marven S, Owen A. Contemporary postnatal surgical management strategies for congenital abdominal wall defects. *Semin Pediatr Surg.* 2008;17:222–235.

42. Broemling N, Campbell F. Anesthetic management of congenital tracheoesophageal fistula. *Paediatr Anaesth.* 2011;21:1092–1099.

43. Orford J, Cass DT, Glasson MJ. Advances in the treatment of oesophageal atresia over three decades: The 1970s and the 1990s. *Pediatr Surg Int.* 2004;20(6): 402–407.

44. Andropoulos DB, Rowe RW, Betts JM. Anaesthetic and surgical airway management during tracheo-oesophageal fistula repair. *Paediatr Anaesth.* 1998;8:313–319.

45. de Buys Roessingh AS, Dinh-Xuan A. Congenital diaphragmatic hernia: Current status and review of the literature. *Eur J Pediatr.* 2009;168:393–406.

46. Malviya MN, Ohlsson A, Shah SS. Surgical versus medical treatment with cyclooxygenase inhibitors for symptomatic patent ductus arteriosus in preterm infants (review). *Cochrane Database Syst Rev.* 2013;3:CD003951.

47. Sathanandam SK, Gutfinger D, O'Brien L, Forbes TJ, Gillespie MJ, Berman DP, et al. Amplatzer Piccolo Occluder clinical trial for percutaneous closure of the patent ductus arteriosus in patients 700 grams. *Catheter Cardiovasc Interv.* 2020;96:1266–1276.

48. Sylvester CL. Retinopathy of prematurity. *Semin Ophthalmol.* 2008;23: 318–323.

49. Thompson DN. Postnatal management and outcome for neural tube defects including spina bifida and encephaloceles. *Prenat Diagn.* 2009;29:412–419.

50. Sanz Cortes M, Lapa DA, Acacio GL, et al. Proceedings of the First Annual Meeting of the International Fetoscopic Myelomeningocele Repair Consortium. *Ultrasound Obstet Gynecol.* 2019;53:855–863.

51. Taghavi K, Powell E, Patel B, McBride CA. The treatment of pyloric stenosis: Evolution in practice. *J Paediatr Child Health.* 2017;53:1105–1110.

52. Kamata M, Cartabuke RS, Tobias JD. Perioperative care of infants with pyloric stenosis. *Pediatr Anesth.* 2015;25:1193–1206.

53. Bissonnette B, Sullivan PJ. Pyloric stenosis. *Can J Anaesth.* 1991;38:668–676.

54. Kelay A, Hall NJ. Perioperative complications of surgery for hypertrophic pyloric stenosis. *Eur J Pediatr Surg.* 2018;28:171–175.

55. Cartabuke RS, Tobias JD, Rice J, Tumin D. Current perioperative care of infants with pyloric stenosis: Comparison of survey results. *J Surg Res.* 2018;223:244–250 e3.

56. Andropoulos DB, Heard MB, Johnson KL, et al. Postanesthetic apnea in full-term infants after pyloromyotomy. *Anesthesiology.* 1994;80:216–219.

57. Virani SS, Alonso A, Aparicio HJ, et al. Heart Disease and Stroke Statistics-2021 update: A report from the American Heart Association. *Circulation.* 2021;143:e254–e743.

58. Andopoulos DB, Stayer SA, Mossad EB, Miller-Hance WC. *Anesthesia for Congenital Heart Disease.* 3rd ed. Hoboken: Wiley-Blackwell; 2015.

59. Whiting D, DiNardo JA, Odegard KC. Anesthesia for congenital heart disease. In: Andropoulos DB, Gregory GA, eds. *Gregory's Pediatric Anesthesia.* 6th ed. Hoboken: Wiley-Blackwell; 2020.

60. Coté CJ, Zaslavsky A, Downes JJ, et al. Postoperative apnea in former preterm infants after inguinal herniorrhaphy: A combined analysis. *Anesthesiology.* 1995;82(4):809–822.

61. Mason KP. Sedation trends in the 21st century: The transition to dexmedetomidine for radiological imaging studies. *Paediatr Anaesth.* 2010;20:265–272.

62. Campbell K, Torres L, Stayer S. Anesthesia and sedation outside the operating room. *Anesthesiol Clin.* 2014;32:25–43.

63. De Buck F, Deprest J, Van de Velde M. Anesthesia for fetal surgery. *Curr Opin Anaesthesiol.* 2008;21:293–297.

64. Lin EE, Tran KM. Anesthesia for fetal surgery. *Semin Pediatr Surg.* 2013;22:50–55.

65. Brusseau R, Mizrahi-Arnaud A. Fetal anesthesia and pain management for intrauterine therapy. *Clin Perinatol.* 2013;40:429–442.

66. Loepke AW, Soriano SG. An assessment of the effects of general anesthetics on developing brain structure and neurocognitive function. *Anesth Analg.* 2008;106:1681–1707.

67. McCann ME, de Graaff JC, Dorris L, et al. Neurodevelopmental outcome at 5 years of age after general anaesthesia or awake-regional anaesthesia in infancy (GAS): An international, multicentre, randomised, controlled equivalence trial. *Lancet.* 2019;393:664–677.

68. Sun LS, Li G, Miller TL, Salorio C, Byrne MW, Bellinger DC, et al. Association between a single general anesthesia exposure before age 36 months and neurocognitive outcomes in later childhood. *JAMA.* 2016;315: 2312–2320.

69. Warner DO, Zaccariello MJ, Katusic SK, et al. Neuropsychological and behavioral outcomes after exposure of young children to procedures requiring general anesthesia: The Mayo Anesthesia Safety in Kids (MASK) Study. *Anesthesiology.* 2018;129:89–105.

IV

35 GERIATRICS

Tyler Seth Chernin

INTRODUCTION

The proportion of the U.S. population over the age of 65 continues to grow (Fig. 35.1). This segment of the population is expected to double between the years 2020 and 2060, and the number of people aged 80 and over is expected to triple within this time frame.[1] Globally, the population aged 65 years and over is the fastest-growing age group, and in most parts of the world, survival beyond age 65 years continues to improve.[2] Not surprisingly, more and more anesthetics are being administered to the elderly, who are increasingly presenting for surgical procedures of varying complexity and invasiveness. In 2015 35% of all surgeries performed in the United States were for patients aged 65 and older.[3,4]

The practicing anesthesia provider must have a solid understanding of the anesthetic considerations unique to the elderly patient. The preoperative assessment should focus on how best to optimize the older patient for a surgical procedure (also see Chapter 13). Issues such as frailty, cognitive function, nutritional status, and functional independence are more likely to affect perioperative outcomes in this age group. The safe delivery of anesthesia care to an older patient requires an appreciation of the many physiologic changes that accompany normal aging, in addition to the significant differences in the pharmacokinetics and pharmacodynamics of the most commonly used anesthetic agents. An increased understanding of the neurobiology of perioperative neurocognitive disorders may allow anesthesia providers to lessen the risk of postoperative delirium (POD) and cognitive decline. Despite the recognized importance of these geriatric-specific anesthetic considerations, a 2020 survey study sent to American Society of Anesthesiologists (ASA) members suggested low adherence to best practices in the anesthetic care of geriatric populations.[5] For example, survey respondents reported low rates of preoperative geriatric evaluations, preoperative screening for frailty or cognitive

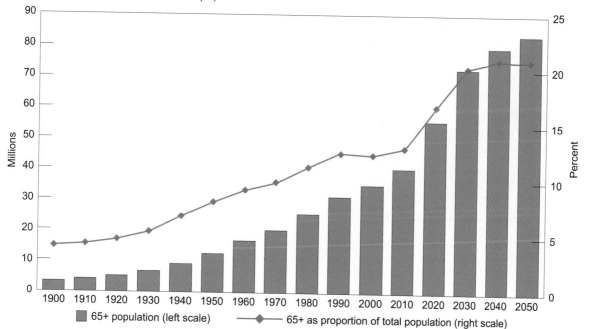

Population Aged 65 and Over: 1900 to 2050
(For information on confidentiality protection, nonsampling error, and definitions, see
www.census.gov/prod/cen2010/doc/sf1/pdf)

■ 65+ population (left scale) ◆ 65+ as proportion of total population (right scale)

Sources: 1900 to 1940, and 1960 to 1980, U.S. Bureau of the Census, 1983: 1950. U.S. Bureau of the Census, 1953: 1990. U.S. Bureau of the Census. 1990: 2000. U.S. Census Bureau. 2001; 2010, U.S. Census Bureau, 2011; 2020 to 2050, U.S. Census Bureau, 2012a: 1900 to 2010. decennial census: 2020 to 2050. *2012 National Population Projections*, Middle series.

Fig. 35.1 The projected aging of the U.S. population. Bars represent the total number of persons aged 65 or older (millions), and the graphical line represents the data as a proportion of the total U.S. population (%). (Reproduced from United States Census Bureau. West LA, Cole S, Goodkind D, et al. 65+ in the United States: 2010. June 2014. https://www.census.gov/content/dam/Census/library/publications/2014/demo/p23-212.pdf. Accessed January 3, 2021.)

IV

disorders, and POD screening in their care of patients over 65 years old.

THE PHYSIOLOGIC CHANGES OF AGING

In the 1940s the American physiologist Walter Cannon coined the term *homeostenosis* to explain the overarching principle that as a person ages, their ability to respond to physiologic stressors and shift back to a state of homeostasis is impaired.[6] This concept provides a helpful framework through which to consider the physiologic changes that accompany normal aging. For the most part, basal physiologic processes remain intact, while physiologic reserves are progressively diminished over time. Once those reserves are exhausted, a person is more predisposed to disease, a concept referred to as *frailty* (Fig. 35.2). In this section we will consider the main physiologic changes of aging most relevant to the anesthesia provider caring for the elderly surgical patient. Most importantly, it is essential to distinguish between the normal physiologic processes that occur with aging

from the disease states that are more common in this population. Indeed, disease is *not* a normal part of the aging process (Table 35.1).

Cardiovascular System

One characteristic change that accompanies the aging process is the decrease in elastin production that begins to occur around the fourth decade of life. Within the cardiovascular system, this leads to fibrosis within the media of the aorta and other large muscular arteries and reduced compliance within both the arterial and venous systems.[7] Approximately 80% of blood volume is normally stored in the venous system, which is a useful adaptive mechanism to help maintain cardiac output (CO) when preload is reduced. Decreased compliance ("stiffening") of venous capacitance vessels makes them less effective at compensating for reductions in preload. This is one of the reasons why elderly patients often experience labile blood pressure during anesthesia.[8] Changes in the vascular endothelial layer include alterations in nitric oxide metabolism that predispose to vasoconstriction,

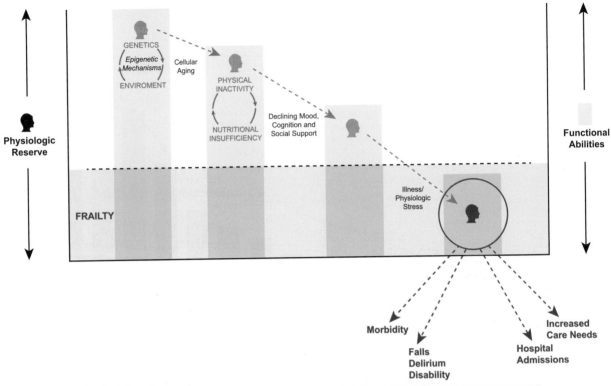

Fig. 35.2 A conceptual model of physiologic reserve, functional ability, and frailty. As the aging process occurs (*dashed, arrowed line*), physiologic reserves and functional abilities normally decline. A multitude of other factors and processes (genetics, environment, cellular aging, nutritional status, physical inactivity, mood and social support) may hasten or slow down this process. At a certain point, the aging process or an acute physiologic stressor causes the individual to enter into a state of frailty (*dashed, horizontal line*), at which point they are at risk of poor outcomes, such as morbidity, falls, cognitive decline, and increased health care needs. These outcomes may further worsen the conditions of frailty. (Reproduced with permission from Khan KT, Hemati K, Donovan AL. Geriatric physiology and the frailty syndrome. *Anesthesiol Clin.* 2019;37[3]:453–474.)

platelet aggregation, and endothelial dysfunction. Progressive calcific deposits within valvular structures and fibrosis within the cardiac conduction system increase the risk of dysrhythmias. Taken together, these changes lead to an increase in systolic blood pressure, systemic vascular resistance, and pulse pressure while diastolic blood pressure tends to decrease.[9]

Because of the progressive increase in left ventricular afterload, the left ventricle hypertrophies with age and becomes less compliant, impairing early ventricular filling and resulting in higher filling pressures, a reliance on atrial systole, and a tendency toward diastolic dysfunction (Fig. 35.3). Total cardiac myocyte number decreases, but the resulting myocytes hypertrophy, which is further enhanced by a reduction in the process of cellular autophagy, an intracellular mechanism whereby by-products of cell turnover are normally degraded by lysosomal activity.[10] There are also changes to cardiac calcium currents, which impair ventricular relaxation. These structural and functional changes

lead to a less compliant, hypertrophied left ventricle predisposed to myocardial ischemia in the setting of hypotension, especially within the subendocardial layer.[9] The elderly patient is less able to compensate for conditions of hypovolemia and hypervolemia. Although early studies suggested that ejection fraction (EF) and CO decreased with age, aging is clearly a risk factor for developing cardiovascular disease. It is likely that many prior studies inadvertently included subjects with latent coronary artery disease that caused systolic dysfunction.[9] Therefore it is now generally accepted that resting EF and CO do not decrease with aging; however, the ability to augment CO under conditions of increased demand is decreased.[10]

Resting heart rate (HR) and maximum HR steadily decline with age. This is partly because of fibrous and fatty infiltration within the sinoatrial node and a loss of pacemaker cells.[10] Although sympathetic nervous system (SNS) output increases with age, with higher levels of circulating norepinephrine and epinephrine, SNS

Table 35.1 Selected Physiologic Effects of Aging by Organ System

Organ System	Structural Changes	Functional Changes
Body composition	Decreased muscle mass Decreased water content Increased fat content	Reduced Vd for hydrophilic agents Increased Vd for lipophilic agents
Cardiovascular	Fibrosis within vascular media layer Fibrosis of conduction system Calcification of valvular structures Reduced myocyte number LV hypertrophy	Increased LV afterload Increased SBP, Increased PP Decreased DBP Increased LV filling pressures Decreased PNS tone Increased SNS output Desensitized B-adrenergic receptors Decreased resting HR and max HR Decreased ability to augment EF/CO Endothelial dysfunction
Pulmonary	Decreased elastin within lung parenchyma Decreased alveolar surface area Decreased thoracic vertebral column height Relative flattening of diaphragm	Increased lung compliance Decreased CW compliance Increased A-a gradient, reduced Pao_2 Increased dead space and shunt Increased CC and CV Blunted response to hypoxemia/hypercarbia Decreased mucociliary function Unchanged TLC Increased RV and FRC Decreased ERV, VC, FEV_1, FVC
Renal	Renal cortical atrophy Decreased number of nephrons	Decreased GFR Decreased RBF Renal vascular dysautonomy Decreased RAAS activity Decreased ability to conserve/excrete sodium Decreased ability to reabsorb free water Diminished tubular function Decreased drug clearance
Nervous	Brain atrophy, decreased number of neurons Increased CSF volume Reduced dopamine, serotonin, acetylcholine, glutamate, BNF signaling More permeable blood brain barrier Demyelination of peripheral nerve fibers	Diminished executive function Diminished short-term memory Decreased CBF Increased sensitivity to sedative agents Increased risk of perioperative neurocognitive disorders
Gastrointestinal/hepatic	Decreased esophageal muscle compliance Hepatic atrophy	Decreased LES tone Increased aspiration risk Prolonged gastric emptying Decreased gastric bicarbonate/PG production Decreased HBF Decreased albumin production Decreased drug clearance
Hematologic	Decreased bone marrow mass Increase in some circulating clotting factors	Increased platelet adhesiveness Increased risk for DVT Immunosenescence

BNF, Brain neurotrophic factor; *CBF*, cerebral blood flow; *CC*, closing capacity; *CO*, cardiac output; *CV*, closing volume; *CW*, chest wall; *DBP*, diastolic blood pressure; *DVT*, deep venous thrombosis; *EF*, ejection fraction; *ERV*, expiratory reserve volume; FEV_1, forced expired volume in 1 second; *FRC*, functional residual capacity; *FVC*, forced vital capacity; *GFR*, glomerular filtration rate; *HBF*, hepatic blood flow; *HR*, heart rate; *LES*, lower esophageal sphincter; *LV*, left ventricle; *PG*, prostaglandin; *PNS*, parasympathetic nervous system; *PP*, pulse pressure; *RAAS*, renin–angiotensin–aldosterone system; *RBF*, renal blood flow; *RV*, residual volume; *SBP*, systolic blood pressure; *SNS*, sympathetic nervous system; *VC*, vital capacity; *Vd*, volume of distribution.

IV

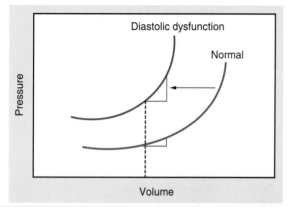

Fig. 35.3 Depiction of the diastolic function. (From Barnett SR. Elderly patients. In Pardo MC, Miller RD, eds. *Basics of Anesthesia*. 7th ed. Philadelphia: Elsevier; 2018:610.)

responsiveness is reduced because of both a downregulation in the number of beta-adrenergic receptors and reduced receptor responsiveness as a result of changes to adenylate cyclase signaling pathways.[10] Parasympathetic nervous system (PNS) regulation also decreases with a blunting of the normal HR variability at rest seen in younger patients and a less robust increase in HR in response to anticholinergic medications.[10] As such, maximum HR tends to decrease by one beat per minute per year over the age of 50.[7] Similarly, the effectiveness

of the HR component of the baroreceptor response is reduced, further predisposing to hypotension in the setting of vasodilation.

Pulmonary System

Lung function tends to decline beginning around the third decade of life. This is caused in part by age-related loss of elastin within the lung parenchyma, in addition to progressive anatomic changes to the chest wall, respiratory musculature, and airway that occur with aging.[11] Resting arterial partial pressure of oxygen (Pao_2) steadily declines with a widening of the A-a gradient. This is explained by a steady loss of alveolar and pulmonary capillary surface area, leading to redistribution of pulmonary blood flow, worsening V/Q mismatch, and increasing anatomic dead space.[8] As elasticity declines within the lung itself, the tendency of smaller airways to collapse increases at lower lung volumes, increasing shunt fraction and further contributing to resting hypoxemia. This is illustrated by an increase in closing capacity (CC) with age, which tends to exceed supine functional residual capacity (FRC) around the age of 45 and sitting FRC by age 65[12] (Fig. 35.4). This loss of elasticity also leads to an increase in lung compliance and a physiologic state of functional emphysema, with a tendency toward air trapping.[11] There is also a significant blunting of the normal physiologic compensatory responses to both hypoxemia

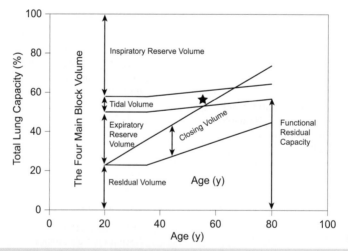

Fig. 35.4 Age-related changes in selected lung volumes. This figure illustrates the main changes to lung volumes that occur during the aging process (x-axis). A number of changes to the lung parenchyma (loss of elastin, increased compliance), chest wall (reduced compliance), and diaphragm (relative flattening) lead to a steady rise in residual volume (RV) and functional residual capacity (FRC), with a reduction in expiratory reserve volume (ERV), inspiratory reserve volume (IRV), and vital capacity (VC = ERV + Tidal volume + IRV). Total lung capacity is generally unchanged. Importantly, closing volume (CV) and closing capacity (CV + RV) also steadily rise. When lung volumes decrease below CC (depicted by the star), small airways start to close, shunting increases, and hypoxemia ensues. CC tends to exceed FRC when supine around the age of 45 and when sitting by age 65 (not depicted in this image). (Image reproduced with permission from Zaugg M, Lucchinetti E. Respiratory function in the elderly. *Anesthesiol Clin North Am.* 2000;18[1]:47-vi.)

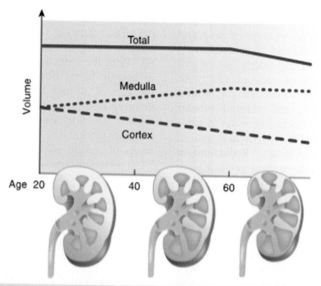

Fig. 35.5 The aging kidney. Renal cortical atrophy begins around the age of 30 (10% loss per decade above age 30), accompanied by a reduction in renal blood flow (10% per decrease over above age 40) and a progressive decline in renal function. Medullary volume initially increases, which may be compensatory, a process that ceases around the age of 60. (Reproduced with permission from O'Neill CW. Structure, not just function. *Kidney Int.* 2014;85[3]:503–505.)

and hypercarbia; however, the ability to excrete carbon dioxide is generally well-maintained.[6]

The chest wall becomes less compliant because of stiffening of the muscles and joints of the thorax. Combined with loss of thoracic vertebral disc space height, overall chest wall remodeling leads to a relative flattening of the diaphragm, which makes contraction less efficient.[6] There is also a reduction in the number of type 2 fast-twitch fibers, which may lead to diaphragmatic fatigue.[11] Altogether, this leads to an increase in work of breathing for the elderly patient under conditions of exercise or stress. Total lung capacity (TLC) tends to remain unchanged, partly because of opposite changes in compliance between the chest wall (reduced) and lung (increased). Although not considered a normal part of the aging process, restrictive lung physiology is common in the elderly in the setting of significant spinal kyphosis. The following lung volumes increase with age: residual volume (RV) by 5% to 10% per decade and FRC by 1% to 3% per decade. Lung volumes that decrease with age include vital capacity (VC) (40% decrease between the ages of 20 and 70),[8] forced vital capacity (FVC), and forced expiratory volume in 1 second (FEV$_1$).[11] Oxygen diffusing capacity (DL$_{CO}$) also steadily declines at about 5% per decade.[6]

Loss of pharyngeal muscle tone and blunting of the normal protective airway reflexes predispose to airway obstruction and pulmonary aspiration.[8] Mucociliary function also becomes less effective with age, and impaired pulmonary macrophage and neutrophil activity can increase the risk of infectious complications and subsequent tissue injury.[13]

Renal System

Renal cortical atrophy appears to be a normal part of the aging process (Fig. 35.5). This loss of renal mass is accompanied by a progressive decline in renal function.[14] At the microscopic level, there are fewer functioning nephrons because of progressive nephrosclerosis with renal tubular atrophy. The remaining nephrons tend to hypertrophy, which may represent a compensatory response. At the macroscopic level, in addition to cortical loss, there tends to be a higher incidence of renal cysts and benign tumors.[14] Renal blood flow (RBF) also decreases with age as a result of anatomic changes within the renal vasculature, a 10% decrease per decade over the age of 40.[8] This makes the kidneys less responsive to changes in volume status, which is further exacerbated by a decrease in activity of the renin–angiotensin–aldosterone system (RAAS) and other autonomic reflexes within the kidney, a term referred to as *renal vascular dysautonomy*.[15] By age 60, there are lower circulating levels of renin and aldosterone.[8] This places the elderly patient at particularly high risk for ischemic complications in the setting of hypotension. In addition, there is a diminished reserve among renal tubular cells for regeneration after ischemic insults.[15]

Glomerular filtration rate (GFR) declines with age, with some estimates showing a decrease of 1 mL/year over the age of 50.[14] However, serum creatinine levels remain normal because of a parallel reduction in muscle mass.[16] The ability to conserve and excrete sodium and to concentrate and dilute urine is impaired, and with it

IV

the ability to rapidly compensate for changes in volume status, predisposing to conditions of hypovolemia and hypervolemia and hyponatremia and hypernatremia.[12] Thirst response is diminished in the elderly, which can further aggravate hypovolemia. A reduced ability to reabsorb free water is caused by a lower tonicity within the renal medulla, lower GFR, and reduced tubular activity. The ability to excrete excess free water is similarly impaired, which predisposes to hyponatremia in the setting of hypoosmolar fluid loads.[15] Reductions in GFR and in renin and aldosterone activity predispose to hyperkalemia. This also leads to changes in the ability to excrete and reabsorb many types of medications.[8]

Nervous System

Although a complete discussion of the neurologic effects of aging is beyond the scope of this chapter, the most notable change is a progressive loss of brain mass and nervous system function. The process of progressive brain atrophy appears to begin earlier in men but occurs at a more rapid pace in women.[8] Volume loss within the central nervous system (CNS) appears more pronounced in the prefrontal cortex and medial temporal lobes, affecting white matter more than gray matter—at a rate of 5% per decade over the age of 40.[17] These anatomic changes may explain why many elderly patients experience impairments in attention and executive function and short-term memory.[12] Parallel changes are seen with increasing cerebrospinal fluid (CSF) volume over time and decreasing cerebral blood flow (CBF) by 5% to 20%.[6] At the microscopic level, there is a reduction in the number of neurons and levels of many neurotransmitters, such as dopamine, serotonin, acetylcholine, glutamate, and brain neurotrophic factor.[17] Neuronal synapses decrease along with specific reductions in cholinergic and muscarinic neurons.[18] The blood–brain barrier tends to become more permeable, and there is a loss of capillary networks and signs of arteriosclerosis and intimal thickening within the intracerebral vessels.[8] On a more global level, the aging patient experiences multiple impairments in processing of sensory inputs across many systems that present notable risk factors for perioperative complications. This is manifested by an increased risk for falls, POD, and cognitive impairment.

Gastrointestinal System

As noted earlier, the elderly patient is at greater risk for aspiration. From a gastrointestinal perspective, there is reduced esophageal muscle compliance and lower esophageal sphincter tone with advancing age, in addition to prolonged gastric emptying.[8] Although gastric acid production likely remains normal, there is reduced gastric prostaglandin and bicarbonate production, which may predispose to gastritis and a higher risk of gastric

irritation from nonsteroidal antiinflammatory drugs (NSAIDs).[6] Similar to other organ systems, the liver atrophies with age by up to 20% to 40% by the age of 80.[8] With the reduction in liver mass comes a reduction in hepatic blood flow (HBF)—a 50% decrease between the ages of 30 and 100, according to some estimates.[19] Reduced HBF places the liver at greater risk of ischemia. Hepatic function also steadily declines, with decreased albumin production, which may lead to higher plasma levels of certain acidic drugs. Additionally, cytochrome P450 metabolism is less effective with aging.[12]

Hematologic System

Hematopoietic reserves decline with aging as bone marrow mass decreases and fat content increases.[20] Advanced age can be considered a prothrombotic state, as there is increased platelet adhesiveness combined with slightly higher levels of certain clotting factors, such as fibrinogen; factors V, VII, and IX; high-molecular-weight kininogen; and prekallikrein. There is also reduced activity of the antithrombotic plasminogen activator inhibitor-1.[6] This may explain why geriatric patients are at greater risk of deep venous thrombosis (DVT). The term *immunosenescence* refers to the fact that the aging immune system is less effective at recognizing and mounting a robust immune response to novel antigens, which seems to impair lymphocytic responses in particular.[6]

PHARMACOLOGIC CONSIDERATIONS

Many unique pharmacodynamic (PD) and pharmacokinetic (PK) changes to commonly administered anesthetic drugs accompany the aging process. Elderly patients are, in general, more sensitive to most anesthetic agents, which may in part be explained by changes at the receptor level. From a PK standpoint, the physiologic changes of aging described earlier lead to notable differences in the absorption, volume of distribution (Vd), metabolism, and clearance of many medications. Oral bioavailability may be affected by changes in gastric pH and gastric emptying and by reductions in gastrointestinal tract and HBF that may affect the amount of drug that reaches the systemic circulation.[21] Total body water (TBW) decreases by 10% to 15%, with a reduction in muscle mass and an increase of 20% to 40% in fat mass. As a result, the Vd for hydrophilic agents is reduced with a resultant increase in their plasma concentration; the opposite is true for lipophilic agents[21,15] (Fig. 35.6). Additionally, serum albumin, which normally binds to acidic drugs, steadily decreases with age, which increases the unbound fraction of drug in the bloodstream.[15] On the other hand, levels of alpha-1-acid glycoprotein, which normally binds basic drugs, increase with age and subsequently reduce the levels of unbound drug.[21] With

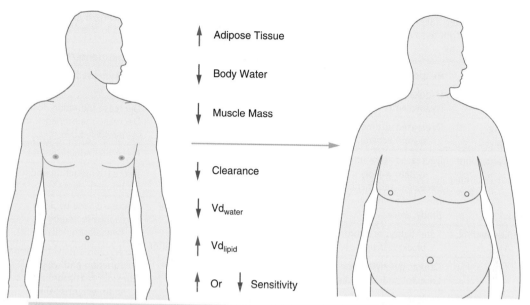

Fig. 35.6 Changes in body composition in elderly patients. *Vd,* Volume of distribution. (From Rivera R, Antognini JF. Perioperative drug therapy in elderly patients. *Anesthesiology.* 2009;110[5]:1176–1181.)

the reduction in HBF and hepatic enzymatic activity comes a reduced clearance for medications that depend on hepatic metabolism and potentially higher plasma levels and a prolongation of action. A similar process occurs for drugs that depend on renal clearance because of reductions in RBF and GFR.[12] Considering that many common comorbid conditions of the elderly, in addition to polypharmacy and nutritional status, also markedly affect drug sensitivity, it is difficult to make universal recommendations for drug dosing that neatly apply to all geriatric patients undergoing anesthesia. The general consensus, though, is that nearly all drug doses should be initially reduced, with potentially longer timing between repeated dosing, and should always be titrated to clinical effect (Tables 35.2 and 35.3).

Pharmacology of Specific Anesthetic Medications in the Elderly

Volatile Anesthetics (Also See Chapter 7)

The minimum alveolar concentration (MAC) for volatile anesthetics is reduced by 6% per decade over the age of 40, with a reduction of 8% per decade for nitrous oxide.[15,21] This is likely explained by PD changes in the CNS, such as neuronal loss, in addition to changes in neurotransmitter levels and functional connectivity.[15,22]

Propofol (Also See Chapter 8)

Induction doses of propofol should generally be reduced by at least 20% and maintenance infusions by 30% to 50%, though dosing should always be titrated to clinical effect.[23] Elderly patients are more sensitive to the effects of propofol and may exhibit reduced clearance because of reductions in hepatic metabolism.[24] In one study of healthy volunteers 75-year-old subjects required roughly half the dose of their 20-year-old counterparts for the same clinical endpoint. In addition, the former were found to achieve deeper anesthetic states as measured by electroencephalogram (EEG), which took longer to reach and recover from.[25]

Etomidate (Also See Chapter 8)

There is a reduction in both clearance and Vd for etomidate in the elderly. Although no known PD changes accompany aging, induction doses should be reduced by up to 50% to 66% in patients aged 80 and older.[15,21] Etomidate boluses produce less hypotension and can be helpful in avoiding postinduction hypotension but can produce myoclonus and adrenal suppression.

Ketamine (Also See Chapter 8)

Some of the benefits of ketamine include less respiratory depression and hypotension, which is ideal given the exaggerated hypotensive response often seen in elderly patients, especially during induction. The transient increase in HR and blood pressure can be of concern in patients with coronary artery disease or stenotic valvular lesions. Concern regarding the dysphoric side effects and potential for worsening delirium have been raised regarding its use in the geriatric population. Despite this, evidence of a pro-delirium effect appears to be mixed,[21] and a cautious reduction in both induction and maintenance dosing is recommended, though exact guidelines are lacking in the literature. Ketamine

IV

Table 35.2	Drugs Often Taken by Elderly Patients That May Contribute to Adverse Effects or Drug Interactions

Drug/Drug Class	Response
Diuretics	Hypokalemia Hypovolemia
Centrally acting antihypertensives	Decreased autonomic nervous system activity
β-Adrenergic antagonists	Decreased autonomic nervous system activity Decreased anesthetic requirements Bronchospasm Bradycardia
Cardiac antidysrhythmics	Potentiation of neuromuscular blocking drugs
Digitalis	Cardiac dysrhythmias Cardiac conduction disturbances
Tricyclic antidepressants	Anticholinergic effects
Antibiotics	Potentiation of neuromuscular blocking drugs
Oral hypoglycemics	Hypoglycemia
Alcohol	Increased anesthetic requirements Delirium tremens

From Barnett SR. Elderly patients. In Pardo MC, Miller RD, eds. *Basics of Anesthesia*. 7th ed. Philadelphia: Elsevier; 2018:610.

Table 35.3	Medication Dosing Adjustments and Other Considerations in the Elderly

Drug/Drug Class	Adjustments/Considerations[a]
Volatile anesthetics	6% decreased MAC per decade over age 40
Propofol	Decrease induction dose by 20% Decrease maintenance infusion dose by 30%–50%
Etomidate	Decrease induction dose
Ketamine	Decrease induction and maintenance infusion doses[b]
Dexmedetomidine	Decrease dose by 33% Possibly affected by hypoalbuminemia
Acetaminophen	No adjustments with normal hepatic function and weight Consider maximum daily dose of 2 g with weight <50 kg
Opioids	Decrease doses by 50% Consider avoiding morphine/meperidine because of renally cleared metabolites Remifentanil—Decrease bolus dose by 50%, maintenance dose by 66%
NSAIDs	Decrease dose by 25%–50% Avoid with GFR <60 Possibly increased risk of GI bleeding and cardiac complications
Benzodiazepines	Decrease dose significantly Prolonged effects Contributes to delirium and cognitive dysfunction Midazolam—Decrease bolus dose by at least 50%
Gabapentinoids	Decrease dose May have synergistic effects with opioids on respiratory depression
Local Anesthetics (LAs)—Neuraxial/Regional Route	Decrease dose May have prolonged effects Amide LAs hepatically metabolized Higher risk of local anesthetic systemic toxicity (LAST)
Neuromuscular Blocking Drugs	Effects may be prolonged No significant pharmacodynamic changes Careful monitoring of depth of blockade recommended to avoid residual effects
Sugammadex	May have slower onset and longer time for full reversal

GFR, Glomerular filtration rate; *MAC*, minimum alveolar concentration.
[a]General dosing recommendations. Drugs should always be titrated to clinical effect.
[b]Exact dosing recommendations in the elderly not available.

is metabolized in the liver to norketamine, which is an active metabolite.[24]

Benzodiazepines (Also See Chapter 8)
Benzodiazepines should be used with caution in the elderly because of their observed tendency to cause and/or worsen delirium. If administered, their doses should be significantly reduced because of both PD-related increases in sensitivity and PK-related changes that reduce their metabolism and potentially prolong their effects. They also have a synergistic effect on respiratory depression when administered with opioids.[21] The midazolam dosage should likely be reduced by at least 50% in the elderly.[15,21] The active metabolite of midazolam, hydroxymidazolam, is renally excreted.[15,21] Lorazepam undergoes glucuronidation, with no active metabolites, but may exhibit a delayed peak and prolonged effect.[24]

Opioids (Also See Chapter 9)
Elderly patients are more sensitive to both the analgesic and respiratory effects of opioids, and most sources recommend a dose reduction of approximately 50%.[12,15] Again, this is the result of both PD- and PK-related

changes in the geriatric patient. Of note, opioids that depend on renal clearance are best avoided, namely meperidine and morphine, both of which are converted to active metabolites (normeperidine, morphine-6-glucu-ronide, and morphine-3-glucuronide, respectively) that are excreted by the kidneys and may accumulate.[21,26] Meperidine may contribute to delirium because of its anticholinergic effects. Fentanyl can be an ideal agent because there are fewer PK-related considerations and no active metabolites, though older patients are more sensitive to its effects.[24] Remifentanil can also be advantageous, because its metabolism by nonspecific tissue and plasma esterases does not depend on end-organ function, though it does appear to have reduced clearance in the elderly and a slower onset and offset. Remifentanil bolus doses should be reduced by 50% and infusion rates by up to two-thirds.[15]

Dexmedetomidine (Also See Chapter 8)

Elderly patients are likely more sensitive to the effects of the alpha$_2$-agonist dexmedetomidine, with dose reductions of up to one-third recommended by some sources as a result of reduced drug clearance.[27] Lower albumin levels may also affect the amount of free drug in the plasma. The potential role of dexmedetomidine infusion in preventing PD is a subject of ongoing investigation.[24]

Acetaminophen

Acetaminophen is a centrally acting cyclooxygenase inhibitor that is well-tolerated by most patients. Significant hepatic dysfunction is the main contraindication in any patient, and generally no dose adjustments are needed in the elderly.[28]

Nonsteroidal Antiinflammatory Drugs

NSAIDs should be used with caution in the elderly because of their side effect profile. As inhibitors of the cyclooxygenase enzyme, they have analgesic and antiinflammatory effects but can precipitate renal failure, cause gastrointestinal bleeding, and possibly increase the risk of cardiac disease. Doses should generally be reduced by 25% to 50% and avoided in patients with GFR <60 mL/min.[28]

Local Anesthetics (Also See Chapter 10)

The degree of systemic absorption of local anesthetics (LAs), and hence risk for toxicity, depends on many factors such as site of injection, degree of local vascularity, dose and volume, and presence of adjunctive agents. The amount of absorption from the neuraxial space may be lower in the elderly because of reduced vascularity.[24] Amide LAs are hepatically metabolized, so doses should be reduced, given the risk for higher plasma concentrations in the setting of reduced HBF. Alpha-1-acid glycoprotein binds many LAs, and as mentioned earlier, its levels tend to rise with aging, though the clinical significance of this to dosing remains unclear.[24]

Neuromuscular Blocking Agents (Also See Chapter 11)

No significant PD-related changes to neuromuscular blocking agents occur with the aging process. However, age-related reductions in hepatic and renal function can prolong the effect of certain agents, such as rocuronium.[21] Cisatracurium, which is metabolized by Hoffmann elimination, is an attractive option. Regardless of the choice of agent, it is important to judiciously monitor the level of neuromuscular blockade, as even small residual effects can lead to clinically significant respiratory compromise. Sugammadex appears to have a slower onset of action and time for full recovery, as demonstrated by train-of-four (TOF) monitoring.[29]

PREOPERATIVE ASSESSMENT AND RISK MANAGEMENT (ALSO SEE CHAPTER 13)

The goal of preoperative assessment is to analyze relevant information obtained through history, physical examination, medical record review, and preoperative testing in order to formulate an anesthetic plan that best balances patient safety with the specific needs of the procedure. In the geriatric patient the following issues arise more frequently and should be evaluated prospectively: cognitive function and decision-making capacity, functional capacity, nutritional status, frailty, and polypharmacy. Elderly patients are more likely to present with comorbidities that may significantly affect the choice of anesthetic, and some geriatric patients may not be able to provide a reliable history because of cognitive decline, hearing or vision impairment, or other factors. As a result, the preoperative assessment of the geriatric patient may not be a straightforward process, and care should be taken to ensure that the patient and other relevant decision-makers have a thorough understanding of the procedure and the risks involved.

There are many published tools for assessing cognitive function.[30] Examples include the Mini Mental Status Exam (MMSE), Mini-Cog, and others (Box 35.1). This is important both to assess baseline cognitive function for the purposes of capacity and decision-making ability and to help guide a patient through the perioperative process with the necessary support structures to ensure optimal recovery and rehabilitation. A 2019 metaanalysis showed that preoperative deficiencies as measured by the MMSE correlated with POD, in-hospital mortality, and 1-year mortality.[31] Having a sense of baseline cognition is also an important part of the process for diagnosing and managing perioperative neurocognitive disorders, which are discussed later. Decision-making capacity in a medical context is defined by proficiency in four major areas: the ability to *understand* the various treatment options, an *appreciation* of the type and severity of disease and its consequences, the ability to *reason* between the various treatment options offered, and finally, the

IV

Box 35.1 Cognitive Assessment With the Mini-Cog Test: Three-Item Recall and Clock Draw

1. Get the patient's attention, then say:
   "I am going to say three words that I want you to remember now and later. The words are: *banana, sunrise, chair*. Please say them for me now." Give the patient three tries to repeat the words. If unable after three tries, go to the next item.
2. Say all the following phrases in the order indicated:
   "Please draw a clock in the space below. Start by drawing a large circle. Put all the numbers in the circle and set the hands to show 11:10 (10 past 11)." If the subject has not finished clock drawing in 3 minutes, discontinue and ask for recall items.
3. Say:
   "What were the three words I asked you to remember?"

Scoring
- Three-item recall (0–3 points); clock draw (0 or 2 points)
- 1 point for each correct word; 0 points for abnormal clock; 2 points for normal clock
- A normal clock has all of the following elements:
  - All numbers 1 to 12, each only once, are present in the correct order and direction (clockwise) inside the circle.
  - Two hands are present, one pointing to 11 and one pointing to 2.
  - Any clock missing any of these elements is scored abnormal. Refusal to draw a clock is scored abnormal.
- Total score of 0, 1, or 2 suggests possible impairment.
- Total score of 3, 4, or 5 suggests no impairment.

From Mini-Cog.com. Copyright S. Borson (soob@uw.edu), used with permission.

Box 35.2 Activities of Daily Living and Instrumental Activities of Daily Living[a]

Activities of Daily Living
Bathing
Dressing
Toileting
Transferring
Eating

Instrumental Activities of Daily Living
Use of telephone
Use of public transportation
Shopping
Preparation of meals
Housekeeping
Taking medications properly
Managing personal finances

[a]From Barnett SR. Elderly patients. In Pardo MC, Miller RD, eds. *Basics of Anesthesia*. 7th ed. Philadelphia: Elsevier; 2018:610.

Box 35.3 Assessment of Gait and Mobility Limitations With the Timed Up and Go (TUG) Test

Patients should sit in a standard armchair with a line 10 feet in length in front of the chair. They should use standard footwear and walking aids and should not receive any assistance.
   Have the patient perform the following commands:
- Rise from the chair (if possible, without using the armrests)
- Walk to the line on the floor (10 feet)
- Turn
- Return to the chair
- Sit down again

From Centers for Disease Control and Prevention. The Timed Up and Go (TUG) Test. http://www.cdc.gov/steadi/pdf/tug_test-a.pdf/. Accessed June 1, 2016.

---

ability to make an *informed choice*.[32] Assessing for mood disorders such as depression is also an essential part of the process, as is evaluating for substance use disorders, the latter of which is commonly screened using the CAGE questionnaire.[33] Often, subclinical impairments in these domains can be challenging to identify but can have important consequences during the perioperative period.

Functional capacity is broadly assessed by evaluating a patient's ability to carry out activities of daily living (ADLs) and instrumental activities of daily living (IADLs) (Box 35.2). Impairments in preoperative functional status correlate with a number of postoperative complications. The recovery plan for an elderly patient may require specific attention to nutritional support, physical therapy and rehabilitation, fall prevention, or other issues found during the preoperative assessment.[32] Deficits in hearing, vision, and swallowing ability should be documented, as they may also affect postoperative care. Falls are often of particular concern to the elderly patient, who may present with baseline deficiencies in balance and coordination, which can be aggravated by anesthetic and analgesic medications given perioperatively. The Timed Up and Go Test is one available tool for assessing mobility and can be used to define risk level for falls[32] (Box 35.3).

Poor nutritional status is associated with a number of perioperative complications, including surgical site infections, pneumonia, and urinary tract infections.[30,32] Objective measures such as albumin level <3 g/dL, body mass index <18.5 kg/m^2, or an unexplained loss of 10% to 15% of body weight within the preceding 6 months are notably worrisome signs and may be indications for delaying elective procedures when targeted interventions are feasible.[34]

Frailty is defined by a global reduction in physiologic reserve that limits a patient's ability to respond to physiologic stressors and return to a state of homeostasis (see Fig. 35.2). Although not strictly a condition of the elderly, increasing age is a major contributor to the frail state. There is no uniformly accepted method for measuring frailty; however, multiple tools are available for quantifying it. The two main tools include frailty phenotype models (e.g., Fried Index) or deficit accumulation approaches (e.g., Modified Frailty Index)[30] (Table 35.4).

Table 35.4 Selected Frailty Assessment Methods in the Perioperative Setting

Name	Description	
Modified Frailty Index (mFI)[a]	Compilation of deficits/impairments into an index based on symptoms, signs, laboratory values, disease states, and disabilities based on NSQIP database	mFI-11—11 factors used mFI-5—5 factors used
Hopkins Frailty Score[b]	Five domains: weight loss, grip strength/weakness, exhaustion, low physical activity, slowed walking speed	Score: 0, nonfrail; 1–2, prefrail; 3–5, frail
Edmonton Frail Scale[c]	Standardized assessment of cognition, general health, functional independence and performance, social support, medication usage, nutritional status, mood, continence	Scored out of 17, higher scores associated with increasing frailty
FRAIL Scale[d]	Five domains: fatigue, resistance, ambulation, illnesses, weight loss	Score: 0, nonfrail; 1–2, prefrail; 3–5, frail
Groningen Frailty Indicator[e]	15-item questionnaire, 8 indicators: mobility, physical fitness, vision, hearing, nutrition, morbidity, cognition, psychosocial	Score out of 15, 4 or greater indicative of frailty

NSQIP, National Surgical Quality Improvement Program.

Reproduced with permission from Khan KT, Hemati K, Donovan AL. Geriatric physiology and the frailty syndrome. *Anesthesiol Clin.* 2019;37(3):453-474.

[a]Farhat JS, Velanovich V, Falvo AJ, et al. Are the frail destined to fail? Frailty index as predictor of surgical morbidity and mortality in the elderly. *J Trauma Acute Care Surg.* 2012;72(6):1526-1530 and Subramaniam S, Aalberg JJ, Soriano RP, et al. New 5-Factor Modified Frailty Index using American College of Surgeons NSQIP data. *J Am Coll Surg.* 2018;226(2):173-181.e8.

[b]Fried LP, Tangen CM, Walston J, et al. Cardiovascular Health Study Collaborative Research Group. Frailty in older adults: Evidence for a phenotype. *J Gerontol A Biol Sci Med Sci.* 2001;56(3):M146-M156.

[c]Rolfson DB, Majumdar SR, Tsuyuki RT, et al. Validity and reliability of the Edmonton Frail Scale. *Age Ageing.* 2006;35(5):526-529.

[d]Morley JE, Malmstrom TK, Miller DK. A simple frailty questionnaire (FRAIL) predicts outcomes in middle aged African Americans. *J Nutr Health Aging.* 2012;16(7):601-608.

[e]Steverink N, Slaets JPJ, Schuurmans H, et al. Measuring frailty: Development and testing of the Groningen Frailty Indicator (GFI). *Gerontologist.* 2001;41(special issue 1):236-237.

Overall, frailty is best viewed as an overall assessment of risk based on age and disease-related factors across multiple organ systems.[35] Multiple studies have shown that increasing frailty is associated with higher morbidity and mortality, an association that may be stronger than simply considering age alone.[36] A 2018 study among ambulatory surgical patients using the American College of Surgeons National Surgical Quality Improvement Program (NSQIP) database found that a modified frailty index (mFI) tool correlated strongly with perioperative adverse outcomes, independent of age and comorbidities. The authors argue that access to care for elderly surgical patients, even at extremes of age, should not be limited simply by a blanket assessment of risk based on chronologic age.[37] Assessing preoperative frailty, like functional capacity and cognitive function, can be an important part of the anesthetic and surgical planning process by helping to guide what specific interventions might present the least risk to the patient. Finally, studies are underway to determine what effect frailty has on the risk of developing postoperative neurocognitive disorders. A 2020 retrospective analysis of elective hip arthroplasties found that baseline frailty index (using the Edmonton Frailty Scale) correlated well with the risk of cognitive decline at 3 and 12 months postoperatively.[36]

About 40% of patients over the age of 65 use five or more medications, with 12% to 19% taking ten or more medications.[38] The issue of polypharmacy is thus extremely relevant to the geriatric patient and necessitates a thorough review of all prescription and over-the-counter medications being used by the patient before undergoing surgery. The preoperative period is also an opportunity to assess compliance with, and appropriateness of, prescribed medications. Clear instructions should be given to elderly patients or their caregivers regarding which medications should be discontinued in the preoperative period. Polypharmacy can contribute to poor outcomes, including falls, increased incidence of adverse drug reactions, hospital length of stay, and mortality[38] (see Table 35.2). Although not unique to the geriatric patient, patients should generally be instructed to continue β-blockers and statins,[30] with most clinicians recommending discontinuation of angiotensin-converting enzyme (ACE) inhibitors and angiotensin receptor blockers (ARBs) on the day of surgery to avoid intraoperative hypotension. To help reduce the risk of delirium, elderly patients should avoid benzodiazepines and anticholinergic medications whenever possible, especially during the perioperative period.[32]

Optimizing an elderly patient before surgery can be challenging because the geriatric patient is more likely to present with one or more significant comorbidities. Additionally, geriatric patients are at a greater risk for perioperative complications.[39] A thorough assessment

IV

of cardiac, pulmonary, and renal systems should be performed at a minimum before any procedure. No specific preoperative studies are recommended solely on the basis of age. Providers should order laboratory, imaging, and other tests as required by the patient's medical conditions and the risks posed by the procedure (also see Chapter 13). Efforts to mitigate the risk of major adverse cardiac events (MACEs) often involve the 2014 American College of Cardiology/American Heart Association (ACC/AHA) Guideline on Perioperative Cardiovascular Evaluation and Management of Patients Undergoing Noncardiac Surgery for managing preoperative cardiac testing.[40] The guideline is a useful tool for adult patients of any age, though cognitive and functional limitations may make subjective assessments of exercise tolerance difficult. Generally, routine electrocardiograms are recommended only for patients with a history of, or risk factors for, cardiac disease or those undergoing intermediate- to high-risk procedures.[30] Preoperative pulmonary optimization for patients with chronic lung disease may involve pulmonary function testing (PFT), preoperative inspiratory muscle training, smoking cessation, and chest x-ray (CXR).[32] A Comprehensive Geriatric Assessment (CGA) is a formalized evaluation by a geriatric specialist that provides a more global assessment of the elderly patient and can be useful before a planned procedure. A geriatrician may then make recommendations for specific modifiable interventions, namely those related to polypharmacy, nutritional status, prehabilitation, and

postoperative planning.[30] Exercise prehabilitation, ideally in the form of regular aerobic and strength training at least 2 weeks before surgery, may significantly reduce the risk of complications and functional decline among elderly, frail patients. In addition, malnutrition can be targeted during prehabilitation programs with focused nutritional programs.[35] Finally, efforts to reduce the risk of POD are essential, as discussed later.

INTRAOPERATIVE CONSIDERATIONS

The choice between general anesthesia, regional anesthesia, and monitored anesthesia care is often heavily influenced by the type of procedure being performed (also see Chapter 14). When options exist between various types of anesthetics or a combination thereof, anesthesia providers must carefully balance the safety of the geriatric patient during the procedure with the goal of ensuring a successful recovery and avoidance of common postoperative problems, such as delirium and cardiopulmonary complications. Much research has focused on the choice between general anesthesia and neuraxial anesthesia in the elderly, especially within the hip fracture population. To date, few trials have shown conclusive evidence that one technique is significantly superior to another, except for a possible reduction in DVT incidence within the neuraxial group in a 2016 Cochrane review on the subject[41] (Table 35.5). There are many possible explanations

Table 35.5 Considerations Regarding Regional Versus General Anesthesia in the Elderly

	General Anesthesia	Regional Anesthesia
Technical Considerations	Difficult mask ventilation in edentulous patients Neck stiffness reducing ROM Exaggerated hemodynamic response to laryngoscopy	Neuraxial techniques may be challenging; ligament ossification, positioning Greater LA spread in neuraxial space
Risk of Deep Venous Thrombosis (DVT)	Variable	May be reduced with neuraxial techniques
Polypharmacy	May contribute to drug–drug interactions perioperatively	Regional techniques are often opioid-sparing Fewer systemic medications needed Elderly patients at higher risk of LAST
Risk of Perioperative Neurocognitive Disorders	No conclusive evidence of one technique being superior. May be confounded by depth of sedation used during regional anesthetics.	
Hemodynamic (HD) Stability	Variable	Hypotension common with neuraxial techniques PNBs under sedation may provide superior HD stability
Perioperative Use of Anticoagulant/ Antiplatelet Medications	May present surgery-specific contraindications	Frequently contraindicates neuraxial and certain PNB procedures Epidural catheters may complicate postoperative DVT prophylaxis/anticoagulation
Pain Control	Variable	Often superior

LA, Local anesthetic; *LAST,* local anesthetic systemic toxicity; *PNB,* peripheral nerve block; *ROM,* range of motion

for this, including significant variability in the depth of sedation used in the regional/neuraxial groups, which can at times approach that of a general anesthetic and confound the results. Furthermore, the presence of comorbidities and frequency of anticoagulant medication usage may often prevent a given patient from receiving a neuraxial technique who would have otherwise benefited.

Despite this, there are many potential benefits to avoiding general anesthesia in the elderly. Regional techniques are opioid-sparing, have the potential to limit polypharmacy and its associated complications in the perioperative period, and may better attenuate the physiologic stress response to pain.[24,42] Although neuraxial techniques have the potential for hypotension, overall hemodynamics during a regional anesthetic may provide superior cardiovascular stability.[24] Further research is needed to define specific blood pressure targets; however, hypotension should be avoided at all times. Several studies have shown a greater risk of myocardial, cerebrovascular, and renal complications with mean arterial pressure (MAP) below 65 mm Hg or significant deviations from baseline MAP.[43] Neuraxial procedures can be more challenging to perform in the elderly because of ossification of ligaments, altered alignment of the vertebral column, presence of kyphosis, or difficulties in achieving optimal positioning.[24] Older patients are more sensitive to LAs, and the lower compliance of the epidural space may lead to greater spread during bolus administration.[42] Similarly, LAs administered into the subarachnoid space tend to block higher dermatomal levels and produce more profound blockade because of the overall decreased CSF volume and increased CSF specific gravity.[24] Peripheral nerve blocks (PNBs) are an excellent choice in elderly, frail patients and often avoid some of the contraindications and complications inherent with neuraxial procedures (e.g., anticoagulant medications, hypotension). Age-related demyelination of peripheral nerve fibers makes them more susceptible to blockade by LAs, and given doses may last longer because of reduced vascularity of the nerve fibers and surrounding tissues.[24] Despite the safety profile of PNBs performed under ultrasound guidance, elderly patients are at greater risk of local anesthetic systemic toxicity (LAST), which may be related to higher free fractions of LA in the bloodstream and slower hepatic metabolism of amide local anesthetics.[24,42]

The approach to airway management in the geriatric patient is similar to a younger patient, with some unique considerations. Because of ligament ossification and joint stiffening, older patients may have significantly reduced range of motion of the cervical spine. Edentulous patients can be more difficult to mask ventilate without an oral airway, and loss of protective airway reflexes makes the elderly patient at higher risk of pulmonary aspiration. There may also be an exaggerated hemodynamic response to laryngoscopy, although this response can be attenuated with short-acting β-blockers.[12]

POSTOPERATIVE MANAGEMENT

Acute Pain (Also See Chapter 40)

There is no evidence that subjective pain perception is affected by the aging process. In fact, pain is often undertreated and underreported in the elderly. This is especially true for those with underlying dementia, in whom pain assessment can be challenging.[28,42] A number of pain scoring systems are widely used in health care settings, with some specifically designed for patients presenting along the spectrum of cognitive impairment, namely the Critical Care Pain Observation Tool (CPOT) and the Faces Pain Scale[28] (Table 35.6). When available, information from family members and caregivers can provide valuable insight into a patient's subjective experience of pain, as many elderly patients who cannot self-report their pain may exhibit behavioral changes that tend to be underappreciated by an unfamiliar provider.

Overall, there is no doubt that acute postoperative pain control in the elderly patient can be challenging. The physiologic changes of aging detailed earlier result in PK and PD alterations that make geriatric patients more susceptible to the adverse effects of many common classes of analgesics.[28,44] This is compounded by the issue of polypharmacy and the presence of comorbidities that may further narrow the therapeutic index. Elderly patients are often at greater risk of respiratory depression from opioids in addition to injuries from falls related to sedative agents.[16,28,42] On the other hand, uncontrolled pain can lead to delirium, an inability to participate in physical therapy and rehabilitation, and chronic pain syndromes. The physiologic effects of pain can also lead to SNS stimulation that may adversely affect underlying cardiovascular disease.

Patient-controlled analgesia (PCA), the mainstay of inpatient acute postsurgical pain management in many health care settings, is likely of limited use in an elderly patient with dementia. Taken together, the best strategy is a multidisciplinary approach that involves all members of the perioperative team along with geriatric expertise to help devise multimodal pain regimens that balance the comfort and safety of the patient. Using a combination of medications may contribute to polypharmacy but may also allow reduced dosages of each agent to help limit their individual side effects. Providers should use adjunctive medications with fewer CNS side effects, such as scheduled acetaminophen or reduced-dose NSAIDs, combined with opioids and other potent analgesics that are dosed appropriately for age and any end-organ dysfunction. Use of regional anesthetic strategies should be emphasized whenever possible. Ultimately, there is no "one size fits all" method for managing acute pain in the elderly, medically complex patient.

IV

Table 35.6	Common Pain Scoring Tools	
Tool	**Assessment**	**Ideal Population**
Visual Analog Scale	Patient places mark on graded line representing pain scale	Cognitively intact patients with difficulty speaking
Numeric Rating Scale	Pain score of 0-10	Cognitively intact, but validated in mild to moderate cognitively impaired patients
Verbal Descriptor Scale	Patient describes pain as "mild, moderate or severe"	Cognitively intact, but validated in mild to moderate cognitively impaired patients
Faces Scale	Patient chooses face that describes level of pain (frowning to smiling)	Validated in mild to moderate cognitively impaired patients
Pain Assessment Checklist for Seniors With Limited Ability to Communicate (PACSLAC)[a]	Observer scored assessment on a wide variety of scales of behavior, movement, facial expression	Validated in severe cognitively impaired patients
Pain Assessment in Advanced Dementia (PAINAD)[b]		
Doloplus-2[c]	Observer-scored assessment of somatic, psychomotor, and psychosocial parameters	

Data from Falzone E, Hoffmann C, Keita H. Postoperative analgesia in elderly patients. *Drugs Aging*. 2013;30(2):81–90; and Gagliese L, Katz J. Age differences in postoperative pain are scale dependent: A comparison of measures of pain intensity and quality in younger and older surgical patients. *Pain*. 2003;103(1-2):11-20. Modified from McKeown JL. Pain management issues for the geriatric surgical patient. *Anesthesiol Clin*. 2015;33(3):563-576.
[a]Fuchs-Lacelle S, Hadjistavropoulos T. Development and preliminary validation of the pain assessment checklist for seniors with limited ability to communicate (PACSLAC). *Pain Manag Nurs*. 2004;5(1):37-49.
[b]Warden V, Hurley AC, Volicer L. Development and psychometric evaluation of the Pain Assessment in Advanced Dementia (PAINAD) scale. *J Am Med Dir Assoc*. 2003;4(1):9-15.
[c]Lefebvre-Chapiro S. The DOLOPLUS 2 scale—Evaluating pain in the elderly. *Eur J Palliat Care*. 2001;8:191-194.

Hypoxemia

Hypoxemia in the postoperative period is common in many older patients. The physiologic effects of aging on the pulmonary system detailed earlier in this chapter lead to a higher propensity for V/Q mismatch and shunting. Combined with a reduced hypoxic ventilatory drive and a propensity for pulmonary aspiration, providers must maintain their vigilance when monitoring elderly patients in the postanesthesia care unit (PACU) (also see Chapter 39). Pulse oximetry should be maintained at all times, along with supplemental oxygen and the use of incentive spirometry when patients are sufficiently alert to participate.[16,22]

Fluid Management (Also See Chapter 24)

Fluid management throughout the perioperative period is complicated by the fact that the aging kidney is less efficient at responding to conditions of hypervolemia and hypovolemia, in addition to alterations in serum sodium levels.[12,15] Older patients are also more likely to have coexisting congestive heart failure, which may further complicate the assessment of volume status. Measurement of urine output alone may not accurately reflect volume status. Providers should consider physical examination findings, such as mucus membrane moisture and orthostatic blood pressure changes, along with data from laboratory

tests (e.g., lactate, electrolytes) and bedside transthoracic echocardiogram to evaluate ventricular filling to make better-informed decisions regarding fluid therapy.

CHRONIC PAIN IN THE ELDERLY (ALSO SEE CHAPTER 44)

Chronic pain is unfortunately common in the elderly and likely underreported, partly because of widely held and erroneous beliefs that pain is a normal part of the aging process.[44] Causes of chronic pain in the older patient are often the result of degenerative processes such as osteoarthritis, but may also be a result of cancer and neuropathy.[44] Similarly to the issues surrounding self-reporting of acute, postsurgical pain, diagnosing chronic pain in the elderly patient with cognitive decline can be a challenge. Providers should also consider coexisting mental health problems, such as depression, which are common in the elderly and may contribute to certain chronic pain syndromes. Focusing treatment strategies on pharmacotherapy, physical therapy, and interventional pain procedures is one approach to managing chronic pain in the older patient.[44] It is also important to consider how the treatment plan will improve the patient's functional status, as opposed to pain scores alone. Tricyclic antidepressants

(TCAs) and serotonin–norepinephrine reuptake inhibitors (SNRIs) can be effective adjuncts for many chronic pain syndromes, and it is important to continue these medications throughout the perioperative period whenever possible to avoid withdrawal symptoms.[42] The disadvantage of TCAs are their anticholinergic effects, which can potentiate cognitive dysfunction, and their tendency to cause orthostatic hypotension and potentially lead to falls. SNRIs have better safety profiles but can also potentially lead to falls. Gabapentinoids are widely used to treat both acute and chronic pain but can cause sedation and should be titrated slowly in the elderly. They may also cause synergistic respiratory depression when coadministered with opioids.[44] Interventional procedures, such as epidural steroid, facet joint, and sacroiliac joint injections, can be very helpful in improving pain and function while also helping to reduce polypharmacy. Finally, physical therapy and rehabilitation programs have been shown to improve strength and mobility[45] and even have positive effects on mood, all of which lead to enhanced quality of life.

PERIOPERATIVE NEUROCOGNITIVE DISORDERS

Cognitive dysfunction in the postoperative period is one of the most frequent complications seen in the elderly surgical patient.[46] The nomenclature for describing the various perioperative cognitive syndromes was revised in 2018 to better standardize definitions across the fields of psychiatry, neurology, geriatrics, and surgery. The umbrella term *perioperative neurocognitive disorder (PND)* now uses the diagnostic criteria already described in the *DSM-5* with respect to cognitive disorders. The various subgroups are further defined by their temporal relationship to the surgical event. The older term *postoperative cognitive dysfunction (POCD)* was largely a research term used in the anesthesia literature, and the heterogeneity in defining POCD made comparison across different studies inconsistent. Although a universally accepted neuropsychiatric testing method to diagnose PNDs has yet to be defined, the hope is that this new clinical framework will foster enhanced collaboration across disciplines.

According to these new guidelines, *preoperative neurocognitive disorders* are, by definition, present before surgery or anesthesia (Table 35.7). *Delayed neurocognitive recovery* is a new cognitive impairment in the postoperative period that resolves by postoperative day 30. A *postoperative neurocognitive disorder* (abbreviated here pNCD and formerly referred to as POCD) is any cognitive deficit that persists beyond postoperative day 30 but resolving by 12 months. Cognitive decline beyond 12 months is defined as the same as it would be during the preoperative period.[47] *Delirium* is a separate clinical entity that is sometimes further defined as *emergence* or *postoperative* depending on its specific timing relative to surgery, and

| Table 35.7 | Revised Nomenclature for Perioperative Neurocognitive Disorders |

Period	Old Nomenclature	New Nomenclature
Before surgery	Preexisting cognitive impairment	Mild and major NCD
Between surgery and hospital discharge	POD	POD
Between hospital discharge and 30 days postdischarge	POCD	dNCR
Between 30 days postdischarge and 1 year postdischarge	POCD	Mild and major postoperative NCD
After 1 year postdischarge	POCD	Mild and major NCD

Adapted from Evered LA, Vitug S, Scott DA, et al. Preoperative frailty predicts postoperative neurocognitive disorders after total hip joint replacement surgery. *Anesth Analg.* 2020;131(5):1582–1588.
dNCR, Delayed neurocognitive recovery; *DSM-5, Diagnostic and Statistical Manual of Mental Disorders,* 5th ed.; *NCD,* neurocognitive disorder; *POCD,* postoperative cognitive dysfunction; *POD,* postoperative delirium.

The new nomenclature for perioperative neurocognitive disorders (NCD) contrasted with the older term postoperative cognitive dysfunction (POCD). The newer terminology incorporates existing clinical definitions used in the *DSM-5* with respect to cognitive disorders and defines the type of postoperative NCD based on the timing postsurgery. Delayed neurocognitive recovery (dNCR) refers to a new cognitive deficit occurring up to 30 days postoperatively, and postoperative NCD refers to deficits arising after 30 days and up to 12 months postoperatively. Deficits occurring outside of these timelines are simply referred to as mild or major NCDs based on existing *DSM-5* criteria.

for the purposes of this chapter will be considered separately from the term pNCD (Table 35.8).

With respect to defining cognitive impairment, *mild cognitive dysfunction* is defined as one to two standard deviations from normal (as assessed by neuropsychiatric testing) with intact ADLs. *Major cognitive dysfunction* requires more than two standard deviations from normal plus some objective impairment in ADLs. In both cases, there must also be an element of "cognitive concern," a subjective assessment of cognitive dysfunction reported by the patient, caregiver, or clinician.[48] All of the aforementioned PNDs are graded as *mild* or *major* according to these criteria.

Postoperative Delirium

Delirium is defined by an acute, fluctuating disturbance in consciousness characterized by alterations in awareness, attention, and cognition that develops over a short period and is not ascribed to a previous cognitive

Table 35.8	Common Delirium Screening Tools			
Tool	**Sensitivity (%)**	**Specificity (%)**	**Criteria**	
Confusion Assessment Method (CAM)[a]	94–100	90–95	Nine criteria from *DSM-III-R*: acute onset and fluctuating course, inattention, disorganized thinking, altered level of consciousness, disorientation, memory impairment, perceptual disturbances, increased or decreased psychomotor activity, sleep–wake cycle disturbance	
CAM-ICU[b]	95–100	89–93	Four items: acute onset or fluctuating course, inattention, disorganized thinking, altered level of consciousness	
Delirium Symptom Interview[c]	90	80	Seven criteria from *DSM-III*: disorientation, consciousness, sleep–wake cycle, perceptual disturbance, speech, psychomotor activity, fluctuating behavior	
Nursing Delirium Screening Scale[d]	86	87	Five items: disorientation, behavior, communication, hallucinations, psychomotor retardation	

Reproduced with permission from Schenning KJ, Deiner SG. Postoperative delirium in the geriatric patient. *Anesthesiol Clin*. 2015;33(3):505–516.
[a]Inouye SK, van Dyck CH, Alessi CA, et al. Clarifying confusion: The Confusion Assessment Method. A new method for detection of delirium. *Ann Intern Med*. 1990;113(12):941–948.
[b]Ely EW, Margolin R, Francis J, et al. Evaluation of delirium in critically ill patients: Validation of the Confusion Assessment Method for the Intensive Care Unit (CAM-ICU). *Crit Care Med*. 2001;29(7):1370–1379.
[c]Albert MS, Levkoff SE, Reilly C, et al. The delirium symptom interview: An interview for the detection of delirium symptoms in hospitalized patients. *J Geriatr Psychiatry Neurol*. 1992;5(1):14–21.
[d]Gaudreau JD, Gagnon P, Harel F, et al. Fast, systematic, and continuous delirium assessment in hospitalized patients: The nursing delirium screening scale. *J Pain Symptom Manage*. 2005;29(4):368–375.

disorder.[47,49] Although the distinction between *emergence delirium* and *postoperative delirium (POD)* can be challenging, the former is usually defined by a very early onset before or at arrival in the PACU.[50] Clinically, POD is often formally diagnosed using the Confusion Assessment Method (CAM) or Riker Sedation Agitation Scale[49,50] and can present as *hyperactive, hypoactive,* or *mixed* types in terms of the perceived level of agitation of the patient, with hypoactive delirium carrying the worst prognosis for subsequent morbidity and mortality[47] (see Table 35.7; also see Chapter 41). One of the strongest predictors for POD is preexisting cognitive impairment, with other notable risk factors being advanced age, number of medical comorbidities, frailty, higher ASA score, prolonged mechanical ventilation, and uncontrolled pain.[51] In addition, many commonly used perioperative medications are known to precipitate delirium, such as benzodiazepines, anticholinergic agents, and steroids.[49] POD is common in the elderly, with estimates ranging from 26% to 35%[46] and is most common after cardiac, vascular, and hip fracture surgeries.[49] Although the specific type of anesthetic does not seem to affect the incidence, emerging literature suggests that deeper planes of anesthesia as measured by EEG or processed EEG may carry the highest risk.[47,51] The exact biologic basis for delirium is unknown, but a neuroinflammatory state precipitated by the physiologic stress of surgery combined with a more permeable blood–brain barrier in the elderly patient is a leading theory.[51] Unfortunately, the presence of POD increases the risk of morbidity and mortality at 6 to 12 months and is also a strong predictor of the eventual development

of permanent cognitive dysfunction and dementia.[22,47,49] Strategies for preventing this complication include frequent reorienting of elderly patients in the postoperative period, early provision of visual and hearing aids, avoidance of urinary catheters and restraints, and proactive geriatric consultation. The initial approach to treatment should always focus on addressing any underlying causes, such as pain, physiologic derangements (e.g., hypoxemia, electrolyte imbalances, hypovolemia), effects from medication interactions or polypharmacy, and substance withdrawal. Pharmacologic intervention, usually in the form of antipsychotic medications like haloperidol, should be reserved for extreme cases when patients are at risk of harming themselves or others.[12,49,51] Numerous studies have also examined the effects of intraoperative dexmedetomidine and ketamine on preventing POD, with mixed results. Ultimately, the most successful strategy is likely one that involves a coordinated and consistent effort among caregivers, employing evidence-based pharmacologic and behavioral tools.[50]

Postoperative Neurocognitive Disorders

Unlike delirium, delayed neurocognitive recovery and postoperative neurocognitive disorders are characterized by deficits in memory, learning, language, motor, and executive functions.[51] Many original studies of POCD found incidences of around 16% to 21% at 3 months postoperatively,[52] with some studies finding rates as high as 30% to 60%.[47] Much of this heterogeneity may be explained by a lack of consistency in the definitions and diagnosis of POCD. These syndromes can also be more challenging to diagnose because they require dedicated neuropsychiatric testing, a more time-consuming process than many of the delirium screening tools that are widely available. Additionally, clearly demonstrating a relationship to surgery or anesthesia also requires an assessment of preoperative baseline cognitive function, which may not be available. The fact that elderly patients are inherently at risk for developing dementia irrespective of surgery can confound the diagnostic process. Although pNCDs are not exclusive to the elderly population, advanced age is clearly a strong risk factor.[47] In fact, many established risk factors for the development of pNCD overlap with POD, including advanced age and preoperative cognitive impairment.[47] Other risks include presence of cerebrovascular disease, lower educational level, and POD itself.[51] Further similarities to POD include an association with a greater risk for postoperative complications such as mortality and functional decline. Initial theories suggested an association with intraoperative insults such as hypotension and hypoxemia, but there does not seem to be a clear causal relationship there, nor with specific types of anesthetic techniques or agents. A neuroinflammatory state generated by the stress of surgery, combined with specific patient-related factors, seems to offer the best explanation for why certain patients develop cognitive decline.[53] Strategies that may offer some benefit in preventing pNCD include prehabilitation programs for high-risk patients and educational programs for patients and caregivers.[47,51] Because POD is an established risk factor for pNCD, *avoiding* the following triggers for delirium may be effective: uncontrolled pain, use of benzodiazepines and anticholinergic medications, disruption of sleep–wake cycles, and deep planes of anesthesia.[47,51]

SUMMARY

Globally, elderly segments of the population are expanding rapidly and are increasingly presenting for surgical procedures in both the inpatient and ambulatory settings. Anesthesia providers must have a solid understanding of the physiologic effects of aging and the many comorbid conditions that often accompany the aging process in order to safely and effectively tailor their anesthetics to meet the needs of this growing patient population. Future research is needed to elucidate many of the neurobiologic mechanisms behind how the anesthetic state and the physiologic effects of surgery affect the aging brain and contribute to the spectrum of PNDs frequently encountered in the elderly. Improved understanding will hopefully lead to more specific interventions for safe perioperative care and improved functional and cognitive independence afterward.

ACKNOWLEDGMENT

The editors and publisher would like to thank Dr. Sheila Barnett for contributing to this chapter in the previous edition of this work. It has served as the foundation for the current chapter.

IV

REFERENCES

1. Mather M, Jacobsen LA, Pollard KM. *Population Bulletin: Aging in the United States*. 2015;70(2). https://www.prb.org/wp-content/uploads/2016/01/aging-us-population-bulletin-1.pdf. [Accessed January 4th, 2021].
2. United Nations. Department of Economic and Social Affairs, Population Division. *World Population Ageing*. 2019;*2019 Highlights* (ST/ESA/SER.A/430).
3. Deiner S, Westlake B, Dutton RP. Patterns of surgical care and complications in elderly adults. *J Am Geriatr Soc*. 2014;62:829–835.
4. Lee PHU, Gawande AA. The number of surgical procedures in an American lifetime in 3 states. *J Am Coll Surg*. 2008;207(3):S75.
5. Deiner S, Fleisher LA, Leung JM, et al. Adherence to recommended practices for perioperative anesthesia care for older adults among US anesthesiologists: Results from the ASA Committee on Geriatric Anesthesia-Perioperative Brain Health Initiative ASA member survey. *Perioper Med (Lond)*. 2020;9:6. Published 2020 Feb 25.
6. Taffet GE, Schmader KE. Normal aging. In: Post TW, ed. *UpToDate*. Waltham: UpToDate; 2020.
7. Rooke GA. Autonomic and cardiovascular function in the geriatric patient. *Anesthesiol Clin North America*. 2000;18(31,46):v–vi.
8. Alvis BD, Hughes CG. Physiology considerations in geriatric patients. *Anesthesiol Clin*. 2015;33(3):447–456.
9. Cheitlin MD. Cardiovascular physiology-changes with aging. *Am J Geriatr Cardiol*. 2003;12(1):9–13.
10. Obas V, Vasan RS. The aging heart. *Clin Sci (Lond)*. 2018;132(13):1367–1382.
11. Tran D, Rajwani K, Berlin DA. Pulmonary effects of aging. *Curr Opin Anaesthesiol*. 2018;31(1):19–23.
12. Deiner S, Silverstein JH. Anesthesia for geriatric patients. *Minerva Anestesiol*. 2011;77(2):180–189.
13. Hearps AC, Martin GE, Angelovich TA, et al. Aging is associated with chronic innate immune activation and dysregulation of monocyte phenotype and function. *Aging Cell*. 2012;11:867–875.
14. Denic A, Glassock RJ, Rule AD. Structural and functional changes with the aging kidney. *Adv Chronic Kidney Dis*. 2016;23(1):19–28.
15. Akhtar S, Ramani R. Geriatric pharmacology. *Anesthesiol Clin*. 2015;33(3):457–469.
16. Monarch S, Wren K. Geriatric anesthesia implications. *J Perianesth Nurs*. 2004;19(6):379–384.
17. Brown EN, Purdon PL. The aging brain and anesthesia. *Curr Opin Anaesthesiol*. 2013;26(4):414–419.
18. Schliebs R, Arendt T. The cholinergic system in aging and neuronal degeneration. *Behav Brain Res*. 2011;221:555.
19. McLean AJ, Le Couteur DG. Aging biology and geriatric clinical pharmacology. *Pharmacol Rev*. 2004;56:163.

20. French RA, Broussard SR, Meier WA, et al. Age-associated loss of bone marrow hematopoietic cells is reversed by GH and accompanies thymic reconstitution. *Endocrinology.* 2002;143:690.

21. Andres TM, McGrane T, McEvoy MD, Allen BFS. Geriatric pharmacology: An update. *Anesthesiol Clin.* 2019;37(3):475–492.

22. Society American Geriatrics. New Frontiers in Geriatrics Research: An Agenda for Surgical and Related Medical Specialties. Cook DJ. *Geriatric Anesthesia.* 2021. Accessed January 5th. http://newfrontiers.americangeriatrics.org/chapter.php?ch=2.

23. Shafer SL. The pharmacology of anesthetic drugs in elderly patients. *Anesthesiol Clin North America.* 2000;18(1):1–29, v.

24. Lin C, Darling C, Tsui BCH. Practical regional anesthesia guide for elderly patients. *Drugs Aging.* 2019;36(3):213–234.

25. Schnider TW, Minto CF, Shafer SL, et al. The influence of age on propofol pharmacodynamics. *Anesthesiology.* 1999;90:1502–1516.

26. Smith HS. Opioid metabolism. *Mayo Clin Proc.* 2009;84(7):613–624.

27. Wang C, Zhang H, Fu Q. Effective dose of dexmedetomidine as an adjuvant sedative to peripheral nerve blockade in elderly patients. *Acta Anaesthesiol Scand.* 2018;62:848–856.

28. Rajan J, Behrends M. Acute pain in older adults: Recommendations for assessment and treatment. *Anesthesiol Clin.* 2019;37(3):507–520.

29. Muramatsu T, Isono S, Ishikawa T, et al. Differences of recovery from rocuronium-induced deep paralysis in response to small doses of sugammadex between elderly and nonelderly patients. *Anesthesiology.* 2018;129(5):901–911.

30. Barnett SR. Preoperative assessment of older adults. *Anesthesiol Clin.* 2019;37(3):423–436.

31. Cao SJ, Chen D, Yang L, Zhu T. Effects of an abnormal mini-mental state examination score on postoperative outcomes in geriatric surgical patients: A meta-analysis. *BMC Anesthesiol.* 2019;19(1):74.

32. Nakhaie M, Tsai A. Preoperative assessment of geriatric patients. *Anesthesiol Clin.* 2015;33(3):471–480.

33. Ewing JA. Detecting alcoholism. The CAGE questionnaire. *JAMA.* 1984;252(14):1905–1907.

34. Chow WB, Rosenthal RA, Merkow RP, et al. American College of Surgeons National Surgical Quality Improvement Program, American Geriatrics Society. Optimal preoperative assessment of the geriatric surgical patient: A best practices guideline from the American College of Surgeons National Surgical Quality Improvement Program and the American Geriatrics Society. *J Am Coll Surg.* 2012;215(4):453–466.

35. McIsaac DI, MacDonald DB, Aucoin SD. Frailty for perioperative clinicians: A narrative review. *Anesth Analg.* 2020;130(6):1450–1460.

36. Evered LA, Vitug S, Scott DA, Silbert B. Preoperative frailty predicts postoperative neurocognitive disorders after total hip joint replacement surgery. *Anesth Analg.* 2020;131(5):1582–1588.

37. Seib CD, Rochefort H, Chomsky-Higgins K, et al. Association of patient frailty with increased morbidity after common ambulatory general surgery operations. *JAMA Surg.* 2018;153(2):160–168.

38. Barnett SR. Polypharmacy and perioperative medications in the elderly. *Anesthesiol Clin.* 2009;27:377–389.

39. Khan KT, Hemati K, Donovan AL. Geriatric physiology and the frailty syndrome. *Anesthesiol Clin.* 2019;37(3):453–474.

40. Fleisher LA, Fleischmann KE, Auerbach AD, et al. 2014 ACC/AHA guideline on perioperative cardiovascular evaluation and management of patients undergoing noncardiac surgery: A report of the American College of Cardiology/American Heart Association Task Force on Practice Guidelines. *J Am Coll Cardiol.* 2014;64(22):e77–e137.

41. Guay J, Parker MJ, Gajendragadkar PR, Kopp S. Pain management issues for the geriatric surgical patient. *Cochrane Database Syst Rev.* 2016;2:CD000521.

42. McKeown JL. Pain management issues for the geriatric surgical patient. *Anesthesiol Clin.* 2015;33(3):563–576.

43. Aucoin S, McIsaac DI. Emergency general surgery in older adults: A review. *Anesthesiol Clin.* 2019;37(3):493–505.

44. Schwan J, Sclafani J, Tawfik VL. Chronic pain management in the elderly. *Anesthesiol Clin.* 2019;37(3):547–560.

45. de Vries NM, van Ravensberg CD, Hobbelen JSM, et al. Effects of physical exercise therapy on mobility, physical functioning, physical activity and quality of life in community-dwelling older adults with impaired mobility, physical disability and/or multi-morbidity: A meta-analysis. *Ageing Res Rev.* 2012;11(1):136–149.

46. Subramaniyan S, Terrando N. Neuroinflammation and perioperative neurocognitive disorders. *Anesth Analg.* 2019;128(4):781–788.

47. Olotu C. Postoperative neurocognitive disorders. *Curr Opin Anaesthesiol.* 2020;33(1):101–108.

48. Evered L, Silbert B, Knopman DS, et al. Recommendations for the nomenclature of cognitive change associated with anaesthesia and surgery-2018. *Anesthesiology.* 2018;129(5):872–879.

49. Schenning KJ, Deiner SG. Postoperative delirium in the geriatric patient. *Anesthesiol Clin.* 2015;33(3):505–516.

50. Donovan AL, Whitlock EL. Intraoperative dexmedetomidine to prevent postoperative delirium: In search of the magic bullet. À la recherche du remède miracle: administration peropératoire de dexmédétomidine pour prévenir le delirium postopératoire. *Can J Anaesth.* 2019;66(4):365–370.

51. Rengel KF, Pandharipande PP, Hughes CG. Special considerations for the aging brain and perioperative neurocognitive dysfunction. *Anesthesiol Clin.* 2019;37(3):521–536.

52. Evered L, Scott DA, Silbert B, Maruff P. Postoperative cognitive dysfunction is independent of type of surgery and anesthetic. *Anesth Analg.* 2011;112:1179–1185.

53. Evered LA, Silbert BS. Postoperative cognitive dysfunction and noncardiac surgery. *Anesth Analg.* 2018 Aug;127(2):496–505.

36 ORGAN TRANSPLANTATION

Randolph H. Steadman, Victor W. Xia

Patients waiting for a transplantable organ share a hope for the future that is predicated on the availability of an organ donor. Donor death must be declared before organ procurement.[1] Donation after brain death (DBD) is the most common setting in which donation occurs. Organ shortages have led to the resurgence of interest in donation after cardiac death (DCD).[2] The ethical considerations related to DCD donation are challenging, yet DCD donation is increasing in response to the national organ shortage.[3]

CONSIDERATIONS FOR ORGAN TRANSPLANTATION

Because of the shortage of available organs, not all potential recipients on the waiting list survive long enough to undergo a transplant procedure. Those who do typically wait a year or more. Prelisting assessments may be outdated by the time an organ is identified, and supplemental testing may be indicated. This testing may necessitate a deferral of the scheduled transplant, which must be weighed against the risk of further deterioration that can preclude transplantation. Untreated systemic infection, incurable malignancy, untreated substance abuse, and lack of sufficient social support to comply with posttransplant care can preclude transplantation.

Once the decision is made to proceed with transplantation, coordination between the donor procedure and multiple recipient hospitals may be involved. Because not all donor organs are suitable for transplantation, the recipient operation should not begin until visual or biopsy-based confirmation of organ suitability has been made. During the time between the identification of the donor and the procurement surgery, the recipient's latest laboratory values should be reviewed. If necessary, dialysis can be performed. The anesthetic plan should be reviewed with the patient and family as part of the consent process before surgery.

Box 36.1 Kidney Transplantation Facts

- The kidney is the most frequently transplanted solid organ.
- More than 16,000 deceased donor and 6000 live donor kidney transplant procedures were performed in the United States in 2018.
- Five-year posttransplantation survival rates are 92% for recipients of live donor grafts and 83% for deceased donor recipients.
- Transplantation provides significant quality-of-life and mortality benefits over dialysis for the treatment of end-stage kidney disease.

From Hart A, Smith JM, Skeans MA, et al. OPTN/SRTR 2018 annual data report: Kidney. *Am J Transplant.* 2020;20(Suppl s1):20-130.

Box 36.2 Kidney Transplant Recipient: Preoperative Assessment

Cardiovascular
Ischemic heart disease
Congestive heart failure
Hypertension

Diabetes

Renal
Hyperkalemia
Acidosis
Anemia
Dialysis history (route and frequency)

KIDNEY TRANSPLANTATION

Kidney transplantation confers a survival advantage and cost saving over dialysis for the management of renal failure[4] (Box 36.1). Quality of a graft can be assessed by kidney donor risk index (KDRI), which is calculated from several donor characteristics.[5] There is a higher risk of graft failure in donors with advanced age, hypertension, diabetes, in grafts with prolonged ischemia times, and in recipients with high panel reactive antibodies (PRAs) levels, which indicate sensitization to human leukocyte antigens.

Preoperative Assessment

The number of kidney transplants has been increasing in the United States and the number of patients waiting for a kidney transplant has been declining. However, a severe mismatch between organ need and supply remains. For deceased donor kidney transplant, 60% of candidates wait more than 5 years.[6] This makes it challenging to maintain an up-to-date pretransplant assessment. Currently approximately one-third of kidney transplants are living-related, which significantly shortens the waiting time and facilitates scheduling preoperative evaluation.

Almost all living donations are performed laparoscopically; few are converted to open procedures.[6]

Diabetes is the most common cause of end-stage renal disease, followed by hypertension and glomerulonephritis (Box 36.2). These three causes account for over two-thirds of the cases of renal failure. Patients with these conditions should be medically managed to achieve treatment goals while on the waiting list (also see Chapter 28).

Although cardiovascular disease is the leading cause of death in patients receiving dialysis, cardiovascular risk factors are often undertreated.[7] After transplant, the cardiovascular risk diminishes from a 10-fold to a twofold increase compared with that of normal patients. Accordingly, the preoperative assessment should focus on screening for ischemic heart disease and management of hypertension, diabetes, and dyslipidemia. Ischemic heart disease may be silent, particularly in diabetic patients. As a result of preexisting vasodilatation stress, echocardiography is probably superior to thallium imaging in predicting postoperative cardiac events, although false-positive and false-negative findings occur with both techniques.[8] Coronary angiography, accompanied by therapeutic intervention for significant lesions, should be considered in patients with reversible cardiac ischemia or in those with significant risk.

Congestive heart failure is prevalent in dialysis patients, but in the absence of ischemic heart disease does not preclude safe transplantation. Ejection fraction typically improves after transplantation. The preoperative focus is on optimal medical management of heart failure and maintenance of intravascular fluid balance.

Anemia may increase cardiovascular risk, particularly in patients with ischemic heart disease. Erythropoietin, when used to correct anemia to levels of 12 g/dL or less, lessens the risk of blood transfusion (see Chapter 25).

Hyperkalemia is common in patients with renal insufficiency and may be associated with increased risks during transplant surgery, particularly during reperfusion. However, mild increases in potassium may reflect normal homeostasis for renal failure, and potassium levels of 5.0 to 5.5 mEq/L are acceptable in this population. Dialysis-dependent patients may benefit from dialysis immediately before transplantation; however, a reduced intravascular central volume may offset the benefits of reduced potassium levels.

Intraoperative Management

Donor kidneys are usually implanted in the iliac fossa. Vascular anastomoses are most frequently to the external iliac artery and vein, and the ureter is anastomosed directly to the bladder (Fig. 36.1). Chronic renal disease can affect drug excretion via the kidney but also through changes in plasma protein binding or hepatic metabolism. When the protein binding is diminished, the free fraction

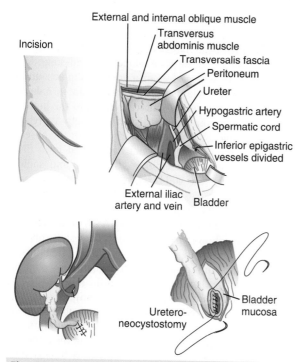

External and internal oblique muscle
Transversus abdominis muscle
Transversalis fascia
Peritoneum
Ureter
Hypogastric artery
Spermatic cord
Inferior epigastric vessels divided
Incision
External iliac artery and vein
Bladder
Ureteroneocystostomy
Bladder mucosa

Fig. 36.1 Kidney recipient operation. (From Townsend CM Jr, Beauchamp RD, Evers BM, et al., eds. *Sabiston Textbook of Surgery.* 18th ed. Philadelphia: Saunders Elsevier; 2007, used with permission.)

of the drug is increased. This results in an increase in the volume of distribution and the clearance. The net effect for the unbound fraction is similar to that in normal patients.

Some drugs require particular caution when administered in patients with renal failure. They include neuromuscular blocking (NMB) drugs (also see Chapter 11) and certain opioids (also see Chapter 9). Long-acting NMB agents that are excreted via the kidneys (e.g., pancuronium) are best avoided. Even intermediate-duration NMBs that are hepatically metabolized, such as vecuronium and rocuronium, may have a prolonged action in patients with renal failure. Cisatracurium's duration of action is more predictable because of spontaneous breakdown (also see Chapter 11). Although atracurium undergoes similar elimination, it is less potent than cisatracurium, so its breakdown product, laudanosine, is found in higher concentrations. Laudanosine can cause seizures at high concentrations; however, such concentrations are unlikely to occur after clinical administration.

Since its introduction in the US market in 2015, sugammadex has gained popularity as a reversal agent for aminosteroid NMB agents. Because the sugammadex–NMB complex is renally excreted, it is not US Food and Drug Administration approved for use in patients with end-stage renal disease because of concerns of recurring paralysis if the complex dissociates. However,

sugammadex has been safely administered to patients with end-stage renal disease.[9]

The 6-glucuronide metabolite of morphine has clinical activity that can result in a prolonged duration of action. Meperidine should be avoided because of the seizure-inducing potential of its metabolite, normeperidine.

Inhaled anesthetics can be used in renal failure patients. Although sevoflurane's metabolite, compound A, is nephrotoxic in rats, similar effects have not been seen in humans. Serum fluoride concentrations of 30 µmol occur in humans after sevoflurane administration, but do not produce renal damage. Isoflurane is metabolized to fluoride, but the extent of metabolism is so small that fluoride levels are negligible. Desflurane is not contraindicated in renal failure, but like the other volatile anesthetics, it produces a decrease in renal blood flow and glomerular filtration rate in a dose-dependent manner.

Intravascular fluid balance should be maintained in patients undergoing kidney transplantation. Typically, crystalloid is used for this purpose, with colloids preferred by some centers. In an intensive care unit (ICU) population (also see Chapter 41) balanced salt solutions (e.g., lactated Ringer's solution, Plasma-Lyte) are preferred over hyperchloremic crystalloids such as normal saline. These balanced salt solutions are associated with a lower incidence of acute kidney injury and a reduced need for renal replacement.[10] Paradoxically, their effect on serum potassium levels is less than that of potassium-free hyperchloremic solutions, which are more likely to increase serum blood potassium concentrations by generating a hyperchloremic acidosis. Albumin is the typical colloid of choice; hydroxyethyl starch solution is associated with a more frequent risk of acute kidney injury.[11]

Monitoring arterial blood pressure via an arterial catheter is avoided in some centers in order to preserve arterial access for dialysis, whereas other centers use arterial monitoring regularly in an aging recipient population with increasingly common comorbid conditions. Central venous pressure (CVP) monitoring is now recognized as a poor monitoring method of preload and fluid responsiveness.[12] Placement of a central venous line should be reserved for medications that require administration into a high-flow vein such as rabbit antithymocyte globulin, an immunosuppression induction drug. Induction of immunosuppression is increasingly common as efforts to increase the living donor pool include the use of unrelated living donors, nondirected donors, and donor exchange programs.

Delayed graft function and acute tubular necrosis can lead to renal replacement therapy after transplantation. The factors responsible include donor hemodynamics, graft warm ischemia, and recipient hemodynamics. Adequate hydration reduces the incidence of acute tubular necrosis. There are few data to support the intraoperative use of diuretics, and there is considerable variability between surgeons regarding the intraoperative use of

IV

Box 36.3 Liver Transplant Recipient: Preoperative Assessment

- Neurologic
  - Encephalopathy
  - Cerebral edema (acute liver failure)
- Cardiovascular
  - Hyperdynamic circulation
  - Cirrhotic cardiomyopathy
  - Portopulmonary hypertension
- Pulmonary
  - Restrictive lung disease
  - Ventilation-perfusion mismatch
  - Intrapulmonary shunts
  - Hepatopulmonary syndrome
- Gastrointestinal
  - Portal hypertension
  - Variceal bleeding
  - Ascites
- Renal/metabolic
  - Hepatorenal syndrome
  - Acid-base abnormalities
- Hematologic
  - Coagulopathy
  - Anemia
- Musculoskeletal
  - Muscle atrophy

---

diuretics.[13] Although of unproven benefit in preventing acute kidney injury in a general perioperative population, administration of osmotic diuretics, such as mannitol, during transplantation may be helpful.[14]

Postoperative Management

Maintaining renal perfusion is an important consideration and is best accomplished by maintaining an adequate intravascular volume. Dopamine, large-dose diuretics, and osmotic diuretics are of no proven benefit in the postoperative period. Postoperative analgesia can be achieved by epidural infusion, although many centers prefer intravenously administered patient-controlled analgesia with fentanyl or morphine (also see Chapter 40). Nonsteroidal antiinflammatory drugs should be avoided.

Enhanced recovery after surgery (ERAS) pathways that include discontinuation of opioids after the first postoperative day have been demonstrated to accelerate recovery and decrease length of hospital stay after renal transplantation.[15]

LIVER TRANSPLANTATION

The liver is second to the kidney as the most frequently transplanted solid organ. The number of deceased donor liver transplants increased by 26% over the last 5 years.[16]

Patients with liver failure have no alternatives to liver transplantation. Currently the median time to transplant for waiting list candidates is 11 months. For the highest-acuity recipients, those with Model for End-stage Liver Disease (MELD) scores of 35 or more (a group accounting for a fifth of transplants), median wait time is 7 days.[17] The MELD score is used to allocate grafts to the highest-acuity candidate on the wait list; it is directly correlated with the recipient's 90-day mortality risk in the absence of transplantation. International normalized ratio (INR) of prothrombin time, creatinine, bilirubin, and sodium are used to derive the MELD score. Online tools are available for this calculation.[18] Currently the most common indications for liver transplantation in the United States are nonalcoholic steatohepatitis (NASH) and alcoholic liver disease, followed by malignancy, cholestatic disease, hepatitis C, and acute liver failure. (ALF)[17] Hepatitis C, the most common indication for transplantation over the previous decade, has decreased significantly because of antiviral agents introduced in 2013. NASH, a diagnosis associated with metabolic syndrome and obesity, is an increasingly prevalent indication for transplantation.

An ongoing shortage of donors has led to the increased use of marginally viable grafts, defined as organs from elderly donors; DCD donors; donors with steatotic livers, obesity, malignancy, prolonged ICU stays, bacterial infection, or high-risk lifestyle; donors on multiple vasopressor infusions; or those who had suffered cardiac arrest.[19]

Preoperative Assessment

The proportion of liver transplant candidates over the age of 65 has doubled over the last decade and now accounts for a quarter of those on the wait list.[17] A higher percentage are hospitalized and have comorbid conditions (also see Chapter 28). Liver transplant candidates have many symptoms ranging from fatigue to multiple organ failure (Box 36.3). Encephalopathy, common in end-stage liver disease (ESLD), can lead to sensitivity to sedative and analgesic medications, increased risk of aspiration of gastric contents, and the need for endotracheal intubation to protect the airway.

The pretransplant cardiac evaluation includes an assessment for ischemic heart disease and screening for portopulmonary hypertension (PPHTN). Dobutamine stress echocardiography and nuclear scans are common screening tests to rule out coronary artery disease; however, they are associated with both false-positive and false-negative results.[8] In older patients with diabetes multiple risk factors, or a history of coronary disease, left-sided heart catheterization may be indicated (also see Chapter 26 and 35). More than two-thirds of ESLD patients have a hyperdynamic circulation characterized by a high cardiac output and low systemic vascular resistance (SVR), most likely because of circulating vasoactive substances not cleared by the liver. This hyperdynamic state can be confused with sepsis and is exacerbated by graft reperfusion.

Resting echocardiography is the test of choice in screening for PPHTN. An estimated right ventricular systolic pressure of less than 50 mm Hg by echocardiography rules out significant PPHTN. Right-sided heart catheterization is indicated if estimated right ventricular pressure exceeds 50 mm Hg. The definitive diagnosis of PPHTN is made when the mean pulmonary artery (PA) pressure is more than 25 mm Hg in the presence of an increased transpulmonary gradient (mean PA minus PA occlusion pressure >12) and an increased pulmonary vascular resistance (>3 Wood units, or >240 dynes-sec/cm^5). Moderate PPHTN (mean PA pressure >35 mm Hg, pulmonary vascular resistance [PVR] >5 Wood units) is associated with increased perioperative mortality, and treatment before transplant should be considered. Severe PPHTN (mean PA pressure >45 to 50 mm Hg) is considered a contraindication to liver transplantation at many centers.[20]

Hepatopulmonary syndrome (resting, room air Pao_2 <70 mm Hg in the presence of an intrapulmonary shunt on bubble echocardiography) resolves after transplantation; however, Pao_2 levels less than 50 mm Hg while breathing room air are associated with increased acuity, longer postoperative hospital stays, and, in some studies a higher postoperative mortality rate.

Renal disease is common in patients who present for liver transplantation. If not long-standing, hepatorenal syndrome may resolve after transplantation. Before transplantation, excessive intravascular volume, acidosis, or hyperkalemia may necessitate renal replacement therapy. The coagulopathy of ESLD is multifactorial and requires correction in the presence of active bleeding. Despite abnormal clotting tests (prolonged INR, hypofibrinogenemia, and thrombocytopenia), patients with ESLD should not be considered "auto-anticoagulated," as levels of endogenous anticoagulants may be more significantly reduced than clotting factors, leading to thrombosis.[21]

ALF accounts for less than 5% of liver transplants. ALF is distinct from chronic liver disease because of the potential for cerebral edema, which is the most common cause of death in ALF.[22] Cerebral edema is managed similarly to other causes of increased intracranial pressure (also see Chapter 30). The cause of ALF often predicts whether spontaneous recovery without transplant is likely. The survival rate in those receiving transplants is similar to the posttransplant survival rate in patients with chronic liver disease.

Intraoperative Management

Intraoperative management requires a consideration of the effects of liver failure on drug metabolism. Preoperative anxiolytic medication should be used sparingly in patients with a history of encephalopathy. The

---

> **Box 36.4** Liver Transplantation: Unique Aspects of Case Preparation
>
> **Transfusion**
> Red blood cells: 6-10 units for adults
> Fresh frozen plasma: 6-10 units for adults
> Rapid infusion device
>
> **Medication**
> Vasopressors: phenylephrine, epinephrine (10 and 100 µg/mL), vasopressin
> Calcium chloride: for infusion and bolus
> Insulin: for infusion (e.g., for poststeroid hyperglycemia and/ or hyperkalemia unresponsive to diuretics)
>
> **Monitors**
> Arterial line
> Central venous pressure catheter
> Pulmonary artery catheter
> Transesophageal echocardiography

---

chosen anesthetic should maintain SVR. The intermediate-duration NMB drugs metabolized by the liver can have a prolonged duration of action; however, after reperfusion, evidence of liver function typically occurs and metabolism of these drugs improves. Alternatively, cisatracurium, which undergoes Hofmann elimination, can be selected to avoid these concerns. Seizures can also be caused by an accumulation of normeperidine, so meperidine should be avoided. The metabolite of morphine, 6-glucuronide morphine, can accumulate and cause a prolonged effect. Fentanyl and the other synthetic opioids are safe choices. Volatile anesthetics have similar, mild effects on hepatic blood flow. Sevoflurane undergoes metabolism by the liver, but the metabolite, compound A, is not toxic to the liver or kidneys in humans.

Intraoperative monitoring varies among medical centers (Box 36.4). An arterial line is placed, followed by a central venous catheter (CVC) and pulmonary artery catheter (PAC), or CVC alone. Continuous cardiac output measurement from arterial waveform analysis may not accurately reflect cardiac output in liver recipients as a result of low SVR, high cardiac output, and vasopressor administration. Stroke volume and pulse pressure variation, although more accurate than CVP monitoring for predicting fluid responsiveness, are less accurate during mechanical ventilation with smaller tidal volumes (<8 mL/kg) and in the presence of cardiac arrhythmias (also see Chapter 20).[23] Transesophageal echocardiography (TEE) is often used, which may obviate the need for PAC monitoring in the operating room. TEE represents the gold standard for cardiac preload monitoring; however, interpretation is operator dependent, and monitoring into the postoperative period is not feasible.

Venovenous bypass, using an extracorporeal circuit to reroute blood from the inferior vena cava (IVC) and portal venous systems to the upper body, is used in some

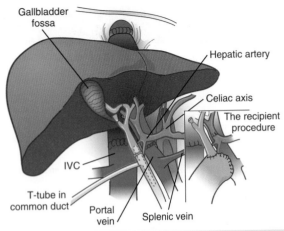

Fig. 36.2 Liver recipient operation. Illustrated are the anastomoses of the donor and recipient suprahepatic IVC, infrahepatic IVC, portal vein, hepatic artery, and duct-to-duct biliary anastomosis, which can be performed with or without T-tube placement. Alternatively *(inset)*, in the presence of disease of the bile duct, biliary drainage is via a choledochojejunostomy. *IVC*, Inferior vena cava. (From Townsend CM Jr., Beauchamp RD, Evers BM, et al., eds. *Sabiston Textbook of Surgery*. 18th ed. Philadelphia: Saunders Elsevier; 2007, used with permission.)

Box 36.5 Liver Transplantation: Treatment for the Physiologic Changes of Reperfusion

- *Hyperkalemia*: calcium, bicarbonate, insulin, and glucose
- *Acidosis*: bicarbonate, other buffers such as tris (hydroxymethyl) aminomethane
- *Decreased SVR*: α-agonists
- *Hypothermia*: warm saline peritoneal lavage

SVR, Systemic vascular resistance.

---

centers to attenuate the effects of IVC clamping on intravascular volume; however, it has risks and adds to the length of the procedure.

The operation is divided into three phases: preanhepatic, anhepatic, and neohepatic. In the preanhepatic phase dissection and preparation for the native hepatectomy occur. This phase is associated with blood loss, particularly in the presence of varices and prior abdominal surgery. Vascular isolation of the native liver (cross-clamping of the IVC, portal vein, and hepatic artery) begins the anhepatic phase. Excision of the native liver occurs next and is followed by implantation of the donor graft. The implantation involves anastomoses of the suprahepatic IVC, the infrahepatic IVC, and the portal vein (Fig. 36.2). An alternative "piggyback" technique involves anastomosis of the donor hepatic veins to the recipient vena cava, followed by portal anastomosis. The anhepatic period is typically quiescent from a hemodynamic perspective. Reperfusion follows portal anastomoses and begins the neohepatic period. Reperfusion is the most precarious event during the procedure because of the release of cold, acidotic effluent from the graft and lower extremities (Box 36.5). *Reperfusion syndrome* is characterized by a decrease in systemic blood pressure and SVR.[24] The portal effluent contains vasoactive peptides that reduce SVR and can increase pulmonary resistance. Hyperkalemia can be life threatening. If hyperkalemia is a concern, dialysis is helpful if started early in the preanhepatic period. Insulin is effective if given at least 10 to 15 minutes before reperfusion; infusions are preferred to repeated bolus dosing. Calcium given immediately before reperfusion blunts the effect of hyperkalemia on the myocardium. α-Adrenergic agonists and alkalizing drugs may be required to maintain SVR and pH, respectively.

During the neohepatic phase, fibrinolysis can occur, resulting in ongoing oozing as a result of microvascular bleeding. If fibrinolysis is not self-limited, antifibrinolytic drugs can be administered. Metabolic acidosis, which worsens during the anhepatic phase and peaks after reperfusion, should improve when the liver starts functioning. Additional signs of liver function include increased core temperature and decreasing calcium requirement (indicating citrate metabolism by the liver). On occasion, oliguric patients with hepatorenal syndrome may show an increase in urine output in the operating room.

Postoperative Management

Posttransplant patient survival rates are 89% at 1 year and 77% at 5 years.[16] Thrombosis of the hepatic artery in the early postoperative period usually necessitates retransplantation. Infection is a major threat to survival in the initial months after transplant.

HEART TRANSPLANTATION

Heart transplantation is the definitive treatment for patients with advanced heart failure. Currently, the two most common indications for heart transplantation are idiopathic dilated cardiomyopathy and ischemic cardiomyopathy, which account for nearly 90% of heart transplants.[25] Congenital heart disease and retransplantation each account for less than 5% of heart transplants. Over 3000 heart transplants are performed annually in the United States, and 1-year survival is about 90%.[25]

Preoperative Evaluation

Although patients undergo extensive multidisciplinary evaluation before being listed, a detailed preanesthetic evaluation is often challenging because of the urgent nature of the surgery, the complex clinical presentation, and multiple comorbid conditions (also see

Chapter 13).[26] Many patients require inotropic drugs or mechanical support at the time of heart transplantation. Preoperative evaluation should focus on medications (particularly the need for inotropic and anticoagulant drugs) and current cardiac status, including dependence on a pacemaker, implantable cardiac defibrillator, and/or mechanical support (intraaortic balloon pump, venoarterial extracorporeal membrane oxygenation [VA-ECMO], or ventricular assist device). The patient should not have severe, irreversible pulmonary hypertension or an active infectious disease. For patients with multiple organ failure, combined heart transplantation with other organs (e.g., lung, kidney, liver) may be considered.

Intraoperative Management

In addition to standard monitors, invasive hemodynamic monitors (arterial lines, CVCs, and PACs) are routinely inserted for heart transplantation.[27] The right internal jugular vein remains a preferred site despite a concern that it may jeopardize postoperative biopsies. The PAC needs to be withdrawn to the jugular vein before the native heart is excised. Alternatively, the PAC is inserted at the central venous position and is advanced after the donor heart is implanted. In some institutions a PAC with capability of continuous monitoring of mixed venous O_2 saturation and cardiac output is also used. TEE plays an important role in assessing intravascular volume status, contractility, and valvular function, while monitoring for thromboembolism.

Patients who are having a heart transplant often have a full stomach because of the urgency of the procedure; therefore a rapid-sequence induction of anesthesia is appropriate. The choice of anesthetic is dictated by the patient's cardiac status. A failing heart is dependent on preload and sensitive to afterload. Even small changes in venous return, vascular resistance, rhythm, heart rate, and contractility can lead to hemodynamic collapse. Anesthetics with minimal hemodynamic impact are often chosen to induce anesthesia. Etomidate is a reasonable selection. Maintenance of anesthesia is often achieved by administration of a combination of a volatile anesthetic and an opioid. A large-dose opioid technique can be used as well.

Management goals during heart transplantation are dictated by the underlying congestive heart failure and the need to avoid conditions that increase PA pressure (Box 36.6). Weaning from cardiopulmonary bypass for heart transplantation is managed similarly to other cardiac surgeries. Patients are rewarmed. Acid–base and electrolytes should be in the normal range, the lungs are ventilated with 100% oxygen, and the cardiac chambers are free of air.

Several intraoperative issues are unique to heart transplantation. First, the transplanted heart is denervated, and bradycardia can occur after reperfusion. The

> **Box 36.6** Heart Transplantation: Perioperative Goals
>
> - Maintain systemic blood pressure to maintain coronary filling
> - Optimize preload
> - Reduce afterload to improve ejection fraction
> - Avoid pulmonary vasoconstriction
>   - Maintain oxygenation
>   - Avoid hypercapnia
>   - Avoid high tidal volumes
>   - Correct acid–base abnormalities
>   - Avoid nitrous oxide
> - Support contractility
>   - Pharmacologic drugs
>   - Intraaortic balloon pump
>   - Assist devices

heart rate response to hemodynamic changes is absent, and drugs acting indirectly on the heart are ineffective. Bradycardia can be treated with pacing (usually 80 to 100 beats/min) or chronotropic drugs such as isoproterenol. Second, failure to wean from cardiopulmonary bypass is often caused by right-sided heart failure. Several possible mechanisms are related to right-sided heart failure during heart transplantation: preexisting pulmonary hypertension can be worsened during reperfusion of the donor heart, and the right ventricle is particularly prone to ischemia/reperfusion injury. The primary treatment goals for right-sided heart failure during heart transplantation are to increase contractility of the right ventricle and decrease PA resistance. Failure to respond may necessitate mechanical right ventricular support. Worsening pulmonary hypertension during heart transplantation is multifactorial. An increase in cardiac output, pulmonary vessel spasm, and blood or air embolism are all possible causes. Adequate ventilation and oxygenation, with avoidance of hypoxia and hypercarbia, can prevent an increase in pulmonary vasculature resistance. Treatment of pulmonary hypertension with nonselective vasodilators such as nitroglycerin and sodium nitroprusside can decrease SVR and result in systemic hypotension. Selective vasodilators such as inhaled nitric oxide, aerosolized iloprost (a carbacyclin analog of prostaglandin I_2), and sildenafil (inhaled or infused) may be helpful.

Postoperative Management

Postoperative management targets adequate oxygenation, ventilation, intravascular volume, pulmonary and systemic pressures, coagulation, and body temperature. Extubation of the trachea is considered when stable hemodynamics and adequate spontaneous ventilation have been achieved. Some patients require permanent pacemaker implantation because of the loss of sinus node function.[27] Most patients require inotropic and chronotropic support in the first few days after heart

IV

transplant. Posttransplant bleeding and a nonfunctional graft are life threatening and need to be identified and managed emergently. Coronary allograft vasculopathy and immunosuppression-related side effects, including malignancy, are the most common threats to long-term survival after heart transplantation.[26]

LUNG TRANSPLANTATION

Currently, over 2000 lung transplants are performed annually in the United States. Posttransplant survival is gradually improving; 1-year posttransplant survival is currently 89%.[28] Chronic obstructive lung disease, bronchiectasis, and interstitial lung disease are common indications for adult lung transplantation.[29] In children cystic fibrosis is the most common indication for lung transplantation. Bilateral lung transplant is the most common type (75%) of transplant performed.[28] Typically bilateral lung transplant involves two sequential single-lung transplants during a single surgery, which allows contralateral lung ventilation during implantation and may avoid cardiopulmonary bypass.[29] The decision to perform a single lung transplant versus a bilateral lung transplant is made based upon the underlying diagnosis, comorbidities, and potential effects of the native lung on the allograft.

Preoperative Evaluation

The preoperative evaluation should focus on the severity of lung disease, the baseline function of other vital organs, the airway, and interval changes since the last examination (also see Chapter 13). The preoperative administration of anxiolytic drugs should be performed with caution, as too much sedation or uncontrolled anxiety can worsen pulmonary hypertension. Supplemental oxygen is administered cautiously because most lung transplant patients depend on their hypoxic drive. Epidural analgesia should be considered in lung transplant patients for postoperative pain control (also see Chapter 40).

Intraoperative Management

In addition to standard monitors, arterial catheters, CVCs, and PACs are usually placed. In some institutions a PAC with continuous mixed venous O_2 saturation and cardiac output monitoring is used. Endobronchoscopy is necessary during lung transplantation. In addition to assessing the position of the double-lumen endotracheal tube, endobronchoscopy can examine the airway anastomoses for stenosis, bleeding, and obstruction secondary to blood or sputum. TEE is often used during lung transplantation. Induction of anesthesia needs to balance the risk of aspiration of gastric contents with hypoxia and hemodynamic instability. Positive-pressure ventilation can cause a decreased venous blood return. Patients with severe pulmonary hypertension are at risk of cardiac arrest during induction of anesthesia. Emergent cardiopulmonary bypass is established in this situation. Positive-pressure ventilation can cause further damage to diseased lungs and worsen hypoxia and hypercarbia. Air trapping and barotrauma should be avoided. Protective ventilation strategies, including small tidal volumes, should be considered.[30]

The most challenging intraoperative issues associated with lung transplantation involve ventilation-reperfusion mismatch and pulmonary hypertension. Strategies to treat hypoxemia during lung transplant are similar to those seen in thoracic surgery (also see Chapter 27). At the time of PA clamping, increased PA pressure is often encountered. Methods to reduce PA pressure include intravascular fluid restriction and nonselective and selective pulmonary vasodilators in both intravenous and inhaled forms. Excessive intravascular fluid administration should be avoided because noncardiogenic pulmonary edema is a frequent development in lung transplant patients.

Postoperative Management

Special care for lung transplant patients in the postoperative period is provided to avoid barotrauma/volutrauma and anastomotic dehiscence during positive-pressure mechanical ventilation. Denervation of the allograft leads to a loss of normal cough reflexes, predisposing to infection. Anastomotic dehiscence and respiratory failure caused by sepsis or rejection are the primary causes of post–lung transplantation mortality.[29]

PANCREAS TRANSPLANTATION

The most common indication for pancreas transplantation is type 1 diabetes. However, in recent years, more transplants are being performed in patients with type 2 diabetes.[31] The transplanted pancreas can provide endogenous insulin and restore normoglycemia and the glucagon response. Diabetes mellitus affects cardiovascular, autonomic, nervous, renal, gastrointestinal, and metabolic systems (also see Chapter 29). The preoperative evaluation should focus on the functional status of the vital organs. Ischemic heart disease is a primary cause of perioperative death. Diagnosis of coronary artery disease in this patient population is difficult in the presence of neuropathy and silent ischemia. If coronary artery disease is suspected, a preoperative stress test or coronary artery angiogram should be performed. The preoperative evaluation should also include examination of renal function, acid–base status, electrolytes, and hemoglobin. Most pancreas transplants are performed simultaneously with kidney transplantation.[31] Compared with pancreas alone or pancreas after kidney transplant, simultaneous pancreas and kidney transplant recipients experience the best outcomes. However, recent data suggest pancreas transplant after living donor kidney transplant as a reasonable alternative, albeit with the requirement of two separate surgeries.[32]

Pancreas transplantation can be performed with general or regional anesthesia. Invasive monitors should be considered if there is cardiovascular disease. The choice of anesthetic drugs should take into account the possibility of severe postinduction hypotension caused by diabetic autonomic nervous system dysfunction. Administration of NMB drugs not dependent on renal excretion for their elimination is preferred if renal function is impaired (also see Chapter 11). Glucose levels should be closely monitored intraoperatively and postoperatively. Severe

intraoperative hyperglycemia may adversely affect islet function and promote posttransplant infection, and postreperfusion graft function can lead to hypoglycemia.

CONCLUSION

Patients presenting for organ transplantation have end-stage disease of one or more organs, and many are critically ill. Anesthetic management tailored to the patient's comorbid conditions is vital for successful transplant. Vigilant anesthetic care, both before and after the transplant, can have a profound impact on minimizing complications and improving posttransplant outcomes. Successful transplantation reverses organ failure and promotes the recovery of organ systems beyond the transplanted organ.

REFERENCES

1. Xia V, Steadman R. Anesthesia for organ procurement. In: Gropper M, ed. *Miller's Anesthesia*. 9th ed.: Philadelphia: Elsevier; 2020:1993–2005.
2. Israni AK, Zaun D, Hadley N, Rosendale JD, Schaffhausen C, McKinney W, et al. OPTN/SRTR 2018 Annual Data Report: Deceased Organ Donation. *Am J Transplant*. 2020;20(Suppl s1):509–541. https://doi.org/10.1111/ajt.15678.
3. Bernat JL. Conceptual Issues in DCDD Donor Death Determination. *Hastings Cent Rep*. 2018;48(Suppl 4):S26–S28. https://doi.org/10.1002/hast.948.
4. Reese PP, Shults J, Bloom RD, Mussell A, Harhay MN, Abt P, et al. Functional status, time to transplantation, and survival benefit of kidney transplantation among wait-listed candidates. *Am J Kidney*. 2015;66:837–845. https://doi.org/10.1053/j.ajkd.2015.05.015.
5. Zhong Y, Schaubel DE, Kalbfleisch JD, Ashby VB, Rao PS, Sung RS. Reevaluation of the Kidney Donor Risk Index. *Transplantation*. 2019;103:1714–1721. https://doi.org/10.1097/TP.0000000000002498.
6. Hart A, Smith JM, Skeans MA, Gustafson SK, Wilk AR, Castro S, et al. OPTN/SRTR 2018 Annual Data Report: Kidney. *Am J Transplant*. 2020;20(Suppl s1):20–130. https://doi.org/10.1111/ajt.15672.
7. Delville M, Sabbah L, Girard D, Elie C, Manceau S, Piketty M, et al. Prevalence and predictors of early cardiovascular events after kidney transplantation: evaluation of pre-transplant cardiovascular work-up. *PloS One*. 2015;10:e0131237. https://doi.org/10.1371/journal.pone.0131237.
8. Lentine KL, Costa SP, Weir MR, Robb JF, Fleisher LA, Kasiske BL, et al. Cardiac disease evaluation and management among kidney and liver transplantation candidates: a scientific statement

from the American Heart Association and the American College of Cardiology Foundation: endorsed by the American Society of Transplant Surgeons, American Society of Transplantation, and National Kidney Foundation. *Circulation*. 2012;126:617–663. https://doi.org/10.1161/CIR.0b013e31823eb07a.
9. Adams DR, Tollinche LE, Yeoh CB, Artman J, Mehta M, Phillips D, et al. Short-term safety and effectiveness of sugammadex for surgical patients with end-stage renal disease: a two-centre retrospective study. *Anaesthesia*. 2020;75:348–352. https://doi.org/10.1111/anae.14914.
10. Yunos NM, Bellomo R, Hegarty C, Story D, Ho L, Bailey M. Association between a chloride-liberal vs chloride-restrictive intravenous fluid administration strategy and kidney injury in critically ill adults. *JAMA*. 2012;308:1566–1572. https://doi.org/10.1001/jama.2012.13356.
11. Mutter TC, Ruth CA, Dart AB. Hydroxyethyl starch (HES) versus other fluid therapies: effects on kidney function. *Cochrane Database Syst Rev*. 2013:CD007594. https://doi.org/10.1002/14651858.CD007594.pub3.
12. Marik PE, Baram M, Vahid B. Does central venous pressure predict fluid responsiveness? A systematic review of the literature and the tale of seven mares. *Chest*. 2008;134:172–178. https://doi.org/10.1378/chest.07-2331.
13. Hanif F, Macrae AN, Littlejohn MG, Clancy MJ, Murio E. Outcome of renal transplantation with and without intra-operative diuretics. *Int J Surg*. 2011;9:460–463. https://doi.org/10.1016/j.ijsu.2011.04.010.
14. Yang B, Xu J, Xu F, Zou Z, Ye C, Mei C, et al. Intravascular administration of mannitol for acute

kidney injury prevention: a systematic review and meta-analysis. *PloS One*. 2014;9:e85029. https://doi.org/10.1371/journal.pone.0085029.
15. Espino KA, Narvaez JRF, Ott MC, Kayler LK. Benefits of multimodal enhanced recovery pathway in patients undergoing kidney transplantation. *Clin Transplant*. 2018;32. https://doi.org/10.1111/ctr.13173.
16. OPTN/SRTR 2018. Annual Data Report: Introduction. *Am J Transplant*. 2020;20(Suppl s1):9.
17. Kwong A, Kim WR, Lake JR, Smith JM, Schladt DP, Skeans MA, et al. OPTN/SRTR 2018 Annual Data Report: Liver. *Am J Transplant*. 2020;20(Suppl s1):193–299. https://doi.org/10.1111/ajt.15674.
18. Kamath P. MELD Score (12 and older). n.d. https://www.mdcalc.com/meld-score-model-end-stage-liver-disease-12-older (accessed August 13, 2020).
19. Attia M, Silva MA, Mirza DF. The marginal liver donor–an update. *Transpl Int*. 2008;21:713–724. https://doi.org/10.1111/j.1432-2277.2008.00696.x.
20. Krowka MJ, Fallon MB, Kawut SM, Fuhrmann V, Heimbach JK, Ramsay MAE, et al. International Liver Transplant Society Practice Guidelines: Diagnosis and management of hepatopulmonary syndrome and portopulmonary hypertension. *Transplantation*. 2016;100:1440–1452. https://doi.org/10.1097/TP.0000000000001229.
21. Lisman T, Caldwell SH, Burroughs AK, Northup PG, Senzolo M, Stravitz RT, et al. Hemostasis and thrombosis in patients with liver disease: the ups and downs. *J Hepatol*. 2010;53:362–371. https://doi.org/10.1016/j.jhep.2010.01.042.
22. Stravitz RT. Critical management decisions in patients with acute liver failure.

IV

Chest. 2008;134:1092–1102. https://doi.org/10.1378/chest.08-1071.

23. Rudnick MR, Marchi LD, Plotkin JS. Hemodynamic monitoring during liver transplantation: A state of the art review. *World J Hepatol.* 2015;7:1302–1311. https://doi.org/10.4254/wjh.v7.i10.1302.

24. Paugam-Burtz C, Kavafyan J, Merckx P, Dahmani S, Sommacale D, Ramsay M, et al. Postreperfusion syndrome during liver transplantation for cirrhosis: outcome and predictors. *Liver Transplant.* 2009;15:522–529. https://doi.org/10.1002/lt.21730.

25. Colvin M, Smith JM, Hadley N, Skeans MA, Uccellini K, Goff R, et al. OPTN/SRTR 2018 Annual Data Report: Heart. *Am J Transplant.* 2020;20(Suppl s1):340–426. https://doi.org/10.1111/ajt.15676.

26. Ramsingh D, Harvey R, Runyon A, Benggon M. Anesthesia for Heart Transplantation. *Anesthesiol Clin.* 2017;35:453–471. https://doi.org/10.1016/j.anclin.2017.05.002.

27. Neethling E, Moreno Garijo J, Mangalam TK, Badiwala MV, Billia P, Wasowicz M, et al. Intraoperative and early postoperative management of heart transplantation: anesthetic implications. *J Cardiothorac Vasc Anesth.* 2020;34:2189–2206. https://doi.org/10.1053/j.jvca.2019.09.037.

28. Valapour M, Lehr CJ, Skeans MA, Smith JM, Uccellini K, Lehman R, et al. OPTN/SRTR 2017 Annual Data Report: Lung. *Am J Transplant.* 2019;19(Suppl 2):404–484. https://doi.org/10.1111/ajt.15279.

29. Deshpande R, Kurup V. Chapter 3 - Restrictive Respiratory Diseases and Lung Transplantation editors. In: Hines R, Marschall K, eds. *Stoeltings Anesthesia and Co-Existing Disease.* 7th ed.: Philadelphia: Elsevier; 2018:33–52.

30. Verbeek GL, Myles PS. Intraoperative protective ventilation strategies in lung transplantation. *Transplant Rev.* 2013;27:30–35. https://doi.org/10.1016/j.trre.2012.11.004.

31. Kandaswamy R, Stock PG, Gustafson SK, Skeans MA, Urban R, Fox A, et al. OPTN/SRTR 2018 Annual Data Report: Pancreas. *Am J Transplant.* 2020;20(Suppl s1):131–192. https://doi.org/10.1111/ajt.15673.

32. Fridell JA, Niederhaus S, Curry M, Urban R, Fox A, Odorico J. The survival advantage of pancreas after kidney transplant. *Am J Transplant.* 2019;19:823–830. https://doi.org/10.1111/ajt.15106.

OUTPATIENT ANESTHESIA

Chihiro Toda, Basem B. Abdelmalak

INTRODUCTION

Ambulatory anesthesia is a rapidly growing field involving three distinct entities: outpatient anesthesia (the primary focus of this chapter), office-based anesthesia (OBA), and non–operating room anesthesia (NORA) (also see Chapter 38). The idea of outpatient anesthesia started over 100 years ago when an ambulatory surgical center (ASC) was opened in Iowa;[1] 50 years later, the first modern ASC was opened in Phoenix, Arizona, in 1970. Since then, indications for outpatient surgery have expanded, and outpatient anesthesia has been performed in many different types of facilities. In 2014 over half of hospital visits (inpatient or ambulatory) that included invasive, therapeutic surgeries were performed in a hospital-owned ambulatory surgery setting.[2]

The Society for Ambulatory Anesthesia (SAMBA)[3] was founded in 1985 to become a resource for providers who practice in settings outside of hospital-based operating rooms. SAMBA periodically issues statements regarding the practice of ambulatory anesthesia and has published an evidence-based guide to the management of ASCs.[4] The American Society of Anesthesiologists (ASA) issued guidelines for ambulatory anesthesia and surgery in 2003; these guidelines were reaffirmed in 2018.[5]

Ambulatory Anesthesia Settings

In ambulatory surgery a patient is anticipated to come to the facility on the day of surgery, undergo a surgery or invasive procedure, and be discharged home on the same day (or within 23 hours). Ambulatory surgery can be performed in several different types of facilities, including an outpatient office, freestanding ASC, freestanding ASC with extended stay (less than 23 hours), ASC within a hospital complex, hospital operating room, and NORA locations (Fig. 37.1). The capabilities at each facility will affect patient selection and the procedures performed.

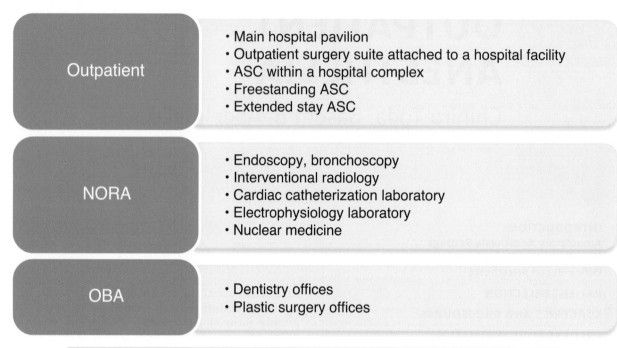

Fig. 37.1 Examples of different ambulatory anesthesia settings. *ASC*, Ambulatory surgery center; *NORA*, non-operating room anesthesia; *OBA*, office-based anesthesia.

Non-Operating Room Anesthesia

Historically known as *remote anesthesia* or *out-of-operating room anesthesia*, NORA is an anesthesia service provided in a hospital unit, albeit away from the regular operating rooms. Common NORA procedures include cardiac catheterization, electrophysiology procedures, gastrointestinal endoscopy, interventional radiology procedures, and others (also see Chapter 38). Challenges of the NORA setting include the following: (1) patients who are deemed "too sick" for an invasive surgery with general anesthesia and are now offered a minimally invasive alternative; (2) limited physical access to patients because of obstacles such as fluoroscopy equipment; and (3) limited availability of medication, staff, or rescue equipment. Compared with patients undergoing procedures in the main operating room, patients receiving NORA are older, and monitored anesthesia care (MAC) is the more common anesthesia choice.[6]

Office-Based Anesthesia

Surgery and other procedures can also be performed outside a hospital or ASC setting at small offices. These procedures are generally elective surgeries of short duration with minimal estimated blood loss; examples include cosmetic plastic surgery, complex dental procedures, podiatric procedures, and certain vascular surgical procedures (e.g., varicose vein treatment).

Office-based surgery facilities have generally been less regulated than ASCs. However, patient safety concerns have led to increasing state legislation and professional society guidelines by organizations including the American College of Surgeons and ASA.[7] Demand for office-based surgery (and anesthesia) has been increasing. Some offices are equipped with an established anesthesia machine and recovery room; in others, the anesthesia providers must transport their own equipment and medications from one office to another as they provide this unique service. The logistical issues regarding management of Drug Enforcement Administration (DEA)–controlled medications provide a challenge to anesthesia practice in the office-based setting. However, OBA providers experience a different professional environment than a hospital-based provider. Many work closely with specific surgery office teams and have greater flexibility in their scheduling and financial arrangements.

PATIENT SELECTION

Careful selection and optimization of patients are essential for safe outpatient anesthesia. In addition, the type of facility should be appropriate for the procedure and patient comorbidities. For example, a patient with multiple medical comorbidities may be better suited for care in the outpatient surgery suite within the main operating room of a hospital or a NORA location versus an office-based practice. Other patients can safely undergo their procedure in a free-standing ASC or an OBA practice setting. The preoperative evaluation and optimization process should proceed in the same manner as a patient scheduled for inpatient surgery (also see Chapter 13). The ASA Practice Guidelines for Postanesthetic Care recommend that a responsible individual should accompany a patient home after surgery.[8]

SURGERIES AND PROCEDURES

The most commonly performed ambulatory surgery procedures are listed in Box 37.1. In addition, certain procedures are performed on an ambulatory basis over 90% of the time (Box 37.2). The spectrum of ambulatory surgeries has been expanding, coincident with the substantial growth in equipment, techniques, and expertise in performing minimally invasive surgeries. More recently, freestanding ASCs have embarked on performing major joint surgeries, such as knee and hip arthroplasty, as an outpatient procedure. These programs use strict patient selection criteria and an anesthetic regimen that facilitates early mobility and adequate pain control. The success of an outpatient major joint program depends on a dedicated ASC team and a protocol that spans the perioperative period starting with patient selection (ideally, a medically stable, motivated patient), surgical scheduling,

---

Box 37.1 Ten Most Common Ambulatory Procedures in the United States[2]

1. Lens and cataract procedures
2. Muscle, tendon, and soft tissue operating room procedures (most commonly rotator cuff repair and trigger finger surgery)
3. Incision or fusion of joint or destruction of joint lesion (most commonly knee and shoulder arthroscopies)
4. Cholecystectomy and common duct exploration
5. Excision of semilunar cartilage of knee
6. Inguinal and femoral hernia repair
7. Repair of diaphragmatic, incisional, and umbilical hernia
8. Tonsillectomy and/or adenoidectomy
9. Decompression of peripheral nerve
10. Operating room procedures of the skin and breast, including plastic procedures on breast

Analysis of data from hospital-based ambulatory surgery settings and hospital inpatient settings. Procedures were defined as those involving incision, excision, manipulation, or suturing of tissue that breaks the skin; typically requiring operating room use; and requiring sedation, regional, or general anesthesia to control pain.

Box 37.2 Procedures Performed in an Ambulatory Setting More Than 90% of the Time[2]

Operations on the eye
Tympanoplasty and myringotomy
Excision of semilunar cartilage of knee
Inguinal and femoral hernia repair
Tonsillectomy and/or adenoidectomy
Decompression of peripheral nerve
Lumpectomy or quadrantectomy of breast
Bunionectomy or repair of toe deformities
Plastic procedures on nose
Varicose vein stripping (lower limb)

Data analysis same as in Box 37.1.

---

preoperative nutrition, patient education, discharge planning, and postoperative pain management and physical therapy regimen.[9]

PREOPERATIVE EVALUATION

Although many ambulatory procedures are of short duration and associated with lesser physiologic impact than those performed in hospital operating rooms, preoperative evaluation follows the same principles (also see Chapter 13). However, the following conditions can present specific challenges in ambulatory anesthesia.

Obstructive Sleep Apnea (also see Chapter 48)

Obstructive sleep apnea (OSA) represents the most common sleep-related breathing disorder. Concerns about OSA for patients undergoing ambulatory surgery include the risk of difficult airway management, intraoperative hypoxemia, need for tracheal reintubation, unanticipated hospital admission, and even hypoxemic brain injury and death. A 2012 SAMBA consensus statement recommended the use of the STOP-BANG screening questionnaire for preoperative screening; other comorbid conditions such as hypertension, arrhythmias, heart failure, cerebrovascular disease, and metabolic syndrome should be evaluated as well.[10] Opioids are likely to exacerbate OSA in the perioperative period, so painful ambulatory surgery that is not amenable to nonopioid analgesia techniques should be reconsidered or rescheduled as an inpatient surgery. Finally, the SAMBA statement notes that a majority of patients with known OSA used continuous positive airway pressure (CPAP) or bilevel positive airway pressure (BiPAP) postoperatively, which likely contributes to a safe perioperative course. If the patient is not able (or is not willing) to use CPAP or BiPAP postoperatively, they may not be suitable for an outpatient procedure.[10] In terms of specific STOP-BANG scores, a 2018 metaanalysis showed that patients with a

IV

STOP-BANG score ≥3 were associated with an increased risk of postoperative complications.[11]

The ASA has also published practice guidelines for perioperative management of OSA. The ASA Task Force recommends that the following factors be considered when determining whether inpatient or outpatient care is most appropriate for a patient with OSA who requires surgery: (1) sleep apnea status, (2) anatomic and physiologic abnormalities, (3) status of coexisting diseases, (4) nature of surgery, (5) type of anesthesia, (6) need for postoperative opioids, (7) patient age, (8) adequacy of postdischarge observation, and (9) capabilities of the outpatient facility.[12]

Obesity

Obesity has been a much-debated issue in outpatient anesthesia. A 1999 observational study of over 17,000 patients undergoing ambulatory surgery found that patients with obesity (body mass index [BMI] >30 kg/m²) had an increased likelihood of developing intraoperative and postoperative respiratory events.[13] Other concerns associated with obesity and ambulatory surgery include the increased risk of OSA, difficult airway management, use of vasopressors, and risk of unplanned admission or readmission.[14] Facility logistics may include operating room bed capacity, equipment requirements, and presence of a lift team and other resources. As with patients with OSA, a multimodal approach should be taken for postoperative analgesia to reduce opioid administration that can suppress respiratory drive.[12,15]

Most freestanding ASCs have developed their own criteria for accepting obese patients. Some use BMI cutoffs, most commonly BMI >50 kg/m², whereas others use a lower BMI limit of 40 kg/m². Other factors relevant to BMI limits for ambulatory surgery include type of obesity (central vs. peripheral), type of procedure, availability of specialized equipment and personnel, and options for an extended postoperative stay.

Chronic Kidney Disease

A patient with end-stage renal disease (ESRD) on dialysis can safely undergo surgery in an ambulatory setting as long as reasonable precautions are followed. Preoperative considerations for patients with ESRD are described in detail in Chapter 28. Issues include timing and method of dialysis in addition to attention to other comorbidities such as hypertension, coronary artery disease, diabetes mellitus, electrolyte abnormalities, altered volume status, and platelet dysfunction. Anesthesia providers should consider using anesthesia agents with minimal dependence on renal excretion. Although succinylcholine causes the same rise in potassium for patients with or without ESRD and is convenient for short surgeries, other muscle relaxants can be considered if the baseline potassium is not known to be normal. Regional anesthesia is an attractive option for these patients; however, even patients with ESRD receiving regular dialysis may exhibit uremic platelet dysfunction.

Implanted and Other Medical Devices

Patients with implanted medical devices such as a pacemaker, implantable cardioverter-defibrillator (ICD), spinal cord or peripheral nerve stimulator, or insulin pump[16] can safely undergo ambulatory surgery. However, these devices need to be evaluated preoperatively; considerations include the medical condition being addressed and any specific testing required. For example, patients with a pacemaker or ICD require regular device interrogation. Pacemakers and ICDs may require reprogramming depending on the location of the planned procedure (also see Chapter 26). This may require coordination with a cardiologist, who may not be readily available at a freestanding ASC.

Difficult Airway Management

Patients with a history of difficult airway management, or anticipated difficulty with airway management, do not represent an absolute contraindication to having the surgery at a freestanding ASC. However, an anesthesia provider may consider this a relative contraindication depending on the planned procedure, nature of airway difficulty, availability of specialized airway equipment, and skills of the anesthesia provider. One option is to avoid airway management altogether by a carefully executed regional anesthetic technique with a judicious plan for sedation. Regardless of whether a freestanding ASC accepts patients with potential difficult airway management, the ASC should have the equipment to manage an unanticipated difficult airway if encountered.

Substance Use Disorders

Patients with acute intoxication are not suitable for ambulatory surgery, but those with substance use disorders may be cared for at ambulatory surgical facilities. Potential issues for patients with opioid use disorder include postoperative pain management, including opioid tolerance or use of medication-assisted treatment with buprenorphine (also see Chapter 40). Multimodal analgesia, including nonopioid analgesics and peripheral nerve block when feasible, may be required to minimize complications such as respiratory depression.

ANESTHETIC TECHNIQUES

Choice of anesthesia technique is discussed in detail in Chapter 14. For outpatient surgeries, the most common risk of general anesthesia that results in prolonged stay is postoperative nausea and vomiting (PONV). Spinal anesthesia can be used for lower extremity orthopedic surgeries. The potential benefits of spinal anesthesia for outpatient surgery include no need for airway instrumentation (unless complicated by a total spinal) and decreased risk of PONV.[17] Although spinal anesthesia also provides postoperative analgesia, prolonged motor blockade can delay discharge (also see Chapter 17).

Peripheral nerve blocks can provide surgical anesthesia, postoperative analgesia, or both. In either case a peripheral nerve block as a part of a multimodal analgesia strategy can reduce the total amount of opioids (also see Chapter 18). This is especially important because postoperative opioid use is a significant risk factor for PONV (Box 37.3).

MAC is a term used to describe a specific anesthesia service in which an anesthesiologist has been requested to participate in the care of a patient undergoing a diagnostic or therapeutic procedure. This service could range from monitoring without administering any medication at all, to managing hemodynamics, and inducing varying degrees of sedation on the depth-of-sedation continuum, up to and including providing general anesthesia. However, the term is commonly used to describe deep sedation or general anesthesia in a spontaneously breathing patient without a secured airway. When this technique is used to avoid inhaled anesthesia, the risk of PONV is reduced. Disadvantages of this approach include an unsecured airway and occasionally patient discomfort if the anesthesia provider is concerned that additional analgesic medication would cause excessive respiratory depression. Although MAC is often considered easier and safer than general anesthesia, closed claim analysis documents significant potential complications, most notably respiratory complications that may have been preventable with proper monitoring.[18,19]

POSTOPERATIVE CARE

Postoperative recovery can be divided into three phases. Phase I is the early stage of recovery and typically occurs in a postanesthesia care unit (PACU). During this phase, the patient awakens from the sedative effects of anesthesia medications, physiologic reflexes return, and issues such as pain management and nausea/vomiting are managed. Once the patient is awake, is hemodynamically stable, and has minimal PONV or pain, phase II recovery begins and continues until the patient is ready to go home (so-called street readiness). Phase II recovery can occur in the PACU or in a different area. Scoring systems such as the modified Aldrete score, which consists of activity, respiration, circulation, consciousness, and oxygenation, are commonly used to determine PACU discharge readiness[20] (also see Chapter 39).

Improvements in surgical techniques and short-acting anesthesia drugs enable patients to recover from anesthesia faster—some patients meet the criteria to transfer from phase I to phase II as they are leaving the operating room. In that case the patient can be directly admitted to phase II, an approach called *fast-tracking.* Phase III recovery occurs at home after PACU discharge.

Postdischarge nausea and vomiting (PDNV)[21] is recognized as an important issue after ambulatory surgery. Additional research now address this entity as ambulatory anesthesiologists extend their expertise in the management of PONV.[22] The incidence of PDNV was reported to be 37% in the first 48 hours after discharge. Independent predictors of PDNV are listed in Box 37.4.[23,24]

QUALITY IMPROVEMENT

Minor adverse events are common after ambulatory surgery and anesthesia. Postdischarge symptoms can include drowsiness, headache, nausea, emesis, myalgia, and sore throat.[25] Other important measures to track after ambulatory surgery include escalation of care, unplanned hospital admission, and readmission after discharge from a freestanding ASC.

Analysis of closed malpractice claims is an approach to studying anesthesia-related safety concerns that was started by the ASA and the University of Washington at Seattle in 1984. Using a similar methodology, a 2017 study analyzed closed claims from the medical malpractice insurer The Doctors Company.[26] The study compared claims related to anesthesia care in ASCs compared with

---

Box 37.3 Simplified Apfel Score to Predict PONV

Risk Factors for PONV
1. Female gender
2. Nonsmoker status
3. Postoperative opioid use
4. History of PONV/motion sickness

PONV, Postoperative nausea and vomiting.
Simplified risk score used to predict PONV after general anesthesia. Each factor adds roughly 20% to the risk of PONV.[17]

Box 37.4 Risk Factors for Postdischarge Nausea and Vomiting[23,24]

Female gender

Age <50 years old

History of PONV

Use of opioids in PACU

Nausea in PACU

PACU, Postoperative anesthesia care unit; *PONV,* postoperative nausea and vomiting.

hospital operating rooms. ASC claims were more likely to be classified as medium severity than hospital operating room claims and were more likely to involve dental damage or pain. However, ASC claims were less likely to involve death or respiratory or cardiac arrest, and mean indemnity payment was significantly lower for ASC claims, averaging $87,888 versus $107,325 for operating room claims.[26] The limitations of closed claims analysis apply to this study, which include their retrospective nature and inability to truly compare the event rates in the two groups because the denominator for risk calculation is unknown.

The Centers for Medicare and Medicaid Services (CMS) has developed a payment incentive program to encourage providers to provide better care and improve the quality of their services. The ASA Committee on Performance and Outcome Measures has formed a Technical Expert Panel for the development of quality measures for ambulatory anesthesia. Leadership of ambulatory anesthesia providers is needed to monitor quality metrics and develop plans to improve patient care in this setting.

ADVANCES AND NEW TRENDS IN OUTPATIENT ANESTHESIA

Developments in pharmacology have led to new medications that may have a role in outpatient anesthesia, including long-acting local anesthetics using microtechnology, sedatives, and antiemetics. For example, liposomal bupivacaine is bupivacaine hydrochloride encapsulated within multiple nonconcentric lipid bilayers. This allows the medication to diffuse slowly over an extended period. Compared with bupivacaine, which lasts approximately 8 hours, liposomal bupivacaine can last up to 72 hours. However, its efficacy and cost-effectiveness have not clearly been demonstrated over standard local anesthetics.[27,28]

Remimazolam is an ultra-short-acting intravenous benzodiazepine used in anesthesia and procedural sedation.[29] It is rapidly metabolized into its pharmacologically inactive metabolite by nonspecific tissue esterase.[30] Because of its rapid onset and predictable recovery, remimazolam may have an advantage over other sedatives (also see Chapter 8).

Other trends in ambulatory surgery include patient access and financial implications of care at an ASC versus a hospital outpatient setting. In general, ASC procedure costs are lower than those for hospital-based outpatient surgery. In addition, many hospitals have long wait times for surgical scheduling compared with an ASC, which may translate into improved access for patients undergoing surgery at an ASC.

CONCLUSION

Demand for ambulatory anesthesia is increasing, and anesthesia providers will care for higher-risk patients undergoing more complex procedures in the ambulatory settings. Proper selection of patients and facilities is essential to provide safe anesthesia care and enhance recovery while minimizing complications and cost.

REFERENCES

1. Waters RM. The downtown anesthesia clinic. *Am J Surg.* 1919;33(7):71–77.
2. Statistical Brief #223. Healthcare Cost and Utilization Project (HCUP). July 2020. Agency for Healthcare Research and Quality, Rockville, MD. www.hcup-us.ahrq.gov/reports/statbriefs/sb223-Ambulatory-Inpatient-Surgeries-2014.jsp Accessed November 9, 2021.
3. Society of Ambulatory Anesthesia (SAMBA). https://sambahq.org/. Accessed November 9, 2021
4. Rajan N. (ed) *Manual of Practice Management for Ambulatory Surgery Centers Book: An Evidence-Based Guide*: Springer Nature Switzerland; 2020.
5. American Society of Anesthesiologists (ASA) Guidelines for Ambulatory Anesthesia and Surgery. https://www.asahq.org/standards-and-guidelines/guidelines-for-ambulatory-anesthesia-and-surgery Accessed November 9, 2021
6. Chang B, Kaye AD, Diaz JH, Westlake B, Dutton RP, Urman RD. Interventional procedures outside of the operating room: Results from the National Anesthesia Clinical Outcomes Registry. *J Patient Saf.* 2018 Mar 14(1):9–16. doi:10.1097/PTS.0000000000000156 PMID: 29461406.
7. Osman BM, Shapiro FE. Office-based anesthesia: A comprehensive review and 2019 Update. *Anesthesiol Clin.* 2019;37(2):317–331.
8. Apfelbaum JL, Silverstein JH, Chung FF, Connis RT, Fillmore RB, Hunt SE, Nickinovich DG, Schreiner MS, Silverstein JH, Apfelbaum JL, Barlow JC, Chung FF, Connis RT, Fillmore RB, Hunt SE, Joas TA, Nickinovich DG, Schreiner MS. American Society of Anesthesiologists Task Force on Postanesthetic Care. Practice guidelines for postanesthetic care: An updated report by the American Society of Anesthesiologists Task Force on Postanesthetic Care. *Anesthesiology.* 2013 Feb 118(2):291–307. doi:10.1097/ALN.0b013e31827773e9 PMID: 23364567.
9. Amundson AW, Panchamia JK, Jacob AK. Anesthesia for same-day total joint replacement. *Anesthesiology Clinics.* 2019;37(2):251–264.
10. Joshi GP, Ankichetty SP, Gan TJ, Chung F. Society for Ambulatory Anesthesia consensus statement on preoperative selection of adult patients with obstructive sleep apnea scheduled for ambulatory surgery. *Anesth Analg.* 2012 Nov 115(5):1060–1068. doi:10.1213/ANE.0b013e318269cfd7 Epub 2012 Aug 10. PMID: 22886843.
11. Nagappa M, Subramani Y, Chung F. Best perioperative practice in management of ambulatory patients with obstructive sleep apnea. *Curr Opin Anaesthesiol.* 2018;31(6):700–706 Dec.
12. American Society of Anesthesiologists. Practice guidelines for the perioperative management of patients with obstructive sleep apnea. Practice guidelines for the perioperative management of patients with obstructive sleep apnea: An updated report by the American Society of Anesthesiologists Task Force on perioperative management of patients with obstructive sleep apnea. *Anesthesiology.* 2014;120:268–286.
13. Chung F, Mezei G, Tong D. Pre-existing medical conditions as predictors of adverse

events in day-case surgery. *Br J Anaesth.* 1999;83:262–270.

14. Stierer TL, Wright C, George A, Thompson RE, Wu CL, Collop N. Risk assessment of obstructive sleep apnea in a population of patients undergoing ambulatory surgery. *J Clin Sleep Med.* 2010 Oct 15;6(5):467–472.

15. Prabhakar A, Helander E, Chopra N, Kaye AJ, Urman RD, Kaye AD. Preoperative assessment for ambulatory surgery. *Curr Pain Headache Rep.* 2017 Aug 31;21(10):43.

16. Abdelmalak B, Ibrahim M, Yared JP, Modic MB, Nasr C. Perioperative glycemic management in insulin pump patients undergoing noncardiac surgery. *Curr Pharm Des.* 2012;18(38):6204–6214.

17. Apfel CC, Läärä E, Koivuranta M, Greim CA, Roewer N. A simplified risk score for predicting postoperative nausea and vomiting: Conclusions from cross-validations between two centers. *Anesthesiology.* 1999 Sep 91(3):693–700.

18. Bhananker SM, Posner KL, Cheney FW, Caplan RA, Lee LA, Domino KB. Injury and liability associated with monitored anesthesia care: A closed claims analysis. *Anesthesiology.* 2006;104(2):228–234.

19. Metzner J, Posner KL, Domino KB. The risk and safety of anesthesia at remote locations: The US closed claims analysis.

20. Aldrete JA. The post-anesthetic recovery score revisited. *J Clin Anesth.* 1995;7:89–91.

21. Chinnappa V, Chung F. Post-discharge nausea and vomiting: An overlooked aspect of ambulatory anesthesia?. *Can J Anaesth.* 2008;55(9):565–571. English, French. doi:10.1007/BF03021429. PMID: 18840585.

22. Gan TJ, Belani KG, Bergese S, Chung F, Diemunsch P, Habib AS, Jin Z, Kovac AL, Meyer TA, Urman RD, Apfel CC, Ayad S, Beagley L, Candiotti K, Englesakis M, Hedrick TL, Kranke P, Lee S, Lipman D, Minkowitz HS, Morton J, Philip BK. Fourth consensus guidelines for the management of postoperative nausea and vomiting. *Anesth Analg.* 2020 Aug 131(2):411–448.

23. Apfel CC, Philip BK, Cakmakkaya OS, et al. Who is at risk for postdischarge nausea and vomiting after ambulatory surgery?. *Anesthesiology.* 2012;117: 475–486.

24. Odom-Forren J, Jalota L, Moser DK, Lennie TA, Hall LA, Holtman J, Hooper V, Apfel CC. Incidence and predictors of postdischarge nausea and vomiting in a 7-day population. *J Clin Anesth.* 2013 Nov 25(7):551–559.

Curr Opin Anaesthesiol. 2009;22(4): 502–508.

25. Wu CL, Berenholtz SM, Pronovost PJ, Fleisher LA. Systematic review and analysis of postdischarge symptoms after outpatient surgery. *Anesthesiology.* 2002;96(4):994–1003.

26. Ranum D, Beverly A, Shapiro FE, Urman RD. Leading causes of anesthesia-related liability claims in ambulatory surgery centers. *J Patient Saf.* 2017 Nov 16.

27. Hamilton TW, Athanassoglou V, Trivella M, Strickland LHH, Mellon S, Murray D, Pandit HG. Liposomal bupivacaine peripheral nerve block for the management of postoperative pain. *Cochrane Database of Syst Rev.* 2016;8. doi:10.1002/14651858 Art. No.: CD011476CD011476.pub2. Accessed 09 November 2021.

28. Ilfeld BM, Eisenach JC, Gabriel RA. Clinical effectiveness of liposomal bupivacaine administered by infiltration or peripheral nerve block to treat postoperative pain. *Anesthesiology.* 2021; 134(2):283–344.

29. Keam SJ. Remimazolam: First approval. *Drugs.* 2020 Apr 80(6):625–633.

30. Rogers WK, McDowell TS. Remimazolam, a short-acting GABA(A) receptor agonist for intravenous sedation and/ or anesthesia in day-case surgical and non-surgical procedures. *IDrugs.* 2010 Dec 13(12):929–937.

IV

38 ANESTHESIA FOR PROCEDURES IN NONOPERATING ROOM LOCATIONS

Wilson Cui, Chanhung Z. Lee

Procedures performed outside the operating room (OR) fall under the term *nonoperating room anesthesia (NORA)*, which refers to providing anesthesia care at any location away from traditional OR suites (Box 38.1). In response to the need for minimally invasive interventions in addition to the rapid advancement in imaging and other technologies, the number of NORA procedures has markedly increased in many medical and surgical specialties. Even as more hybrid ORs are being built inside or close to the main operating suites, NORA is increasingly becoming a significant part of anesthesia care. Data from the National Anesthesia Clinical Outcomes Registry (NACOR) has shown that the proportion of NORA cases increased from 28% to 36% of all anesthesia cases in the period 2010–2014.[1] Knowledge and skills for providing anesthesia in NORA locations has recently become part of the core curriculum of residency training required by the Accreditation Council for Graduate Medical Education, given the need for specific preparation of anesthesiologists in this fast-growing area.[2]

Many patients treated in NORA locations are deemed "too sick" to undergo traditional surgical interventions. The NACOR data analysis has also revealed a higher mean age and higher proportion of patients with American Society of Anesthesiologists (ASA) Physical Status class III-IV in the NORA group compared with the OR group.[1] As with most anesthetics, both patient

---

Box 38.1 NORA Locations That Commonly Require Anesthesia Services

Radiology and Nuclear Medicine
Diagnostic radiology and nuclear medicine
    Computed tomography
    Fluoroscopy
Therapeutic radiology
    Interventional body angiography (can involve embolization
      or stent placement)
    Interventional neuroangiography (can involve embolization
      or stent placement)
Magnetic resonance imaging
Positron emission tomography (PET) scan

Radiation Therapy
Standard x-ray therapy with collimated beams
Gamma knife x-ray surgery for brain tumors and arteriovenous
    malformations
CyberKnife x-ray surgery for central nervous system, body
    tumors, and arteriovenous malformations
Electron beam radiation therapy (usually intraoperative)

Cardiology
Cardiac catheterization with or without electrophysiologic studies

Cardioversion
Structural cardiac intervention

Gastroenterology
Upper gastrointestinal endoscopy
Colonoscopy
Endoscopic retrograde cholangiopancreatography

Pulmonary Medicine
Tracheal and bronchial stent placement
Bronchoscopy
Pulmonary lavage

Psychiatry
Electroconvulsive therapy

Urology
Extracorporeal shock wave lithotripsy
Nephrostomy tube placement

General Dentistry and Oral and Maxillofacial Surgery

Reproductive Health
In vitro fertilization procedures

---

and procedure factors must be considered (Table 38.1). Anesthesia-related concerns include (1) maintenance of patient comfort, immobility, and physiologic stability; (2) perioperative management of anticoagulation; (3) readiness for sudden unexpected complications during the procedure; (4) provision of smooth and rapid emergence from anesthesia and sedation at appropriate times (which may even be required during the procedure); and (5) appropriate postprocedural monitoring and management during transport. Another study of the NACOR database compared anesthetic complications between NORA and OR locations.[3] Although NORA procedures have overall lower morbidity and mortality rates compared with OR procedures, the incidence of death in the subgroup of NORA cardiology and NORA radiology locations (0.05%) was slightly higher than the OR (0.04%).

Table 38.1 Factors Considered for the Involvement of Anesthesia Services

Patient	Procedure
History of anxiety	Duration
Chronic opiate dependency	Nonsupine position
High oxygen requirement	Breath holding
Sleep apnea	Immobilization
Altered mental status	Degree of invasiveness
Inability to follow commands	
Comorbid conditions	

This chapter emphasizes the unique aspects of working in some of the common NORA locations, which often include special medical, procedural, and safety concerns, and corresponding anesthesia approaches.

CHARACTERISTICS OF NORA LOCATIONS

Importance of Communication

Remote locations are structured differently from the typical OR, but clear communication is prudent for efficient and safe practice in either site. With clear communication, the actions of anesthesia personnel can be integrated with those of the procedural team involved in the NORA intervention. The anesthesia provider should have a detailed plan for communicating with more centrally located anesthesia colleagues and technicians in case help is urgently required. For instance, an unexpected difficult airway can be especially challenging because of the remote NORA location. Additional anesthesia personnel and resources should be immediately available if needed. Sometimes the anesthesia providers in NORA locations feel isolated from the facilities available to OR personnel. The lack of mutual experience and vocabulary presents challenges for anesthesia providers and other staff working in NORA locations. Anesthesia providers and proceduralists should have a shared understanding of the specifics and challenges in the procedures in addition to those in medical care. Anesthesia providers working in an unfamiliar remote location must keep track of the identity and role of personnel participating in the

IV

interventional procedure or patient care. During times when the anesthesia provider may need experienced medical assistance (e.g., tracheal intubation, placement of an invasive monitor, or intravenous access), the availability of qualified staff members must be identified. Readily available preoperative documents for all patients in remote locations must include patient history and physical examination by the attending proceduralist. Patient arrival and check-in arrangements should be similar to those for patients undergoing procedures in a traditional OR setting.

Standard of Care and Equipment

Anesthesia care provided in remote locations must adhere to the same standards as those for the OR. The ASA has issued a Statement on Nonoperating Room Anesthetizing Locations that posts minimal guidelines for NORA procedures. In summary, the statement recommends adequate monitoring capabilities, the means to deliver supplemental oxygen via a facemask with positive-pressure ventilation, the availability of suction, the equipment for providing controlled mechanical ventilation, an adequate supply of anesthetic drugs and ancillary equipment, and supplemental lighting for procedures that involve darkness. The same perioperative precautions for infectious diseases must be followed in NORA locations to protect the health and safety of patients and health care workers. During the coronavirus disease 2019 (COVID-19) pandemic, mitigating the risk of airborne transmission poses extra challenges because an isolation room may not be readily available in every NORA location. One option is to perform airway management (intubation and extubation) in a designated negative-pressure room for patients with confirmed or suspected COVID-19 infection.[4]

It is not always possible to place the anesthesia workstation in close proximity to the patient owing to the presence of essential, specialized equipment such as fluoroscopy systems. The additional distance and material between the anesthetized patient and the provider pose further safety concerns for both parties. There are frequently additional hazards, such as exposure to radiation, loud sound levels, and heavy mechanical equipment. Advance preparation should be made to ensure all the necessary safety equipment are available, such as personal radiation protective garments, portable radiation shields, and eye and ear protection. If anesthetic gases are to be used, scavenging must be sufficient to ensure that trace amounts are below the upper limits set by the Occupational Safety and Health Administration (OSHA) (also see Chapter 49). After the procedure, one often has to travel longer distances to the postanesthesia care unit (PACU). To do so safely and expeditiously, these remote locations should have available sufficient supplies of supplemental oxygen, transport monitors, and elevator access keys. The anesthesia provider should always know the location of the nearest defibrillator, fire extinguisher, gas shutoff valves, and exits.

SAFETY AND CONCERNS IN RADIOLOGY SUITES

Imaging-related procedures for both diagnostic and interventional purposes represent a major component of NORA anesthetizing locations.

Radiation Safety Practices

Ionizing radiation and radiation safety issues are commonly encountered in NORA locations.[5] Radiation intensity and exposure decrease with the inverse square of the distance from the emitting source. Frequently, the anesthesia provider can be located immediately behind a portable lead-glass shield. Regardless of whether this is possible, the anesthesia provider should wear a lead apron and a lead thyroid shield and remain at least 1 to 2 m away from the radiation source. Radiation-induced cataracts are a recognized hazard for interventional cardiologists and radiologists. A 2017 study of eye lens dosimetry in anesthesiology highlighted the importance of maintaining radiation safety standards and adequate eye protection for anesthesia providers working for a significant time in the radiology suite.[6] Clear communication between the radiology and anesthesia teams is crucial for limiting radiation exposure.

Monitoring the Radiation Dose

Anesthesia providers, like all other health care workers who are at risk for radiation exposure, can monitor their monthly dosage by wearing radiation exposure badges. The physics unit of measurement for a biologic radiation dose is the sievert (Sv): 100 rem = 1 Sv. Because some types of ionizing radiation are more injurious than others, the biologic radiation dose is a product of the type-specific radiation weighting factor (or "quality factor") and the ionizing energy absorbed per gram of tissue. Radiation exposure can be monitored with one or more film badges. In the United States the average annual dose from cosmic rays and naturally occurring radioactive materials is about 3 mSv (300 mrem). Patients undergoing a chest radiograph receive a dose of 0.04 mSv, whereas those undergoing a computed tomography (CT) scan of the head receive 2 mSv. Federal guidelines set a limit of 50 mSv for the maximum annual occupational dose.

Adverse Reactions to Contrast Materials

Contrast materials are used in more than 10 million diagnostic radiology procedures performed each year. In 1990 fatal adverse reactions after the intravenous administration of contrast media were estimated to occur approximately once every 100,000 procedures, whereas serious adverse reactions were estimated to occur 0.2% of the time with ionic materials and 0.4% of the time with low-osmolarity materials. Radiocontrast materials can trigger anaphylaxis in sensitive patients, and such reactions necessitate aggressive intervention, including the administration of oxygen, intravenous fluids, and epinephrine, with epinephrine being the essential component of therapy (also see Chapter 45).[7]

Adverse drug reactions are more common after the injection of iodinated contrast agents (used for x-ray examinations such as CT) than after gadolinium contrast agents (used for magnetic resonance imaging [MRI]). The signs and symptoms of anaphylaxis can be mild (nausea, pruritus, diaphoresis), moderate (faintness, emesis, urticaria, laryngeal edema, bronchospasm), or severe (seizures, hypotensive shock, laryngeal edema, respiratory distress, cardiac arrest). Premedication can be used to inhibit the activation of mast cells and basophils, which release inflammatory cytokines such as histamine, serotonin, and bradykinin and cause severe vasodilation and possible shock. The mainstays of treatment include steroids and antihistamines, administered on the night before and the morning of the procedure, with a typical regimen of 40 mg prednisone, 20 mg famotidine, and 50 mg diphenhydramine for an adult. Patients undergoing contrast procedures usually have induced diuresis from the intravenous osmotic load presented by the contrast agent. Adequate hydration of these patients is important to prevent worsening of coexisting hypovolemia or azotemia. Chemotoxic reactions to contrast media are typically dose-dependent (unlike anaphylactic reactions) and related to the osmolarity and ionic strength of the contrast agent.

A serious adverse reaction called *nephrogenic systemic fibrosis (NSF)* can occur after exposure to gadolinium-based MRI contrast agents.[8] In NSF there is fibrosis of the skin, connective tissue, and sometimes internal organs. The severity can range from mild to fatal. However, NSF apparently occurs only when severe renal impairment (e.g., dialysis-dependent renal failure) also exists. Anesthesia providers and radiologists should not unnecessarily administer gadolinium-containing MRI contrast agent to patients with renal disease.

MAGNETIC RESONANCE IMAGING

MRI is a standard diagnostic tool that can supplement or replace conventional x-ray techniques. However, scanning sequences and acquisition time can be long, up to several hours, and image degradation is more common because of motion artifact. The MRI "bore," where the patient is positioned, is a tube with a diameter of only 60 to 70 cm and a length of approximately 120 cm. Thus patient cooperation and inability to remain motionless

are the primary indication for sedation or general anesthesia. Patients who routinely require anesthesia services for MRI include children or adults with claustrophobia, severe pain, or critical illness.

MRI Safety Considerations

Although MRI does not involve ionizing radiation, other safety issues are prominent in the magnet suite. Hearing loss may occur from high sound levels during the scan. Electrical burns can occur if incompatible monitoring equipment is attached to the patient. Similarly, patients with ferromagnetic implants should never be placed inside a large magnetic field, as device heating and malfunction can result in patient injury. Finally, missile injury can occur if ferromagnetic objects are brought within the vicinity of the magnetic field.

Objects in the magnet room need to be both MRI safe and MRI compatible. The term "MR conditional" was defined by the American Society for Testing and Materials to describe an item that poses no known hazards in a specified MRI environment (based on the static magnetic field strength and spatial gradient field generated by the MRI model). Before entering the magnet room, one needs to ensure the patient has been screened and cleared by MRI technicians to rule out the presence of susceptible metal objects such as incompatible orthopedic hardware, cardiac implantable electronic devices (CIEDs), or catheters with ferromagnetic material. Only an MRI-compatible fiber-optic pulse oximeter should be used; otherwise, burns can result at the point of skin contact with a standard pulse oximeter. Similar concerns pertain to any other monitoring or management devices that make patient contact. Of note, some popular brands of athletic clothing contain metallic microfibers that can result in skin burns during MRI.

Missile injury in an MRI suite is a serious and life-threatening risk. The superconducting electrical currents that generate an MRI scanner's large magnetic field are always "on." Therefore MRI scanners are always surrounded by large magnetic field gradients (up to 6 m away). Magnetic field gradients can pull metallic objects into the magnet with alarming speed and force. Certain metals such as nickel and cobalt are dangerous because they are magnetic, whereas other metals such as aluminum, titanium, copper, and silver do not pose a missile danger. These metals are used to make MRI-compatible intravenous poles, fixation devices, and nonmagnetic anesthesia workstations. MRI-compatible intravenous infusion pumps are clinically available. If one must bring susceptible metal items such as infusion pumps into the MRI magnet room, they should be safely located and fixed, preferably bolted to a wall or floor. The additional equipment should be placed and verified as secure before the patient enters the MRI scanner. In the event that an object is pulled into the magnet causing patient injury and equipment damage the superconducting magnet can be turned off immediately. This process, called *quenching,* should only be performed by MRI technicians. The superconducting magnet of an MRI operates at cryogenic temperatures near absolute zero and requires coolant (cryogen) such as liquid helium to maintain the low temperature. The quenching process involves a rise in temperature of the superconducting magnet with escape of cryogen into a venting system outside the MRI room. However, cryogen can escape into the MRI room and displace oxygen, which can cause cold injury and asphyxiation.

Monitoring Issues in MRI Suites

Many anesthesia providers prefer to be outside the magnet room during the scan. This practice is acceptable as long as the provider (1) has access to all vital sign monitor displays and (2) can view the patient through a window or video camera. Critically ill patients undergoing MRI may require an arterial line for blood pressure monitoring. If the pressure transducer is classified as "MR conditional" for the particular MRI scanner, then it may be used during the procedure along with an MRI-compatible pressure cable and monitoring system. Otherwise, a long extension of pressure tubing must be added so that pressure transducers and their electrical cables can be located far from the magnet, preferably outside the magnet room. The radiofrequency pulse from an MRI can cause the pressure transducer, and the pulse oximeter, to generate artifacts that can be misleading. Fortunately, visual inspection of the waveforms allows rapid recognition. The use of IV extensions and stopcocks in vascular access lines increases the risk of inadvertent disconnection; these connections should be tightened and verified as secure before imaging.

Compatible Equipment

Typically, a patient requiring general anesthesia for MRI is anesthetized using a primary anesthesia workstation outside the magnet room. A second anesthesia workstation inside the magnet room must be MRI safe and have fully functioning suction, physiologic monitoring, and ventilator capabilities. If a critical event occurs during MRI, the scan is stopped immediately, and the patient must be promptly transferred from the magnet room back to the primary workstation so that optimal care and additional help can be provided.

ANESTHESIA FOR NONINVASIVE IMAGING PROCEDURES

Because noninvasive imaging procedures do not cause pain, most adult patients do not need sedation or general anesthesia. The ASA has described a continuum of depth of sedation that includes progressive levels of sedation, including minimal sedation (anxiolysis), moderate sedation (so-called "conscious sedation"), deep sedation, and general anesthesia (also see Chapter 14). For those adult patients who require sedation, anxiolysis (pharmacologic or nonpharmacologic) may be all that is required. In many medical centers minimal sedation and moderate sedation can be provided by appropriately trained nonanesthesia personnel, whereas deep sedation and general anesthesia must be administered by anesthesia providers. For pediatric patients, deep sedation or general anesthesia is often required to facilitate the imaging procedure. In addition to the requirements for sedation, comorbidities such as airway compromise, severe cardiopulmonary disease, or morbid obesity may require an anesthesia provider to assure maintenance of adequate oxygenation, hemodynamic stability, patient immobility, and minimization of pain and anxiety during the procedure.

Physiologic Monitoring

The ASA Standards for Basic Anesthetic Monitoring (also see Chapter 20) are applicable to all noninvasive imaging procedures. Commonly available nasal cannulas incorporate an integrated CO_2 sampling line. The resulting capnography can provide the respiratory rate and pattern, though the expired CO_2 waveform and concentration are more difficult to interpret in a nonintubated patient. If capnography is not possible, ventilation must be assessed by continuous visual inspection, auscultation, or both.

Oxygen Administration

Supplemental oxygen via a nasal cannula should come from a dedicated flowmeter instead of the anesthesia workstation common gas outlet. This approach permits more rapid deployment of the anesthesia workstation breathing circuit for delivering noninvasive oxygen or positive-pressure ventilation if the patient develops hypoventilation, hypoxemia, or apnea. For procedures of long duration, humidified oxygen should be given via nasal cannula to promote patient comfort by minimizing drying of the nasal and pharyngeal mucosa. Certain patients, including infants and small children, will not tolerate a nasal cannula but can receive oxygen with a blow-by method.

Pharmacologically Induced Sedation

Many medications can be used to provide sedation for imaging procedures (also see Chapters 8 and 9). For brief procedures, a small dose of a rapid-onset, short-acting opioid such as remifentanil or alfentanil is often an appropriate selection. Lengthier sedation can usually be managed successfully with a continuous propofol infusion, with or without supplemental intravenous opioids or benzodiazepines (or both). Dexmedetomidine is another useful drug, primarily in procedures lasting more than an hour. Because dexmedetomidine is less likely to cause respiratory depression compared with propofol, it is especially useful for patients with severe pulmonary hypertension or those who require frequent assessment of mental status.

Management of Anesthesia for CT

CT is often used for intracranial imaging and for studies of the thorax and abdomen. Because CT is painless, non-invasive, and generally of short duration, adult patients undergoing elective diagnostic scans rarely require more than emotional support. In addition, the bore of the CT scan is much more open than an MRI, so claustrophobia is rarely an issue. CT scanning is a crucial diagnostic tool in several acute settings, including traumatic injury (head and abdominal), acute stroke, and acute altered mental status of unknown cause. CT scanning is also used for urgent assessment of gastrointestinal integrity or acute pulmonary embolism in critically ill patients, who may require complex care during ICU transport. Sedation or general anesthesia is often essential for such patients and for children and adults who have difficulty remaining motionless.

Management of Anesthesia for MRI

For pediatric patients (also see Chapter 34), a common technique consists of (1) inhaled induction of anesthesia with sevoflurane; (2) placement of intravenous catheter; (3) intravenous infusion of propofol; and (4) either nasal cannula, laryngeal mask airway, or endotracheal tube for airway management, based on patient comorbid conditions. For adults who require general anesthesia for MRI, the body region being imaged may influence airway management choice. For example, in some patients spontaneously breathing with a supraglottic airway, even slight airway obstruction can cause excessive motion during brain MRI scan, which can be avoided with an endotracheal airway.

INTERVENTIONAL RADIOLOGY

Interventional radiology (IR) is a rapidly changing field as a result of continuing improvement in imaging quality and technologic advances. The ability to combine real-time, noninvasive imaging with minimally invasive, often catheter based, interventions offers great benefits to patients who otherwise have to experience the stress of an open surgery and possibly lengthier recovery. Interventional neuroradiology (INR), also called *endovascular neurosurgery,* mixes traditional neurosurgery with neuroradiology while also including certain aspects of

head and neck surgery. Body IR mixes general surgery with general radiology. In angiographic procedures the relevant blood vessel trees are imaged, after which a decision is made to advance to one or more therapeutic interventions via drugs, devices, or both. The list of IR procedures is extensive and continues to grow.

Interventional Neuroradiology

Anesthesia Choice
Most medical centers routinely use general endotracheal anesthesia for complex procedures or those of long duration, but there is no clearly superior anesthetic technique.[9] The specific choice of anesthesia may be guided primarily by the procedure needs and cardiovascular and cerebrovascular considerations.[10] Advantages of general anesthesia include control of ventilation and immobility, which improves image quality. Intermittent apnea may be requested by the interventional team to even further reduce motion artifact during digital subtraction angiography. Mechanical ventilation goals include maintenance of normocapnia or slight hypocapnia as long as intracranial pressure is normal. A patient with increased intracranial pressure may benefit from mild hyperventilation before anesthesia induction and during maintenance of anesthesia in order to counteract inhaled anesthetic-induced cerebral vasodilation (also see Chapter 30). As an alternative to general anesthesia, minimal or moderate sedation has the advantage of allowing assessment of neurologic function during the procedure. A variety of medications can be used for sedation based on the experience of the provider and the goals of anesthetic management.

Access and Monitoring
The INR suite requires multiple imaging screens and a large fluoroscopy C-arm device that is capable of extensive movement around the patient. As a result, the distance from the intravenous catheter to the intravenous fluid bag can be twice as long as normal. The tubing extensions must be securely connected and of sufficient length to prevent accidental dislodgement. Infusions of intravenous anesthetics or vasoactive drugs should be connected as close to the intravenous catheter as possible to minimize tubing dead space. For procedures involving the blood supply to the central nervous system (CNS), arterial line placement for continuous blood pressure monitoring may be prudent. A significant volume of fluid (e.g., heparinized flush solution and radiographic contrast agent) can be administered through catheters placed by the interventional team, in addition to the fluid administered by the anesthesia provider. Foley catheter placement will facilitate assessment of urine output and assist in fluid management decisions and will promote patient comfort by avoiding bladder distention.

IV

Arterial Blood Pressure Management

Baseline arterial blood pressure and cardiovascular reserve should be assessed carefully because blood pressure manipulation is commonly required during INR procedures and treatment-related perturbations regularly occur. Maintenance of arterial blood pressure within a predetermined range is particularly important in patients with cerebrovascular disease. Arterial blood pressure targets should always be discussed preoperatively with the interventional team. Deliberate hypertension, that is, maintaining a higher-than-normal arterial blood pressure, is used in INR patients with occlusive cerebrovascular disease to promote collateral cerebral blood flow. Such cases include patients undergoing emergency thrombolysis[11] and patients with aneurysmal subarachnoid hemorrhage in whom vasospasm has developed. Maintaining normal or supranormal arterial pressure is also important in patients with tumors that compromise blood flow to the spinal cord, kidneys, and other organs. Conversely, prevention of arterial hypertension may be critical in certain patients, including those with recently ruptured intracranial aneurysms or recently obliterated intracranial arteriovenous malformation. Patients who have undergone cerebrovascular angioplasty and stent placement in extracranial conductance vessels such as the carotid artery are susceptible to posttreatment cerebral hyperperfusion injury and require careful monitoring and timely intervention of arterial blood pressure after the procedure (also see Chapter 30). Besides traditional approaches to blood pressure control within fixed ranges, the use of near-infrared spectroscopy (a measure of brain tissue oxygenation) or neuroangiographic findings may lead to individual-specific blood pressure targets in the postintervention period to avoid both hypoperfusion and hyperperfusion.[12,13]

Management of Neurologic and Procedural Crises

Crisis management during an INR procedure requires a well-thought-out plan coupled with rapid and effective communication between the anesthesia and radiology teams. The initial responsibility of the anesthesia provider is to assure that airway patency, gas exchange, and hemodynamic status remain intact. Then the anesthesia provider should communicate with the procedural team and determine whether the INR problem is hemorrhagic or occlusive.

In the setting of vascular occlusion the goal is to increase distal perfusion by augmentation of arterial blood pressure with or without direct thrombolysis. This may require preparation and administration of a vasopressor infusion.

If the problem is hemorrhage, the anesthesia provider should discuss with the interventional team whether to immediately cease heparin administration and administer reversal with protamine. Complications of protamine administration include hypotension, anaphylaxis, and pulmonary hypertension. Most cases of vascular rupture can be managed in the angiography suite. The INR team can attempt to seal the rupture site via endovascular approach and may abort the originally planned procedure. In addition, a ventriculostomy catheter may be placed emergently in the angiography suite if elevated intracranial pressure is suspected. Patients with suspected rupture will require emergent head CT scan; emergent craniotomy may be needed depending on imaging findings.

Body Interventional Radiology

Interventional radiologists use x-rays, CT, ultrasound, MRI, and other imaging modalities to perform image-guided procedures throughout the body. These procedures are usually performed using needles and catheters, which are regarded as minimally invasive compared with traditional surgery. This section highlights the general approaches and challenges of anesthesia management for the most common image-guided procedures, such as diagnostic procedures, catheter drainage, stent placement, tumor ablation, vascular angioplasty and embolization treatment, and site-specific delivery of therapeutic agents (Table 38.2). The transjugular intrahepatic portosystemic shunt (TIPS) procedure deserves special recognition because of the severity of illness in its patient population.[14]

Table 38.2 List of Common Interventional Radiology Procedures

Vascular	Liver/Biliary	Cancer	Miscellaneous
Angiography	Biliary drainage and stenting	Percutaneous (needle) biopsy	Abscess drainage
Balloon angioplasty	Transjugular liver biopsy	Chemoembolization	Chest tube
Embolization	Transjugular intrahepatic portosystemic shunt	Radiofrequency ablation	Percutaneous nephrostomy tube
Central venous/hemodialysis access			Gastrostomy tube
Thrombolysis			
Vena cava filter			

Anesthesia Evaluation and Management

The anesthesia requirements of patients undergoing IR procedures can vary greatly. Because of the minimally invasive nature, many procedures in the IR suites are performed with minimal sedation without an anesthesia provider present. However, a number of factors can prompt the involvement of the anesthesia provider (see Table 38.1). The presence of an anesthesia provider allows the proceduralists to focus their complete attention on the intervention at hand. A clear and detailed discussion should take place among the team members so the proceduralists can specify their intraprocedural needs and the anesthesia provider can describe any anesthetic concerns.

The preprocedural evaluation by the anesthesia provider follows the same approach as with any other anesthetic (also see Chapter 13). The choice of anesthetic technique follows the same principles outlined earlier in this chapter (also see Chapter 14). Patients who have altered mental status or cognitive dysfunction—dementia, delirium, encephalopathy, or developmental delay—may not be candidates for sedation if they are expected to cooperate and breath-hold during the procedure. The medication list should be reviewed. Special concerns for body interventional procedures include therapy with the oral antihyperglycemic metformin, which may cause lactic acidosis if administered with intravenous contrast agent in the setting of renal failure. Lactic acidosis is extremely rare when a patient with normal renal function receives both metformin and intravenous contrast agent. ASA Practice Guidelines for Preoperative Fasting should be followed, as with any other elective procedure.

If general anesthesia is not the initial anesthetic choice, the anesthesia provider should be prepared to escalate the level of sedation as needed, up to and including general anesthesia. Therefore all necessary equipment, monitors, and medications should be available.

Transjugular Intrahepatic Portosystemic Shunt

Patients who are scheduled to undergo the TIPS procedure have significant liver disease and complications of portal hypertension, which can include variceal bleeding, ascites, and hepatorenal syndrome. The Model for End-Stage Liver Disease (MELD) score serves as a marker of liver disease severity and is a predictor of short-term mortality risk in these patients, who may be candidates for liver transplantation. Anesthetic evaluation should focus on the multisystem effects of liver failure, including cardiovascular, pulmonary, neurologic, renal, and hematologic manifestations (also see Chapter 28). Hepatic encephalopathy is a common finding in this patient population and is a contraindication for TIPS. Coagulopathy and thrombocytopenia may increase bleeding risk and require correction before the procedure.

The anesthetic management of a patient undergoing the TIPS procedure can be quite challenging. Because of the presence of cardiopulmonary comorbid conditions, coagulopathy, and the unpredictable length of the procedure, most proceduralists prefer general anesthesia. Medications that have significant liver metabolism and biliary clearance should be avoided or minimized. The presence of tense ascites and gastroesophageal reflux are obvious risk factors for pulmonary aspiration of gastric contents. An endotracheal tube is preferred for airway management (as opposed to a supraglottic airway) because the neck must be rotated to provide internal jugular venous access. Lastly, the anesthesia provider must be aware of several important post-TIPS complications: altered mental status because of post-TIPS encephalopathy, massive hemorrhage from intrahepatic bleeding or vascular injury, and worsening liver failure from decreased portal vein blood flow.

Challenges: Hemostasis and Anticoagulation

Many IR procedures involve access of the arterial tree with large-diameter catheters. To minimize the risk of thromboembolic complication, the anesthesia provider is often asked to maintain intraprocedural anticoagulation. This is usually achieved with intravenous heparin, and the degree of anticoagulation is monitored with whole-blood activated clotting time (ACT). Heparin has the advantage of a short half-life and reliable reversal with protamine. For patients with heparin or protamine allergy or heparin-induced thrombocytopenia, direct thrombin inhibitors are alternatives. However, there is no reliable reversal for these drugs. They are metabolized by the liver, and the plasma half-life of bivalirudin, shortest in the group, is 25 minutes.

Frequently IR embolization is performed as urgent therapy for acute hemorrhage. Common applications include gastrointestinal, uterine, or other intraabdominal bleeding. Diagnostic angiography is performed to identify the site and mechanism of bleeding. Often, coils and thrombotic agents can be injected into the culprit arterial branch to stop the bleeding. To safely induce anesthesia and to rapidly secure the airway in a bleeding patient can be challenging. The patient's vital signs may further deteriorate after induction of anesthesia, and resuscitation is required with medication, fluid, and blood transfusion (also see Chapters 24 and 25). In addition to acute anemia, coagulopathy and thrombocytopenia are common, either as the cause of the initial hemorrhage or as the result of dilution from fluid replacement or factor consumption. The correction of coagulopathy should ideally be guided by laboratory data and a treatment algorithm. However, timely data may not be available during an emergency. The decision whether to transfuse will depend on the patient's medical history (e.g., presence of hematologic and hepatic diseases), recent medications (e.g., anticoagulant or antiplatelet therapy), physical findings (e.g., of disseminated intravascular coagulopathy), and the clinician's judgment. In addition to platelets,

IV

plasma, and cryoprecipitate, recombinant factors and factor concentrates may offer the benefit of correcting factor deficiency without the risk of transfusion-related complications.

ENDOSCOPY AND ENDOSCOPIC RETROGRADE CHOLANGIOPANCREATOGRAPHY

Endoscopy is frequently performed for the diagnosis and screening of gastrointestinal conditions. Indications for upper endoscopy (esophagogastroduodenoscopy [EGD]) include gastroesophageal reflux, bleeding, dysphagia, protracted pain or nausea, accidental ingestion, and abnormal imaging. Additionally, therapeutic interventions such as treatment of bleeding source, ablation of Barrett esophagus, biopsy and removal of abnormal growth, dilation and stenting of stricture, and feeding tube placement can be performed. The development of high-frequency endoscopic ultrasound (EUS) using a small-caliber catheter through the biopsy channel of the endoscope can provide high-resolution images of benign and neoplastic lesions in the gastrointestinal tract.

For EGD, the patient is typically placed in a left lateral position with the neck flexed. The usual sequence of events includes (1) application of topical anesthesia to the patient's pharynx with either lidocaine or benzocaine; (2) placement of a plastic mouth guard to minimize risk of damage to teeth or endoscope; (3) administration of medications to achieve minimal to moderate sedation; (4) insertion of endoscope through mouth into esophagus; (5) examination of esophagus, gastroesophageal junction, stomach, pylorus, and duodenum as required; and (6) performance of therapeutic maneuvers when necessary.

Endoscopic retrograde cholangiopancreatography (ERCP) is often performed for the diagnosis and possible treatment of bile duct and pancreatic duct diseases. ERCP requires specialized equipment, including a dedicated fluoroscopy system. Common indications include jaundice, acute biliary pancreatitis, chronic pancreatitis of unknown cause, pancreatic pseudocyst, suspected biliary or pancreatic malignancy, sphincter of Oddi disorders, duct stricture, and postoperative bile leak. ERCP interventions include sphincterotomy, dilation, stenting (e.g., bile duct, fistulas, stricture, bile leak), drain placement, EUS, and tissue biopsy. The patient is typically placed in a left lateral or prone position with the head turned toward the endoscopist. The first portion of the procedure is similar to EGD whereby the endoscope is advanced past the pharynx and is inserted into the esophagus. Once the endoscope is in the duodenum, it is rotated to face the papilla. A cannula is inserted into the papilla, contrast agent is injected, and the duct is visualized under fluoroscopy. Excessive intestinal motility can impede endoscopic examination and can be inhibited by the administration of either anticholinergic drugs or glucagon.

Anesthesia Evaluation and Management

Anesthesia providers are often asked to care for patients requiring procedures in the gastrointestinal endoscopy suite.[15] The standard approach to preprocedural evaluation (also see Chapter 13) and anesthetic choice (also see Chapter 14) applies in this setting. Simple EGD and ERCP in otherwise healthy patients can be performed with minimal or moderate sedation administered by a trained nonanesthesia provider. However, anesthesia services (whether monitored anesthesia care or general anesthesia) may be requested if the procedure is expected to be challenging or prolonged, patient immobility is desired, or the patient's history suggests airway difficulty or other comorbid conditions. Hepatobiliary dysfunction is common in patients who require ERCP. These patients may have coagulopathy because of decreased synthesis of coagulation factors and thrombocytopenia (also see Chapter 28). Blood product transfusion may be necessary before the endoscopy, especially for the more invasive ERCP.

The choice of anesthetic technique requires clear communication between the patient, endoscopist, and anesthesia provider. Although minimal or moderate sedation is the most common technique for uncomplicated EGD, deep sedation or general anesthesia may be necessary for EGD based on patient comorbid conditions or severity of clinical status (e.g., critically ill patient with massive hematemesis). A short-acting anxiolytic, midazolam, combined with an analgesic, fentanyl, used by anesthesia and nonanesthesia providers alike, can be quite effective in providing mild to moderate sedation for routine endoscopy. Propofol is a commonly used agent by anesthesia providers to provide a deeper level of anesthesia, favored for its rapid onset and short duration of action.

ERCP is considered to be a riskier procedure compared with EGD, based on the nature of the procedure and the typical patient population. The patient is most often in the prone position, and the anesthesia provider has limited access to the patient's airway because the endoscopist stands next to the patient's head. Finally, the room is darkened to allow better viewing of the fluoroscopy screen, and the provider must wear protective lead shields to minimize exposure to ionizing radiation. Factors that may increase the risk of adverse events include ASA class >3, Mallampati airway score of 4, ascites, obesity, sleep apnea, chronic lung disease, and significant alcohol use. General anesthesia with endotracheal intubation may be safer in such patients.[16] Many patients undergo repeat ERCP and have developed a preference for monitored anesthesia care versus general anesthesia based on their experience.

Challenges and Complications

Complications of EGD or ERCP can generally be grouped by sedation and airway, procedure, and patient-related factors (Table 38.3). The most common complications are adverse respiratory events—hypoxemia, hypercapnia, aspiration, loss of airway, and cardiopulmonary arrest. Although the goal in the sedated patient is to maintain spontaneous respiration, airway obstruction and an inability to ventilate can occur with very little warning. It is often more prudent to continually assess the effectiveness of ventilation with direct observation and monitoring with capnography than to rely solely on pulse oximetry, as hypoxemia can be a late sign of hypoventilation. The anesthesia provider's ability to intervene is further complicated by the shared airway during upper endoscopy. Topical benzocaine administration can lead to methemoglobinemia (also see Chapter 10).

Procedure-related complications, such as esophageal perforation, are rare but can be life threatening. Esophageal perforation is more likely to occur in patients with a history of stricture, previous perforation, previous surgery, or other anatomic abnormalities. Symptoms may include neck, chest, or abdominal pain. Clinical signs are often nonspecific (e.g., tachycardia, tachypnea, hypotension, abdominal distention, and even sepsis). Clinical suspicion should be raised especially if the symptoms do not resolve or are self-limited. The diagnosis of perforation is usually made radiographically, often with the use of water-soluble contrast material. Depending on the lesion, some perforations can be managed medically, whereas others constitute surgical emergencies. Another rare but potentially fatal complication is gas embolism, which is more common during ERCP than other GI endoscopy procedures. Whereas minor cases are likely subclinical and underreported, large venous gas embolisms can cause dyspnea, right heart strain or failure, and even cardiopulmonary collapse.

Both the endoscopist and the anesthesia provider must remain vigilant for this possibility.

The anesthetic management of a patient with upper gastrointestinal bleeding can be especially challenging. Tracheal intubation may be complicated by ongoing hematemesis. Large-bore, possibly central, venous access is required to continue resuscitation with fluid, blood, and vasopressors. Often the patient may be coagulopathic, either because of a preexisting underlying cause or ongoing blood loss. A typical example is a patient who has end-stage liver disease with deficiency in coagulation factors, thrombocytopenia, portal hypertension, and variceal bleeding. For anesthesia providers caring for such critically ill patients, anesthesia management is further complicated by the location outside the operating suite, where resources and help are often far away.

CATHETER-BASED CARDIOLOGY PROCEDURES

Adult Cardiac Catheterization

Patients needing coronary artery or peripheral artery angiography usually show evidence of coronary ischemia on noninvasive cardiac stress tests or other clinical manifestations of atherosclerosis. Preprocedural assessment and preparation should be focused on their cardiopulmonary functional status, airway, relevant medications, and other common comorbid conditions such as diabetes mellitus and renal insufficiency.

Percutaneous coronary intervention (PCI) usually involves the cannulation of one or more peripheral arteries, such as the radial, brachial, or femoral. A noninvasive arterial blood pressure monitor should be placed on an extremity that is not involved with the procedure. The cardiologist will inject local anesthetic at the site of cannulation supplemented by intravenous sedation using midazolam

IV

Table 38.3	Complications of Esophagogastroduodenoscopy (EGD) or Endoscopic Retrograde Cholangiopancreatography (ERCP)		

Sedation and Airway-Related	Procedure-Related	Patient-Related
Hypoxemia	Bleeding	Bleeding
Excessive secretion	Perforation	Coagulopathy
Aspiration	Pancreatitis (ERCP)	Thrombocytopenia
Laryngospasm	Air embolism (insufflation of air by endoscopist)	Cardiac arrhythmia (e.g., if epinephrine is injected into gastrointestinal mucosa to stop hemorrhage)
Bronchospasm	Hypercarbia (CO_2 insufflation may be used by endoscopist to improve visibility)	
Methemoglobinemia (from topical benzocaine, if used)	Contrast agent allergy	

ERCP, Endoscopic retrograde cholangiopancreatography.

and fentanyl. PCI is usually well tolerated by the patient with light sedation. Anesthesia care is requested when the patient has a history of severe anxiety, an inability to lie flat because of chronic pain or orthopnea, or high-grade coronary stenosis such as chronic total occlusion (CTO). PCI in CTO lesions is more technically challenging, and therefore longer in duration, and has a higher risk of complications. Sometimes, a PCI may require mechanical device support, such as intraaortic balloon pump, extracorporeal circulatory life support (ECLS), or percutaneous ventricular assist device. In these clinical situations a dedicated anesthesia provider is invaluable in providing sedation, managing the airway, and supporting hemodynamic stability.

General anesthesia is rarely indicated unless the patient is unable to cooperate and remain still, there is ongoing need for pulmonary resuscitation (e.g., from hypoxemia or hypercarbia), or a surgical exposure for ECLS cannulation is planned. The risk of hemodynamic instability during general anesthesia is clearly high. Because the procedure duration is usually short, an opiate-based induction of anesthesia is not desirable. A small dose of propofol, etomidate, ketamine, or an inhaled induction of anesthesia may be appropriate. Either a low concentration of inhaled anesthetic or intravenous anesthetic infusion is usually sufficient to maintain anesthesia. The use of vasoconstrictors may be needed to maintain systemic vascular resistance, and inotropic drugs such as dobutamine, epinephrine, or dopamine may be needed in patients with severely depressed left ventricular ejection fraction. Finally, as with any NORA location, the anesthesia provider may be emergently called to the catheterization suite to help resuscitate a patient, including securing the airway and possibly organizing transport to the intensive care unit (ICU) or OR.

Electrophysiology Studies

Catheter-Based Ablation

Electrophysiology (EP) covers the diagnosis of cardiac dysrhythmias, detailed mapping of their circuitry, and treatment with catheter-based ablation.[17] With rapid advancements in cardiac monitors, CT, MRI, and catheter technologies, a wide variety of dysrhythmias—atrial fibrillation (AF), supraventricular tachyarrhythmias (SVTs), and ventricular tachycardia (VT)—are amendable to EP study and treatment. The characteristics of patients undergoing EP studies and ablation can vary greatly, ranging from healthy young adults with isolated dysrhythmia to those with end-stage heart failure with left ventricular assist devices. Preprocedural evaluation of these patients should focus on their cardiopulmonary reserve (particularly signs and symptoms when dysrhythmias occur), airway, comorbid conditions, and relevant medications, especially anticoagulants such as heparin, warfarin and the newer direct factor Xa inhibitors, and direct thrombin inhibitors.

The intracardiac catheters are usually placed via the femoral and internal jugular veins, unless a retrograde approach to the left side of the heart via the femoral artery is planned. Endocardial mapping studies are performed with stimulation and recording from the internal and external electrodes, followed by catheter ablation of the endocardium (usually with radiofrequency energy) to produce a scar that disrupts dysrhythmia generation or propagation. Generous subcutaneous injection of local anesthetics and intravenous administered sedation medications during cannulation is sufficient for most patients. The anesthetic plan and monitoring should take into consideration the patient's comfort and cooperation, clinical stability, and the need for successful EP study and ablation of dysrhythmia of interest.[17,18] An EP study can be time-consuming and requires the patient to lie flat and remain motionless for an extended period, which can be challenging for anyone but especially those with chronic anxiety or pain. During the study, the patient may become unstable because of induction of tachyarrhythmia or from ventricular pacing. A history of syncope or angina during a tachycardic episode or preexisting cardiomyopathy may suggest depressed cardiac output and significant hypotension in the setting of tachycardia, and invasive arterial pressure monitoring may be warranted. A successful EP study requires stable catheter-tissue contact, which can be negatively affected by cardiac, respiratory, and patient motion. Some arrhythmias are more difficult to induce than others.

The ideal anesthetic regimen would provide the following: (1) patient comfort, (2) patient immobility, (3) predictable respiratory pattern, (4) unchanged autonomic tone, (5) unchanged inducibility of arrhythmia, and (6) unchanged intrinsic pacemaker (PM) function and conduction propagation. However, an ideal anesthetic agent does not exist.[16] For example, propofol and dexmedetomidine decrease sympathetic tone, and remifentanil decreases sinus and atrioventricular (AV) node function. For most EP studies, the patient receives deeper sedation during the initial cannulation and catheter insertion and minimal sedation thereafter to ensure minimal suppression of catecholamine-dependent arrhythmias such as SVT, paroxysmal AF, or VT.

For patients with chronic AF, the success rate of ablation is higher for patients receiving general anesthesia.[17] The AF ablation procedure typically involves endocardial ablation that isolates pulmonary vein ostia from the rest of the left atrium. General anesthesia allows predictable respiratory movement during ablation, monitoring of esophageal temperature to avoid left atrial perforation, and detection of any phrenic nerve stimulation. For procedures involving catheters in the left-sided chambers of the heart, anticoagulation is usually achieved with intravenous heparin to avoid thromboembolic complications.[17] Finally, vascular sheaths are continually flushed to remain patent and ablation catheters are cooled with irrigated fluid to avoid thrombus buildup. Because the amount of fluid can be substantial over a long procedure, patients with a history of heart failure may require a diuretic to avoid excessive intravascular volume.

Cardiac Implantable Electronic Devices

Another common group of procedures performed in the EP suite is the placement of CIEDs, such as implantable cardioverter-defibrillators (ICDs) and PMs. The anesthesia provider should understand the indication of the device, whether it is heart block, primary prevention for sudden cardiac death in cardiomyopathy, secondary prevention for a history of VT, or biventricular pacing for cardiac resynchronization therapy. Transcutaneous pacing and defibrillator devices should be attached to the patient, and the anesthesia provider should understand how to operate these devices to institute emergency pacing or defibrillation. Again, the procedure can be performed successfully with subcutaneous local anesthetic injection and intravenous sedation and analgesia medications. However, the anesthesia provider may decide that general anesthesia may be safer, for example, in a patient with altered mental status. The cardiologist may choose to perform a defibrillation threshold test, in which fibrillation is intentionally induced and the device's ability to sense and terminate fibrillation is confirmed. In some patients, such as those with severe systolic left ventricular dysfunction (e.g., ischemic cardiomyopathy), the brief loss of cardiac output and perfusion, even for seconds, may be poorly tolerated. For these patients, invasive pressure monitoring is advisable to facilitate timely treatment of hypotension. Before the test, administration of oxygen and a small intravenous dose of a short-acting anesthetic to produce amnesia is appropriate.

Cardioversion

The anesthesia provider is frequently involved in caring for patients who are undergoing cardioversion for atrial fibrillation or atrial flutter.[17] Because of the risk of thromboembolic disease in these patients, cardioversion is often immediately preceded by a transesophageal echocardiogram (TEE) to examine the left atrium for thrombus. TEE may be bypassed if the patient has been receiving therapeutic anticoagulation.

For cardioversion without TEE, the patient first undergoes a few minutes of preoxygenation. Then, a small dose of hypnotic, such as propofol, is given to render the patient amnestic. After cardioversion, the anesthesia provider monitors the patient, relieves any airway obstruction, and provides additional oxygen until satisfactory recovery of mentation and airway reflexes before PACU transport.

For TEE before cardioversion, the echocardiographer may choose to topicalize the upper airway with local anesthetics to suppress gag reflex during probe insertion. The drawback with topicalization is that the loss of airway reflex may linger beyond the procedure and limit the patient's ability to manage excessive secretions. A common anesthetic choice is a short-acting hypnotic such as propofol infusion. Supplemental oxygen is started before TEE probe insertion. Sedatives are titrated to accommodate the passage of the probe; typically, a lower dose is required for the rest of the examination. Maneuvers such as jaw thrust, chin lift, or pharyngeal suctioning may be necessary to avoid obstruction or clear secretions.

Structural Heart Disease Intervention

Catheter-based intervention for the treatment of structural heart diseases is a rapidly evolving field. Balloon valvuloplasty or even valve replacement can be performed on all of the intracardiac valves. Atrial septal defect (ASD), patent foramen ovale (PFO), ventricular septal defect (VSD), and coronary fistula can be closed with expandable devices. These procedures are performed using fluoroscopy with additional guidance using echocardiography. Because a significant proportion of this patient population has had previous sternotomy for cardiac surgery, the transcatheter approach avoids the morbidity and risk of repeat sternotomy and inadvertent cardiac injury.

General anesthesia has a number of advantages: an immobile patient, controlled ventilatory movement, ease of continuous TEE examination, and a secured airway in the case of hemodynamic instability or when open surgery is needed. The induction of anesthesia may be challenging, however, given the implications of the cardiac lesion being treated. Pediatric patients with cyanotic heart lesions or adult patients with palliative treatment of congenital heart diseases may be especially challenging. A thorough preprocedural discussion is required between the anesthesia provider, congenital cardiologist, interventional cardiologist, and cardiac surgeon to address the cardiac anatomy, surgical history, and potential anesthetic concerns.

Pediatric Studies

Caring for neonates, infants, and children who are undergoing invasive cardiac studies and procedures is one of the most challenging tasks faced by the anesthesia provider (also see Chapter 34). To safely anesthetize these patients requires a deep understanding of the neonatal cardiopulmonary physiology, complex anatomy of cardiac lesions, pharmacology, pediatric airway, and other coexisting congenital diseases. Because of their age and cognitive development, most pediatric patients require either general anesthesia or deep sedation for these procedures. Special attention must be paid to the possibility of a difficult airway, the rapidity of ventilation problems adversely affecting cardiovascular stability,

IV

the pharmacodynamic and pharmacokinetic properties of anesthetic drugs, and the avoidance of hypothermia. The onset of intravenous and inhaled anesthetics will be significantly altered owing to the presence of intracardiac or extracardiac shunts. Similarly, the onset of medication effect can be delayed as a result of congestive heart failure and low cardiac output. The following conditions should be avoided because they can lead to increased pulmonary vascular resistance and right-sided heart failure: hypoxemia, hypercapnia, excessive positive airway pressure, metabolic acidosis, hypothermia, and painful stimulation without adequate analgesia. However, in patients with intracardiac shunts, hyperoxia and resulting pulmonary vasodilation may promote excessive left-to-right shunt and cause systemic hypotension. Also, cyanotic patients often develop secondary polycythemia to compensate for chronic oxygen deprivation. This places them at a higher risk of thrombotic complications during the procedures. The rule of thumb is to have the cyanotic patient remain at preanesthetic hemodynamic and oxygenation baseline, which can be a considerable challenge during anesthesia.

Challenges and Complications

Providing anesthetic care in interventional cardiology locations can be challenging. The typical arrangement of a room designed for the interventional cardiologist frequently places the anesthesia provider far away from the patient, with other equipment serving as obstacles. The anesthesia provider should always be prepared to escalate the depth of anesthesia, secure the airway, and provide resuscitation in case of emergency. The most common complications with interventional cardiology procedures are related to vascular access that include bleeding, hematoma, pneumothorax, and vascular injury. In addition, intracardiac catheters can trigger arrhythmia and heart blocks, which may cause significant cardiovascular changes.

Rarely, cardiac perforation can occur, resulting in pericardial effusion and tamponade. Clinical signs include persistent hemodynamic instability unrelated to the induced arrhythmia and refractory to routine administration of vasoconstrictors and intravenous fluids. The procedural team should be informed if perforation is suspected. The diagnosis can be confirmed with echocardiography. Blood products should be ordered immediately. Perhaps anticoagulation should be reversed after a consultation with the proceduralist. One or more of the venous sheaths can be used for intravascular volume resuscitation. The management options for a new pericardial effusion in this setting could include the following: (1) a "wait-and-watch" approach if the effusion is small and self-limiting, (2) emergent pericardial drain placement, or (3) rapid mobilization for surgical decompression of tamponade. Thus communication

and understanding of the procedural plan between the anesthesia provider and the cardiologist are crucial. The cardiologist's specialty expertise can be an asset during a cardiovascular emergency, including the rapid placement of invasive lines for monitoring and fluid resuscitation.

ELECTROCONVULSIVE THERAPY

Electroconvulsive therapy (ECT) is an effective treatment for patients suffering from severe depression (both unipolar and bipolar types), psychotic depression, and schizophrenia.[19] For severe depression, ECT has the following advantages compared with antidepressant medication alone: more rapid remission, decreased acute suicide risk, and reduced relapse rate. Most guidelines recommend ECT for patients who have failed medical therapy with antidepressants, have depression with severe psychotic features (e.g., catatonia), or patients at risk of suicide who need a rapid, definitive treatment response. The American Psychiatric Association also recommends its use as maintenance therapy. ECT exerts its therapeutic effect by inducing a generalized seizure. The efficacy of ECT for depression is influenced by technique-related factors such as electrode placement, length of convulsion, and number of ECT treatments. Generalized seizures likely change the neurobiology of depression by increasing CNS γ-aminobutyric acid (GABA) concentration, normalizing serotonin function, and suppressing hypothalamic–pituitary–adrenal axis hyperactivity.[19]

Electrically Induced Seizures

A trained ECT physician produces a generalized seizure by placing two electrodes in bifrontotemporal (bilateral), right unilateral, or bifrontal positions on the patient's head. The right unilateral or bifrontal position is often chosen over the bilateral position to minimize side effects of ECT such as short-term cognitive dysfunction. On the other hand, the bilateral electrode position has the advantages of ease of use, lower energy requirement, and higher efficacy (i.e., lower remission rate). A brief (0.5 to 2 ms) or an ultra-brief (<0.5 ms) pulse of electrical charge, usually 100 to 600 µC (microcoulombs) is applied with the goal to trigger a seizure of at least 15 seconds duration. Seizure threshold can either be determined empirically during the initial ECT treatment or based on the patient's age (for bilateral position). Threshold can be affected by a number of factors (e.g., chronic medication, blood pH) and may increase over the course of the treatment series. The electrical duration of the seizure is monitored with single-channel electroencephalography (EEG). Motor seizure activity can also be followed; however, motor activity typically stops before the electrical activity. Seizures shorter than 15 seconds or a complete lack of seizure may be subtherapeutic, whereas prolonged seizures (>120 seconds) may be harmful. Adjustment of stimulation by the ECT physician and possible intervention by the anesthesia provider may be necessary. A typical therapeutic course may involve three treatments per week and a total of 6 to 20 treatments.

Anesthesia Evaluation

Before starting ECT, a patient should undergo a full medical evaluation by the ECT physician and the anesthesia provider (also see Chapter 13).[20] Any interval change in health and side effects from previous treatments should be elicited during subsequent visits. Because of the CNS and cardiovascular changes associated with the induced seizure, special attention should be given to the presence of coexisting cardiovascular and CNS disease. Approximately one-third of patients undergoing ECT are aged 65 years or older, with an increased incidence of cardiopulmonary conditions (also see Chapter 35). Patients with unstable cardiac disease, such as malignant hypertension, decompensated heart failure, or hemodynamically significant arrhythmia, should be evaluated and optimized by a cardiologist. Patients with CIEDs can undergo ECT safely with certain precautions in place, as described later. Patients with unstable fractures may be at risk owing to motor seizure activity, though the risk is mitigated with adequate neuromuscular blockade.

Standard preoperative fasting guidelines should be followed. Chronic medication for cardiovascular or pulmonary diseases should usually be continued. One exception is the bronchodilator drug theophylline, which can increase the risk of status epilepticus. Chronic anticoagulation (e.g., warfarin) should be continued, as the risk of bleeding is minimal. Chronic medications for gastroesophageal reflux disease should be taken, but there is no evidence for routine prophylactic use of an antacid, H_2 antagonist, or proton pump inhibitor in an asymptomatic patient.[20]

Psychotropic Medications

Many ECT patients are receiving psychotropic medications. Lithium, anticonvulsants, and benzodiazepines, which may shorten seizure duration, may be tapered under the direction of the ECT physician. However, many psychotropic medications (e.g., monoamine oxidase inhibitors, serotonin reuptake inhibitors, tricyclic antidepressants, lithium, and benzodiazepines) have sympathomimetic, anticholinergic, and CNS effects and can cause serious drug–drug interactions with commonly used perioperative medications.[20]

Management of Anesthesia and Seizure

The steps in anesthesia management are described in Table 38.4.[20] If the patient has an ICD, the defibrillation function should be temporarily deactivated, typically with a magnet, so that the device does not misinterpret the ECT electrical stimulus as a tachyarrhythmia. For a patient who is PM-dependent, a magnet placed over the PM usually converts it to an asynchronous mode. This is required because the electrical artifact from the ECT stimulus and resulting motor movement can cause PM inhibition, leading to severe bradycardia or asystole. An external defibrillator machine with PM capabilities should be immediately available for those patients with CIEDs.

The most common induction drug is intravenous methohexital (0.5 to 1.5 mg/kg), a short-acting barbiturate. By contrast, propofol is a potent anticonvulsant that may increase seizure threshold and shorten seizure duration when used during ECT.[20] An alternative is intravenous etomidate (0.2 to 0.3 mg/kg),[21] which has the advantage of maintaining hemodynamic stability and can decrease seizure threshold and augment seizure duration in some patients. However, etomidate can induce nonepileptic myoclonic activity and cause adrenal insufficiency with just a single dose. Ketamine is another alternative, but its use is controversial, as it may cause posttreatment confusion.[21] If a patient has undergone prior ECT, the anesthesia provider should determine what induction drug and dose were administered, the resulting seizure duration, and the presence of any adverse effects. A subtherapeutic seizure may prompt a dose adjustment or a change of the induction drug, in consultation with the ECT physician. A prolonged seizure (>2 minutes) can be terminated by a small propofol bolus.

Once the patient loses consciousness, the manual blood pressure cuff on the distal limb is inflated (see Table 38.4). A fast-acting neuromuscular blocker, usually succinylcholine (0.5 to 1.5 mg/kg), is then administered. For patients with a contraindication to succinylcholine, rocuronium can be substituted, which can be rapidly reversed after the seizure with sugammadex (see Chapter 11).

Physiologic Responses to Seizure and Treatment

The electrically induced seizure can have profound effects on the patient's vital signs.[20] The first (tonic) phase is characterized by profound parasympathetic discharge that can lead to bradycardia, AV block, atrial arrhythmia, premature atrial or ventricular contraction, hypotension, or even asystole. Treatment with atropine or glycopyrrolate may be necessary for profound bradycardia. However, the tonic phase is rapidly followed by the second (clonic) phase of sympathetic overstimulation characterized by tachycardia and hypertension, which can also be profound. This may be exacerbated by hypoventilation and the resultant hypercarbia. Although the hemodynamic response usually subsides quickly after seizure termination, persistent hypertension and tachycardia, especially in patients with significant cardiovascular

IV

Table 38.4 Steps in Anesthesia Management for Electroconvulsive Therapy

Management Step	Description	Comment
1. Monitoring	Standard monitors plus the monitors described later.	Invasive pressure monitoring is rarely indicated.
	Additional manual BP cuff on distal limb with EMG leads attached to ECT machine.	Manual BP cuff is inflated before NMB administration so that the distal extremity can display muscle movement and EMG activity of the induced seizure.
	ECT leads attached to patient's head.	ECT leads will record EEG seizure activity.
	Peripheral nerve stimulator (PNS).	PNS can assess onset and duration of NMB
2. Preoxygenation	Preoxygenation by facemask.	Thorough preoxygenation is necessary because the patient will be apneic during the seizure.
3. Induction of anesthesia	Methohexital or etomidate are the most common agents.	See text for details.
4. Inflation of manual BP cuff on distal extremity	Inflation of the manual cuff above systolic blood pressure prevents NMB from reaching the distal extremity.	Seizure-related motor movement and EMG activity can be recorded distal to the manual BP cuff.
5. Neuromuscular blockade	Succinylcholine is given unless there is a contraindication.	NMB minimizes side effects from seizure-related motor activity such as myalgia or lactic acidosis. Also, NMB reduces oxygen consumption from muscle metabolism that would be increased during a generalized tonic-clonic seizure.
6. Hyperventilation	Mask ventilation and hyperventilation.	Hypocapnia from hyperventilation can lower seizure threshold and facilitate ECT.
7. Electrical stimulation and induced seizure	A bite block is placed before electrical stimulation.	Bite block reduces the risk of tongue laceration during seizure.
	When succinylcholine fasciculations stop, NMB should be adequate for treatment.	If rocuronium is used or if fasciculations are not well seen, peripheral nerve stimulation can confirm NMB.
	Electrical and motor monitoring of seizure duration.	EEG monitoring for electrical activity and EMG or observation of distal extremity is recorded for the duration.
8. Assess physiologic effects of seizure	Cardiovascular manifestations can include bradycardia, tachycardia, and hypertension.	See text for details.
9. Monitor respiratory, neuromuscular, and mental status	PNS monitoring for recovery after NMB. Airway obstruction may require chin lift/jaw thrust or oral airway placement. The level of consciousness begins to return several minutes after seizure ends.	Spontaneous respirations will become stronger as NMB abates. Supraglottic airway may be useful if airway obstruction persists despite mask ventilation with oral airway. Endotracheal intubation is rarely needed.

BP, Blood pressure; *ECT*, electroconvulsive therapy; *EEG*, electroencephalography; *EMG*, electromyography; *NMB*, neuromuscular blockade; *PNS*, peripheral nerve stimulator.

diseases at risk for ischemia, may require treatment such as β-adrenergic antagonists (e.g., esmolol or labetalol) and other antihypertensives (e.g., hydralazine).

Side Effects

Side effects of ECT are common. If a patient has had prior ECT treatments, the anesthesia provider should review the prior anesthesia record to determine the intraoperative hemodynamic response and post-ECT experience of the patient. If the patient had an excessive sympathetic response during past treatments, the anesthesia provider may choose to administer prophylactic β-adrenergic antagonists immediately before seizure induction. Post-ECT symptoms such as headache, muscle pain, or nausea may be treated with small doses of opiates, acetaminophen, nonsteroidal antiinflammatory drugs, or antiemetics.

REFERENCES

1. Nagrebetsky A, Gabriel RA, Dutton RP, et al. Growth of nonoperating room anesthesia care in the United States: a contemporary trends analysis. *Anesth Analg.* 2017;124:1261–1267.

2. Boggs SD, Luedi MM. Nonoperating room anesthesia education: Preparing our residents for the future. *Curr Opin Anaesthesiol.* 2019;32:490–497.

3. Chang B, Kaye AD, Diaz JH, et al. Interventional procedures outside of the operating room: results from the National Anesthesia Clinical Outcomes Registry. *J Patient Saf.* 2018;14:9–16.

4. Wax RS, Christian MD. Practical recommendations for critical care and anesthesiology teams caring for novel coronavirus (2019-nCoV) patients. *Can J Anaesth.* 2020;67:568–576.

5. Orme NM, Rihal CS, Gulati R, et al. Occupational health hazards of working in the interventional laboratory: a multisite case control study of physicians and allied staff. *J Am Coll Cardiol.* 2015;65:820–826.

6. Vaes B, Van Keer K, Struelens L, et al. Eye lens dosimetry in anesthesiology: a prospective study. *J Clin Monit Comput.* 2017;31:303–308.

7. Rosado Ingelmo A, Doña Diaz I, Cabañas Moreno R, et al. Clinical Practice Guidelines for Diagnosis and Management of Hypersensitivity Reactions to Contrast Media. *J Investig Allergol Clin Immunol.* 2016;26:144–155.

8. Woolen SA, Shankar PR, Gagnier JJ, et al. Risk of nephrogenic systemic fibrosis in patients with stage 4 or 5 chronic kidney disease receiving a group II gadolinium-based contrast agent: a systematic review and meta-analysis. *JAMA Intern Med.* 2020;180:223–230.

9. Talke P, Dowd CF, CZ Lee. Interventional neuroradiology: anesthetic management*Cottrell and Patel's Neuroanesthesia.* : Elsevier 2016 6th ed..

10. Schönenberger S, Hendén PL, Simonsen CZ, et al. Association of general anesthesia vs procedural sedation with functional outcome among patients with acute ischemic stroke undergoing thrombectomy: a systematic review and meta-analysis. *JAMA.* 2019;322:1283–1293.

11. Businger J, Fort AC, Vlisides PE, et al. Management of acute ischemic stroke-specific focus on anesthetic management for mechanical thrombectomy. *Anesth Analg.* 2020;131:1124–1134.

12. Ghuman M, Tsang ACO, Klostranec JM, et al. Sentinel angiographic signs of cerebral hyperperfusion after angioplasty and stenting of intracranial atherosclerotic stenosis: a technical note. *AJNR Am J Neuroradiol.* 2019;40:1523–1525.

13. Petersen NH, Silverman A, Strander SM, et al. Fixed compared with autoregulation-oriented blood pressure thresholds after mechanical thrombectomy for ischemic stroke. *Stroke.* 2020;51:914–921.

14. Chana A, James M, Veale P. Anaesthesia for transjugular intrahepatic portosystemic shunt insertion. *BJA Educ.* 2016;16:405–409.

15. Bhavani S. Non-operating room anesthesia in the endoscopy unit. *Gastrointest Endosc Clin N Am.* 2016;26:471–483.

16. Smith ZL, Mullady DK, Lang GD, et al. A randomized controlled trial evaluating general endotracheal anesthesia versus monitored anesthesia care and the incidence of sedation-related adverse events during ERCP in high-risk patients. *Gastrointest Endosc.* 2019;89:855–862.

17. Fujii S, Zhou JR, Dhir A. Anesthesia for cardiac ablation. *J Cardiothorac Vasc Anesth.* 2018;32:1892–1910.

18. Mittnacht AJ, Dukkipati S, Mahajan A. Ventricular tachycardia ablation: a comprehensive review for anesthesiologists. *Anesth Analg.* 2015;120:737–748.

19. Lisanby SH. Electroconvulsive therapy for depression. *N Engl J Med.* 2007;357:1939–1945.

20. Bryson EO, Aloysi AS, Farber KG, et al. Individualized anesthetic management for patients undergoing electroconvulsive therapy: a review of current practice. *Anesth Analg.* 2017;124:1943–1956.

21. Soehle M, Bochem J. Anesthesia for electroconvulsive therapy. *Curr Opin Anaesthesiol.* 2018;31:501–505.

IV

THE RECOVERY PERIOD

39 POSTANESTHESIA RECOVERY

Matthias R. Braehler, Ilan Mizrahi

The postanesthesia care unit (PACU) is managed by anesthesiologists, who provide general medical supervision and coordination of patient care. Historically, PACUs did not become a standard part of hospital design until the late 1940s, after an influential study of mortality within 24 hours of anesthesia induction noted a significant number of deaths resulting from inadequate nursing care and respiratory obstruction in the immediate postoperative period. In contemporary practice the PACU serves as the location for patients to safely transition from anesthesia (of any type) to lower levels of care, including the hospital ward or home. The PACU staff must be prepared to identify and manage early complications of anesthesia and surgery, which will be described later. In addition, the PACU can be the site of care for complex, critically ill, mechanically ventilated postoperative patients who require short-term intensive care (also see Chapter 41).

ADMISSION TO THE POSTANESTHESIA CARE UNIT

The PACU is staffed by specially trained nurses skilled in the prompt recognition of postoperative complications. Upon arrival at the PACU, a member of the anesthesia team provides the PACU nurse with an information hand-off including pertinent details of the patient's history, medical condition, anesthesia management, and surgery. The American Society of Anesthesiologists (ASA) Standards for Postanesthesia Care[1] emphasize that particular attention should be directed toward monitoring oxygenation, ventilation, circulation, level of consciousness, and temperature. Although a vital sign frequency is not stated in the ASA Standards for Postanesthesia Care, a common practice is to record them at least every 15 minutes while the patient is in the unit. Vital signs and other pertinent information are recorded as part of the patient's medical record. More specific recommendations regarding evaluation and interventions in the PACU can be found in the ASA Practice Guidelines for Postanesthesia Care.[2]

EARLY POSTOPERATIVE PHYSIOLOGIC CHANGES

Emergence from general anesthesia and surgery may be accompanied by a number of physiologic disturbances that affect multiple organ systems (Box 39.1).

Box 39.1 Physiologic Disorders Manifested in the Postanesthesia Care Unit

Neurologic
Delayed awakening
Emergence agitation
Delirium
Nausea and vomiting
Pain

Respiratory
Upper airway obstruction
Arterial hypoxemia
Hypoventilation

Cardiovascular
Hypotension
Hypertension
Cardiac arrhythmias

Renal
Oliguria

Hematologic
Bleeding
Coagulopathy

Metabolic
Decreased body temperature
Electrolyte and acid–base abnormalities

In a prospective study of more than 18,000 consecutive admissions to the PACU the complication rate was found to be as high as 24%. Nausea and vomiting (10%), the need for upper airway support (7%), and hypotension (3%) were the most common.[3] Despite the significant incidence of nausea and vomiting in the PACU, the most serious adverse outcomes occur with airway/respiratory and cardiovascular compromise. A 2002 analysis of the Australian Incident Monitoring Study (AIMS) database (a voluntary self-report of actual or potential anesthesia incidents) contained over 8000 reports, with approximately 6% occurring in the recovery area. Of these incidents, the most common problems included airway (21%), respiratory (23%), cardiovascular (24%), and drug error (11%).[4] These reports highlight the vulnerability of patients during transport from the operating room to the PACU. Airway obstruction and hypoventilation can be difficult to detect clinically; therefore increased vigilance is required during this phase of care.

UPPER AIRWAY OBSTRUCTION

Loss of Pharyngeal Muscle Tone

The most frequent cause of airway obstruction in the immediate postoperative period is the loss of pharyngeal muscle tone in a sedated or obtunded patient. The persistent effects of inhaled and intravenous (IV) anesthetics, neuromuscular blocking drugs, and opioids all contribute to the loss of pharyngeal tone in this setting.

In an awake patient opening of the upper airway is facilitated by the contraction of the pharyngeal muscles at the same time that negative inspiratory pressure is generated by the diaphragm. As a result, the tongue and soft palate are pulled forward, tenting the airway open during inspiration. This pharyngeal muscle activity is depressed during sleep, and the resulting decrease in tone can promote airway obstruction. A vicious cycle then ensues wherein the collapse of compliant pharyngeal tissue during inspiration produces a reflex compensatory increase in respiratory effort and negative inspiratory pressure that promotes further airway obstruction.

The effort to breathe against an obstructed airway is characterized by a paradoxical breathing pattern consisting of retraction of the sternal notch and exaggerated abdominal muscle activity. Collapse of the chest wall and protrusion of the abdomen with inspiratory effort produce a rocking motion that becomes more prominent with increasing airway obstruction. Obstruction secondary to loss of pharyngeal tone can be relieved by simply opening the airway with the "jaw thrust maneuver" or continuous positive airway pressure (CPAP) applied via a facemask (or both). Support of the airway is needed until the patient has adequately recovered from the effects of drugs administered during anesthesia. If the airway obstruction cannot be overcome by the afore-mentioned approach, placement of an oropharyngeal or nasopharyngeal airway, a supraglottic airway device, or an endotracheal tube (ETT) may be required.

Residual Neuromuscular Blockade

Postoperative residual neuromuscular blockade is very common, with reported incidences between 20% and 40%.[5] A 2015 study even found that 56% of patients (the majority of whom received neostigmine for neuromuscular blockade reversal) had residual neuromuscular blockade upon arrival in the PACU.[6] When evaluating upper airway obstruction in the PACU, the possibility of residual neuromuscular blockade should be considered in any patient who received neuromuscular blocking drugs during anesthesia. Residual neuromuscular blockade may not be evident upon arrival in the PACU because the diaphragm recovers from neuromuscular blockade before the pharyngeal muscles do. With an ETT in place, end-tidal carbon dioxide concentrations and tidal volumes may indicate adequate ventilation while the ability to maintain a patent upper airway and clear upper airway secretions remains compromised. The stimulation associated with tracheal extubation, followed by the activity of patient transfer to the gurney and subsequent encouragement to breathe deeply, may keep the airway open during transport to the PACU. Only after the patient is calmly resting in the PACU does upper airway obstruction become evident. Even patients treated with intermediate- and short-acting neuromuscular blocking drugs may manifest residual paralysis in the PACU despite what was deemed clinically adequate pharmacologic reversal in the operating room.

The recovery from neuromuscular blockade and the assessment of residual blockade can be done by clinical assessment and by using a nerve stimulator (also see Chapter 11). Measurement of the train-of-four (TOF) ratio is a subjective assessment that is often misleading when done by touch or observation alone. The use of quantitative TOF measurement is the most reliable indicator of adequate reversal. Significant signs and symptoms of clinical weakness persist up to a ratio of 0.7, whereas pharyngeal function is not restored to normal until an adductor pollicis TOF ratio is greater than 0.9.

Qualitative TOF measurement and 5-second sustained tetanus at 50 Hz are insensitive and will not detect residual paralysis. In an awake patient clinical assessment of reversal of neuromuscular blockade is preferred to the application of painful TOF or tetanic stimulation. Clinical evaluation includes grip strength, tongue protrusion, ability to lift the legs off the bed, and the ability to lift the head off the bed for a full 5 seconds. Of these maneuvers, the 5-second sustained head lift has been considered to be the standard, reflecting not only generalized motor strength but, more importantly, the patient's ability to maintain and protect the airway. However, studies have shown that the 5-second head lift is remarkably insensitive and should not routinely be used to assess recovery from neuromuscular blockade. The ability to strongly oppose the incisor teeth against a tongue depressor is a more reliable indicator of pharyngeal muscle tone. This maneuver correlates with an average TOF ratio of 0.85.

When a PACU patient demonstrates signs and/or symptoms of muscular weakness in the form of respiratory distress and/or agitation, one must suspect that there could be residual neuromuscular blockade, and prompt review of possible etiologic factors is indicated (Box 39.2). Common factors include respiratory acidosis and hypothermia, alone or in combination. Upper airway obstruction as a result of the residual depressant effects of volatile anesthetics or opioids (or both) may result in progressive respiratory acidosis after the patient is admitted to the PACU and external stimulation is minimized.

Box 39.2 Causes of Prolonged Neuromuscular Blockade (also see Chapter 11)

Factors Contributing to Prolonged Nondepolarizing Neuromuscular Blockade
Drugs
  Inhaled anesthetic drugs
  Local anesthetics (lidocaine)
  Cardiac antiarrhythmics (procainamide)
  Antibiotics (polymyxins, aminoglycosides, lincosamides, metronidazole, tetracyclines)
  Corticosteroids
  Calcium channel blockers
  Dantrolene
  Furosemide
Metabolic and physiologic states
  Hypermagnesemia
  Hypocalcemia
  Hypothermia
  Respiratory acidosis
  Hepatic/renal failure
  Myasthenia syndromes

Factors Contributing to Prolonged Depolarizing Neuromuscular Blockade
Excessive dose of succinylcholine
Reduced plasma cholinesterase activity
  Decreased levels
  Extremes of age (newborn, old age)
  Disease states (hepatic disease, uremia, malnutrition, plasmapheresis)
  Hormonal changes
  Pregnancy
  Contraceptives
  Glucocorticoids
Inhibited activity
  Irreversible (echothiophate)
  Reversible (edrophonium, neostigmine, pyridostigmine)
Genetic variant (atypical plasma cholinesterase)

Simple measures such as warming the patient, airway support, and correction of electrolyte abnormalities can facilitate recovery from neuromuscular blockade.

A 2016 study of one institution's surgical database found that patients who had received neuromuscular blocking drugs but did not receive reversal agents had a 2.3 times greater risk of developing postoperative pneumonia compared with those who did receive reversal agents.[7] The introduction of sugammadex may have a major impact on residual paralysis in patients who received aminosteroid neuromuscular blocking drugs. Although reversal with neostigmine requires a baseline twitch response and the time until the patient has a TOF ratio of ≥0.9 is highly variable, sugammadex can be administered at any depth of neuromuscular blockade and most commonly produces full recovery (TOF ratio ≥0.9) within several minutes after administration (also see Chapter 11). The increased availability and use of sugammadex as an alternative to neostigmine will result in a decreased incidence of residual neuromuscular blockade in the PACU. Indeed, a 2020 study comparing sugammadex with neostigmine for neuromuscular blockade reversal confirmed that the risk of postoperative pneumonia, respiratory failure, and other major complications is significantly lower with sugammadex.[8]

Laryngospasm

Laryngospasm refers to a sudden spasm of the vocal cords that completely occludes the laryngeal opening via forceful contractions of the laryngeal muscles. It typically occurs in the transitional period when the extubated patient is emerging from general anesthesia. Although laryngospasm is most likely to occur in the operating room at the time of extubation, patients who arrive in the PACU asleep after general anesthesia are also at risk for laryngospasm upon awakening, triggered by airway irritants such as secretions or blood. Treatment of laryngospasm involves suctioning to remove the stimulus and applying a jaw thrust with CPAP (up to 40 cm H_2O) to *break* the laryngospasm. However, if this fails, immediate skeletal muscle relaxation can be achieved with succinylcholine (0.1 to 1 mg/kg intravenously or 4 mg/kg intramuscularly [IM]). If laryngospasm persists, one should proceed with emergent intubation with a full dose of an induction agent and intubating dose of a muscle relaxant. Because of the risk of causing glottic injury, the anesthesia provider should not attempt to forcibly pass an ETT through a glottis that is closed because of laryngospasm.

Airway Edema or Hematoma

Airway edema is a possible complication of prolonged procedures in the prone or Trendelenburg position, procedures involving the airway and neck (including thyroidectomy, carotid endarterectomy, and cervical spine procedures), and those with large-volume resuscitation. Although facial and scleral edema is an important physical sign that can alert the clinician to the presence of airway edema, visible external signs may not accompany significant edema of pharyngeal tissue. Patients who had a difficult intubation or repeated airway instrumentation may also have increased airway edema. If extubation is to be attempted in these patients in the PACU, evaluation of airway patency must precede removal of the ETT. This is commonly done with a leak test.[9] The patient's ability to breathe around the ETT can be evaluated by suctioning the oral pharynx and deflating the ETT cuff. With occlusion of the proximal end of the ETT, the patient is then asked to breathe around the tube. Satisfactory air movement suggests that the patient's airway will remain patent after tracheal extubation. An alternative method measures the intrathoracic pressure required to produce a leak around the ETT with the cuff deflated. Lastly, when ventilating patients in the volume control mode, one can measure the exhaled tidal volume before and after cuff deflation. The presence of a cuff leak demonstrates the likelihood of successful extubation, but is not a guarantee, just as a failed cuff leak does not rule out a successful extubation. The cuff leak test should not take the place of sound clinical judgment when deciding to safely extubate the patient. If concern for airway compromise is significant, the patient can be extubated with a tracheal tube exchange catheter left in place as a conduit to reintroduce an ETT.

If airway edema is deemed significant enough to preclude extubation, the following measures can facilitate resolution of edema: (1) sitting the patient upright to ensure venous drainage and reduce any component of dependent edema, (2) diuretic administration; and (3) IV dexamethasone to decrease airway swelling.

External airway compression is most often caused by hematomas after thyroid, parathyroid, or carotid surgeries. Patients may complain of pain and/or pressure and dysphagia and can demonstrate signs of respiratory distress. Mask ventilation may not be possible in a patient with a large hematoma. An attempt can be made to decompress the airway by releasing the clips or sutures on the wound and evacuating the hematoma. If emergency tracheal intubation is required, then difficult airway equipment and surgical backup to perform an emergency tracheostomy are crucial; one should assume increased difficulty secondary to laryngeal and airway edema and possible tracheal deviation or compression. If the patient is able to spontaneously ventilate, then awake intubation is preferred because visualization of the vocal cords by direct laryngoscopy may not be possible.

Obstructive Sleep Apnea (also see Chapter 48)

Obstructive sleep apnea (OSA) is an often-overlooked cause of airway obstruction in the PACU, given that the vast majority of patients are undiagnosed at the time of surgery. Patients with OSA have more frequent cardiopulmonary complications and need for intensive care unit (ICU) transfer.[10]

Patients with OSA are particularly prone to airway obstruction and should not be extubated until they are fully awake and following commands. Once in the PACU, a patient with OSA is exquisitely sensitive to opioids, and, when possible, continuous regional anesthesia and multimodal opioid-sparing analgesic (acetaminophen, nonsteroidal anti-inflammatory drugs [NSAIDs], dexmedetomidine) techniques should be used[11] (also see Chapter 40). Benzodiazepines can have a greater effect on pharyngeal muscle tone than opioids, and the use of benzodiazepines in the perioperative setting can significantly contribute to airway obstruction in the PACU.

When caring for a patient with OSA, plans should be made preoperatively to provide CPAP in the immediate postoperative period. Patients should be asked to bring their own CPAP machines with them on the day of surgery to enable the equipment to be set up before the patient's arrival in the PACU.[12,13] Patients who do not routinely use CPAP at home or who do not have their machines with them may require additional attention from the respiratory therapist to ensure proper fit of the CPAP delivery device (mask or nasal airways) and to determine the amount of positive pressure needed to prevent upper airway obstruction. Patients with known or suspected OSA should have continuous pulse oximetry monitoring in the postoperative period.

DIFFERENTIAL DIAGNOSIS OF ARTERIAL HYPOXEMIA IN THE PACU (ALSO SEE CHAPTER 5)

Atelectasis and alveolar hypoventilation are the most common causes of transient postoperative arterial hypoxemia in the immediate postoperative period. Clinical correlation should guide the workup of a postoperative patient who remains persistently hypoxemic. Review of the patient's history, operative course, and clinical signs and symptoms will direct the workup to rule in possible causes (Box 39.3).

Alveolar Hypoventilation

Review of the alveolar gas equation demonstrates that hypoventilation alone is sufficient to cause hypoxemia in a patient breathing room air (Box 39.4). At sea level, a normocapnic patient breathing room air will have an alveolar oxygen pressure (P_{AO_2}) of 100 mm Hg. Thus a healthy patient without a significant alveolar-arterial gradient will have a Pa_{O_2} near 100 mm Hg. In the same patient an increase in Pa_{CO_2} from 40 to 80 mm Hg (from alveolar hypoventilation) results in a P_{AO_2} of 50 mm Hg. Hence, even a patient with normal lungs will become

---

Box 39.3 Factors Contributing to Postoperative Arterial Hypoxemia by Mechanism of Hypoxemia

Right-to-Left Intrapulmonary Shunt or Ventilation-Perfusion Mismatch
Atelectasis (with decreased functional residual capacity, e.g., postsurgical or from obesity)
Pulmonary edema (e.g., from fluid overload, postobstructive edema, transfusion-related lung injury, acute respiratory distress syndrome)
Aspiration of gastric contents
Pneumothorax
Pulmonary embolus (can also cause reduced cardiac output)

Alveolar Hypoventilation
Residual effects of anesthetics and/or neuromuscular blocking drugs

Venous Admixture
Reduced cardiac output
Congestive heart failure

Diffusion Hypoxia
From nitrous oxide administration (though unlikely if patient receiving supplemental oxygen)

Increased Oxygen Consumption
Shivering

Decreased Oxygen Delivery
Unrecognized disconnection of oxygen source
Empty oxygen tank

Box 39.4 Hypoventilation as a Cause of Arterial Hypoxemia

$$P_{AO_2} = F_{IO_2}(PB - PH_2O) - \frac{Pa_{CO_2}}{RQ}$$

Pa_{CO_2} = 40 mm Hg

$$P_{AO_2} = 0.21(760 - 47) - \frac{40}{0.8} = 150 - 50 = 100 \ mm \ Hg$$

Pa_{CO_2} = 80 mm Hg

$$P_{AO_2} = 0.21(760 - 47) - \frac{80}{0.8} = 150 - 100 = 50 \ mm \ Hg$$

FIO_2, Fraction of inspired oxygen concentration; P_{AO_2}, alveolar oxygen pressure; PB, barometric pressure; PH_2O, vapor pressure of water; RQ, respiratory quotient.

---

hypoxemic if significant hypoventilation occurs while breathing room air.

Arterial hypoxemia secondary to hypercapnia can be reversed by administering supplemental oxygen or by normalizing the patient's Pa_{CO_2} by external stimulation to awaken the patient, pharmacologic reversal of opioid or benzodiazepine effect, or controlled mechanical ventilation.

Decreased Alveolar Partial Pressure of Oxygen

Diffusion hypoxia refers to the rapid diffusion of nitrous oxide into alveoli at the end of a nitrous oxide anesthetic (also see Chapter 7). Nitrous oxide dilutes the alveolar gas and produces a transient decrease in P_{AO_2} and P_{ACO_2}. In a patient breathing room air the resulting decrease in P_{AO_2} can produce arterial hypoxemia, whereas a decreased P_{ACO_2} can depress the respiratory drive. In the absence of supplemental oxygen administration diffusion hypoxia can persist for 5 to 10 minutes after discontinuation of a nitrous oxide anesthetic; therefore it may contribute to arterial hypoxemia in the initial minutes in the PACU.

Ventilation-Perfusion Mismatch and Shunt

Hypoxic pulmonary vasoconstriction refers to the attempt of normal lungs to optimally match ventilation and perfusion (also see Chapter 5). This response constricts vessels in poorly ventilated regions of the lung and directs pulmonary blood flow to well-ventilated alveoli. In the PACU the residual effects of inhaled anesthetics and vasodilators, such as nitroprusside and dobutamine, will blunt hypoxic pulmonary vasoconstriction and contribute to arterial hypoxemia.

Unlike ventilation-perfusion mismatch, a true shunt will not respond to supplemental oxygen. Causes of postoperative pulmonary shunt include atelectasis, pulmonary edema, gastric aspiration, pulmonary emboli, and pneumonia. Of these, atelectasis is probably the most common cause of pulmonary shunting in the immediate postoperative period. Mobilization of the patient to the sitting position, incentive spirometry, and positive airway pressure by facemask can be effective in treating atelectasis.

Increased Venous Admixture

Increased venous admixture typically refers to low cardiac output states. It is caused by the mixing of desaturated venous blood with oxygenated arterial blood. Normally, only 2% to 5% of cardiac output is shunted through the lungs, and this shunted blood with a normal mixed venous saturation has a minimal effect on PaO_2. In low cardiac output states blood returns to the heart severely desaturated. Additionally, the shunt fraction increases significantly in conditions that impede alveolar oxygenation, such as pulmonary edema and atelectasis. Under these conditions, mixing of desaturated shunted blood with saturated arterialized blood decreases PaO_2.

Decreased Diffusion Capacity

A decreased diffusion capacity may reflect the presence of underlying lung disease such as emphysema, interstitial lung disease, pulmonary fibrosis, or primary pulmonary hypertension. In this regard the differential diagnosis of arterial hypoxemia in the PACU must include the contribution of any preexisting pulmonary condition.

PULMONARY EDEMA IN THE PACU

Pulmonary edema in the immediate postoperative period is often cardiogenic in nature, secondary to intravascular volume overload or congestive heart failure. Other causes of noncardiogenic pulmonary edema include postobstructive pulmonary edema (secondary to airway obstruction), sepsis with acute respiratory distress syndrome, or transfusion-related acute lung injury (TRALI) (also see Chapter 41).

Postobstructive Pulmonary Edema

Postobstructive pulmonary edema (also referred to as *negative pressure pulmonary edema, NPPE*) is a rare, but significant, consequence of laryngospasm (or, less commonly, other upper airway obstruction) that may follow extubation. The etiology of NPPE is multifactorial but is clearly correlated with the generation of exaggerated negative intrathoracic pressure during inspiration against a closed glottis. The resulting negative intrathoracic pressure augments venous return, which in turn increases pulmonary hydrostatic pressures, promoting the movement of fluid into the interstitial and alveolar spaces from the pulmonary capillaries. Patients who are muscular are at increased risk of postobstructive pulmonary edema secondary to their ability to generate significant inspiratory force.

The resulting arterial hypoxemia develops quickly (usually within 90 minutes of the upper airway obstruction) and is accompanied by dyspnea, pink frothy sputum, and bilateral fluffy infiltrates on the chest radiograph. Treatment is generally supportive and includes supplemental oxygen, diuresis, and, in severe cases initiation of positive-pressure ventilation. These patients should be monitored for 2 to 12 hours postoperatively. When recognized and treated immediately, NPPE typically resolves within 12 to 48 hours; however, if diagnosis and therapy are delayed, mortality rates can reach 40%. Although uncommon, pulmonary hemorrhage and hemoptysis have been observed.[14]

Transfusion-Related Acute Lung Injury

The differential diagnosis of pulmonary edema in the PACU should include TRALI in any patient who intraoperatively received blood products. TRALI usually manifests within 2 to 4 hours after the transfusion of plasma-containing blood products, including packed red blood cells, whole blood, fresh frozen plasma, or platelets. TRALI occurs when recipient neutrophils become activated by donor plasma and then release inflammatory mediators, which cause increased pulmonary vascular permeability resulting in pulmonary edema. Clinical manifestations include fever, pulmonary infiltrates on chest radiograph, cyanosis, and systemic hypotension. The sudden onset of hypoxemic respiratory failure can occur up to 6 hours after the conclusion of the transfusion, and TRALI may first present when the patient is in the PACU.[15]

Treatment is supportive and includes supplemental oxygen and diuresis. Approximately 80% of patients will recover within 48 to 96 hours.[16] Mechanical ventilation may be needed to support hypoxemia and respiratory failure, and vasopressors may be required to treat refractory hypotension.

MONITORING AND TREATMENT OF HYPOXEMIA

Oxygen Supplementation

In the era of cost containment one could argue that the routine delivery of supplemental oxygen to all patients recovering from general anesthesia is a costly and unnecessary practice. The argument against the use of routine oxygen supplementation relies on the fact that continuous pulse oximetry, now a PACU standard, readily identifies those patients who will require oxygen therapy. Moreover, the majority of patients after general anesthesia do not develop hypoxemia. However, a significant percentage of patients will become hypoxemic at some point during their PACU stay. Thus the safe practice of postanesthesia care without oxygen supplementation requires ideal conditions at all times—functioning oxygen delivery apparatus at every bedside and sufficient personnel for observation and immediate intervention. The degree of vigilance is likely unrealistic, and the risk of adverse outcome to even a small number of patients is unwarranted.

Limitations of Pulse Oximetry

The ASA Standards for Postanesthesia Care require a quantitative method of assessing oxygenation such as pulse oximetry. However, pulse oximetry does not reflect the adequacy of ventilation, especially in patients receiving supplemental oxygen. When monitoring ventilation in the PACU, pulse oximetry is not a substitute for close observation by trained personnel.

Oxygen Delivery Systems (also see Chapter 41)

The degree of hypoxemia, the surgical procedure, and patient compliance determine the oxygen delivery system of choice in the PACU. Regardless of the delivery system, oxygen should be humidified in order to prevent the subsequent dehydration of the nasal and/or oral mucosa. Patients who have undergone head and neck surgery

may not be candidates for facemask oxygen because of the risk of pressure necrosis on incision sites and microvascular muscle flaps, whereas nasal packing prohibits the use of nasal cannulas after other procedures. Face tent oxygen or blow-by setups are viable alternatives in cases in which tight-fitting masks and straps are contraindicated.

The delivery of oxygen through a traditional nasal cannula with bubble humidifier is usually limited to a maximum flow of 6 L/min to minimize the discomfort and complications that result from inadequate humidification. As a general rule, each liter per minute of oxygen flow through nasal cannula increases the FiO_2 by 0.04, with 6 L/min delivering an FiO_2 of approximately 0.44.

Simple facemasks are generally used in the postoperative setting in patients who are breathing spontaneously yet require a higher oxygen concentration to maintain their oxygen saturation. Oxygen flow rates should be at least 5 L/min in order to prevent rebreathing of exhaled CO_2.

Maximum oxygen delivery to extubated patients traditionally required delivery by facemask through a nonrebreather system or high-flow nebulizer. However, these systems can be inefficient, and inadequate mask fit and/or high-minute ventilation requirements can result in significant entrainment of room air. Newer high-flow nasal cannula (HFNC) devices can comfortably deliver oxygen at 60 L/min, 37°C, and 99.9% relative humidity. The delivery of high-flow oxygen directly to the nasopharynx produces an FiO_2 equal to that delivered by traditional mask devices. The efficacy of these devices may be enhanced by a CPAP effect resulting from the high gas flow.[17] A 2017 metaanalysis evaluated the use of HFNC (or noninvasive ventilation) compared with conventional oxygen therapy in ICU or emergency department patients with hypoxemic respiratory failure. In this population HFNC reduced the need for intubation and mechanical ventilation compared with conventional oxygen therapy but was equivalent to noninvasive ventilation for preventing these outcomes.[18]

Continuous Positive Airway Pressure

As discussed earlier, respiratory failure in the immediate postoperative period is often the result of transient and rapidly reversible conditions such as splinting from pain, diaphragmatic dysfunction, muscular weakness, and pharmacologically depressed respiratory drive. Readily reversible hypoxemia may be caused by hypoventilation, atelectasis, or volume overload. The application of CPAP can decrease hypoxemia resulting from atelectasis by recruiting alveoli and can reduce work of breathing.[19]

One surgical population at increased risk of postoperative pulmonary complications is patients undergoing major abdominal surgery. A 2014 Cochrane review of postoperative CPAP in this setting provided very low-quality evidence that CPAP may reduce atelectasis,

V

pneumonia, and reintubation, with uncertain effects on hypoxemia, need for invasive ventilation, or mortality.[20] Many patients with obesity undergoing gastric bypass surgery have OSA and would benefit significantly from postoperative CPAP therapy. Yet surgeons may be hesitant to embrace this modality for fear that applying positive pressure to the airway would inflate the stomach and proximal intestine and result in anastomotic disruption.

Noninvasive Positive-Pressure Ventilation

Even with the application of CPAP in the PACU, a number of patients will require additional ventilatory support. Noninvasive positive-pressure ventilation (NIPPV) can be an effective alternative to endotracheal intubation in the ICU setting (also see Chapter 41). Although the use of NIPPV for patients with specific causes of acute or chronic respiratory failure is well established, its application in the PACU is more limited.

Careful consideration of both patient and surgical factors must guide the decision to use noninvasive modes of ventilation in the PACU. Relative contraindications include hemodynamic instability or life-threatening arrhythmias, altered mental status, high risk of aspiration, inability to use nasal or facial mask (e.g., for head and neck procedures), and refractory hypoxemia.[21]

NIPPV can be delivered by facemask using the pressure support mode of a mechanical ventilator. Alternatively, the use of a biphasic positive airway pressure machine allows the delivery of positive pressure with nasal pillows, nasal mask, or facemask.

NIPPV should be considered postoperatively in patients with OSA, chronic obstructive pulmonary disease (COPD), and cardiogenic pulmonary edema. In the immediate postoperative period using PPV or HFNC in patients with hypoxemia after extubation (or risk factors for worsening hypoxemia) may help prevent acute respiratory failure and the need for reintubation.[22]

HEMODYNAMIC INSTABILITY

Hemodynamic compromise in the PACU patient can manifest in a number of ways—systemic hypertension, hypotension, tachycardia, or bradycardia—alone or in combination. Hemodynamic instability in the PACU has a negative impact on long-term outcome. Interestingly, postoperative systemic hypertension and tachycardia are associated with an increased risk of unplanned critical care admission and a higher mortality than hypotension and bradycardia.

Systemic Hypertension

Patients with a history of essential hypertension are at greatest risk for significant systemic hypertension in the PACU, especially if they did not take their morning antihypertensive medications. Additional factors are listed in Box 39.5. The surgical procedures most commonly associated with postoperative hypertension include carotid endarterectomy and intracranial procedures.

Systemic Hypotension

Postoperative hypotension can be attributed to the following mechanisms: (1) hypovolemic (decreased preload), (2) distributive (decreased systemic vascular resistance), (3) cardiogenic (intrinsic pump failure), and/or (4) extracardiac/obstructive (Box 39.6). Prolonged hypotension of any cause can lead to shock, a state of circulatory failure characterized by cellular or tissue hypoxia and vital organ dysfunction (also see Chapter 41).

The underlying cause of hypotension and/or shock must be identified and treated. Fluids, blood products, and vasopressors can be used as needed to restore intravascular volume and support organ perfusion while the patient is being assessed or undergoing a subsequent therapeutic procedure.

Hypovolemic Shock

Systemic hypotension in the PACU is often the result of decreased intravascular volume and preload and, as such, responds favorably to IV fluids. Common causes of decreased intravascular volume in the immediate postoperative period include ongoing third-space translocation or loss of fluid, inadequate intraoperative fluid

---

Box 39.5 Factors Leading to Postoperative Hypertension

Cardiovascular
Preoperative hypertension
Hypervolemia

Respiratory
Arterial hypoxemia
Hypercapnia

Neurologic
Pain
Emergence agitation
Shivering
Nausea/vomiting
Increased intracranial pressure
Increased sympathetic nervous system activity

Drug-related
Withdrawal from β-blocker, clonidine
Withdrawal from opioids, benzodiazepines
Alcohol withdrawal
Substance use (e.g., cocaine, methamphetamine, phencyclidine)

Gastrointestinal/genitourinary
Bowel distention
Urinary retention

replacement, and loss of sympathetic nervous system tone as a result of neuraxial blockade.

Patients in hypovolemic shock often have typical clinical signs, including tachycardia, tachypnea, mottled skin, and decreased urine output.

Ongoing bleeding and hemorrhagic shock should be ruled out in patients who have undergone a surgical procedure in which significant blood loss was possible. Tachycardia may not be a reliable indicator of hypovolemia or anemia if the patient is taking β-blockers or calcium channel blockers. Regardless of the estimated intraoperative blood loss, if the patient is unstable, then point-of-care hemoglobin can be measured at the bedside to eliminate laboratory turnover time.

Distributive Shock

Iatrogenic sympathectomy secondary to regional or neuraxial anesthetic techniques is an important cause of hypotension in the perioperative period. A high sympathetic block (to T4) will decrease vascular tone and block the cardioaccelerator fibers. If not treated promptly, the resulting bradycardia in the presence of severe hypotension can lead to cardiac arrest even in young healthy patients. Vasopressors, including phenylephrine and ephedrine, are pharmacologic treatments of hypotension caused by sympathetic nervous system blockade.

Patients who are critically ill may rely on increased sympathetic tone to maintain systemic blood pressure and heart rate. In these patients even minimal doses of inhaled anesthetics, opioids, or sedative-hypnotics can decrease sympathetic nervous system tone and produce significant systemic hypotension.

Allergic (anaphylactic) reactions may be the cause of hypotension in the PACU (also see Chapter 45). In addition to profound hypotension, patients experiencing an allergic reaction often present with associated rash/hives, bronchospasm/wheezing, stridor, and facial edema. Patients should be treated immediately, with prompt removal of the offending agent, steroids, H1 and H2 blockers, fluids, and vasopressors. Epinephrine is the drug of choice to treat hypotension secondary to an allergic reaction. Increased serum tryptase concentration can confirm the occurrence of an allergic reaction. However, the blood specimen for tryptase determination must be obtained within 30 to 120 minutes after the allergic reaction, and the results are not typically available for several days. Neuromuscular blocking drugs are the most common cause of anaphylactic reactions in the surgical setting, followed by natural rubber latex, antibiotics, and others.[23]

If sepsis is suspected as the cause of hypotension in the PACU, blood cultures should be obtained, and empiric antibiotic therapy initiated as soon as possible. Urinary tract manipulation and biliary tract procedures can result in a sudden onset of severe systemic hypotension secondary to sepsis. Although fluid resuscitation is the most important immediate intervention, vasopressor support is often required. Norepinephrine is the pressor of choice in septic patients (also see Chapter 41).

Cardiogenic Shock

Significant cardiogenic causes of postoperative hypotension include myocardial ischemia and infarction, cardiomyopathy, and cardiac arrhythmias. Myocardial ischemia and cardiac arrhythmias are discussed separately in the next section of this chapter. The differential diagnosis of cardiogenic shock depends on the surgical procedure and the patient's preoperative cardiac risk and medical condition. To determine the cause of hypotension, central venous pressure monitoring, echocardiography, and, rarely, pulmonary artery catheter monitoring may be required. The mortality rate for those in cardiogenic shock is remarkably high, reaching up to 70%. Patients may require immediate postoperative placement of an intraaortic balloon pump (IABP), cardiac catheterization and stenting, echocardiography, or a surgical procedure for a mechanical/valvular abnormality.

The potential for local anesthetic toxicity must be considered when assessing perioperative hypotension. For example, a patient may have received local or regional anesthetic at the end of surgery immediately before PACU transfer. Central nervous system signs (including tinnitus, confusion, altered mental status, and ultimately seizures) may not always precede cardiovascular collapse. Once recognized, supportive therapy should be immediately provided to support cardiovascular function. Twenty percent lipid emulsion therapy should be initiated—bolus 1.5 cc/kg IV over 2 to 3 minutes followed by a continuous rate of 0.25 cc/kg per minute. Repeated boluses can be given every 5 minutes if cardiovascular collapse continues[24] (also see Chapter 10).

Extracardiac/Obstructive Shock

Impaired diastolic filling, which ultimately results in decreased preload, can lead to shock if not promptly recognized and treated. Inferior vena cava (IVC) compression, tension pneumothorax, cardiac tamponade, constrictive pericarditis, and excessive positive end-expiratory pressure (PEEP) can lead to diminished filling and compromised venous return. Intrathoracic tumor and tension pneumothorax typically present similarly to hypovolemic shock—tachycardia and hypotension, possibly with associated distended neck veins.

Patients may need to undergo emergent needle thoracostomy and chest tube placement for a tension pneumothorax, a pericardiocentesis for tamponade, or thrombolysis/embolectomy for a pulmonary embolism. Point-of-care ultrasound can be very helpful in both the diagnosis and management of these conditions (also see Chapter 21).

Myocardial Ischemia

Detection of myocardial ischemia in the PACU can be challenging because of the patient's inability to identify or communicate symptoms related to cardiac ischemia. In one study of patients over 45 years of age undergoing noncardiac surgery only 35% of patients with postoperative myocardial infarction complained of typical chest pain.[25] The ASA Practice Guidelines for Postanesthesia Care discuss routine pulse, blood pressure, and electrocardiographic monitoring during emergence and recovery.[2] Although there are certain categories of patients or procedures for whom routine electrocardiographic monitoring may not be necessary, there was agreement that these monitoring modalities can detect cardiovascular complications and reduce adverse outcomes.

Low-Risk Patients

ST-segment changes on the electrocardiogram (ECG) in the PACU should be interpreted in light of the patient's cardiac history and risk index. In low-risk patients (<45 years of age, no known cardiac disease, only one risk factor), postoperative ST-segment changes on the ECG do not usually indicate myocardial ischemia. Relatively benign causes of ST-segment changes in these low-risk patients include anxiety, esophageal reflux, hyperventilation, and hypokalemia. In general, low-risk patients require only routine PACU observation unless associated signs and symptoms warrant further clinical evaluation. A more aggressive evaluation is indicated if the changes are accompanied by cardiac rhythm disturbances, hemodynamic instability, angina, or associated symptoms.

High-Risk Patients

In contrast to low-risk patients, ST-segment and T-wave changes on the ECG in high-risk patients can be significant even in the absence of typical signs or symptoms of myocardial ischemia. In this patient population any ST-segment, T-wave, or rhythm changes that are compatible with myocardial ischemia should prompt further evaluation to rule out myocardial ischemia. Determination of serum troponin levels is indicated when myocardial ischemia or infarction is suspected in the PACU. Once blood samples for measurement of troponin and a 12-lead ECG are completed, arrangements must be made for the appropriate cardiology follow-up.

Even small increases of troponin in the postoperative period are associated with an increased short- and long-term mortality rate, and there is currently no defined management strategy for these patients.[26-29] As a result, current American Heart Association/American College of Cardiology (AHA/ACC) guidelines cite insufficient evidence regarding routine postoperative 12-lead ECG or troponin measurements in patients at high risk for perioperative myocardial ischemia but without ongoing signs or symptoms. These guidelines recommend against routine screening of an unselected patient population using troponin measurements.[30]

Cardiac Arrhythmias

Perioperative cardiac arrhythmias are frequently transient and multifactorial in cause. Box 39.7 lists several factors that may increase a patient's risk of arrhythmia. Appropriate diagnosis and treatment of these conditions are often necessary to restore baseline cardiac rhythm and maintain hemodynamic stability.

Tachyarrhythmias

Sinus tachycardia is the most common tachyarrhythmia in the PACU. Although all the causes in Box 39.7 may contribute to sinus tachycardia, the most common in the PACU include postoperative pain, agitation, hypoventilation, hypovolemia, shivering, and stimulation of the ETT in an intubated patient.

The incidence of new postoperative atrial arrhythmias may be as high as 10% after major noncardiothoracic surgery. The incidence is even higher after cardiac and thoracic procedures when the cardiac arrhythmia is often attributed to atrial irritation. These new-onset atrial arrhythmias are not benign because they are associated

---

Box 39.7 Factors Leading to Postoperative Cardiac Arrhythmias

Cardiovascular
Preoperative cardiac arrhythmias
Myocardial ischemia
Hypertension
Intravascular volume shifts

Respiratory
Hypoxemia
Hypercarbia (respiratory acidosis)

Neurologic
Pain
Agitation
Substance withdrawal

Metabolic
Hypothermia
Hyperthermia
Electrolyte abnormalities
Anemia

Medication-Related
Anticholinesterases
Anticholinergics
Vasopressors (especially catecholamines)
Digitalis intoxication

---

with a longer hospital stay and increased mortality rate.[31]

For a patient with new-onset atrial fibrillation, control of the ventricular response rate is the immediate goal. Hemodynamically unstable patients may require prompt electrical cardioversion, but most patients can be treated pharmacologically with an IV β-blocker or calcium channel blocker.[32] Ventricular rate control with these drugs will often facilitate restoration of sinus rhythm in the postoperative patient whose arrhythmia may be catecholamine driven. If the goal of therapy is chemical cardioversion, an amiodarone infusion can be initiated in the PACU.

In the PACU setting premature ventricular contractions (PVCs) and ventricular bigeminy are common. PVCs often reflect increased sympathetic nervous system stimulation, which may occur around tracheal extubation and with transient hypercapnia. True ventricular tachycardia generally reflects the presence of underlying cardiac disease. For patients with polymorphic ventricular tachycardia from torsades de pointes, QT-interval prolongation on the ECG may be intrinsic or drug related (e.g., from amiodarone, procainamide, methadone, haloperidol, or droperidol).

Bradyarrhythmias

Bradycardia in the PACU is often iatrogenic. Drug-related causes include β-adrenergic blocker therapy, neostigmine reversal of neuromuscular blockade, opioid administration, and treatment with dexmedetomidine. Procedure- and patient-related causes include bowel distention, increased intracranial or intraocular pressure, and spinal anesthesia. A high spinal block of cardioaccelerator fibers originating from T1 through T4 can produce severe bradycardia. The resulting sympathectomy, and possible intravascular volume depletion and associated decreased venous return, can result in sudden cardiac arrest, even in young healthy patients.

Treatment

The urgency of treatment of a cardiac arrhythmia depends on the physiologic consequences (principally systemic hypotension and myocardial ischemia). Tachyarrhythmia decreases diastolic and coronary perfusion time and increases myocardial oxygen consumption. Its impact depends on the patient's underlying cardiac function, and it is most harmful in patients with coronary artery disease. Bradycardia is more deleterious in patients with a fixed stroke volume, such as infants and patients with restrictive pericardial disease or cardiac tamponade. The specific management of both bradyarrhythmias and tachyarrhythmias is described further in the AHA Guidelines Update for Cardiopulmonary Resuscitation and Emergency Cardiovascular Care 2020[32] (also see Chapter 45).

RENAL DYSFUNCTION

The differential diagnosis of postoperative renal dysfunction includes prerenal, intrarenal, and postrenal etiologies (Box 39.8). Frequently, the cause of renal insufficiency in the postoperative periods is multifactorial,

---

Box 39.8 Postoperative Renal Dysfunction

Prerenal
Hypovolemia (bleeding, sepsis, third-space fluid loss, inadequate volume resuscitation)
Hepatorenal syndrome
Low cardiac output
Renal vascular obstruction or disruption
Intraabdominal hypertension

Renal
Ischemia (acute tubular necrosis)
Radiographic contrast dyes
Rhabdomyolysis
Tumor lysis
Hemolysis

Postrenal
Surgical injury to the ureters
Obstruction of the ureters with clots or stones
Mechanical (urinary catheter obstruction or malposition)

V

with an intraoperative insult exacerbating preexisting renal insufficiency.[33] In the PACU diagnostic efforts should focus on the identification and treatment of readily reversible causes of oliguria (i.e., urine output less than 0.5 mL/kg/hr). For example, urinary catheter obstruction or dislodgment is easily remedied and often overlooked. When appropriate, one should confer with the surgical team regarding the details of the surgical procedure to rule out anatomic obstruction or disruption of the ureters, bladder, or urethra.

Patient-related factors play a role in the development of acute kidney injury (AKI) in the postoperative period. Comorbidities such as preexisting renal insufficiency, diabetes mellitus, hypertension, morbid obesity, male sex, and old age are a number of issues that should be considered when identifying if a patient is at an increased risk of perioperative renal dysfunction. In addition to nonmodifiable patient risk factors, the surgical procedure itself comprises an independent risk factor in the development of perioperative renal dysfunction, with cardiac surgery, emergency surgery, and major surgery (vascular, transplant, thoracic) all serving to increase the probability.

A number of perioperative events may alter renal perfusion. Angiography can result in ischemic injury secondary to renal vasoconstriction and direct renal tubular injury from contrast agents. Perioperative volume depletion can exacerbate acute tubular necrosis caused by sepsis. The surgical procedure itself can alter renal vascular patency, decreasing renal perfusion. Finally, increased intraabdominal pressure (IAP) can impair renal perfusion.

Judicious intraoperative fluid management is of utmost importance during the perioperative period (also see Chapter 24). Hemodynamics must be monitored to ensure that relative intravascular volume is sufficient to allow for adequate tissue perfusion. Crystalloid solutions are ubiquitous in the operating room and PACU. Balanced solutions (lactated Ringer's [LR], PlasmaLyte) may be superior to chloride-only-containing solutions (NaCl), as hyperchloremia is associated with the development of AKI. A 2018 study of critically ill adult patients randomized to receive balanced crystalloid or saline revealed that saline had an increased risk of renal replacement therapy or persistent renal dysfunction compared with balanced solutions.[34] In general, hydroxyethyl starch solutions (HES) should be avoided, as there are no clear benefits to their use.

The risk of developing postoperative AKI was increased when mean arterial pressure (MAP) <60 mm Hg for >20 minutes or MAP <55 mm Hg for >10 minutes.[35] Vasopressors may be needed as an adjunct to fluid therapy in hypotensive patients. To date, there is no evidence that one vasopressor is superior to the other. Although low-dose dopamine can increase urine output, there is no evidence that it is renoprotective, and it is not a recommended treatment strategy for prevention or treatment of AKI.

Oliguria

Intravascular Volume Depletion

The most common cause of oliguria in the immediate postoperative period is intravascular volume depletion. If the patient also demonstrates signs of hypovolemia, a fluid challenge (500 to 1000 mL of crystalloid) is usually effective in restoring urine output. Patients with a history of hypertension may require higher MAPs to produce adequate urine output. Volume resuscitation to maximize renal perfusion is particularly important to prevent ongoing ischemic injury and the development of acute tubular necrosis.

If a fluid challenge is contraindicated or oliguria persists, assessment of intravascular fluid volume status and cardiac function is indicated to differentiate hypovolemia from sepsis and low cardiac output states. A fractional excretion of sodium <1% can be useful in suggesting prerenal etiology, assuming that diuretics have not been given. However, the diagnosis of prerenal azotemia will not differentiate hypovolemia, congestive heart failure, or hepatorenal syndrome. Further evaluation with central venous monitoring or echocardiography may facilitate the differential diagnosis.

Postoperative Urinary Retention

Ultrasonography can measure bladder volume and identify urinary retention in the PACU.[36] Using this technique, urinary retention is generally defined as bladder volume greater than 600 mL in conjunction with an inability to void within 30 minutes. The strongest predictive factors are age older than 50 years and intraoperative fluid more than 750 mL. Bladder ultrasound is an efficient and accurate method to identify patients at high risk of urinary retention. The ASA Practice Guidelines for Postanesthetic Care do not recommend a routine requirement for urination before PACU discharge, although this may be necessary for selected ambulatory surgery patients.

Contrast Nephropathy

An increasing number of patients receive IV contrast for angiographic procedures for aortic, peripheral vascular, or cerebral vascular disease. In these patients contrast nephropathy should always be considered in the differential diagnosis of postoperative renal dysfunction. Prompt diagnosis is crucial, as contrast nephropathy, in general, is one of the reversible causes of postoperative AKI. The creatinine tends to increase within 24 to 48 hours after the administration of contrast media, typically returning to the patient's baseline within 1 week. Perioperative attention to adequate hydration is indicated in any patient who has received an IV contrast agent. Intravascular volume expansion with isotonic saline is the single most effective means of protection against contrast nephropathy.[37] AKI prevention strategies such as routine administration of acetylcysteine or alkalinization of the urine with a sodium bicarbonate infusion have not definitively demonstrated benefit and are not recommended.[37]

Intraabdominal Hypertension

Intraabdominal hypertension (IAH) should be considered in any patient with oliguria and a tense abdomen after abdominal surgery. Elevated intraabdominal pressure (IAP) can impede renal perfusion and lead to renal ischemia and postoperative renal dysfunction. Normal IAP in a patient who is not obese is approximately 5 mm Hg. IAH is defined as a sustained IAP greater than 12 mm Hg, with abdominal compartment syndrome (ACS) defined as a sustained IAP greater than 20 mm Hg associated with new organ dysfunction/failure.[38]

Elevation of IAP impairs venous drainage from the kidney secondary to the increased vascular resistance that ensues when the renal vein is compressed. When IAPs reach 15 mm Hg, oliguria tends to develop, whereas anuria is not common until pressures reach approximately 30 mm Hg. Bladder pressure, an indirect assessment of IAP, should be measured in patients in whom IAH is suspected, to ensure the initiation of prompt intervention to relieve the pressure and therefore restore renal perfusion.[39]

Medical management of increased IAP includes measures to improve abdominal wall compliance, evacuation of intraluminal gastrointestinal contents (e.g., nasogastric decompression), and correction of positive fluid balance.[38] For a patient with primary ACS, however, surgical decompression of the abdomen may be required.

Rhabdomyolysis

Rhabdomyolysis may complicate the postoperative course of patients who have suffered major crush or thermal injury. Patients may complain of myalgias, abdominal pain, nausea, and weakness. Myoglobinuria may be present, and creatine kinase (CK) levels are elevated. The incidence is also significantly increased in morbidly obese patients undergoing bariatric surgery. Risk factors include increased body mass index (BMI) and the length of the surgery. Patient history and the operative course should guide the decision to measure CK in the PACU. Early aggressive hydration to maintain urine output is the mainstay of treatment. Electrolyte abnormalities, including hyperkalemia, hyperphosphatemia, and hypocalcemia, must be detected and corrected immediately. Loop diuretics can be administered if volume overload occurs. The infusion of mannitol to enhance the elimination of myoglobin casts from the renal tubules and bicarbonate to protect against renal tubular myoglobin toxicity is commonly practiced but may not provide further benefit.

POSTOPERATIVE HYPOTHERMIA AND SHIVERING

Postoperative hypothermia, defined as a core temperature <36°C, is a detrimental and unpleasant condition that can occur after general and neuraxial anesthesia. The ASA Practice Guidelines for Postanesthesia Care recommend that patient temperature be periodically assessed during emergence and recovery and that normothermia should be a goal during this time.[2] Mild to moderate hypothermia (33°C to 35°C) inhibits platelet function, coagulation factor activity, and drug metabolism.[40] Hypothermia may also exacerbate postoperative bleeding, prolong neuromuscular blockade, and delay awakening. Whereas these immediate consequences are associated with a prolonged PACU stay, long-term deleterious effects can include an increased incidence of myocardial ischemia and myocardial infarction and delayed wound healing. Postoperative shivering also often occurs after general and neuraxial anesthesia and can be uncomfortable for patients. The incidence of postoperative shivering may be as high as 66% after general anesthesia. Independent risk factors include young age, endoprosthetic (joint replacement) surgery, and core hypothermia.

Mechanism

Postoperative hypothermia occurs secondary to redistribution and heat loss during surgery. Postoperative shivering is usually, but not always, associated with hypothermia. Although thermoregulatory mechanisms can explain shivering in the hypothermic patient, a number of different mechanisms have been proposed to explain shivering in normothermic patients. One proposed mechanism is based on the observation that the brain and spinal cord do not recover simultaneously from general anesthesia. The more rapid recovery of spinal cord function is thought to result in uninhibited spinal reflexes manifested as clonic activity. This theory is supported by the fact that doxapram, a central nervous system stimulant, is somewhat effective in abolishing postoperative shivering.

Treatment

Patients who are hypothermic upon arrival in the PACU should be actively warmed using a forced air warmer or warm blankets to avoid both immediate and delayed complications of hypothermia. Accurate core body temperature can be obtained at the tympanic membrane; however, this may be technically challenging—oral and axillary temperatures are usually close to core temperature and can be reasonably used for patients recovering from anesthesia.[41] A number of opioids and α_2-adrenergic agonists have been shown to be effective in abolishing shivering once it has started. Of those, meperidine (12.5–25 mg IV) is the most commonly used agent in adults.

V

POSTOPERATIVE NAUSEA AND VOMITING

Without prophylactic intervention, roughly one-third of patients who undergo inhalational anesthesia will develop postoperative nausea and vomiting (PONV) (range, 10%–80%).[42] The consequences of PONV include delayed discharge from the PACU, unanticipated hospital admission, increased incidence of pulmonary aspiration, and significant postoperative discomfort. The ability to identify high-risk patients for prophylactic intervention can significantly improve the quality of patient care and satisfaction in the PACU. From a patient's perspective, PONV may be more uncomfortable than postoperative pain.

Prevention and Treatment

The likelihood of a patient experiencing PONV depends on several risk factors and increases with the number of those risk factors (Fig. 39.1). These factors can be divided into patient-related, anesthesia-related, and surgery-related risk factors. As for patient-related risk factors, female gender, nonsmoking status, history of PONV and/or motion sickness, the need for postoperative opioids, and young age (<50 years) have been identified

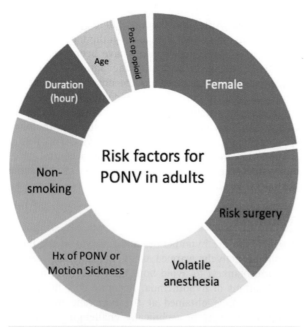

Fig. 39.1 PONV risk factor summary. Intraoperative and postoperative risk factors of PONV in adults; the size of each segment is proportional to the odds ratios of PONV associated with each risk factor. *PONV*, Postoperative nausea and vomiting. (Figure reused with permission from the American Society for Enhanced Recovery.)

as independent risk factors.[43] Anesthesia-related risk factors are the use of volatile anesthetics and nitrous oxide, in addition to the administration of higher doses of perioperative opioids and neostigmine for reversal of neuromuscular blockade. As for surgery-related risk factors, the length of surgery and certain surgical procedures (cholecystectomy, laparoscopy, gynecologic surgery) have been identified as significant contributing factors.

Prophylactic measures to prevent PONV include modification of anesthetic technique and pharmacologic intervention. Whenever feasible, a regional anesthesia technique should be used, the use of volatile anesthetics and nitrous oxide should be restricted, and measures to reduce the postoperative use of opioids (e.g., multimodal analgesia) should be used. As for pharmacologic interventions, multiple drugs are available for prophylaxis and treatment of PONV. Box 39.9 lists different recommended antiemetic medications commonly administered for both prophylaxis and treatment of PONV, which should be chosen tailored to the individual patient.

An international panel of experts just published the Fourth Consensus Guidelines for the Management of Postoperative Nausea and Vomiting.[42] These advocate a very liberal approach to prophylaxis and recommend giving two antiemetic agents to all patients with one or two risk factors and giving three to four antiemetic agents to all patients with more than two risk factors. If an adequate number and dose of antiemetic drugs given at the appropriate time are ineffective, simply giving more of the same class of drug in the PACU is unlikely to produce any significant benefit. It is not recommended to redose any medication of the same class within 6 hours after the initial dose. Therefore a drug from another class that has not previously been administered should be chosen for treatment of PONV in the PACU.

DELIRIUM

Postoperative delirium (POD) is defined as an acute and fluctuating alteration of mental state of reduced awareness and disturbance of attention (also see Chapter 35). POD often starts in the recovery room but can occur up to 5 days after surgery. The incidence of POD depends on preoperative and intraoperative risk factors and is highly variable, with incidences between 4% and 75% reported in the literature. It is important to distinguish between the hyperactive and the hypoactive subtype of delirium, because the latter may easily go unnoticed and therefore untreated. Multiple studies across different surgical specialties in both elective and emergency cases have shown that POD is associated with worse surgical outcomes, increased hospital length of stay, functional decline, higher rates of institutionalization, higher mortality, and higher cost and resource utilization.[44]

Box 39.9 Commonly Used Antiemetics, With Adult Doses

Anticholinergics
Scopolamine: transdermal patch, 1.5 mg
  Apply to a hairless area behind the ear before surgery; remove 24 hours postoperatively

Antihistamines
Hydroxyzine: 12.5-25 mg IM

Phenothiazines
Promethazine: 6.25-12.5 mg IV/IM
Prochlorperazine: 2.5-10 mg IV/IM

Butyrophenones
Droperidol: 0.625-1.25 mg IV
  See black box warning regarding torsades de pointes: monitor the ECG for prolongation of the QT interval for 2-3 hs after administration—preoperative 12-lead ECG recommended
Haloperidol: 0.5 to <2 mg IM/IV
  Use with caution if prolonged QT interval present in ECG

Nk-1 Receptor Antagonists
Aprepitant: 40 mg PO before induction of anesthesia
Casopitant: 150 mg PO before induction of anesthesia

Prokinetic
Metoclopramide: 10-20 mg IV
  Minimal antiemetic properties, avoid in patients with any possibility of gastrointestinal obstruction

Serotonin Receptor Antagonists
Ondansetron: 4 mg IV 30 minutes before conclusion of surgery
Granisetron: 0.35-3 mg IV near the conclusion of surgery
Tropisetron: 2 mg IV near the conclusion of surgery
Ramosetron: 0.3 mg IV near the conclusion of surgery
Palonosetron: 0.075 mg IV with induction of anesthesia
Dolasetron: 12.5 mg IV 15-30 minutes before conclusion of surgery (no longer marketed in the United States because of risk of QTc prolongation and torsades de pointes)

Corticosteroids
Dexamethasone: 4-8 mg IV with induction of anesthesia
Methylprednisolone: 40 mg IV with induction of anesthesia

ECG, Electrocardiogram; *IM*, intramuscularly; *IV*, intravenously; *PO*, by mouth.

Risk Factors

POD has been linked to multiple risk factors. These are commonly distinguished between predisposing factors (inherent to the patient) and precipitating factors (triggering the onset of delirium)[44] (Box 39.10). Major predisposing patient risk factors include age >65 years, cognitive impairment, severe illness or comorbidity burden, hearing or vision impairment, and presence of infection. In the perioperative context the performed surgical procedure acts as a physiologic stressor, with the extent of surgery having a major impact on the likelihood of developing delirium. The highest-risk procedures include cardiac surgery, vascular surgery, and hip fracture surgery. Risk assessment is a shared clinical responsibility and should ideally be implemented in a perioperative clinical pathway.

Prophylaxis and Management

Patients at increased risk of POD should ideally be identified before entering the operating room by using a delirium risk screening tool (e.g., the AWOL-S delirium risk stratification tool).[45] Patients who screen as high risk for developing delirium should ideally be put on a delirium reduction pathway to decrease their likelihood of developing delirium in the postoperative phase. Such a pathway should include recommendations for the preoperative, intraoperative, and postoperative care of the patient. Once the patient is in the recovery room, any deliriogenic medications should be avoided (e.g., anticholinergics, sedative-hypnotics, meperidine),[46] unless the specific needs for any of these medications outweigh their potential risks (e.g., benzodiazepines for seizures or for benzodiazepine/alcohol withdrawal). Simple measures, such as frequent reorientation, sensory enhancement (ensuring glasses, hearing aids, or listening amplifiers are available upon arrival in the PACU), pain control, cognitive stimulation, simple communication standards and approaches to prevent the escalation of behaviors, and keeping the patients in their circadian rhythm can decrease the incidence of developing POD by 30% to 40%.[47] Screening for delirium in the PACU should be performed before the patient leaves the unit (e.g., with the Nursing Delirium Screening Scale [NuDESC] or Confusion Assessment Method [CAM] score). If prevention has failed and the patient screens positive, prompt evaluation of possible precipitating factors should occur (see Box 39.10).[44] Treatment of causative factors and symptoms has a major impact on reducing the duration of delirium and should therefore be initiated immediately. Generally, multicomponent nonpharmacologic interventions described earlier should be used for all patients with delirium. Pharmacologic interventions should only be used in the lowest effective dose for patients with agitated delirium when other interventions have failed and the patients pose a substantial harm to themselves or others. The medication of choice is haloperidol starting at 0.5 to 1 mg IM/IV.

Emergence Agitation

Persistent POD should not be confused with emergence agitation, which is a transient confusional state that is associated with emergence from general anesthesia. Emergence agitation is common in children, with more than 30% experiencing agitation or delirium at some period during their PACU stay (also see Chapter 34). It usually occurs within the first 10 minutes of recovery but can have an onset later in children who are brought to the recovery room asleep. The peak age of emergence

V

Box 39.10 Risk Factors for Delirium

Predisposing (Baseline)
Cognitive impairment (e.g., dementia)
Age >65 years
Sensory impairment (vision, hearing)
Severe illness (e.g., requiring ICU admission)
Presence of infection
Poor functional status (e.g., frailty, limited mobility)
Alcohol abuse
Malnutrition

Precipitating
Medications or medication withdrawal: Psychotropic medications (antidepressants, antiepileptics, antipsychotics, benzodiazepines), anticholinergics, muscle relaxants, antihistamines, GI antispasmodics, opioid analgesics, antiarrhythmics, corticosteroids, more than six total medications, more than three new inpatient medications
Pain
Hypoxemia
Hypoglycemia
Electrolyte abnormalities
Malnutrition
Dehydration
Environmental change (e.g., ICU admission)
Sleep–wake cycle disturbances
Urinary catheter use
Restraint use
Infection

GI, Gastrointestinal; *ICU*, intensive care unit.

Box 39.11 Causes of Delayed Emergence From General Anesthesia[48,49]

Residual anesthetic drug effects
Substance use (alcohol, others)
Central anticholinergic syndrome
Serotonin syndrome
Neurologic disorders
  Cerebral hypoxia
  Acute stroke (embolic, ischemic, hemorrhagic)
  Seizures (with postictal state)
  Elevated intracranial pressure
Metabolic disturbances
  Hypothermia
  Electrolyte imbalances (especially sodium disorders)
  Hypoglycemia
  Liver dysfunction (causing hepatic encephalopathy)

---

agitation in children is between 2 and 4 years. Unlike delirium, emergence agitation typically resolves quickly and is followed by uneventful recovery. In contrast to children, the incidence of emergence agitation in adults is estimated to only be between 3% and 5%. In children emergence agitation is most frequently associated with rapid "wake up" from inhalational anesthesia. Other possible etiologic factors include intrinsic characteristics of the anesthetic, postoperative pain, type of surgery, age, preoperative anxiety, underlying temperament, and adjunct medications. Awareness of these contributors allows one to identify and treat children who are at increased risk.

DELAYED AWAKENING

Even after prolonged surgery and anesthesia, a response to stimulation should occur within 60 to 90 minutes. If emergence has not taken place by that time, there are multiple potential causes. Residual anesthetic drug effects are the most frequent cause of delayed emergence. The most common drugs to consider are benzodiazepines, opioids, and neuromuscular blocking drugs; however, after a very long anesthetic, propofol and volatile anesthetics can also cause a delay in emergence. Other causes of delayed emergence are listed in Box 39.11.[48–51]

Treatment

For a patient in the PACU with delayed emergence, the initial management includes the following steps: (1) confirm airway, breathing, and circulatory status; (2) ensure that all anesthetic agents have been discontinued; (3) check core temperature and begin rewarming if necessary; (4) perform a neurologic examination to detect focal findings; (5) evaluate for residual neuromuscular blockade and treat if required; (6) consider laboratory tests with rapid turnaround such as glucose (to rule out hypoglycemia) and arterial blood gas with electrolytes (to evaluate for hypercarbia, sodium disorders).[48,49] The following reversal medications can be considered depending on clinical context: (1) naloxone 40 mcg every 2 minutes up to 200 mcg (for suspected residual opioid effect), (2) flumazenil 0.1 to 0.2 mg every 1 minute up to 1 mg (for suspected residual benzodiazepine effect), (3) physostigmine 1 to 4 mg (for suspected central anticholinergic syndrome). If there is concern for acute stroke, consider "code stroke" activation with a neurologist, which will require a stat brain computed tomography (CT). If the patient remains unresponsive despite these management steps, admission to the ICU for further neurologic monitoring and evaluation is indicated.

DISCHARGE CRITERIA

Although specific PACU discharge criteria may vary, certain general principles are universally applicable (Box 39.12). Patient mental status should be clear or at baseline level. Hemodynamic criteria are based on the patient's baseline hemodynamics without specific systemic blood pressure and heart rate requirements. Discharge criteria should be designed to minimize the risk of cardiorespiratory or central nervous system depression after leaving the PACU.[2]

Box 39.12 General Principles for Discharge From the Postanesthesia Care Unit

1. Patients should be observed until they are no longer at increased risk for cardiorespiratory depression.
2. Patients should be routinely required to have a responsible person accompany them home after outpatient surgery.
3. Requiring patients to urinate before discharge should not be part of a routine discharge protocol and may be necessary only in selected patients.
4. The demonstrated ability to drink and retain clear fluids should not be part of a routine discharge protocol but may be appropriate for selected patients.
5. A minimum mandatory stay in the unit should not be required.

Adapted from Practice guidelines for postanesthetic care. Anesthesiology. 2013;118:291-307.

Table 39.1 Criteria for Determining Release From the Postanesthesia Care Unit: The Modified Aldrete Score

Variable Evaluated	Score
Activity	
Able to move four extremities on command	2
Able to move two extremities on command	1
Able to move no extremities on command	0
Breathing	
Able to breathe deeply and cough freely	2
Dyspnea	1
Apnea	0
Circulation (systemic blood pressure)	
Within 20% of the preanesthetic level	2
20%–49% of the preanesthetic level	1
≥50% of the preanesthetic level	0
Consciousness	
Fully awake	2
Arousable	1
Not responding	0
Oxygen Saturation (pulse oximetry)	
>92% while breathing room air	2
Needs supplemental oxygen to maintain saturation >90%	1
<90% even with supplemental oxygen	0

Adapted from Aldrete JA. The post anaesthesia recovery score revisited. *J Clin Anesth*. 1995;7:89–91.
Score ≥ 9 required for discharge.

POSTANESTHESIA SCORING SYSTEMS

To standardize and facilitate discharge from PACU, several different scoring systems have been developed and updated over time. The most commonly used postanesthesia scoring system to monitor recovery from anesthesia is the Aldrete score, which was first described in 1970. In its latest version it assigns a number of 0, 1, or 2 to five variables: activity, respiration, circulation, consciousness, and oxygen saturation (Table 39.1). Another system, the Postanesthesia Discharge Scoring System (PADS), was designed to determine when a patient can be discharged home after outpatient surgery (Table 39.2).[52]

Table 39.2 Criteria for Determination of Discharge Score for Release Home to a Responsible Adult: The Postanesthesia Discharge Scoring System (PADS)

Variable Evaluated	Score[a]
Vital signs (stable and consistent with age and preanesthetic baseline)	
Systemic blood pressure and heart rate within 20% of the preanesthetic level	2
Systemic blood pressure and heart rate 20%–40% of the preanesthetic level	1
Systemic blood pressure and heart rate >40% of the preanesthetic level	0
Activity Level	
Steady gait without dizziness or meets the preanesthetic level	2
Requires assistance	1
Unable to ambulate	0
Nausea and Vomiting	
None to minimal	2
Moderate	1
Severe (continues after repeated treatment)	0
Pain (minimal to no pain, controllable withoral analgesics)	
Yes	2
No	1
Surgical Bleeding (consistent with that expected for the surgical procedure)	
Minimal (does not require dressing change)	2
Moderate (up to two dressing changes required)	1
Severe (more than three dressing changes required)	0

[a]Patients achieving a score of at least 9 are ready for discharge.
Modified from Marshall SI, Chung F. Discharge criteria and complications after ambulatory surgery. Anesth Analg. 1999;88:508-517.

V

The ASA Standards for Postanesthesia Care require that a physician accept responsibility for the discharge of patients from the PACU.[1] This is the case even when the decision to discharge the patient is made at the bedside by the PACU nurse in accordance with hospital-sanctioned discharge criteria or scoring systems. If discharge criteria are to be used, they must first be approved by the department of anesthesia and the hospital medical staff.[53] A responsible physician's name must be noted on the record.

REFERENCES

1. American Society of Anesthesiologists; Standards for Postanesthesia Care, Approved by the ASA House of Delegates on Oct. 27, 2004 and last amended on Oct. 23, 2019. https://www.asahq.org/standards-and-guidelines/standards-for-postanesthesia-care. Accessed February 4, 2021.
2. Apfelbaum JL, Silverstein JH, Chung FF, et al. American Society of Anesthesiologists Task Force on Postanesthetic Care. Practice guidelines for postanesthetic care: An updated report by the American Society of Anesthesiologists Task Force on Postanesthetic Care. *Anesthesiology.* 2013;118(2):291–307.
3. Hines R, et al. Complications occurring in the postanesthesia care unit: A survey. *Anesth Analg.* 1992;74(4):503–509.
4. Kluger MT, Bullock MF. Recovery room incidents: A review of 419 reports from the Anaesthetic Incident Monitoring Study (AIMS). *Anaesthesia.* 2002;57(11):1060–1066.
5. Brull SJ, Kopman AF. Current status of neuromuscular reversal and monitoring: Challenges and opportunities. *Anesthesiology.* 2017;126(1):173–190.
6. Fortier LP, McKeen D, Turner K, et al. The RECITE Study: A Canadian prospective, multicenter study of the incidence and severity of residual neuromuscular blockade. *Anesth Analg.* 2015;121(2):366–372.
7. Bulka CM, Terekhov MA, Martin BJ, et al. Nondepolarizing neuromuscular blocking agents, reversal, and risk of postoperative pneumonia. *Anesthesiology.* 2016;125(4):647–655.
8. Kheterpal S, Vaughn MT, Dubovoy TZ, et al. Sugammadex versus neostigmine for reversal of neuromuscular blockade and postoperative pulmonary complications (STRONGER): A multicenter matched cohort analysis. *Anesthesiology.* 2020;132(6):1371–1381.
9. Kuriyama A, Jackson JL, Kamei J. Performance of the cuff leak test in adults in predicting post-extubation airway complications: A systematic review and meta-analysis. *Crit Care.* 2020;24:640.
10. Abdelsattar ZM, Hendren S, Wong SL, Campbell Jr DA, Ramachandran SK. The impact of untreated obstructive sleep apnea on cardiopulmonary complications in general and vascular surgery: A cohort study. *Sleep.* 2015;38(8):1205–1210.
11. Lam KA, Kunder S, Wong J, Doufas A, Chung F. Obstructive sleep apnea, pain, and opioids. *Curr Opin Anaesthesiol.* 2016;29:134–140.
12. Chung F, Memtsoudis SG, Ramachandran SK, Nagappa M, Opperer M, Cozowicz C, et al. Society of Anesthesia and Sleep Medicine guidelines on preoperative screening and assessment of adult patients with obstructive sleep apnea. *Anesth Analg.* 2016;123:452–473.
13. Nagappa M, Mokhlesi B, Wong J, Wong D, Kaw R, Chung F. The effects of continuous positive airway pressure on postoperative outcomes in obstructive sleep apnea patients undergoing surgery. *Anesth Analg.* 2015;120:1013–1023.
14. Bhattacharya M, Kallet RH, Ware LB, Matthay MA. Negative-pressure pulmonary edema. *Chest.* 2016;150(4):927–933.
15. Semple JW, Rebetz J, Kapur R. Transfusion-associated circulatory overload and transfusion-related acute lung injury. *Blood.* 2019;133(17):1840–1853.
16. Vlaar AP, Toy P, Fung M, Looney MR, Juffermans NP, Bux J, et al. A consensus redefinition of transfusion-related acute lung injury. *Transfusion.* 2019;59:2465–2476.
17. Chaudhuri D, Granton D, Wang DX, Burns KEA, Helviz Y, Einav S, et al. High-flow nasal cannula in the immediate postoperative period: A systematic review and meta-analysis. *Chest.* 2020;158(5):1934–1946.
18. Zhao, et al. High-flow nasal cannula oxygen therapy is superior to conventional oxygen therapy but not to noninvasive mechanical ventilation on intubation rate: A systematic review and meta-analysis. *Critical Care.* 2017;21:184.
19. Chung F, Nagappa M, Singh M. Mokhlesi CPAP in the perioperative setting. *Chest.* 2016;149:586–597.
20. Ireland CJ, Chapman TM, Mathew SF, Herbison GP, Zacharias M. Continuous positive airway pressure (CPAP) during the postoperative period for prevention of postoperative morbidity and mortality following major abdominal surgery. *Cochrane Database Syst Rev.* 2014;2014(8):CD008930.
21. Jaber S, Chanques G, Jung B, Riou B. Postoperative noninvasive ventilation. *Anesthesiology.* 2010;112:453–461.
22. Stéphan F, Barrucand B, Petit P, Rézaiguia-Delclaux S, Médard A, Delannoy B, et al. High-flow nasal oxygen vs noninvasive positive airway pressure in hypoxemic patients after cardiothoracic surgery: A randomized clinical trial. *JAMA.* 2015;313(23):2331–2339.
23. Hepner DL, Castells MC. Anaphylaxis during the perioperative period. *Anesth Analg.* 2003;97(5):1381–1395.
24. Neal JM, Barrington MJ, Fettiplace MR, et al. The Third American Society of Regional Anesthesia and Pain Medicine Practice Advisory on Local Anesthetic Systemic Toxicity: Executive summary 2017. *Reg Anesth Pain Med.* 2018;43:113–123.
25. Hepner DL, Castells MC. Anaphylaxis during the perioperative period. *Anesth Analg.* 2003;97(5):1381–1395.
26. Devereaux PJ, Xavier D, Pogue J, et al. Characteristics and short-term prognosis of perioperative myocardial infarction in patients undergoing noncardiac surgery: A cohort study. *Ann Intern Med.* 2011;154(8):523–528.
27. Beaulieu RJ, Sutzko DC, Albright J, Jeruzal E, Osborne NH, Henke PK. Association of high mortality with postoperative myocardial infarction after major vascular surgery despite use of evidence-based therapies. *JAMA Surg.* 2020;155(2):131–137.
28. Verbree-Willemsen L, Grobben RB, van Waes JA, et al. Causes and prevention of postoperative myocardial injury. *Eur J Prev Cardiol.* 2019;26(1):59–67.
29. Vascular Events In Noncardiac Surgery Patients Cohort Evaluation (VISION) Study InvestigatorsDevereaux PJ, Chan MT, Alonso-Coelho P, et al. Association between postoperative troponin levels and 30-day mortality among patients undergoing noncardiac surgery. *JAMA.* 2012;307(21):2295–2304.
30. Botto F, Alonso-Coello P, Chan MT, et al. Myocardial injury after noncardiac surgery: A large, international, prospective cohort study establishing diagnostic criteria, characteristics, predictors, and 30-day outcomes. *Anesthesiology.* 2014;120(3):564–578.
31. Fleisher LA, Fleischmann KE, Auerbach AD, et al. 2014 ACC/AHA guideline on perioperative cardiovascular evaluation and management of patients undergoing noncardiac surgery: Executive summary:

A report of the American College of Cardiology/American Heart Association Task Force on Practice Guidelines. *Circulation*. 2014;130(24):2215–2245.

32. Bhave PD, Goldman LE, Vittinghoff E, et al. Incidence, predictors, and outcomes associated with postoperative atrial fibrillation after major noncardiac surgery. *Am Heart J*. 2012;164(6):918–924.

33. Panchal AR, Bartos JA, Cabañas JG, et al. Part 3: Adult Basic and Advanced Life Support: 2020 American Heart Association Guidelines for Cardiopulmonary Resuscitation and Emergency Cardiovascular Care. *Circulation*. 2020;142:S366–S468.

34. Bhave PD, Goldman LE, Vittinghoff E, et al. Incidence, predictors, and outcomes associated with postoperative atrial fibrillation after major noncardiac surgery. *Am Heart J*. 2012;164(6):918–924.

35. Baldini G, Bagry H, Aprikian A, Carli F, Warner DS, Warner MA. Postoperative urinary retention: Anesthetic and perioperative considerations. *Anesthesiology*. 2009;110:1139–1157.

36. Semler MW, et al. Balanced crystalloids versus saline in critically ill adults. *N Engl J Med*. 2018;378(9):829–839.

37. Sun LY, Wijeysundera DN, Tait GA, Beattie WS. Association of intraoperative hypotension with acute kidney injury after elective noncardiac surgery. *Anesthesiology*. 2015;123:515–523.

38. Kowalik U, Plante MK. Urinary retention in surgical patients. *Surg Clin North Am*. 2016;96(3):453–467.

39. Mehran R, Dangas GD, Weisbord SD. Contrast-associated acute kidney injury. *N Engl J Med*. 2019;380(22):2146–2155.

40. Kirkpatrick AW, Roberts DJ, De Waele J, Jaeschke R, Malbrain ML, De Keulenaer, et al. Intra-abdominal hypertension and the abdominal compartment syndrome: Updated consensus definitions and clinical practice guidelines from the World Society of the Abdominal Compartment Syndrome. *Intensive Care Med*. 2013;39(7):1190–1206.

41. Murphy PB, Parry NG, Sela N, Leslie K, Vogt K, Ball I. Intra-abdominal hypertension is more common than previously thought: A prospective study in a mixed medical-surgical ICU. *Crit Care Med*. 2018;46(6):958–964.

42. Sessler DI. Perioperative thermoregulation and heat balance. *Lancet*. 2016;387:2655–2664.

43. Sessler DI. Perioperative temperature monitoring. *Anesthesiology*. 2021;134:111–118.

44. Gan TJ, Belani KG, Bergese S, et al. Fourth consensus guidelines for the management of postoperative nausea and vomiting. *Anesth Analg*. 2020;131(2):411–448.

45. Apfel CC, Philip BK, Cakmakkaya OS, Shilling A, Shi YY, Leslie JB, Allard M, Turan A, Windle P, Odom-Forren J, Hooper VD, Radke OC, Ruiz J, Kovac A. Who is at risk for postdischarge nausea and vomiting after ambulatory surgery?. *Anesthesiology*. 2012;117:475–486.

46. Mohanty S, Rosenthal RA, Russell MM, et al. Optimal perioperative management of the geriatric patient: A best practices guideline from the American College of Surgeons NSQIP and the American Geriatrics Society. *J Am Coll Surg*. 2016;222(5):930–947.

47. Whitlock EL, Braehler MR, Kaplan JA, Finlayson E, Rogers SE, Douglas V, Donovan AL. Derivation, validation, sustained performance, and clinical impact of an electronic medical record-based perioperative delirium risk stratification tool. *Anesth Analg*. 2020;131(6):1901–1910.

48. By the 2019 American Geriatrics Society Beers Criteria® Update Expert Panel. American Geriatrics Society 2019 Updated AGS Beers Criteria® for Potentially Inappropriate Medication Use in Older Adults. *J Am Geriatr Soc*. 2019;67(4):674–694.

49. The American Geriatrics Society Expert Panel. Postoperative delirium in older adults: Best practice statement from the American Geriatrics Society. *J Am Coll Surg*. 2015;220(2):136–148.

50. Tzabazis A, Miller C, Dobrow MF, Zheng K, Brock-Utne JG. Delayed emergence after anesthesia. *J Clin Anesth*. 2015;27(4):353–360. doi:10.1016/j.jclinane.2015.03.023 Epub 2015 Apr 23. PMID: 25912729.

51. Misal US, Joshi SA, Shaikh MM. Delayed recovery from anesthesia: A postgraduate educational review. *Anesth Essays Res*. 2016;10(2):164–172.

52. Aldrete JA. The post anaesthesia recovery score revisited. *J Clin Anesth*. 1995;7:89–91.

53. Marshall SI, Chang F. Discharge criteria and complications after ambulatory surgery. *Anesth Analg*. 1999;88:508–517.

V

40 PERIOPERATIVE PAIN MANAGEMENT

Heather A. Columbano, Robert W. Hurley, Meredith C.B. Adams

Postoperative pain is a complex physiologic reaction to tissue injury. For many patients, the primary concern about surgery is how much pain they will experience after the procedure. Similarly, postoperative pain management is an integral part of anesthesia care. Postoperative pain is directly related to patient satisfaction, which has evolved into an important measure for high-quality health care. Postoperative pain produces acute adverse physiologic effects with manifestations in multiple organ systems, leading to significant morbidity (Box 40.1). Catecholamines released in response to pain may result in tachycardia and hypertension, which may induce myocardial ischemia in susceptible patients. Pain after upper abdominal or thoracic surgery often leads to hypoventilation from splinting. This promotes atelectasis, which impairs ventilation-to-perfusion relationships and increases the likelihood of arterial hypoxia and pneumonia. Pain that limits postoperative ambulation combined with a stress-induced hypercoagulable state may contribute to an increased incidence of deep vein thrombosis. In a 2015 observational study 54% of patients experienced moderate to extreme acute postoperative pain at the time of their discharge from the hospital.[1] This represents an improvement in postoperative pain management as compared with an earlier study in which 64% of patients had the same level of pain at hospital discharge.[2] However, it is concerning that in the more recent study 46% reported a moderate to extreme level of postoperative pain 2 weeks after discharge.

Factors that positively correlate with increased postoperative pain include preoperative opioid intake, increased body mass index, anxiety, depression, pain intensity level, characteristics of fibromyalgia, and the duration of surgical operation.[3] Factors that negatively correlate include increased patient age and the level of the surgeon's operative experience. Despite these findings being replicated in numerous studies, the immediate postoperative pain assessment may suffer from significant observer bias. In addition to the previous factors positively and

Box 40.1 Adverse Physiologic Effects of Postoperative Pain

Pulmonary System
Atelectasis
Decreased lung volumes
Ventilation-to-perfusion mismatching
Arterial hypoxemia
Hypercapnia
Pneumonia

Cardiovascular System
Sympathetic nervous system stimulation
Systemic hypertension
Tachycardia
Myocardial ischemia
Cardiac dysrhythmias

Endocrine System
Hyperglycemia
Sodium and water retention
Protein catabolism

Immune System
Decreased immune function

Coagulation System
Increased platelet adhesiveness
Decreased fibrinolysis
Hypercoagulation
Deep vein thrombosis

Gastrointestinal System
Ileus

Genitourinary System
Urinary retention

negatively associated with the postoperative pain, the factor that was most highly associated with the first postoperative pain score was which nurse was performing the assessment.[4]

A perioperative plan reflecting risk factors should be developed to decrease patients' postoperative pain.[5-7] But other comorbidities may affect the design of the "ideal" postoperative pain plan. For example, despite having a lower predictive risk for postoperative pain, elderly patients can present with significant management challenges. Elderly patients are at higher risk for cognitive dysfunction in the perioperative period because of various factors, including increased sensitivity to drugs and other medical comorbidities (also see Chapter 35). Patients taking opioids for chronic pain relief preoperatively have higher pain scores, higher opioid consumption, and lower pain thresholds in the immediate postoperative period.[8,9] Perioperative management plans that incorporate these variables may favor the use of regional anesthesia because of the decreased mortality rate and infrequent incidence of postoperative cognitive dysfunction and pain. Preoperative regional analgesia may enhance pain control, decrease adverse cognitive effects, and improve postoperative recovery overall.[10] Well-controlled pain

postoperatively will enhance postoperative rehabilitation, which may improve short- and long-term recovery in addition to the quality of life after surgery.[11]

Beyond the perioperative period, postoperative pain may have long-term consequences as well. Poorly controlled postoperative pain may be an important predictive factor for the development of chronic postsurgical pain (CPSP),[12] defined as pain after a surgery lasting longer than the normal recuperative healing time. CPSP is a largely unrecognized problem that may occur in 10% to 65% of postoperative patients, with 2% to 10% of these patients experiencing severe CPSP.[13] Transition from acute to chronic pain occurs very quickly, and long-term behavioral and neurobiologic changes occur much earlier than previously anticipated.[14] CPSP is relatively common after surgical procedures such as limb amputation (30% to 83%), thoracotomy (22% to 67%), sternotomy (27%), breast surgery (11% to 57%), and gallbladder surgery (up to 56%).[15]

Improved understanding of the epidemiology and pathophysiology of postoperative pain has increased the use of multimodal management of pain in an effort to improve patient comfort, decrease perioperative morbidity, and reduce cost. Cost reduction is primarily achieved by shortening the time spent in postanesthesia care units (PACUs), intensive care units (ICUs), and hospitals. Multimodal approaches involve the use of multiple mechanistically distinct medications with the application of peripheral nerve or neuraxial analgesia. The added complexity of a true multimodal approach to perioperative pain requires the formation of perioperative pain management services, most often directed by an anesthesiologist or pain medicine physician.

COMMON TERMINOLOGY

- *Pain (nociception):* Pain is described as an unpleasant sensory and emotional experience caused by actual or potential tissue damage or described in terms of such damage.[16]
- *Acute pain:* Acute pain follows injury to the body and generally recedes when the bodily injury heals. For instance, acute pain occurs during the time needed for inflammation to subside or for acute injuries, such as lacerations or incisions, to repair with the union of separated tissues. It is often, but not always, associated with objective physical signs of autonomic nervous system activity (e.g., increased heart rate).
- *Chronic (persistent) pain:* Chronic pain is pain that has persisted beyond the time of healing.[16] The length of time is determined by the nature of the injury or surgical operation, but the pain is considered to be chronic (persistent) when it exceeds 3 months (or half the days in a 6-month period) in duration. Of note, CPSP is now a diagnosis in the International Classification of Diseases (ICD-11).[17]

V

- *Pain management:* Pain management is the clinical practice of relieving acute, subacute, and chronic (persistent) pain through the implementation of psychological, physical therapeutic, pharmacologic, and interventional (procedural) methods. Physicians, advanced practice clinicians (nurse practitioners and physician assistants), physical therapists, and psychologists commonly participate in pain management in inpatient and outpatient settings.

In-Hospital (Inpatient) Pain Service

- *Perioperative (acute) pain medicine service:* The perioperative pain medicine service is a team of highly specialized members who practice acute pain medicine and regional analgesic interventions for the patient who is about to undergo surgery, undergoing surgery, and in the process of recovery from surgery and in trauma-induced pain. The role of the perioperative pain physician is to reduce the pain resulting from surgery and minimize the period of recuperation and to inhibit the development of chronic (persistent) pain through early intervention. A revival of the concept of a transitional pain service is meant to provide overlap for acute pain in patients with chronic pain (acute on chronic pain) as they transition to ambulatory (outpatient) care.[18]
- *Chronic (persistent) pain medicine service:* The chronic pain medicine service is a multidisciplinary team of providers who treat chronic (persistent pain) and cancer pain using diverse treatment modalities, including psychological interventions, analgesic medications, and regional analgesic and chronic pain procedural interventions. The patient population served includes the perioperative patient with preoperative chronic/persistent pain issues, the inoperable patient with chronic/persistent pain issues, and patients who have not undergone surgery but have comorbid persistent pain. The role of the inpatient chronic pain physician is to attenuate the patient's pain, provide rationalized pain medication care, and transition the patient to outpatient pain care.
- Many institutions do not make the distinctions noted earlier and treat all patients within the hospital with pain regardless of modality of treatment, etiology of pain, or duration of pain. These institutions may call the service an inpatient pain service, and it can be staffed by regional anesthesiologists, pain physicians, advanced practice clinicians, or a combination of these individuals.

NEUROBIOLOGY OF PAIN

Nociception

Nociception involves the recognition and transmission of painful stimuli. Stimuli generated from thermal, mechanical, or chemical tissue damage may activate nociceptors, which are free afferent nerve endings of myelinated Aδ and unmyelinated C fibers. These peripheral afferent nerve endings send axonal projections into the dorsal horn of the spinal cord, where they synapse with second-order afferent neurons. Axonal projections of second-order neurons cross to the contralateral side of the spinal cord and ascend as afferent sensory pathways (e.g., spinothalamic tract) to the level of the thalamus.[19] Along the way, these neurons divide and send axonal projections to the reticular formation and periaqueductal gray matter. In the thalamus second-order neurons synapse with third-order neurons, which send axonal projections into the sensory cortex.

Surgical incision produces tissue injury, with consequent release of histamine and inflammatory mediators, such as peptides (e.g., bradykinin), lipids (e.g., prostaglandins), neurotransmitters (e.g., serotonin), and neurotrophins (e.g., nerve growth factor).[20] The release of inflammatory mediators activates peripheral nociceptors, which initiate transduction and transmission of nociceptive information to the central nervous system. Noxious stimuli are transduced by peripheral nociceptors and transmitted by Aδ and C nerve fibers from peripheral visceral and somatic sites to the dorsal horn of the spinal cord, where integration of peripheral nociceptive and descending inhibitory modulatory input (i.e., serotonin, norepinephrine, γ-aminobutyric acid [GABA], and enkephalin) or descending facilitatory input (i.e., cholecystokinin, excitatory amino acids, dynorphin) occurs. Further transmission of nociceptive information is determined by complex modulating influences in the spinal cord. Some impulses pass to the ventral and ventrolateral horns to initiate spinal reflex responses. These segmental responses may be associated with increased skeletal muscle tone, inhibition of phrenic nerve function, or even decreased gastrointestinal motility. Other signals are transmitted to higher centers through the spinothalamic and spinoreticular tracts, where they produce cortical responses to ultimately generate the perception of pain.

Modulation of Nociception

The question of how the disease of chronic pain develops from the symptom of acute pain remains unanswered. The traditional dichotomy between acute and chronic pain is somewhat arbitrary, as animal and clinical studies demonstrate that acute pain may become chronic pain. However, the duration of painful or noxious stimuli, type of stimuli, genetic or phenotypic makeup, or other possible factors leading to the transition from the symptom of acute pain to the disease of chronic pain remains unclear.

Noxious stimuli can produce expression of new genes (the basis for neuronal sensitization) in the dorsal horn of the spinal cord within 1 hour, and these changes are sufficient to alter behavior within the same time frame.[21,22]

Box 40.2 Endogenous Mediators of Inflammation
Prostaglandins (PGE$_1$ > PGE$_2$)
Histamine
Bradykinin
Serotonin
Acetylcholine
Lactic acid
Hydrogen ions
Potassium ions
PGE$_1$, PGE$_2$, prostaglandins E$_1$ and E$_2$

Box 40.3 Examples of Pain-Modulating Neurotransmitters
Excitatory
Glutamate
Aspartate
Vasoactive intestinal polypeptide
Cholecystokinin
Gastrin-releasing peptide
Angiotensin
Substance P
Inhibitory
Enkephalins
Endorphins
Somatostatin

Additionally, the intensity of acute postoperative pain is a significant predictor of chronic postoperative pain.[15] Continuous release of inflammatory mediators in the periphery sensitizes functional nociceptors and activates dormant nociceptors (Box 40.2).[14] Sensitization of peripheral nociceptors results in a decreased threshold for activation, increased discharge rate with activation, and increased rate of spontaneous discharge. Intense noxious input from the periphery may also produce central sensitization and hyperexcitability. Central sensitization is the development of "persistent post-injury changes in the central nervous system that result in pain hypersensitivity."[23] Hyperexcitability is the "exaggerated and prolonged responsiveness of neurons to normal afferent input after tissue damage."[23] Noxious input can trigger the cascade that leads to functional changes in the dorsal horn of the spinal cord and other sequelae. Ultimately, these changes may later cause postoperative pain to be perceived as more painful than would otherwise have been experienced. The neural circuitry in the dorsal horn is extremely complex, and we are just at the beginning of understanding the specific role of the various neurotransmitters and receptors in the process of nociception.[20,22]

Key receptors (e.g., N-methyl-D-aspartate [NMDA]) may play a significant role in the development of chronic pain after an acute injury. Neurotransmitters or second messenger effectors (e.g., substance P, protein kinase C-γ) may also play important roles in spinal cord sensitization and chronic pain (Box 40.3).[21] Our understanding of the neurobiology of nociception includes the dynamic integration and modulation of nociceptive transmission at several levels. Still, the specific roles of various receptors, neurotransmitters, and molecular structures in the process of nociception are not fully understood.

Preventive Analgesia

The development of central or peripheral sensitization after traumatic injury or surgical incision can result in amplification of postoperative pain.[3] Therefore preventing the establishment of altered central processing by analgesic treatment may, in the short term reduce postprocedural or traumatic pain and accelerate recovery. In the long term the benefits may include a reduction in chronic pain and improvement in the patient's quality of recovery and life satisfaction. Although the concept of preventive analgesia in decreasing postinjury pain is valid, the findings of clinical trials are mixed.[24-26]

The precise definition of preventive analgesia is one of the major controversies in perioperative pain medicine, contributing to the confusion regarding its clinical relevance. Preemptive analgesia can be defined as an analgesic intervention initiated before the noxious stimulus develops in order to block peripheral and central pain transmission.[27] Preventive analgesia can be functionally defined as an attempt to block pain transmission before the injury (incision), preventing the establishment of altered, and after the injury and throughout the recovery period. Preventive analgesia has been examined in trials of Enhanced Recovery After Surgery (ERAS).[28,29] Confining the definition of preemptive analgesia to only the immediate preoperative or early intraoperative (incisional) period may not be clinically relevant or appropriate because the inflammatory response may last well into the postoperative period and continue to maintain peripheral sensitization. However, preventive analgesia is a clinically relevant phenomenon. Katz and McCartney[12] described an analgesic benefit of preventive analgesia but no such benefit with the preemptive strategy. Maximal clinical benefit is observed when there is complete blockade of noxious stimuli, with extension of this blockade into the postoperative period. Central sensitization and persistent pain after surgical incision are predominantly maintained by the incoming barrage of sensitized peripheral pain fibers throughout the perioperative period,[30] which extend into the postsurgical recovery period. By preventing central sensitization and its prolongation by peripheral input, preventive analgesia, along with intensive multimodal analgesic interventions, could, theoretically, reduce acute postprocedure pain/hyperalgesia and therefore chronic pain after surgery.[15]

V

Multimodal Approach to Perioperative Recovery

A multimodal approach to analgesia is a broad definition that may include a combination of interventional analgesic techniques (epidural or peripheral nerve catheter or peripheral nerve block) and a combination of systemic pharmacologic therapies (nonsteroidal antiinflammatory drugs [NSAIDs], α-adrenergic agonists, NMDA receptor antagonists, membrane stabilizers, and opioid administration). Postprocedural or posttraumatic pain is best managed through this multimodal approach.[31]

The principles of a multimodal strategy include a sufficient improvement of the patient's pain to instill a sense of control over their pain, enable early mobilization, allow early enteral nutrition, and attenuate the perioperative stress response. The secondary goal of this approach is to maximize the benefit (analgesia) while minimizing the risk (side effects of the medication being used). These goals are often achieved through regional anesthetic techniques and a combination of analgesic medications. In amenable pain conditions epidural anesthesia and analgesia is an integral part of the multimodal strategy because of the superior analgesia and physiologic benefits conferred by epidural analgesia.[32] A multimodal approach involving a combination of neuraxial analgesia and systemic analgesics during recovery from radical prostatectomy resulted in a reduction of opioid use, lower pain scores, and decreased length of stay.[33] Patients undergoing major abdominal or thoracic procedures managed with a multimodal strategy have a reduction in hormonal and metabolic stress, preservation of total-body protein, shorter times to tracheal extubation, lower pain scores, earlier return of bowel function, and earlier achievement of criteria for discharge from the ICU.[34] Integrating the most recent data and techniques for surgery, anesthesiology, and pain treatment, the multimodal approach is an extension of clinical pathways or fast-track protocols by revamping traditional care programs into effective postoperative rehabilitation pathways.[34] This approach may decrease perioperative morbidity, decrease the length of hospital stay, and improve patient satisfaction without compromising safety. However, the widespread implementation of these programs requires multidisciplinary collaboration, changes in the traditional principles of postoperative care, additional resources, and expansion of the traditional acute pain service, all of which may be difficult in the current medical-economic climate.

Opioid-Induced Hyperalgesia

Short-term administration of opioids in the perioperative setting may lead to a paradoxical increase in the patient's pain severity and decrease in their pain tolerance.[9] This has been demonstrated in humans who received intraoperative opioid infusion for operative analgesia and in human and animal experimental models.[35] Although the clinical impact of opioid-induced hyperalgesia (OIH) has not been fully elucidated, the possibility of it contributing to acute postoperative pain should be considered. OIH has also been implicated as a risk for the development of CPSP, and the pro-nociceptive process involves the activation of the NMDA receptor.[35]

Opioid-Sparing Versus Opioid-Free Techniques

The desire for improved postoperative analgesic outcomes along with concern that short-term opioid use may lead to chronic opioid therapy in some patients in light of the opioid crisis has led to increasing interest in opioid-sparing and even opioid-free analgesic techniques. A recent review of opioid-sparing versus opioid-free approaches in the perioperative period concluded that although complete opioid sparing is possible in some contexts and procedures, there is no evidence that opioid-free strategies have lasting benefits above and beyond opioid-sparing techniques.[36] In fact, the risk of persistent postoperative opioid use was not found to differ between the opioid-sparing versus opioid-free approaches.[37]

Multimodal analgesic approaches can clearly reduce pain and opioid consumption in some settings. However, adjuvant medications are not free of undesirable effects or additional risks. For example, gabapentinoids, benzodiazepines, and "muscle relaxants" (e.g., baclofen) can produce additive or, in fact, potentiate opioid-induced respiratory depression. In a 2020 meta analysis of 281 randomized controlled trials comparing gabapentinoids with controls no clinical difference in acute, subacute, or chronic pain was observed, and the adverse events of dizziness and visual disturbance were greater with gabapentinoid use.[38]

The need to tailor the perioperative analgesic plan specific to the needs of the individual patient is critical. A patient's comorbidities and preoperative pain medication regimen, in addition to the specific surgical procedure being performed, should be taken into account when formulating an analgesic plan. The goal is to develop multimodal analgesia regimens that provide long-lasting benefit with improved recovery trajectories while optimizing drug selection to limit risks and side effects. Additional trials are needed to evaluate the short- and long-term benefits and risks of the perioperative use of opioid-sparing (and opioid-free) techniques.

ANALGESIC DELIVERY SYSTEMS

The traditional delivery systems for the management of perioperative pain include oral and parenteral on-demand administration of analgesics. Based on consensus guidelines and/or hospital-driven protocols, continuous

Table 40.1 Oral and Parenteral Analgesics for Treatment of Perioperative Pain

Agent	Route of Administration	Dose (mg)	Half-life (hr)	Onset (hr)	Analgesic Action (hr)	Peak Duration (hr)
Opioids and Opioid Derivatives						
Morphine	Intravenous	2.5–15	2–3.5	0.25	0.125	2–3
	Intramuscular	10–15	3	0.3	0.5–1.5	3–4
	Oral	30–60	3	0.5–1	1–2	4
Codeine	Oral	15–60	4	0.25–1	0.5–2	3–4
Hydromorphone	Intravenous	0.2–1.0	2–3	0.2–0.25	0.25	2–3
	Intramuscular	1–4	2–3	0.3–0.5	1	2–3
	Oral	1–4	2–3	0.5–1	1	3–4
Fentanyl	Intravenous	20–50 (µg)	0.5–1	5–10 min	5 min	1–1.5
	Transmucosal*	200–1600 (µg)	2–12	0.1–0.25	0.5–1	0.25–0.5
	Transdermal	12.5–100 (µg)	20–27	12–24	20–72	72
Oxymorphone	Oral	5–10	3.3–4.5	0.5	1	2–6
	Intravenous	0.5–1	3–5	0.15	0.25	3–6
	Subcutaneous	1–1.5	3–5	0.15	0.25	3–6
	Intramuscular	1–1.5	3–5	0.15	0.25	3–6
Hydrocodone	Oral	5–7.5	2–3	30	90	3–4
Oxycodone	Oral	5	3–5	0.5	1–2	4–6
Methadone	Oral	2.5–10	3–4	0.5–1	1.5–2	4–8
Other						
Tramadol†	Oral	50–100	5–6	0.5–1	1–2	4–6

*Transmucosal fentanyl is most appropriately reserved for breakthrough malignant (cancer) pain.
†Not classified by the U.S. Food and Drug Administration as an opioid; however, tramadol possesses naloxone partial-reversal analgesia.

intravenous (IV) infusions of analgesics such as ketamine and lidocaine are increasingly being used.[39] A patient-controlled analgesia (PCA) mechanism can be delivered via oral, IV, subcutaneous (SC), epidural, and intrathecal routes and by peripheral nerve catheter (Tables 40.1 to 40.3). This medication delivery technique is based on improved understanding of the neurophysiology of pain and the potential deleterious effects of postoperative pain. The formation of perioperative pain management services, directed by anesthesiologists with expertise in the pharmacology of analgesics and regional analgesia, has facilitated the widespread application of these techniques and improved the care of the postoperative patient.

Patient-Controlled Analgesia

When compared with traditional methods of intermittent intramuscular (IM) or IV injections of opioids to manage perioperative pain, PCA provides better analgesia with more safety, less total drug use, less sedation, fewer nocturnal sleep disturbances, and more rapid return to physical activity.[40] PCAs are designed to safely allow patient-administered analgesic medications. Upon activation of the delivery system, limits are placed on the number of doses per unit of time that will be administered to the patient. There is also a minimum time interval that must elapse between dose administrations (lockout interval). Also, a continuous background infusion superimposed on patient-controlled boluses can be implemented. Most patients determine a level of pain that is acceptable, and their dosage requirements taper as they recover. Patient acceptance of PCA is high because it restores the patient's autonomy. Some institutions employ pulse oximetry monitoring to assess the respiratory depression associated with opioid administration. Although better than having no specific monitor at all, pulse oximetry may not capture the relationship between respiratory depression and opioid administration. The addition of supplemental oxygen lowers the detection sensitivity of pulse oximetry as a monitor for respiratory depression and renders this monitor ineffective (also see Chapter 20). Capnography and respiratory rate are more

V

Table 40.2 Guidelines for Delivery Systems Used in Intravenous Patient-Controlled Analgesia

Drug Concentration	Size of Bolus*	Lockout Interval (min)	Continuous Infusion
Agonists			
Morphine (1 mg/mL)			
Adult	0.5–2.5 mg	5–10	—
Pediatric	0.01–0.03 mg/kg (max, 0.15 mg/kg/hr)	5–10	0.01–0.03 mg/kg/hr
Fentanyl (0.01 mg/mL)			
Adult	10–20 µg	4–10	—
Pediatric	0.5–1 µg/kg (max, 4 µg/kg/hr)	5–10	0.5–1 mg/kg/hr
Hydromorphone (0.2 mg/mL)			
Adult	0.05–0.25 mg	5–10	—
Pediatric	0.003–0.005 mg/kg (max, 0.02 mg/kg/hr)	5–10	0.003–0.005 mg/kg/hr
Alfentanil (0.1 mg/mL)	0.1–0.2 mg	5–8	—
Methadone (1 mg/mL)	0.5–2.5 mg	8–20	—
Oxymorphone (0.25 mg/mL)	0.2–0.4 mg	8–10	—
Sufentanil (0.002 mg/mL)	2–5 µg	4–10	—
Agonist-Antagonists			
Buprenorphine (0.03 mg/mL)	0.03–0.1 mg	8–20	—
Nalbuphine (1 mg/mL)	1–5 mg	5–15	—
Pentazocine (10 mg/mL)	5–30 mg	5–15	—

*All doses are for adult patients unless noted otherwise. Units vary across agents for size of the bolus (mg versus mg/kg vs. µg vs. µg/kg) and continuous infusion (mg/kg/hr versus mg/kg/hr). The anesthesia provider should proceed with titrated intravenous loading doses if necessary to establish initial analgesia. Individual patient requirements vary widely, with smaller doses typically given to elderly or critically ill patients. Continuous infusions are not initially recommended for opioid-naive adult patients.
Modified from Wu HE, Elkassabany, Wu. *Miller Anesthesia* 9th ed.

specific monitors of respiratory depression. However, capnography is not readily available in all institutions and is not needed universally for patients receiving opioid therapy. Capnography is best reserved for patients with substantial comorbidities that increase the risks associated with opioid therapy.

SYSTEMIC THERAPY

Oral Administration

Oral administration of analgesics is not optimal for the management of moderate to severe perioperative pain, primarily because of the nil per os (NPO) status of patients in the immediate postoperative period. Traditionally, postoperative patients are switched to oral analgesics (aspirin, acetaminophen, COX-1/COX-2 inhibitors, opioids) when pain has diminished to the extent that the need for rapid adjustments of analgesia level is unlikely.

The increased complexity of outpatient surgical procedures has introduced the need for perioperative analgesia plans that enable moderate to severe postoperative pain to be effectively treated in the outpatient setting. NSAIDs, although not effective when given alone preoperatively, are effective for acute postsurgical pain and CPSP when given as part of a preoperative polypharmacologic regimen. Preoperative administration of acetaminophen may improve acute postoperative pain but has not been shown to reduce CPSP. Amine reuptake inhibitors such as tricyclic antidepressants and serotonin-norepinephrine reuptake inhibitors (e.g., duloxetine) have received mixed evidence about their efficacy in acute postoperative pain or the prevention of CPSP. In a recent study of elective orthopedic surgery patients adding perioperative duloxetine 60 mg to a multimodal analgesia regimen significantly lowered total postoperative opioid consumption and reduced pain without significant adverse effects.[41] Preoperative and postoperative vitamin C has been found to reduce the incidence of complex regional

Table 40.3 Neuraxial Analgesics

Drug	Intrathecal or Subarachnoid Single Dose	Epidural Single Dose	Epidural Continuous Infusion
Opioid*			
Fentanyl	5-25 µg	50-100 µg	25-100 µg/hr
Sufentanil	2-10 µg	10-50 µg	10-20 µg/hr
Alfentanil	—	0.5-1 mg	0.2 mg/hr
Morphine	0.1-0.3 mg	1-5 mg	0.1-1 mg/hr
Hydromorphone	—	0.5-1 mg	0.1-0.2 mg/hr
Extended-release morphine†	Not recommended	5-15 mg	Not recommended
Local Anesthetic†			
Bupivacaine	5-15 mg	25-150 mg	1-25mg/hr
Ropivacaine	Not recommended	25-200 mg	6-20 mg/hr
Adjuvant Medications			
Clonidine	Not recommended	100-900 µg	10-50 µg/hr

*Doses are based on use of a neuraxial opioid alone. No continuous intrathecal or subarachnoid infusions are provided. Smaller doses may be effective when administered to the elderly or when injected in the cervical or thoracic region. Units vary across drugs for single dose (mg versus µg) and continuous infusion (mg/hr vs. µg/hr).

†Most commonly used in combination with an opioid, in which case the total dose of local anesthetic is reduced.
Modified from "Wu HE, Elkassabany, Wu. *Miller Anesthesia* 9th ed.

pain syndrome (CRPS) after orthopedic extremity surgery. A systematic review found moderate-level evidence supporting the use of a 2-g preoperative dose of vitamin C as an adjunct for reducing postoperative morphine consumption and high-level evidence supporting perioperative vitamin C supplementation of 1 g per day for 50 days for CRPS I prevention.[42]

The use of gabapentinoids, which were heavily used in multimodal analgesia protocols, has since been challenged. The evidence of harm and risk has grown without significant gains in benefit. Perioperative gabapentinoid use has been found to be associated with greater postoperative respiratory depression, noninvasive ventilation, and naloxone use.[43] In fact, when gabapentinoids are combined with opioids, the risk of respiratory depression is even greater than when opioids are administered alone. Thus the routine use of perioperative gabapentinoids for treatment of postoperative pain is no longer supported.[38] This change in practice highlights the need for further evidence-based studies of nonopioid analgesics in the perioperative setting.

Intravenous Administration

Intermittent IV administration of small doses of opioids (see Table 40.1 and Table 40.2) is commonly used to treat acute and severe pain in the PACU or ICU, where continuous nursing surveillance and monitoring are available. With a small IV dose of an opioid, the time delay for analgesia and the variability in plasma concentrations

characteristic of IM injections are minimized. Rapid redistribution of the opioid produces a shorter duration of analgesia after a single IV administration than after an IM injection.

Ketamine is traditionally recognized as an intraoperative anesthetic; however, it is also effective in small (subanesthetic or analgesic—up to 15 µg/kg/min) dose infusions for postoperative analgesia partly because of its direct analgesic properties through antagonism of the NMDA receptor. Ketamine also reduces the OIH associated with intraoperative opioid infusion.[35] Patients receiving large doses of opioids may experience hyperalgesia, resulting in increased excitatory amino acid release in the spinal cord. Ketamine directly inhibits the actions of the excitatory amino acids and reverses OIH, leading to improved postoperative pain. A preoperative IV ketamine bolus dose of 0.5 mg/kg followed by an intraoperative infusion of subanesthetic (4 to 5 µg/kg/min) ketamine reduces postoperative pain and CPSP. This indirect antihyperalgesic effect may occur through suppression of central sensitization.[44] The benefit of subanesthetic dosing of ketamine also includes a decrease in postoperative nausea or vomiting, with minimal adverse effects. Subanesthetic ketamine infusions do not cause hallucinations or cognitive impairment. The incidence of side effects, such as dizziness, itching, nausea, or vomiting, is comparable to that seen with opioids. Therefore, the use of perioperative ketamine in patients, especially at high risk for the development of CPSP, is warranted.[29,39]

V

Lidocaine, with its short half-life of 90 to 120 minutes, is the local anesthetic of choice for continuous IV infusions for both intraoperative anesthetic and postoperative analgesia. However, caution must be used in patients with delayed elimination because of hepatic or renal insufficiency, which may cause drug accumulation and lead to local anesthetic toxicity. The reported benefits of perioperative lidocaine infusions have included reductions in pain scores, nausea, ileus duration, opioid requirements, and length of hospital stay. Lidocaine's mechanism of action for postoperative analgesic benefits is not fully understood, but likely goes beyond its function as a sodium channel blocker, given its persistent effects for many hours or even days after termination of the infusion. Lidocaine is likely involved in inflammatory signaling through the blockade of the priming of the polymorphonuclear granulocyte in addition to neuronal effects by blocking the excitatory responses of glycine in wide-dynamic-range neurons.[45] Perioperative lidocaine infusions are commonly used in doses ranging from 1.5 to 3 mg/kg/hr or 40 µg/kg/min after an induction bolus of 1.0 mg/kg intraoperatively. Postoperative infusions are commonly run at 0.5 to 1.0 mg/min. Current meta analyses have shown that perioperative lidocaine infusions are likely beneficial, but also suggest that their clinical effectiveness differ based on the surgical procedure.[45] Toxicity from perioperative lidocaine infusion in these dose ranges is rare but may present with symptoms of tinnitus, perioral numbness, and cardiac dysrhythmias.

Acetaminophen can be given IV in addition to orally and rectally. This has increased the ability to provide additional nonopioid analgesia to patients who are NPO but refuse rectal administration. Despite assumptions that IV preparations are more potent or effective, to date no clinical trial has demonstrated a difference in efficacy between oral and IV formulations.[46] Although the formulations differ in bioavailability and time to onset of analgesia, IV dosing has not been associated with improved efficacy and is associated with increased cost.

Preoperative administration of dexamethasone decreases acute postoperative pain scores and decreases opioid consumption.[47] There appears to be dose dependence of this benefit with increased efficacy at doses >10 mg. Intraoperative administration of clonidine decreases postoperative pain, but bradycardia and hypotension limit the benefits of its modest analgesic properties. Intraoperative magnesium administration is associated with reduction of postoperative pain or opioid requirements.[48] The mechanism of action is thought to be through the accentuation of blockade of the NMDA receptor.

Subcutaneous Administration

SC administration of select medications (e.g., hydromorphone) is highly efficacious and is a practical approach for providing analgesia in patients without IV access or those in need of long-term, home-based analgesic care. Hydromorphone exhibits the same pharmacokinetics whether it is administered subcutaneously or intravenously. This route of administration is primarily used in palliative care populations.

Transmucosal Administration

Transmucosal delivery of analgesics, such as fentanyl, may serve as an alternative to the oral administration of NSAIDs and opioids, especially when a rapid onset of drug effect is desirable. However, these medications rarely have a role in the management of postoperative pain because IV, IM, SC, or PO delivery routes are sufficient for the delivery of analgesic medications.

Perioperative Management of Buprenorphine

In light of the opioid epidemic, an increasing number of patients are receiving medication-assisted treatment for opioid use disorder (OUD). The U.S. Food and Drug Administration (FDA) has approved three medications for the treatment of opioid dependence: methadone, naltrexone, and buprenorphine. This section addresses the challenges in perioperative pain management of patients receiving buprenorphine for OUD and/or chronic pain. Patients taking buprenorphine-containing medications have similar challenges to the opioid-tolerant patient in the perioperative setting, but also present challenges related to the partial mu-opioid agonist pharmacodynamics of buprenorphine. Although buprenorphine is a partial agonist, when given in conjunction with a full mu-opioid agonist, it functions as a pharmacologic antagonist (also see Chapter 9). Buprenorphine also possesses variable time to dissociation from the opioid receptor; therefore when used in combination with a full agonist (e.g., morphine, hydromorphone, oxycodone), its action as an antagonist may abate unpredictably. This can develop a dangerous situation in which previously appropriate dosages of one of the full agonists is now enough to result in respiratory depression or other dose-related adverse events.

Although it is ideal to discontinue buprenorphine 3-5 days in advance of surgery in patients taking it for chronic pain treatment, it is often not feasible in many of our surgical settings in which patients are first seen by the anesthesia provider immediately before the operation. Discontinuing buprenorphine in a patient with OUD can precipitate withdrawal symptoms, and substitution of a full opioid agonist may provoke OUD relapse. In patients with OUD, presurgical planning is necessary to avoid major complications from resultant full agonist opioid therapy, including precipitating patient cravings and subsequent relapse.[49] If a patient has not discontinued their buprenorphine therapy well in advance of surgery, they should receive their baseline buprenorphine via sublingual or transdermal routes.

Alternatively, and if necessary, the provider can convert the patient's buprenorphine requirements to the IV equivalent dose of buprenorphine while the patient is in the immediate perioperative period. While the patient is maintained on a stable dosage of buprenorphine, additional full agonist opioids may be titrated to pain reduction. Alternatively, nonopioid adjuvants, including clonidine, ketamine,[50,51] lidocaine, or dexmedetomidine, can be used instead of opioids for the patient's postoperative pain. In patients with OUD Some authors suggest stopping buprenorphine preoperatively and switching to a short-acting opioid or methadone to prevent withdrawal symptoms if the surgery is major and will generate severe pain. The choice of methadone is a reasonable one, as it is an effective full opioid agonist but also has a long half-life, thereby providing benefit for continuation of medication-assisted therapy.

Regardless of the approach, coordinated communication between the pain team, surgical service, and the primary buprenorphine prescriber should take place to make sure that the patient eventually goes back to their prescribed buprenorphine dose.[50] Sometimes, the logistics of this process can be difficult. Therefore more often than not, anesthesia providers opt to continue buprenorphine perioperatively and optimize all components of multimodal analgesia for postoperative pain management. Regional anesthesia and local infiltration techniques should be used whenever feasible in these patients (Table 40.4).[51]

NEURAXIAL ANALGESIA (ALSO SEE CHAPTER 17)

A variety of neuraxial (intrathecal and epidural) and peripheral regional analgesic techniques are employed for postoperative pain. In general, when compared with systemic opioids, neuraxial and peripheral regional analgesia techniques can provide superior analgesia, especially when local anesthetics are applied; furthermore, these techniques may decrease morbidity and mortality rates.[52] Clinical judgment is required when using these techniques in the presence of various anticoagulants (see later discussion). The benefits and risks of the analgesic techniques used for each patient must be weighed based on the patient's medical history, including preoperative opioid and nonopioid pain medication use in addition to the specific surgery being performed.

Table 40.4 Perioperative Management of Buprenorphine

Preoperative Assessment	Intraoperative Plan	Postoperative Management	Hospital Discharge
- Past medical history, including chronic pain history - Medications: to include buprenorphine dose and route - Physical examination - Timing of surgery (>3 days consider holding buprenorphine) - If **cannot** discontinue buprenorphine therapy well in advance of surgery, the patient should receive their **baseline** buprenorphine via sublingual or transdermal routes - Buprenorphine prescribing provider - Establish goals of care	- Continue buprenorphine therapy as needed based on the preoperative assessment and plan - If necessary, convert the patient's buprenorphine requirements to the intravenous equivalent of buprenorphine for increased post operative pain needs - Multimodal analgesia strategies (regional, NSAIDs/acetaminophen, ketamine, lidocaine, PCA, etc.) - Full opioid agonists with caution, as may require higher dose	- Continue buprenorphine therapy as needed based on the preoperative assessment and plan - If necessary, convert the patient's buprenorphine requirements to the intravenous equivalent of buprenorphine - Multimodal analgesia strategies (regional, NSAIDs/acetaminophen, ketamine, lidocaine, PCA, etc.) - Full opioid agonists with caution, as may require higher dose - Consider converting buprenorphine to methadone if able to prevent acute withdrawal - Coordinated communication between the acute pain team, surgical service, and the primary buprenorphine prescriber	- Continue on preoperative buprenorphine dose - Continue multimodal analgesia pain management - Establish follow-up with pain team/buprenorphine prescribing provider - Confirm strong social support in place for patient - Provide written instructions for pain regimen and contact phone numbers - Rediscuss goals of care

Intrathecal Administration

Intrathecal administration of an opioid can provide short-term to intermediate-length postoperative analgesia after a single injection. The intrathecal route offers the advantage of precise and reliable placement of low concentrations of the drug near its site of action. The onset of analgesic effects after intrathecal opioid administration is directly proportional to the lipid solubility of the drug. Duration of effect is longer with more hydrophilic compounds. Morphine produces peak analgesic effects in 20 to 60 minutes and postoperative analgesia for 12 to 36 hours. Adding a small dose of fentanyl to the morphine-containing opioid solution may speed the onset of analgesic effect. For lower abdominal procedures performed with spinal anesthesia (e.g., cesarean section), morphine may be added to the local anesthetic solution to increase the duration of analgesia.

The primary disadvantage of an intrathecal opioid injection is the lack of flexibility inherent to a single-shot modality. Clinicians must either repeat the injection or consider other options when the analgesic effect of the initial dose diminishes. The practical aspects of leaving a catheter in the intrathecal space for either continuous or repeated intermittent opioid injections is controversial, especially in view of reports of cauda equina syndrome after continuous spinal anesthesia with hyperbaric local anesthetic solutions injected through a small-diameter catheter.

Epidural Administration

Continuous infusion of a local anesthetic through an epidural catheter is a common method of providing perioperative analgesia. Epidural infusion of local anesthetic alone may be used for postoperative analgesia and may be done to avoid opioid-related side effects. However, there is a significant failure rate (from regression of sensory block and inadequate analgesia) and relatively frequent incidence of motor block and hypotension. Pain control is generally more effective with combined local anesthetic and opioid epidural infusion.

The benefit of opioid monotherapy (i.e., without local anesthetic) in epidural infusions is that they generally do not cause motor block or hypotension from sympathetic blockade. There are mechanistic differences between continuous epidural infusions of lipophilic (e.g., fentanyl, sufentanil) and hydrophilic (e.g., morphine, hydromorphone) opioids. The analgesic site of action (spinal vs. systemic) for continuous epidural infusions of lipophilic opioids is not clear, although several randomized clinical trials suggest that it is systemic[53] because there were no differences in plasma concentrations, side effects, or pain scores between those who received IV or epidural infusions of fentanyl. A continuous infusion rather than an intermittent bolus of epidural opioids may provide superior analgesia with fewer side effects. Hydrophilic opioid epidural infusions have a spinal mechanism of action.

The impact of epidural analgesia with local anesthetics is dependent on the total dose administered rather than the volume or concentration; therefore a higher-concentration local anesthetic delivered in a small volume is functionally equivalent to that of a low concentration in a higher volume.

Clinical efficacy of epidural analgesia (local anesthetic with and without opioids) for abdominal surgeries has demonstrated superior pain relief in the initial postoperative period, with fewer gastrointestinal-related side effects compared with systemic opioid therapy; however, there is an increased incidence of pruritus. Epidural analgesia is beneficial for major joint surgery of the lower extremity but has the associated disadvantages of neuraxial analgesia. Thoracic epidural analgesia has been the mainstay of analgesia for thoracotomy, but paravertebral blockades may be just as effective with a more favorable side effect profile.[54] One of the primary benefits of epidural analgesia for traumatic rib fractures is the decreased duration of mechanical ventilation when compared with using a local anesthetic alone (e.g., intercostal nerve block).

Side Effects of Neuraxial Analgesic Drugs

Many medication-related (opioid and local anesthetic) side effects can occur with postoperative epidural analgesia. When side effects are suspected, the patient's overall clinical status should be evaluated so that serious comorbidities are not inappropriately attributed to epidural analgesia. The differential diagnosis for a patient with neuraxial analgesia and hypotension should also include hypovolemia, bleeding, and a decreased cardiac output. Patients with respiratory depression should also be evaluated for acute stroke, pulmonary edema, and evolving sepsis. Standing orders and nursing protocols for analgesic regimens, neurologic monitoring, treatment of side effects, and physician notification about critical variables should be required for all patients receiving neuraxial and other types of postoperative analgesia.

Most Common Side Effects

The most frequent side effects of neuraxial analgesia are described in Box 40.4. Although respiratory depression and hypotension are the most life-threatening of the side effects, the others can be particularly troublesome to patients.

Anticoagulants

The concurrent use of anticoagulants with neuraxial anesthesia and analgesia has always been a controversial

---

Box 40.4 Most Common Side Effects of Neuraxial Analgesia for Perioperative Pain Management

- *Urinary retention* (10%-30%): Epidural administration of local anesthetics and/or opioids is associated with urinary retention.
- *Nausea, vomiting, and pruritus* (15%-18%): Pruritus is one of the most common side effects of epidural or intrathecal administration of opioids, with an incidence of approximately 60% compared with about 15%-18% for local epidural anesthetic administration or systemic opioids.
- *Motor block* (2%-3%): In most cases motor block resolves within 2 hr after discontinuing the epidural infusion. Persistent or increasing motor block should be promptly evaluated, and spinal hematoma, spinal abscess, and intrathecal catheter migration should be considered as part of the differential diagnosis.
- *Hypotension* (0.3%-7%): Local anesthetics used in an epidural analgesic regimen may block sympathetic fibers and contribute to postoperative hypotension.
- *Respiratory depression* (0.1%-0.9%): Neuraxial opioids administered in appropriate doses are not associated with a more frequent incidence of respiratory depression than that seen with systemic administration of opioids. Risk factors for respiratory depression with neuraxial opioids include larger dose, geriatric age group, concomitant administration of systemic opioids or sedatives, the possibility of prolonged or extensive surgery, the presence of comorbidities, and thoracic surgery.

---

issue in anesthesia management. Traditionally, the incidence of spinal hematoma is estimated at approximately 1 in 150,000 for epidural block, with a less frequent incidence of 1 in 220,000 for spinal blocks.[55] Low-molecular-weight heparin was used in Europe without significant problems before its introduction in North America. However, the incidence of spinal hematoma increased to as frequent as 1 in 40,800 for spinal anesthetics and 1 in 6600 for epidural anesthetics (1 in 3100 for postoperative epidural analgesia) in the United States between 1993 and 1998. The estimate of the more frequent incidence of spinal hematomas after epidural catheter removal is based in part on the FDA's MedWatch data, which suggest that epidural catheter removal may be a traumatic event, although this is still a relatively controversial issue.

The different types and classes of anticoagulants vary in pharmacokinetic properties that affect the timing of neuraxial catheter or needle insertion and catheter removal. Despite a number of observational and retrospective studies investigating the incidence of spinal hematoma in the setting of various anticoagulants and neuraxial techniques, there is no definitive conclusion regarding the absolute safety of neuraxial anesthesia with anticoagulation.

The American Society of Regional Anesthesia and Pain Medicine (ASRA) lists a series of consensus statements, based on the available literature, for the administration (insertion and removal) of neuraxial techniques in the presence of various anticoagulants, including oral anticoagulants (warfarin), antiplatelet agents, fibrinolytics-thrombolytics, standard unfractionated heparin, and low-molecular-weight heparin. The ASRA consensus statements include the concepts that (1) the timing of neuraxial needle or catheter insertion or removal should reflect the pharmacokinetic properties of the specific anticoagulant, (2) frequent neurologic monitoring is essential, (3) concurrent administration of multiple anticoagulants may increase the risk of bleeding, and (4) the analgesic regimen should be tailored to facilitate neurologic monitoring, which may be continued in some cases for 24 hours after epidural catheter removal. An updated version of the ASRA consensus statements on neuraxial anesthesia and anticoagulation[56,57] can be found on their website (www.asra.com), with some of these statements addressing the newer anticoagulants.

Infection

Infection associated with postoperative epidural analgesia may result from exogenous or endogenous sources. Serious infections (e.g., meningitis, spinal abscess) associated with epidural analgesia are rare (<1 in 10,000), although some researchers report a more frequent incidence (approximately 1 in 1000 to 1 in 2000).[58] Closer examination of the studies that report a more frequent incidence of epidural abscesses reveal that the patients had a relatively longer duration of epidural analgesia or the presence of coexisting immunocompromising or complicating diseases (e.g., malignancy, trauma). Use of epidural analgesia in the general surgical population, with a typical duration of postoperative catheterization of approximately 2 to 4 days, is generally not associated with epidural abscess formation. A trial of postoperative epidural analgesia (mean catheterization of 6.3 days) in more than 4000 surgical cancer patients did not reveal any abscesses.

SURGICAL SITE (INCISION) INFILTRATION

Surgical site infiltration with local anesthetic before incision and before tissue closure is recommended for the reduction of postoperative pain.[59] Liposomal bupivacaine was approved in 2011 for surgical site administration after bunionectomy and hemorrhoidectomy. Although this extended-release formulation is designed to slowly release bupivacaine to surrounding tissues over 96 hours, it was superior to placebo only for the first 24 hours after administration.[60]

INTRAARTICULAR ADMINISTRATION

Intraarticular injection of opioids may provide analgesia for up to 24 hours postoperatively and prevent the development of CPSP. Opioid receptors are found in the peripheral terminals of primary afferent nerves, which may explain this improved analgesia despite the lack of response with the addition of opioids to perineural anesthetic injections. The analgesic benefit of intraarticular opioids over systemic administration has not been demonstrated, and the systemic analgesic effect of these injections has not been excluded. Extended-release bupivacaine was found to be less effective than traditional local anesthetic and opioid infiltration in one study and no different from traditional bupivacaine alone in another.[60] Glenohumeral intraarticular continuous catheters have been associated with chondrolysis when bupivacaine is used and therefore should be avoided.[61]

PARAVERTEBRAL BLOCKS

The increased use of paravertebral blockade can be directly correlated with the beneficial effects for patients undergoing breast surgery. This block provides an effective mechanism for controlling acute pain associated with this procedure but has also demonstrated benefit in decreasing the development of CPSP over other analgesic regimens.[62] This technique can be performed as a single-shot technique or as a continuous catheter infusion to provide ongoing perioperative analgesia. This use of this technique has expanded to thoracic, cardiac, and pediatric applications.[63]

PERIPHERAL NERVE BLOCK

Peripheral nerve blockade can provide analgesia as part of an autonomous or multimodal pain regimen (also see Chapter 18). Single-shot injections can provide coverage for intraoperative pain control. However, many providers feel that the risk of the intervention warrants the prolonged benefit, which includes postoperative pain control, and have driven the need for flexible duration of action. Intermediate-term pain relief (<24 hours) can be achieved with a combination of a local anesthetic and adjuvant drugs in a single injection. Longer-acting pain control may be indicated by the surgical technique, rehabilitation needs, and patient comorbidities and can be achieved by using perineural catheters for continuous local anesthetic infusions.

Techniques

Nerve blocks can be inserted using anatomic landmarks, nerve stimulation, and ultrasound guidance. The efficacy between ultrasound-guided techniques and nerve stimulation varies, depending on the skill of the provider, primarily resulting in differences in comfort during placement and procedural time of the blockade. Nonetheless, these techniques provide a comparable quality of analgesia and similar complication profile.[64]

Adjuvant Drugs

Commonly used adjuvant drugs include epinephrine, clonidine, dexmedetomidine, and opioids.[65] Epinephrine for peripheral nerve blockade significantly increases the duration of the blockade with minimal side effects. The mechanism of this effect is primarily through vasoconstriction. Epinephrine can also increase the sensitivity of intravascular injection; concentrations of 2.5 to 5 µg/mL are generally used. Opioids probably should not be added to a peripheral nerve blockade. Clonidine is beneficial in extending the duration of preoperative blockade but has less value with perineural catheters. The mechanism is most likely peripheral α_2-adrenergic receptor–mediated and dose-dependent. Clonidine is a better preemptive analgesic when added to a local anesthetic block than when used as a single drug. Side effects, including hypotension, bradycardia, and sedation, are less likely to occur in doses <1.5 µg/kg.[66] The use of clonidine increases the duration of analgesia and motor blockade by approximately 2 hours. More recently, the addition of dexmedetomidine to peripheral nerve blocks has been shown to improve analgesia duration and opioid reduction.[67]

REGIONAL ANALGESIA

Efficacy and safety are the primary limiting factors in the implementation of any therapeutic measure. Regional analgesia is an effective technique for perioperative pain control and a multimodal analgesic plan. The advantages, disadvantages, and technical details are discussed in detail in Chapter 18. This section focuses on the utility and comparative efficacy of these blocks in perioperative pain management.

Catheter Versus Single-Shot Techniques

Upper Extremity
Continuous interscalene blockade allows for a longer duration of action compared with single-shot techniques. This technique has increased utility with the posterior interscalene approach for moderate to severely painful shoulder surgeries. The continuous administration allows for increased pain relief, with minimal opioid supplementation and increased patient satisfaction and sleep quality.[68]

Lower Extremity

Lower extremity orthopedic surgeries resulting in moderate to severe perioperative pain also benefit from long-acting regional techniques. Lower extremity perineural catheters are used for major joint surgery of the hip, knee, ankle, and foot. This type of catheter may decrease clinical signs of inflammation for some lower extremity procedures, although inflammation is not decreased at the cellular level. Epidural catheters are used to provide good analgesia for major joint surgeries of the lower extremities, but expose patients to neuraxial analgesia risks and generally have bilateral effects (whereas surgery is typically limited to one extremity only). Lumbar plexus catheters have been used as part of a multimodal regimen, with better pain scores at rest and with physical therapy than multimodal regimens that include PCA with or without femoral catheters for unilateral hip repairs.[69] Patients undergoing major foot and ankle surgeries under continuous perineural blockade are not only potentially able to obtain pain relief comparable to single-shot and systemic analgesia but also are discharged from PACUs in a shorter period.[70]

TRANSVERSUS ABDOMINIS PLANE BLOCK

For many abdominal procedures, the use of neuraxial analgesia techniques has been replaced by the transversus abdominis plane (TAP) block. Theoretical advantages of this technique over other modalities include avoidance of both neuraxial involvement and lower extremity blockade, decreased urinary retention, and decreased systemic side effects. Compared with placebo blocks, TAP block provided increased analgesia and decreased systemic medication requirements as part of a multimodal analgesic regimen for total abdominal hysterectomy, cesarean section, and laparoscopic cholecystectomy. Moreover, guidance by ultrasound has made this a more reliably efficacious treatment modality.[71]

REFERENCES

1. Buvanendran A, Fiala J, Patel KA, Golden AD, Moric M, Kroin JS. The incidence and severity of postoperative pain following inpatient surgery. *Pain Med.* 2015;16:2277–2283.
2. Apfelbaum JL, Chen C, Mehta SS, Gan TJ. Postoperative pain experience: Results from a national survey suggest postoperative pain continues to be undermanaged. *Anesth Analg.* 2003;97:534–540.
3. Glare P, Aubrey KR, Myles PS. Transition from acute to chronic pain after surgery. *Lancet.* 2019;393:1537–1546.
4. Wanderer JP, Shi Y, Schildcrout JS, Ehrenfeld JM, Epstein RH. Supervising anesthesiologists cannot be effectively compared according to their patients' postanesthesia care unit admission pain scores. *Anesth Analg.* 2015;120:923–932.
5. The Lancet. Best practice in managing postoperative pain. *Lancet.* 2019;393:1478.
6. Chou R, Gordon DB, de Leon-Casasola OA, et al. Management of postoperative pain: A clinical practice guideline from the American Pain Society, the American Society of Regional Anesthesia and Pain Medicine, and the American Society of Anesthesiologists' Committee on Regional Anesthesia, Executive Committee, and Administrative Council. *J Pain.* 2016;17:131–157.
7. Eisenach JC, Brennan TJ. Pain after surgery. *Pain.* 2018;159:1010–1011.
8. Sceats LA, Ayakta N, Merrell SB, Kin C. Drivers, beliefs, and barriers surrounding surgical opioid prescribing: A qualitative study of surgeons' opioid prescribing habits. *J Surg Res.* 2020;247:86–94.
9. Colvin LA, Bull F, Hales TG. Perioperative opioid analgesia-when is enough too much? A review of opioid-induced tolerance and hyperalgesia. *Lancet.* 2019;393:1558–1568.
10. Scholz J, Yaksh TL. Preclinical research on persistent postsurgical pain: What we don't know, but should start studying. *Anesthesiology.* 2010;112:511–513.
11. Kent ML, Tighe PJ, Belfer I, et al. The ACTTION-APS-AAPM Pain Taxonomy (AAAPT) multidimensional approach to classifying acute pain conditions. *J Pain.* 2017;18:479–489.
12. Katz J, McCartney CJ. Current status of preemptive analgesia. *Curr Opin Anaesthesiol.* 2002;15:435–441.
13. Kehlet H, Jensen TS, Woolf CJ. Persistent postsurgical pain: Risk factors and prevention. *Lancet.* 2006;367:1618–1625.
14. Carr DB, Goudas LC. Acute pain. *Lancet.* 1999;353:2051–2058.
15. Perkins FM, Kehlet H. Chronic pain as an outcome of surgery. A review of predictive factors. *Anesthesiology.* 2000;93:1123–1133.
16. Merskey H. Pain and psychological medicine. In: Wall PD, Melzack R, eds. *Textbook of Pain.* 3rd ed. New York: Churchill Livingstone; 1994:903–920.
17. Treede RD, Rief W, Barke A, et al. Chronic pain as a symptom or a disease: The IASP Classification of Chronic Pain for the International Classification of Diseases (ICD-11). *Pain.* 2019;160:19–27.
18. Katz J, Weinrib A, Fashler SR, et al. The Toronto General Hospital Transitional Pain Service: Development and implementation of a multidisciplinary program to prevent chronic postsurgical pain. *J Pain Res.* 2015;8:695–702.
19. Basbaum AI, Fields HL. Endogenous pain control systems: Brainstem spinal pathways and endorphin circuitry. *Annu Rev Neurosci.* 1984;7:309–338.
20. Julius D, Basbaum AI. Molecular mechanisms of nociception. *Nature.* 2001; 413:203–210.
21. Basbaum AI. Spinal mechanisms of acute and persistent pain. *Reg Anesth Pain Med.* 1999;24:59–67.
22. Besson JM. The neurobiology of pain. *Lancet.* 1999;353:1610–1615.
23. Kissin I. Preemptive analgesia. *Anesthesiology.* 2000;93:1138–1143.
24. Moiniche S, Kehlet H, Dahl JB. A qualitative and quantitative systematic review of preemptive analgesia for postoperative pain relief: The role of timing of analgesia. *Anesthesiology.* 2002;96: 725–741.
25. Dahl JB, Moiniche S. Pre-emptive analgesia. *Br Med Bull.* 2004;71:13–27.
26. Ong CK, Lirk P, Seymour RA, Jenkins BJ. The efficacy of preemptive analgesia

V

for acute postoperative pain management: A meta-analysis. *Anesth Analg.* 2005;100:757–773.

27. Chidambaran V, Ashton M, Martin LJ, Jegga AG. Systems biology-based approaches to summarize and identify novel genes and pathways associated with acute and chronic postsurgical pain. *J Clin Anesth.* 2020;62:109738.

28. Beverly A, Kaye AD, Ljungqvist O, Urman RD. Essential elements of multimodal analgesia in Enhanced Recovery After Surgery (ERAS) guidelines. *Anesthesiol Clin.* 2017;35:e115–e143.

29. Gelman D, Gelmanas A, Urbanaitė D, et al. Role of multimodal analgesia in the evolving Enhanced Recovery After Surgery pathways. *Medicina (Kaunas).* 2018;54:20.

30. Pogatzki-Zahn EM, Zahn PK. From preemptive to preventive analgesia. *Curr Opin Anaesthesiol.* 2006;19:551–555.

31. Kehlet H. Multimodal approach to control postoperative pathophysiology and rehabilitation. *Br J Anaesth.* 1997;78:606–617.

32. Block BM, Liu SS, Rowlingson AJ, Cowan AR, Cowan JA Jr., Wu CL. Efficacy of postoperative epidural analgesia: A meta-analysis. *JAMA.* 2003;290:2455–2463.

33. Ben-David B, Swanson J, Nelson JB, Chelly JE. Multimodal analgesia for radical prostatectomy provides better analgesia and shortens hospital stay. *J Clin Anesth.* 2007;19:264–268.

34. Kehlet H, Wilmore DW. Multimodal strategies to improve surgical outcome. *Am J Surg.* 2002;183:630–641.

35. Joly V, Richebe P, Guignard B, et al. Remifentanil-induced postoperative hyperalgesia and its prevention with small-dose ketamine. *Anesthesiology.* 2005;103:147–155.

36. Kharasch ED, Clark JD. Opioid-free anesthesia: Time to regain our balance. *Anesthesiology.* 2021;134:509–514.

37. Shanthanna H, Ladha KS, Kehlet H, Joshi GP. Perioperative opioid administration. *Anesthesiology.* 2021;134:645–659.

38. Verret M, Lauzier F, Zarychanski R, et al. Perioperative use of gabapentinoids for the management of postoperative acute pain: A systematic review and meta-analysis. *Anesthesiology.* 2020;133:265–279.

39. Schwenk ES, Viscusi ER, Buvanendran A, et al. Consensus Guidelines on the Use of Intravenous Ketamine Infusions for Acute Pain Management from the American Society of Regional Anesthesia and Pain Medicine, the American Academy of Pain Medicine, and the American Society of Anesthesiologists. *Reg Anesth Pain Med.* 2018;43:456–466.

40. Egbert AM, Parks LH, Short LM, Burnett ML. Randomized trial of postoperative patient-controlled analgesia vs intramuscular narcotics in frail elderly men. *Arch Intern Med.* 1990;150:1897–1903.

41. Branton MW, Hopkins TJ, Nemec EC. Duloxetine for the reduction of opioid use in elective orthopedic surgery: A systematic review and meta-analysis. *Int J Clin Pharm.* 2021. doi:10.1007/s11096-020-01216-9. Jan 18, In Press.

42. Chen S, Roffey DM, Dion C-A, Arab A, Wai EK. Effect of perioperative vitamin C supplementation on postoperative pain and the incidence of chronic regional pain syndrome. *Clin J Pain.* 2016;32:179–185.

43. Kharasch ED, Clark JD, Kheterpal S. Perioperative gabapentinoids. *Anesthesiology.* 2020;133:251–254.

44. De Kock M, Lavand'homme P, Waterloos H. "Balanced analgesia" in the perioperative period: Is there a place for ketamine? *Pain.* 2001;92:373–380.

45. Dunn LK, Durieux ME. Perioperative use of intravenous lidocaine. *Anesthesiology.* 2017;126:729–737.

46. Jibril F, Sharaby S, Mohamed A, Wilby KJ. Intravenous versus oral acetaminophen for pain: Systematic review of current evidence to support clinical decision-making. *Can J Hosp Pharm.* 2015;68:238–247.

47. Nielsen RV, Siegel H, Fomsgaard JS, et al. Preoperative dexamethasone reduces acute but not sustained pain after lumbar disk surgery: A randomized, blinded, placebo-controlled trial. *Pain.* 2015;156:2538–2544.

48. De Oliveira GS Jr, Castro-Alves LJ, Khan JH, McCarthy RJ. Perioperative systemic magnesium to minimize postoperative pain: A meta-analysis of randomized controlled trials. *Anesthesiology.* 2013;119:178–190.

49. Sritapan Y, Clifford S, Bautista A. Perioperative management of patients on buprenorphine and methadone: A narrative review. *Balkan Med J.* 2020;37:247–252.

50. Anderson TA, Quaye ANA, Ward EN, Wilens TE, Hilliard PE, Brummett CM. To stop or not, that is the question: Acute pain management for the patient on chronic buprenorphine. *Anesthesiology.* 2017;126:1180–1186.

51. Lembke A, Ottestad E, Schmiesing C. Patients maintained on buprenorphine for opioid use disorder should continue buprenorphine through the perioperative period. *Pain Med.* 2019;20:425–428.

52. Wu CL, Fleisher LA. Outcomes research in regional anesthesia and analgesia. *Anesth Analg.* 2000;91:1232–1242.

53. Loper KA, Ready LB, Downey M, et al. Epidural and intravenous fentanyl infusions are clinically equivalent after knee surgery. *Anesth Analg.* 1990;70:72–75.

54. Gulbahar G, Kocer B, Muratli SN, et al. A comparison of epidural and paravertebral catheterisation techniques in post-thoracotomy pain management. *Eur J Cardiothorac Surg.* 2010;37:467–472.

55. Tryba M. Epidural regional anesthesia and low molecular heparin: Pro. *Anasthesiol Intensivmed Notfallmed Schmerzther.* 1993;28:179–181.

56. Horlocker TT, Wedel DJ, Rowlingson JC, et al. Regional anesthesia in the patient receiving antithrombotic or thrombolytic therapy: American Society of Regional Anesthesia and Pain Medicine Evidence-Based Guidelines (Third Edition). *Reg Anesth Pain Med.* 2010;35:64–101.

57. Narouze S, Benzon HT, Provenzano D, et al. Interventional Spine and Pain Procedures in Patients on Antiplatelet and Anticoagulant Medications (Second Edition): Guidelines from the American Society of Regional Anesthesia and Pain Medicine, the European Society of Regional Anaesthesia and Pain Therapy, the American Academy of Pain Medicine, the International Neuromodulation Society, the North American Neuromodulation Society, and the World Institute of Pain. *Reg Anesth Pain Med.* 2018;43:225–262.

58. Horlocker TT, Wedel DJ. Neurologic complications of spinal and epidural anesthesia. *Reg Anesth Pain Med.* 2000;25:83–98.

59. Group TPW. PROSPECT (Procedure Specific Postoperative Pain Management). http://www.postoppain.org/. Published 2015. Accessed October, 1, 2015.

60. Uskova A, O'Connor JE. Liposomal bupivacaine for regional anesthesia. *Curr Opin Anaesthesiol.* 2015;28:593–597.

61. Busfield BT, Romero DM. Pain pump use after shoulder arthroscopy as a cause of glenohumeral chondrolysis. *Arthroscopy.* 2009;25:647–652.

62. Vila H Jr, Liu J, Kavasmaneck D. Paravertebral block: New benefits from an old procedure. *Curr Opin Anaesthesiol.* 2007;20:316–318.

63. Wardhan R. Update on paravertebral blocks. *Curr Opin Anaesthesiol.* 2015;28:588–592.

64. Fredrickson MJ, Ball CM, Dalgleish AJ, Stewart AW, Short TG. A prospective randomized comparison of ultrasound and neurostimulation as needle end points for interscalene catheter placement. *Anesth Analg.* 2009;108:1695–1700.

65. Prabhakar A, Lambert T, Kaye RJ, et al. Adjuvants in clinical regional anesthesia practice: A comprehensive review. *Best Pract Res Clin Anaesthesiol.* 2019;33:415–423.

66. Neal JM, Gerancher JC, Hebl JR, et al. Upper extremity regional anesthesia: essentials of our current understanding, 2008. *Reg Anesth Pain Med.* 2009;34:134–170.

67. Fritsch G, Danninger T, Allerberger K, et al. Dexmedetomidine added to ropivacaine extends the duration of interscalene brachial plexus blocks for elective shoulder surgery when compared with ropivacaine alone: A single-center, prospective, triple-blind, randomized controlled trial. *Reg Anesth Pain Med.* 2014;39:37–47.

68. Mariano ER, Afra R, Loland VJ, Sandhu NS, Bellars RH, Bishop ML, Cheng GS, Choy LP, Maldonado RC, Ilfeld BM. Continuous interscalene brachial plexus block via an ultrasound-guided posterior approach: A randomized, triple-masked, placebo-controlled study. *Anesth Analg.* 2009 May;108(5):1688–1694.

69. Marino J, Russo J, Kenny M, et al. Continuous lumbar plexus block for postoperative pain control after total hip arthroplasty. A randomized controlled trial. *J Bone Joint Surg Am.* 2009;91:29–37.

70. Hunt KJ, Higgins TF, Carlston CV, Swenson JR, McEachern JE, Beals TC. Continuous peripheral nerve blockade as postoperative analgesia for open treatment of calcaneal fractures. *J Orthop Trauma.* 2010;24:148–155.

71. El-Dawlatly AA, Turkistani A, Kettner SC, et al. Ultrasound-guided transversus abdominis plane block: Description of a new technique and comparison with conventional systemic analgesia during laparoscopic cholecystectomy. *Br J Anaesth.* 2009;102:763–767.

V

CONSULTANT ANESTHETIC PRACTICE

41 CRITICAL CARE MEDICINE

Ashish Agrawal, Anne L. Donovan

ICU DEFINITIONS, INTERPROFESSIONAL CARE, AND PHYSICIAN STAFFING

Intensive care units (ICUs), as defined by The Joint Commission, are geographically separated nursing care areas that provide intensive observation, diagnosis, and therapeutic procedures for patients who are critically ill. Though the first modern ICU was started in 1953 to provide mechanical ventilation to patients with polio, they have since evolved to allow for monitoring and support of critically ill patients with a wide variety of life-threatening disease. Complexity of care has increased over time, as a result of both patient factors (i.e., patients living with more serious comorbidity) and the development of more specialized therapies.

Provision of modern critical care medicine therefore relies on the collective expertise of providers from many health care professions working together toward a common goal, which is known as *interprofessional care*. A robust body of literature suggests that patient outcomes are improved when ICU care is provided by an interprofessional team. Providers integral to the care of critically ill patients include (but are not limited to) nurses, pharmacists, respiratory care practitioners, rehabilitation specialists, dieticians, spiritual care providers, case managers, social workers, advance practice providers, intensivist physicians, and nonintensivist physician consultants. Patients and family members are at the center of the care team and should be engaged as partners in their care.[1]

Physicians are an important part of this interprofessional critical care team, but physician staffing in the ICU can vary between hospitals. Larger, primarily academic, centers may consistently staff critical care–trained intensivists who manage all aspects of a patient's care 24 hours a day, whereas at the other extreme smaller community hospitals may depend on nonintensivist physicians who would otherwise manage the patient on a general ward. Studies of the various physician models have shown that the involvement of an intensivist in a patient's daily care can reduce mortality and length of stay,[2] though the benefit of overnight or continuous intensivist staffing is still being evaluated.

ORGAN FAILURE AND SUPPORT

Although patients admitted to the ICU can vary in their diagnoses or severity of illness, most have some degree of organ dysfunction or failure. In complex patients a single diagnosis such as sepsis can lead to multiple organ failures, including shock, respiratory failure, and acute renal failure (ARF). Severity scores, such as the Sequential Organ Failure Assessment (SOFA), can predict increased mortality in patients with multiple organ involvement of their disease process. Diagnosing and treating the common problems that affect organ systems in the ICU, and understanding how they might interrelate, is an important skill for a critical care provider.

Neurologic: Encephalopathy and Delirium

Encephalopathy, defined as a neurologic process that causes altered levels of consciousness or sensorium, is common in the ICU. Primary causes of encephalopathy can include neurologic injury from stroke, seizures, tumors, or traumatic brain injury. Secondary encephalopathy includes patients with altered mentation resulting from extracranial causes, such as metabolic derangements, sepsis-associated encephalopathy, or ICU delirium.

ICU delirium affects greater than 30% of patients in the ICU and up to 80% of mechanically ventilated patients. It is diagnosed based on the acute onset of waxing and waning mental status, inattention, disorganized thinking, and altered level of consciousness. Although it is most easily recognized in its hyperactive form manifesting as patient agitation and restlessness, the majority of patients have a hypoactive or mixed syndrome reflected by flat affect and apathy along with cognitive dysfunction. Because of these varying presentations and the difficulty diagnosing patients with a hypoactive form of delirium, routine use of an objective delirium screening tool is recommended. The most commonly used tool is the Confusion Assessment Method for the ICU (CAM-ICU).[3]

Delirium can prevent patients from engaging in their care, and at its most extreme can lead to patient harm by interfering with important therapies or necessitating physical or chemical restraints. As such, the presence of delirium is associated with a threefold increase in 6-month mortality and a twofold increase in length of hospital stay, as well as a higher risk of persistent cognitive dysfunction at 1 year after discharge.[4] Factors that predispose patients to delirium include both nonmodifiable (e.g., advanced age, preexisting cognitive dysfunction, multiorgan dysfunction, infection or sepsis, and mechanical ventilation) and modifiable (e.g., immobility, pain, sleep deprivation, dehydration, electrolyte abnormalities, and use of high-risk medications including benzodiazepines and anticholinergics) risk factors.

Evidence-based treatment for delirium involves primarily nonpharmacologic strategies, including frequent reorientation, restoring day/night and sleep cycles, presence of family members, physical therapy or activity out of bed, and use of appropriate sensory aids such as glasses and hearing aids, and avoiding known delirium triggers, such as benzodiazepines. Pharmacologic treatment with melatonin may treat delirium and restore sleep,[5] and haloperidol or atypical antipsychotics can help control symptoms of agitated delirium, though they do not shorten its course. No pharmacologic therapy has yet consistently prevented ICU delirium.

Cardiovascular: Shock

Shock is a state where there is insufficient delivery of oxygen to the body's critical organs and tissues to maintain normal function. Though low blood pressure is often associated with shock, it is neither necessary nor sufficient to diagnose a patient with shock. These patients must be treated for the underlying cause emergently, as untreated shock decompensates into multiorgan failure and death. Shock can be categorized based on its underlying cause: hypovolemic, cardiogenic, obstructive, and distributive (Table 41.1, Fig. 41.1).

Table 41.1	Characteristics of Various Shock States				
Shock Type	Cardiac Output	Systemic Vascular Resistance	Central Venous Pressure	Pulmonary Capillary Wedge Pressure	Mixed Venous Oxygen Saturation
Hypovolemic	↓	↑	↓	↓	↓
Cardiogenic	↓	↑	↑	↑*	↓
Obstructive	↓	↑	↑	↓**	↓
Distributive	↑ or even	↓	↓	↓	↑ or even

*Pulmonary capillary wedge pressure is normal to low in right ventricular failure.
**Pulmonary capillary wedge pressure is elevated in cardiac tamponade.

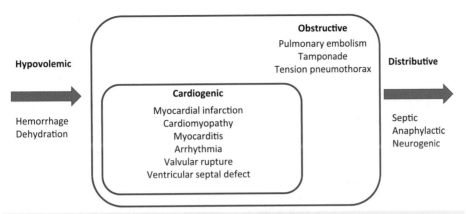

Fig. 41.1 Categories and Etiologies of Shock. This figure suggests a semi anatomic framework to help conceptualize the four broad categories of shock. **Hypovolemic shock** occurs when insufficient preload is delivered to the heart to maintain adequate cardiac output. **Cardiogenic shock** occurs when the heart itself (represented by the inner oval) is unable to produce sufficient cardiac output because of ischemia, arrhythmia, valvular disease, or poor contractility. In **obstructive shock** something external to the heart (represented by the outer oval) presents a physical obstruction to ventricular ejection. **Distributive shock** occurs as a result of vasodilation in the systemic arterial system. Examples of specific etiologies within each category are listed.

Hypovolemic Shock

Hypovolemic shock occurs when the body's circulating blood volume is inadequate to return blood to the right side of the heart, resulting in a decrease in preload (left ventricular end-diastolic volume) and subsequently a decrease in cardiac output. Although compensatory mechanisms can offset small decreases in blood volume, large volume shifts will result in shock. Most causes of acute hypovolemic shock are caused by bleeding, often the result of trauma, surgery, or gastrointestinal hemorrhage. However, severe dehydration or fluid loss caused by diarrhea, vomiting, or profuse sweating can also lead to hypovolemic shock.

Clinical Manifestations

Acute blood loss, or hypovolemia, initially results in the translocation of interstitial fluid into the circulating blood volume to transiently restore cardiac output. The activation of the renin–angiotensin–aldosterone system results in sodium conservation by the kidneys and reduction of additional fluid loss. A decrease in circulating blood volume of 15% or more will trigger the baroreceptor reflex to increase heart rate and maintain cardiac output, and sympathetic stimulation and catecholamines will vasoconstrict blood vessels away from skin, skeletal muscle, and splanchnic circulation to maintain perfusion to vital organs. Ongoing loss of circulating volume, which outstrips these compensation mechanisms, results in hypotension and shock.

Patients in hypovolemic shock can present with physical examination findings of dry mucous membranes and decreased skin turgor. As a result of vasoconstriction, their skin can be cold and clammy. They may be tachycardic with mild to moderate hypovolemia, though hypotension is usually a delayed sign with severe hypovolemia.

Treatment

Adequate intravascular volume resuscitation and source control are key to the treatment of hypovolemic shock. Intravenous access must be obtained quickly, ideally with short, large-bore (16-gauge or greater) intravenous peripheral catheters, which can be used to administer intravenous fluid or blood. Central venous access or intraosseous catheters can be considered if peripheral access is challenging, though intraosseous catheters should be removed and replaced with intravenous access as soon as possible because of concerns about compartment syndrome with extravasation.

The choice of resuscitation fluid should depend on the presumed cause of hypovolemia. Severe or ongoing bleeding caused by trauma or gastrointestinal hemorrhage should be replaced by blood products in a 1:1:1 ratio of packed red blood cells, fresh frozen plasma, and platelets[6] (also see Chapter 25). Massive transfusion protocols should be activated for patients who are expected to receive 10 units of packed red blood cells in 24 hours or 4 units in 1 hour, and where available, rapid transfusion devices should be used. Replacement of calcium and maintenance of normothermia in these patients will reduce ongoing coagulopathy, and tranexamic acid can reduce fibrinolysis and mortality for traumatically injured patients when given within 3 hours of injury.[7]

Of note, in patients who present with massive bleeding resuscitation should be started based on clinical assessments of the patient and should target a low-normal

VI

blood pressure until the source of bleeding has been controlled, a technique known as *permissive hypotension.* Initial hematocrit values may be misleading if compensatory mechanisms or crystalloid resuscitation has not yet led to the dilution of remaining red blood cell mass. Laboratory values therefore should not be used immediately on presentation as a sole guide for resuscitation, but can be used to target and guide later resuscitation.

For patients who are hypovolemic but not bleeding, resuscitation should be initiated with isotonic, balanced crystalloid such as Plasma-Lyte or lactated Ringer's solution. Normal saline should be avoided because of the risk of iatrogenic hyperchloremic metabolic acidosis (also see Chapter 24). Vasopressors can be used as a temporizing measure in patients with hypovolemic shock but should never be used as a substitute for adequate fluid resuscitation.

Cardiogenic Shock

Cardiogenic shock results when either the left or the right ventricle is unable to fill with volume or contract effectively to generate an adequate stroke volume. These processes are referred to as heart failure with preserved ejection fraction (diastolic) or heart failure with reduced ejection fraction (systolic), respectively. Causes of cardiogenic shock can include acute myocardial infarction, severe cardiomyopathy, myocarditis, arrhythmia, valvular rupture, or ventricular septal defect. Regardless of the initial cause, cardiogenic shock can occur on an acute, chronic, or acute-on-chronic basis classified by whether it occurs soon after an injury, chronically as the heart reaches its limits of adaptation, or because of an acute decompensation or exacerbation in an otherwise chronically compensated heart.

Clinical Manifestations

The development of cardiogenic shock depends on a complex interplay between myocardial work and oxygen demand. In a normal heart the ventricles pump blood to supply oxygen to both itself and to the rest of the body. Any process that decreases oxygen supply to the heart (e.g., acute coronary syndromes) or increases oxygen demand (e.g., tachycardia or hypertension) may result in a supply–demand mismatch interrupting this finely calibrated balance.

With mild disruption, the heart can compensate and adapt. By gradually thickening the left ventricular walls or by increasing its left ventricular end-diastolic volume, the heart can find a new balance on the Frank-Starling curve to increase its stroke volume and maintain cardiac output. However, these adaptations have a natural limit, as thicker walls and higher left ventricular end-diastolic pressure decrease perfusion to the endocardium, making the heart more susceptible to ischemia and increasing the risk of decompensation into acute heart failure and cardiogenic shock. Furthermore, whereas the left ventricle

generally can compensate given time to remodel, the right ventricle is more susceptible to ischemia and has fewer adaptation mechanisms and thus can be the source of considerable morbidity and mortality.

The symptoms of cardiogenic shock can vary depending on which ventricle is primarily involved. In left ventricular failure end-diastolic volume rises, leading to overdistension of the ventricle, decreased cardiac output, and the development of pulmonary edema. In right ventricular failure signs of inadequate forward flow of blood often include distended neck veins, peripheral edema, and hepatic congestion. Biventricular failure can result when the pulmonary congestion from left ventricular failure leads to pulmonary arterial hypertension and concomitant right ventricular failure. Both forms of heart failure can lead to cold and poorly perfused extremities caused by peripheral vasoconstriction and decreased cardiac output.

Treatment

Immediate interventions should be targeted toward improving cardiac output, decreasing cardiac filling pressures, and restoring balance between myocardial oxygen supply and demand. Inotropes (e.g., dobutamine) may be used to improve cardiac output. In hypotensive patients a vasopressor such as norepinephrine may be needed to counteract the vasodilatory effect of dobutamine to maintain normotension. In hypertensive patients vasodilators (e.g., nitroglycerin or nitroprusside) may help to decrease afterload and preload and improve forward flow. In fluid-overloaded patients careful diuresis may optimize cardiac filling pressures. Patients with isolated right heart failure can sometimes acutely decompensate as a result of hypoxia, hypercarbia, and positive-pressure ventilation. In select cases pulmonary vasodilators such as epoprostenol or inhaled nitric oxide may be appropriate.

Soon after initial stabilization, any reversible causes of cardiogenic shock should be identified and treated. For patients with cardiogenic shock complicating an acute myocardial infarction, early revascularization with angiography or fibrinolytic therapy can improve mortality.[8] Treating tachyarrhythmias can improve cardiac filling and forward flow. Other underlying contributors, such as systemic infection, should be treated rapidly.

Mechanical Circulatory Support

Despite optimal management of cardiogenic shock, there will be a subset of patients for whom there is insufficient cardiac function to maintain other end-organ functions. In these cases various forms of mechanical circulatory support can be considered. Although an in-depth discussion of these techniques is beyond the scope of this chapter, the following devices may be used in specialized centers.

Intraaortic Balloon Pump

An intraaortic balloon pump (IABP) is a percutaneously placed balloon inserted through the femoral artery and positioned in the aorta. Using helium gas, it is quickly inflated during diastole and deflated during systole, thus augmenting diastolic blood pressure and cardiac perfusion while decreasing systolic pressure and left ventricular afterload. An IABP is thought to improve cardiac perfusion while decreasing cardiac work and is usually considered for patients with myocardial ischemia for whom increased cardiac work is poorly tolerated. Despite the physiologic basis for utility in these patients, large randomized controlled trials have not shown mortality benefits for the use of IABP in cardiogenic shock.[9]

Extracorporeal Membrane Oxygenation

In patients for whom the heart is severely damaged a device that replaces the function of all or a part of the heart may be needed. Extracorporeal membrane oxygenation (ECMO) is a device that removes deoxygenated blood from a large vein, processes the blood through a pump and oxygenator, and returns it to either a large artery (venoarterial or VA-ECMO) or a large vein (venovenous or VV-ECMO). VA-ECMO can replace the function of both the heart and the lungs, whereas VV-ECMO replaces the function of the lung as an oxygenator but does not improve cardiac contractility.

Ventricular Assist Devices

A left ventricular assist device (LVAD), a surgically implanted pump to move blood from the left ventricle to the aorta, is an option for patients who require ongoing assistance with ventricular function. These devices can allow patients to live outside the hospital while they await definitive treatment such as a heart transplant (i.e., as a "bridge to transplant"). Alternatively, an LVAD can be implanted to improve quality of life in end-stage heart failure (i.e., as "destination therapy"). LVADs can strain damaged right ventricles, and patients may require continuous inotrope infusions or dual left- and right-sided VADs to support the function of both ventricles.

Impella

The Impella is a short-term, catheter-based, miniaturized VAD that can be percutaneously placed across the aortic valve to augment left ventricular flow. The most common indication is for short-term left ventricular support during high-risk percutaneous coronary interventions. Further study is needed to determine whether this device can improve outcomes in patients with cardiogenic shock.[10]

Obstructive Shock

Obstructive shock occurs when there is a physical obstruction to flow either within the heart or the large vessels of the pulmonary or systemic circulation. The most common causes of obstructive shock are massive pulmonary embolism, pericardial tamponade, and tension pneumothorax.

Clinical Manifestations

In many ways patients with obstructive shock appear to have a form of cardiogenic shock. The obstructive process causes a decrease in left ventricular filling, resulting in decreased stroke volume and cardiac output. This results in compensatory tachycardia, peripheral vasoconstriction, and increased systemic vascular resistance (SVR). The resistance to forward flow can also lead to elevated central venous pressures (CVPs) along with signs of venous congestion such as elevated jugular venous pressure and hepatomegaly.

Point-of-care ultrasound can be an important technique to diagnose obstructive shock (also see Chapter 21). Pneumothorax may be visible on examination of the lung, and a pericardial effusion or tamponade may be evident on examination of the heart. Though a pulmonary embolism can rarely be seen directly, associated signs such as right ventricular dysfunction or septal flattening from pressure overload can be suggestive of this diagnosis.

Treatment

Treatment of obstructive shock usually involves emergent targeted treatment of the specific cause, along with measures to increase cardiac output. Massive pulmonary embolism can be treated with fibrinolytic therapy. Pericardial tamponade is treated with pericardiocentesis or a surgical pericardial window. Tension pneumothorax is treated with emergent needle thoracostomy, usually followed by chest tube placement.

Until definitive treatment can be completed, providers should be careful to avoid changing physiologic variables that compensate for the obstruction. Because these patients require adequate preload to maintain stroke volume, the change from spontaneous to positive-pressure ventilation can cause hemodynamic instability. Tachycardia is another compensatory mechanism to maintain cardiac output. Administration of medications that decrease heart rate, contractility, or preload (e.g., β-blockers, diuretics) may lead to cardiac arrest and death.

Distributive Shock

Distributive shock also called *vasodilatory shock*, results from profound dilation of the arterial vascular system leading to decreased SVR and hypotension. Distributive shock can be broken down into three main types: septic, anaphylactic, and neurogenic shock.

Sepsis and Septic Shock

Sepsis is the most common reason for admission to the ICU and is the leading cause of ICU mortality. It is defined as life-threatening organ dysfunction resulting from a dysregulated host response to infection.

Clinical Manifestations

Diagnostic criteria for sepsis were updated in 2016 to place greater emphasis on the organ dysfunction that

Box 41.1 qSOFA

Suspected infection + 2 out of 3 qSOFA criteria:
Altered mental status (GCS <15)
Respiratory rate ≥ 22
Systolic blood pressure ≤100

GCS, Glasgow Coma Scale.

contributes to mortality. As such, the current definition requires the presence of an infection or suspected infection along with a 2-point increase in the SOFA score.[11] However, because SOFA scores cannot be calculated quickly as a result of the instrument's complexity, the quick SOFA (qSOFA) screening tool was developed to identify patients with infections who are at high risk of death or needing an ICU (Box 41.1).

Treatment

Despite extensive study of multiple therapeutics over many years (e.g., activated protein C, glucocorticoids), no definitive therapy exists to treat sepsis. In 2001 a landmark clinical trial showed improved mortality with early goal-directed therapy (EGDT), which focused on (1) intravascular fluid resuscitation, (2) vasopressors to achieve a mean arterial pressure goal, and (3) packed red blood cell transfusion or dobutamine infusion to improve central venous oxygen saturation ($Scvo_2$).[12] Whereas the first two components were adopted broadly, central venous catheters (CVCs), blood transfusions, and inotropes remained controversial. To isolate the role of these more controversial components of EGDT, three subsequent multicenter randomized controlled trials compared EGDT with usual care or protocol-based standard care.[13] All three trials showed no decrease in mortality rate from EGDT compared with modern management of sepsis, which did not mandate $Scvo_2$ monitoring, blood transfusions, or inotropes.

With these new data, optimal treatment of sepsis can be distilled to these fundamentals: early recognition, rapid fluid resuscitation, prompt antibiotic administration, and treatment of the infectious source. Monitoring of fluid resuscitation should rely on composite endpoints, which include the clinical examination, fluid responsiveness, and lactate clearance, rather than focusing on a single number such as CVP or $Scvo_2$. Vasopressors should be used to support organ perfusion after intravascular volume repletion. Norepinephrine is considered to be the vasopressor of choice, followed by vasopressin or epinephrine. Dopamine, in particular, is associated with arrhythmias and poor outcomes. Central lines should not be inserted in all patients unless indicated clinically.

Finally, although goal-directed fluid administration during the acute phase of sepsis is an important core of treatment, some evidence suggests that excess fluid beyond what is needed can be harmful. In the Fluid and Catheter Treatment Trial (FACTT), which included patients with acute lung injury (mostly caused by pneumonia or sepsis), patients in the "conservative fluid" (i.e., minimal use of fluids) management group had improved lung function; improved central nervous system (CNS) function; and a decreased need for sedation, mechanical ventilation, and intensive care when compared with a liberal fluid group without increased complications such as organ failure or shock.[14]

Anaphylactic Shock
Clinical Manifestations

Anaphylactic shock is the most severe manifestation of anaphylaxis, which is a systemic, immediate hypersensitivity reaction mediated by immunoglobulin E (IgE) that results in basophil and mast cell degranulation. Anaphylaxis involves multiple organ systems, inducing mucocutaneous symptoms (urticaria, pruritis, flushing, angioedema), respiratory symptoms (wheezing, stridor, upper airway obstruction), gastrointestinal symptoms (nausea, vomiting), or cardiovascular compromise (hypotension and shock).[15] These symptoms are mediated by histamine and other molecules released by mast cells and basophils that increase capillary leak and further amplify an inflammatory cascade. Capillary leak can lead to decreased intravascular volume, which compounds hypotension because of arterial vasodilation and a decrease in SVR. To compensate, patients develop tachycardia, though this rarely maintains adequate cardiac output in serious cases.

Treatment

Patients with suspected anaphylactic shock should be treated immediately with epinephrine. The α-adrenergic effect of epinephrine helps reverse arterial vasodilation, and $β_2$-adrenergic receptors can relax bronchospasm and respiratory symptoms of anaphylaxis. Other management priorities include addressing impending upper airway obstruction and discontinuing any suspected triggering agents.

Further treatment of hypotension should include intravenous fluids and repeated doses or infusions of epinephrine to maintain tissue perfusion. Adjunct therapy for anaphylaxis can include corticosteroids and antihistamines to reverse or neutralize the inflammatory response and albuterol or other bronchodilators for persistent bronchospasm.

Neurogenic Shock
Clinical Manifestations

Neurogenic shock generally follows a traumatic injury to the brain or spinal cord, resulting in interruption to sympathetic outflow to the periphery and leading to unopposed parasympathetic tone. The pooling of blood in vascular beds from increased venous capacitance and low

SVR leads to hypotension and circulatory failure. Spinal cord injury above the fourth thoracic level may also be associated with bradycardia caused by interruption of cardiac accelerator fibers.

Treatment

Early neurosurgical intervention can improve outcomes after spinal cord injury. To prevent secondary ischemic injury, early treatment goals are to maintain blood flow and perfusion pressure to the brain and spinal cord by avoiding hypotension and, in many cases, targeting a higher-than-physiologic mean arterial pressure of >85 mm Hg for 3 to 7 days.[16] To achieve this, fluid resuscitation with a balanced crystalloid solution can replace some of the pooled volume in vascular beds, but some patients require supplementation with a vasopressor such as norepinephrine to improve SVR, inotropy, and chronotropy. Once out of the window for secondary neurologic injury, some patients will continue to need blood pressure support with an oral α-agonist such as midodrine.

Hemodynamic Monitoring

Given the complexity of patients in shock, appropriate monitoring plays a key role in treatment. Intensive care settings not only allow for more frequent monitoring but also for the placement of continuous invasive monitors (e.g., arterial, central, and pulmonary artery catheters [PACs]). This section will focus on use of these monitors in critically ill patients (also see Chapter 20).

Arterial Catheter

Arterial catheters are the most commonly inserted invasive monitors in the ICU. Besides obtaining beat-to-beat information regarding arterial blood pressure, arterial waveform analysis has gained acceptance as a tool to predict a patient's hemodynamic response to intravascular volume expansion. Parameters derived from the arterial line include systolic pressure variation (SPV) and pulse pressure variation (PPV). PPV is more accurate than measurements of cardiac filling pressures (CVP, pulmonary artery occlusion pressure [PAOP]) to predict intravascular fluid responsiveness[17] (also see Chapter 24).

Central Venous Catheter

CVP, which is generally recorded at the junction of the superior vena cava and the right atrium, has traditionally been used to monitor preload and to guide fluid therapy. However, CVP is a poor predictor of fluid responsiveness, and thus CVP measurement alone is an insufficient reason to place a CVC.[18] ($Scvo_2$ measurement can be helpful in patients with unclear etiology of cardiogenic shock or as a means to track improvement in cardiac function. Oxygen uptake by the body can be estimated by the difference between $Scvo_2$ and the arterial oxygen saturation. This difference depends partially on cardiac output. A lower $Scvo_2$ (i.e., <50%) indicates greater oxygen extraction, usually because of lower cardiac output. Slower flow through the capillary beds in low cardiac output states allows more time for tissues to extract oxygen from the blood. In contrast, higher $Scvo_2$ (i.e., >65%) would imply either higher cardiac output (e.g., distributive shock) or inability for tissues to extract oxygen from the blood (e.g., mitochondrial dysfunction in sepsis). $Scvo_2$ is subject to error for a number of reasons, and the data should only be one part of a global clinical assessment of the patient.

Pulmonary Artery Catheter

In the past PACs were commonly used in ICU patients to measure cardiac output and to estimate left ventricular preload. After multiple randomized clinical trials of PAC monitoring did not demonstrate a mortality benefit, their use has decreased markedly.[19] In addition, placement of PACs has significant risk of morbidity caused by arrhythmias or pulmonary artery injury, and they have higher rates of infection than other CVCs. There are rare patients for whom PACs may still be helpful, including ICU patients with dual cardiogenic and septic shock, though greater emphasis is being placed on noninvasive measures of cardiac output and fluid responsiveness.

Noninvasive Cardiac Output Monitors

Because of the risks of invasive monitors, several noninvasive cardiac output monitors have been introduced to the ICU. These methods can include arterial pulse contour analysis, esophageal Doppler, bioimpedance, bioreactance, pulse wave transit time, and analysis of an arterial waveform using the volume clamp method or radial artery applanation tonometry. Research is still ongoing to determine the accuracy and clinical benefit for these tools in critically ill patients.[20]

Point-of-Care Ultrasonography

Point-of-care ultrasonography is a powerful tool in the ICU for both differentiation of the various causes of shock and monitoring the response to treatment. Though the accuracy of ultrasound is dependent on operator skill, it is now routinely taught in critical care fellowship programs. Its main benefits include the rapidity of a focused assessment to answer a specific clinical question and its ability to be repeated in real time as a patient's clinical picture evolves (also see Chapter 21).

Pulmonary: Respiratory Failure

Respiratory failure remains a common indication for ICU admission. It can be categorized based on the acuity of the process (e.g., acute vs. chronic) and the physiologic perturbation present (e.g., hypercapnia vs. hypoxemia).

VI

Such distinctions help to direct appropriate treatment and supportive care. However, multiple processes can occur simultaneously. For example, a patient may have acute-on-chronic respiratory failure with the presence of both hypoxemia and hypercapnia.

Hypoxemic Respiratory Failure

Hypoxemic respiratory failure can be characterized by either pathophysiology or etiology. The former framework often distinguishes between the presence or absence of a difference between alveolar (A) and arterial (a) oxygen partial pressures, known as the *A-a gradient*. The presence of an A-a gradient indicates a problem with oxygen diffusion between the alveolus and arterial capillary (e.g., from pulmonary edema or pulmonary fibrosis), ventilation/perfusion (V/Q) mismatch (e.g., from pulmonary embolism), or shunting (e.g., from atelectasis). The absence of an A-a gradient in a patient with hypoxemia indicates normal oxygen movement across the alveolar membrane (e.g., from hypoventilation or inhalation of a hypoxic gas mixture). In clinical practice most patients with hypoxemia have an increased A-a gradient. Disease processes causing hypoxemia include acute respiratory distress syndrome (ARDS), sepsis, pneumonia, pulmonary embolism, cardiogenic or noncardiogenic pulmonary edema, trauma, and obstructive lung disease, among others (also see Chapter 5).

ARDS

ARDS is an important cause of hypoxemic respiratory failure. It is caused by a diffuse, inflammatory injury of the lung, resulting in the development of noncardiogenic pulmonary edema with resultant V/Q mismatch, hypoxemia, and decreased pulmonary compliance. ARDS is defined by the Berlin definition[21] (Box 41.2). ARDS typically follows within 1 week of an inciting event that can lead to direct or indirect lung injury (Table 41.2). Our understanding of the triggers of ARDS is constantly evolving. For example, in late 2019 the severe acute respiratory syndrome coronavirus 2 (SARS-CoV-2) virus emerged as a new cause of ARDS, triggering a global pandemic responsible for millions of deaths worldwide in the first years after its detection.

Although the underlying cause of lung injury may predict outcome, patient-specific factors such as age, immunocompromised status, and organ dysfunction are stronger predictors for survival. In some patients ARDS resolves after the acute phase; however, others experience a chronic alveolitis leading to pulmonary fibrosis. Such patients often experience continued hypoxemia, increased physiologic dead space, and decreased compliance with chronic ventilator dependence.

Treatment

In addition to treating the underlying cause of ARDS, management is largely supportive with a focus on lung-protective (ARDSnet) ventilation to prevent ventilator-associated lung injury (i.e., barotrauma, volutrauma, and atelectrauma). The central tenets of lung-protective ventilation include lower tidal volumes (i.e., 6 mL/kg of ideal body weight), limited plateau pressure (i.e., <30 cmH_2O), using higher positive end-expiratory pressure (PEEP), and accepting lower PaO_2 and higher $PaCO_2$

Box 41.2 Berlin Definition of Acute Respiratory Distress Syndrome

Timing	Within 1 week of a known clinical insult or new or worsening respiratory symptoms
Oxygenation	Mild: PaO_2/FiO_2 >200 ≤300 mm Hg with PEEP or CPAP ≥5 cmH_2O
	Moderate: PaO_2/FiO_2 >100 ≤200 mm Hg with PEEP ≥5 cmH_2O
	Severe: PaO_2/FiO_2 ≤100 mm Hg with PEEP ≥5 cmH_2O
Chest Radiograph	Bilateral opacities not fully explained by effusions, lobar/lung collapse, or nodules
Edema	Respiratory failure not fully explained by cardiac failure or fluid overload
Risk Factor	If no risk factor for lung injury identified, then need objective assessment such as echocardiography to exclude hydrostatic edema

Adapted from Acute respiratory distress syndrome: The Berlin definition. *JAMA.* 2012;307(23). *ARDS,* Acute respiratory distress syndrome; *CPAP,* continuous positive airway pressure; *FiO_2,* fraction of inspired oxygen; *PaO_2,* arterial partial pressure of oxygen; *PEEP,* positive end-expiratory pressure.
Modified from Liu LL, Gropper MA: Critical care anesthesiology. Ch 101. In Miller RD (ed): Miller's Anesthesia, 8e. Philadelphia: Elsevier, 2015.

Table 41.2 Triggers of Acute Respiratory Distress Syndrome

Causes of Direct Lung Injury	Causes of Indirect Lung Injury
Pneumonia	Sepsis
Aspiration of gastric contents	Severe trauma
Pulmonary contusion	Cardiopulmonary bypass
Reperfusion pulmonary edema	Drug overdose
Amniotic fluid embolus	Acute pancreatitis
Inhalational injury	Near-drowning
	Transfusion-related acute lung injury

Data from Ware LB, Matthay MA. The acute respiratory distress syndrome. *N Engl J Med.* 2000;342:1334–1349.

values ("permissive" hypoxemia and hypercapnia). In the landmark ARDSnet trial use of this ventilation strategy resulted in a mortality reduction from 40% to 31% when compared with usual care at the time.[22] Other evidence-based supportive care strategies for patients with ARDS include restrictive fluid management, neuromuscular blockade (in carefully selected patients), and prone positioning. Many additional therapies, including inhaled pulmonary vasodilators and ECMO, have been trialed in ARDS without clear mortality benefit but may be used on a case-by-case basis as rescue therapies for patients with refractory hypoxemia.

Hypercapnic Respiratory Failure

Causes of hypercapnic respiratory failure include hypoventilation (e.g., from drug intoxication or neuromuscular weakness) or increased dead space (e.g., from chronic obstructive pulmonary disease [COPD] or asthma). Hypercapnia may also be present in severe forms of an infiltrative pulmonary process such as ARDS.

Respiratory Support

Both hypercapnic and hypoxemic respiratory failure may require respiratory support, which can be provided through noninvasive or invasive means. Decision making around ventilatory support requires knowledge of the underlying pathophysiology of the patient's diagnosis and the indications and contraindications for specific supportive modalities.

Supplemental Oxygen

Supplemental oxygen can be provided by low-flow (e.g., nasal cannula, simple facemask, nonrebreather mask) or high-flow (e.g., high-flow nasal cannula [HFNC]) devices. For low-flow devices, the maximum fraction of inspired oxygen (FiO_2) provided depends on both the location and flow rate at which the oxygen is delivered and also, importantly, on the patient's respiratory effort. Delivery of oxygen through these devices creates an oxygen reservoir in the patient's nasopharynx. Patients who are breathing quietly will inspire higher oxygen concentrations from the nasopharyngeal reservoir, whereas patients who are tachypneic and/or breathing at a higher peak inspiratory flow rate will entrain more room air and inspire a lower oxygen concentration with each breath.

HFNC uses heated and humidified oxygen that is delivered at high flow rates through a nasal cannula, which provides a functionally larger nasopharyngeal reservoir and more consistent delivery of inspired oxygen. At very high flow rates, HFNC provides a small amount of positive airway pressure and reduces dead space by flushing expired carbon dioxide from the upper airways. Most patients find HFNC to be more comfortable than noninvasive positive-pressure ventilation (NIPPV) via a facemask. In a multicenter trial comparing outcomes in patients with acute hypoxemic, nonhypercarbic

respiratory failure, patients treated with HFNC had reduced mortality compared with patients treated with standard oxygen therapy or noninvasive ventilation, although there was no difference in the rate of tracheal intubation.[23]

Noninvasive Positive-Pressure Ventilation

NIPPV, which includes both continuous positive airway pressure (CPAP) and bilevel positive airway pressure (BiPAP), delivers positive-pressure breaths via a facemask, nasal pillows, or helmet without an endotracheal tube (ETT) present. For patients with COPD and acute hypercapnic respiratory failure, appropriate use of NIPPV can reduce mortality rate, avoid endotracheal intubation, improve dyspnea, and reduce hospital length of stay. Other established indications for NIPPV include acute cardiogenic pulmonary edema, postoperative respiratory failure, and hypoxemic respiratory failure in immunocompromised patients (e.g., organ and bone marrow transplant recipients). NIPPV is most beneficial in patients who have a potentially rapidly reversible pulmonary process that requires some ventilator support. Potential drawbacks to using NIPPV include the potential for aspiration, the inability to control tidal volume and airway pressure in patients with ARDS, and potential delays in endotracheal intubation, which can lead to less controlled circumstances if an emergent procedure is required. Contraindications for using NIPPV are listed in Box 41.3.

Mechanical Ventilation

Though respiratory support can be delivered through noninvasive means, mechanical ventilation typically refers to positive-pressure ventilation delivered through an invasive approach (i.e., via ETT or tracheotomy). The goals of mechanical ventilation include (1) decreasing the work of breathing, (2) improving oxygen delivery, (3) facilitating carbon dioxide removal, and (4) minimizing ventilator-associated lung injury. Modern ICU ventilators are controlled by microprocessors that allow for high flow rates,

Box 41.3 Contraindications for Noninvasive Positive-Pressure Ventilation
Impaired neurologic state (coma, seizures, encephalopathy)
Respiratory arrest or upper airway obstruction
Shock or severe cardiovascular instability
Severe upper gastrointestinal bleeding
Recent gastroesophageal surgery
Vomiting
Excessive airway secretions
Facial lesions that prevent proper fit of nasal or facial masks

VI

Table 41.3 Modes of Mechanical Ventilation

		CMV (AC)		IMV (SIMV)		Spontaneous
Name		**AC-VC**	**AC-PC**	**SIMV-VC**	**SIMV-PC**	**PSV**
Target		Volume	Pressure	Volume[a]	Pressure[a]	Pressure
Parameters	Set	- V_T - Flow rate - f - PEEP - FiO_2	- PIP - I:E ratio or I-time - f - PEEP - FiO_2	- V_T - Flow rate - f - PEEP - FiO_2 - Spont breath support	- PIP - I:E ratio or I-time - f - PEEP - FiO_2 - Spont breath support	- Driving P (PIP and PEEP) - FiO_2 - Flow or pressure trigger
	Variable	PIP	V_T, V_E	PIP	V_T, V_E	V_T, V_E
Trigger		Time	Time	Time	Time	Flow or pressure
Cycle		Volume	Time	Volume	Time	Flow
Limit		Volume and pressure	Pressure	Volume	Pressure	Pressure

[a]Target for controlled breaths delivered by ventilator. Spontaneous breaths may be either unsupported or supported by pressure support or volume support.

AC, assist control; *CMV,* controlled mandatory ventilation; *f,* respiratory rate (frequency); *FiO_2,* fraction of inspired oxygen; *I:E,* inspiratory:expiratory; *IMV,* intermittent mandatory ventilation; *I-time,* inspiratory time; *PC,* pressure control; *PEEP,* positive endexpiratory pressure; *PIP,* peak inspiratory pressure; *PSV,* pressure support ventilation; *SIMV,* synchronized intermittent mandatory ventilation; *Spont,* spontaneous; *VC,* volume control; *V_T,* tidal volume; *V_E,* minute ventilation.

carefully controlled tidal volumes and airway pressures, fine control over flow characteristics, hybrid ventilation modes, and advanced monitoring that facilitates delivery of protective ventilation to severely diseased lungs.

In the most basic sense mechanical ventilation is delivered in one of three modes: continuous mandatory ventilation (CMV), intermittent mandatory ventilation (IMV), and spontaneous. These modes are defined by whether the ventilator (CMV) or the patient (spontaneous) initiates the breath or whether a combination of the two (IMV) occurs. *Assist control (AC)* is a commonly used type of CMV in which every breath, including those occurring at a set rate and those initiated by the patient, is fully supported by the ventilator. *Synchronized intermittent mandatory ventilation (SIMV)* is the most commonly used form of IMV, in which the ventilator provides volume- or pressure-targeted breaths at a rate set by providers but also allows the patient to breathe spontaneously in between ventilator-delivered breaths. The ventilator synchronizes its controlled breaths with the patient's spontaneous breaths if they occur within a short window of time before a scheduled controlled breath. Spontaneous breaths in SIMV may be either supported (with pressure or volume support) or unsupported. *Pressure support ventilation (PSV)* is the most common type of spontaneous mode, in which the ventilator delivers a set pressure only when the patient initiates a breath.

The type of support the ventilator provides in each mode is defined by the *target* set by providers for the breath. If the ventilator is set to target a particular tidal volume, the type of support is termed *volume control ventilation (VCV)* whereas if the ventilator is set to deliver a specific airway pressure, it is termed *pressure control ventilation (PCV)*. What triggers (or starts) the breath and what cycles (or stops) the breath may vary in each type of support (Table 41.3).

In each mode some parameters are set by the provider, whereas other parameters vary (see Table 41.3). The physical concept of lung compliance (Box 41.4), which describes how much volume enters the lung when a specific amount of pressure is applied, enables better understanding of these modes. When providers specify a tidal volume to be delivered by the ventilator in VCV, the airway pressure needed to provide that volume varies according to the patient's lung compliance. The inverse is also true; in PCV when the ventilator delivers a breath targeted to achieve a specific airway pressure, the tidal volume of that breath varies depending on the patient's lung compliance (and may even vary breath to breath in the same patient). Because minute ventilation equals tidal volume times respiratory rate, a patient's minute ventilation is also variable in PCV. In addition to the ventilator target, providers must specify other parameters for each

Box 41.4 Formula for Lung Compliance

Compliance = ΔVolume/ΔPressure

Table 41.4 Mechanical Ventilator Orders

Example	Ventilator Orders Written	Additional Settings That Can Be Ordered	Explanation
Example 1: Assist control–volume control (AC-VC)	Mode AC/VC Rate 10 V_T 500 mL PEEP 5 cmH$_2$O Fio$_2$ 1.0	Flow rate: typically 60 L/ min Trigger: flow or pressure	Ventilator will deliver the preset tidal volume of 500 mL 10 times a minute; if the patient's respiratory rate is greater than 10, each breath will also be 500 mL
Example 2: Assist control– pressure control (AC-PC)	Mode AC/PC Rate 10 PIP 20 cmH$_2$O PEEP 5 cmH$_2$O Fio$_2$ 1.0	I:E ratio: typically 1:2 Inspiratory time Trigger: flow or pressure	Ventilator will deliver 10 breaths per minute; each breath will reach a peak pressure of 20 cmH$_2$O; if the patient's respiratory rate is greater than 10, each breath will also reach a peak pressure of 20 cmH$_2$O
Example 3: Synchronized intermittent mandatory ventilation–volume control (SIMV-VC)	Mode SIMV-VC Rate 10 V_T 500 mL Pressure support 5 cmH$_2$O PEEP 5 cmH$_2$O Fio$_2$ 0.5	Flow rate: typically 60 L/ min Trigger: flow or pressure (this applies to all the breaths, SIMV, or pressure support)	Ventilator will deliver 10 breaths per minute with tidal volume 500 mL; if the patient's respiratory rate is greater than 10, those nonmandatory breaths will receive inspiratory pressure support to peak pressure 5 cmH$_2$O above the PEEP of 5 cmH$_2$O
Example 4: Pressure support ventilation (PSV)	Mode PSV Driving pressure 8 cmH$_2$O PEEP 5 cmH$_2$O Fio$_2$ 0.5	Trigger: flow or pressure	Patient must be breathing spontaneously; each breath will receive inspiratory pressure support to peak pressure 8 cmH$_2$O above the PEEP of 5 cmH$_2$O

Fio$_2$, Fraction of inspired oxygen; *I:E*, inspiratory to expiratory ratio; *PEEP*, positive end-expiratory pressure; *PIP*, peak inspiratory pressure; *V$_T$*, tidal volume.

type of ventilation, which may include PEEP, respiratory rate (f), FiO$_2$, flow rate, inspiratory:expiratory ratio, and limit/alarm settings (Table 41.4).

Hybrid modes of mechanical ventilation, which allow for control of more than one parameter at the same time, also exist. These modes are typically given proprietary names by ventilator manufacturers. A combined mode that targets both pressure and volume (known as *pressure-regulated volume control* [PRVC] or *pressure control ventilation-volume guaranteed* [PCV-VG] by different manufacturers) is a general example. In this type of mode the provider specifies both tidal volume and airway pressure targets. The ventilator automatically adjusts the amount of pressure delivered on a breath-by-breath basis to achieve the desired tidal volume without exceeding the pressure limit. This allows a minute ventilation to be achieved in a pressure-targeted mode, which cannot be done using classic PCV.

Weaning From Mechanical Ventilation

Weaning may account for more than 40% of the patient's time on mechanical ventilation. Initiation of an efficient, standardized weaning process as soon as a patient recovers from the initial cause of respiratory failure should decrease the duration of mechanical ventilation and the risk of complications such as ventilator-associated pneumonia (VAP). No single algorithm can accurately predict

successful tracheal extubation in all cases, but reasonable criteria are listed here. The average rate of failed tracheal extubation (i.e., inadequate ventilation after extubation of the trachea) in surgical ICUs is 5% to 8%, whereas in medical and neurologic ICUs, the rate is 17%.

Criteria for Weaning Trial

Oxygenation The patient should have adequate oxygenation, usually defined as PaO$_2$/FiO$_2$ more than 150 mm Hg with PEEP less than 8 cm H$_2$O. This amount of oxygen is chosen because this level can be reliably delivered via facemask or nasal cannula. These numbers are general guidelines, and the ultimate decision for an individual patient requires clinical judgment and experience.

Ventilation Patients should be able to adequately eliminate carbon dioxide without the help of mechanical ventilation. A V$_T$ greater than 5 to 6 cc/kg (with spontaneous breathing or minimal ventilatory support) and a minute ventilation less than 10 L/min are commonly used criteria for extubation readiness.

Respiratory Mechanics

Rapid shallow breathing index (RSBI): RSBI, the ratio of respiratory rate (breaths/min) to tidal volume (in liters), is the most extensively studied and commonly used predictor of extubation success. Though an RSBI less than 105 breaths/min/L is somewhat associated with weaning success, an RSBI more

VI

than 105 breaths/min/L is likely better at identifying patients who will fail.

Maximum inspiratory force (MIF): Patients must have the respiratory muscle strength to generate an adequate tidal volume. Although an MIF more negative than -20 cmH$_2$O (normal: -100 cmH$_2$O) indicates little or no increase in the probability of weaning success, an MIF less negative than -20 cmH$_2$O predicts a small increase in the probability of weaning failure. The challenge of obtaining an accurate measurement in a spontaneously breathing patient is one reason for the poor predictive ability of the MIF. MIF is not routinely measured before weaning from ventilation in most ICUs, though if a patient is not progressing in the weaning process, measurement of an MIF may suggest a cause such as muscle weakness or deconditioning.

Other Criteria Other factors that may affect the success of weaning from mechanical ventilation are described in Box 41.5.

Box 41.5 Factors Affecting Weaning From Mechanical Ventilation

- Secretions: The nature and amount of airway secretions and the ability to clear secretions, which involves the gag reflex and cough strength.
- Upper airway patency:
  - The presence of upper airway edema can lead to airway obstruction and hypoxemia after tracheal extubation. The degree of airway edema can be measured with the cuff leak test. Both volume and pressure approaches for measuring cuff leak have been described.
    - In the volume approach the leak is defined as the difference between the expired tidal volume in volume control mode with the cuff inflated and with the cuff deflated, as a percentage of set tidal volume. A leak of greater than 15% is predictive of successful extubation.
    - In the pressure approach the ETT cuff is deflated and positive pressure is delivered through the ETT until an air leak is heard. A leak pressure of less than 10 cmH$_2$O suggests the absence of airway edema, whereas a leak pressure greater than 20 cmH$_2$O may indicate significant airway edema.
  - Ongoing anatomic obstructions such as upper airway masses may play a role in determining whether to remove an ETT.
- Mental status: Patients should have an adequate level of consciousness to protect their airway from aspiration of gastric contents.
- Hemodynamic stability: Patients should be hemodynamically stable, because discontinuation of positive-pressure ventilation can lead to increased work of breathing and alter left ventricular preload and afterload.
- Clinical course: Resolution or improvement of the process for which the patient was intubated should be considered.

ETT, endotracheal tube.

Weaning Strategies

All mechanically ventilated patients should undergo a daily assessment of extubation readiness.[24] If the patient is deemed ready, a spontaneous breathing trial (SBT) is performed. If the factors described previously (e.g., respiratory mechanics, mental status, hemodynamics) remain adequate throughout the SBT, a decision for tracheal extubation can be made. Protocol-based weaning by nurses and respiratory therapists allows more rapid tracheal extubation compared with physician-directed weaning. The SBT can be conducted with different ventilation modes, including PSV or T-piece trial. No specific ventilation mode has yet been shown to be superior to others.[25] However, for an individual patient, a specific mode may have clinical advantages. For example, in patients with heart failure and reduced left ventricular ejection fraction the change from positive-pressure ventilation to negative-pressure ventilation can increase left ventricular afterload and worsen cardiovascular strain. This patient may benefit from a T-piece trial for the SBT, because even low levels of positive pressure and PEEP may provide afterload reduction. If the patient does not develop signs of pulmonary edema during the T-piece trial, the decision for tracheal extubation can proceed.

The optimal duration of an SBT is unknown, but most range from 30 minutes to 2 hours. Longer periods may be required for patients with chronic respiratory failure or for patients who fail their initial SBT. In select patients weaning strategies that include NIPPV can reduce the rate of mortality, VAP, and weaning failure without increasing the risk of tracheal reintubation.[26] This approach may be considered in patients who do not have difficult-to-manage airways, excessive secretions, or an impaired mental status and should be coupled with an early decision regarding tracheal reintubation if the patient remains tachypneic or in distress. Tracheal reintubation, especially if delayed, is associated with increased mortality rate, longer hospital stay, and lower likelihood of returning home.

Tracheotomies

A small proportion of patients may require prolonged mechanical ventilation during their critical illness. A tracheotomy may facilitate rehabilitation and allow for weaning of sedation. The timing of tracheotomy remains a controversial topic. Early tracheotomy ($\leq$4 days) does not result in decreased mortality or ICU length of stay when compared with late tracheotomy ($\geq$10 days).[27] Physicians are poor at predicting those patients requiring prolonged mechanical ventilation. Only 45% of the patients who were predicted to require more than 7 days of mechanical ventilation actually required a tracheotomy; the remaining 55% were successfully extubated. Because of this, tracheotomies are often deferred until 10 to 14 days after tracheal intubation.

Placement of tracheotomies can lead to the loss of mean airway pressure and derecruitment of alveolar units, so the procedure should be deferred in unstable patients and those with high PEEP and oxygen requirements. Inadvertent dislodgement of the tracheostomy tube during the first 7 days after placement is a potentially life-threatening problem. In this circumstance blind tracheotomy tube advancement may result in passage through a false subcutaneous tract rather than into the trachea. When feasible, orotracheal intubation should be the first maneuver to obtain a secure airway. Otherwise, a pediatric laryngoscope blade or a fiber-optic scope may be inserted into the stoma, and a new tracheotomy tube or ETT can be inserted under direct visual identification of tracheal rings.

Gastrointestinal: Nutrition

The goal of nutrition in the ICU is to preserve lean body mass and avoid malnourishment, which can lead to increased mortality rate, prolonged hospital stays, poor wound healing, and increased risk for infection. However, there are no reliable laboratory markers to determine the patients at risk, because of fluctuating volume status and impaired protein synthesis associated with critical illness and multiorgan failure. Therefore identification of patients at risk requires careful history taking and a targeted nutritional physical examination.

Estimates of daily caloric requirements can be calculated from various equations. The Harris Benedict equation estimates basal energy expenditure based on weight, height, age, and sex. An additional adjustment must then be made for the increased metabolism associated with underlying disease processes such as infections, multisystem organ dysfunction, trauma, and burns. A quick method to estimate whether the patient is receiving enough calories based on weight and level of stress or illness is described in Table 41.5. Sometimes, a simple nutritional plan can be started based on these estimates, and then further tests (e.g., nitrogen balance study) can be obtained to assess the adequacy of the protein-based calories.

Enteral nutrition is always preferred to parenteral nutrition in order to maintain gut integrity and reduce the risk of gastrointestinal bleeding. However, achieving goal rate or goal calories is not urgent, at least for the first week in otherwise well-nourished patients.[28] Vomiting and aspiration of gastric contents have long been

Table 41.5	Quick Estimate of Caloric Needs
Level of Illness/Stress	**Estimated Caloric Need**
Maintenance or minimal	25–30 kcal/kg/day
Moderate	30–35 kcal/kg/day
Severe	35–40 kcal/kg/day

The nutritional intake composition should be 1.2–2 g/kg/day protein, 15%–30% of calories should be from lipids, and the remainder of the calories should be from carbohydrates (30%–70%).

concerns for critically ill patients fed via a feeding tube. In the past feedings were often reduced or held for minimal gastric residual volume, leading patients to receive only a small portion of their estimated caloric requirement over time. Current literature does not support this practice, so significantly larger residual volumes are now accepted (500 mL or more).[29]

Patients undergoing frequent surgeries (like burn debridements) may end up malnourished from frequent nutritional holds that start at midnight or 8 hours before surgery.[30] With increased emphasis on continuing enteral nutrition, there has been a shift toward decreasing or eliminating fasting times for critically ill patients having surgical procedures. At some institutions all enteral feeding in intubated patients can be continued until transport to the operating room, whereas others enforce longer fasting intervals for gastric feeding tubes versus postpyloric or jejunal feeding tubes. Some providers recommend aspiration of any residual gastric contents before transfer. Most institutions continue to recommend 6 to 8 hours fasting before procedures involving manipulation of the ETT (such as tracheostomies or laryngectomies). No definitive data exist to guide practice, and ultimately the decision is based on a hospital's practice and the clinical discretion of the anesthesia provider.

Renal: Acute Kidney Injury

Epidemiology

The incidence of acute kidney injury (AKI) in the ICU is as high as 35%. Despite improvements in renal replacement technology, ARF requiring dialysis in the ICU is associated with in-hospital mortality of more than 50%.

Diagnosis

Multiple criteria exist in the literature to define AKI.[31] The Acute Dialysis Quality Initiative (ADQI) group, an alliance of experts consisting of nephrologists and intensivists, proposed the RIFLE criteria (Table 41.6), which stands for risk, injury, failure, and two outcome classes (loss and end-stage kidney disease).[32] For each increasing RIFLE class, there is a stepwise increase in mortality rate independent of other comorbidities. Therefore strategies to prevent even mild AKI may improve survival.

ARF is normally categorized by prerenal, renal, and postrenal causes (Box 41.6). The workup should include careful physical examination and assessment of intravascular volume status in order to differentiate hypovolemia leading to prerenal azotemia versus hypervolemia from oliguria. Laboratory evaluations should include serum and urine electrolytes, urinalysis, and examination of urinary sediment. Urine sodium concentration and fractional excretion of sodium can help identify prerenal azotemia. In patients who have received a diuretic the fractional excretion of urea may be a more sensitive test than fractional excretion of sodium.

VI

Table 41.6 The RIFLE Criteria

RIFLE Category	GFR Criteria	UO Criteria	OR Hospital Mortality
Risk	Cr increased × 1.5 or GFR decreased >25%	<0.5 mL/kg/ hr × 6 hr	2.2 (95% CI 2.17–2.3)
Injury	Cr increased × 2 or GFR decreased >50%	<0.5 mL/kg/ hr × 12 hr	6.1 (95% CI 5.74–6.44)
Failure	Cr increased × 3 or GFR decreased >75% or Cr >4 mg/dL	<0.3 mL/kg/ hr × 24 hr or Anuria × 12 hr	8.6 (95% CI 8.07–9.15)
Loss	Complete loss of renal function for >4 weeks		
ESRD	End-stage renal disease		

Cr, Creatinine; ESRD, end-stage renal disease; GFR, glomerular filtration rate; OR, odds ratio; UO, urine output.
Data modified from KDI Global, OKAKIW Group. Kidney Disease Improving Global Outcomes (KDIGO) clinical practice guideline for acute kidney injury. Kidney Int. 2012;(Suppl 2):1–138.

Box 41.6 Causes of Acute Renal Failure

Prerenal

Hypovolemia

Low effective circulating volume (e.g., from decompensated heart failure or liver disease)

Renal

Glomerulonephritis

Toxins (e.g., NSAIDs, cisplatin, aminoglycosides, contrast agent, myoglobin, hemoglobin)

Vasculitis (e.g., TTP/HUS)

AIN (e.g., from PCN, cephalosporins, cimetidine, SLE, sarcoidosis)

Tubular disease (e.g., ATN, tumor lysis syndrome)

Postrenal

Obstructive nephropathy

AIN, Acute interstitial nephritis; ATN, acute tubular necrosis; NSAIDs, nonsteroidal antiinflammatory drugs; PCN, penicillin; SLE, systemic lupus erythematosus; TTP/HUS, thrombotic thrombocytopenic purpura/hemolytic uremic syndrome.

Treatment

Supportive care should be focused on maintenance of euvolemia, avoidance of nephrotoxic drugs such as non-steroidal antiinflammatory drugs (NSAIDs) or contrast,

medication dose adjustments for creatinine clearance, and electrolyte and acid–base monitoring. Platelet dysfunction may occur as a result of uremia and require desmopressin (DDAVP) for support if bleeding is problematic. Pharmacologic approaches to improve renal function such as low-dose dopamine, diuretics, and N-acetylcysteine have not shown benefit.

Dialysis

Dialysis is often required in patients with advanced renal failure to help with excessive intravascular volume and electrolyte disturbances. In the ICU dialysis can be offered as intermittent hemodialysis (iHD) or continuous renal replacement therapy (CRRT), which is itself divided into versions that rely on hemodialysis (CVVHD) or hemofiltration (CVVH). Although CRRT has several theoretical advantages over iHD in hemodynamically unstable patients or those at risk of injury with rapid fluid or electrolyte shifts, randomized trials have not supported its superiority.[33]

Fluid Status Assessment

Management of critically ill patients often involves assessment of fluid status. Whether a patient is hypovolemic or hypervolemic can alter management in many disease processes, including AKI and hyponatremia. Because no single data point can accurately predict volume status, a global assessment of the patient is needed. This can include physical examination findings (mucous membranes, peripheral edema), ultrasound (inferior vena cava [IVC] examination), static measurements (CVP, pulmonary capillary wedge pressure), and dynamic measurements (SPV on arterial lines, straight-leg raise)[17] (also see Chapter 24).

Infectious Disease: Hospital-Acquired Infections

While community-acquired infections are far more prevalent in ICU patients than hospital-acquired infections (HAIs), some HAIs can be reduced or prevented by the introduction of evidence-based bundles of care. Successfully reducing these infections can improve patient outcomes by reducing complications and reduce cost for the hospital, which does not receive reimbursement for treatment provided for HAIs. The most common HAIs in ICUs are urinary tract infections (31%), followed by pneumonia (27%), and primary bloodstream infections (19%).

Catheter-Associated Urinary Tract Infection

No single strategy prevents catheter-associated urinary tract infections (CAUTIs). The only recommendations have been to use aseptic techniques for placement and to limit the duration of indwelling urinary catheters by assessing for daily need. Asymptomatic bacteriuria is often confused for a CAUTI, so urine cultures are only recommended when symptoms or a urinalysis suggest infection or inflammation.

Ventilator-Associated Pneumonia

Evidence-based bundles to reduce the incidence of VAP include elevation of the head of the bed to 30 degrees, use of ETTs with subglottic suctioning, and daily use of spontaneous awakening trials (SATs) and SBTs to assess ongoing need for mechanical ventilation. Excessive use of medications for stress ulcer prophylaxis increases gastric pH and the risk for VAP, so they should be discontinued when patients lack an indication for their use.[34]

Catheter-Related Bloodstream Infection

Catheter-related bloodstream infections (CRBSIs) are usually associated with central venous access. Bundles that ensure sterile placement of these central lines along with daily assessment of their ongoing need can reduce rates of CRBSIs. These bundles include skin preparation with chlorhexidine, chlorhexidine sponge for site dressing, antimicrobial-impregnated central lines, maximal sterile barrier use during line placement, and hand hygiene during line placement.[35]

Endocrine: Glucose Management

Based on a landmark 2001 study, intensive insulin therapy to achieve a blood glucose level between 80 and 110 mg/dL was previously thought to be essential for improving survival in the ICU.[36] However, more recent data have shown that intensive insulin therapy does not improve survival and actually increases the risks of hypoglycemia and mortality.[37,38] Given these findings, current ICU management goals include minimizing severe hypoglycemia (less than 40 mg/dL) and hyperglycemia (more than 200 mg/dL) by targeting a moderate glucose range between 140 and 180 mg/dL. The optimal glucose target for an individual patient may vary from this range based on the patient's baseline blood glucose or unique clinical situation.

Prophylaxis

Venous Thromboembolism

Critically ill patients are at increased risk for venous thromboembolisms (VTEs), including deep vein thrombosis (DVT) and pulmonary embolism. Along with risk factors for the general population such as immobility, independent risk factors specific to critically ill patients include mechanical ventilation, central venous catheterization, and vasopressor administration.

Randomized controlled trials reveal that chemoprophylaxis with unfractionated heparin (UFH) or low-molecular-weight heparin (LMWH) significantly reduces the occurrence of DVTs.[39] The American College of Chest Physicians recommends either UFH or LMWH in patients with moderate risk for VTE, whereas high-risk patients, such as trauma and orthopedic patients, should receive LMWH. In patients at increased risk for bleeding complications mechanical thromboprophylaxis (e.g., graduated compression stockings, intermittent pneumatic compression devices) provides some level of protection against VTE, but it is less effective than chemoprophylaxis and is generally ineffective as dual therapy in patients already receiving chemoprophylaxis.[40]

Gastrointestinal Prophylaxis

Gastrointestinal stress ulcers occur in critically ill patients because of an increase in gastric acid production in conjunction with a functionally impaired mucosal barrier. Gastrointestinal bleeding occurs more frequently in patients who are mechanically ventilated for more than 48 hours and in those with a coagulopathy (Box 41.7), especially in patients unable to tolerate enteral feeding. Prophylaxis with a proton pump inhibitor or an H$_2$ blocker can reduce rates of gastrointestinal bleeding in these high-risk patients, with the data somewhat favoring proton pump inhibitors; however, neither reduce mortality.[41] Patients who receive gastrointestinal prophylaxis may have increased risks of developing hospital-associated pneumonia or *Clostridium difficile* infection because of an increased gastric pH. Thus prophylaxis should be discontinued as soon as patients are no longer at high risk of gastrointestinal bleeding or once they tolerate any enteral nutrition.[42]

A-F BUNDLE

There is a well-established connection between common critical care diagnoses (such as sepsis or delirium) and long-term impairment in cognition and/or physical function in survivors of critical illness. The term

Box 41.7 Indications for Stress Ulcer Prophylaxis
History of GI bleed within last year
Mechanical ventilation >48 hours
Coagulopathy not from pharmacologic anticoagulation (platelet count <50 × 10^9/L, INR >1.5, or PTT >2 × control)
Trauma
Spinal cord injury
Severe traumatic brain injury
Extensive thermal injury or burns
High-dose steroids in patients with severe sepsis or septic shock

GI, Gastrointestinal; *INR,* international normalized ratio; *PTT,* partial thromboplastin time.

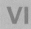

VI

"post–intensive care syndrome" (PICS) has been developed to describe a constellation of physical, cognitive, or psychological symptoms that persist in critically ill patients or their family members after an ICU stay.[43]

The A-F bundle[44] is a care strategy that was developed to help prevent or ameliorate the long-term cognitive, physical, and psychological impairments associated with PICS. Successful bundle implementation requires collaboration among members of the interprofessional ICU care team and application of many of the concepts previously discussed in this chapter. Hospitals that have implemented this bundle report increased hospital survival and increased delirium-free and coma-free days.[45] Elements of the bundle include the following components.

A: Assess, Prevent, and Manage Pain

Pain affects nearly all ICU patients whether they are capable of communicating it or not. Therefore regular pain assessment using a validated assessment tool is critical. Scales relying on self-reporting of pain are preferred (i.e., Numeric Rating Scale), but validated tools also exist for those who are unable to communicate (i.e., Behavioral Pain Scale or Critical Care Pain Observation Tool). Opioid pain medications are recommended as first-line agents to treat pain in ICU patients, but nonopioid adjuncts and nonpharmacologic techniques such as relaxation and music should also be considered when appropriate. Pain should be controlled preemptively if an upcoming procedure is expected to cause discomfort (also see Chapter 40).

B: Both SAT and SBT

Reducing the amount of time a patient receives mechanical ventilation is an important goal. Performing a daily coordinated SAT together with an SBT reduces the duration of mechanical ventilation.[46] An SAT should not be performed in patients with contraindications to stopping continuous sedation, including neuromuscular blockade, alcohol withdrawal, seizures, or elevated intracranial pressure. During an SAT, continuous sedative infusions are paused, and the patient's pain and agitation levels are assessed. A validated sedation scale such as the Richmond Agitation-Sedation Scale (RASS) should be used for assessment. If the patient remains calm, continuous sedation should not be restarted, and pain should be treated, as noted earlier. If the patient becomes agitated, continuous sedation should be restarted at the lowest dose necessary to achieve a calm, cooperative patient. This sedation strategy focuses on providing the lightest possible sedation level necessary to facilitate mechanical ventilation. Light sedation can help diminish long-term psychological consequences of ICU admission, such as posttraumatic stress disorder.[47] Protocolized management of SAT and SBT by non physicians has been shown to decrease time to extubation.[48]

C: Choice of Sedation and Analgesia

Before starting continuous sedation, pain should be controlled aggressively, usually with intermittent intravenous opioids. If pain has been optimally controlled and the patient remains agitated or has delirium, these issues should be targeted next. Propofol or dexmedetomidine are the preferred agents for continuous sedative infusions when they are needed. Light sedation levels (i.e., RASS 0 or -1) should be targeted in most patients. Because benzodiazepine sedation in the ICU is associated with increased mortality and duration of mechanical ventilation, continuous infusions of these medications should generally be avoided when other options are available.[49] Common sedative and analgesic agents are listed in Table 41.7.

Table 41.7 Sedatives and Analgesics

Drug	Elimination Half-Time	Peak Effect[a]	Suggested Dose	
			Bolus	Infusion
Morphine	2–4 hr	30 min	1–4 mg	1–10 mg/hr
Fentanyl	2–5 hr	4 min	25–100 µg	25–200 µg/hr
Hydromorphone	2–4 hr	20 min	0.2–1 mg	0.2–5 mg/hr
Ketamine	2–3 hr	30–60 s		1–5 µg/kg/min
Midazolam	3–5 hr	2–5 min	1–2 mg	0.5–10 mg/hr
Lorazepam	10–20 hr	2–20 min	1–2 mg	0.5–10 mg/hr
Propofol	20–30 hr	90 s		25–100 µg/kg/min
Dexmedetomidine	2 hr	1–2 min		0.2–0.7 µg/kg/hr

[a]With intravenous administration.

D: Delirium: Assess, Prevent, and Manage

Delirium affects up to 80% of mechanically ventilated patients in the ICU and can lead to a number of long-term consequences. Methods to assess, prevent, and manage delirium are discussed earlier in this chapter.

E: Early Mobility

Patients in the ICU experience rapid deterioration of muscle strength and function. Early mobility is safe in mechanically ventilated patients and in those with invasive lines and monitors and has been associated with improved outcomes, including increased ventilator-free days, reduced duration of delirium, and improved functional status at the time of discharge.[50]

F: Family Engagement and Empowerment

Providing patient- and family-centered care is increasingly a quality focus in the ICU. These terms acknowledge the importance of patient and family values and preferences in shared medical decision making. Many structures have been proposed to facilitate patient- and family-centered care. A few examples include patient and family inclusion on rounds, extended visiting hours, and family presence during procedures. Patients report many benefits from this type of care, including decreased anxiety, confusion, and agitation and increased satisfaction.

ACKNOWLEDGMENT

The editors and publisher would like to thank Drs. John Turnbull and Linda Liu for contributing to this chapter in the previous edition of this work. It has served as the foundation for the current chapter.

REFERENCES

1. Donovan AL, Aldrich JM, Gross AK, et al. Interprofessional care and teamwork in the ICU. *Crit Care Med.* 2018;46(6):980–990.
2. Pronovost PJ, Angus DC, Dorman T, Robinson KA, Dremsizov TT, Young TL. Physician staffing patterns and clinical outcomes in critically ill patients: A systematic review. *JAMA.* 2002;288(17):2151–2162.
3. Ely EW, Inouye SK, Bernard GR, et al. Delirium in mechanically ventilated patients: Validity and reliability of the Confusion Assessment Method for the Intensive Care Unit (CAM-ICU). *JAMA.* 2001;286(21):2703–2710.
4. Ely EW, Shintani A, Truman B, et al. Delirium as a predictor of mortality in mechanically ventilated patients in the intensive care unit. *JAMA.* 2004;291(14):1753–1762.
5. Hatta K, Kishi Y, Wada K, et al. Preventive effects of ramelteon on delirium: A randomized placebo-controlled trial. *JAMA Psychiatry.* 2014;71(4):397–403.
6. Holcomb JB, Tilley BC, Baraniuk S, et al. Transfusion of plasma, platelets, and red blood cells in a 1:1:1 vs a 1:1:2 ratio and mortality in patients with severe trauma: The PROPPR randomized clinical trial. *JAMA.* 2015;313(5):471–482.
7. Shakur H, Roberts I, et al. CRASH-2 Trial Collaborators Effects of tranexamic acid on death, vascular occlusive events, and blood transfusion in trauma patients with significant haemorrhage (CRASH-2): A randomised, placebo-controlled trial. *Lancet.* 2010;376(9734):23–32.
8. Hochman JS, Sleeper LA, Webb JG, et al. Early revascularization in acute myocardial infarction complicated by cardiogenic shock. SHOCK Investigators. Should We Emergently Revascularize Occluded Coronaries for Cardiogenic Shock. *N Engl J Med.* 1999;341(9):625–634.
9. Thiele H, Zeymer U, Neumann F-J, et al. Intraaortic balloon support for myocardial infarction with cardiogenic shock. *N Engl J Med.* 2012;367(14):1287–1296.
10. Schrage B, Ibrahim K, Loehn T, et al. Impella support for acute myocardial infarction complicated by cardiogenic shock. *Circulation.* 2019;139(10):1249–1258.
11. Cecconi M, Evans L, Levy M, Rhodes A. Sepsis and septic shock. *Lancet.* 2018;392(10141):75–87.
12. Rivers E, Nguyen B, Havstad S, et al. Early goal-directed therapy in the treatment of severe sepsis and septic shock. *N Engl J Med.* 2001;345(19):1368–1377.
13. PRISM InvestigatorsRowan KM, Angus DC, et al. Early, goal-directed therapy for septic shock—A patient-level meta-analysis. *N Engl J Med.* 2017;376(23):2223–2234.
14. National Heart, Lung, and Blood Institute Acute Respiratory Distress Syndrome (ARDS) Clinical Trials NetworkWiedemann HP, Wheeler AP, et al. Comparison of two fluid-management strategies in acute lung injury. *N Engl J Med.* 2006;354(24):2564–2575.
15. LoVerde D, Iweala OI, Eginli A, Krishnaswamy G. Anaphylaxis. *Chest.* 2018;153(2):528–543.
16. Hadley MN, Walters BC, Grabb PA, et al. Blood pressure management after acute spinal cord injury. *Neurosurgery.* 2002;50(3 Suppl):S58–S62.
17. Bentzer P, Griesdale DE, Boyd J, MacLean K, Sirounis D, Ayas NT. Will this hemodynamically unstable patient respond to a bolus of intravenous fluids?. *JAMA.* 2016;316(12):1298–1309.
18. Marik PE, Baram M, Vahid B. Does central venous pressure predict fluid responsiveness? A systematic review of the literature and the tale of seven mares. *Chest.* 2008;134(1):172–178.
19. Rajaram SS, Desai NK, Kalra A, et al. Pulmonary artery catheters for adult patients in intensive care. *Cochrane Database Syst Rev.* 2013(2):CD003408.
20. Teboul J-L, Saugel B, Cecconi M, et al. Less invasive hemodynamic monitoring in critically ill patients. *Intensive Care Med.* 2016;42(9):1350–1359.
21. Acute respiratory distress syndrome: The Berlin definition. *JAMA.* 2012;307(23).
22. RG Brower, Matthay MA, et al. Acute Respiratory Distress Syndrome Network Ventilation with lower tidal volumes as compared with traditional tidal volumes for acute lung injury and the acute respiratory distress syndrome. *N Engl J Med.* 2000;342(18):1301–1308.
23. Frat J-P, Thille AW, Mercat A, et al. High-flow oxygen through nasal cannula in acute hypoxemic respiratory failure. *N Engl J Med.* 2015;372(23):2185–2196.
24. McConville JF, Kress JP. Weaning patients from the ventilator. *N Engl J Med.* 2012;367(23):2233–2239.

VI

25. Ladeira MT, Vital FMR, Andriolo RB, Andriolo BNG, Atallah AN, Peccin MS. Pressure support versus T-tube for weaning from mechanical ventilation in adults. *Cochrane Database Syst Rev.* 2014(5):CD006056.

26. Burns KEA, Meade MO, Premji A, Adhikari NKJ. Noninvasive positive-pressure ventilation as a weaning strategy for intubated adults with respiratory failure. *Cochrane Database Syst Rev.* 2013(12):CD004127.

27. Young D, Harrison DA, Cuthbertson BH, Rowan K, Collaborators TracMan. Effect of early vs late tracheostomy placement on survival in patients receiving mechanical ventilation: The TracMan randomized trial. *JAMA.* 2013;309(20):2121–2129.

28. Rice TW, Wheeler AP, et al. National Heart, Lung, and Blood Institute Acute Respiratory Distress Syndrome (ARDS) Clinical Trials Network Initial trophic vs full enteral feeding in patients with acute lung injury: The EDEN randomized trial. *JAMA.* 2012;307(8):795–803.

29. Casaer MP, Van den Berghe G. Nutrition in the acute phase of critical illness. *N Engl J Med.* 2014;370(13):1227–1236.

30. Pham CH, Collier ZJ, Webb AB, Garner WL, Gillenwater TJ. How long are burn patients really NPO in the perioperative period and can we effectively correct the caloric deficit using an enteral feeding "Catch-up" protocol?. *Burns J Int Soc Burn Inj.* 2018;44(8):2006–2010.

31. Palevsky PM, Liu KD, Brophy PD, et al. KDOQI US commentary on the 2012 KDIGO Clinical Practice Guideline for Acute Kidney Injury. *Am J Kidney Dis Off J Natl Kidney Found.* 2013;61(5):649–672.

32. Bellomo R, Kellum JA, Ronco C. Defining and classifying acute renal failure: From advocacy to consensus and validation of the RIFLE criteria. *Intensive Care Med.* 2007;33(3):409–413.

33. Vinsonneau C, Camus C, Combes A, et al. Continuous venovenous haemodiafiltration versus intermittent haemodialysis for acute renal failure in patients with multiple-organ dysfunction syndrome: A multicentre randomised trial. *Lancet.* 2006;368(9533):379–385.

34. Hellyer TP, Ewan V, Wilson P, Simpson AJ. The Intensive Care Society recommended bundle of interventions for the prevention of ventilator-associated pneumonia. *J Intensive Care Soc.* 2016;17(3):238–243.

35. Pronovost PJ, Goeschel CA, Colantuoni E, et al. Sustaining reductions in catheter related bloodstream infections in Michigan intensive care units: Observational study. *BMJ.* 2010;340:c309.

36. van den Berghe G, Wouters P, Weekers F, et al. Intensive insulin therapy in critically ill patients. *N Engl J Med.* 2001;345(19):1359–1367.

37. NICE-SUGAR Study InvestigatorsFinfer S, Chittock DR, et al. Intensive versus conventional glucose control in critically ill patients. *N Engl J Med.* 2009;360(13):1283–1297.

38. Annane D, Cariou A, et al. COIITSS Study Investigators Corticosteroid treatment and intensive insulin therapy for septic shock in adults: A randomized controlled trial. *JAMA.* 2010;303(4):341–348.

39. Minet C, Potton L, Bonadona A, et al. Venous thromboembolism in the ICU: Main characteristics, diagnosis and thromboprophylaxis. *Crit Care.* 2015;19:287.

40. Arabi YM, Al-Hameed F, Burns KEA, et al. Adjunctive Intermittent Pneumatic Compression for Venous Thromboprophylaxis. *N Engl J Med.* 2019;380(14):1305–1315.

41. Krag M, Marker S, Perner A, et al. Pantoprazole in patients at risk for gastrointestinal bleeding in the ICU. *N Engl J Med.* 2018;379(23):2199–2208.

42. Huang H-B, Jiang W, Wang C-Y, Qin H-Y, Du B. Stress ulcer prophylaxis in intensive care unit patients receiving enteral nutrition: A systematic review and meta-analysis. *Crit Care.* 2018;22(1):20.

43. Needham DM, Davidson J, Cohen H, et al. Improving long-term outcomes after discharge from intensive care unit: Report from a stakeholders' conference. *Crit Care Med.* 2012;40(2):502–509.

44. Ely EW. The ABCDEF Bundle: Science and Philosophy of How ICU Liberation Serves Patients and Families. *Crit Care Med.* 2017;45(2):321–330.

45. Barnes-Daly MA, Phillips G, Ely EW. Improving hospital survival and reducing brain dysfunction at seven California community hospitals: Implementing PAD Guidelines via the ABCDEF Bundle in 6,064 patients. *Crit Care Med.* 2017;45(2):171–178.

46. Girard TD, Kress JP, Fuchs BD, et al. Efficacy and safety of a paired sedation and ventilator weaning protocol for mechanically ventilated patients in intensive care (awakening and breathing controlled trial): A randomised controlled trial. *Lancet.* 2008;371(9607):126–134.

47. Treggiari MM, Romand J-A, Yanez ND, et al. Randomized trial of light versus deep sedation on mental health after critical illness. *Crit Care Med.* 2009;37(9):2527–2534.

48. Ely EW, Baker AM, Dunagan DP, et al. Effect on the duration of mechanical ventilation of identifying patients capable of breathing spontaneously. *N Engl J Med.* 1996;335(25):1864–1869.

49. Jakob SM, Ruokonen E, Grounds RM, et al. Dexmedetomidine vs midazolam or propofol for sedation during prolonged mechanical ventilation: Two randomized controlled trials. *JAMA.* 2012;307(11):1151–1160.

50. Schweickert WD, Pohlman MC, Pohlman AS, et al. Early physical and occupational therapy in mechanically ventilated, critically ill patients: A randomised controlled trial. *Lancet.* 2009;373(9678):1874–1882.

42 PERIOPERATIVE MEDICINE

Matthew D. McEvoy, Jeanna D. Blitz, Emilee Borgmeier

INTRODUCTION

The practice of anesthesiology historically focused on the care of an individual patient undergoing surgery. The specialty has an impressive track record for improving quality and safety in patient care (also see Chapter 46). Although anesthesia practice continues to evolve, patients undergoing major surgery still experience adverse outcomes related to their physiologic reserve and the metabolic and inflammatory response to the surgical intervention. The focus on the nonoperative care of patients undergoing major surgery has led to the concept of perioperative medicine. Two leaders in the field have stated that "Perioperative Medicine is the future of anesthesia, if our specialty is to thrive."[1] Others acknowledge the importance of perioperative medicine as a means to promote value-based, patient-centered care.[2,3]

The evolution of perioperative medicine has come a long way, and yet is still in its infancy. Other medical specialties have also experienced exponential growth and a distinct area of focus, including the evolution of interventional radiology within radiology and hospital-based medicine in internal medicine.

One estimate of the average number of operations that an average American will undergo in an 85-year lifetime is nine procedures.[4] Of these, three were non–operating room procedures (e.g., colonoscopy), three were outpatient procedures (e.g., cataracts, minor orthopedic surgery), and three were inpatient procedures. The most common operating room procedures in men were coronary angioplasty (percutaneous transluminal coronary angioplasty [PTCA]), wound debridement, and groin hernia; for women, the most common operating room procedures were cesarean section, cholecystectomy, and lens and cataract procedures. As such, the preoperative, intraoperative, and postoperative anesthesia and surgical management is a major health concern. This chapter will describe the emerging domain of perioperative medicine, which spans the period beginning with preoperative assessment and nonsurgical patient optimization, the surgical procedure itself, and subsequent care until the patient returns to their primary care and other longitudinal providers after recovery from surgery.

THE PERIOPERATIVE MEDICINE CONSULTANT

The perioperative medicine consultant, who may someday be called a "perioperativist", is a physician specifically trained to optimize patient health in order to improve postoperative outcomes. Although there is overlap with many medical subspecialties, perioperative medicine is a distinct medical discipline with a unique focus on preparing patients for the stress of surgery, anesthesia, and recovery throughout the postoperative period.[2,5] Although it is possible that physicians from surgical or medical disciplines could provide this care, the anesthesiologist is uniquely suited for this role (Box 42.1). The core training focuses on the immediate perioperative period; however, the expansion of anesthesia care to include optimization of patient care for long-term outcome improvement represents a natural extension of the specialty.[6]

IMPROVING PERIOPERATIVE OUTCOMES AND OPERATIONALIZING PERIOPERATIVE MEDICINE

For many decades, the immediate perioperative period was the focus for improving patient safety and outcomes. As safety vastly improved in the intraoperative

---

Box 42.1 The Anesthesiologist as Perioperative Physician

The skills, experience, and training of anesthesiologists are suitable for the perioperative medicine role, including the following perspectives:

- Unique understanding of the physiologic and psychological stress of surgery and anesthesia
- Expertise in acute care medicine related to the perioperative period, with training in the postanesthesia care unit (PACU) and intensive care unit
- Training in residency to focus on the nonsurgical aspects of patient care, including preanesthesia assessment, and an understanding of how optimization of medical comorbidities can be accomplished in conjunction with surgical planning
- Understanding of how chronic medical conditions interface with the resource constraints of an ambulatory surgery center (ASC) and criteria for candidacy for surgery at an ASC.

---

and immediate postoperative period, the focus widened to include in-hospital complications and then the first 30 days after surgery.[7] Most recently, clinical advances have afforded the ability to focus even further to include outcomes at 1 year after surgery and beyond.[8] Those advances have enabled perioperative care teams to study and focus more and more on the patient from a holistic perspective, including functional capacity, social interactions, pain interference, sleep disturbances, and more.[9] This expanded focus involves three distinct phases of care: prehabilitation, immediate perioperative care, and recovery/rehabilitation.

When considering the work of the perioperative medicine consultant, one metaphor relates the perioperative period to traversing a dangerous mountain. The novice traveler, the patient in this metaphor, has a better chance of safe passage (good outcome) if assisted by someone more familiar with the trail, the perioperative consultant (Fig. 42.1). The ascent is focused on prehabilitation and medical optimization for surgery, as the current focus of perioperative medicine is largely on the preoperative period. However, the descent (postoperative period) is more dangerous, as the most serious outcomes, including death, are more likely to occur in this phase of care. Future studies will need to focus on helping vulnerable patients safely descend from the stressful summit of surgery and anesthesia. A timeline of the perioperative management of the conditions discussed here will be provided at the end of this chapter.

VALUE-ADDED PREOPERATIVE SCREENING AND TESTING

Indications for preoperative testing are evolving. Campaigns such as the American Board of Internal Medicine (ABIM) Foundation's Choosing Wisely[10] and the United Kingdom's National Institute for Health and Care Excellence (NICE) guidelines[11] emphasize selection of testing that is evidence based and that supports a value-based care paradigm. Risk prediction tools have become more readily accessible, refined, and patient-specific. This has resulted in a shift away from routine preoperative testing toward a balanced, systems-based approach targeting the identification of *modifiable* factors.[12] The current American Society of Anesthesiologists Practice Advisory for the preanesthesia evaluation recommends that preoperative testing be based on patient risk factors and surgical severity, as opposed to the provision of routine screening in the absence of clinical indications.[12] Examples of routine testing to be avoided include electrocardiograms (ECGs) in asymptomatic patients simply based on age or medical history (e.g., hypertension), chest x-rays in asymptomatic patients with normal physical examination, and urinalysis.[12]

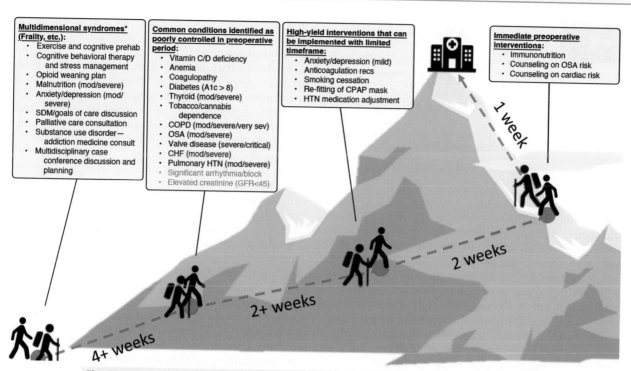

Multidimensional syndromes* (Frailty, etc.):
- Exercise and cognitive prehab
- Cognitive behavioral therapy and stress management
- Opioid weaning plan
- Malnutrition (mod/severe)
- Anxiety/depression (mod/ severe)
- SDM/goals of care discussion
- Palliative care consultation
- Substance use disorder— addiction medicine consult
- Multidisciplinary case conference discussion and planning

Common conditions identified as poorly controlled in preoperative period:
- Vitamin C/D deficiency
- Anemia
- Coagulopathy
- Diabetes (A1c > 8)
- Thyroid (mod/severe)
- Tobacco/cannabis dependence
- COPD (mod/severe/very sev)
- OSA (mod/severe)
- Valve disease (severe/critical)
- CHF (mod/severe)
- Pulmonary HTN (mod/severe)
- Significant arrhythmia/block
- Elevated creatinine (GFR<45)

High-yield interventions that can be implemented with limited timeframe:
- Anxiety/depression (mild)
- Anticoagulation recs
- Smoking cessation
- Re-fitting of CPAP mask
- HTN medication adjustment

Immediate preoperative interventions:
- Immunonutrition
- Counseling on OSA risk
- Counseling on cardiac risk

1 week

2 weeks

2+ weeks

4+ weeks

Fig. 42.1 Optimizing Patients for the Perioperative Journey—The Ascent.
*Multidimensional syndromes are those that span multiple domains that affect perioperative and long-term health outcomes, including physical, physiologic, psychological, cognitive, financial, and social. The interventions and resources required are very patient dependent, and the perioperative plan of care is often made on a case-by-case basis. Proposed timelines are based on the amount of time typically needed to fully assess and manage a new diagnosis or finding of poor control of the specific condition in the optimization clinic, but these must be balanced with the time-sensitive nature of surgery. *CAD,* Coronary artery disease; *CHF,* congestive heart failure; *COPD,* chronic obstructive pulmonary disease; *GFR,* glomerular filtration rate; *HTN,* hypertension; *mod,* moderate; *OSA,* obstructive sleep apnea; *SDM,* shared decision making.

Instead, a history and physical examination that is focused through the lens of the perioperative specialist serves as the basis of the preoperative evaluation. Those foundational elements are enhanced when used alongside validated screening tools to identify relevant, potentially modifiable clinical conditions such as the STOP-BANG for obstructive sleep apnea, preoperative nutrition screening (PONS) for malnutrition, or a clinical frailty scale.[13,14] Results generated by this multifaceted examination can direct necessary preoperative testing, focused upon identification and diagnosis of modifiable medical conditions that affect perioperative outcomes.[12] The result is an appropriate use of preoperative testing in a select population, including tests such as cardiac biomarkers, hemoglobin A_{1C}, and studies to determine the etiology of anemia.

This increase in optimization-focused testing is counterbalanced by a reduction in ubiquitous testing in all patients where no such opportunity to affect outcomes or change perioperative management is likely to occur (also see Chapter 13).

MEDICAL MANAGEMENT OF THE MOST COMMON COMORBIDITIES

Anemia

Preoperative anemia, defined in Table 42.1, is common, and any degree of anemia should be evaluated and corrected before elective surgery. The prevalence of preoperative anemia is highest in the orthopedic, gynecologic, and colorectal surgical populations, affecting >50% of surgical patients.[15] This is of profound importance because anemia increases overall perioperative risk, specifically a 16-fold increased mortality risk and doubled risk of perioperative complications like acute kidney injury, major adverse cardiac events, and length of hospitalization.[16]

The most common cause of preoperative anemia is iron deficiency. Diagnosis of iron deficiency anemia (IDA) is made by the presence of transferrin saturation <30%, a ferritin level of <100 μg/L, and/or reticulocyte hemoglobin content <30%, although these numbers are

VI

Table 42.1	World Health Organization (WHO) Anemia Threshold		
	Mild	**Moderate**	**Severe**
Male	11–13 g/dL	8–11 g/dL	<8 g/dL
Female	11–12 g/dL	8–11 g/dL	<8 g/dL

The World Health Organization definition of anemia differs by biologic sex and is commonly used in perioperative management protocols.
From https://www.who.int/vmnis/indicators/haemoglobin.pdf. Accessed November 10, 2021.

not absolute, and clinical context is important for interpretation.[17] Absolute iron deficiency may still contribute to the etiology of anemia in cases of functional iron deficiency (e.g., anemia of inflammation, also called *anemia of chronic disease*) for which the diagnosis is made when the transferrin saturation is >20% and serum ferritin level is 100 to 400 µg/L in the presence of normal or elevated values for folate, B_{12}, reticulocyte count, and renal function.[18] In these cases intravenous (IV) iron is most effective when combined with an erythropoiesis-stimulating agent (ESA) such as epoetin alpha.[19]

The goal of iron repletion therapy is correction of preoperative anemia in order to improve postoperative outcomes. The total iron deficit is calculated using the Ganzoni equation (Box 42.2) and is used to determine the repletion dose.[20] Iron repletion may be given either orally or intravenously, depending on factors such as time to surgery, patient preference, the degree of anemia, and the presence of chronic inflammation.[17] Oral replacement therapy is inexpensive, readily accessible, and safe; it may be effective in cases of mild anemia if initiated 4 to 8 weeks before surgery. Current dosing recommendations are 80 to 100 mg of oral iron every other day. The addition of vitamins C and D is recommended to increase absorption. Major limitations of oral iron therapy include lack of compliance because of gastrointestinal (GI) side effects (in >70% of patients), lack of absorption in patients with GI diseases or inflammation (because of hepcidin dysregulation), and the need for at least a 1-month interval before surgery for effectiveness. Alternatively, IV iron therapy has demonstrated increased efficacy, efficiency, and reduction of GI side effects when compared with oral replacement strategies, with recent improvements in the safety profile and variety of formulations. Response to IV iron begins within 1 week (50% response) after dosing, with maximum response 3

to 4 weeks after infusion.[21] The rate and magnitude of response depend on the patient's bone marrow functional reserve and use of an ESA.[19]

Numerous retrospective or pre/postintervention studies have shown a significant benefit to implementing standardized patient blood management programs.[22,23] However, a prospective randomized controlled trial (PREVENTT) demonstrated that administration of a single, standardized preoperative dose of IV iron to anemic patients but without confirmation of iron deficiency and within 2 weeks of surgery does not effectively correct anemia or reduce transfusions and postoperative complications. But this study did show that correction of iron deficiency may lead to a reduction in readmission after surgery.[24] Another trial that evaluated the implementation of a preoperative anemia clinic concluded that the implementation of preoperative anemia and iron screening and treatment were associated with a 50% reduction in transfusion, reduced length of stay by 15%, and reduced hospital costs for colorectal surgery patients.[25] Current evidence suggests that preoperative screening for and treatment of IDA should be pursued.[26]

When considering ESAs and the indications and contraindications for their use, several points are worth noting. First, many guidelines propose that ESAs should not be used in the setting of active cancer when chemotherapy is not being used *and* when the intention of oncologic treatment is curative.[27] However, in the preoperative period some institutions report using short courses of ESAs (one to two doses) even in the setting of cancer. There is also some concern for use in the setting of cardiac or vascular surgery, although this is debated. ESAs have also been associated with an increased risk of thromboembolism, although a recent meta analysis demonstrated no increased risk of thromboembolic complications with use in the preoperative period.[19] Thromboprophylaxis recommendations are based on patient history, and dosing strategies need to be adjusted based on renal function.

ESAs can be used in the setting of anemia for which there has been a lack of response to or no indication for iron, folate, and vitamin B_{12}. A recommended dosing schedule of epoetin alfa-epbx (Retacrit) is 40,000u subcutaneously every week for 2 to 4 weeks with a hemoglobin check before each dose. In summary, administering an ESA within 4 weeks of surgery can improve hemoglobin and may increase the efficacy of IV iron if used concomitantly.

Nutritional Optimization

Malnutrition is common in the adult presurgical population, affecting at least 50% of patients presenting for major surgery, with the highest rates in patients presenting for GI surgery.[13] If left untreated, malnutrition is associated with poor postoperative outcomes such as

Box 42.2	Ganzoni Equation for Calculating Iron Deficit

Total Iron Deficit = Weight (kg) × (Target Hgb – Actual Hgb) × 2.4 + Iron Stores (mg)
Note: Iron Stores = 500 mg, If Weight >35 kg

wound infection, prolonged hospitalization, and mortality. Yet in the absence of a formalized screening initiative less than 10% are identified and provided with an appropriate nutritional intervention before surgery.[28] Thus all patients should be screened for risk of malnutrition preoperatively, especially those with frailty syndrome, where malnutrition is both prevalent and highly detrimental.[29]

The diagnosis of malnutrition is made by the Global Leadership Initiative on Malnutrition (GLIM) criteria, which includes the presence of subnormal body mass index (BMI), weight loss, reduced muscle mass, decreased food intake, and disease burden.[30] The goal of preoperative nutritional therapy with oral nutritional supplementation (ONS) and immunonutrition (IMN) is to ensure adequate protein intake to achieve anabolism. Both high-protein ONS and IMN are available without a prescription; however, barriers to implementation of nutritional supplementation include lack of knowledge and cost.

The PONS[29] (Box 42.3) and the Malnutrition Universal Screening Tool (MUST)[28] (Table 42.2) are simple, validated tools used to screen for risk of malnutrition in the preoperative population. An abbreviated form of the MUST, known as the *Malnutrition Screening Tool (MST)*, is also available (Table 42.3).[31]

Current recommendations suggest that all "at-risk" patients be offered a preoperative regimen of high-protein ONS plus IMN.[13] Guidance on dietary choices to ensure adequate protein intake of >1.5 g/kg/day should be provided and combined with high-protein ONS when indicated. Patient-oriented educational materials on protein intake are available from the Academy of Nutrition and Dietetics.[32] High-protein ONS is most effective when initiated at least 2 to 4 weeks before surgery.[13] IMN supplements include a combination of arginine, omega-3 fatty acids, glutamine, and nucleotides. Current guidelines recommend 7 days of IMN before surgery; however, benefits from as few as 3 days have been demonstrated in patients with malnutrition and GI cancer.[33] Further evaluation of the patient's nutritional status and

consultation with a registered dietitian for a diagnosis of malnutrition may be indicated.

An important consideration when assessing a patient's preoperative nutritional status includes evaluation for specific vitamin deficiencies. Nutritional deficiencies are commonly seen in patients who are frail, who are chronically ill, who do not have access to fresh food sources, and who

Table 42.2 Malnutrition Universal Screening Tool (MUST)

Body Mass Index (BMI) Score	Weight Loss Score	Acute Disease Effect Score
BMI >20 kg/m² = 0 points	Weight loss <5% = 0 points	If patient has been or is likely to have no nutritional intake for > 5 days = 2 points
BMI 18.5 kg/m² to 20 kg/m² = 1 point	Weight loss 5%–10% = 1 point	
BMI <18.5 kg/m² = 2 points	Weight loss >10% = 2 points	

The MUST is specifically validated for use in the geriatric population and those patients who reside in long-term care facilities. A score ≥2 is considered "at risk" of malnutrition.

From Stratton RJ, Hackston A, Longmore D, et al. Malnutrition in hospital outpatients and inpatients: Prevalence, concurrent validity and ease of use of the "malnutrition universal screening tool" ("MUST") for adults. Br J Nutr. 2004;92(5):799-808.

Table 42.3 Malnutrition Screening Tool (MST)

Question	Points
Have you lost weight recently without trying?	
No	0
Unsure	2
If yes, how much weight (kilograms) have you lost?	
1–5	1
6–10	2
11–15	3
>15	4
Unsure	2
Have you been eating poorly because of a decreased appetite?	
No	0
Yes	1

The Malnutrition Screening Tool was developed in an adult acute care hospital. A score of 2 or more points indicates a patient at risk of malnutrition.

From Ferguson M, Capra S, Bauer J, et al, Development of a valid and reliable malnutrition screening tool for adult acute hospital patients. Nutrition. 1999;15(6):458-434.

Box 42.3 Perioperative Nutrition Screen (PONS)

The PONS score is based on four commonly used malnutrition criteria:

Screening question 1: Have you lost ≥10% of body weight in the last 6 months without trying?

Screening question 2: Have you been eating <50% of your normal diet in the preceding week?

Measurement: Is body mass index (BMI) <18.5 (or <20 if age >65 years)?

Laboratory test: Is albumin <3 g/dL?

  Each question is assigned 1 point for a "yes" answer. A PONS score of ≥1 is considered "at risk" for malnutrition.

From Williams DGA, Villalta E, Aronson S, et al. Tutorial: Development and implementation of a multidisciplinary preoperative nutrition optimization clinic. J Parenter Enteral Nutr. 2020;44(7):1185-1196.

Table 42.4	Impact of Smoking Cessation on Specific Organ Systems	
Organ System	**Impact of Smoking Cessation**	**Time Course**
Wound healing, bone healing	Improvement in inflammatory cell migration and killing of oxidative bacteria	4 weeks
	Improved proliferative phase of wound healing	>3 months
Cardiovascular[a]	Reduced nicotine levels	Half-life: 1 hour
	Reduced carbon monoxide levels	Half-life: 4 hours
Respiratory[b]	Decreased postoperative pulmonary complications (e.g., pneumonia, unplanned reintubation, prolonged mechanical ventilation)	4 weeks, though abstinence of 8 weeks provides greater risk reduction

Cigarette smoke contains many toxic chemicals, including nicotine, carbon monoxide, hydrogen cyanide, and nitric oxide. For some perioperative complications, the duration of smoking cessation required to demonstrate benefit is unknown.
[a]Limited data do not show significant differences in postoperative cardiovascular complications in patients who are current smokers compared with former smokers with less than 8 weeks abstinence or never smokers.
[b]There is no evidence of increased postoperative pulmonary complications with smoking abstinence durations of less than 4 weeks.
From Yousefzadeh A, Chung F, Wong DT, et al. Smoking cessation: The role of the anesthesiologist. Anesth Analg. 2016;122(5):1311–1320.

are current smokers. Because malnutrition and vitamin deficiencies often coexist, patients at risk for vitamin deficiencies may be effectively screened for using malnutrition screening tools or by specific laboratory evaluation. This chapter will focus on vitamins C and D.

Vitamin D has several key intracellular roles and has been implicated in worsened all-cause mortality after hospital admission, with improvement in mortality if supplementation is provided to those who are deficient.[34] A single study of admitted patients who screened positive for malnutrition had laboratory values consistent with vitamin D deficiency in 58% of patients, with 22% demonstrating severe deficiency. Likewise, vitamin C plays a vital role in cellular protection from reactive oxygen species and synthesis of endogenous pressors and is implicated in the maintenance of endothelial barriers in the presence of oxidative stress.[35] Vitamin C is quickly depleted even during brief periods of poor dietary intake and may play a role in decreasing length and severity of critical illness, although research to date is inconclusive.

Vitamin C supplementation may improve outcomes in the critically ill,[36] but so far there is no evidence that the

Box 42.4 Current Cigarette Smoking in U.S. Adults

The following groups were more likely to be current cigarette smokers in 2019:
Education level of general education development (GED) certificate—35% (vs. 7% of adults with undergraduate degree or 4% of adults with a graduate degree)
Severe generalized anxiety disorder—35% (vs. 12% of adults with no or minimal anxiety)
Lack of health insurance—23% or Medicaid—25% (vs. 9% of adults with Medicare only)
Annual household income <$35,000—21% (vs. 7% of adults with annual income >$100,000)
Lesbian/gay/bisexual orientation—19% (vs. 14% of heterosexual/straight orientation)
Geographic location in Midwest—16% (region with lowest current smoking rate is West, at 10%)
Men—15% (vs. 12% of women)
According to the Centers for Disease Control and Prevention (CDC), 14% of the U.S. adult population is smoking cigarettes in 2019, a decline from 21% in 2005.

From Centers for Disease Control and Prevention. Current Cigarette Smoking Among Adults in the United States. https://www.cdc.gov/tobacco/data_statistics/fact_sheets/adult_data/cig_smoking/index.htm. Accessed November 11, 2021.

same benefits occur in the perioperative patient. Supplementation of vitamins C and D is inexpensive, is easily accessible, and can generally be recommended without significant risk to the patient.

Smoking Cessation

Cigarette smoking is a modifiable risk factor, and cessation may improve short- and long-term patient outcomes. The Centers for Disease Control and Prevention (CDC) estimates that approximately 14% of the adult population in the United States is currently smoking cigarettes[37] (Box 42.4). From a general medicine perspective, patients who smoke have increased rates of chronic obstructive pulmonary disease (COPD), pneumonia, stroke, diabetes, cataracts, obstetric complications (e.g., preterm labor, stillbirth), and cancer. Overall, more than two-thirds of all deaths among current smokers over the age of 45 to 55 years are associated with smoking.[38,39] Patients who are current smokers at the time of surgery are at a 20% increased risk for perioperative mortality and 40% increased risk of postoperative complications, including wound infection, pneumonia, prolonged intubation (>48 hours), stroke, pulmonary embolism, sepsis, septic shock, myocardial infarction, and cardiac arrest.[40,41]

Despite this remarkable increase in risk and the known benefits of smoking cessation, many perioperative health care providers, including preoperative assessment clinics managed by anesthesiologists, do not routinely provide smoking cessation interventions. This should be of particular interest to anesthesia providers because, much like anemia and malnutrition, this is a modifiable risk factor that can have a major impact in the perioperative period and in personal and population health. However, achieving abstinence is difficult, and simply advising a patient to stop smoking is not effective. Rates of abstinence in the general population vary according to the intensity of the intervention: self-directed (<5%), provider advice/treatment (10%), hotline/quitline counseling (15%), specialized treatment including nicotine replacement therapy (NRT), cognitive behavioral counseling (CBC), and other pharmacologic agents (e.g., varenicline and bupropion) (40%–50%).[42]

When smoking cessation is achieved, multiple smoking-induced pathologic changes begin to improve[41] (see Table 42.4). Considering these benefits, several consensus guidelines have been published with almost identical recommendations[40-42] (Box 42.5). Although the evidence for increased risk with smoking is clear and there are numerous barriers to implementing routine screening and treatment, continued research is needed to identify the best strategies to achieve large-scale implementation. Additionally, there is insufficient evidence to determine whether e-cigarettes should be used for perioperative smoking cessation.

Glycemic Control (also see Chapter 29)

Although the underlying mechanisms relating hyperglycemia to poor outcomes are not completely understood, it seems clear that physiologic changes in the

---

Box 42.5 Recommendations for Perioperative Smoking Cessation

Smoking cessation should be attempted at any time before surgery

Proven models should be used routinely in preoperative clinics: for example, AAR[a] (ask, advise, refer) or 5 A's[†] (ask, advise, assess, assist, arrange)

High-intensity interventions (including NRT, CBC, and varenicline) reduce risk of postoperative complications *and* increase long-term postoperative abstinence rates

Data from Pierre S, Rivera C, Le Maitre B, et al. Guidelines on smoking management during the perioperative period. Anaesth Crit Care Pain Med. 2017;36(3):195–200; Yousefzadeh A, Chung F, Wong DT, et al. Smoking cessation: The role of the anesthesiologist. Anesth Analg. 2016;122(5):1311–1320; and Wong J, An D, Urman RD, et al. Society for Perioperative Assessment and Quality Improvement (SPAQI) consensus statement on perioperative smoking cessation. Anesth Analg. 2020;131(3):955–968.

CBC, Cognitive behavioral counseling; *NRT,* nicotine replacement therapy.

[a]AAR: **Ask** to identify all tobacco users at every visit; **Advise** tobacco users briefly to quit and offer cessation assistance via the quitline; **Refer** tobacco users to quitline-delivered counseling and provide them with quitline numbers.

[†]Five A's: **Ask** to identify all tobacco users at every visit; **Advise** tobacco users in a clear and personalized manner to quit at every visit; **Assess** their willingness to make a quit attempt; **Assist** them through offering medications and providing counseling; **Arrange** for follow-up meeting beginning the first week after the quit date.

---

hyperglycemic state are indeed associated with worse outcomes.[43] Hyperglycemia is known to alter neutrophil function while also increasing the production of inflammatory mediators (cytokines/chemokines by macrophages), reactive oxygen species, and free fatty acids. These pathophysiologic changes contribute to impaired immune function (i.e., increasing risk of infection) and also cause direct cellular damage and vascular dysfunctions.

A large and growing body of literature demonstrates a clear association between perioperative hyperglycemia and adverse clinical outcomes.[43,44] Long-term glycemic control (i.e., A_{1C} level) is associated with an increased risk for perioperative mortality and postoperative complications, including hyperglycemia (as ≥180 mg/dL) on admission and during the hospital stay.[44] The perioperative complications most associated with hyperglycemia are wound infection and poor wound healing.

In the preoperative setting assessment for and management of diabetes mellitus (DM, A_{1C} ≥6.5) and impaired fasting glucose (A_{1C} >5.7 and <6.5) are both very important. Guidelines have been published for assessing patients for diabetes before surgery and for managing medications for DM,[44] which is a field that is constantly evolving. However, routine use of testing in preoperative assessment clinics is rare. Yet as with smoking cessation, this screening represents an important target for assessing and modifying the risk of patients, especially before major surgery. At one of the author's institutions, a hemoglobin A_{1C} is obtained on patients presenting for major inpatient surgery who have any of the following risk factors: BMI >25 kg/m², age >45 years, history of gestational diabetes, certain ethnic groups (African American, Hispanic), family history of DM, or history of DM type 1 or 2 without an A_{1C} level in the past 3 months. If a new diagnosis of DM is made and the A_{1C} is <8, the patient is recommended for an inpatient consult from the Glucose Management Service after surgery. If the A_{1C} is ≥8, the patient is either referred back to their endocrinologist for improved glycemic control or, if they had no prior established care with an endocrinologist, a referral is made to a specialized outpatient diabetes clinic for preoperative optimization.

In the perioperative setting correction of hyperglycemia with insulin administration reduces hospital complications and decreases mortality in both cardiac and general surgery patients. Although optimal glucose management during the perioperative period is widely debated, it is clear that frequent glucose checks and structured sliding-scale or infusion protocols to achieve a moderate glucose level (e.g., 140–180 mg/dL or 120–160 mg/dL) are associated with better outcomes while avoiding episodes of severe hypoglycemia. Additionally, optimization of preoperative glycemic control may have the potential to decrease same-day cancellations because of severe hyperglycemia.

VI

Obstructive Sleep Apnea and Chronic Obstructive Pulmonary Disease (also see Chapters 48 and 27)

Preventing postoperative pulmonary complications (PPCs) is an important goal in the perioperative period. PPCs are dangerous to the patient and costly to the health system, adding an average of $25,000+ per episode for significant complications (e.g., pneumonia, pleural effusion, reintubation, prolonged intubation).[45] Several calculators can estimate the perioperative risk of PPC for a given patient, and use of these can inform discussions with the surgeon concerning perioperative case planning.[46-48] Only one of the calculators includes the presence of COPD as a risk factor, and neither of the major PPC risk calculators includes obstructive sleep apnea (OSA) as a risk factor. However, as these conditions are highly prevalent and are often undiagnosed, patients should routinely be assessed for both of these conditions before surgery as part of a comprehensive assessment of pulmonary health.[14,49]

COPD is more likely in patients with a smoking history ≥40 pack-years and age ≥45 years. COPD should be suspected in patients with risk factors (primarily a history of smoking) who report dyspnea at rest or with exertion, chronic cough with or without sputum production, or a history of wheezing. COPD may be suspected based on findings from the history and physical examination. However, spirometry (to detect airflow obstruction) is required to establish the diagnosis. Patients who present for major surgery with pulmonary symptoms and a clear smoking history may require pharmacotherapy for COPD and an intervention to promote smoking cessation, as described earlier.

In the medical management of COPD guidelines recommend starting monotherapy (inhaled bronchodilator or antimuscarinic agent) and advancing to combination therapy as needed.[50] At the recommendation of pulmonologists at the authors' institution, because time before surgery is often <1 month, we routinely start combination therapy for patients who are newly diagnosed as GOLD III/IV (Box 42.6) or who are GOLD B, C, or D according to the most recent guidelines.

Another modifiable risk factor for PPCs is OSA. OSA is defined as repeated partial or complete obstruction of the upper airway during sleep, which is terminated by cortical arousals or awakenings. Numerous adverse cardiovascular, pulmonary, and metabolic sequelae can result. It is estimated that 80% to 90% of moderate to severe OSA may be undiagnosed and untreated. That degree of severity is known to increase perioperative risk for poor cardiac and respiratory outcomes, such as postoperative desaturation, respiratory failure, cardiac events, and intensive care unit (ICU) transfer.[51] As such, screening for OSA is important, and simple tools such as the STOP-BANG are able to guide perioperative risk assessment, planning, and ordering of formal polysomnography (PSG) in select individuals.[52]

> **Box 42.6** Global Initiative for Chronic Obstructive Lung Disease (GOLD) Classification of Airflow Limitation Severity in COPD
>
> GOLD 1: Mild, FEV_1 ≥80% predicted
> GOLD 2: Moderate, 50% ≤FEV_1 <80% predicted
> GOLD 3: Severe, 30% ≤FEV_1 <50% predicted
> GOLD 4: Very Severe, FEV_1 <30% predicted
>
>   This classification of airflow limitation severity is based on specific spirometry cut-points and should be assessed after an adequate dose of at least one short-acting inhaled bronchodilator. It applies to patients with an FEV_1/FVC <0.70. In the 2011 GOLD update the ABCD assessment tool was created to incorporate patient-reported symptoms, including dyspnea (e.g., MRC Dyspnea Scale), health status impairment (COPD Assessment Test [CAT]), and outcomes such as exacerbations and hospital admissions.

From Global Initiative for Chronic Obstructive Lung Disease. Global Strategy for the Diagnosis, Management, and Prevention of Chronic Obstructive Pulmonary Disease (2021 Report). https://goldcopd.org/wp-content/uploads/2020/11/GOLD-REPORT-2021-v1.1-25Nov20_WMV.pdf. Accessed November 11, 2021.

Patients with a known diagnosis of OSA who use a continuous positive airway pressure (CPAP) device at home should be advised to bring their device to the hospital on the day of surgery. Patients with a known diagnosis of OSA who have declined to use CPAP can proceed to surgery but should be placed on a monitored ward for at least the first 24 to 48 hours after anesthesia, as the risk of postoperative hypoxemia and other complications related to OSA is greatest during that period. Patients with a STOP-BANG ≥5 or STOP-BANG ≥3 and serum bicarbonate ≥28 should be referred for PSG unless the surgery is time-sensitive. If PSG cannot occur, they should be treated as high risk of OSA, recovered in a monitored unit, and initiation of perioperative CPAP should be recommended for any episodes of hypoxemia or observed apnea.[53]

Prehabilitation

The specific combination of nutritional optimization, physical exercise, and psychological preparation is commonly referred to as *prehabilitation*. The major aim of prehabilitation is to improve the patient's ability to withstand the stress of the perioperative period from both a physiologic and psychological perspective.[54] Emerging evidence suggests that multidimensional syndromes such as frailty are best addressed via patient-specific, multimodal preoperative interventions, such as physical exercise, psychological intervention (e.g., anxiety reduction), and nutrition supplementation.[54,55] Prehabilitation interventions are often resource- and time-intensive, and further research on optimal timing, duration, and combination of interventions is warranted. To date, the data are mixed on the efficacy of prehabilitation programs for all surgical patients because of a wide variety in the heterogeneity of possible interventions.[56,57] However, patients in specific surgical populations such as colorectal,[58,59] esophageal, prostate,[60] and some orthopedic surgeries may benefit. Ongoing trials may indicate whether prehabilitation has definitive benefit in high-risk surgical patients.

Physical Exercise Regimen

The patient's mobility may be assessed in the preoperative period using a timed up and go (TUG) test and 6-minute walk test (6MWT). TUG requires a patient to rise from a seated position in an armchair, walk to a line 10 feet away, turn, and return to sitting. Patients who require >12 seconds to complete the test are considered at risk for impaired mobility and falls. A 6MWT is performed by asking the patient to ambulate a 15-meter stretch of level ground for 6 minutes at a tiring pace. Distance traveled is compared with the average score for patients of the same age and gender. 6MWT is used as an assessment of functional exercise capacity; this test strongly correlates with maximal oxygen consumption on cardiopulmonary exercise testing (CPET).[61] Weak grip strength is commonly measured using a handheld dynamometer and is used as an estimate of overall muscle function and changes in body composition.[62] The 1-minute sit to stand test (1-MSTST) can also be used to assess mobility and functional capacity.[63] Patients are asked to rise from a seated position and return to a seated position as many times as possible within 1 minute.

Patients with slow gait speed, poor grip strength, and/or decreased balance may benefit from preoperative home-based or supervised exercise regimens depending on their baseline function.[61,64] The primary components of a prehabilitation-focused exercise regimen include aerobic activity for 30 minutes per day, strength training (1–2 sets, 8–15 repetitions per set), and exercises to promote balance and flexibility. Deep breathing exercises or formal inspiratory muscle training may be recommended for patients at high risk of PPCs. Inspiratory muscle training is associated with decreased pulmonary complications if initiated within 6 weeks of surgery.[55]

Although an exercise regimen may not definitively decrease perioperative complications, the evaluation of a patient's physical abilities compared with age-group norms (e.g., with the 6MWT and TUG) provides valuable information about baseline functional status. Based on this information, concrete recommendations for targeted activities may lead to improved aerobic capacity and strength before surgery.

PSYCHOLOGICAL STATE: ASSESSMENT AND INTERVENTIONS

Anxiety and depression are common in patients facing a new diagnosis and preparing for surgery. These conditions are prevalent and undertreated in the general population, especially among the elderly. When left untreated, anxiety and depression represent barriers to successful engagement in preoperative optimization. Patients with psychiatric comorbidities may avoid seeking care because of fear of stigmatization or prior negative experiences in a health care setting. Other medical comorbidities may then go unidentified or be poorly managed.[65] The presence of anxiety, depression, posttraumatic stress disorder, or another psychiatric comorbidity in the preoperative period is associated with postoperative complications ranging from increased and prolonged pain and opioid use, longer hospitalization, and increased risk of in-hospital mortality.[65]

Examples of screening tools for preoperative psychological distress include the Hospital Anxiety and Depression (HADS) Score and the Patient Health Questionnaire (PHQ).[65,66] The 14-question HADS tool screens for both anxiety and depression, whereas the PHQ is specific to depression and exists in both two- and nine-question variations. In high-risk patients, such as those with opioid use disorder and a psychiatric condition, preoperative consultation with a pain management specialist may be required in order to formulate an individualized perioperative optimization plan[65,67] (also see Chapter 40).

Psychological preparation describes strategies aimed at modifying a patient's thoughts and perceptions of an experience.[68] The most effective strategies for psychological preparation are nonpharmacologic, low-cost, and tailored to the individual patient.[68,69] Providing patient-centered procedural information (what, when, and how events will occur) and sensory information (expected sensations, sounds, and smells) are effective strategies for decreasing preoperative anxiety related to uncertainty. Procedural and sensory information, when combined, are associated with the greatest improvement in patient-reported outcomes.[68] Relaxation-based interventions demonstrate the greatest reduction in postoperative pain, as compared with other anxiety reduction techniques such as procedural and sensory information. A well-studied relaxation technique is the use of music therapy. Music activates the limbic system; reduces heart rate; and can decrease sympathetic output via regulation of endogenous opioids, oxytocin, cortisol, and catecholamines.[70] The impact of music therapy is greatest when the patient selects the playlist and uses it throughout the preoperative, intraoperative, and postoperative period (postanesthesia care unit [PACU]).[71]

Participation in cognitive behavioral therapy (CBT) for 4 to 8 weeks before surgery is associated with faster recovery and improved postoperative pain control.[65,66] CBT is also a common component of smoking cessation therapy. CBT interventions to address the behavioral aspect of tobacco dependence aim to assist the patient with developing a new approach to stress management. Despite demonstrating positive results, CBT is

VI

time-intensive and requires specially trained providers, which has implications for cost and scalability of a CBT program for patients.[65]

COGNITIVE SCREENING AND INTERVENTIONS (ALSO SEE CHAPTER 35)

The primary goal of preoperative cognitive screening is to identify patients at increased risk of postoperative delirium. A common instrument used in the preoperative evaluation clinic is the Mini-Cog, derived from the Montreal Cognitive Assessment (MoCA). Benefits of this tool include brevity and established reliability.[72-74] The Mini-Cog involves three-word recall and a clock-drawing test. Scores of 0, 1, and 2 designate patients at high risk for postoperative delirium. It can be administered in <5 minutes, making it more feasible to use in the preoperative clinic than the more extensive and time-consuming MoCA or mini-mental status exams (MMSEs).

Patients identified as high risk for delirium should receive information regarding signs and symptoms of delirium and have a discussion with family members who will be present during the hospital stay regarding potential prevention and mitigation strategies. Deliriogenic medications should be weaned preoperatively whenever possible.[75] Benzodiazepines, anticholinergics, medications to prevent muscle spasms, sleep aids, opioids, and multiple psychotropic medications may negatively affect cognition and increase the risk of postoperative delirium.[75] Deprescribing should be done in a stepwise fashion, using a validated framework in consultation with, or with expert opinion from, a geriatrician.[76]

Positive screening test results or a diagnosis of postoperative delirium should be communicated to the patient's primary care physician or geriatrician to ensure longitudinal follow-up.

HEALTH LITERACY AND SHARED DECISION MAKING

Patients at highest risk for surgical complications often have a poor understanding of their health status and overestimate their ability to manage their medical conditions. Low health literacy level is a risk factor independently associated with longer hospitalization after major surgery.[77,78] A key pillar of the Geriatric Surgical Verification program is improved communication with patients and their families through goals-of-care conversations and shared decision making.[79] Shared decision making is most effective when the patient has a clear understanding of both the benefits and risks of the proposed surgery, procedure, and/or anesthetic and the risks and benefits of alternatives to the proposed therapy, including foregoing further treatment. Health literacy occurs when health information and services match the patient's ability to understand and use them.

The four-question version of the Brief Health Literacy Screen (BHLS) is commonly used, although consensus regarding the best preoperative screening tool has not been established. Responses are scored on a Likert scale from 1 (always) to 5 (never) and correlated with basic health literacy. The use of a single question, "How confident are you in filling out medical forms?" has also been validated for reliability.[80]

Patients with lower health literacy levels often benefit from face-to-face discussions, repeated oral instructions, and preoperative information that is presented via video or infographics.[81] Use of the "teach-back method" method is another proven strategy to enhance retention and to identify existing gaps in understanding.[82] Although screening for health literacy remains controversial in the context of perioperative optimization, the goal is to ensure adequate communication, patient engagement, and equitable care delivery.

Creation of a standardized discussion template to facilitate the shared decision-making process during the preoperative evaluation clinic visit is valuable, even in the absence of a formal assessment of health literacy level. Key elements include asking permission and introducing the topic, ascertaining the patient's understanding of his or her illness, exploring goals of care and fears, and identifying an alternative decisionmaker.[72]

OTHER OPPORTUNITIES TO IMPROVE PERIOPERATIVE OUTCOMES

Table 42.5 summarizes the perioperative management of the conditions discussed earlier. Many other important comorbidities should be assessed in the perioperative period, including cardiac, thyroid, and renal dysfunction (also see Chapters 13 and 26). However, screening for elevations of cardiac biomarkers (troponin and B-type natriuretic peptide [BNP/NT-proBNP]) and derangements in thyroid function (low or high thyroid-stimulating hormone [TSH]) have utility in selected, high-risk patient populations, as alterations in these hormones are associated with worse perioperative outcomes.[83,84] Also, assessing renal function and perioperative risk of acute kidney injury is important when creating a perioperative care plan for high-risk patients[85,86] (also see Chapter 28).

FUTURE DIRECTIONS IN PERIOPERATIVE MEDICINE: SOCIAL DETERMINANTS OF HEALTH

Recent population-based studies of health in the United States have catalyzed an increased awareness of social and economic factors that contribute to poor health

Table 42.5 Perioperative Management of Selected Conditions

Modifiable Condition	Screening and Diagnostic Tools	Interventions: Time Frame/Phase of Care
Malnutrition, nutritional deficiency	PONS, MST, MUST scores	**Preop:** Immunonutrition (IMN) and oral nutrition supplementation (ONS) × ≥1 week **In-hospital:** Continuation of IMN and ONS, early feeding, total parental nutrition (TPN) when indicated
Anemia	TSAT, ferritin, folate, B_{12}, GFR, CHr	**Preop:** PO or IV iron depending on time frame and patient factors, epoetin alfa, folate, B_{12} × 2–4 weeks **In-hospital:** TXA, Cell-saver, postoperative IV iron, epoetin-alfa
Frailty phenotype: Slow gait speed, decreased functional status, weak grip strength	6-minute walk test (6MWT), timed up and go test (TUG), chair sit to stands, cardiopulmonary exercise testing (CPET), hand grip strength	**Preop:** Prehabilitation regimen (cardio training, strength training, mobility, and balance exercises) × 4–6 weeks **In-hospital:** Early mobility, physical therapy
Postoperative delirium, postoperative neurocognitive disorders	Mini Cog, Montreal Cognitive Assessment (MoCA), St Louis University Mental Status Exam (SLUMS), Mini-Mental Status Exam (MMSE), Telephone Interview for Cognitive Status (TICS)	**Preop:** Patient and family counseling about delirium, wean deliriogenic medications, tailor anesthetic plan, establish care with geriatrician **In-hospital:** Tailor anesthetic plan, multimodal analgesia, glasses/hearing aids, reorientation, clock, sleep hygiene, bowel regimen, mobility, blood pressure within target, geriatric comanagement
Anxiety/depression/poor coping skills	Self-reported, Hospital Anxiety and Depression Scale (HADS), Patient Health Questionnaire (PHQ-2/9), Pain Catastrophizing Scale (PCS), Patient Reported Outcome Measures (PROMS)	**Preop:** Provision of patient-specific procedural and sensory information (≥1 day before), relaxation-based techniques (music therapy, guided positive imagery 1 day to 2 weeks), motivational interviewing, cognitive behavioral therapy (CBT) × 4–8 weeks **In hospital:** Music therapy, relaxation techniques
Health literacy	BRIEF tool	**Preop:** Face-to-face education with diagrams, teach-back method, videos
Social determinants of health	Social history of electronic health record	**Preop:** Proactive case management, nurse navigator support **In-hospital:** Case management, social work referral, referral to community aid organizations
Tobacco dependence	Self-reported, "5 A's," serum cotinine level	**Preop physiologic dependence:** Varenicline, Wellbutrin, nicotine replacement therapy (NRT) × 1–4 weeks **Preop psychological dependence:** CBT, "quit for a bit," smokers quitline × 1 day to 4 weeks **In-hospital:** Referral to smoking cessation services postdischarge, NRT, pharmacotherapy, CBT
Obstructive sleep apnea (OSA)	STOP-BANG	**Preop:** CPAP adherence, sleep study (can be done at home × 1 day to 4 weeks), change CPAP mask **In-hospital:** Multimodal analgesia, postoperative monitoring/CPAP, optimization of other comorbidities
Diabetes mellitus, poor glycemic control	Spot serum glucose, A_{1c}, fructosamine (if anemic)	**Preop:** Treatment initiation or adjustment, dietary changes, fast-track referral to endocrinology: 1–4 weeks **In-hospital:** Initiation or titration of insulin
Chronic obstructive pulmonary disease (COPD)	Pulmonary function testing (PFT), patient-reported history	**Preop:** Diagnosis, medication initiation or adjustment, inspiratory muscle training, smoking cessation: 1 day to 4 weeks **In-hospital:** Lung-protective ventilation, tailoring anesthetic plan, incentive spirometry use

VI

outcomes.[87,88] Vulnerability to perioperative stress is now understood to result from the confluence of physical, physiologic, psychological, and social factors.[89]

Causes of health disparities have not been completely elucidated but are likely multifactorial. Patients from historically marginalized populations may avoid health care because of prior experiences of discrimination by health care providers.[81] Racial discordance between the patient and physician is a commonly cited contributing factor. Patients from historically marginalized populations report both overt discrimination and more subtle mistreatment such as low expectations for adherence with recommendations and less empathy from providers. These experiences are thought to result in disengagement by the patient and deferral of necessary therapies.[90]

Provider-facing initiatives that result in an awareness of implicit bias and a deeper understanding of the impact of race, gender, and socioeconomic factors on perioperative outcomes may result in greater health equity.[90] Health disparities in individuals who have experienced incarceration are well documented. Poorly controlled chronic diseases, mental health conditions, substance use disorders, and social isolation are prevalent among the incarcerated patient population. The effects of incarceration on an individual are far-reaching, and previously incarcerated individuals often lack an established relationship with a primary care physician.[91,92] Additionally, incarceration serves as a risk multiplier for elderly and frail individuals.[93]

Further research is needed to identify interventions that mitigate perioperative risk related to severe deficits in the patient's social, economic, and physical environment. Achievement of optimal outcomes in vulnerable patient populations will likely require an emphasis on early and frequent care coordination initiatives across the entire perioperative continuum.

The COVID-19 pandemic catalyzed a period of rapid evolution within perioperative medicine. The need for social distancing, implementation of preoperative COVID testing, and a pause on all but critical surgeries required immediate changes to our care delivery framework. Although changes in health care initiated by the pandemic may have been rapid and painful, there is increased attention on caring for vulnerable populations in a manner that is less burdensome and costly. Virtual optimization visits via telemedicine may allow expansion of prehabilitation and perioperative medicine initiatives that previously required in-person care.

REFERENCES

1. Grocott MP, Pearse RM. Perioperative medicine: The future of anaesthesia? *Br J Anaesth.* 2012;108(5):723–726.
2. Vetter TR, Bader AM. Continued evolution of perioperative medicine: Realizing its full potential.. *Anesth Analg.* 2020;130(4):804–807.
3. Beutler S, McEvoy MD, Ferrari L, Vetter TR, Bader AM. The future of anesthesia education: Developing frameworks for perioperative medicine and population health. *Anesth Analg.* 2020;130(4):1103–1108.
4. Lee PH, Gawande AA. The number of surgical procedures in an American lifetime in 3 states. *J Am Coll Surg.* 2008;207(3):S75.
5. King AB, McEvoy MD, Fowler LC, Wanderer JP, Geiger TM, Furman WR, et al. Disruptive education: Training the future generation of perioperative physicians. *Anesthesiology.* 2016;125(2):266–268.
6. McEvoy MD, Lien CA. Education in anesthesiology: Is it time to expand the focus? *A A Case Rep.* 2016;6(12):380–382.
7. Li G, Warner M, Lang BH, Huang L, Sun LS. Epidemiology of anesthesia-related mortality in the United States, 1999-2005. *Anesthesiology.* 2009;110(4):759–765.
8. Myles PS. Measuring quality of recovery in perioperative clinical trials. *Curr Opin Anaesthesiol.* 2018;31(4):396–401.
9. Abola RE, Bennett-Guerrero E, Kent ML, Feldman LS, Fiore Jr JF, Shaw AD, et al. American Society for Enhanced Recovery and Perioperative Quality Initiative Joint Consensus Statement on Patient-Reported Outcomes in an Enhanced Recovery Pathway. *Anesth Analg.* 2018;126(6):1874–1882.
10. Choosing Wisely. An Initiative of the ABIM Foundation. https://www.nice.org.uk/guidance/ng180 Accessed November 2021
11. Perioperative care in adults. NICE guideline [NG180]: https://www.nice.org.uk/guidance/ng180 (accessed November 2021)
12. Committee on Standards and Practice ParametersApfelbaum JL, Connis RT, Nickinovich DGAmerican Society of Anesthesiologists Task Force on Preanesthesia Evaluation, Pasternak LR, Arens JF, Caplan RA, Connis RT, Fleisher LA, Flowerdew R, Gold BS, Mayhew JF, Nickinovich DG, Rice LJ, Roizen MF, Twersky RS. Practice advisory for preanesthesia evaluation: An updated report by the American Society of Anesthesiologists Task Force on Preanesthesia Evaluation. *Anesthesiology.* 2012;116(3):522–538.
13. doi:10.1097/ALN.0b013e31823c1067. MarPMID: 22273990.
13. Wischmeyer PE, Carli F, Evans DC, Guilbert S, Kozar R, Pryor A, et al. Association of STOP-Bang Questionnaire as a Screening Tool for Sleep Apnea and Postoperative Complications: A systematic review and Bayesian meta-analysis of prospective and retrospective cohort studies. *Anesth Analg.* 2018;126(6):1883–1895.
14. Nagappa M, Patra J, Wong J, Subramani Y, Singh M, Ho G, et al. Association of STOP-Bang Questionnaire as a Screening Tool for Sleep Apnea and Postoperative Complications: A Systematic Review and Bayesian Meta-analysis of Prospective and Retrospective Cohort Studies. *Anesth Analg.* 2017;125(4):1301–1308.
15. Shander A. Preoperative anemia and its management. *Transfus Apher Sci.* 2014;50(1):13–15.
16. Musallam KM, Tamim HM, Richards T, Spahn DR, Rosendaal FR, Habbal A, et al. Preoperative anaemia and postoperative outcomes in non-cardiac surgery: A retrospective cohort study. *Lancet.* 2011;378(9800):1396–1407.
17. Warner MA, Shore-Lesserson L, Shander A, Patel SY, Perelman SI, Guinn NR. Perioperative anemia: Prevention, diagnosis, and management throughout the

spectrum of perioperative care. *Anesth Analg.* 2020;130(5):1364–1380.

18. Kansagra AJ, Stefan MS. Preoperative anemia: Evaluation and treatment. *Anesthesiol Clin.* 2016;34(1):127–141.

19. Cho BC, Serini J, Zorrilla-Vaca A, Scott MJ, Gehrie EA, Frank SM, et al. Impact of preoperative erythropoietin on allogeneic blood transfusions in surgical patients: Results from a systematic review and meta-analysis. *Anesth Analg.* 2019;128(5):981–992.

20. Koch TA, Myers J, Goodnough LT. Intravenous iron therapy in patients with iron deficiency anemia: Dosing considerations.. *Anemia.* 2015;2015:763576.

21. Peters F, Ellermann I, Steinbicker AU. Intravenous iron for treatment of anemia in the 3 perisurgical phases: A review and analysis of the current literature.. *Anesth Analg.* 2018;126(4):1268–1282.

22. Heller LB, Shander A. Preoperative anemia management: Value-based care for orthopedic surgery. *Techniques in Orthopaedics.* 2020;35(1):7–14.

23. Gani F, Cerullo M, Ejaz A, Gupta PB, Demario VM, Johnston FM, et al. Implementation of a blood management program at a tertiary care hospital: Effect on transfusion practices and clinical outcomes among patients undergoing surgery. *Ann Surg.* 2019;269(6):1073–1079.

24. Richards T, Baikady RR, Clevenger B, Butcher A, Abeysiri S, Chau M, et al. Preoperative intravenous iron to treat anaemia before major abdominal surgery (PREVENTT): A randomised, double-blind, controlled trial. *Lancet.* 2020;396(10259):1353–1361.

25. Trentino KM, Mace H, Symons K, Sanfilippo FM, Leahy MF, Farmer SL, et al. Associations of a Preoperative Anemia and Suboptimal Iron Stores Screening and Management Clinic in Colorectal Surgery With Hospital Cost, Reimbursement, and Length of Stay: A net cost analysis. *Anesthesia & Analgesia.* 2021;132(2):344–352.

26. Warner MA, Goobie SM. Preoperative anemia screening and treatment: Is it worth the return on investment? *Anesth Analg.* 2021;132(2):341–343.

27. Bohlius J, Bohlke K, Castelli R, Djulbegovic B, Lustberg MB, Martino M, et al. Management of cancer-associated anemia with erythropoiesis-stimulating agents: ASCO/ASH clinical practice guideline update. *J Clin Oncol.* 2019;37(15):1336–1351.

28. Williams DGA, Villalta E, Aronson S, Murray S, Blitz J, Kosmos V, et al. Tutorial: Development and implementation of a multidisciplinary preoperative nutrition optimization clinic: Development and Implementation of a Multidisciplinary Preoperative Nutrition Optimization Clinic. *JPEN J Parenter Enteral Nutr.* 2020;44(7):1185–1196.

29. Stratton RJ, Hackston A, Longmore D, Dixon R, Price S, Stroud M, et al. Malnutrition in hospital outpatients and inpatients: Prevalence, concurrent validity and ease of use of the "malnutrition universal screening tool" ("MUST") for adults. *Br J Nutr.* 2004;92(5):799–808.

30. Cederholm T, Jensen GL, Correia M, Gonzalez MC, Fukushima R, Higashiguchi T, et al. GLIM criteria for the diagnosis of malnutrition—A consensus report from the global clinical nutrition community. *J Cachexia Sarcopenia Muscle.* 2019;10(1):207–217.

31. Ferguson M, Capra S, Bauer J, Banks M. Development of a valid and reliable malnutrition screening tool for adult acute hospital patients. *Nutrition.* 1999;15(6): 458–434.

32. Academy of Nutrition and Dietetics. How Much Protein Should I Eat? https://www.eatright.org/food/nutrition/dietary-guidelines-and-myplate/how-much-protein-should-i-eat Accessed November 10, 2021.

33. Adiamah A, Skorepa P, Weimann A, Lobo DN. The impact of preoperative immune modulating nutrition on outcomes in patients undergoing surgery for gastrointestinal cancer: A systematic review and meta-analysis. *Ann Surg.* 2019;270(2):247–256.

34. Merker M, Amsler A, Pereira R, Bolliger R, Tribolet P, Braun N, et al. Vitamin D deficiency is highly prevalent in malnourished inpatients and associated with higher mortality: A prospective cohort study. *Medicine (Baltimore).* 2019;98(48):e18113.

35. Hill A, Wendt S, Benstoem C, Neubauer C, Meybohm P, Langlois P, et al. Vitamin C to improve organ dysfunction in cardiac surgery patients-Review and pragmatic approach. *Nutrients.* 2018;10(8).

36. Langlois PL LF. Vitamin C for the critically ill: Is the evidence strong enough? *Nutrition.* 2019;60.

37. Centers for Disease Control and Prevention. Current Cigarette Smoking Among Adults in the United States. https://www.cdc.gov/tobacco/data_statistics/fact_sheets/adult_data/cig_smoking/index.htm Accessed November 11, 2021.

38. Banks E, Joshy G, Weber MF, Liu B, Grenfell R, Egger S, et al. Tobacco smoking and all-cause mortality in a large Australian cohort study: Findings from a mature epidemic with current low smoking prevalence.. *BMC Med.* 2015;13:38.

39. Thun MJ, Carter BD, Feskanich D, et al. 50-year trends in smoking-related mortality in the United States. *N Engl J Med.* 2013;368(4):351–364.

40. Pierre S, Rivera C, Le Maitre B, Ruppert AM, Bouaziz H, Wirth N, et al. Guidelines on smoking management during the perioperative period. *Anaesth Crit Care Pain Med.* 2017;36(3):195–200.

41. Yousefzadeh A, Chung F, Wong DT, Warner DO, Wong J. Smoking cessation: The role of the anesthesiologist. *Anesth Analg.* 2016;122(5):1311–1320.

42. Wong J, An D, Urman RD, Warner DO, Tonnesen H, Raveendran R, et al. Society for Perioperative Assessment and Quality Improvement (SPAQI) consensus statement on perioperative smoking cessation. *Anesth Analg.* 2020;131(3):955–968.

43. Duggan EW, Klopman MA, Berry AJ, Umpierrez G. The Emory University perioperative algorithm for the management of hyperglycemia and diabetes in non-cardiac surgery patients. *Curr Diab Rep.* 2016;16(3):34.

44. Duggan EW, Carlson K, Umpierrez GE. Perioperative hyperglycemia management: An update. *Anesthesiology.* 2017;126(3):547–560.

45. Fleisher LA, Linde-Zwirble WT. Incidence, outcome, and attributable resource use associated with pulmonary and cardiac complications after major small and large bowel procedures. *Perioper Med (Lond).* 2014;3:7.

46. Canet J, Sabate S, Mazo V, Gallart L, de Abreu MG, Belda J, et al. Development and validation of a score to predict postoperative respiratory failure in a multicentre European cohort: A prospective, observational study. *Eur J Anaesthesiol.* 2015;32(7):458–470.

47. Canet J, Gallart L, Gomar C, Paluzie G, Valles J, Castillo J, et al. Prediction of postoperative pulmonary complications in a population-based surgical cohort. *Anesthesiology.* 2010;113(6):1338–1350.

48. Gupta H, Gupta PK, Fang X, Miller WJ, Cemaj S, Forse RA, et al. Development and validation of a risk calculator predicting postoperative respiratory failure. *Chest.* 2011;140(5):1207–1215.

49. Nagappa M, Wong J, Singh M, Wong DT, Chung F. An update on the various practical applications of the STOP-Bang questionnaire in anesthesia, surgery, and perioperative medicine. *Curr Opin Anaesthesiol.* 2017;30(1):118–125.

50. Global Initiative for Chronic Obstructive Lung Disease. Global Strategy for the Diagnosis, Management, and Prevention of Chronic Obstructive Pulmonary Disease (2021 Report). https://goldcopd.org/wp-content/uploads/2020/11/GOLD-REPORT-2021-v1.1-25Nov20_WMV.pdf Accessed November 11, 2021.

51. Kaw R, Chung F, Pasupuleti V, Mehta J, Gay PC, Hernandez AV. Meta-analysis of the association between obstructive

VI

sleep apnoea and postoperative outcome. *Br J Anaesth.* 2012;109(6):897–906.

52. Chung F, Yang Y, Brown R, Liao P. Alternative scoring models of STOP-bang questionnaire improve specificity to detect undiagnosed obstructive sleep apnea. *J Clin Sleep Med.* 2014;10(9):951–958.

53. Fernandez-Bustamante A, Bartels K, Clavijo C, Scott BK, Kacmar R, Bullard K, et al. Preoperatively screened obstructive sleep apnea is associated with worse postoperative outcomes than previously diagnosed obstructive sleep apnea. *Anesth Analg.* 2017;125(2):593–602.

54. Carli F. Prehabilitation for the anesthesiologist. *Anesthesiology.* 2020;133(3):645–652.

55. Norris CM, Close JCT. Prehabilitation for the frailty syndrome: Improving outcomes for our most vulnerable patients. *Anesth Analg.* 2020;130(6):1524–1533.

56. Carli F, Bousquet-Dion G, Awasthi R, Elsherbini N, Liberman S, Boutros M, et al. Effect of multimodal prehabilitation vs postoperative rehabilitation on 30-day postoperative complications for frail patients undergoing resection of colorectal cancer: A randomized clinical trial. *JAMA Surg.* 2020;155(3):233–242.

57. Cabilan CJ, Hines S, Munday J. The effectiveness of prehabilitation or preoperative exercise for surgical patients: A systematic review. *JBI Database System Rev Implement Rep.* 2015;13(1):146–187.

58. Trepanier M, Minnella EM, Paradis T, Awasthi R, Kaneva P, Schwartzman K, et al. Improved disease-free survival after prehabilitation for colorectal cancer surgery. *Ann Surg.* 2019;270(3):493–501.

59. Gillis C, Buhler K, Bresee L, Carli F, Gramlich L, Culos-Reed N, et al. Effects of nutritional prehabilitation, with and without exercise, on outcomes of patients who undergo colorectal surgery: A systematic review and meta-analysis. *Gastroenterology.* 2018;155(2):391–410 e4.

60. Santa Mina D, Hilton WJ, Matthew AG, Awasthi R, Bousquet-Dion G, Alibhai SMH, et al. Prehabilitation for radical prostatectomy: A multicentre randomized controlled trial. *Surg Oncol.* 2018;27(2):289–298.

61. Kow AW. Prehabilitation and its role in geriatric surgery. *Ann Acad Med Singap.* 2019;48(11):386–392.

62. Kilgour RD, Vigano A, Trutschnigg B, Lucar E, Borod M, Morais JA. Handgrip strength predicts survival and is associated with markers of clinical and functional outcomes in advanced cancer patients. *Support Care Cancer.* 2013;21(12):3261–3270.

63. Bohannon RW, Crouch R. 1-Minute Sit-to-Stand Test: Systematic review of procedures, performance, and clinimetric properties. *J Cardiopulm Rehabil Prev.* 2019;39(1):2–8.

64. Tew GA, Ayyash R, Durrand J, Danjoux GR. Clinical guideline and recommendations on pre-operative exercise training in patients awaiting major non-cardiac surgery. *Anaesthesia.* 2018;73(6):750–768.

65. Doan LV, Blitz J. Preoperative assessment and management of patients with pain and anxiety disorders. *Curr Anesthesiol Rep.* 2020;10(1):28–34.

66. Ohkura Y, Shindoh J, Ichikura K, Udagawa H, Ueno M, Matsushima E. Perioperative risk factors of psychological distress in patients undergoing treatment for esophageal cancer. *World J Surg Oncol.* 2020;18(1):326.

67. Edwards DA, Hedrick TL, Jayaram J, Argoff C, Gulur P, Holubar SD, et al. American Society for Enhanced Recovery and Perioperative Quality Initiative Joint Consensus Statement on Perioperative Management of Patients on Preoperative Opioid Therapy. *Anesth Analg.* 2019;129(2):553–566.

68. Freeman SC, Scott NW, Powell R, Johnston M, Sutton AJ, Cooper NJ. Component network meta-analysis identifies the most effective components of psychological preparation for adults undergoing surgery under general anesthesia. *J Clin Epidemiol.* 2018;98:105–116.

69. Powell R, Scott NW, Manyande A, Bruce J, Vogele C, Byrne-Davis LM, et al. Psychological preparation and postoperative outcomes for adults undergoing surgery under general anaesthesia. *Cochrane Database Syst Rev.* 2016;(5):CD008646.

70. Wu PY, Huang ML, Lee WP, Wang C, Shih WM. Effects of music listening on anxiety and physiological responses in patients undergoing awake craniotomy. *Complement Ther Med.* 2017;32:56–60.

71. Carter JE, Pyati S, Kanach FA, Maxwell AMW, Belden CM, Shea CM, et al. Implementation of perioperative music using the consolidated framework for implementation research. *Anesth Analg.* 2018;127(3):623–631.

72. Cooper L, Abbett SK, Feng A, Bernacki RE, Cooper Z, Urman RD, et al. Launching a geriatric surgery center: Recommendations from the Society for Perioperative Assessment and Quality Improvement. *J Am Geriatr Soc.* 2020;68(9):1941–1946.

73. Culley DJ, Flaherty D, Fahey MC, Rudolph JL, Javedan H, Huang CC, et al. Poor performance on a preoperative cognitive screening test predicts postoperative complications in older orthopedic surgical patients. *Anesthesiology.* 2017;127(5):765–774.

74. O'Reilly-Shah VN, Hemani S, Davari P, Glowka L, Gebhardt E, Hill L, et al. A preoperative cognitive screening test predicts increased length of stay in a frail population: A retrospective case-control study. *Anesth Analg.* 2019;129(5):1283–1290.

75. By the 2019 American Geriatrics Society Beers Criteria® Update Expert Panel. American Geriatrics Society 2019 Updated AGS Beers Criteria® for Potentially Inappropriate Medication Use in Older Adults. *J Am Geriatr Soc.* 2019 Apr;67(4):674-694.

76. Scott IA, Hilmer SN, Reeve E, Potter K, Le Couteur D, Rigby D, et al. Reducing inappropriate polypharmacy: The process of deprescribing. *JAMA Intern Med.* 2015;175(5):827–834.

77. Chew LD, Bradley KA, Flum DR, Cornia PB, Koepsell TD. The impact of low health literacy on surgical practice. *Am J Surg.* 2004;188(3):250–253.

78. Halleberg Nyman M, Nilsson U, Dahlberg K, Jaensson M. Association between functional health literacy and postoperative recovery, health care contacts, and health-related quality of life among patients undergoing day surgery: Secondary analysis of a randomized clinical trial. *JAMA Surg.* 2018;153(8):738–745.

79. American College of Surgeons Geriatric Surgery Verification Program. https://www.facs.org/Quality-Programs/geriatric-surgery Accessed November 11, 2021.

80. Chew LD, Bradley KA, Boyko EJ. Brief questions to identify patients with inadequate health literacy. *Fam Med.* 2004;36(8):588–594.

81. Blitz J, Swisher J, Sweitzer B. Special considerations related to race, sex, gender, and socioeconomic status in the preoperative evaluation: Part 1: Race, history of incarceration, and health literacy. *Anesthesiol Clin.* 2020;38(2):247–261.

82. Ha Dinh TT, Bonner A, Clark R, Ramsbotham J, Hines S. The effectiveness of the teach-back method on adherence and self-management in health education for people with chronic disease: A systematic review. *JBI Database System Rev Implement Rep.* 2016;14(1):210–247.

83. Vacante M, Biondi A, Basile F, Ciuni R, Luca S, Di Saverio S, et al. Hypothyroidism as a Predictor of Surgical Outcomes in the Elderly. *Front Endocrinol (Lausanne).* 2019;10:258.

84. Ruetzler K, Khanna AK, Sessler DI. Myocardial injury after noncardiac surgery: Preoperative, intraoperative, and postoperative aspects, implications, and directions. *Anesth Analg.* 2020;131(1):173–186.

85. Weiss R, Meersch M, Pavenstadt HJ, Zarbock A. Acute kidney injury: A frequently underestimated problem in perioperative medicine. *Dtsch Arztebl Int.* 2019;116(49):833–842.

86. Meersch M, Schmidt C, Zarbock A. Perioperative acute kidney injury: An under-recognized problem. *Anesth Analg.* 2017;125(4):1223–1232.

87. Jerath A, Austin PC, Ko DT, Wijeysundera HC, Fremes S, McCormack D, et al. Socioeconomic status and days alive and out of hospital after major elective noncardiac surgery: A population-based cohort study. *Anesthesiology.* 2020;132(4):713–722.

88. Qi AC, Peacock K, Luke AA, Barker A, Olsen MA, Joynt Maddox KE. Associations between social risk factors and surgical site infections after colectomy and abdominal hysterectomy. *JAMA Netw Open.* 2019;2(10):e1912339.

89. McIsaac DI, MacDonald DB, Aucoin SD. Frailty for perioperative clinicians: A narrative review. *Anesth Analg.* 2020;130(6):1450–1460.

90. Nelson A. Unequal treatment: Confronting racial and ethnic disparities in health care. *J Natl Med Assoc.* 2002;94(8):666–668.

91. Trotter RT 2nd, Lininger MR, Camplain R, Fofanov VY, Camplain C, Baldwin JA. A survey of health disparities, social determinants of health, and converging morbidities in a county jail: A cultural-ecological assessment of health conditions in jail populations. *Int J Environ Res Public Health.* 2018;15(11):2500.

92. Bai JR, Befus M, Mukherjee DV, Lowy FD, Larson EL. Prevalence and predictors of chronic health conditions of inmates newly admitted to maximum security prisons. *J Correct Health Care.* 2015;21(3):255–264.

93. Williams BA, Lindquist K, Sudore RL, Strupp HM, Willmott DJ, Walter LC. Being old and doing time: Functional impairment and adverse experiences of geriatric female prisoners. *J Am Geriatr Soc.* 2006;54(4):702–707.

VI

43 ANESTHESIA FOR TRAUMA

Marc P. Steurer, Benn Lancman

INTRODUCTION

Background

Injury is the leading cause of fatality worldwide, causing more than 5 million deaths—9% of the world's deaths—each year.[1] According to the Centers for Disease Control and Prevention (CDC), trauma accounted for nearly 230,000 U.S. deaths in 2018, costing over $400 billion in health care and lost productivity. Trauma is the most frequent cause of fatality in those aged 1 to 44 years, accounting for 54% of deaths in age group 1 to 9 years, 85% in the age group 10 to 24 years, and 57% in the age group 25 to 44 years.[2] The disease of trauma disproportionately affects younger age groups, with trauma responsible for over 36% of potential years of life lost in people younger than 65 years old.[3]

During the past decades, mortality trends have continued to decrease as care for the severely injured patient has improved. Emergent care for the severely injured is aggregated at designated trauma centers, which are independently verified by strict criteria stipulated by the American College of Surgeons. The most specialized trauma centers, designated as Level I, have the ability to deliver 24-hour specialized multidisciplinary care. Trauma care delivered at Level I trauma centers decreases overall mortality risk by 25% when compared with nontrauma centers.[4] Anesthesia providers, in particular, play a vital role in the acute resuscitation and early management of severely injured patients. In this chapter, the basics of trauma care for anesthesia providers will be discussed.

Physiology in Trauma

Physiologic derangements in patients who have suffered trauma-induced injuries depend on the mechanism and severity of injury. Most commonly, hypotension in trauma is the result of severe blood loss or hemorrhagic shock, which is the main cause of fatality in critically injured patients. After sources of hemorrhagic shock are investigated, the following causes of shock must also be considered when encountering hypotension in the trauma setting: relative hypovolemia from obstructed venous return (e.g., from tension pneumothorax or cardiac tamponade), cardiogenic shock, and neurogenic shock.

The initial presenting arterial blood pressure values of a trauma patient may be misleading in early hemorrhage. The degree of hemorrhage can be masked by compensatory reflexes via the sympathetic nervous system, carotid sinus and aortic arch baroreceptors, and other low-pressure receptors. The renin–angiotensin system and vasopressin secretion from the pituitary play a later compensatory role. These responses allow sympathetic vasoconstriction of the arterioles to increase total peripheral resistance, venoconstriction to increase venous return, and an increase in heart rate. With extreme hypoxia and acidosis, the central nervous system also provides additional sympathetic stimulation.

Hemorrhagic shock can generally be divided into a compensated and progressive phase. Each phase has different characteristics depending on the acuity and volume of blood lost (Table 43.1).

In compensated hemorrhage, physiologic compensatory mechanisms that are intact may be adequate to sustain systemic perfusion without clinical intervention. About 10% to 15% of blood loss may be adequately compensated for by physiology alone. As blood loss continues, hemorrhagic shock progresses. If inadequate perfusion persists, generalized tissue and cellular necrosis, cardiac dysfunction, and metabolic acidosis occur. This can ultimately lead to multiorgan failure.

Hemorrhagic shock and tissue hypoperfusion subsequently lead to complex interactions between inflammatory factors, intrinsic anticoagulants, and other cellular dysfunctions that can cause an acute traumatic coagulopathy after injury. This coagulopathy is attributed to factor deficiency, hyperfibrinolysis, and platelet dysfunction. Iatrogenic factors of resuscitation can further disrupt the coagulation process. These factors include hemodilution, hypocalcemia, hypothermia, and acidosis. This is known as *trauma-induced coagulopathy*. All of these processes lead to a positive feedback loop that eventually ends in death. Hypothermia, coagulopathy, and acidosis are commonly termed the *triad of death* or *lethal triad* (Fig. 43.1). Hemorrhagic shock may cross a threshold at which it becomes irreparable despite blood transfusions and other therapies owing to severe, irreversible multiorgan failure.

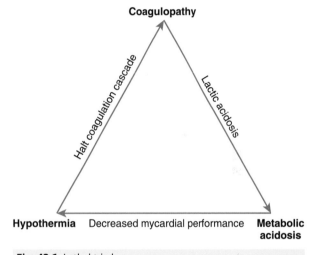

Fig. 43.1 Lethal triad.

Table 43.1	Classes of Hemorrhagic Shock in Adults			
	Class I	**Class II**	**Class III**	**Class IV**
Blood loss[a] (mL)	Up to 750	750–1500	1500–2000	>2000
Blood loss (% blood volume)	Up to 15%	15%–30%	30%–40%	>40%
Pulse rate (BPM)	<100	100–120	120–140	>140
Systolic BP	Normal	Normal	Decreased	Decreased
Pulse pressure	Normal or increased	Decreased	Decreased	Decreased
Respiratory rate	14–20	20–30	30–40	>35
Urine output (mL/h)	>30	20–30	5–15	Negligible
CNS/mental status	Slightly anxious	Mildly anxious	Anxious, confused	Confused, lethargic

[a]For 70-kg adult.
Modified from the Advanced Trauma Life Support (ATLS) program.
BP, Blood pressure; *BPM*, beats per minute; *CNS*, central nervous system.

VI

INITIAL MANAGEMENT

Successfully managing a patient who has suffered a major trauma requires a coordinated systematic approach to history, mechanism, examination, diagnosis, and treatment. Furthermore, these processes must run swiftly and in parallel. Often initial management is commenced before a definitive diagnosis has been established.

Each patient has a unique constellation of injuries and mechanisms, and when combined with their premorbid status, there are an immeasurable number of potential presentations. To prepare for the unpredictability of trauma, many of the initial assessment and management processes are standardized, and clinicians must be familiar with their local institution's policies and guidelines.

This section will focus on the initial management of a major trauma patient, focusing primarily on the time in the emergency department. The initial management can significantly influence intraoperative care. The components of a mature trauma system can be divided into prearrival, the trauma bay, adjuncts, and definitive care.

Prearrival Preparation

Preparation for the arrival of an intensely injured patient enables the trauma team to deliver rapid, effective care, which is essential for a positive outcome to occur. This involves more than just confirming that essential equipment is present and functioning. Although these checks are very important, organizational and patient-specific preparations also need to be considered.

Universal Organization/Preparation

Caring for a major trauma patient requires the mobilization and deployment of a large and diverse range of health care resources to a single point. Preparations include considering the following questions: (1) Is there a designated trauma bay in the emergency department? (2)Who attends the trauma call, and how are they notified? (3) What are the policies and protocols for activation of emergency radiology services, emergency operating room (OR) use, massive blood transfusion, and patient transport? (4) What are the referral pathways to internal and external providers?

These issues should be addressed before the arrival of a critically ill patient. Because of the unpredictable nature of trauma, a novel set of circumstances can overwhelm or bypass an organization's existing preparation. In these situations, the clinicians involved—as members of a learning organization—must notify and alert the individuals who can provide the required resources.

Patient-Specific Preparation

This should occur immediately before the arrival of an individual major trauma patient. Information regarding the patient's injury and status should be provided to

Box 43.1 IMIST—Paramedic Handover Tool	
Identification of the patient	Age Gender Name (if known)
Mechanism/medical complaint	What happened?
Injuries/information relative to the complaint	Known/suspected injuries
Signs (vital signs and Glasgow Coma Scale score)	Presence of breath sounds Tracheal deviation
Treatment and trends/ response to treatment	Vital signs Drugs Fluids Splints

emergency department staff by the ambulance service to facilitate resource mobilization.

Most ambulance services around the world use a standardized handover tool to provide essential information in a succinct and efficient manner. An example of this tool is IMIST, a mnemonic for *I*dentification of the patient, *M*echanism/medical complaint, *I*njuries/information relative to the complaint, *S*igns (including vital signs and Glasgow Coma Scale [GCS] score), and *T*reatment and trends/response to treatment (Box 43.1).[5] With this information, the health care team can anticipate the patient's clinical needs and prepare accordingly.

Prearrival Briefing

The purpose of this briefing is to optimize team efficiency and performance. This enables all members of the team to introduce themselves, develop group situational awareness about the known condition of the patient, and assign appropriate team roles.

Trauma Bay

Primary Survey

Once the patient arrives, the focus of the team shifts to rapid and simultaneous diagnosis and treatment of life-threatening conditions.

The Advanced Trauma Life Support (ATLS) approach was developed by the American College of Surgeons Committee on Trauma. ATLS was first introduced in 1980 and has since been widely adopted throughout the world. It is structured into primary, secondary, and tertiary surveys. This chapter will only address the primary survey. The ATLS course is highly recommended as an introduction to trauma management. Most importantly, it provides a common language and framework to organize thinking required for optimal individual and team performance.

The purpose of the primary survey is to identify and treat immediately life-threatening injuries. It is organized into the ABCDE mnemonic (Box 43.2).

Box 43.2	Primary Survey
A	Airway and cervical spine control
B	Breathing and oxygenation
C	Circulation and hemorrhage control
D	Disability
E	Exposure

Modified from the Advanced Trauma Life Support (ATLS) program.

Airway and Oxygenation (Also See Chapter 16)

Establishment of a patent airway is of paramount importance to ensure a positive outcome for the patient. Rapid assessment is most easily achieved by asking the patient some simple questions. If the patient can speak, then the airway at the time of assessment is usually patent. Intervention may still be required, but there is time to plan the safest treatment.

Management of the Airway and Trauma

The trauma patient may require a definitive patent airway (a cuffed endotracheal tube) for many reasons (Box 43.3). Induction of anesthesia before tracheal intubation may be a high-risk and dangerous procedure. The top priority is always to maintain adequate tissue oxygenation. If a patent airway is maintained with simple airway maneuvers, then there is time to optimize the patient's physiology and properly prepare for the intubation attempt. If the clinical situation allows, performing a focused neurologic assessment before anesthesia induction can provide invaluable information that would be difficult to obtain in the sedated, endotracheally intubated patient.

There are several differences in the approach to intubating the trachea in a trauma patient in the emergency department as compared with an elective surgical patient in the OR.

Preoxygenation (Administration of Oxygen Before Induction of Anesthesia)

Preoxygenation in the patient who has injuries from trauma can be challenging. The objective of preoxygenation is to "denitrogenate" the lung, thus providing a reservoir of oxygen in the patient's functional residual capacity (FRC) to prevent desaturation (hypoxemia) during the

Box 43.3 Trauma Patients Who May Require Endotracheal Intubation
• Maxillofacial trauma
• Major hemodynamic instability
• Low SaO$_2$
• Burns
• Head injury
• Intoxicated/behavioral/safety issues
• Transport (radiology/OR/ICU/external)

ICU, Intensive care unit; *OR*, operating room.

apneic phase of tracheal intubation. However, many injuries sustained by trauma patients prevent this process from being effective. Specifically, any injury that reduces FRC or creates a shunt (lung units that are perfused but not ventilated) will increase the likelihood of desaturation despite technically adequate preoxygenation. Examples of such injuries include direct lung parenchymal injury, hemothorax or pneumothorax, pulmonary aspiration of blood or gastric contents, intraabdominal bleeding, diaphragmatic injury, and rib fractures. Addition of an alternative oxygen source to provide apneic oxygenation throughout the peri-intubation period has been evaluated in the emergency department literature.[6] Despite a theoretical benefit, as a result of all the issues with preoxygenation in trauma patients, no benefit has been demonstrated in experienced laryngoscopists' hands.[7] The best defense against desaturation is reducing total apneic time.

Fasting

All trauma patients should be assumed to have a "full stomach" even when many hours have elapsed since their last oral intake. As such, a rapid-sequence induction (RSI) is considered standard practice. The use of cricoid pressure is common clinical practice but may worsen the view at laryngoscopy. A review of the evidence is presented in Chapter 16.

Altered Physiology

Major trauma patients who require emergent tracheal intubation are often the most critically ill patients in the hospital. The justification for endotracheal intubation and the impact of that physiologic insult on their response to laryngoscopy must be clearly defined. For example, if the reason for endotracheal intubation is respiratory distress from a major lung injury, then optimal preoxygenation may still result in rapid desaturation after apnea occurs.

Hemodynamic Status

The hemodynamic response to anesthetics given to induce anesthesia is often exaggerated for two main reasons. First, acute intravascular volume loss from bleeding results in an inability to maintain arterial blood pressure and cardiac output in the face of the vasodilatory effects of anesthetic drugs. Second, sympathetic stimulation caused by pain and distress can mask the true intravascular volume state; if so, induction of anesthesia can cause marked hemodynamic instability. This can usually be anticipated by the appropriate intravascular administration of fluids (i.e., crystalloids, blood, colloids) and the availability of vasopressors.

Anesthetic Drug Choices

The choice of drugs to induce anesthesia in the critically ill patient is an area of much controversy (also see Chapter 8). Propofol and etomidate are often the primary choice, with some opting for ketamine in certain

VI

situations. The hemodynamic impact and stability are more a reflection of drug dosing rather than the choice of agent. Most important is for the clinician to be very familiar with the anesthetic drugs they plan to use rather than using a new, unfamiliar drug. In general, the dose of anesthetic drug should be decreased because of a relatively reduced volume of distribution of drugs in a very ill or hypovolemic patient. Preferential perfusion to essential organs, such as the brain, heart, and kidneys, occurs in such patients. A vasopressor should be immediately available to manage any transient hypotension caused by the anesthetic drugs.

Manual In-Line Stabilization

The process of laryngoscopy can produce an unacceptable amount of force through the cervical spine. Attempts should always be made to reduce this force. Any patient with a suspected spinal injury should be placed in a hard collar. The front of the collar should be opened at the time of laryngoscopy and the head and neck stabilized by an additional clinician. Ideally, the manual in-line stabilization (MILS) of the neck is performed by a second provider standing at the patient's torso, so as to not interfere with the laryngoscopist (Fig. 43.2). When the intubation and laryngoscopy are done in the OR with the patient prepped and draped, MILS needs to be performed with the person stabilizing the neck standing (or squatting) directly next to the laryngoscopist (Fig. 43.3). In this case, the person attempts to stabilize the neck while allowing the optimal position for the laryngoscopist. The objective is to minimize movement of the cervical spine during laryngoscopy. A pragmatic approach is required during MILS because a failed endotracheal intubation attempt presents a much greater immediate risk to the patient (i.e., hypoxia) than the risk of small neck movements. In the event of poor visualization of the glottic structures, consideration should be given to relaxing MILS to facilitate endotracheal intubation before replacing the hard cervical collar. The use of video laryngoscopy may facilitate adequate intubating conditions while minimizing unnecessary neck movement and should be considered as a first-line device in these patients where available.

Choice of Laryngoscope

Video laryngoscopy has transformed the way airways are managed in the emergency department and OR. The advantages of video laryngoscopy include the following: (1) gives an adequate tracheal intubating view with reduced pressure and force; (2) provides group situational awareness of progress and difficulty of laryngoscopy; (3) improves visualization of the larynx in more difficult

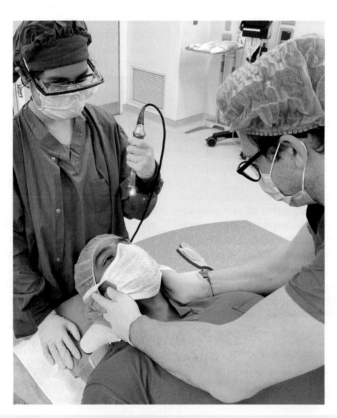

Fig. 43.2 Manual in-line stabilization of the neck from below.

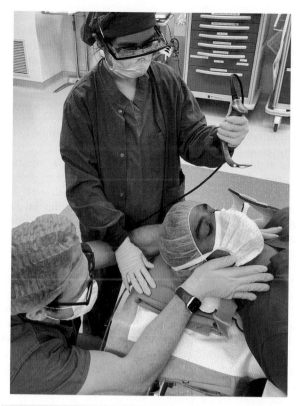

Fig. 43.3 Manual in-line stabilization of the neck from above.

patients without the need to change equipment; and (4) allows supervisors and trainers to provide dynamic feedback throughout the laryngoscopy.

Failed Endotracheal Intubation Drills

Failed endotracheal intubations are rare. Nevertheless, management of the unanticipated difficult airway is more likely in the trauma patient. Several factors contribute to the increased difficulty of airway management: cervical spine precautions, blood or foreign body in the airway, and the stress experienced by the person performing the intubation. Plans for failed intubation must be made explicit, such as what equipment will be needed, its location, and the immediate availability of staff who are assisting with intubation before induction of anesthesia. Staff who work outside the OR environment may not be familiar with airway equipment such as laryngeal masks or surgical airway kits, and their comfort with using this type of equipment should be known in advance.

Posttracheal Intubation Care

Endotracheal intubation is a mechanism for providing physiologic support—it is not therapeutic treatment itself. The focus of the emergency department team needs to remain on the patient's transition to definitive care. Several issues need to be managed immediately after intubation (Box 43.4).

Special Groups

Several special circumstances need to be considered when making a decision on the management of the trauma patient's airway:

1. Airway burns: Patients with airway burns require expedited management of their airway. Within a very short time, they can progress from minimal or no respiratory distress to a completely occluded airway because of edema expansion. Warning signs of potential airway burns include facial burns, soot in mouth/nose, carbonaceous sputum, explosive injuries to the upper body, and stridor.
2. Oral trauma: Blood is often found in the upper airway of trauma patients. Bleeding can range from a minor nuisance to a life-threatening hemorrhage. It is important to recognize this situation (i.e., blood in the airway) because induction of anesthesia can result in the rapid loss of a patent airway. Video laryngoscopes and fiber-optic scopes do not perform well when blood obscures the field of view. An additional suction source is mandatory, and a surgical airway team should be immediately available.
3. Direct airway injury: Although uncommon, tracheal trauma should be suspected in any patient with direct penetrating or blunt trauma to the neck. Warning signs such as stridor and subcutaneous emphysema may be present. These airways should be managed only by experienced clinicians with early involvement of a head and neck surgeon. Advancing the cuff of the endotracheal tube past a confirmed or suspected lesion is a critical concept in these scenarios.

Circulation and Hemorrhage

Adequate circulation and perfusion need to be reestablished to ensure sufficient oxygen delivery to essential organs. The first priority is to stop any bleeding. This can be achieved through a combination of interventions performed in the emergency department (direct pressure, suturing wounds), surgical intervention, or angioembolization. Simultaneously, the anesthesia provider must ensure adequate oxygen delivery to essential organs such as the brain and heart. Damage control resuscitation

---

Box 43.4 Postintubation Issues in the Trauma Patient

- Ongoing sedation—postintubation hypertension is common and should be avoided because of its effect on uncontrolled bleeding and intracerebral physiology
- Ventilator and settings
- Disposition—where is the patient going next? To the computed tomography (CT) scanner, the operating room (OR), or the intensive care unit (ICU)?
- Additional intravenous or arterial access, or both—these procedures should not delay any movement to definitive care

VI

(DCR) is the term given to a resuscitative strategy that provides circulatory support sufficient to prevent permanent end-organ damage while avoiding the pitfalls of excessive resuscitation. Hypothermia, acidosis, and hypocalcemia represent additional clinical issues that often arise in managing the hypotensive trauma patient.

Disability

The assessment of the neurologic system should identify potentially catastrophic injuries that require prompt management. This rapid assessment is based on the GCS score, pupillary response, and gross limb function. Intubation is usually required for patients with a GCS score less than 8 (Box 43.5).

Exposure

To avoid missing major injuries that are not visible, the patient must be exposed and inspected on all sides, including the back, for other injuries. However, prolonged patient exposure for many minutes contributes to hypothermia, which adversely affects coagulation, oxygen consumption, and mortality risk.

Adjuncts and Investigations

Any tests or investigations that are ordered should have an impact on diagnosis and management. Because clinical events can change rapidly and dramatically in trauma

patients, timely access to information can be a considerable challenge. Results that are especially useful have a rapid turnaround time, are performed serially to follow trends, and correlate with possible treatments that can improve outcome (Box 43.6).

Definitive Care and Transport

Definitive care is the process of fixing the underlying physiologic problem. Examples include stopping a bleeding source, plating a fracture, or removing a ruptured spleen. Some components of definitive care should be performed emergently, whereas others can wait for the patient's condition to improve. Depending on the patient's injuries and the capabilities of individual institutions, definitive care may require transfer to another health care facility. Either way, the patient will need to transfer out of the emergency department.

Setting Priorities: What Is Next?

Conflict often arises when trying to decide the most appropriate location to treat the patient. Depending on the injuries sustained, there can be disagreement about the most clinically urgent injury, and thus the most appropriate location for treatment. The logistical barriers to treatment can make it impossible to do everything the patient needs in a single location.

An example is a patient who sustains major pelvic and neurosurgical trauma. The most appropriate place for management of neurosurgical trauma is the OR; however, current guidelines for pelvic trauma recommend angioembolization. The decision about which injury to prioritize is a difficult one and should be made on the clinical nuances of that individual patient. Many Level I trauma centers now have hybrid ORs where both angiographic and operative interventions can be performed; thus the treatment comes to the patient rather than vice versa.

Box 43.5 The Glasgow Coma Scale (GCS) Score[a]

Eyes (E)
- 4—Open spontaneously
- 3—Open to voice
- 2—Open to pain
- 1—Do not open

Verbal (V)
- 5—Oriented
- 4—Confused
- 3—Inappropriate words
- 2—Incomprehensible sounds
- 1—No sounds

Motor (M)
- 6—Obeys commands
- 5—Localizes to pain
- 4—Withdraws to pain
- 3—Abnormal flexion to pain
- 2—Abnormal extension to pain
- 1—No response

Total score = best responses for eyes, verbal, and motor
- E = 4
- V = 5
- M = 6
- Total GCS score = 15

The Glasgow Coma Scale score is the sum of the best scores in each of the three categories: eye opening, verbal response, and motor response. The 15-point scale is the predominant one in use.
[a]Best response used.

Box 43.6 Initial Investigations

Minimum "standard" major trauma investigations:
- Complete blood count
- Electrolytes/BUN
- Blood gas (preferably arterial)
- Chest radiograph
- Pelvis radiograph
- Coagulation testing—ideally viscoelastic testing (ROTEM/TEG)
- Blood group and antibody screen

Additional investigations to consider:
- ECG
- CT scan
- General radiograph

BUN, Blood urea nitrogen; *CT*, computed tomography; *ECG*, electrocardiogram; *ROTEM*, rotational thromboelastometry; *TEG*, thromboelastography.

A reasonable alternative for many conditions is conservative management during the acute phase. This allows time for restoration of normal physiology, clarification of medical history, and a more complete assessment of the extent of injuries. Providing intensive-care-level observation and a regular review of conditions is an extremely appropriate and responsible course of action.

Local Care Versus Transfer

Once a patient's clinical needs exceed the services provided by the institution, the process for timely transfer begins. A key management principle is to seek help from the accepting hospital early in the process. Moving a critically ill patient takes time, and timely communication with the accepting hospital enables the required resources to be mobilized. Regardless of the ultimate destination, the patient's clinical status can be optimized by regular reassessment via ATLS primary and secondary surveys. When transporting critically ill patients, the level of care received at the hospital should be continued during transfer to the new facility. Specific equipment, staff skill mix, routes, and oxygen supplies should all be considered before initiating a transfer.

Decision Making in Trauma

Mature and complex systems such as health care and trauma require multiple individuals with different and complementary skill sets to work together toward the common goal of achieving the best patient outcomes. Some simple strategies can be employed to optimize team performance and bring order to the potential chaos of a major trauma (Box 43.7).

Leadership and Followership

Traditional medical teaching reinforces the need for a clearly defined leader to ensure that any resuscitation runs smoothly. The role of the leader is to act as a central point for information and decision making (Box 43.8). Conversely, what makes a good follower is less often discussed. Although each team will have only one leader at any time, there will be several followers. The qualities of a good follower support the leader in the ability to make the right decisions at any given point in time (Box 43.9).

Box 43.7 Questions to Ask Locally to Be an Effective Part of a Trauma Team

- How do we alert a major trauma?
- How do we define a major trauma?
- Who responds to trauma calls?
- What is our massive transfusion protocol?
- How do we get more help if we need it?
- What are the limits of what we can deal with locally?

Box 43.8 Leadership

Qualities of a good leader:
- Listens to the team
- Provides clear direction and expectations for patient care
- Shares uncertainty
- Delegates appropriately
- Stands back and maintains "big picture" situational awareness

Good leaders do NOT need to:
- Know the most
- Be the most experienced clinician
- Always be right

Box 43.9 Followership

Qualities of a good follower:
- Uses closed-loop communication (e.g., clarify instructions, report back when task is complete)
- Offers suggestions (e.g., would you like me to ...)
- Alerts the leader to changes in clinical status of patient (e.g., hypotension)
- Provides feedback on personal limitations, skills, experience
- Uses communication techniques such as graded assertiveness (see Box 43.10)

Graded Assertiveness

Graded assertiveness is one technique for communicating personal concerns about decision making or priorities to the team leader in a way that maintains constructive group performance. It assumes that poor decision making is based on incorrect or insufficient information. Followers are able to see the situation from a unique perspective and can communicate their concerns. They can then use the Probe, Alert, Challenge, and Emergency action (PACE) technique (described in Box 43.10) to communicate their concerns in a constructive manner.[8] The team leader is very important and is usually aware of information that the follower may not be, and as such those concerns may not be the priority at that point in time.

Box 43.10 Graded Assertiveness—PACE

Probe
"I thought our goal was to keep the arterial blood pressure higher than 90 mm Hg."

Alert
"Did you realize the arterial blood pressure is low? Would you like me to give some blood?"

Challenge
"Is there a reason you are tolerating hypotension in this patient?"

Emergency action
"The arterial blood pressure is dangerously low. I am going to treat it now."

VI

INTRAOPERATIVE MANAGEMENT

The spectrum of patients who need to go to the OR for surgical or interventional procedures because of trauma is vast. It encompasses injuries of all levels of magnitude in all organs and structures of the human body. Some are very minor and simple, and others involve specific organs with explicit consequences and treatment. The latter group consists of life-threatening injury to one or multiple organs and is the main focus of this section. All current concepts that should be applied to the severely injured and bleeding patient can be applied to the lesser injured to varying degrees.

The severely injured and massively bleeding patient usually presents in hemodynamic shock and is in need of lifesaving interventions. The differential diagnosis of a trauma patient in shock consists of massive hemorrhage, tension pneumothorax, cardiac tamponade, severe cardiac contusion, and neurogenic shock. Underlying medical conditions can lead to exaggeration of the degree of shock (Table 43.2).

The management of severely injured patients with massive hemorrhage can be divided into three discrete phases. This distinction is based on different physiologic aspects, a varying approach, and management principles. Early in the first phase, patients suffer from uncontrolled hemorrhage. The second phase begins when at least partial control of the hemorrhage has been achieved. The third and last phase is reached when the patient's physiology starts to normalize (e.g., arterial blood pressure). The breakdown into these three phases takes into account the different treatment goals for each phase plus the varying angle and pragmatism of the approach. It allows the provider to appreciate the specific goals for the given phase. These three phases exist in a continuum, and the borders are very fluid (Table 43.3).

Table 43.2	Differential Diagnosis of Shock in the Trauma Patient
Medical Condition	**Investigation Modalities**
Massive hemorrhage	Clinical examination Bedside TTE—assess volume status FAST scan—abdominal source
Tension pneumothorax	Clinical examination (percussion/trachea) Lung ultrasound
Cardiac tamponade	TTE (subcostal view best)
Severe cardiac contusion	TTE

FAST, Focused assessment with sonography for trauma; *TTE,* transthoracic echocardiogram.

Phase 1: Uncontrolled Hemorrhage

The medical team has one goal only for trauma patients with massive hemorrhage that warrants emergent surgical procedures in the OR—to stop the bleeding as soon as possible. Everyone involved facilitates that aim by all means. There is no time to wait for study results, to order additional tests, or for consultation with other specialists. The anesthesia team's role is to facilitate achievement of hemostasis as quickly as possible. Massively bleeding patients who come to the OR for resuscitation and hemostasis present a challenge to the anesthesia providers, who are faced with a very hectic and dynamic situation. Additional personnel can be very helpful but have to be managed, ideally in a standardized fashion. Having too many team members can be a hindrance and may prevent the team from functioning efficiently. The airway has to be secured and the patient should be ventilated with 100% oxygen. Details and consideration of airway management can be found in the section, "Initial Management," earlier in this chapter and in Chapter 16. The use of high fraction of inspired oxygen (Fio_2) restores the oxygen delivery to a certain extent by compensating for lost Hb via an increase of the dissolved oxygen fraction. Another important institutional protocol to have in place is the massive transfusion protocol (MTP) (also see Chapter 25). The MTP facilitates communication, optimizes the response time of the blood bank, and minimizes errors. Although these procedures are essential to taking care of such patients, the absolute mainstay of this phase is the hemostatic resuscitation of the patient. As prehospital care systems have matured and evolved, there has been an increasing opportunity to transport critically unstable patients directly from the ambulance into the OR. This direct-to-OR pathway has demonstrated improved survival in major penetrating trauma and should be explored within the constraints of local resources.[9]

Historically, the anesthesia provider would deploy large volumes of crystalloids early in order to aggressively restore the circulating volume and restore normal arterial blood pressure values. This can lead to a direct escalation in the bleeding rate by increasing cardiac output in addition to both the arterial and venous pressures. This abandoned practice would also lead to a dilution of coagulation factors and hypothermia, further increasing the bleeding. Over the past 10 to 15 years, the initial resuscitation has been revolutionized and the concept entirely changed.[10] The main goal of the initial resuscitation is on bridging the patient for as long as possible until the bleeding can be stopped. DCR is the term used to describe the new concept[11] (Box 43.11).

Damage Control Resuscitation

Permissive hypotension, limited use of crystalloids and colloids, and early use of blood products represent the cornerstones of DCR.[11]

Table 43.3 Phases of Major Traumatic Resuscitation

	Phase 1	Phase 2	Phase 3
Clinical status	Life-threatening uncontrolled hemorrhage	Ongoing hemorrhage—not immediately life threatening— partial surgical control	Hemorrhage controlled

Clinical priorities	• STOP THE BLEEDING
	• Call for HELP
	• Control airway, FiO₂ 100%
	• Damage control resuscitation (DCR)
	  - SBP <100 mm Hg
	  - MAP 50-60 mm Hg
	  - Consider modifications if TBI, carotid stenosis, CAD
		• TAILORED RESUSCITATION
		• Place supportive lines (arterial/CVC)
		• Prevent hypothermia
		  - Esophageal temperature probe
		  - Warmed fluids
		  - Warming blankets (upper and lower body)
		  - Increase room temperature
			• RESTORE PHYSIOLOGY
			• Rapid intravascular filling
			• Stepwise deepening of anesthesia
			  - Fentanyl boluses
			  - Increased volatile anesthetics
			  - Additional lines (urinary catheter, nasogastric tube)
			  - Communicate with all team members and ICU

Blood products	• Activate massive transfusion protocol (MTP) • Consider emergency (unmatched) blood products • Early use • Empiric 1:1:1 transfusion ratio	• TEG/ROTEM to guide coagulation products • ABG to guide red blood cell transfusion	• Only as required on testing • Deactivate MTP when appropriate
Crystalloids/colloids	• Cautious use	• Use for hypovolemia with normal coagulation/Hb • Use serial lactate/BE to guide fluid requirements	• Attempt to normalize BE/ lactate
Special points	• Consider CaCl₂ 1 g for every three blood products • Large bore IV access (>16 g) or CVC • Rapid infusing system (e.g., Belmont) • Avoid vasoconstrictors	• Consider cell salvage • Aim to repeat TEG/ROTEM/ ABG every 30 min • Consider TEE for difficult cases	• Consider vasoactive infusions if necessary

ABG, Arterial blood gas; *BE,* base excess; *CAD,* coronary artery disease; *CVC,* central venous catheter; *ICU,* intensive care unit; *IV,* intravenous; *MAP,* mean arterial pressure; *MTP,* massive transfusion protocol; *ROTEM,* rotational thromboelastometry; *SBP,* systolic blood pressure; *TBI,* traumatic brain injury; *TEE,* transesophageal echocardiography; *TEG,* thromboelastography.

Box 43.11 Principles of Damage Control Resuscitation (DCR)

Permissive hypotension
Stop bleeding early—pressure, angiography, operating room
Early use of hemostatic products
Minimize crystalloid use

Permissive hypotension aims to use the body's physiologic response to hemorrhage. The resulting low venous and arterial blood pressures and the decrease in cardiac output lead to a reduction in the driving force behind the bleeding. At the same time, the providers can take advantage of the normal response to blood loss: vasoconstriction in nonvital regions and redirection of the blood flow to the most important organs. The ultimate goal is to benefit from this compensatory mechanism for as long as possible. Unfortunately, there are no direct and accurate measures of when this mechanism is at its limits and the oxygenation of vital organs is starting to be impaired. Systolic blood pressure (SBP, invasive or noninvasive) continues to serve as a very basic surrogate variable, even though there is no reliable correlation between SBP and organ microcirculation. Animal models of shock demonstrate that resuscitation to 60% of the baseline mean arterial pressure (MAP) does not reduce the regional organ perfusion compared with normotensive resuscitation, but the less aggressive resuscitation does lead to a decreased blood loss. At the same time, brain perfusion was not different between the two groups. Consequently, there is some expert consensus to tolerate SBP around 80 to 90 mm Hg in actively hemorrhaging patients until

VI

hemostasis is achieved with adjustment to the patient's age, preexisting medical conditions, and injury pattern. For example, on one extreme, there is the young and healthy patient with a massive abdominal bleed. In that case, SBP in the 60 mm Hg range can be tolerated for a short duration. On the other end of the spectrum, keeping SBP well above 100 mm Hg for elderly patients with multiple medical conditions and multisystem trauma involving the brain should be considered. These measures are only temporarily in place until hemostasis is achieved or the patient's condition further deteriorates. In the latter case, the intravascular volume has to be replenished.

At the point when the patient needs additional intravascular fluids, crystalloids and colloids should be avoided in this early phase.[12] Otherwise, the cardiac output and intravascular pressures will increase, as will the rate of bleeding; coagulation factors will continually be consumed in an effort to clot the bleeding sites; and their plasma levels will rapidly decline. All of these conditions will negatively affect a patient's ability to survive a disastrous bleeding episode. Restoring vital signs to normal values will bring a short period of better physiology before the disastrous combination of an increased bleeding rate and rapid deterioration of the patient's coagulation capability significantly worsen the overall situation. In addition, large volumes of crystalloids will worsen reperfusion injury and augment inflammatory response. Administration of synthetic colloids will even further increase coagulopathy by impairing both fibrinogen polymerization and platelet function.

As a result, the use of crystalloids and colloids has been restricted in the setting of severe hemorrhage. Instead, blood products are the fluids of choice for the resuscitation of massively bleeding patients (also see Chapter 25). Packed red blood cells (PRBCs), fresh frozen plasma (FFP), and platelets are the mainstays for the initial resuscitation.

Evidence is emerging that demonstrates the pragmatic and early use of these blood products in a fixed ratio (i.e., 1:1:1, PRBC:FFP:platelets).[13] The benefit of using this approach is that the oxygen-carrying capacity is maintained or restored with the PRBCs, and the patient's ability to form clots is supported with the plasma factors in the FFP and platelet infusions. When transfusing large amounts of this combination of blood products, one should consider the additional supplementation of fibrinogen in the form of cryoprecipitate, as fibrinogen is one of the key components of hemostasis. Fig. 43.4 provides an example of blood products provided as part of a MTP. Cryoprecipitate is consumed much faster than can be resynthesized by the liver under such circumstances, and as a result, tranexamic acid, an antifibrinolytic, is given for preventing coagulopathy in severely injured hypotensive patients early in their course.[14,15] In recent years, the use of whole blood early in the context of expected massive transfusion has gained momentum in both the prehospital and intrahospital contexts. Conceptually, the use of whole blood not only simplifies the approach, but it also offers less dilution of red blood cells, platelets, and coagulation factors compared with component therapy.[16] See Fig 43.5. The use of whole blood has been established as safe, and it may even be associated with improved outcomes, at least in military settings.[17]

As an alternative, or in addition, to fractionated products, fibrinogen concentrate or prothrombin complex concentrate (PCC) can be administered. These also have the advantage of not requiring crossmatching and are shelf stable. There is some early evidence that combined use of four-factor PCC combined with FFP can reduce total transfusion volume and improve coagulation laboratory values.[18] A persisting concern is the potential for an increased risk of clinically significant thrombosis. Although this has not been born out in the literature at this stage, the authors recommend pairing their use with viscoelastic hemostatic assays (VHAs) to ensure their administration is tailored to the patient's needs. The role of vasopressors for hemodynamic support in this phase remains largely controversial. They should generally be avoided, because in an already severely hypovolemic state further vasoconstriction may compromise the blood flow to vital organs.

Access for Intravascular Resuscitation

To deploy adequate resuscitation in a severely bleeding patient, proper access to the patient's vascular system needs to be obtained. Every patient with significant trauma or mechanism of trauma should have two large-bore peripheral intravenous (PIV) lines placed. They should be 16-gauge or larger and preferably inserted in the upper extremities. The integrity and the time to meaningful venous access are of equal importance. It is better to quickly obtain a well-functioning 18-gauge PIV than to waste valuable time on obtaining an elusive 14-gauge PIV.

Cooler #	Contents
1st Cooler	4 units PRBC 4 units FFP
2nd Cooler	4 units PRBC 4 units FFP 6 units platelets (1 pooled)
3rd Cooler	As 1st
4th Cooler	As 2nd
Repeat	Consider adding cryoprecipitate after 4th cooler or if fibrinogen <1

Fig. 43.4 Example of a massive transfusion protocol.

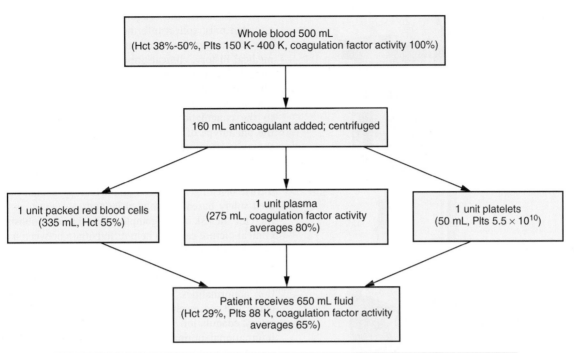

Fig. 43.5 Dilution and storage loss reduce the effectiveness of component blood product therapy compared with fresh whole blood. (Redrawn from Dutton R. Haemostatic resuscitation. Br J Anaesth. 2012;109[Suppl 1]:i39–i46.) *FFP*, Fresh frozen plasma; *PRBC*, packed red blood cells.

Prolonged or significant massive transfusions usually benefit from large-bore central access. Classically, a large-bore (e.g., 8.5 Fr) catheter introducer sheath is placed in either the femoral, internal jugular, or subclavian vein. If the circumstances permit, this is performed with ultrasound guidance.

Intraosseous (IO) access is suitable as a first-line access if PIV access is poor or delayed. Although an IO line cannot be used for rapid volume resuscitation, it can serve as a line to administer medications. With better overall flow rates and the proximity to the heart, the humeral approach is the preferable location for an IO line in adults.

The use of a modern rapid infuser system is of paramount importance. The rapid infuser provides the anesthesia team with the capability to deliver large amounts of warmed blood products very quickly and safely. Rapid infuser systems are highly capable, and the patient and the clinical situation should be closely monitored to avoid excessive resuscitation (Fig. 43.6).

When all the aforementioned measures and techniques are properly deployed, the anesthesia team can provide the patient and surgical team with the valuable extra time needed until hemostasis can be achieved. Once the bleeding is mostly under control, the priorities and speed of approach change and phase 2 of resuscitation begins.

Phase 2: Controlled Hemorrhage

In phase 2 after the major aspects of the bleeding source have been controlled, the anesthesia team should focus on a more individualized, tailored approach. Depending on the dynamics of a given case and the number and experience of anesthesia providers available, phase 2 items can happen earlier and in parallel with phase 1.

Invasive monitoring should begin at this point. The insertion should never delay or distract from the massive transfusion, the placement of intravenous lines, and the surgical hemostasis. Additionally, it is technically much easier to place an arterial line in a properly resuscitated patient.

In phase 2 the dynamics of the case slow down, the process becomes less blind, and the patient's needs should be reanalyzed. A mainstay during phase 2 is the utilization of point-of-care testing (POCT) to guide the resuscitation.[19] To do so, one has to reflect on the main physiologic goals of resuscitation: guaranteeing adequate oxygen delivery and coagulation function. Oxygen delivery depends mostly on the oxygen-carrying capacity and normal intravascular filling. The first is measured via hemoglobin (Hb) concentration or the hematocrit (Hct) in the patient's blood. Depending on the patient's age, comorbid conditions, and injuries, Hct values between

VI

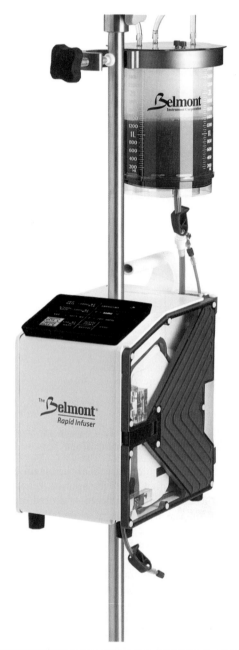

Fig. 43.6 The Belmont rapid infuser. (Courtesy of Belmont Instrument Corporation, Billerica, MA.)

18% and 28% are targeted. The intravascular volume status can be assessed by a combination of a multitude of clinical clues, such as vital signs, urine output, and, if applicable, direct observation of the patient's heart and major vessels. In more challenging cases (e.g., suspected cardiac comorbid conditions, cardiac contusions, arrhythmias), a transesophageal echocardiogram (TEE) can further quantify the intravascular volume.

To best assess the coagulation status of a patient, the clinician must collect information from the four main pillars of perioperative coagulation monitoring: the patient's medical history, clinical presentation, standard laboratory coagulation tests, and point-of-care coagulation tests. If obtainable, the patient's medical history can provide information on medications and medical conditions relevant to the coagulation system. The clinical presentation of the phenotype of bleeding is a simple but critical tool for the existence and differential diagnosis of coagulopathy. Any abnormal coagulation test needs to be correlated to the clinical presentation. Without any clinically relevant diffuse bleeding, no procoagulant therapy should be initiated solely based on isolated laboratory values, as it will increase the risk of any complications (i.e., thrombosis). The clinical picture can also help differentiate between a surgical versus nonsurgical origin of the bleeding. Nonsurgical bleeding presents itself with a diffuse and more widespread pattern and must be addressed by correcting the coagulation abnormalities. In contrast, surgical bleeding must be controlled via mechanical hemostasis. The standard laboratory coagulation tests consist of prothrombin time and international normalized ratio (PT/INR), activated partial thromboplastin time (aPTT), platelet count, and fibrinogen concentration. These tests come with significant limitations such as sensitivity, specificity, validity, and timeliness that render them virtually useless early in dynamic massive transfusion scenarios (also see Chapter 23).

Viscoelastic Testing

Over the past decade, viscoelastic point-of-care coagulation tests have become a mainstay for timely assessment of the situations previously described. The thromboelastograph (TEG) and rotational thromboelastometry (ROTEM) are standard tools to assess the magnitude and nature of the coagulation disturbance and help guide interventions (Fig. 43.7). Both devices provide the clinician with a graphical output that can guide the procoagulant interventions. The readout of TEG/ROTEM can be divided into parts: (1) preclot formation phase, (2) clot formation phase, and (3) clot stability phase (Fig. 43.8). The first phase, preclot formation, starts with the addition of reagents that trigger the plasma coagulation cascade and activate the platelets. This phase lasts less than 5 minutes and can inform the anesthesia provider about the coagulation cascade. If there are deficiencies in this phase, PCC and FFP can be given. The second phase starts with the beginning of the clot formation and ends when the maximum clot firmness is reached. This phase reflects the functional platelet mass and the availability of fibrinogen. Defects in the second phase can be corrected with the transfusion of cryoprecipitate, fibrinogen concentrate, or platelet concentrates. The third and last phase reflects the stability of the clot, allowing fibrinolysis to be detected and quantified. When identified, it can be effectively treated with an antifibrinolytic drug.

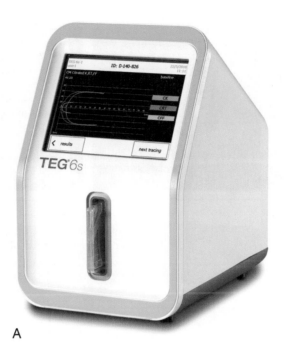

A

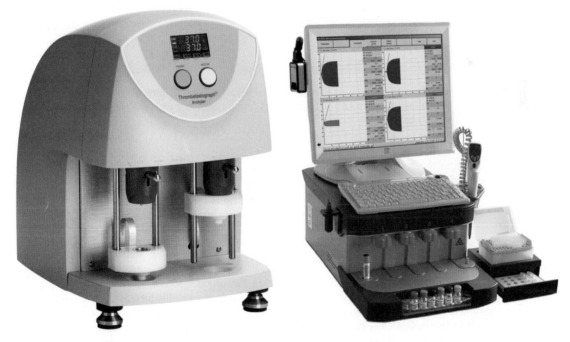

B   **TEG 5000, Haemoneics Corp.**   **ROTEM Delta, TEM Systems**

Fig. 43.7 Tools for viscoelastic point-of-care coagulation testing. *Left,* Thromboelastograph (*TEG*). *Right,* Rotational thromboelastometry (*ROTEM*).

VI

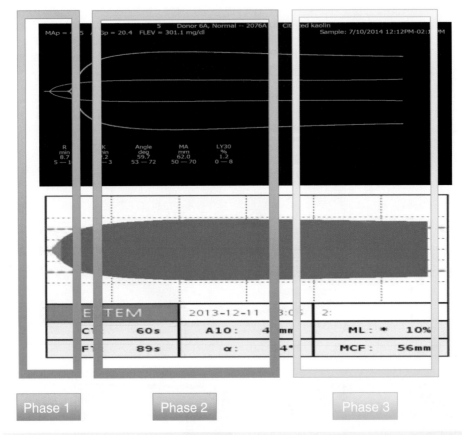

Fig. 43.8 Three phases of viscoelastic tests: phase 1 (preclot), phase 2 (formation), and phase 3 (stability). TEG tracing in top panel and ROTEM tracing in bottom panel. *ROTEM*, Rotational thromboelastometry; *TEG*, thromboelastograph.

With the information from the four pillars of coagulation monitoring, the treatment can be tailored using a goal-directed approach and predefined algorithms. This approach also must consider that any procoagulant therapy always has to be used with caution. A coagulopathy should never be excessively corrected; otherwise, the risk for serious thromboembolic events can increase (Fig. 43.9).

After hemorrhage has been controlled, frequent analysis of POCT (Hb/Hct, arterial blood gases, electrolytes) should be obtained because they help guide PRBC transfusions and adjustments in ventilation to the patient's needs. Additionally, electrolyte disturbances (e.g., hypocalcemia and hyperkalemia) frequently occur and warrant consideration.

During resuscitation, hypothermia should be prevented. This is mainly achieved by only administering warmed fluids, increasing the room temperature, and the use of forced air warmers. The insertion of an esophageal temperature probe helps the clinician to monitor the success of these interventions and serves as a reminder to try to achieve normothermia.

Phase 3: Restoration of Physiology

The third and final resuscitation phase includes the fine-tuning and restoration of the patient's physiology. This should occur once the surgical hemostasis is complete and the dynamic of the resuscitation is under control. The DCR principles no longer apply, as the potential for harm likely outweighs the benefits. The intravascular volume is replenished during this phase. Additional cardiac output monitoring devices can help guide the process. If not already achieved, the anesthetic should be incrementally increased to a level near 1 MAC. Low-dose vasoactive infusions can be considered to counteract anesthesia-induced vasodilation but should not be used to compensate for inadequate intravascular volume resuscitation. Continued serial POCT (i.e., arterial blood gas analysis, thromboelastometry) is useful in determining the success of the resuscitation. Normalizing serum lactate and base deficit levels are excellent indicators for this achievement.

Anesthetics

For patients with life-threatening uncontrolled hemorrhage, the administration of even low-dose anesthetics

SFGH ROTEM guideline

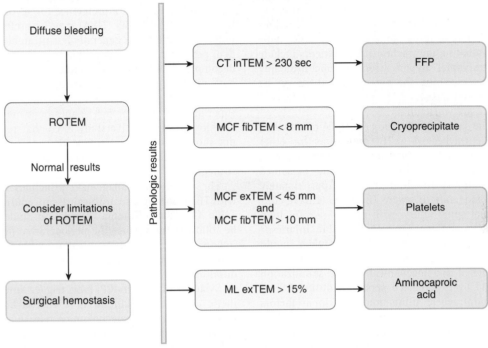

Fig. 43.9 An example of a rotational thromboelastometry (*ROTEM*) treatment algorithm for use in trauma. (Courtesy of San Francisco General Hospital and Trauma Center.)

may contribute to worsening hypotension. Once blood and fluid resuscitation begin to restore intravascular volume and tissue blood flow, administration of additional anesthetics is appropriate. A stepwise approach to restoring adequate anesthetic levels uses arterial blood pressure values as a guide to increasing anesthetic depth. Thus slow administration of anesthetics should be started in phase 2. The stepwise deepening of the anesthetic can be achieved by either repeated boluses of opioids or increasing inhaled anesthetic concentrations in an incremental manner.[20]

SPECIAL CONSIDERATIONS

Traumatic Brain Injury

Traumatic brain injury (TBI) is defined as injury to the head that disrupts normal brain function (also see Chapter 30). In the United States, over 15 million people are seen in emergency departments for TBI each year, and TBI contributes to 30% of trauma deaths.[21] Long-term effects of TBI may lead to cognitive and functional impairment, disability, and an overall reduction in quality of life.

Primary neurologic injury is irreversible, occurring at the moment of injury and causing immediate neuronal damage. The magnitude of the primary injury is a significant prognostic factor of TBI. Secondary injury is the subsequent injury to the brain after the primary injury occurs. Common causes of secondary injury include intracranial hypertension, arterial hypotension, hypoxia, hyperthermia, coagulopathy, hyperglycemia or hypoglycemia, and acidosis. The focus of TBI management for the anesthesia provider is to optimize patient physiology and limit secondary injury in the perioperative period to achieve the best possible neurologic outcome.

Neurologic manifestations of TBI largely depend on the mechanism, severity, and type of injury that have occurred. Types of injuries include skull fractures; intracerebral, subdural, and epidural hematomas; hemorrhagic contusions; and diffuse axonal injuries. These injuries may be focal or diffuse. The GCS is commonly used to initially assess and classify TBI patients, though iatrogenic intoxication (e.g., sedatives or analgesics administered prior to evaluation) and other factors may sometimes lead to misclassification. GCS score should be reported for each of the three components (eye, verbal, motor) separately. Untestable components of GCS should be documented. Early computed tomography (CT) scan is critical in delineating the type and extent of injury.

Like other trauma patients, the initial evaluation begins with ATLS. An early definitive airway should be established in a TBI patient who does not have the ability to maintain a patent airway owing to loss of reflexes and inadequate oxygenation or ventilation. These factors are usually related to a deteriorating GCS score—usually 8 or less—or other concurrent injuries. Nasal airways (and nasogastric tubes) should be avoided if possible in TBI patients with facial or suspected skull base fractures because of the risk of intracranial insertion. Other indications for intubating the trachea of TBI patients include signs of intracranial hypertension or uncontrollable seizure activity. Securing the airway should always be considered before transport if the patient's mental status and GCS score are worsening.

Many of the same considerations must be taken when intubating the trachea of a TBI patient as for other trauma patients, such as inadequate fasting, hypoxia, uncertain intravascular volume status, and presumed cervical spine injury in blunt trauma. Approximately 4% to 8% of moderate to severe TBI patients have concurrent cervical spine injury, with greater risk for high cervical injuries and mechanically unstable injuries.[22] Of particular attention to the anesthesia provider should be the integrity of the cervical spine. Cervical collars should be opened and mechanical in-line stabilization should be held by experienced personnel during RSI of anesthesia and tracheal intubation. Additional factors such as increased intracranial pressure (ICP) or pending herniation, concurrent airway injuries, uncooperative patients, and combativeness should also be considered. It is not clear whether video laryngoscopy is superior to intubation with conventional laryngoscopy. Video laryngoscopy may produce slightly less cervical spine motion and obtain better glottis visualization, but at the cost of a slightly longer time to endotracheal intubation in an experienced laryngoscopist's hands.[23,24] Selection of the intubation method should be based on speed of establishing a definitive airway and experience of the laryngoscopist, but video laryngoscopy is quickly, and appropriately, establishing itself as the first-line choice in high-acuity situations.

The use of anesthetics should focus on hemodynamic stability to maintain cerebral perfusion pressure (CPP). Propofol and etomidate are commonly selected as induction agents for their reduction in cerebral blood flow (CBF), which is coupled to a reduction in cerebral metabolic rate of oxygen ($CMRO_2$) requirement (also see Chapter 8). Although once considered controversial, use of ketamine in this population has not led to increases in ICP or worsened outcomes.[25] Nondepolarizing neuromuscular blocking drugs have no significant effect on cerebral hemodynamics. Succinylcholine may theoretically increase ICP, but this effect has not been demonstrated to be clinically significant and may be attenuated with a defasciculating dose of a nondepolarizing drug (also see Chapter 11).

Emergent neurosurgical management may sometimes be indicated. Volatile anesthetics may increase CBF while decreasing $CMRO_2$, known as "uncoupling" (also see Chapter 7). Increased CBF does not generally occur below 0.5 MAC, or below 1 MAC for sevoflurane specifically. If volatile anesthetics are used, less than 1 MAC should be administered, with a preference for sevoflurane. Total intravenous anesthesia (TIVA) may be preferred because it decreases ICP but is generally less titratable during sudden, profound hypotension that may occur during dural decompression. Although volatile anesthetics and TIVA have different effects on cerebral hemodynamics, there is no definitive prospective outcome study demonstrating superiority of one approach to anesthetic maintenance. In addition, a retrospective study in combat-related TBI did not show significant difference between neurologic outcomes at discharge when comparing the two anesthetic strategies.[26,27]

The anesthesia management principles for a patient with TBI requiring a neurosurgical procedure are listed in Table 43.4. Brain Trauma Foundation guidelines should be followed throughout the perioperative period.[28] Most importantly, close communication with the operative team must be maintained before decompression and dural opening.

Systemically, high ICP may trigger intense sympathetic activity to maintain CPP. This is known as the *Cushing reflex.* The catecholamine release and increased systemic vascular resistance may mask intravascular volume depletion. Sudden, profound hypotension may sometimes occur after decompression and normalization of ICP, especially in patients who are not adequately volume resuscitated. It is hence critical to restore euvolemia before dural decompression. Additionally, anesthetic drugs should be gradually decreased and vasopressors and inotropes should be available for administration before major decompression.

The decision for postoperative intubation vs. immediate tracheal extubation should be discussed with the surgeon. Many TBI patients remain tracheally intubated owing to the risks of postoperative hypoventilation, hypoxia, depressed level of consciousness, other concurrent injuries, and the need for further diagnostic studies or therapies. These patients should be transported with full monitoring. Sedation and a transport ventilator are usually necessary if the patient remains intubated. Before transporting TBI patients, a small-dose muscle relaxant may be considered to reduce episodes of agitation, bucking, or coughing. The use of large-dose muscle relaxation at the end of the procedure or for transport may delay postoperative neurologic examination and is not recommended. TBI guidelines mentioned earlier should continue to be followed throughout the immediate perioperative period.[28]

Spinal Cord Injury

Spinal cord injury (SCI) occurs when acute trauma disrupts normal sensory, motor, or autonomic function. In the United States, 12,500 new patients sustain an SCI per

Table 43.4 Anesthesia Management Principles for TBI Patients Requiring Neurosurgical Procedures

Organ System/ Issue	Management Principle	Comments
Patient position	Patient is usually placed in reverse Trendelenburg or head of bed elevated to 30 degrees.	Facilitates cerebral venous drainage.
Monitoring/lines	Large-bore intravenous access is necessary for intraoperative fluid administration. An arterial line should be inserted for continuous arterial blood pressure monitoring and withdrawal of blood for serial laboratory analysis.	
Fluid/blood	Blood should be checked for availability of transfusion. Intravascular fluid administration/resuscitation is usually required to achieve euvolemia, especially after administration of mannitol. Isotonic crystalloid is usually preferred. The use of albumin may increase mortality risk in the resuscitation of ICU brain-injured patients when compared with crystalloid.[27]	Surgery for compound depressed skull fractures near venous sinuses are at particularly intense risk for massive hemorrhage. Coagulopathy should be ruled out with viscoelastometric testing and traditional laboratory coagulation panel. Blood should be immediately available for sudden, abrupt bleeding.
Cardiovascular	Hypotension should be promptly treated to maintain a cerebral perfusion pressure (CPP) of at least 50–70 mm Hg.	
Respiratory	Hypoxemia should be avoided. Attention should be paid to peak inspiratory pressure and positive end-expiratory pressure to avoid obstruction of cerebral venous drainage.	Hyperventilation is not recommended within the first 24 hours of injury unless treating impending herniation.
Seizure prophylaxis	Prophylactic administration of mannitol and antiseizure administration is recommended.	
Metabolic	Glucose should be monitored regularly. Hyperglycemia and hypoglycemia should be treated to avoid exacerbation of secondary injury.	General recommendations are to treat blood glucose levels above 180 mg/dL.

year, and over 200,000 people currently live with SCI.[29] The most common causes of injury are motor vehicle accidents, falls, and assault.

The presentation of SCI depends largely on the extent, severity, and level at which injury occurs. An injury may be described as "complete" if the patient has no motor or sensory function below the level of injury. Incomplete SCIs describe partial injury to the cord that results in varying degrees of residual sensory and motor function. The American Spinal Injury Association (ASIA) classification is the preferred impairment scale to describe findings of neurologic examinations. The ASIA scale uses muscle function and sensation of light touch and pin prick at multiple body locations to generate a grade of A (complete injury), B (sensory incomplete), C (motor incomplete), D (motor incomplete), or E (normal).[30]

Spinal cord precautions should be immediately undertaken when suspecting an injury, including a cervical collar and strict logroll precautions whenever transporting or moving patients. Adequacy of ventilation and oxygenation should be quickly evaluated. Cervical spine injuries, especially those with complete injuries, may result in diaphragm impairment and weakness. This leads to decreased vital capacity and the inability to cough and clear secretions. Concurrent lung injury associated with trauma or chronic lung disease may exacerbate the patient's ability to ventilate and oxygenate. Signs of inadequate ventilation may include rapid, shallow breathing; increased work of breathing; and paradoxical abdominal movement. These signs may appear with thoracic and high lumbar injuries affecting intercostal and abdominal muscles. The airway should be secured with an endotracheal tube in a similar fashion as with TBI patients. Up to 16% of patients admitted with SCI are diagnosed with concurrent TBI. In this population with concurrent diagnoses, the cervical spine was most frequently injured.[31] Succinylcholine may be used to safely provide neuromuscular blockade in an SCI patient within the first 24 hours of injury. However, it should be avoided after 48 hours of injury because of the risk of severe hyperkalemia that may result with administration. Exaggerated bradycardic response and hypotension have been reported with direct laryngoscopy and intubation of the trachea of patients with cervical or high thoracic injuries.

During the acute phase, high thoracic (usually T4 and above) and cervical SCIs may result in significant bradyarrhythmia and atrioventricular block (AV block) owing to disruption of sympathetic cardiac accelerator fibers leading to unopposed parasympathetic innervation. Sympathetic blockade may also lead to systemic vasodilation

VI

and result in severe hypotension. In addition to the motor and sensory findings below the level of injury, this physiologic constellation has been referred to as "neurogenic shock." Treatment is supportive and includes administration of isotonic fluid, vasopressors, and inotropes.

MAP should be kept at 85 to 90 mm Hg for patients with SCI to maintain adequate spinal cord perfusion, unless otherwise contraindicated by concurrent injuries. Administration of methylprednisolone is no longer recommended by the American Association of Neurological Surgeons, as there is evidence that large-dose steroids are associated with mostly negative effects, including death.[32]

Burns

Major burns can occur in isolation or in combination with other forms of traumatic injury. Patients with major burns can decline rapidly and require systematic advanced trauma management. This section will focus on special considerations in the immediate management of a major acute burn patient.

Burn Severity

Burns are categorized based on their severity as superficial, partial-thickness, or full-thickness burns (Table 43.5).

Estimating Burn Surface Area

The patient's clinical management, including the decision to transfer to a tertiary center, is based on the percentage of body surface area (BSA) affected by burns. One approach to estimating the affected BSA is the "rule of nines" (Fig. 43.10).

Types of Burns: Thermal, Chemical, and Electrical

The first priority in managing the burn is to halt the burning process. Remove any clothing that can be removed easily. The subsequent approach depends on the type of burn, as detailed further in Table 43.6.

Fluid Management

Fluid management is an important cornerstone of modern burn management; however, controversy still exists about the correct amount of fluid to give and the appropriate endpoints to be monitoring. There is increasing recognition of the adverse effects of excessive intravenous fluid resuscitation and the increased risk of precipitating acute respiratory distress syndrome (ARDS) 3 to 5 days after injury.

Multiple formulas can be used for estimating fluid resuscitation requirements. Most were developed over 30 years ago. One of the most common is the modified Parkland formula: 4 mL/kg/% burn (adults) over the first 24 hours after burn injury.

Only crystalloid fluid is used for the first 24 hours, as the amount of protein leak into the interstitial space is thought to be greatest during this period, thus rendering colloids ineffective. The most commonly used fluid is a balanced salt solution such as lactated Ringer's solution or PlasmaLyte. These formulas should be taken as a guide only, and current best practice is to tailor the exact fluid administered to the patient's physiologic response. Hourly urine output measured via a Foley catheter is considered the most helpful metric of adequacy of fluid resuscitation. Other values that are often trended include Hct, cardiac output, osmolarity, electrolytes, albumin, calcium, and glucose.[34]

Airway (Also See Chapter 16)

Burns are characterized by erythema and the rapid onset of edema in affected tissues. When this happens in the upper airway, the swelling can result in total airway obstruction and death. Clinicians must anticipate this possibility for patients with burns affecting the airway and prepare for tracheal intubation early—before swelling makes it impossible. Some warning signs are presented in Box 43.12. Consider inserting an endotracheal tube 0.5 to 1 mm internal diameter smaller than usual to allow for the expected tissue swelling.

Table 43.5	Burn Severity
Burn Type	**Comment**
Superficial	This burn affects the epidermis only (e.g., sunburn). It does not require any specific treatment other than first aid. Superficial burns are not included in the calculation of percentage body surface area (%BSA) affected.
Partial thickness	This burn involves all of the epidermis and part of the dermis. It can further be divided into superficial dermal, mid-dermal, and deep dermal. These burns change in appearance as the burn destroys more of the dermis and vasculature; the pain ranges from minimal to extreme; color can be red to pale/white; and exudates can be high fluid to relatively dry. Blisters are often present. They may require surgical management.
Full thickness	This burn involves complete destruction of all of the epidermis and dermis. It is white, insensate, and has a waxy or leathery appearance. This type of skin is called an *eschar*.

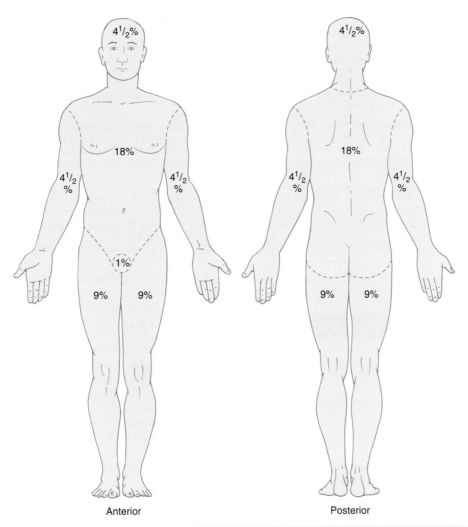

Anterior   Posterior

Fig. 43.10 The rule of nines—used to calculate percentage of body surface area (BSA) burns. This rule is most useful for patients with localized burns to a particular body part. However, this rule overestimates the percentage of BSA in a patient with morbid obesity. Another approach is to use the patient's palmar surface area, which represents approximately 1% of total BSA.

Pain (Also See Chapter 40)

Depending on the severity of the burn, pain can be a major issue. Analgesia should be provided for all patients as required. A regimen based on opiates, with the addition of ketamine if necessary, usually provides sufficient relief for the majority of patients. Because of the prolonged nature and significant amount of pain associated with the treatment of burns, these patients are at notably greater risk of developing opiate tolerance. Consultation from a specialist pain service should be sought early in their recovery.

Inhalation

In addition to the actual burn injury, the products of combustion can produce gases that are toxic to the human body. The most common is carbon monoxide (CO). CO has a much higher binding affinity for Hb compared with oxygen. Thus CO-poisoning can result in a significant reduction in the oxygen-carrying capacity of the blood. The only way to detect CO poisoning is through CO-oximetry performed on a blood gas sample. Standard pulse oximetry monitors are unable to detect CO poisoning and will read a normal value even in the presence of profound tissue hypoxemia. The application of high-concentration oxygen significantly reduces the half-life of CO in the blood, and any patient with suspected CO inhalation should be provided with high-concentration oxygen as an initial measure.

Infection

Infection is a major cause of delayed morbidity and death. Although empiric antibiotics addressing skin flora are sufficient for the immediate management, coverage

VI

Table 43.6 Special Considerations of Specific Burn Types

Burn Type	Special Considerations
Thermal burns	Remove source of heat as soon as possible (e.g., burning clothing). Continue prolonged irrigation with cold fluid, but beware of causing hypothermia. Be suspicious for associated injuries (inhalational, other forms of trauma).
Chemical burns	Irrigate the area thoroughly with running water. Prevent irrigation fluid from running across unaffected skin. Continue irrigation until skin pH or fluid pH is neutral (use litmus paper). Adequate irrigation may take several hours with some chemical burns. DO NOT use water for elemental metal burns (lithium, magnesium, potassium, sodium), as they react with water, worsening the burn; use mineral oil instead in this setting.
Electrical burns	Look for entry and exit points because injury has occurred along that trajectory. Beware of underlying muscle damage; there is the risk of compartment syndrome and rhabdomyolysis. There is a slightly increased fluid requirement. Beware of arrhythmias caused by the electric current, because ventricular fibrillation is the most common cause of death after an electrical shock.[33]

Box 43.12 Signs of Potential Airway Burns

- Carbonaceous sputum
- Stridor
- Voice changes
- Facial burns
- Explosive injuries involving upper torso/head
- Prolonged entrapment in fire

of the burn surface with sterile dressings is essential to reestablish the external barrier to organisms. Overresuscitation with fluids is also associated with increased risk of infectious complications.

Escharotomies

The eschar of full-thickness burns significantly reduces the compliance of body tissues. If the eschars are circumferential around any part, it can result in a compartment-like syndrome. This is particularly concerning around the torso, where ventilation can be impeded. If this occurs, escharotomies may need to be performed. The preferred location for incisions is outlined in Fig. 43.11.

Transfer of Burn Patients

In general, most regions have a burn center or unit that provides specialized treatment of burn patients; expert care in these centers is associated with improved outcomes. The decision to transfer to a dedicated burn center requires consideration of other associated injuries and where these can best be managed. Sometimes it may be appropriate to stabilize the major visceral injuries at the trauma center before transferring care to the burn unit at a later stage. Commonly used transfer criteria are listed in Box 43.13.

Extremes of Age

Pediatric Trauma (Also See Chapter 34)

Trauma is the most common cause of major morbidity and fatality in the pediatric population (Box 43.14). The presentation of an injured child to a hospital is usually a source of anxiety for most clinicians. By delivering high-quality advanced trauma care, the burden of the child's injury can be lessened and an improved outcome attained.

This section will present a brief overview of some of the issues that are unique to trauma in the pediatric patient. The fundamental principles of ATLS form the basis of management in this patient population.

Special Considerations

Nonaccidental injury

This differential diagnosis should always be considered in pediatric injury. The majority of jurisdictions have mandatory reporting for child abuse. Warning signs are listed in Box 43.15.

Pediatric physiology

Children are able to mask significant hemodynamic compromise because of their robust physiology. There are also confounders for signs such as tachycardia, pain, and a fear or stress response. Beware of rapid deterioration once a compensatory threshold is reached.

Vascular access

Pediatric venous cannulation can present a challenge even in a well-hydrated patient. In the presence of hemorrhagic shock, intravenous catheter placement can be almost impossible. The priority should be restoring circulating intravascular volume, and early IO access is advocated. A rule of thumb used by some institutions is two attempts at a PIV line in two locations before you transition to the IO approach.

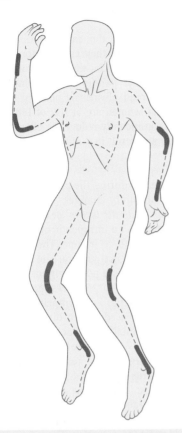

Fig. 43.11 Locations for escharotomy incisions.

Box 43.13 Criteria for Transfer of Patients to a Tertiary Burn Center (American Burn Association)

- >10% total BSA partial-thickness burns
- Full-thickness burns in any age group
- Burns involving sensitive areas (hands, feet, perineum, face, genitals, major joints)
- Inhalation injuries
- Electrical/lightning burns
- Circumferential burns to limbs or torso
- Significant chemical burn risking cosmetic or functional outcome
- Major preexisting comorbid conditions

BSA, Body surface area.

Box 43.14 Common Injuries in Pediatrics

- Simple fractures—falls from height/play equipment, sports
- Pedestrian versus car—more chest/head injuries—especially with SUVs
- More major visceral injury without overlying fractures

SUVs, Sport-utility vehicles.

Box 43.15 Warning Signs of Child Abuse

- Injury pattern inconsistent with developmental milestones (e.g., a 2-month-old rolling off the diaper changing table)
- Multiple injuries (especially if these appear to have been inflicted over time)
- Frequent presentations
- Inconsistent history of incident

Drug dosing

Because the majority of drug doses and fluids are weight based, it is essential to get an accurate estimation of the child's weight. The clinician's choices are to ask a caregiver or parent or to use a tool such as the Broselow Pediatric Emergency Tape to get an estimate. Visual aids and age-stratified charts can serve as excellent tools to help with choosing the right-sized equipment and administering appropriate drug doses. The considerations for dose reduction of some drugs in the trauma patient still apply to pediatrics.

Behavior

Health care visits of any kind can be emotionally and psychologically traumatic for pediatric patients. Thus a child's openness and compliance with diagnosis and treatment will vary depending on their age and clinical circumstances. There should be consideration for the appropriateness of diagnostic tests such as CT and the requirement for the child to be still. Anesthesia and tracheal intubation may be required to facilitate the diagnostic and treatment process.

Blood administration and dosing (Box 43.16)

Small children have a substantially reduced circulating blood volume, and a small amount of blood loss can be significant. In a 20-kg 4-year-old child the estimated circulating blood volume is only 1600 mL. Loss of 375 mL (equivalent to a 12-oz can of soft drink) represents over 20% of the total circulating volume. It is important to be vigilant for occult sources of bleeding and intervene early. Transfusing red blood cells will increase Hb by 2 to 2.5 g/dL for every 10 mL/kg administered.

Geriatric Trauma (Also See Chapter 35)

As with pediatrics the elderly trauma patient also requires some unique considerations for management. Although trauma is not a major contributor to morbidity and

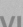

VI

Box 43.16 Blood Volume Estimations

- Preterm neonate—95 mL/kg
- Full-term neonate—85 mL/kg
- Infant—80 mL/kg
- Adult (male)—75 mL/kg
- Adult (female)—65 mL/kg

mortality in the geriatric population, their physiologic age, coexisting diseases, and chronic medications make this group more susceptible to poor outcomes if their care is not of the highest standards. The principles of advanced trauma management remain paramount and the basis of all interventions. This section will briefly outline some of the unique considerations for the trauma patient of advanced age.

Special Considerations

Preexisting illness and physiologic reserve

With advancing age comes the potential for a variety of medical conditions that may affect a patient's ability to survive a major trauma. This combines with the decline in physiologic reserve that occurs with healthy aging, placing these patients at serious risk of major morbidity or mortality.

Medications

Medications, such as antihypertensives, for relatively minor and well-controlled conditions can exacerbate hemodynamic instability after a trauma. β-Adrenergic blocking drugs can mask the tachycardia associated with blood loss.

Minimal impact trauma

Relatively minor mechanisms can result in significant injuries. Geriatric patients are more prone to fractures and head injuries. Subdural hematomas are particularly common.

Elder abuse

An increasingly recognized cause of injury to the geriatric population in long-term care facilities is abuse. This should be considered and explored, especially in patients who are in care facilities and have reduced mobility or cognitive function.

End-of-life care

It is important to consider what is appropriate when providing an intervention to a patient. When possible, determine the patient's wishes and any preexisting limitation of treatment orders. Remain focused on interventions that can return the patient to a level of function that she or he would find fulfilling. This can be very difficult in the chaos of a major trauma, but when there is an opportunity, discuss this with the patient, or the family, or both.

Trauma in Pregnancy

Fundamentally, the management of a pregnant patient is the same as that of any other trauma victim. A focus on delivering advanced trauma management will optimize the outcomes for both the mother and the fetus. Still some specific issues need to be considered when managing a pregnant trauma patient. This section will focus on clinical aspects of managing a pregnant trauma patient.

Causes of Trauma

Pregnant women suffer the same types of trauma as nonpregnant women, yet they can be more vulnerable to injury. There are a few special situations worth considering. For example, intimate partner violence increases during pregnancy and should always be actively considered. In addition, pregnant women are at risk of improper seatbelt use, which can significantly reduce the effectiveness of this countermeasure and result in a different injury pattern.

Anatomy of Injury

As the fetus develops during the pregnancy, the nature of maternal and fetal injury changes.

First trimester (0 to 13 weeks' gestational age)

The uterus remains an intrapelvic organ; thus it is well protected from blunt force trauma. There are the "usual" adult injuries to abdominal viscera. The embryo is nonviable; vaginal bleeding is a poor prognostic sign.

Second trimester (14 to 26 weeks' gestational age)

The uterus moves into an extrapelvic position. There is a progressive, increased risk of direct fetal injury. The maternal organs gradually become more shielded.

Third trimester (27 to 40 weeks' gestational age)

The maternal organs are relatively protected from injury by the uterus and fetus. Exception—the bladder is at increased risk. There is an increased likelihood of precipitating early labor.

Special Considerations

Maternal Physiology

Maternal physiology undergoes significant change to accommodate the growing fetus (also see Chapter 33). The following physiologic changes have the greatest impact on treatment: (1) increased circulating blood volume that can mask significant blood loss; (2) compensated respiratory alkalosis with normal carbon dioxide partial pressure (Pco_2) of about 30 mm Hg; and (3) increased clotting factors or hypercoagulable state toward the end of pregnancy (e.g., at term, a fibrinogen of 300 mg/dL would be abnormally low).

Aortocaval Compression

Starting at approximately 20 weeks gestational age, the increasing mass of the uterus and fetus can apply compression to the inferior vena cava and abdominal aorta, causing a drop in cardiac output of up to 30%. To prevent this phenomenon, a wedge can be placed under the right hip to achieve a left tilt of approximately 15 to 30 degrees. Or a spine board can be used to rotate the patient an appropriate amount (Fig. 43.12). An alternative approach during a resuscitation is to have an assistant manually displace the uterus to the patient's left.

Maternal Airway

Difficult tracheal intubation is more likely in a pregnant patient (also see Chapter 33). This is caused by the following

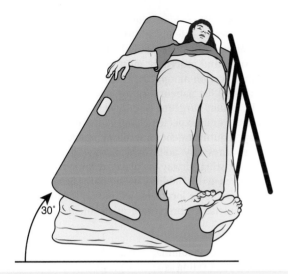

Fig. 43.12 Left tilt of pregnant patient on spine board.

30°

changes in anatomy and biomechanics: (1) increased generalized soft tissue edema that affects pharyngeal/laryngeal structures; (2) increased breast size affecting chest compliance and positioning in the supine position and spatial interference with laryngoscopy; (3) reduced FRC, resulting in relatively rapid desaturation; and (4) lower esophageal sphincter incompetence, resulting in higher risk of aspiration. Because of these factors, the approach to the maternal airway requires increased attention in the trauma setting. As with nonpregnant patients, airway considerations include potential spinal immobilization and availability of equipment such as video laryngoscopy.

Anti-D Immunoglobulin

For women with Rh (rhesus)-negative blood type, there is a risk of isoimmunization with fetal Rh-positive antigen. Pregnant patients with major trauma, and particularly any with injuries that involve the abdomen, should be considered at risk of contact between maternal and fetal circulations. To prevent longer-term impact on future pregnancies, an Rh-negative mother should be given anti-D immunoglobulin. This can be given any time after maternal blood group is determined but should be less than 72 hours after the trauma.

Radiation Exposure

Understandably, great effort is made to reduce radiation exposure to pregnant women. In the context of a major trauma, the insult most likely to cause morbidity or fatality to the patient and her fetus is delayed diagnosis of major life-threatening conditions. If a diagnostic modality is immediately available that uses less radiation (e.g., ultrasound), then it is appropriate to use it. The objective is to minimize the use of ionizing radiation but ensure the diagnosis is not delayed.

Fetal Monitoring

Fetal monitoring should not be commenced until maternal stability has been achieved. Monitoring should be performed by those with appropriate skills and training to interpret the information. Continuous fetal monitoring is usually not recommended for a fetus younger than 24 weeks unless there are plans to offer full resuscitation and neonatal intensive care support. The duration of monitoring is controversial, but most authorities recommend an initial 2 to 4 hours. The perfusion to the uteroplacental unit is not autoregulated. As such, any reduction in maternal cardiac output, even if asymptomatic, can cause a significant reduction in perfusion to the fetus. Any deterioration in fetal condition should prompt reassessment of maternal hemodynamics.

Delivery

It may be necessary to expedite delivery of the fetus to optimize maternal or fetal survival. Delivery of the fetus may be the only way to control massive uterine or placental bleeding and ensure a successful resuscitation. Consultation with obstetric and pediatric colleagues should be sought before undertaking any operative delivery. In the event of sustained cardiac arrest, a perimortem cesarean section should be considered if 5 minutes have elapsed without return of spontaneous circulation.[35]

Specific Differential Diagnoses (Also See Chapter 33)

The following diagnoses are unique to the pregnant patient and should always be considered in addition to standard differential diagnoses: (1) *Amniotic fluid embolus* can cause potentially life-threatening hemodynamic collapse. (2) *Placental abruption* is the process of inappropriate separation of the placenta from the uterine wall. The effect on the mother and fetus depends on the size and location of the disruption. Large disruptions can result in massive hemorrhage and fetal hypoxia. (3) *Uterine rupture* can result from major trauma with loss of containment of the fetus in the uterine cavity. This results in fetal parts being in the mother's abdominal cavity—a life-threatening obstetric emergency for both mother and fetus. Women who have had previous cesarean sections are at greater risk. (4) *Eclampsia* is a rare disorder but should be considered in any pregnant woman with an altered level of consciousness. It is usually associated with hypertension (i.e., arterial blood pressure more than 140/90 mm Hg) and proteinuria.

Care for Trauma Patients in Non-OR Settings

Many procedures that are performed on trauma patients outside the OR require anesthesia care (also see Chapter 38). These procedures occur at varying stages of resuscitation. Care in the non-OR environment can present unique challenges because of the unfamiliarity with surroundings, equipment, and staff. Patients are often evaluated in the CT scanner before further triage. Other locations of care

VI

may include radiologic suites, such as magnetic resonance imaging (MRI) or interventional radiology (IR), or the ICU.

Equipment considerations at non-OR locations include availability of emergency airway equipment along with medications for anesthetic induction and hemodynamic support. Suction should also be available in each location, particularly if thoracostomy tubes have been placed. Interventions performed in IR that require the presence of an anesthesia provider should have an anesthesia machine available, in addition to a standard OR cart with basic equipment and medications. If the patient is still in the acute phase of care while undergoing a procedure outside the OR, the anesthesia provider must be ready for active cardiopulmonary resuscitation, which may require the availability of blood, fluid warmers, large-bore intravenous access, rapid transfusion machines, and invasive monitoring. The patient's temperature should be monitored and normothermia maintained.

A handoff from one anesthesia provider to another is likely as the patient moves from one location to another. Importantly, a full accounting of the mechanism of trauma in addition to known information of past medical history, injuries, laboratory values, interventions already performed, and the planned procedure should be gathered as time allows. The focus of the anesthesia provider should remain on airway patency and the hemodynamic stability of the patient. Adequate patient monitoring throughout the transport and procedure must be maintained.

Communication among the trauma care team must be maintained as the patient location and status change. For example, trauma surgeons should be notified immediately of any acute or unexpected changes in the patient's status that may require urgent procedural intervention. If the patient requires any additional airway interventions or has a preexisting airway in place, respiratory therapists may be needed for additional support. Because of the remoteness of some locations, additional help from anesthesia technicians, nurses, and other ancillary staff may be critical.

ACKNOWLEDGMENT

The editors and publisher would like to thank Dr. Tony Chang for contributing to this chapter in the previous edition of this work. It has served as a foundation for the current chapter.

REFERENCES

1. World Health Organization. *Injuries and Violence: The Facts 2014*. Geneva: World Health Organization; 2014.
2. Heron M. Deaths: Leading causes for 2011. *Natl Vital Stat Rep*. 2015;64(7):1–96.
3. Centers for Disease Control and Prevention. *Injury Prevention & Control: Data & Statistics (WISQARS)*. Atlanta, GA: Centers for Disease Control and Prevention; 2015.
4. MacKenzie E, Rivara F, Jurkovich G. A national evaluation of the effect of trauma-center care on mortality. *N Engl J Med*. 2006;354:366–378.
5. Dawson S, King L, Grantham H. Improving the hospital clinical handover between paramedics and emergency department staff in the deteriorating patient. *Emerg Med Aust*. 2013(25):393–405.
6. Weingart S, Levitan R. Preoxygenation and prevention of desaturation during emergency airway management. *Ann Emerg Med*. 2012;59(3):165–175.
7. Vourch M, Asfar P, Volteau C. High-flow nasal cannula oxygen during endotracheal intubation in hypoxemic patients: A randomized controlled clinical trial. *Intensive Care Med*. 2015;41(9):1538–1548.
8. Lancman B, Jorm C. Taking the heat in critical situations: Being aware, assertive and heard. In: Iedema R, Piper D, Manidis M, eds. *Communicating Quality and Safety in Healthcare*. Cambridge, England: Cambridge University Press; 2015.
9. Martin, et al. A decade of experience with a selective policy for direct to operating room trauma resuscitations. *Amer J Surg*. 2012;204(2).

10. Spahn D. Management of bleeding and coagulopathy following major trauma: An updated European guideline. *Crit Care*. 2013;17(2):R76.
11. Duchesne JC, McSwain JrNE, Cotton BA, et al. Damage control resuscitation: the new face of damage control. *J Trauma*. 2010;69(4):976–990.
12. Feinman M, Cotton B, Haut E. Optimal fluid resuscitation in trauma: Type, timing, and total. *Curr Opin Crit Care*. 2014;20(4):366–372.
13. Study Group PROPPR, Holcomb JB, Tilley BC, Baraniuk S, et al. Transfusion of plasma, platelets, and red blood cells in a 1:1:1 vs a 1:1:2 ratio and mortality in patients with severe trauma: The PROPPR randomized clinical trial. *JAMA*. 2015;313(5):471–482.
14. Roberts I, Shakur H, Coats T, et al. The CRASH-2 trial: A randomised controlled trial and economic evaluation of the effects of tranexamic acid on death, vascular occlusive events and transfusion requirement in bleeding trauma patients. *Health Technol Assess*. 2013;17(10):1–79.
15. Morrison J, Dubose JJ, Rasmussen TE, et al. Military Application of Tranexamic Acid in Trauma Emergency Resuscitation (MATTERs) study. *Arch Surg*. 2012;147(2):113–119.
16. Armand R, Hess JR. Treating coagulopathy in trauma patients. *Transfus Med Rev*. 2003 Jul;17(3):223–231.
17. Black JA, et al. The evolution of blood transfusion in the trauma patient: Whole blood has come full circle. *Semin Thromb Hemost*. 2020;46:215–220.

18. Jehan F, Aziz H, O'Keeffe T, Khan M, Zakaria ER, Hamidi M, Zeeshan M, Kulvatunyou N, Joseph B. The role of four-factor prothrombin complex concentrate in coagulopathy of trauma: A propensity matched analysis. *J Trauma Acute Care Surg*. 2018 Jul;85(1):18–24. doi:10.1097/TA.0000000000001938 PMID: 29664892.
19. Steurer M, Ganter M. Trauma and massive blood transfusions. *Curr Anesthesiol Rep*. 2014;4:200–208.
20. Dutton R. Haemostatic resuscitation. *Br J Anaesth*. 2012;109(suppl 1):i39–i46.
21. Frieden T, Houry D, Baldwin G. *Report to Congress on Traumatic Brain Injury in the United States: Epidemiology and Rehabilitation*. Atlanta, GA: National Center for Injury Prevention and Control, Division of Unintentional Injury Prevention; 2014.
22. Holly LT, Kelly DF, Counelis GJ, et al. Cervical spine trauma associated with moderate and severe head injury: Incidence, risk factors, and injury characteristics. *J Neurosurg*. 2002;96(3 suppl): 285–291.
23. Robitaille A, Williams SR, Tremblay MH, et al. Cervical spine motion during tracheal intubation with manual in-line stabilization: Direct laryngoscopy versus GlideScope videolaryngoscopy. *Anesth Analg*. 2008;106(3):935–941.
24. Turkstra T, Craen RA, Pelz DM, Gelb AW. Cervical spine motion: A fluoroscopic comparison during intubation with lighted stylet, GlideScope, and Macintosh laryngoscope. *Anesth Analg*. 2005;101(3): 910–915.

25. Zeiler F, Teitelbaum J, West M, Gillman LM. The ketamine effect on ICP in traumatic brain injury. *Neurocrit Care.* 2014;21(1):163–173.

26. Grathwohl K, Black I, Spinella P. Total intravenous anesthesia including ketamine versus volatile gas anesthesia for combat-related operative traumatic brain injury. *Anesthesiology.* 2008;109:44.

27. The SAFE Study Investigators; Australian and New Zealand Intensive Care Society Clinical Trials GroupAustralian Red Cross Blood Service; George Institute for International HealthMyburgh J, Cooper DJ, Finfer S, et al. Saline or albumin for fluid resuscitation in patients with traumatic brain injury. *N Engl J Med.* 2007;357(9):874–884.

28. Carney N, Totten AM, O'Reilly C, Ullman JS, Hawryluk GW, Bell MJ, Bratton SL, Chesnut R, Harris OA, Kissoon N, Rubiano AM, Shutter L, Tasker RC, Vavilala MS, Wilberger J, Wright DW, Ghajar J. Guidelines for the Management of Severe Traumatic Brain Injury, Fourth Edition. Neurosurgery. 2017 Jan 1;80(1):6–15. doi: 10.1227/NEU.0000000000001432. PMID: 27654000

29. National Spinal Cord Injury Statistical Center. *Facts and Figures at a Glance.* Birmingham, AL: University of Alabama; 2013.

30. International Standards for Neurological Classification of Spinal Cord Injury (ISNCSCI) (Revised 2019). American Spinal Injury Association. https://asia-spinalinjury.org/product/international-standards-for-neurological-classification-of-spinal-cord-injury-isncsci-revised-2019/.

31. Ghobrial G, Amenta P, Maltenfort M. Longitudinal incidence and concurrence rates for traumatic brain injury and spine injury—a twenty year analysis. *Clin Neurol Neurosurg.* 2014;123:174–180.

32. Walters B, Hadley M, Hurlbert R. Guidelines for the management of acute cervical spine and spinal cord injuries: 2013 update. *Neurosurgery.* 2013;60(suppl 1):82–91.

33. Pilecky D, Vamos M, Bogyi P, et al. Risk of cardiac arrhythmias after electrical accident: A single-center study of 480 patients. *Clin Res Cardiol.* 2019;108:901–908. https://doi.org/10.1007/s00392-019-01420-2.

34. Haberal M, Sakallioglu Abali AE, Karakayali H. Fluid management in major burn injuries. *Indian J Plast Surg.* 2010;43(Suppl):S29–S36. doi:10.4103/0970-0358.70715.

35. Enlav S, Sela H, Weiniger C. Management and outcomes of trauma during pregnancy. *Anesthesiol Clin.* 2013;31(1):141–156.

VI

CHRONIC PAIN MANAGEMENT

Christopher R. Abrecht

INTRODUCTION

Expertise in pain management is a core element of anesthetic care, and from this expertise there has emerged a distinct distinct medical specialty: pain medicine. Regardless of chronicity, the practice of this medical specialty is inherently multifaceted and multidisciplinary. There are multiple certification pathways for pain medicine. The American Board of Medical Specialties (ABMS) recognizes pain medicine as a distinct medical specialty. The American Board of Anesthesiology (ABA) is responsible for development, administration, and scoring of the certification exam in pain medicine, and physicians with primary training in anesthesiology represent over 80% of board-certified specialists in pain medicine.[1] Other medical specialties are recognized by ABMS for cosponsorship of the certification in pain medicine, and an increasing number of nonanesthesiologists are specializing in this field. These other specialties include the American Board of Psychiatry and Neurology, the American Board of Physical Medicine and Rehabilitation, the American Board of Emergency Medicine, and the American Board of Radiology. The American Board of Family Medicine also offers a certificate in pain medicine, after completion of an ACGME-accredited pain medicine fellowship and passing of the ABA-administered examination. Each of the above medical boards credentials its own candidates, with completion of a fellowship and the ABA-administered examination being among the requirements for certification. This array of physicians pursuing a career in pain medicine reflects the multidisciplinary nature of the specialty.

The following chapter covers key points for a physician trainee rotating in a pain clinic.

CHRONIC PAIN FOUNDATIONS

Terminology

The International Association for the Study of Pain definition of pain is "an unpleasant sensory and emotional experience associated with, or resembling that associated with, actual or potential tissue damage." Pain is thus possible even without evidence of tissue damage. Also noted by this task force was that individuals through their life experiences learn the concept of pain and that the personal experience of pain is influenced to varying degrees by biologic and psychological factors.[2] For pain to be chronic, a period of 3 months is often cited.[3]

Epidemiology

The Centers for Disease Control and Prevention (CDC), citing data from a 2016 survey, has estimated that 20% (50 million) of U.S. adults had chronic pain and 8% (19.6 million) had "high-impact chronic pain," defined as pain that on most days limits life or work activities. This survey also noted that chronic pain and high-impact chronic pain were more common among females, older adults, unemployed adults who previously were employed, and impoverished adults.[4]

Pathophysiology

In a simplified framework nociceptive pain signals are transmitted from the periphery to the brain in a three-neuron pathway. A first-order neuron with a cell body in the dorsal root ganglion (DRG) receives distal input from a nociceptor, which is a sensory receptor for painful stimuli. This input is transmitted to a second-order neuron in the spinal cord. From there, input is transmitted to the thalamus. A third-order neuron in the thalamus then transmits to the cortex, creating a pain perception. The thalamus is the key processing center for pain.

In reality, the system is much more complex. The thalamus connects with the somatosensory cortex, which is responsible for the sensory and discriminative component of pain (e.g., location and intensity of pain). This pathway is often referred to as the *lateral pathway*.

The thalamus also has indirect and direct connections with the amygdala, hippocampus, anterior cingulate cortex, and prefrontal cortex, which are responsible for the emotional or affective component of pain (e.g., the unpleasantness of pain). This pathway is often referred to as the *medial pathway*. These connections are the underpinnings of the biopsychosocial model of pain.

Peripheral sensitization is increased sensitivity to nociceptive input at the terminal ends of first-order neurons (i.e., primary hyperalgesia). Inflammatory molecules released by tissue damage are a driver of this process. Central sensitization is enhanced transmission of pain signals, or transmission of pain signals even in the absence of nociceptive input, at the level of the spinal cord and brain. This process also may involve the expansion of sensory neuron receptor fields, such that nonpainful stimuli result in pain (i.e., allodynia). Ongoing pain, opioid therapy, and other factors may drive this process.[5]

Neuropathic pain is caused by damage to nerve tissue. Typically, damage to the nervous system results in a loss of function, such as numbness or weakness. Neuropathic pain, in contrast, is a maladaptive, pathologic "gain of function" (i.e., pain) response to nervous system damage.[6]

PAINFUL CONDITIONS: SPINE

Lower Back Pain: An Overview

Lower back pain (LBP) is a nonspecific term that could stem from a variety of distinct pain generators. At any given time, the global prevalence of LBP may be 7.8%, meaning that over 500 million people may be experiencing it at any moment. It is the top global cause of disability. In the United States over $100 billion is spent annually on this condition. Noted risk factors for the development of this symptom are obesity, deconditioning, smoking, repetitive bending/twisting/lifting, and depression.[7]

A functional spinal unit is two adjacent vertebrae, the intervertebral disc, facet joints, and spinal ligaments (Fig. 44.1). Approximately, 70% of compression is transmitted by the vertebral body, with the remainder transmitted through the facet joints. In the prone position the L4–L5 intradiscal pressure is about 100 kPA, approximately, the same as a maximumly inflated soccer ball. When standing upright, the pressure in the L4–L5 disc increases to about 500 kPA; when standing and forward flexing the lumbar spine, the pressure increases to about 1300 kPA.[8] Degenerative changes may be the result of mechanical microinsults over time or macroinsults such as trauma, surgery, or inflammatory processes.

Degenerative changes, sometimes also called "age-related changes," are very common on magnetic resonance imaging (MRI) but are nonspecific. In a systematic review of asymptomatic adults undergoing lumbar spine MRI or computed tomography (CT) facet joint degeneration was present in 9% of adults in their thirties and in 83% of adults in their eighties. Disc degeneration was present in 52% of adults in their thirties and in 96% of adults in their eighties.[9] Thus abnormal spine imaging does not necessarily mean a pain generator has been identified, although a pain physician must be intimately familiar with spinal imaging terminology. Important terms to understand include the difference between spondylosis, spondylolysis, and anterolisthesis (Table 44.1). The ability to and practice of personally interpreting spinal imaging is also paramount.

VI

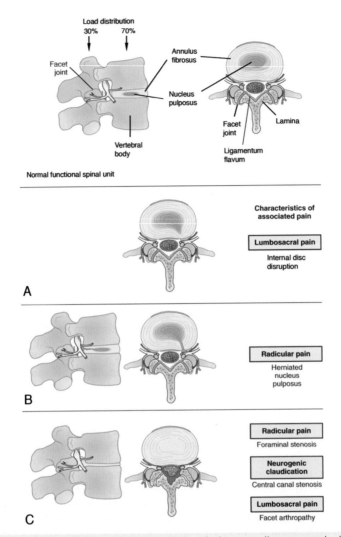

Fig. 44.1 Spinal Anatomy. The functional spinal unit is two adjacent vertebral bodies, the intervertebral disc, the facet joints, and spinal ligaments. Depicted is the lumbar spinal region. (A) An internal disc disrption or degenerative disc disease (DDD) is a common early change in the lumbar spine, sometimes causing axial lumbosacral pain. (B) A herniated nucleus pulposus or disc herniation may cause nerve root irritation. (C) A combination of degenerative changes, of the disc, the facets, and the spinal ligaments may contribute to foraminal stenosis, causing nerve root irritation, and canal stenosis, causing neurogenic claudication.

By the time most patients have been referred to a pain physician, they have already undergone advanced imaging, such as MRI. Both in the primary care clinic and in the specialty pain clinic setting, imaging should be considered if a patient develops LBP with "red flag" symptoms. Symptoms of new urinary retention, bowel incontinence, and saddle anesthesia could reflect cauda equina syndrome and should prompt imaging. Unintended weight loss in a patient with a history of malignancy, in particular, a malignancy with proclivity for bone metastases, could reflect recurrence or progression of cancer in the spine. Fever, especially in a patient who is immunocompromised

or with a history of injection drug use, could reflect an epidural abscess, osteomyelitis, or other spinal infection. Recent trauma, another "red flag," can lead to various neurologic deficits if anatomic stability is not properly assessed.[10]

Lumbosacral Spine Pain: Axial Pain Generators

Potential pain generators for axial LBP include myofascial pain, facet arthropathy, sacroiliac joint (SIJ) dysfunction, discogenic pain, and lumbar spinal stenosis (Table 44.2). Myofascial pain is a common musculoskeletal pain condition

Table 44.1 Common Radiologic Spine Findings Defined

Term	Definition
Spondylosis	General term for arthritis of the spine.
Spondylolysis	Fracture in the pars interarticularis, which is the junction of the vertebral body and the posterior elements.
Anterolisthesis	Anterior displacement of a vertebral relative to the one below.
Retrolisthesis	Posterior displacement of a vertebral body relative to the one below.
Spondylolisthesis	Anterolisthesis secondary to spondylolysis.
Spinal stenosis	Narrowing of the vertebral canal, as by pathology of a disc, facet, or ligamentum flavum.
Scoliosis	Lateral curvature of the spine in the coronal plane, with direction determined by the convexity.
Lordosis	The normal inward curvature of the lumbar and cervical spine. Excessive lordotic curving results in buttocks prominence (swayback).
Kyphosis	The normal outward curvature of the thoracic spine. Excessive kyphotic curving results in hunched shoulders (Scheuermann disease).

From Fardon DF, Williams AL, Dohring EJ, et al. Lumbar disc nomenclature: Version 2.0: Recommendations of the combined task forces of the North American Spine Society, the American Society of Spine Radiology and the American Society of Neuroradiology. Spine J. 2014;14:2525

Table 44.2 Common Pain Generators for Axial Lower Back and Leg Pain

Condition	Signs and Symptoms	Examination Maneuver	Possible Procedural Intervention
Myofascial pain	Trigger points, which are taut bands of muscle and fascia, are palpated on examination. These are also common outside of the lumbar spine, such as in the periscapular region and neck.	Trigger points are palpated along the piriformis muscle.	Trigger point injection
Lumbar facet arthropathy	Tenderness to paraspinal palpation, worse with lumbar extension and lateral rotation, sometimes with posterior referral patterns, but usually not past the knee.	Lumbar extension and lateral rotation.	Facet joint injection or medial branch block followed by radiofrequency ablation

VI

Table 44.2 Common Pain Generators for Axial Lower Back and Leg Pain—cont'd

Condition	Signs and Symptoms	Examination Maneuver	Possible Procedural Intervention
Sacroiliac joint dysfunction	Buttocks and "hip" pain, worse with sitting, more common in women; examination maneuvers include focal pain with palpation at the posterior superior iliac spine.	FABER: Flexion, abduction, and external rotation. Also called Patrick test.	Sacroiliac joint injection
Discogenic pain	Worse with sitting (with inability to find "comfortable" position), worse with coughing, sneezing, and forward flexion. Is somewhat controversial, thought to stem from disc itself, rather than damage to adjacent neural structures.	Bending forward, in particular, when improperly curving the lower back and not engaging the hips.	Lumbar epidural steroid injection, although efficacy is debated
Lumbar radiculopathy	Irritation to the nerve roots, as from a disc herniation, results in pain and possibly loss of deep tendon reflexes and weakness in the distribution of a particular nerve root. A straight leg raise may elicit symptoms.	Straight leg raise is positive if "sciatica," not just hamstring "tightness," is elicited.	Lumbar epidural steroid injection
Lumbar spinal stenosis	Buttocks, low back, and possibly leg pain, worse with standing and walking, improved with sitting and forward flexion of lumbar spine (the "shopping cart" sign). Neurologic examination may be normal; clinical history and imaging findings are useful in coming to this diagnosis.	Pain is relief with forward flexion of lumbar spine, as with favored use of a shopping cart.	Decompressive techniques likely provide more lasting benefit than lumbar epidural steroid injections

sometimes marked by the presence of taut bands of fascia and muscle, called *trigger points (TPs)*. When palpated or injected, these points may result in a "twitch response," wherein the associated muscles contract; when perturbed, these points may also result in a referred pain pattern, usually in the direction of the affected muscles. Often, TPs and myofascial pain exist along with other pathology, such as deeper spondylosis or major joint arthritis. TPs may also stem from overuse and psychological stress.[11,12]

The facet joint, also called the *zygapophyseal joint,* is considered a possible pain generator in a patient with axial pain, tenderness to paraspinal palpation, and with increased severity of symptoms upon loading of the facet joint via standing or maneuvers such as lumbar extension and lateral rotation. Although facet pain is predominantly axial, it can exhibit radiation patterns, usually along the back and posterior thighs but rarely past the knee.[13,14]

The SIJ exists at the junction of the sacrum with the ilium of the pelvis. Forces from the spine are transmitted to this joint, which is also part of the pelvic girdle, with an array of ligamentous attachments such as the lumbosacral ligaments and the sacrospinous ligaments.[15] In some cases dysfunction of the SIJ is related to pathology of the lumbar spine, sometimes called hip-spine syndrome.[16] Pain from the SIJ is thought to manifest as lower back, buttocks, or "hip" pain; worse with sitting; and with a higher incidence in women. A variety of physical examination maneuvers might indicate SIJ pathology, although the weight of the existing evidence is that a number of these findings must be present to reasonably assume the patient has SIJ dysfunction. SIJ pain provocation tests include the following: worse pain with palpation at the posterior superior iliac spine (the Fortin finger test, as the patient indicates pain is located in a focal point); worse pain with femoral abduction and external rotation (the FABER or Patrick test); and worse pain when the patient is in the lateral decubitus position and pressure is applied downward on the lateral iliac crest (the compression test). By some studies, at least three positive tests must be present in order to relatively confidently state a patient has SIJ dysfunction, if making that basis on physical examination alone.[17]

The intervertebral disc consists of an inner nucleus pulposus, which is a gelatinous structure made of proteoglycans and water, and a surrounding annulus fibrosis. When there is a herniation of disc material toward the spinal canal or nerve roots, an intense inflammatory response ensues, with the usual result being lumbosacral radicular pain or neurogenic claudication. In a related but distinct process pathologic changes of the annulus fibrosis itself may induce pain, separate from any effect it might have on the spinal cord or nerve roots.[18] This latter element of "discogenic pain" may manifest as axial lumbosacral pain. It is more common in younger patients; worse with sitting (often with a classic inability to find a

comfortable position); and worse with coughing, sneezing, and lumbar flexion. The latter is a trigger, as it raises the pressure within the intervertebral disc, as discussed in the prior section.[19]

Lumbosacral Radiculopathy

A disc herniation is the presence of disc material outside of the usual margins of the disc space; the herniated contents can be of the central nucleus pulposus, the surrounding annulus fibrosis, or both. Pain from a disc herniation involves both mechanical and biochemical processes; the contact of a nerve root by herniated disc material results in an inflammatory response, which induces pain. Lumbar spondylosis and other processes may also result in a lumbar radiculopathy, which is nerve root disease causing pain, loss of sensation, weakness, and/or other neurologic symptoms[20] (Table 44.3). A time-honored physical examination maneuver in the evaluation of lumbosacral radiculopathy is the straight leg raise. This maneuver, which creates dural tension in the low lumbar and upper sacral area, reproduces radicular pain. Pain should be reproduced with elevation between 30 and 70 degrees in this test, which has greater sensitivity than specificity.[21]

There is ongoing debate about the best treatment for lumbar radiculopathy. Generally, if the lumbar radiculopathy is acute (within 6 weeks of onset) and without a prominent motor deficit, there is general agreement to first explore nonsurgical treatment. For lumbar radiculopathy existing past 6 weeks, however, there is more debate. Studies have compared surgical and nonsurgical management of patients with image-confirmed lumbar radiculopathy present for at least 6 weeks. Surgical management generally results in faster resolution of the lumbar radiculopathy, but patients in both surgical and nonsurgical groups noted substantial improvement over greater than a 2-year period.[22,23] Even in cases where a lumbar radiculopathy present for 6 to 12 weeks involves a motor deficit, surgical treatment results in faster resolution of symptoms but compared with nonsurgical management results in similar outcomes at the 1-year mark.[24] Thus for a patient with a chronic lumbar radiculopathy, a reasonable approach based on the available data is to educate the patient on surgical and nonsurgical treatment pathways, with the trajectory based in part on the patient's preference, and of course also the physician's assessment of the patient's comorbidities. If there has been substantial improvement with conservative management and there is no severe neurologic deficit present, then most physicians will make a stronger recommendation for continued nonsurgical care.[25]

Lumbar Spinal Stenosis

Lumbar spinal stenosis (LSS) is a reduction in the cross-sectional area of the spinal canal. Lumbar disc herniation, facet hypertrophy, epidural lipomatosis, and

VI

Table 44.3 Presentation of Common Lumbosacral Radiculopathies

	Nerve Root		
	L4	L5	S1
Pain dermatomal distribution			
Motor deficit	Quadriceps knee extension impaired	Dorsiflexion impaired	Plantarflexion impaired
Examination	Squatting and rising impaired	Walking on heels impaired	Walking on toes impaired
Reflexes	Knee jerk (patellar) impaired	None reliable	Ankle jerk (Achilles) impaired

ligamentum flavum hypertrophy are among the causes of this condition, which most commonly affects elderly patients. Symptoms of neurogenic intermittent claudication (NIC) include pain in the buttocks, lower back, and legs present with standing or walking and improved with forward flexion of the spine or sitting down. When leaning forward, as when ambulating with a walker or using a shopping cart (sometimes called the "shopping cart sign"), there is an increase in the interlaminar and intra-canal space, such that symptoms are less severe. The mechanism behind NIC is thought to be occlusion of the subarachnoid space resulting in a combination of direct mechanical compression of neural components and downstream epidural venous congestion, resulting in a transient compartment syndrome of the cauda equina.[26] Lumbar epidural steroid injections are commonly performed to treat this condition, although studies suggest they do not provide much long-term benefit.[27] As such, decompressive techniques may be explored.

PAINFUL CONDITIONS: NEUROPATHIC PAIN

Peripheral Neuropathy

The term *peripheral neuropathy* is often used synonymously with *polyneuropathy*, referring to a generalized disorder affecting multiple peripheral nerves, whose distal ends are most prominently affected. Causes of peripheral neuropathy include toxic (e.g., alcohol use disorder) and infectious (e.g., HIV). A typical presentation is bilateral, distal loss of sensation, often with burning sensations, in a "glove and stocking" distribution. The most common peripheral neuropathy is diabetic peripheral neuropathy (DPN), which affects about half of adults with diabetes mellitus.[28] Chemotherapy-induced peripheral neuropathy is another common cause, in particular, as the life expectancy increases for patients with cancer. Some studies estimate that up to one-third of all chemotherapy patients may develop neuropathy symptoms within 6 months of treatment.[29] In all cases treatment of the underlying disease process is a key element of management.

Complex Regional Pain Syndrome

Sympathetically mediated pain is a type of neuropathic pain in which the sympathetic nervous system amplifies pain. Anxiety, stress, and other types of emotional distress, all of which activate the sympathetic nervous system, are thus intimately connected with sympathetically mediated pain. By the same reasoning, the treatment of these conditions *must* be multidisciplinary, including not just pharmacologic and procedural arms but intense psychological care targeting the sympathetic nervous system.

The archetypal chronic pain syndrome thought to have an element of sympathetically mediated pain is complex regional pain syndrome (CRPS). This condition usually manifests with pain disproportionate to any inciting event in a distal extremity, usually after trauma or prolonged immobilization, such as from the use of a cast after orthopedic surgery. Females are more commonly affected, with at least a 2:1 prominence, and at younger ages, with some studies noting peaks in the early twenties and in the mid-thirties. CRPS type 1, representing about 90% of all cases, is present when there is no clear peripheral nerve injury. CRPS type 2, also called *causalgia*, is present when a peripheral nerve injury is identified. Further subtypes include a "warm" CRPS, in which there is a marked increase in skin temperature, perhaps suggesting a prominent inflammatory component, and "cold" CRPS, where there is decreased skin temperature. The condition is usually isolated to one limb, but when severe, it can spread to adjacent limbs.[30] The Budapest Criteria describe the elements required for diagnosis: sensory, vasomotor, sudomotor, and motor (Box 44.1). Treatments for this condition are varied. Commonly used medications include neuropathic analgesics (discussed later); bisphosphonates and ketamine may also provide benefit. Guided motor imagery and mirror therapy are often explored. Procedurally, sympathetic blocks and spinal cord stimulation are the techniques of choice. The purpose of these interventions is to reduce pain to a level that allows the patient to engage in physical therapy, which even more so than other chronic pain syndromes, is essential to treat CRPS.[31]

PAINFUL CONDITIONS: CHRONIC POSTSURGICAL PAIN

Chronic postsurgical pain (CPSP) is pain that develops after a surgical procedure and exists past the usual healing process, often cited as at least 3 months postoperatively.[32] CPSP can occur after any surgical procedure, but is noted particularly after thoracotomy, mastectomy, inguinal herniorrhaphy, knee arthroplasty, and limb amputation. In all of these conditions the incidence of CPSP that is severe, with a numeric pain score of greater than five or causing a pain disability, is about 5% to 10%. CPSP may be multifaceted. In amputation, for instance, a patient may develop residual limb pain from mechanical factors or from neuroma; phantom limb pain, which is a central pain syndrome, may also be present. Noted risk factors for the development of CPSP include young age, female gender, preoperative chronic pain, preoperative opioid use, poorly controlled postoperative pain, and surgical factors (e.g., invasiveness of surgery, presence of nerve damage).[33] Among the strongest predictors of CPSP are the severity of preoperative pain, regardless of whether it is related to the planned surgery, and the severity of postoperative pain. As a result, there is an increasing movement toward the development of a transitional pain service, whereby a physician board-certified in pain medicine oversees a multidisciplinary team to optimize modifiable patient factors preoperatively, oversee perioperative pain plans, and then ensure continued high-level pain care post-discharge.[34]

Box 44.1 Budapest Diagnostic Criteria for Complex Regional Pain Syndrome

Continuing pain, which is disproportionate to any inciting event
Must report at least one symptom in *three of the four* following categories:
  Sensory: reports of hyperesthesia or allodynia
  Vasomotor: reports of temperature asymmetry or skin color changes or skin color asymmetry
  Sudomotor/edema: reports of edema or sweating changes or sweating asymmetry
  Motor/trophic: reports of decreased range of motion or motor dysfunction (weakness, tremor, dystonia) or trophic changes (hair, nail, skin)
Must display at least one sign at time of evaluation in *two or more* of the following categories:
  Sensory: evidence of hyperalgesia (to pinprick) or allodynia (to light touch or deep somatic pressure or joint movement)
  Vasomotor: evidence of temperature asymmetry or skin color changes or asymmetry
  Sudomotor/edema: evidence of edema or sweating changes or sweating asymmetry
  Motor/trophic: evidence of decreased range of motion or motor dysfunction (weakness, tremor, dystonia) or trophic changes (hair, nail, skin)
No other diagnosis better explains the signs and symptoms

PAIN CONDITIONS: ADDITIONAL GENERATORS

Given the limited scope of this chapter, only a selection of chronic pain syndromes will be discussed in detail. Other pain conditions include central pain from dysfunction of the central nervous system (CNS), poststroke pain, multiple sclerosis, and postherpetic neuralgia. Headache conditions, including migraine, trigeminal neuralgia, and others, are another common entity. Fibromyalgia, a pain syndrome marked by widespread pain in multiple points throughout the body with associated somatic symptoms such as fatigue and cognitive blunting, is also commonly seen. Chronic pelvic pain, whether from pelvic floor muscle dysfunction, endometriosis, or other etiologies, is another chronic pain syndrome. Cancer pain is common, often with mixed nociceptive and neuropathic elements, and may be amenable to a variety of interventional pain techniques discussed later.

VI

PSYCHOLOGICAL TREATMENT PILLAR: CATASTROPHIZING

In the biopsychosocial model of chronic pain psychological factors are considered not a reaction to pain, but part of a "bidirectional link." Indeed, anxiety, mood disorders, and negative cognitive processes such as catastrophizing are noted to be among the strongest predictors of "chronification" of pain, that is, of chronic pain vulnerability.[35] Pain catastrophizing is a negative cognitive process described as an "exaggerated negative mental set brought to bear during actual or anticipated painful experience." The Pain Catastrophizing Scale introduced in 1995 assesses for key components, such as excessive worry, rumination, and negative expectations. Some of the questions on this survey are whether a patient thinks: "It's terrible and I think it's never going to get any better," "I become afraid that the pain will get worse," and "I keep thinking about how badly I want the pain to stop." A psychological intervention employed in the management of pain catastrophizing is cognitive behavioral therapy (CBT). This therapy is relatively active and structured, somewhat more so than other modalities such as mindfulness-based stress reduction and open-ended supportive psychological care; CBT focuses on how cognition (distorted thoughts) affects behaviors (actions) and develops an action plan to address both of these elements.[36]

PHYSICAL MEDICINE TREATMENT PILLAR

Almost universally in chronic pain syndromes, there exists a fear, or at least a concern, that particular movements will result in worsening of pain. Thus in addition to receiving psychological care, most patients with chronic pain will benefit from a structured physical therapy program to address fear avoidance and associated deconditioning. Physical therapy is also a treatment in its own right for a variety of musculoskeletal and mixed neuropathic conditions such as fibromyalgia. The particular therapy will vary from patient to patient, although in general any nudge toward movement is generally thought to be beneficial. Structure exercises, yoga, and progressive relaxation are all reasonable exercises.[37] In the same vein many patients will also benefit from integrative medicine or complementary and alternative medicine (CAM). In CAM practices not yet fully embraced in mainstream medical practice ("standard of care") are included in a patient's care plan. These may include acupuncture, transcutaneous electrical nerve stimulation, biofeedback, meditation, massage therapy, and dietary changes. Increasingly, CAM practices are becoming more mainstream, in particular as there is rising interest in nonopioid and cost-effective treatment modalities, and evidence to support their efficacy.

PHARMACOLOGIC TREATMENT PILLAR

Nonopioid Analgesics

In pain medicine there is no overall best pharmacologic treatment, as therapy must be personalized for each patient's particular chronic pain syndrome, medical comorbidities, and other medications. However, some general principles are helpful to consider. In particular, for predominantly nociceptive chronic pain, as from osteoarthritis, acetaminophen and nonsteroidal antiinflammatory drugs (NSAIDs) may be useful. The mechanism of action of acetaminophen remains unclear; NSAIDs inhibit the enzyme cyclooxygenase, thereby reducing prostaglandins, which mediate inflammation and pain. Muscle relaxants (e.g., baclofen) are sometimes employed for long-term management of a variety of chronic pain syndromes, although the data are lacking for most applications, and these agents may cause CNS depression, in particular, when used in combination with other sedating analgesics. In the presence of actual muscular spasticity, such as may occur from multiple sclerosis or other neurologic conditions, muscle relaxants such as baclofen or tizanidine may be of use.

For neuropathic pain, a variety of medications are available. First-line therapy includes antiepileptic gabapentinoids and antidepressant serotonin-norepinephrine reuptake inhibitors (SNRIs) and tricyclic antidepressants (TCAs). Side effects of gabapentin and pregabalin include dizziness, CNS depression, weight gain, and possible respiratory depression when used in combination with opioids. The effective dose of gabapentin is usually 1200 to 3600 mg/day; the effective dose of pregabalin is usually 300 to 600 mg/day. The number needed to treat (NNT) to achieve 50% pain relief is 6.3 for gabapentin and 7.7 for pregabalin. SNRI side effects include nausea and headache but are comparatively well tolerated. The effective dose of duloxetine is usually 60 mg/day, although it sometimes may be up to 120 mg/day; the effective dose of venlafaxine is usually 75 to 225 mg a day. The NNT is about 6.4. TCA side effects include potent anticholinergic effects such as dry mouth, constipation, urinary retention, and lightheadedness. TCAs may not be well tolerated, particularly in elderly patients. Nortriptyline (at the usual effective dose 25–100 mg/day) generally has a more favorable side effect profile than amitriptyline. The NNT is 3.6. Second-line medications for neuropathic pain management include topical lidocaine and capsaicin, which is a substance derived from chili peppers that depletes substance P from the primary afferent neurons with repeated application. Medications further down the line for neuropathic pain include subcutaneous botulinum toxin and tramadol.[38]

There is increased interest in the role of cannabis and cannabinoids in the pharmacologic management of chronic pain. Currently, partly because of their varied legal status, there has not been sufficiently robust clinical research on the efficacy of cannabis and cannabinoids in the management of chronic, noncancer pain. Existing studies looking at a variety of patient populations and a variety of drug formulations have shown mixed results; the long-term effects of these substances also remain unclear.[39]

Other pharmacologic treatment modalities include infusion therapy. Ketamine, an N-methyl-D-aspartate (NMDA) antagonist increasingly explored for the management of depression, is often considered for the management of CRPS and other refractory chronic pain conditions, in particular, if there appears to be a prominent neuropathic element. The data on ketamine infusions in the management of chronic pain remain mixed, with the suggestion that higher doses and longer therapy may result in relief lasting weeks to months.[40] Lidocaine, offered as an outpatient infusion, has also shown some benefit for a heterogenous population of chronic pain syndromes, mostly those with a prominent neuropathic element. As with ketamine therapy, the optimal patient population, dosing, and treatment frequency require additional study.[41]

Opioid Analgesics (Also See Chapter 9)

The opioid epidemic, most notable in the United States but also relevant globally, refers to the rapid increase of opioid prescriptions and opioid-related complications such as overdose and opioid use disorder. There are essentially no data showing that opioids are effective in the management of chronic, noncancer pain, but there is a wealth of data showing that they result in myriad side effects. Among the side effects are depression of the CNS and the gastrointestinal, immunologic, and endocrinologic systems. The CDC published a guideline for the prescription of opioids for chronic, noncancer pain. Among the recommendations from this guideline were that the lowest possible dose be used, ideally below 50 morphine milligram equivalents or more per day; preference for short-acting instead of long-acting formulations; and avoidance of coprescription of an opioid with a benzodiazepine. It was also noted that for patients with opioid use disorder, medication-assisted treatment with buprenorphine or methadone should be offered.[42] As a result of these guidelines, many patients on long-term opioid therapy for noncancer pain, and their prescribers, found themselves uncertain how to get to an "acceptable" regimen. In response, the CDC subsequently published a clarification, noting that opioid therapy should not be abruptly discontinued. Tapering, when deemed appropriate, may need to be very slow, as little as a 10% decrease per month, and may take months to years to achieve a given goal. There is no hard limit on what dose a patient should be prescribed. At higher doses, pain specialist

consultation may be sought.[43] Ideally, patients on chronic opioid therapy should be assessed for continued analgesia, improved activities of daily living, lack of adverse side effects, lack of aberrant drug behaviors, adherence (e.g., via prescription drug monitoring program review, intermittent urine drug toxicology), a signed opioid agreement, and assessment of misuse and potential for adverse reaction (e.g., validated risk assessment surveys, naloxone coprescription, avoidance of concurrent benzodiazepine prescription). Some patients may benefit from switching to buprenorphine-based therapy for their chronic pain, in part because of the generally superior safety profile of buprenorphine (a partial mu receptor agonist) compared with full agonist opioids.

When managing chronic opioid therapy, several related entities must be understood. Opioid tolerance occurs when with repeated exposure to opioids, a decreased therapeutic effect is noted (i.e., higher doses are needed to achieve the same benefit). In this scenario if the opioid dose is increased, the pain will improve temporarily. Opioid-induced hyperalgesia occurs when with repeated exposure to opioids, a paradoxical increase in pain is noted, along with allodynia and hyperalgesia, usually beyond the initial pain area. In this scenario if the opioid dose is increased, the pain will worsen. Physiologic dependence is a natural consequence of opioid therapy. For patients receiving chronic opioid therapy, cessation or reduction of the opioid dose will result in withdrawal symptoms. Opioid addiction, more appropriately referred to as *opioid use disorder,* is a neurobiologic condition wherein patients take opioids in larger amounts and over a longer period than intended, resulting in a persistent desire or unsuccessful attempt to cut down opioid use. In these patients cravings are present and opioid use continues despite adverse consequences.[44] For a patient on chronic opioid therapy, there is also always the possibility of progression of their underlying pain generator. Thus when encountering a patient with "worse pain," a clinician must therefore be able to tease out a variety of related but distinct pain entities.

PROCEDURAL TREATMENT PILLAR

Epidural Steroid Injections

Epidural steroid injections are among the most commonly performed injections in pain medicine. Typically, these are performed to reduce neuraxial inflammation causing pain, such as from a herniated intervertebral disc. The two main techniques are an interlaminar approach and a transforaminal approach. In the interlaminar approach a loss-of-resistance needle is advanced under fluoroscopic guidance between the lamina and a modest volume of medication administered. In the transforaminal approach a spinal needle is directed in an oblique trajectory toward the intervertebral foramen and a generally smaller

VI

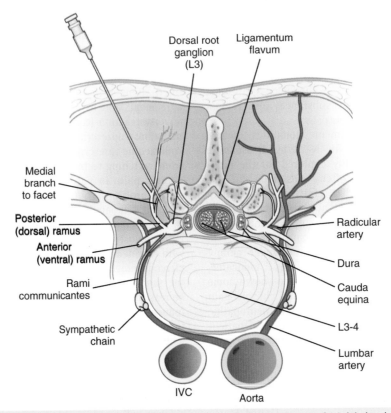

Fig. 44.2 Lumbar Epidural Steroid Injection, the Transforaminal Approach. Axial view is shown. (From Rathmell JP. *Atlas of Image-Guided Intervention in Regional Anesthesia and Pain Medicine.* Philadelphia, PA: Lippincott Williams & Wilkins; 2006:58.)

volume of medication administered (Fig. 44.2). This approach may also be employed not just for therapeutic purposes but also more often for diagnostic purposes, such as for presurgical planning. Epidural steroid injections, in particular, when performed in the cervical spine, are associated with a rare risk of catastrophic neurologic injury. Possible complications include epidural hematoma or neurovascular compromise from direct vascular injury or steroid embolism. Thus particulate steroids should be avoided in cervical transforaminal injections and used with caution in the lumbar spine. Whether to choose an interlaminar or transforaminal approach is the ultimate decision of the treating physician, balancing the patient-specific risks and benefits for a given approach.[45]

results in considerable pain relief, then a radiofrequency ablation (RFA) may be attempted (Fig. 44.3). The RFA procedure includes use of a specialized, insulated needle directed to the location of the medial branch nerve and subsequent coagulation at the desired location. Traditional RFA consists of tissue coagulation via heating at 80°C for 2 minutes. An alternative technique is a facet joint injection, in which local anesthetic and steroid are administered directly into the joint. There is ongoing debate about the preferred treatment approach and the best technique for the RFA procedure.[46] For analogous pain generators such as the SIJ, similar approaches are available, including both intraarticular and denervation techniques.

Facet Injections

The facet joint, which is the articulating bridge between adjacent vertebral bodies, receives innervation via two medial branch nerves from corresponding dorsal rami, one from the spinal nerve above and one from the spinal nerve blow the joint. To perform a single facet block, one must therefore block two nerves. If such a block

Sympathetic Blockade

The sympathetic nervous system derives from the T1–L2 spinal levels and clusters in various ganglia on its path to distal organs (also see Chapter 6). Blockade at sympathetic ganglia may be employed for a variety of chronic pain syndromes, in particular, if there is a sympathetically mediated element as in CRPS. Starting cranially,

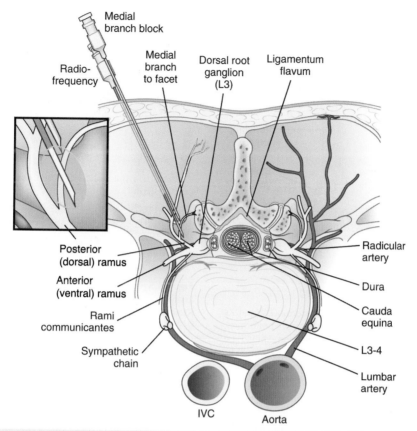

Fig. 44.3 Lumbar Medial Branch Block and Radiofrequency Ablation. Axial view is seen. Note that the needle used for radiofrequency is deeper, so that coagulation is performed along the length of the medial branch nerve. (From Rathmell JP. *Atlas of Image-Guided Intervention in Regional Anesthesia and Pain Medicine*. Philadelphia, PA: Lippincott Williams & Wilkins; 2006:89.)

the stellate ganglion is the fusion of the inferior cervical ganglion and, when present, the first thoracic ganglion. This ganglion is the transmission point for sympathetic input to the head, neck, and upper extremity. A typical indication for stellate ganglion block is CRPS affecting the upper extremity or other conditions, such as Raynaud disease or vascular disease. The stellate ganglion can be blocked at the level of C6, at the anterior tubercle of the transverse process of C6 (Chassaignac tubercle), adjacent to which the vertebral artery is usually contained. The block may also be performed at C7, although there is a slightly higher chance of pneumothorax at this level, given the proximity to the dome of the lung. Although a landmark-based technique is possible, an image-guided approach is now preferred, typically either with fluoroscopy or ultrasound, with the given technique depending on the experience of the physician. With ultrasound guidance, direct visualization of medication administration superficial to the longus colli muscle is the desired outcome (Fig. 44.4). A successful block should result in a Horner syndrome of miosis, ptosis, enophthalmos

(sunken appearance of eye), and anhidrosis. With the block, there should also be unilateral nasal congestion, venodilation, and increase in temperature in the affected limb of 2°C. Spread of local anesthetic may also affect the recurrent laryngeal nerve, resulting in hoarseness or coughing, and the phrenic nerve, resulting in shortness of breath. Complications of this block include vascular injury causing hematoma or stroke or inadvertent intravascular injection causing seizure.

The next sympathetic plexus farther caudad is the celiac plexus, which is located along the anterolateral surface of the aorta at the T12–L1 level. The greater, lesser, and least splanchnic nerves coalesce at this level, receiving input from T5 to T12 and affecting the alimentary tract from the stomach to the transverse colon in addition to the pancreas, liver, and kidneys. Abdominal visceral nociceptive *afferents* accompany sympathetic *efferents,* and thus the celiac ganglion allows blockade of painful nociceptive input, as might occur from pancreatic cancer. Numerous approaches have been described for celiac plexus blockade: fluoroscopic, CT,

VI

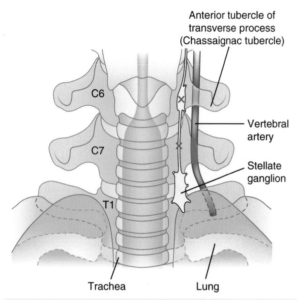

Fig. 44.4 Stellate Ganglion, Relevant Anatomy. The red Xs mark the locations where this procedure is typically performed. Not shown is the longus colli muscle; injection should be lateral and superficial to this structure. (From Rathmell JP. *Atlas of Image-Guided Intervention in Regional Anesthesia and Pain Medicine.* Philadelphia, PA: Lippincott Williams & Wilkins; 2006:116.)

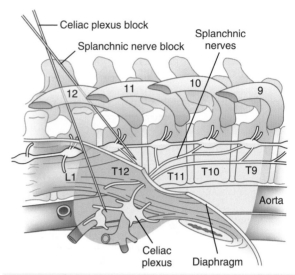

Fig. 44.5 Celiac plexus and splanchnic nerve block, relevant anatomy. (From Rathmell JP. *Atlas of Image-Guided Intervention in Regional Anesthesia and Pain Medicine.* Philadelphia, PA: Lippincott Williams & Wilkins; 2006:124.)

and an endoscopic approach with ultrasound. No one technique has been shown consistently to be the most effective or safe. Rather, it depends on the anatomic and medical considerations of a given patient and the comfort of the procedural physician. The fluoroscopic technique alone has a few approaches. A celiac plexus block using a transcrural approach administers local anesthetic directly on the celiac ganglion; passage of the needle through the aorta may be an element of this approach. For splanchnic nerve block, the needles are posterior to the diaphragmatic crura in close proximity to the T12 vertebral body; in this case the splanchnic nerves are targeted before they coalesce into the plexus (Fig. 44.5). The splanchnic technique may be more appropriate in the case of extensive intraabdominal tumor burden; the celiac technique is considered by some physicians to be less likely to spread medication toward the spinal nerve roots. In either case with blockade of the celiac plexus, the sympathectomy and unopposed parasympathetic activity may result in orthostatic hypotension and diarrhea. A neurolytic technique may also be employed, using alcohol or phenol; this approach is most often performed for patients with pancreatic cancer. A rare but devastating complication from celiac plexus neurolysis is paraplegia from spread of medication toward the spinal segmental arteries, including possibly the artery of Adamkiewicz. Direct injury to the aorta is also possible. In part for those

reasons this neurolytic technique is often reserved for cancer-related pain.

The lumbar sympathetic chain coalesces into paired ganglia that lie over the anterolateral surface of the L2–L4 vertebral bodies. Blockade at this point is often performed for CRPS affecting the lower extremity. Other sympathetic ganglia of relevance in pain medicine include the superior hypogastric plexus (located anterior to the L5 vertebral body and the sacral promontory), which may be relevant to management of pelvic pain, and the ganglion impar (located anterior to the anterior surface of the sacrococcygeal junction), which may be intervened upon in the management of tailbone or perineal pain.

NEUROMODULATION: ADVANCED INTERVENTIONAL PAIN MEDICINE

Advanced interventional pain techniques, sometimes called *"surgical pain" interventions,* include spinal cord stimulation (SCS), intrathecal drug delivery systems (IDDSs), and decompressive procedures. To become facile in these approaches, a pain physician should complete a fellowship with a robust neuromodulation program and start their practice working closely with an experienced colleague. This rapidly advancing area of pain medicine has great potential for the reduction of pain disability. Complications of SCS and IDDS are not uncommon and may be biologic (e.g., surgical site infection, hematoma, seroma, wound dehiscence) or device related (e.g., lead migration or break, catheter leak, device failure). Proper training in neuromodulation is key to minimize complications.[47]

SCS is, in essence, the administration of electrical impulses in lieu of pharmacology in the management of pain. There are likely multiple mechanisms, but one is thought to be the interruption of ascending pain input by the activation of nonpainful signals. Traditional SCS refers to the placement of electrodes in the dorsal epidural space, either by a percutaneous or a surgical paddle lead approach. Implantation of the electrodes along with an implantable pulse generator (IPG) is typically preceded by a trial in which electrodes alone are inserted for several days to determine whether pain relief occurs. The most common indications for SCS are failed back surgery syndrome (postlaminectomy pain syndrome) or CRPS, although it is in practice used for an increasing number of indications. A variety of stimulation programs have also been developed, beyond the traditional paresthesia-based system. Newer programs include high-frequency stimulation at 10,000 Hz and burst stimulation, which consists of bursts of five pulses. Other developments in neurostimulation include the use of DRG stimulation for neuropathic pain centered around a particular dermatome and the use of peripheral nerve stimulation for neuropathic pain centered around a particular peripheral nerve. New stimulation programs and systems are rapidly appearing on the market.[48]

IDDS allow the administration of analgesics from an implanted reservoir directly into the cerebrospinal fluid. This therapy is usually reserved for patients who note benefit from systemic analgesics but are limited by side effects. A common scenario is a patient with spasticity that is improved with baclofen but who cannot tolerate higher doses. Usually, oral baclofen doses greater than 80 mg/day cannot be tolerated, whereas the intrathecal daily dose of baclofen is in the microgram range. IDDS is generally appropriate for patients with intractable pain not responsive to other treatment modalities, in particular, for patients with cancer. The three Food and Drug Administration (FDA) approved medications for intrathecal use are baclofen, morphine, and ziconotide. In practice, a combination of medications is often administered concurrently; the additional medications include bupivacaine, hydromorphone, clonidine, and others.[49]

The minimally invasive lumbar decompression (MILD) procedure is a decompressive technique whereby hypertrophied ligamentum flavum is resected. This percutaneous, fluoroscopically guided technique is performed using a 6 gauge port and is typically performed as an outpatient procedure with local anesthesia alone. Most patients resume normal activity within a day. The MILD procedure is FDA-approved for the treatment of symptomatic LSS Multiple level 1 randomized controlled trials (RCTs) have shown a safety profile similar to that of lumbar epidural steroid injection. The benefit from the MILD procedure is also more substantial: at 1 year after MILD, the average walking distance increased from 246 feet to 3956 feet and the average standing time increased from 8 minutes to 56 minutes.[50] The MILD procedure reflects the growing armamentarium of an appropriately trained pain physician.

There are also many other "advanced" procedures in interventional pain medicine, but given the scope of this introductory chapter, they will not be disused at this time.

SUMMARY

In providing an overview of the breadth of knowledge and expertise needed to practice as a pain physician, this chapter hopefully has succeeded in conveying pain medicine as a distinct career. Pain care is not truly pain care unless it is comprehensive and multidisciplinary. Similarly, pain specialists are not really pain specialists unless they understand the neurobiology of pain; the biopsychological model of pain; and the full spectrum of pharmacologic, rehabilitative, integrative, and procedural modalities available. Pain, that "sensory and emotional experience", is an entity that will touch every person at some point in their lives. It also remains an incompletely understood entity. From my perspective, as someone who went into medicine to better understand and improve the human condition, there can be no more exciting field of medicine to enter.

ACKNOWLEDGMENT

The editors and publisher would like to thank Drs. Omar Hyder and James Rathmell for contributing to this chapter in the previous edition of this work. It has served as a foundation for the current chapter.

VI

REFERENCES

1. Owens W, Abram S. The genesis of pain medicine as a subspecialty in anesthesiology. *J Anesth Hist.* 2020;6(1):13–16.
2. Raja SN, Carr DB, Cohen M, Finnerup NB, Flor H, Gibson S, Keefe FJ, Mogil JS, Ringkamp M, Sluka KA, Song XJ, Stevens B, Sullivan MD, Tutelman PR, Ushida T, Vader K. The revised International Association for the Study of Pain definition of pain: concepts, challenges, and compromises. *Pain.* 2020 May 23.
3. Treede RD, Rief W, Barke A, Aziz Q, Bennett MI, Benoliel R, Cohen M, Evers S, Finnerup NB, First MB, Giamberardino MA, Kaasa S, Kosek E, Lavand'homme P, Nicholas M, Perrot S, Scholz J, Schug S, Smith BH, Svensson P, Vlaeyen JW, Wang SJ. A classification of chronic pain for ICD-11. *Pain.* 2015;156(6):1003–1007.
4. Dahlhamer J, Lucas J, Zelaya C. Prevalence of chronic pain and high-impact chronic pain among adults—Unite States, 2016. *MMWR Morb Mortal Wkly Rep.* 2018;67:1001–1006.
5. Pak D, Yong R, Kaye A, Urman R. Chronification of pain: Mechanisms, current understanding, and clinical implications. *Curr Pain Headache Rep.* 2018;22(9):1–6.

6. Colloca L, Ludman T, Bouhassira D, Baron R, Dickenson AH, Yarnitsky D, Freeman R, Truini A, Attal N, Finnerup NB, Eccleston C, Kalso E, Bennett DL, Dworkin RH, Raja SN. *Neuropathic pain.* *Nat Rev Dis Primers.* 2017;16(3):17002.

7. Buchbinder R, Underwood M, Hartvigsen J, Maher C. *The Lancet* series call to action to reduce low value care for low back pain: An update. *Pain.* 2020;161(1):S57–S64.

8. Kushchayev S, Glushko T, Jarraya M, et al. ABCs of the degenerative spine. *Insights Imaging.* 2018;9:253–274.

9. Brinjiki W, Leutmer PH, Comstock, et al. Systematic literature review of imaging features of spinal degeneration in asymptomatic populations. *Am J Neuroradiol.* 2015;35(4):811.

10. Chou R, Qaseem A, Owens DK, et al. Diagnostic imaging for low back pain: Advice for high-value health care from the American College of Physicians. *Ann Intern Med.* 2011;154:181.

11. Travell JG, Simons DG. Myofascial Pain and Dysfunction*The Trigger Point Manual: Upper Half of Body.* 2nd ed. Baltimore: Lippincott, Williams & Wilkins; 1988.

12. Galasso A, Urits I, An D, Nguyen D, Borchart M, Yazdi C, Manchikanti L, Kaye RJ, Kaye AD, Mancuso KF, Viswanath O. A comprehensive review of the treatment and management of myofascial pain syndrome. *Curr Pain Headache Rep.* 2020;24(8):43.

13. Cohen S, Raja S. Pathogenesis, diagnosis, and treatment of lumbar zygapophysial (facet) joint pain. *Anesthesiology.* 2017;106:591–614.

14. Perolat R, Kastler A, Nicot B. Facet joint syndrome: From diagnosis to interventional management. *Insights Imaging.* 2018;9(5):773–789.

15. Poilliot A, Zwirner J, Doyle T, Hammer N. A systematic review of the normal sacroiliac joint anatomy and adjacent tissues for pain physicians. *Pain Physician.* 2019;22(4):E247.

16. Schneider B, Rosati R, Zheng P, McCormick Z. Challenges in diagnosing sacroiliac joint pain: A narrative review. *PM&R.* 2019;11(1):S40–S45.

17. Lasleet M, April CN, McDonald B, Young SB. Diagnosis of sacroiliac joint pain: Validity of individual provocation test and composites of tests. *Man Ther.* 2005;10(3):207–218.

18. Bogduk N, Aprill C, Derby R. Lumbar discogenic pain: State-of-the-art review. *Pain Med.* 2013;14(6):813–836.

19. ManchikantiL Hirsch J. An update on the management of chronic lumbar discogenic pain. *Pain Manag.* 2015;5(5):373–386.

20. Deyo R, Mirza S. Herniated lumbar intervertebral disk. *NEJM.* 2016;354:1763–1772.

21. Awm van der WIndt D, Simmons E, Riphagen I, et al. Physical examination for lumbar radiculopathy due to disc herniation in patients with low-back pain. *Cochrane Database Syst Rev.* 2010;17(2).

22. Weinstein JN, Tosteson TD, Lurie JD, Tosteson AN, Hanscom B, Skinner JS, Abdu WA, Hilibrand AS, Boden SD, Deyo RA. Surgical vs nonoperative treatment for lumbar disk herniation: The Spine Patient Outcomes Research Trial (SPORT): A randomized trial. *JAMA.* 2006;296(20):2441–2450.

23. Lurie JD, Tosteson TD, Tosteson AN, Zhao W, Morgan TS, Abdu WA, Herkowitz H, Weinstein JN. Surgical versus nonoperative treatment for lumbar disc herniation: Eight-year results for the spine patient outcomes research trial. *Spine (Phila Pa 1976).* 2014;39(1):3–16.

24. Overdevest GM, Vleggeert-Lankamp CL, Jacobs WC, Brand R, Koes BW, Peul WC. Recovery of motor deficit accompanying sciatica—Subgroup analysis of a randomized controlled trial. *Spine J.* 2014;14:1817–1824.

25. Schoenfeld AJ, Kang JD. Decision making for treatment of persistent sciatica. *N Engl J Med.* 2020;382(12):1161–1162.

26. Sandella DE, Haig AJ, Tomkins-Lane C, Yamakawa KS. Defining the clinical syndrome of lumbar spinal stenosis: A recursive specialist survey process. *PM R.* 2013;5(6):491–495.

27. Friedly JL, Comstock BA, Turner JA, et al. A randomized trial of epidural glucocorticoid injections for spinal stenosis. *N Engl J Med.* 2014;371(1):11–21.

28. Hicks CW, Selvin E. Epidemiology of peripheral neuropathy and lower extremity disease in diabetes. *Curr Diab Rep.* 2019;19(10):86.

29. Seretny M, Currie GL, Sena ES, Ramnarine S, Grant R, MacLeod MR, Colvin LA, Fallon M. Incidence, prevalence, and predictors of chemotherapy-induced peripheral neuropathy: A systematic review and meta-analysis. *Pain.* 2014;155(12):2461–2470.

30. Ott S, Maihöfner C. Signs and symptoms in 1,043 patients with complex regional pain syndrome. *J Pain.* 2018;19(6):599–611.

31. Duong S, Bravo D, Todd KJ, Finlayson RJ, Tran Q. Treatment of complex regional pain syndrome: An updated systematic review and narrative synthesis. *Can J Anaesth.* 2018;65(6):658–684.

32. Treede RD, Rief W, Barke A, Aziz Q, Bennett MI, Benoliel R, Cohen M, Evers S, Finnerup NB, First MB, Giamberardino MA, Kaasa S, Kosek E, Lavand'homme P, Nicholas M, Perrot S, Scholz J, Schug S, Smith BH, Svensson P, Vlaeyen JW, Wang SJ. A classification of chronic pain for ICD-11. *Pain.* 2015;156:1003–1007.

33. Schug SA, Bruce J. Risk stratification for the development of chronic postsurgical pain. *Pain Rep.* 2017;2(6):e627.

34. Katz J, Weinrib A, Fashler SR, Katznelzon R, Shah BR, Ladak SS, Jiang J, Li Q, McMillan K, Santa Mina D, Wentlandt K, McRae K, Tamir D, Lyn S, de Perrot M, Rao V, Grant D, Roche-Nagle G, Cleary SP, Hofer SO, Gilbert R, Wijeysundera D, Ritvo P, Janmohamed T, O'Leary G, Clarke H. The Toronto General Hospital Transitional Pain Service: Development and implementation of a multidisciplinary program to prevent chronic postsurgical pain. *J Pain Res.* 2015;8:695–702.

35. Edwards RR, Dworkin RH, Sullivan MD, Turk DC, Wasan AD. The role of psychosocial processes in the development and maintenance of chronic pain. *J Pain.* 2016;17:T70–T92.

36. Gatchel RJ, Neblett R. Pain catastrophizing: What clinicians need to know. *Prac Pain Manag.* 2017;15(6).

37. Chou R, Deyo R, Friedly J, Skelly A, Hashimoto R, Weimer M, Fu R, Dana T, Kraegel P, Griffin J, Grusing S, Brodt ED. Nonpharmacologic therapies for low back pain: A systematic review for an American College of Physicians clinical practice guideline. *Ann Intern Med.* 2017;166(7):493–505.

38. Finnerup NB, Attal N, Haroutounian S, et al. Pharmacotherapy for neuropathic pain in adults: A systematic review and meta-analysis. *Lancet Neurol.* 2015;14(2):162–173.

39. Stockings E, Campbell G, Hall WD, Nielsen S, Zagic D, Rahman R, Murnion B, Farrell M, Weier M, Degenhardt L. Cannabis and cannabinoids for the treatment of people with chronic noncancer pain conditions: A systematic review and meta-analysis of controlled and observational studies. *Pain.* 2018;159(11):1932–1954.

40. Cohen SP, Bhatia A, Buvanendran A, Schwenk ES, Wasan AD, Hurley RW, Viscusi ER, Narouze S, Davis FN, Ritchie EC, Lubenow TR, Hooten WM. Consensus guidelines on the use of intravenous ketamine infusions for chronic pain from the American Society of Regional Anesthesia and Pain Medicine, the American Academy of Pain Medicine, and the American Society of Anesthesiologists. *Reg Anesth Pain Med.* 2018;43(5):521–546.

41. Iacob E, Hagn EE, Sindt J, Brogan S, Tadler SC, Kennington KS, Hare BD, Bokat CE, Donaldson GW, Okifuji A, Junkins SR. Tertiary care clinical experience with intravenous lidocaine infusions for the treatment of chronic pain. *Pain Med.* 2018;19(6):1245–1253.

42. Dowell D, Haegerich TM, Chou R. CDC Guideline for Prescribing Opioids for Chronic Pain-United States, 2016. *JAMA.* 2016;315(15):1624–1645.

43. Dowell D, Haegerich T, Chou R. No shortcuts to safer opioid prescribing. *N Engl J Med.* 2019;380(24):2285–2287.

44. Velayudhan A, Bellingham G, Morley-Forster P. Opioid-induced hyperalgesia. *Br J Anaesth.* 2014;4(3):125–129.

45. Rathmell James P, Benzon Honorio T, Dreyfuss Paul, Huntoon Marc, Wallace Mark, Baker Ray, Riew KDaniel, Rosenquist Richard W, Aprill Charles, Rost Natalia S, Buvanendran Asokumar, Scott Kreiner D, Bogduk Nikolai, Fourney Daryl R, Fraifeld Eduardo, Horn Scott, Stone Jeffrey, Vorenkamp Kevin, Lawler Gregory, Summers Jeffrey, Kloth David, O'Brien David, Tutton Sean. Safeguards to prevent neurologic complications after epidural steroid injections: Consensus opinions from a multidisciplinary working group and national organizations. *Anesthesiology.* 2015;122:974–984.

46. Cohen SP, Bhaskar A, Bhatia A, Buvanendran A, Deer T, Garg S, Hooten WM, Hurley RW, Kennedy DJ, McLean BC, Moon JY, Narouze S, Pangarkar S, Provenzano DA, Rauck R, Sitzman BT, Smuck M, van Zundert J, Vorenkamp K, Wallace MS, Zhao Z. Consensus practice guidelines on interventions for lumbar facet joint pain from a multispecialty, international working group. *Reg Anesth Pain Med.* 2020;45(6):424–467.

47. Abd-Elsayed A, Abdallah R, Falowski S, Chaiban G, Burkey A, Slavin K, Guirguis M, Raslan AM. Development of an educational curriculum for spinal cord stimulation. *Neuromodulation.* 2020;23(5):555–561.

48. Deer TR, Pope JE, Hayek SM, Bux A, Buchser E, Eldabe S, De Andrés JA, Erdek M, Patin D, Grider JS, Doleys DM, Jacobs MS, Yaksh TL, Poree L, Wallace MS, Prager J, Rauck R, DeLeon O, Diwan S, Falowski SM, Gazelka HM, Kim P, Leong M, Levy RM, McDowell II G, McRoberts P, Naidu R, Narouze S, Perruchoud C, Rosen SM, Rosenberg WS, Saulino M, Staats P, Stearns LJ, Willis D, Krames E, Huntoon M, Mekhail N. The Polyanalgesic Consensus Conference (PACC): Recommendations on intrathecal drug infusion systems best practices and guidelines. *Neuromodulation.* 2017 Feb;20(2):96–132. doi:10.1111/ner.12538 Epub 2017 Jan 2. Erratum in: Neuromodulation. 2017 Jun;20(4):405–406. PMID: 28042904.

49. Deer TR, Pope JE, Hayek SM, Bux A, Buchser E, Eldabe S, De Andrés JA, Erdek M, Patin D, Grider JS, Doleys DM, Jacobs MS, Yaksh TL, Poree L, Wallace MS, Prager J, Rauck R, DeLeon O, Diwan S, Falowski SM, Gazelka HM, Kim P, Leong M, Levy RM, McDowell II G, McRoberts P, Naidu R, Narouze S, Perruchoud C, Rosen SM, Rosenberg WS, Saulino M, Staats P, Stearns LJ, Willis D, Krames E, Huntoon M, Mekhail N. The Polyanalgesic Consensus Conference (PACC): Recommendations on Intrathecal Drug Infusion Systems Best Practices and Guidelines. *Neuromodulation..* 2017;20(4):405–406.

50. Jain S, Deer T, Sayed D, Chopra P, Wahezi S, Jassal N, Weisbein J, Jameson J, Malinowski M, Golovac S. Minimally invasive lumbar decompression: A review of indications, techniques, efficacy and safety. *Pain Manag.* 2020;10(5):331–348.

VI

45 CARDIOPULMONARY RESUSCITATION

Joyce Chang, David Shimabukuro

INTRODUCTION

Cardiopulmonary resuscitation (CPR) was initially defined over 50 years ago as the administration of mouth-to-mouth ventilation and closed chest cardiac compressions in a pulseless patient. Since that time, significant advances in CPR and cardiovascular life support have been made. Today, the early descriptions of CPR are termed *basic life support (BLS)*, whereas adult advanced cardiovascular life support (ACLS) and pediatric advanced cardiovascular life support (PALS) include additional invasive techniques by experienced practitioners.

Out-of-hospital resuscitation is well described. Historically, in-hospital resuscitation and life support were less commonly studied. However, in-hospital cardiac arrests (IHCAs) are common and associated with high mortality rates indicating a need for more research. An estimated 290,000 IHCAs arrests occur in the United States annually. Although IHCAs continue to have poor outcomes, recent data suggest improvement over the past 2 decades, which may be the result of increased awareness of the influence of evidence-based clinical management.[1] Cardiac arrest in the perioperative period is unique in that it can frequently be anticipated, and health care providers and resources are immediately available.

EVIDENCE BASED

The American Heart Association (AHA), in conjunction with the International Liaison Committee on Resuscitation (ILCOR), published updated guidelines for the performance of CPR and emergency cardiovascular care (ECC) in 2020. These guidelines, revised from the 2015 version, include added emphasis on enhanced algorithms and visual aids to provide easy-to-remember guidance for BLS and ACLS resuscitation scenarios; the importance of early initiation of CPR by lay rescuers; early administration of epinephrine; optimal post–cardiac arrest care, including neuroprognostication; and debriefing and follow-up for emotional support for lay rescuers, emergency medical services (EMS) providers, and hospital-based health care workers.[2] The 2015 guidelines had added emphasis on systems of care in the prehospital, in-hospital, and post-resuscitation settings and on the continued education of CPR techniques to providers. Going forward, the AHA will continually update new evidence, revise guidelines, and distribute online to providers as needed instead of issuing 5-year overall updates.[3,4]

PRINCIPLES OF MANAGEMENT

Basic Life Support

BLS includes a number of key measures, including recognition of unresponsiveness and cardiac arrest, activation of an emergency response system, early administration of CPR, and early defibrillation if indicated. In the hospital setting a health care provider will perform the following sequence of steps (some steps may be performed by others), as described by the AHA algorithm: (1) verify scene safety; (2) check for responsiveness; (3) activate resuscitation team; (4) retrieve defibrillator (with or without automatic external defibrillation [AED] function) and emergency equipment and code cart; (5) simultaneously check for adequate breathing and pulse; (6) begin CPR; (7) use defibrillator as soon as it is available; and (8) provide two-person CPR as help arrives[5] (Fig. 45.1).

Recognition

Rapid recognition of cardiac arrest is essential in a successful resuscitation. The recognition and management of cardiac arrest in an unresponsive patient differ between laypersons and health care providers. The AHA guidelines recognize this distinction and include increased flexibility in emergency response activation either before or after breathing and pulse assessment for health care providers. Dispatcher-assisted CPR continues to play a large role for laypersons in treating out-of-hospital cardiac arrest (OHCA). It is recommended for laypersons to initiate CPR for presumed cardiac arrest, as the risk of harm is low if the patient is not in cardiac arrest.[2]

Health care providers should check for a pulse while simultaneously evaluating for the adequacy of ventilation. The pulse should be assessed at either the carotid or femoral artery, and the time elapsed for assessment should not exceed 10 seconds to minimize time to start chest compressions. When monitoring respirations, occasional agonal gasps should not be mistaken for normal breathing.

Cardiopulmonary Resuscitation

High-quality chest compressions are important for optimizing outcomes from cardiac arrest. When initiating chest compressions, the heel of the hand is placed longitudinally in the center of the chest on the lower half of the sternum with the other hand atop the first hand. Goals of optimal chest compressions include (1) maintain a rate of 100 to 120 compressions per minute; (2) compress the chest at least 5 cm (2 inches) but no more than 6 cm (2.5 inches); (3) allow for complete chest recoil between compressions; and (4) minimize the frequency and number of interruptions. Rates of compression over 120 per minute can lead to a decrease in the depth of compressions.[6] Excessive compressions over 6 cm have been associated with an increased rate of thoracic injury. Complete chest recoil allows for venous return and is important for effective CPR. Additionally, the AHA recommends performing manual chest compressions on a firm surface when possible. The pattern is 30 compressions to 2 breaths (30:2 equals 1 cycle of CPR), regardless of whether one or two rescuers are present.

Since 2010, the importance of definitive airway management has taken a secondary role to chest compressions. The old mnemonic ABCD (airway, breathing, circulation, and defibrillation) has given way to CAB (compression, airway, breathing). This is because the early initiation of high-quality chest compressions improves the likelihood of a return of spontaneous circulation (ROSC). Airway maneuvers are still attempted, but they should occur quickly, efficiently, and with minimal interruptions in chest compressions. Opening the airway can be achieved by a simple head tilt–chin lift technique (Fig. 45.2). A jaw thrust maneuver can be used in patients with suspected cervical spine injury. If necessary to relieve obstruction, properly sized simple airway devices, such as nasal or oral airways, can be inserted to displace the tongue from the posterior oropharynx.

Although several large out-of-hospital studies have demonstrated that chest compression–alone CPR is not inferior to traditional compression–ventilation CPR, health care providers are still expected to provide assisted ventilation.[7,8] Care should be taken to avoid rapid or forceful breaths in addition to excessive positive-pressure ventilation, as this can reduce preload and cardiac output.[9] Complications may also occur from gastric insufflation and subsequent aspiration of gastric contents. Maximum oxygen concentration is administered in order to provide optimally saturated arterial hemoglobin concentrations. Optimal ventilation includes providing only enough tidal volume to observe chest rise (~400–600 mL), giving each ventilation over 1 second, with a rate of 1 breath every 6 seconds. Hyperventilation is detrimental for neurologic recovery. The decreased minute ventilation is also appropriate because cardiac output is much lower than normal during resuscitation.

Defibrillation

A defibrillator should be attached to the patient as soon as possible. Optimal electrode placement on the chest

VI

Adult Basic Life Support Algorithm for Health Care Providers

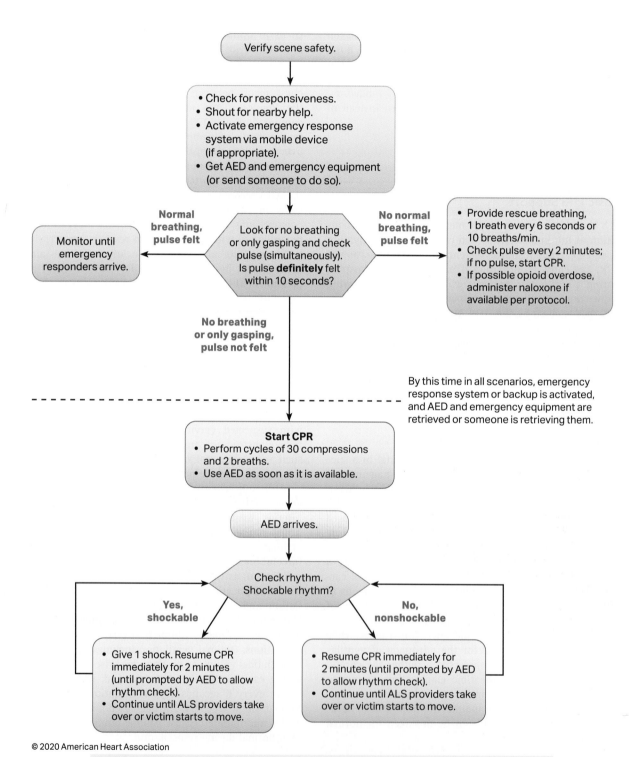

© 2020 American Heart Association

Fig. 45.1 BLS Health Care Provider Adult Cardiac Arrest Algorithm—2020 Update. (From 2020 AHA Guidelines for CPR and ECC: Adult Basic & Advanced Life Support. © 2020 American Heart Association.)

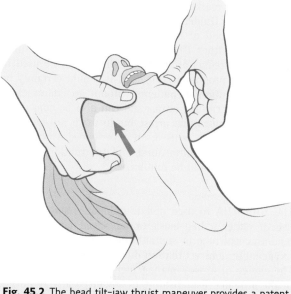

Fig. 45.2 The head tilt–jaw thrust maneuver provides a patent upper airway by tensing the muscles attached to the tongue, thus pulling the tongue away from the posterior pharynx. Forward displacement of the mandible is accomplished by grasping the angles of the mandible and lifting with both hands, which serves to displace the mandible forward while tilting the head backward.

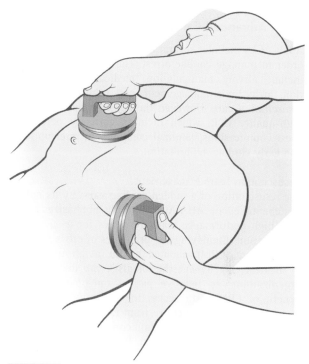

Fig. 45.3 Schematic depiction of the proper placement of paddle electrodes in an adult.

wall is right of the upper sternal border below the clavicle and to the left of the nipple with the center in the midaxillary line (Fig. 45.3). Most electrode pads now come with diagrams showing their correct positioning. Alternative locations include anterior-posterior, anterior-left infrascapular, and anterior-right infrascapular regions. Right anterior axillary-left anterior axillary is not recommended unless there are no other options available.

The amount of energy (joules [J]) delivered is dependent on the type of defibrillator used. Two major defibrillator types, monophasic (less common) and biphasic (more common), are available. Monophasic waveform defibrillators deliver a unidirectional energy charge, whereas biphasic waveform defibrillators deliver an in-series bidirectional energy charge. Based on evidence from implantable defibrillators, bidirectional energy delivery is more successful in terminating ventricular tachycardia (VT) and ventricular fibrillation (VF). In addition, biphasic waveform shocks require less energy than traditional monophasic waveform shocks (120–200 J vs. 360 J, respectively) and may therefore cause less myocardial damage.

The time until defibrillation is critical to survival, especially because most adults who can be saved from cardiac arrest are in VT/VF. Defibrillation should occur as soon as possible when it is recognized as a VT/VF arrest. CPR should be initiated while emergency equipment is

being retrieved. In one study of IHCAs 30% of patients received delayed defibrillation. Patients receiving delayed defibrillation have lower rates of ROSC, lower survival to hospital discharge, and worse long-term survival rates. Furthermore, each additional minute of delay was associated with worse outcomes.[10,11] Chest compressions should be resumed immediately after defibrillation.

Alternative Techniques and Ancillary Devices

The 2015 AHA CPR and ECC committee reviewed the evidence for ancillary devices used during CPR and found insufficient support to recommend any of the following: impedance threshold device, active compression-decompression CPR with impedance threshold device, mechanical piston device for chest compressions, and load-distributing band devices.

In 2019 the AHA published a focused update stating there were insufficient available studies to recommend extracorporeal CPR (venoarterial extracorporeal membrane oxygenation [ECMO]) for patients in cardiac arrest, consistent with the 2015 AHA guidelines. However, it can be considered for carefully selected patients who suffer from witnessed IHCA secondary to reversible causes when conventional CPR efforts are failing. It should only be instituted in settings in which it can be expeditiously implemented and supported by skilled providers.[12]

VI

Adult Advanced Cardiovascular Life Support

Adult ACLS includes several interventions besides BLS in order to manage cardiac arrest. These interventions can include airway manipulation, medication administration, arrhythmia management, and transition to post-resuscitation care. However, the key element of ACLS is high-quality CPR, which includes correctly performed chest compressions, minimal compression interruptions, and early cardiac defibrillation.

Resuscitation Team Management

The resuscitation of a sudden cardiac arrest by its nature is a chaotic event. AHA ACLS training emphasizes effective, high-performance team dynamics for a successful resuscitation. Employing the principles of crisis resource management (CRM), adapted by the aviation industry to medical care by anesthesiologists, can decrease disorganization and improve patient outcomes.[13] A key benefit of CRM is to access the collective knowledge and experience of the entire team rather than rely on a single individual. Two important components of CRM are leadership and communication. Resuscitation teams are often composed of health care providers from different disciplines, who may or may not have worked together before. Role clarity is important, yet can be challenging in this environment. It is imperative to establish a team leader who can take on assigning roles and assuming global management of the resuscitation. Communication during a resuscitation can also be challenging. Two important components are to have closed loop communications and for there to be a single point for all communication (i.e., the team leader). Practically, closed loop communication consists of the following (1) the team leader gives a clear message, order, or assignment to a team member; (2) the team member gives a clear response and eye contact to confirm that they have heard and understood the message; and (3) the team member tells the team leader when the task has been completed. While most decisions will come from the team leader, a good team leader will enlist the collective knowledge and experience of the entire team.

Monitoring Cardiopulmonary Resuscitation

A number of physiologic variables can be used to monitor CPR. Continuous monitoring of end-tidal carbon dioxide ($Petco_2$) with waveform capnography can be beneficial during the resuscitation. In addition to confirmation of advanced airway placement, $Petco_2$ can guide the rescuers in the adequacy of chest compressions.[14] Targeting compressions to $Petco_2$ value at 10 mm Hg or greater may be useful as a marker of CPR quality. Alternative physiologic measures during CPR include arterial relaxation diastolic pressure, arterial pressure monitoring, and central venous oxygen saturation. Targeting an arterial relaxation diastolic pressure of 20 mm Hg or greater may

be useful as a marker of CPR quality. Data from the AHA Get With the Guidelines Resuscitation registry show a higher likelihood of ROSC when CPR quality is monitored using either $Petco_2$ or diastolic blood pressure.[2] A prolonged reduction in $Petco_2$ should not be used in isolation for prognostication, and it should certainly be used with caution in patients without an endotracheal tube. Bedside cardiac ultrasound can also be considered when managing cardiac arrest, but its use is not routinely recommended. If it is used, an experienced sonographer should perform the ultrasound, and interruptions in chest compressions should be minimized.[15]

Airway Management

The 2019 AHA focused update guidelines state that the use of either a bag-mask or advanced airway device (endotracheal tube or supraglottic airway) for providing oxygenation and ventilation during CPR is acceptable.[12] The choice of airway management depends on the skill of the provider. Establishing an advanced airway during an IHCA results in fewer interruptions to chest compressions during CPR.[16] Chest compressions should not be interrupted for longer than 10 seconds during advanced airway placement. Once an endotracheal tube is placed, care should be taken to avoid excessive ventilation, as generation of elevated intrathoracic pressure can lead to reduced preload and reduced cardiac output. If an advanced airway is used, placement should be performed by expert providers trained in these procedures. Frequent experience or frequent retraining is recommended; however, there is insufficient evidence about the ideal frequency of retraining.[12] Insertion of an advanced airway can be deferred until after the patient fails to respond to several cycles of CPR and defibrillation. However, the clinical course of the arrest should be considered. For example, a patient with severe pulmonary edema may benefit from endotracheal intubation sooner rather than later. There are no formal recommendations for the timing of advanced airway placement.

Continuous waveform capnography is recommended as the measurement of choice for the assessment of advanced airway placement. Clinical evaluation should also occur, including auscultation of bilateral breath sounds and visualization of bilateral chest rise. If capnography is not available, alternative methods include esophageal detector device, non waveform capnography, and ultrasound. Once the endotracheal tube is confirmed to be in the trachea, it is secured in place. One breath is delivered every 6 seconds (10 breaths/min) and does not require synchronization with compressions.

Management of Specific Arrhythmias

The additional components of ACLS and specific arrhythmia management will be discussed here. As there were no updates to the bradycardia and tachycardia algorithms, they will not be reviewed in detail.

Bradycardia

Bradycardia is defined as a heart rate <60 beats per minute. However, when bradycardia is the cause of symptoms, the heart rate is usually <50 beats per minute. A slow heart rate may be physiologically normal for some individuals. The AHA bradycardia algorithm focuses on the management of clinically significant (i.e., symptomatic) bradycardia.[17] Fig. 45.4 summarizes the management of a patient with bradycardia.

Tachycardia

Tachycardia is defined as a heart rate >100 beats per minute. However, clinically significant (i.e., symptomatic) tachycardia tends to occur with a heart rate >120 to 150 beats per minute, depending on if it is atrial or ventricular in nature. A rapid heart rate is an appropriate response to a physiologic stress or other underlying conditions. Therefore it is important to determine whether the tachycardia is the cause of the presenting

Adult Bradycardia Algorithm

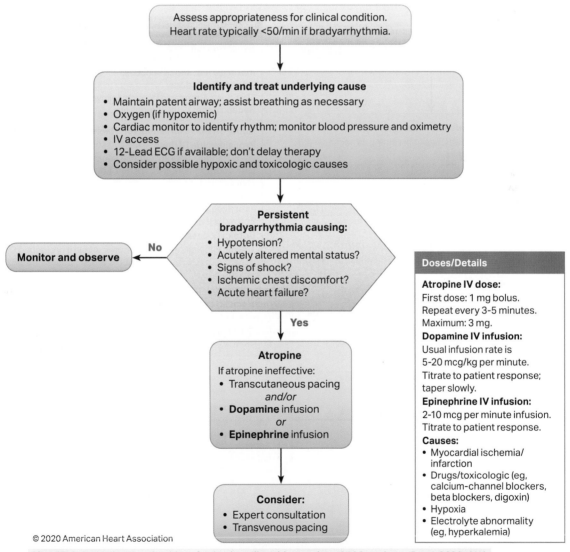

Fig. 45.4 Resuscitation algorithm for bradycardia with a pulse—2020 update. (From 2020 AHA Guidelines for CPR and ECC: Adult Basic & Advanced Life Support. © 2020 American Heart Association.)

VI

symptom or secondary to an underlying condition.[17] Fig. 45.5 summarizes the management of a patient with tachycardia.

Pulseless Arrest

Cardiac dysrhythmias that produce pulseless cardiac arrest are (1) VF, (2) VT, (3) pulseless electrical activity (PEA), and (4) asystole (Fig. 45.6). During pulseless cardiac arrest, the primary goals are to provide effective chest compressions and quick defibrillation if the rhythm is VF or VT. Drug administration is of secondary importance and may be administered after initial defibrillation attempts have failed. In the cardiac arrest patient with a non shockable rhythm it is reasonable to administer epinephrine as soon as feasible.[2] After initiating CPR and defibrillation (when there is a shockable rhythm), rescuers can then establish intravenous access, obtain a more definitive airway, and consider drug therapy (Table 45.1), all while providing continued chest compressions and ventilation. In addition, while performing CPR–defibrillation cycles, the team needs to consider potential inciting causes (Table 45.2).

Adult Tachycardia With a Pulse Algorithm

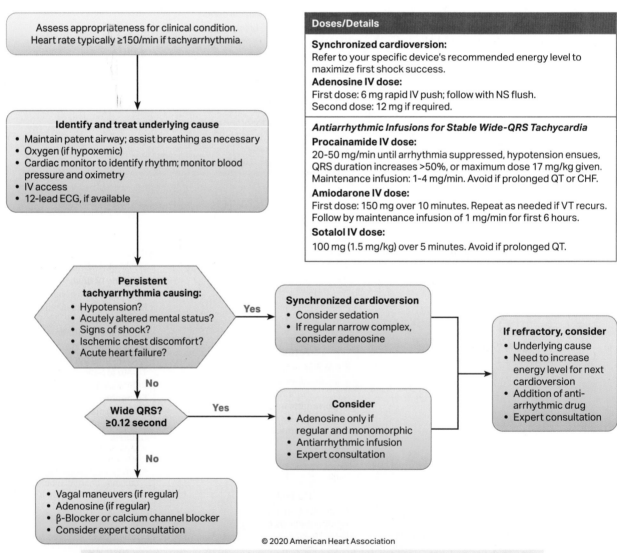

Fig. 45.5 Resuscitation algorithm for tachycardia with a pulse—2020 update. (From 2020 AHA Guidelines for CPR and ECC: Adult Basic & Advanced Life Support. © 2020 American Heart Association.)

Adult Cardiac Arrest Algorithm

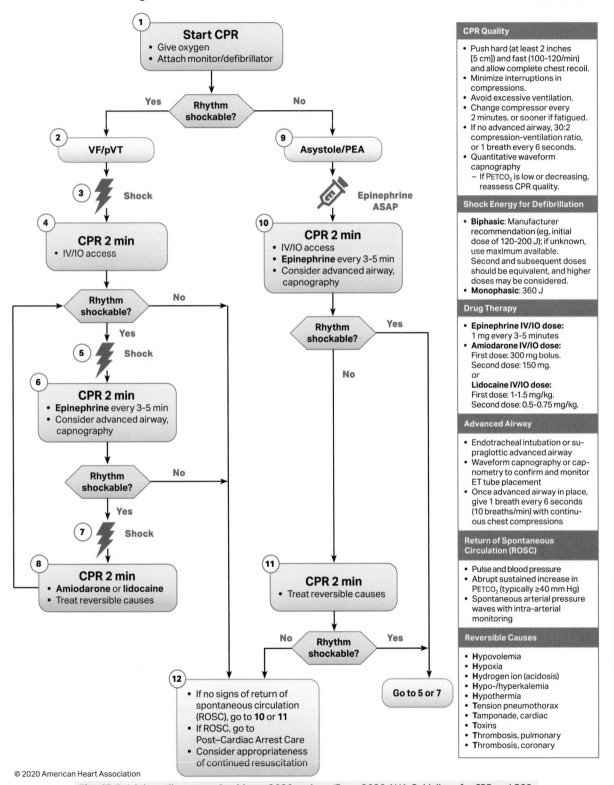

Fig. 45.6 Adult cardiac arrest algorithm—2020 update. (From 2020 AHA Guidelines for CPR and ECC: Adult Basic & Advanced Life Support. © 2020 American Heart Association.)

Table 45.1 Drugs Used During Cardiopulmonary Resuscitation

Drug Name	Dose	Indication
Adenosine	6 mg IV/IO May repeat 12 mg IV/IO (Cut dose in half if using central line)	For stable narrow QRS tachycardia or monomorphic VT (contraindicated with pre-excitation syndrome)
Amiodarone	300 mg IV/IO May repeat 150 mg IV/IO 150 mg IV/IO over 10-min Maintenance infusion of 1 mg/min for 6 hr, then 0.5 mg/min Maximum total dose of 2.2 g/24 hr	For pulseless VT/VF For stable VT or uncertain wide QRS tachycardia and narrow QRS tachycardias
Atropine	0.5-1 mg IV/IO May repeat every 3-5 min Maximum total dose of 3 mg	For bradycardia
Diltiazem	15-20 mg (0.25 mg/kg) IV/IO over 2-min May repeat in 15 min at 20-25 mg (0.35 mg/kg) Maintenance infusion of 5-15 mg/hr	For stable narrow QRS tachycardia (contraindicated with pre-excitation syndrome)
Dopamine	2-10 mcg/kg/min by infusion	For bradycardia instead of a pacer, while awaiting a pacer, or if a pacer is ineffective or not tolerated
Epinephrine	1 mg IV/IO Repeat every 3-5 min 2-10 mcg/min by infusion	For pulseless cardiac arrest For bradycardia instead of a pacer, while awaiting a pacer, or if a pacer is ineffective or not tolerated
Esmolol	0.5 mg/kg IV/IO May repeat 0.5 mg/kg IV/IOMaintenance infusion of 0.05-0.3 mg/kg/min	For stable narrow QRS tachycardias (contraindicated with pre excitation syndrome)
Lidocaine	1-1.5 mg/kg IV/IO May repeat 0.5-0.75 mg/kg Maximum total of 3 doses or 3 mg/kg	For pulseless VT/VF
Magnesium	1-2 g IV/IO	For torsades de pointes
Metoprolol	5 mg IV/IO May repeat every 5 min Maximum total dose of 15 mg	For stable narrow QRS tachycardias (contraindicated with pre excitation syndrome)
Procainamide	20-50 mg/min IV/IO until arrhythmia suppressed Maintenance infusion of 1-4 mg/min Maximum total dose of 17 mg/kg	For stable wide QRS tachycardia
Sotalol	100 mg (1.5 mg/kg) IV/IO over 5 min	For stable wide QRS tachycardia
Verapamil	2.5-5 mg IV/IO over 2-min May repeat 5-10 mg over a 15- to 30-minute period Maximum total dose of 20 mg	For stable narrow QRS tachycardia (contraindicated with pre excitation syndrome)

Ventricular Fibrillation/Ventricular Tachycardia

VF and pulseless VT are nonperfusing rhythms originating from the ventricles. The key management steps to achieving ROSC are high-quality CPR and rapid defibrillation. When sudden cardiac arrest is recognized, immediately start chest compressions while a defibrillator is attached. Once the defibrillator is attached, immediately evaluate to determine if the rhythm is shockable. If the rhythm is VF or VT, resume chest compressions while the defibrillator is charging to the appropriate energy level. Once charged, deliver a shock, then resume CPR immediately and continue for five cycles or 2 minutes, followed by re evaluation of the cardiac rhythm. Repeat defibrillation if they remain in cardiac arrest with a shockable

Table 45.2 Major Causes of Cardiovascular Collapse in the Perioperative Period

8 Hs	8 Ts
Hypovolemia	**T**oxins (anaphylaxis/anesthesia)
Hypoxia	**T**amponade
Hydrogen ions (acidosis)	**T**ension pneumothorax
Hyperkalemia/hypokalemia	**T**hrombosis in coronary artery
Hypoglycemia	**T**hrombus in pulmonary artery
Hypothermia	**T**rauma
Malignant **h**yperthermia	Q**T** interval prolongation
Hypervagal response	Pulmonary hyper**t**ension

rhythm (see Fig. 45.6). A biphasic defibrillator is preferred over monophasic, and a single shock is preferred over sequential (stacked) shocks. If VF or VT persists after at least one CPR–defibrillation cycle, a vasopressor is given. Epinephrine 1 mg intravenously (IV) may be administered every 3 to 5 minutes. Amiodarone and/or lidocaine can be administered to improve the likelihood of restoring and maintaining ROSC. Although the role of antiarrhythmics in improving survival after VF/VT is not completely clear, it is recommended by current ACLS guidelines and may be most useful in witnessed cardiac arrests. Magnesium sulfate may be considered if torsade de pointes is suspected.[18]

Asystole/Pulseless Electrical Activity

Asystole is the absence of any electrical or mechanical cardiac activity; PEA is defined as electrical cardiac activity without sufficient mechanical cardiac activity to generate a palpable pulse. These two cardiac rhythms have been combined as the second part of the pulseless arrest algorithm because of similarities in their management (see Fig. 45.6). These are nonperfusing rhythms and therefore require excellent CPR. Neither will benefit from defibrillation; instead, administer epinephrine as soon as feasible. Epinephrine 1 mg IV is given every 3 to 5 minutes. The primary interventions for successful ROSC include effective CPR with minimal interruptions, identifying and treating reversible causes, and establishing an advanced airway. The administration of high-quality chest compressions can be monitored by Petco_2, diastolic blood pressure, or central venous saturation, if available. If an organized cardiac rhythm is present, the rescuer checks for a pulse. If there is no pulse, CPR should be continued. If there is a pulse, the rescuer identifies the rhythm, and vital signs are obtained while starting

post-resuscitation care as described further below. A bedside cardiac ultrasound may provide valuable information regarding the cause of arrest. Additionally, the absence of ventricular wall motion on ultrasound portends an unlikely ROSC.[19]

Medication Administration

Establishing intravenous access is important for drug administration but should not interfere with CPR or defibrillation. A single, large peripheral intravenous catheter is preferred and is sufficient for resuscitating most pulseless patients. If unable to obtain intravenous access, intraosseous (IO) access can be considered. If neither intravenous nor IO access is feasible, certain medications (epinephrine, lidocaine, atropine, naloxone) can be given via the endotracheal tube. The endotracheal dose is 2 to 10 times the recommended intravenous dose, and the drug is diluted in 5 to 10 mL of sterile water before instillation down the endotracheal tube.

Epinephrine and amiodarone are among the most commonly used drugs in the ACLS algorithm and deserve special attention. Epinephrine is a combined direct α- and β-adrenergic receptor agonist. Several randomized controlled trials demonstrated increased survival to hospital discharge and ROSC.[12] Epinephrine can increase diastolic blood pressure and thereby restore coronary perfusion pressure and blood flow back to the myocardium. However, epinephrine also increases myocardial oxygen consumption by increasing heart rate and afterload.

Amiodarone was initially developed as an antianginal drug in the 1950s but was abandoned because of its side effects. Because it has effects on cardiac sodium and potassium channels, in addition to α- and β-receptors, amiodarone was reinvestigated for its antiarrhythmic effects. In this regard, amiodarone prolongs repolarization and refractoriness in the sinoatrial node, the atrial and ventricular myocardium, the atrioventricular node, and the His–Purkinje cardiac conduction system. Amiodarone can exacerbate or induce arrhythmias, especially torsade de pointes. This drug may interact with volatile anesthetics to produce heart block, profound vasodilation, myocardial depression, and severe hypotension. Amiodarone has many drug interactions and can prolong the effects of oral anticoagulants, phenytoin, digoxin, and diltiazem. Despite its multiple disadvantages, administration of amiodarone improves survival to hospital admission in adults with out-of-hospital VF/VT arrest when compared with placebo.[12] The recommended dose of amiodarone for VF/VT is 300 mg IV. An additional bolus dose of 150 mg IV may be given for persistent pulseless VF/VT.

The routine administration of lidocaine, an antiarrhythmic that blocks sodium channels, was removed from the ACLS algorithm in the 2010 ACLS guideline update. However, in the 2018 AHA focused update lidocaine was reinstated as a drug therapy to consider in refractory

VF/VT. A study of OHCA patients showed favorable results with the administration of lidocaine compared with placebo, but not amiodarone.[12] Vasopressin, a non-adrenergic vasopressor, was removed from the 2015 ACLS guidelines because of a lack of demonstrated benefit when compared with epinephrine.[20] Drugs used for ACLS are associated with ROSC but not with improved survival to hospital discharge or neurologic recovery. Administration of steroids along with vasoactive drugs may improve the likelihood of survival and favorable neurologic outcomes for IHCA; however, there is no recommendation for their routine use.[21] In patients with cardiac arrest secondary to opioid overdose administration of naloxone should be considered.

Pediatric Advanced Life Support

CPR of infants and children follows the same basic principles as those for adults. The AHA offers two courses for health care providers who require resuscitation-related training for pediatric patients: PALS and Pediatric Emergency Assessment, Recognition and Stabilization (PEARS). This section will highlight salient differences in management for these patients. Most pediatric cardiac events are triggered by respiratory deterioration. Therefore airway management and ventilation management are critical to a successful pediatric resuscitation. In contrast, adults tend to experience cardiac arrest as a result of VT or VF secondary to myocardial ischemia. Regardless, pediatric BLS and ACLS follow the similar algorithm of CAB. Naturally, there are several specific differences between adult and pediatric patients. Infants are defined as younger than 1 year in age, whereas children are between the age of 1 year and adolescence. Adult resuscitation guidelines can be used for adolescent children. The elements of high-quality CPR in pediatrics remain unchanged from adults and include (1) adequate chest compression rate, (2) adequate chest compression depth, (3) adequate recoil between chest compressions, (4) minimal interruption to chest compressions, and (5) avoidance of excess ventilation. Key differences include (1) CPR quality: depth > one-third anteroposterior diameter of chest and compression–ventilation ratio of 30:2 (one rescuer) or 15:2 (two rescuers) if there is no advanced airway and one breath every 2 to 3 seconds if there is an advanced airway; (2) shock energy for defibrillation: first shock at 2 J/kg, second shock at 4 J/kg, and subsequent shocks >4 J/kg with a maximum of 10 J/kg or adult dose; and (3) drug therapy dosing that is weight based. Refer to Fig. 45.7 for the AHA pediatric cardiac arrest algorithm.[22]

Circulation

In a child the heel of one or both hands should be placed on the lower half of the sternum, between the nipples, while keeping the fingers off the ribcage and staying above the xiphoid process. In an infant chest compressions are delivered via the two-finger technique (Fig. 45.8) or two-thumb encircling hands technique (Fig. 45.9). Fingers should be placed over the lower half of the sternum just below the intermammary line while keeping above the xiphoid process. For both infants and children, the sternum should be depressed at least one-third to one-half the anteroposterior diameter of the chest (4 cm in infants, 5 cm in children) at a rate of 100 to 120 compressions per minute.

Pulse checks and closed chest compressions are performed slightly differently, depending on whether the patient is a child or an infant. In children the pulse is palpated at the carotid or femoral artery, similar to adults. In infants the pulse is checked at the brachial or femoral artery. As with adults, P_{ETCO_2} can be used to evaluate the quality of CPR. If invasive monitoring, such as an arterial catheter, is already in place, it may also be used to evaluate and guide CPR.

ECMO can be considered in all pediatric cardiac arrest patients who are refractory to standard conventional therapies. It is most beneficial in the ICHA setting with existing ECMO protocols, expertise, and equipment. There is insufficient evidence for its use in the OHCA setting.[23]

Airway and Ventilation Management

The airway of pediatric patients is slightly different from that of an adult, but head tilt–chin lift is still the technique of choice to open the airway (also see Chapter 16). Children tend to have a larger tongue and epiglottis in relation to the mouth and larynx. In addition, they have a larger head in relation to the body. Overextension or excessive flexion of the head can lead to difficulty visualizing the glottic opening during direct laryngoscopy. Straight laryngoscope blades may be preferred over curved blades to lift the epiglottis anteriorly and away from the glottic opening in young children.

Given the likely causes of pediatric cardiopulmonary arrest, conventional CPR (compressions and ventilation) is recommended over compression-only resuscitation. The pattern should be 30 compressions to 2 breaths if there is a single rescuer and 15 compressions to 2 breaths if there are two rescuers.

Defibrillation

In children defibrillation should be performed when a pulseless shockable rhythm (VT, VF) is present. An initial energy of 2 to 4 J/kg should be attempted, regardless of the waveform type. Subsequent defibrillations should be at least 4 J/kg but should not exceed 10 J/kg. Biphasic AEDs can be used in children older than 1 year outside the hospital setting. AHA guidelines recommend the use of a pediatric-dose attenuator system that will decrease the amount of delivered energy. If one is not available, a standard external defibrillator can be substituted.

Pediatric Cardiac Arrest Algorithm

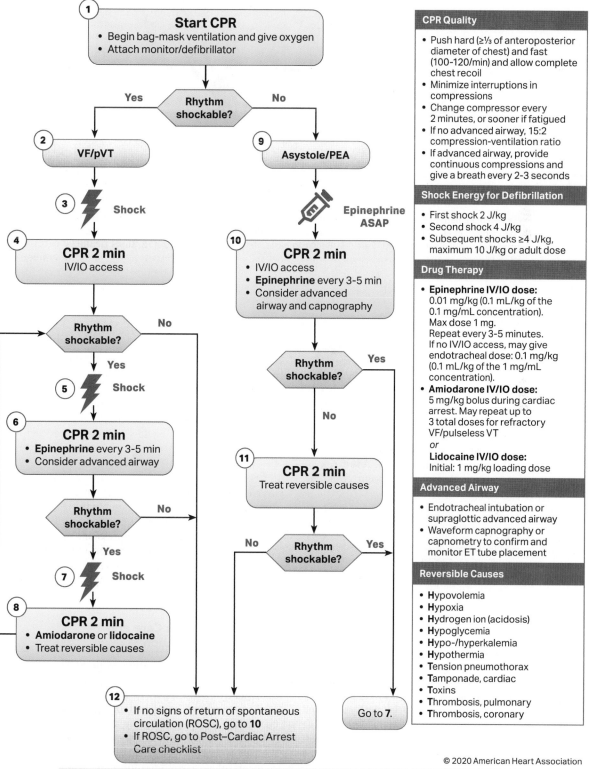

CPR Quality

- Push hard (≥⅓ of anteroposterior diameter of chest) and fast (100–120/min) and allow complete chest recoil
- Minimize interruptions in compressions
- Change compressor every 2 minutes, or sooner if fatigued
- If no advanced airway, 15:2 compression-ventilation ratio
- If advanced airway, provide continuous compressions and give a breath every 2–3 seconds

Shock Energy for Defibrillation

- First shock 2 J/kg
- Second shock 4 J/kg
- Subsequent shocks ≥4 J/kg, maximum 10 J/kg or adult dose

Drug Therapy

- **Epinephrine IV/IO dose:** 0.01 mg/kg (0.1 mL/kg of the 0.1 mg/mL concentration). Max dose 1 mg. Repeat every 3–5 minutes. If no IV/IO access, may give endotracheal dose: 0.1 mg/kg (0.1 mL/kg of the 1 mg/mL concentration).
- **Amiodarone IV/IO dose:** 5 mg/kg bolus during cardiac arrest. May repeat up to 3 total doses for refractory VF/pulseless VT
  or
  Lidocaine IV/IO dose: Initial: 1 mg/kg loading dose

Advanced Airway

- Endotracheal intubation or supraglottic advanced airway
- Waveform capnography or capnometry to confirm and monitor ET tube placement

Reversible Causes

- **H**ypovolemia
- **H**ypoxia
- **H**ydrogen ion (acidosis)
- **H**ypoglycemia
- **H**ypo-/hyperkalemia
- **H**ypothermia
- **T**ension pneumothorax
- **T**amponade, cardiac
- **T**oxins
- **T**hrombosis, pulmonary
- **T**hrombosis, coronary

© 2020 American Heart Association

Fig. 45.7 Pediatric cardiac arrest algorithm—2020 update. (From 2020 AHA Guidelines for CPR and ECC: Adult Basic & Advanced Life Support. © 2020 American Heart Association.)

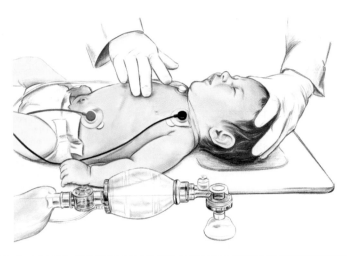

Fig. 45.8 Pediatric chest compressions via two-finger technique. (From Berg MD, Schexnayder SM, Chameides L et al. 2010 American Heart Association guidelines for cardiopulmonary resuscitation and emergency cardiovascular care. Part 13: Pediatric basic life support. 2010;122[18/Suppl 3]:S862–S875.)

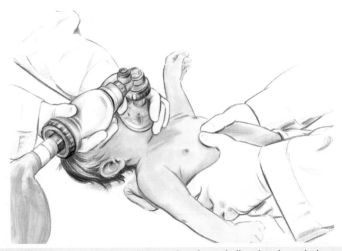

Fig. 45.9 Pediatric chest compressions via two-thumb encircling hands technique. (From 2005 American Heart Association [AHA] guidelines for cardiopulmonary resuscitation [CPR] and emergency cardiovascular care (ECC) of pediatric and neonatal patients: Pediatric advanced life support. *Pediatrics.* 2006:117[5]:e1005–e1028.)

Medications

Most medication dosages are calculated by using current known weight or ideal body weight based on height. Most pediatric units have resuscitation carts divided by weight to facilitate drug administration in an emergency so that calculations do not need to be performed and valuable time is not wasted. As with adults, epinephrine has been associated with an increased rate of ROSC and can be used in cardiac arrest. For refractory VT or pulseless VT, either amiodarone or lidocaine can be administered.

Post-resuscitation Care and Neuroprognostication

After successful resuscitation with ROSC, patients are admitted to a critical care unit for further definitive management and supportive treatment (Fig. 45.10). Post-cardiac arrest care must include optimization of cardiopulmonary function to ensure adequate organ perfusion. It should be consistent, integrated, and multidisciplinary. If arrest occurs at a center that is not equipped to manage elements of post-resuscitation care, transfer to a larger regional center should be considered.[24]

ACLS Health Care Provider
Post–Cardiac Arrest Care Algorithm

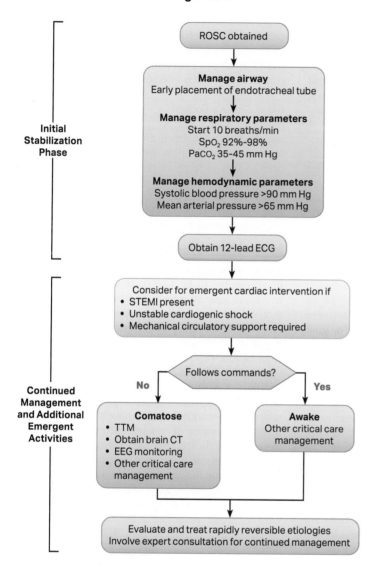

Initial Stabilization Phase

Resuscitation is ongoing during the post-ROSC phase, and many of these activities can occur concurrently. However, if prioritization is necessary, follow these steps:

- Airway management: Waveform capnography or capnometry to confirm and monitor endotracheal tube placement
- Manage respiratory parameters: Titrate FiO_2 for SpO_2 92%-98%; start at 10 breaths/min; titrate to $PaCO_2$ of 35-45 mm Hg
- Manage hemodynamic parameters: Administer crystalloid and/or vasopressor or inotrope for goal systolic blood pressure >90 mm Hg or mean arterial pressure >65 mm Hg

Continued Management and Additional Emergent Activities

These evaluations should be done concurrently so that decisions on targeted temperature management (TTM) receive high priority as cardiac interventions.

- Emergent cardiac intervention: Early evaluation of 12-lead electrocardiogram (ECG); consider hemodynamics for decision on cardiac intervention
- TTM: If patient is not following commands, start TTM as soon as possible; begin at 32-36°C for 24 hours by using a cooling device with feedback loop
- Other critical care management
  - Continuously monitor core temperature (esophageal, rectal, bladder)
  - Maintain normoxia, normocapnia, euglycemia
  - Provide continuous or intermittent electroencephalogram (EEG) monitoring
  - Provide lung-protective ventilation

H's and T's

Hypovolemia
Hypoxia
Hydrogen ion (acidosis)
Hypokalemia/**h**yperkalemia
Hypothermia
Tension pneumothorax
Tamponade, cardiac
Toxins
Thrombosis, pulmonary
Thrombosis, coronary

VI

Fig. 45.10 Post-cardiac arrest algorithm—2020 update. (From 2020 AHA Guidelines for CPR and ECC: Adult Basic & Advanced Life Support. © 2020 American Heart Association.)

When possible, therapies are administered concurrently. Specifically, percutaneous coronary interventions (PCIs) should not be delayed to institute targeted-temperature management (TTM), and the institution of TTM should not delay PCI. Often, vasopressors and inotropes need to be administered during the immediate post-resuscitation period because of the presence of myocardial stunning and hemodynamic instability. Central venous access for drug administration may be necessary, along with an arterial catheter to facilitate hemodynamic monitoring.

Acute Coronary Syndrome

An electrocardiogram is obtained as soon as possible after ROSC in order to evaluate for ST-segment elevation myocardial infarction (STEMI). If acute ST-segment elevation is noted, the patient should be taken for emergent angiography. Some patients with non-ST-segment elevation may also benefit from emergent angiography.[25] These evaluations are made regardless of neurologic status.

Pulmonary and Hemodynamic Goals

After a ROSC, oxygenation and ventilation should be evaluated and optimized. Advanced airway placement may be needed, and hyperventilation is avoided. The goal for oxygenation is a pulse oximetry saturation between 92% and 98%, and for ventilation the goal is a $Paco_2$ of 35 to 45 mm Hg. Hypotension, defined as systolic arterial blood pressure less than 90 mm Hg or mean arterial blood pressure less than 65 mm Hg, should be aggressively treated. This can be achieved with a combined administration of IV fluids and/or vasoactive/inotropic medications. No specific hemodynamic variables, including arterial blood pressure, cardiac output, venous oxygen saturation, or urine output, have been recommended, as these likely vary widely between individual patients. Reversible causes for cardiac arrest are again assessed. An electrocardiogram, echocardiogram, and serial cardiac enzymes are obtained. When applicable, serum or whole-blood lactate and central venous or mixed-venous oxygen saturation are monitored to assess for adequate tissue perfusion.

Neurologic Monitoring

In addition to cardiac recovery, neurologic recovery is of vital importance. The 2020 AHA ACLS guidelines contain significant new clinical data concerning optimal care in the days after cardiac arrest. Refer to Fig. 45.11 for the new multimodal approach to neuroprognostication. To be reliable, neuroprognostication should not be performed until 72 hours after return to normothermia.

Targeted Temperature Management

Temperature should be monitored closely, and hyperthermia is avoided at all times, as this can worsen ischemic brain injury. An advisory statement from the AHA strongly recommends TTM of 32 to 36°C, which is a change from the previous recommendation of 32 to 34°C.[26] Although the evidence is stronger for TTM for OHCA, it is still recommended for IHCA. Complications of therapeutic hypothermia occur at the lower targeted temperature and can include impaired coagulation, hypokalemia, hyperglycemia, worsening of arrhythmias, and an increased risk of infection. Thus patient factors should be taken into consideration when selecting the targeted temperature.

Blood Glucose Control

Increased blood glucose concentrations after resuscitation from cardiac arrest are associated with poor neurologic outcome. Yet tight control of serum glucose has not been shown to improve neurologic outcome. Regardless, glucose levels after resuscitation should be monitored closely to avoid significant hypoglycemia, hyperglycemia, and swings in individual blood glucose values.

Special Perioperative Considerations

The incidence of intraoperative cardiac arrest (ICA) has been reported to be 7.22 in 10,000 surgeries. Intraoperative blood loss, as indicated by the amount of transfusions received by the patient, was the most important predictor of ICA, but anaphylaxis has also been consistently implicated.[27,28] Cardiac arrest during anesthesia is distinct from cardiac arrest in other settings because of anesthetic medication–related alterations to their physiology. In addition, ICA during an anesthesia encounter is usually witnessed and frequently anticipated. The cause is often related to the surgical intervention and may be more easily reversible. Because of this, perioperative cardiac arrests are associated with a higher survival rate and better neurologic outcomes than other in-hospital arrests.[29] The traditional CPR and ECC guidelines do not necessarily translate well into the perioperative setting. In 2008 the American Society of Anesthesiologists (ASA) Committee on Critical Care Medicine published a monograph specific to ACLS for anesthesia providers. In a follow-up publication the authors described common causes of perioperative cardiac arrest, including the following categories and factors[30]:

1. *Medications:* anesthetic overdose, high neuraxial blockade, local anesthetic toxicity, drug administration errors
2. *Respiratory:* hypoxemia, auto–positive end-expiratory pressure (PEEP), acute bronchospasm
3. *Cardiovascular:* vasovagal, hypovolemic/hemorrhagic shock, distributive shock, obstructive shock, right ventricular failure, left ventricular failure, arrhythmia, acute coronary syndrome

The authors suggest several initial interventions when performing resuscitation in the operating room (Box 45.1). Five clinical circumstances that are unique to the intraoperative setting are detailed next.

Neuroprognostication Diagram

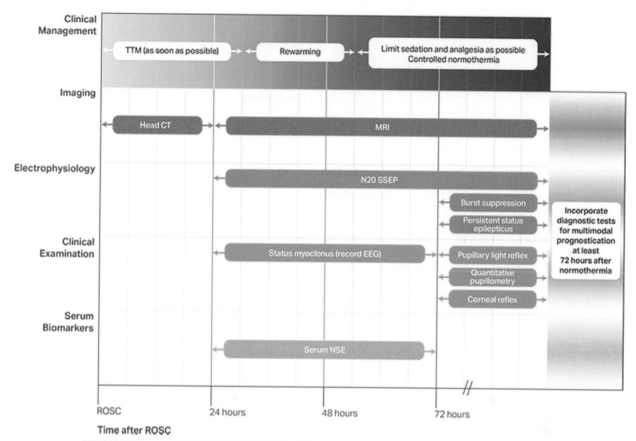

Fig. 45.11 Approach to multimodal neuroprognostication in adults after cardiac arrest. (From 2020 AHA Guidelines for CPR and ECC: Adult Basic & Advanced Life Support. © 2020 American Heart Association.)

Box 45.1   Initial Interventions During Intraoperative Cardiac Arrest

1. Initiate chest compressions
2. Call for help
3. Discontinue anesthetic
4. Check surgical field; hold surgery
5. Retrieve emergency equipment, including defibrillator
6. Increase fraction of inspired oxygen (FiO_2) to 100%
7. Manually ventilate the lungs
8. Open all intravenous lines
9. Use capnography to assess CPR

Anaphylaxis

Minor drug reactions, such as a rash, are a common occurrence in the operating room. Major reactions, such as anaphylactic shock, occur much less often. Common drugs associated with anaphylaxis are latex, β-lactam antibiotics, succinylcholine, all muscle relaxants, and intravenous contrast material. The treatment of anaphylaxis involves the administration of epinephrine to interrupt the cascade of profound vasodilation and significant vascular leak. If possible, the offending drug should be removed and discontinued. Epinephrine and vasopressin can be used to support arterial blood pressure, and steroids and antihistamines are administered to further attenuate the response. Intravenous fluid administration is essential secondary to the vascular leak. CPR and ACLS should be immediately instituted if there is no palpable pulse. In the event of complete cardiovascular collapse larger doses of epinephrine may be required.

Gas Embolism

Although a very rare event, the incidence of gas embolism has the potential to increase in parallel with the worldwide increase in laparoscopic surgical procedures,

VI

posterior spine surgery, and endobronchial laser procedures. The initial management includes cessation of the offending cause (i.e., halt insufflation), occlusion of open veins, and flooding of the surgical field with saline. Patients should be placed in the Trendelenburg position with the left side down to keep the gas in the apex of the right ventricle and allow for filling with blood. Complete circulatory collapse should be treated with CPR and ACLS.

Local Anesthetic Systemic Toxicity (LAST)
(Also See Chapter 10)

Local anesthetics affect sodium channels throughout the body, including the brain and the heart. In general, toxicity occurs in a dose-dependent fashion, with cardiovascular collapse occurring at the end of the spectrum. In non-anesthetized patients central nervous system symptoms are vital to recognize, as they tend to precede cardiac manifestations. The cardiac rhythm can range from premature ventricular contractions to asystole. If possible, the administration of the local anesthetic should be stopped. Intralipid should be given for cardiovascular toxicity. Good neurologic recovery in these patients can occur despite a prolonged resuscitation. Treatment recommendations include the following: (1) stop the local anesthetic; (2) CPR/ACLS if pulseless; (3) 20% intralipid IV with a load of 1.5 mL/kg followed by an infusion of 0.25 ml/kg/hr if less than 70 kg; (3) sodium bicarbonate to maintain pH >7.25; and (4) consider transcutaneous or transvenous pacing for bradycardic rhythms. Vasopressin should be avoided, and epinephrine doses should be decreased (<1 mcg/kg) (Fig. 45.12).

Cardiovascular Collapse From Neuraxial Anesthesia

Cardiovascular collapse from neuraxial anesthesia has been described but is inadequately understood.[31] It seems to occur in younger, otherwise healthy patients undergoing routine surgical procedures with neuraxial anesthesia. Proposed mechanisms causing the cardiac arrest include a shift in autonomic balance toward the parasympathetic system, a decrease in venous return from pooling in the splanchnic circulation, and activation of baroreceptors that stimulate a paradoxical Bezold–Jarisch response. A high level of spinal anesthesia seems to be the most frequent culprit. Regardless, treatment follows standard CPR and ACLS recommendations, including immediate administration of IV epinephrine.

Cardiac Arrest in Pregnancy

The best outcome for mother and fetus is successful maternal resuscitation. Priorities should be high-quality CPR and relief of aortocaval compression. Newly emphasized in the 2020 AHA ACLS guidelines is the importance and prioritization of oxygenation and airway management because of the fact that pregnant patients are more prone to hypoxia. If a pregnant patient with a fundus height at or above the umbilicus has not achieved ROSC with usual resuscitative measures and manual left lateral uterine displacement, it is advised to prepare for perimortem cesarean delivery (PMCD), ideally within 5 minutes after the time of arrest. TTM is recommended for post-resuscitation care with the addition of continuous fetal monitoring.[2]

Debriefing

A new recommendation in the 2020 AHA ACLS guidelines is care for the rescuers. Debriefings and referral for emotional support for lay rescuers, EMS providers, and hospital-based health care providers after a cardiac arrest can be beneficial. Rescuers have been shown to experience anxiety and posttraumatic stress after providing BLS and/or ACLS care. In addition, team debriefing may allow for review of team performance and subsequent improvements in care delivery.[2]

Systems of Care

Health care delivery systems differ significantly between OHCA and IHCA. The AHA discusses both of these distinct systems. A patient at risk of cardiac arrest while in the hospital depends on appropriate surveillance and prevention, prompt recognition and response by a multidisciplinary team, high-quality CPR, prompt defibrillation, and ACLS as needed.[32] The ACLS 2020 updates emphasize post-resuscitation care after ROSC in addition to debriefing and continuous quality improvement.[33] Though recovery from IHCA has improved over the last few decades, there remains considerable variability and room for improvement.

The AHA guidelines recommend the establishment of rapid response teams or medical emergency teams in order to reduce the incidence of cardiac arrest in patients who are at increased risk. These patients should be transferred to a higher-acuity setting, such as an intensive care unit. Discussions with the patient or family members regarding preference for aggressive resuscitation should ideally be conducted before an actual cardiac arrest event. CRM techniques should be used in order to optimize the dynamics among resuscitation team members. These include a designated resuscitation team with predetermined roles and communication strategies and a plan for debriefing after an event.

In 2015 the National Academy of Medicine (formerly the Institute of Medicine) released a report titled "Strategies to Improve Cardiac Arrest Survival: A Time to Act." This report noted the significant morbidity associated with cardiac arrest and the need to improve outcomes.[34,35] The report introduced eight recommendations to improve resuscitative practices: (1) robust data collection and dissemination, (2) improved public response, (3) enhanced EMS capability, (4) updated national accreditation standards, (5) continuous quality improvement, (6) increased research funding in

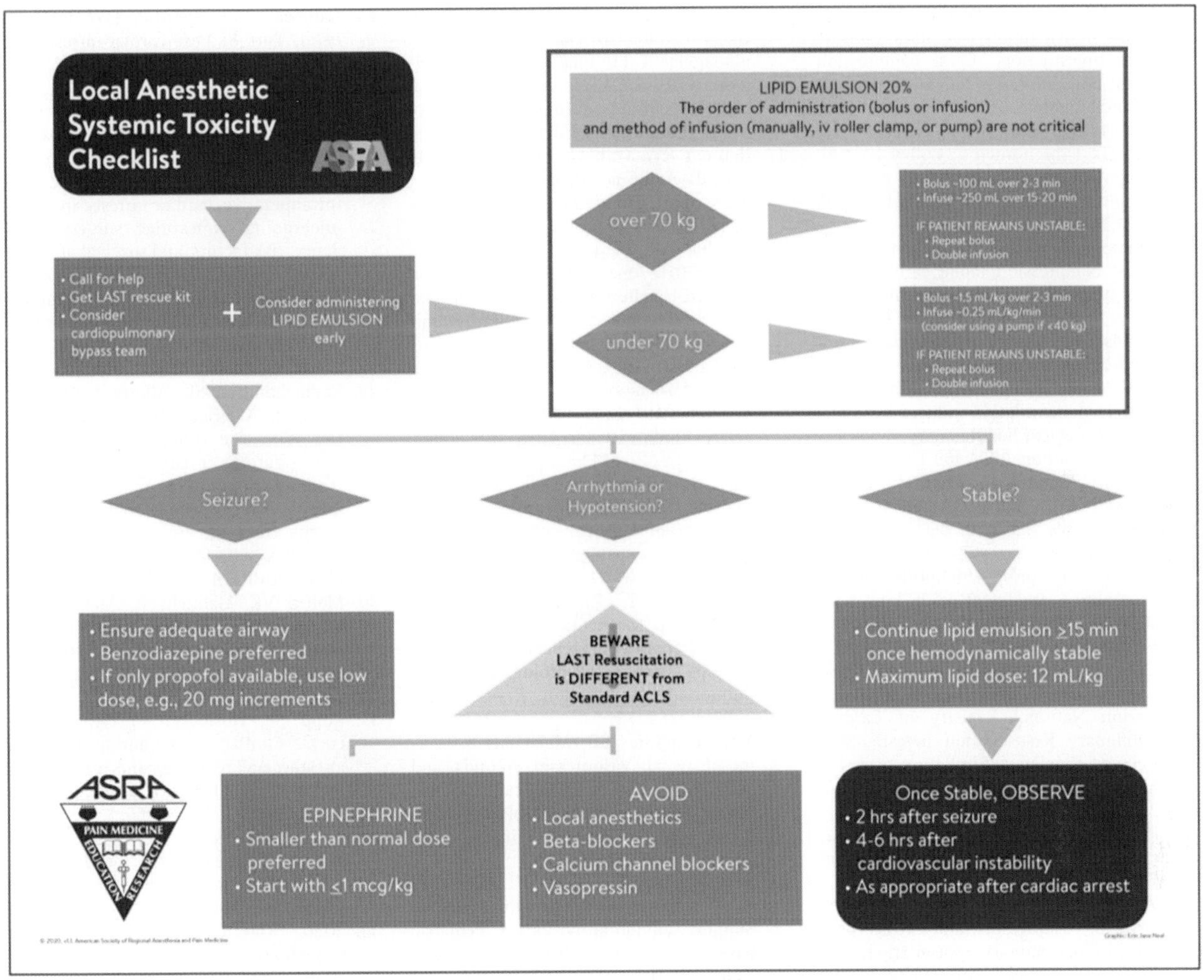

Fig. 45.12 American Society of Regional Anesthesia and Pain Medicine Local Anesthetic Systemic Toxicity Checklist: 2020 version. (Copyright 2020 by the American Society of Regional Anesthesia and Pain Medicine.)

resuscitative science, (7) increased speed in adopting existing strategies, and (8) establishment of a new nationwide cardiac arrest collaborative. The AHA has responded to this call to action by announcing commitments to improve systems of care, resuscitative research, and creation of a national cardiac arrest collaborative.[36]

REFERENCES

1. Andersen LW, Holmberg MJ, Berg KM, Donnino MW, Granfeldt A. In-Hospital cardiac arrest: A review. *JAMA.* 2019;321:1200–1210.
2. Merchant RM, Topjian AA, Panchal AR, et al. Adult Basic and Advanced Life Support, Pediatric Basic and Advanced Life Support, Neonatal Life Support, Resuscitation Education Science, and Systems of Care Writing Groups: Part 1: Executive summary: 2020 American Heart Association Guidelines for Cardiopulmonary Resuscitation and Emergency Cardiovascular Care. *Circulation.* 2020;142:S337–S357.
3. Neumar RW, Shuster M, Callaway CW, et al. Part 1: Executive summary: 2015 American Heart Association guidelines update for cardiopulmonary resuscitation and emergency cardiovascular care. *Circulation.* 2015;132: S315–S367.
4. American Heart Association. CPR ECC Guidelines. http://eccguidelines.heart.org
5. Olasveengen TM, Mancini ME, Perkins GD, et al. Adult Basic Life Support Collaborators: Adult Basic Life Support: 2020 International Consensus on Cardiopulmonary Resuscitation and Emergency Cardiovascular Care Science With Treatment Recommendations. *Circulation.* 2020;142: S41–S91.

VI

6. Idris AH, Guffey D, Pepe PE, Brown SP, et al. Resuscitation Outcomes Consortium Investigators: Chest compression rates and survival following out-of-hospital cardiac arrest. *Crit Care Med.* 2015;43:840–848.

7. Rea TD, Fahrenbruch C, Culley L, et al. CPR with chest compression alone or with rescue breathing. *N Engl J Med.* 2010;363:423–433.

8. Dumas F, Rea TD, Fahrenbruch C, et al. Chest compression alone cardiopulmonary resuscitation is associated with better long-term survival compared with standard cardiopulmonary resuscitation. *Circulation.* 2013;127:435–441.

9. Aufderheide TP, Sigurdsson G, Pirrallo RG, et al. Hyperventilation-induced hypotension during cardiopulmonary resuscitation. *Circulation.* 2004;109:1960–1965.

10. Patel KK, Spertus JA, Khariton Y, Tang Y, Curtis LH, Chan PS. American Heart Association's Get With the Guidelines-Resuscitation Investigators: Association between prompt defibrillation and epinephrine treatment with long-term survival after in-hospital cardiac arrest. *Circulation.* 2018;137:2041–2051.

11. Chan PS, Krumholz HM, Nichol G, Nallamothu BK. American Heart Association National Registry of Cardiopulmonary Resuscitation Investigators: Delayed time to defibrillation after in-hospital cardiac arrest. *N Engl J Med.* 2008;358:9–17.

12. Panchal AR, Berg KM, Hirsch KG, et al. 2019 American Heart Association Focused Update on Advanced Cardiovascular Life Support: Use of advanced airways, vasopressors, and extracorporeal cardiopulmonary resuscitation during cardiac arrest: An update to the American Heart Association Guidelines for Cardiopulmonary Resuscitation and Emergency Cardiovascular Care. *Circulation.* 2019;140:e881–e894.

13. Murray WB, Foster PA. Crisis resource management among strangers: Principles of organizing a multidisciplinary group for crisis resource management. *J Clin Anesth.* 2000;12:633–638.

14. Sheak KR, Wiebe DJ, Leary M, et al. Quantitative relationship between end-tidal carbon dioxide and CPR quality during both in-hospital and out-of-hospital cardiac arrest. *Resuscitation.* 2015;89:149–154.

15. Link MS, Berkow LC, Kudenchuk PJ, et al. Part 7: Adult advanced cardiovascular life support. *Circulation.* 2015;132:S444–S464.

16. Yeung J, Chilwan M, Field R, Davies R, Gao F, Perkins GD. The impact of airway management on quality of cardiopulmonary resuscitation: An observational study in patients during cardiac arrest. *Resuscitation.* 2014;85:898–904.

17. Neumar RW, Otto CW, Link MS, et al. Part 8: Adult advanced cardiovascular life support. *Circulation.* 2010;122:S729–S767.

18. Panchal AR, Berg KM, Kudenchuk PJ, et al. 2018 American Heart Association Focused Update on advanced cardiovascular life support use of antiarrhythmic drugs during and immediately after cardiac arrest: An update to the American Heart Association Guidelines for Cardiopulmonary Resuscitation and Emergency Cardiovascular Care. *Circulation.* 2018;138:e740–e749.

19. Blyth L, Atkinson P, Gadd K, Lang E. Bedside focused echocardiography as predictor of survival in cardiac arrest patients: A systematic review. *Acad Emerg Med.* 2012;19:1119–1126.

20. Mukoyama T, Kinoshita K, Nagao K, Tanjoh K. Reduced effectiveness of vasopressin in repeated doses for patients undergoing prolonged cardiopulmonary resuscitation. *Resuscitation.* 2009;80:755–761.

21. Mentzelopoulos SD, Malachias S, Chamos C, et al. Vasopressin, steroids, and epinephrine and neurologically favorable survival after in-hospital cardiac arrest: A randomized clinical trial. *JAMA.* 2013;310:270–279.

22. Topjian AA, Raymond TT, Atkins D, et al. Pediatric Basic and Advanced Life Support Collaborators: Part 4: Pediatric basic and advanced life support: 2020 American Heart Association Guidelines for Cardiopulmonary Resuscitation and Emergency Cardiovascular Care. *Circulation.* 2020;142:S469–S523.

23. Duff JP, Topjian AA, Berg MD, et al. 2019 American Heart Association Focused Update on Pediatric Advanced Life Support: An update to the American Heart Association Guidelines for Cardiopulmonary Resuscitation and Emergency Cardiovascular Care. *Circulation.* 2019;140:e904–e914.

24. Tagami T, Tosa R, Omura M, Yokota H, Hirama H. Implementation of the fifth link of the Chain of Survival concept for out-of-hospital cardiac arrest. *Crit Care.* 2012;16:P266.

25. Callaway CW, Donnino MW, Fink EL, et al. Part 8: Post–cardiac arrest care. *Circulation.* 2015;132:S465–S482.

26. Donnino MW, Andersen LW, Berg KM, et al. Temperature management after cardiac arrest. *Circulation.* 2015;132:2448–2456.

27. Goswami S, Brady JE, Jordan DA, Li G. Intraoperative cardiac arrests in adults undergoing noncardiac surgery: Incidence, risk factors, and survival outcome. *Anesthesiology.* 2012;117:1018–1026.

28. Constant A-L, Montlahuc C, Grimaldi D, et al. Predictors of functional outcome after intraoperative cardiac arrest. *Anesthesiology.* 2014;121:482–491.

29. Ramachandran SK, Mhyre J, Kheterpal S, et al. American Heart Association's Get With The Guidelines-Resuscitation Investigators: Predictors of survival from perioperative cardiopulmonary arrests: A retrospective analysis of 2,524 events from the Get With The Guidelines-Resuscitation Registry. *Anesthesiology.* 2013;119:1322–1339.

30. Moitra VK, Gabrielli A, Maccioli GA, O'Connor MF. Anesthesia advanced circulatory life support. *Can J Anaesth.* 2012; 59(6):586–603. doi:10.1007/s12630-012-9699-3.

31. Kopp SL, Horlocker TT, Warner ME, et al. Cardiac arrest during neuraxial anesthesia: Frequency and predisposing factors associated with survival. *Anesth Analg.* 2005;100:855–865.

32. Kronick SL, Kurz MC, Lin S, et al. Welsford Michelle: Part 4: Systems of care and continuous quality improvement. *Circulation.* 2015;132:S397–S413.

33. 2020 American Heart Association Guidelines for Cardiopulmonary Resuscitation and Emergency Cardiovascular Care. Part 7: Systems of care. https://cpr.heart.org/en/resuscitation-science/cpr-and-ecc-guidelines/systems-of-care.

34. NASEM. *Treatment of Cardiac Arrest*: National Academy Press; 2015.

35. Becker LB, Aufderheide TP, Graham R. Strategies to improve survival from cardiac arrest: A report from the Institute of Medicine. *JAMA.* 2015;314:223–224.

36. Neumar RW, Eigel B, Callaway CW, et al. American Heart Association: American Heart Association response to the 2015 Institute of Medicine Report on Strategies to Improve Cardiac Arrest Survival. *Circulation.* 2015;132:1049–1070.

46 QUALITY AND PATIENT SAFETY IN ANESTHESIA CARE

Avery Tung

INTRODUCTION

Clinical anesthesia practice is often considered a model for quality and safety in medicine. In 1999 the Institute of Medicine report, "To Err Is Human" specifically identified anesthesia as "an area in which very impressive improvements in safety have been made."[1] Such attention to a specialty comprising approximately 5% of U.S. physicians highlights the many contributions to perioperative quality and safety generated by the specialty of anesthesia. Although unadjusted anesthesia-specific mortality has remained relatively constant for the last several decades,[2] anesthesia providers are also able to care for increasingly older patients with more comorbidities than previously. The principles by which anesthesiologists transformed the inherently dangerous task of blunting human responses to pain and controlling vital life-support functions into a safe and almost routine occurrence are important elements of the anesthesia toolbox and should be familiar to all practicing anesthesia providers.

This chapter reviews the history of anesthesia quality and safety, identifies key approaches and strategies for improvement not only in anesthesia but also in medical specialties, and examines current and future challenges in anesthesia-related quality and safety.

DEFINITIONS: QUALITY VERSUS SAFETY

Quality and safety are related but not identical terms. Safety refers to a lack of harm and focuses on avoiding adverse events. If patient injury is avoided, then the process can be considered safe regardless of other considerations. In contrast, quality refers to the optimal performance of a task, which is multidimensional and may refer to outcome, efficiency, cost, satisfaction, or some other metric of performance in addition to avoiding injury.

It is easy to see how quality and safety do not always overlap. As an example, a process can always be made incrementally safer by installing an additional check or adding extra equipment. In anesthesia practice, for example, an anesthesia provider is arguably not fully safe unless a fiber-optic scope is present in the operating room to facilitate difficult airway management. Another extreme example is having a second (or third) anesthesia provider in the room for the entire case. Clearly, these approaches make anesthesia safer but do not necessarily represent more quality because of their poor risk/reward balance. In contrast, higher-quality care involves an "optimization" element. If a process is changed to produce faster room turnaround, better patient satisfaction, or a shorter length of stay, for example, it may represent higher quality but not necessarily better safety.

In anesthesia practice an example of a strategy that improves both quality and safety is the use of ultrasound to place central lines. By reducing the incidence of carotid puncture,[3] ultrasound clearly improves safety. By reducing the time to successful insertion (and the number of misses), most would agree that ultrasound improves quality as well (some might argue that the additional cost of ultrasound technology mitigates that improvement). Historically, advances in anesthesia performance have affected both quality and safety.

SPECIFIC APPROACHES TO ANESTHESIA SAFETY

Learning From Experience

Because the mechanisms by which most anesthetics exert their effects are not fully understood, and because many intraoperative states (one-lung ventilation, muscle relaxation, cardiopulmonary bypass) are not part of normal human activity, a large component of anesthesia safety is derived from a history of empiric observation and experience. Driven by the goal of reducing perioperative and anesthesia-specific mortality during the early years of anesthesia practice, anesthesia providers have, over time systematically, accumulated an experience base of adverse events. Emery Rovenstine's case series of nine cardiac arrests, published in 1951,[4] is an example of this empiric approach to safety. Although he offered no definitive solutions, practical observations (diagnosing shock versus cardiac standstill can be difficult) allowed anesthesia providers to incrementally and empirically improve anesthesia safety.

Beecher and Todd's exhaustive 1954 study of anesthesia-associated deaths in 10 centers over 4 years is another example of the empiric approach to anesthesia safety.[5] Beecher and Todd tracked the outcomes of 599,548 anesthetics and identified 7977 deaths (more than 1 in 100) and cataloged the causes as from patient disease, surgical error, or anesthesia. Their observation that patients who received neuromuscular blocking drugs during their anesthetic were more likely to have an adverse event remains true today.[6]

Other examples of empirically derived anesthesia safety observations include the surprising difficulty in detecting esophageal intubation (or arterial desaturation), the tendency of some anesthetics (e.g., desflurane) to trigger hypertension and tachycardia,[7] the dangers of circuit disconnection, and the potential for delivery of a hypoxic gas mixture. In all of these the anesthesia approach has been to identify and describe the events, determine how they might occur in clinical practice, develop and test countermeasures, and disseminate the results through technical improvements or education. Taken together, observations such as these have led to reductions in anesthesia-related mortality, with current estimates ranging from 1:250,000 for healthy patients[8] to 1:1500 for those with complex medical problems.[2]

In addition to empiric observations about how best to prevent adverse events related to anesthesia administration, anesthesiologists have evaluated safety issues related to provider performance and how humans interact with the anesthesia delivery system. As in aviation, the human–anesthesia machine interface has been designed specifically to reduce inadvertent errors. In the same way that levers in an airplane for landing gear and flap control have a knob shaped like a wheel and a flap, for example, the knob on an anesthesia machine for oxygen gas flow is shaped differently from knobs controlling air and nitrous oxide and are always located on the right. Interestingly, some newer-generation anesthesia workstations do not have separate physical knobs for controlling individual gases; instead, they allow direct input of total gas flow and inspired oxygen concentration (also see Chapter 15). Similarly, the potentially dangerous delivery of hypoxic gas mixtures is prevented by "linking" the oxygen and nitrous oxide flow controls so that oxygen is always present in fresh gas flow. Nonuniversal connectors to ensure that oxygen is being delivered through the oxygen flowmeter and an oxygen analyzer to serve as a final check on the delivered gas mixture are other examples of safety mechanisms designed to avoid the inadvertent delivery of a hypoxic gas mixture.

Even though adverse events resulting from failure of mechanical ventilation or inadvertent hypoxic gas delivery have almost been eradicated in anesthesia, this process of empiric observation, event detection, risk recognition, and countermeasure development continues today. More recent examples of events recognized from empiric observation include the dangers of anemia during spine surgery (also see Chapter 32),[9] hypotension in the sitting position (also see Chapter 19),[10] or the role of fibrinogen in coagulopathy during maternal hemorrhage (also see Chapter 33).[11]

Adoption of Specialty-Wide Standards

Because anesthesia is normally administered in conjunction with therapeutic or diagnostic procedures, identifying adverse outcomes attributable specifically to the anesthesia component is challenging. An explicit goal of Beecher and Todd was to define "the extent of the responsibility which must be borne by anesthesia for failure in the care of the surgical patient."[5] Because adverse events clearly attributed to anesthesia are rare, promulgating appropriate countermeasures across the specialty is difficult. Nevertheless, anesthesia was the first medical specialty to embrace universally applicable standards, developing and disseminating a set of monitoring recommendations with the goal of reducing anesthesia-related adverse events.[12] These standards were developed from a database of adverse events and included continuous anesthesiologist presence and vital sign monitoring, including blood pressure, heart rate, electrocardiogram (ECG), and breathing system oxygen concentration[12] (Box 46.1).

Although not evidence-based at the time, this monitoring paradigm was declared an intraoperative monitoring standard by the American Society of Anesthesiologists (ASA) 2 months later and has remained one of only three practice standards endorsed by the ASA (the other two being standards for preoperative and postoperative care: https://www.asahq.org/standards-and-guidelines). Since their adoption in 1987, conclusive evidence for the efficacy of these standards has remained elusive, but retrospective observations and clinical experience have suggested benefit. In a 1989 follow-up study the authors of the monitoring standards published a case series of 11 major intraoperative accidents attributable to anesthesia from 1976 to 1988 but found that only one occurred after universal adoption of the monitoring standards.[13] Observations from the ASA Closed Claims Project database also suggest a reduction in the number of claims for death or permanent brain damage during that period.[14]

Whether monitoring standards, better anesthesia training, or (possibly) new technology were responsible for a perceived reduction in adverse events, the willingness of anesthesia providers as a group to adopt practice standards remains an approach almost unique to anesthesiology and an example of the priority anesthesia providers place on eliminating perioperative adverse events.

Patient Safety-Focused Programs

A third element characteristic of the anesthesia approach to patient safety is the formation of patient safety–focused societies. Existing only for the promulgation of safety, these societies play an important role in identifying and disseminating quality and safety lessons to the anesthesia community.

One example is the Anesthesia Patient Safety Foundation (APSF), an independent nonprofit corporation begun in 1985 with the vision "that no patient shall be harmed by anesthesia." Supported by the ASA and corporate sponsors, APSF members include anesthesiologists, nurse anesthetists, manufacturers of equipment and drugs, engineers, and insurers.

The clinical impact of the APSF has been immense. The APSF newsletter, published four times a year (http://apsf.org/resources.php), is dedicated solely to safety and has become one of the most widely circulated anesthesia publications in the world. Identifying aspects of anesthesia practice with potential for adverse events, the APSF newsletter has highlighted diverse issues such as the anesthesia machine checkout, opioid-induced respiratory depression, residual neuromuscular blockade, postoperative visual loss, and emergency manual use. Instructional videos, research grants, and other special conferences are also part of the APSF effort to promote safety.

A second entity with a unique approach to safety is the ASA Closed Claims Project.[14] Operating in cooperation with malpractice lawyers, the Closed Claims Project group reviews data from settled anesthesia lawsuits to identify anesthesia safety concerns that may be amenable to targeted efforts. In a series of academic publications since 1988 and continuing into the present the Closed Claims Project has investigated a wide range of topics (Table 46.1) and focused on rare events difficult to study systematically. Although such analyses cannot estimate incidences, they provide a wealth of descriptive information that has helped anesthesia providers address patient safety issues.[13,15-19] Among these are the recognition that listening to the chest may not be a reliable method of detecting esophageal intubation[14] and that a common factor in adverse outcomes caused by massive hemorrhage is late recognition.[16]

> **Box 46.1** Anesthesia Monitoring Standards Proposed in 1986
>
> - An anesthesiologist should be present in the operating room
> - Arterial blood pressure and heart rate should be monitored at least every 5 minutes where not clinically impractical
> - Electrocardiogram shall be continuously displayed during anesthesia
> - Ventilation and circulation shall be continuously monitored during anesthesia
> - A method for monitoring breathing system disconnect shall be used in every general anesthetic
> - The oxygen concentration in the breathing circuit should be measured with an oxygen analyzer
> - During every administration of general anesthesia, temperature should be measured
>
> From Eichhorn JH, Cooper JB, Cullen DJ, et al. Standards for patient monitoring during anesthesia at Harvard Medical School. JAMA. 1986;256:1017-1020.

Table 46.1	Noteworthy Closed Claims Project Observations		
Year	**Title**	**No. of Claims**	**Notable Finding(s)**
1988	Cardiac arrest during spinal anesthesia[17]	14	• Bradycardia was the most common presenting symptom with hypotension as the second • Epinephrine was not given until 8 minutes (mean) after onset of asystole
1990	Adverse respiratory events in anesthesia[15]	522	• Death/brain damage occurred in 85% of cases • In 48% of esophageal intubations auscultation of breath sounds was performed and documented
1999	Nerve injury associated with anesthesia[18]	670	• Ulnar nerve injuries were most frequent, were associated with general anesthesia, and were predominantly in men
2006	Injury associated with monitored anesthesia care[19]	121	• Monitored anesthesia care claims involved older and sicker patients than general anesthesia claims • Respiratory depression caused by sedative/opioid administration was the most common mechanism of damage (21%) • Electrocautery and oxygen was a recognized mechanism in 17%
2014	Massive hemorrhage[16]	3211	• 30% of claims involved obstetrics, and thoracic/lumbar spine procedures were also overrepresented • Recognition and initiation of transfusion therapy were commonly delayed
2015	Postoperative opioid-induced respiratory depression[20]	357	• 88% of events occurred within 24 hr of surgery, and somnolence was noted in 62% before the event
2017	Situational awareness errors[21]	266	• Anesthesiologist situational awareness errors contributed to 74% of death/brain damage claims • Respiratory system events were more likely to have situational issues (56%)
2019	Difficult tracheal intubation[20,22]	195	• Preoperative predictors were present in 76% of cases, inappropriate airway management occurred in 73%, and surgical airway access was delayed in 39%

The Anesthesia Quality Institute (AQI) is a third patient safety–focused group (www.aqihq.org). Begun in 2008 and sponsored by the ASA, the goal of the AQI was "to be the primary source of information for quality improvement in the clinical practice of anesthesiology." AQI administers and supports an Anesthesia Incident Reporting System (AIRS) and the National Anesthesia Clinical Outcomes Registry (NACOR), which works to identify relevant quality metrics and allows anesthesiologists to report quality metrics as part of merit-based incentive systems. The Multicenter Perioperative Outcomes Group (MPOG) serves a similar function, receiving electronic health systems information from more than 75 hospitals and generating provider-level feedback on both process and outcome metrics (an example of the former is administration of two antiemetics for high-risk patients, and an example of the latter is postoperative acute kidney injury).

FROM SAFETY TO QUALITY: MAKING ANESTHESIA BOTH SAFER AND BETTER

Although most observers believe anesthesia care to be safer today than 50 years ago, whether the quality of anesthesia care has also improved is less clear. Anesthesia quality involves optimization of multiple parameters, including (but not limited to) safety, efficiency, cost, patient comfort, and satisfaction. Technically, first-case start and turnover times can thus represent quality.

Aspects of anesthesia quality related to clinical care delivery can be surprisingly difficult to measure. Because perioperative care is inherently multidisciplinary, identifying the contribution of anesthesia care relative to surgical or perioperative nursing care is challenging. If a patient goes home a day sooner after a colectomy, for example, determining whether that improvement is the result of anesthesia, surgery, or hospital care is difficult.

More than likely, this type of improvement is a result of all disciplines working together.

Process Measures

A major obstacle to anesthesia quality is a clear understanding of how anesthetic interventions affect patient outcomes. Because much of the patient's postoperative course lies outside the operating room, understanding how a patient's clinical course is affected by alterations in anesthesia care has been historically challenging. Early attempts to improve anesthesia quality thus focused on perioperative processes (such as intraoperative glucose levels) rather than outcomes (such as surgical site infections). The United States Surgical Care Improvement Project (SCIP) was conducted by the Centers for Medicare & Medicaid Services from 2006 to 2015 as a national test of this approach. By incentivizing the public reporting of hospital performance on measures such as administering antibiotics in a timely fashion and perioperative administration of perioperative β-adrenergic blockers, policymakers hoped to improve care quality. Unfortunately, although performance on nearly all SCIP process measures improved over the project duration, outcomes[23,24] failed to improve. In addition, some process measures such as preoperative β-adrenergic blockers were recognized as harmful,[25] and several others were rescinded because of concern for adverse outcomes. Among these were how often β-adrenergic blockers were given to patients within 24 hours of admission for myocardial infarction (increases hypotension)[26] and verifying that antibiotics were given within 4 hours of an emergency room visit for pneumonia (leads to inappropriate antibiotic use).[27]

Why implementation of a suite of process measures, all with literature support, did not clearly improve patient outcomes remains a mystery. Clearly, improving quality by mandating specific processes of care is not straightforward and has led quality experts to be reluctant to embrace process measures alone as a method of assessing clinical care.

Structural Measures

The quality of care can also be estimated by the presence or absence of structural elements relevant to quality care. Structure refers to specific organizational features considered to be integral to the provision of high-quality care. If present, such features then suggest that the clinical care is of high quality.

Examples of structural elements that fit this definition include the ready availability of diagnostic radiologic testing, having physicians on call for emergencies, implementing an electronic medical record, and mandating a dedicated intensivist for all critical care units. The presence of an active quality improvement program is also considered a structural feature of high-quality care. Although structural quality is relatively invisible to trainees, other structural examples include hospital rules governing nurse–patient ratios, timely availability of obstetric anesthesia specialists, protocols for hand hygiene, and availability of personal protective equipment.

Although structural measures are generally easy to measure, the link between structure and improved outcomes is often difficult to discern. The availability of in-house critical care attendings at night, for example, is intuitively reasonable and would be an easy structural metric to measure. However, more than one study[28,29] suggests that hospitals that have implemented an in-house night-call system might not clearly see improvements in outcomes.

Outcome Measures

One logical consequence of an inability to identify clinically relevant process measures is to focus instead on outcomes. Logically, the considerable practice variability in anesthesia practice[30,31] should translate into some variability in perioperative outcomes. In principle, by identifying "bright spot" institutions that have better outcomes, the corresponding best practices can be identified and disseminated. Although NACOR is not yet mature enough to allow outcome analysis, surgical databases are approaching that goal. The Society of Thoracic Surgeons (STS) Adult Cardiac Surgery Database is perhaps the best example, capturing data from more than 90% of all cardiac procedures in the United States.[32] Other databases include the National Surgical Quality Improvement Program (NSQIP) and National Inpatient Sample (NIS). Because sufficiently complete data for outcome reporting have historically not been available, few hospitals have routinely made outcome data available to their clinical care staff. In addition, outcome reporting for anesthesia providers can be challenging because different anesthesia subspecialties may have different rates of adverse outcomes such as acute kidney injury or reintubation.

Difficulties in collecting and analyzing intraoperative data are likely to diminish as health care records move to electronic form. In particular, the increasing use of electronic health records for intraoperative management has improved the ability of anesthesia providers to track their performance on process measures accessible to electronic analysis. An example is the Multispecialty Perioperative Outcomes Group (MPOG). MPOG is a privately run consortium of >80 institutions that defines, collects, and analyzes intraoperative (and selected postoperative) outcomes. MPOG members receive monthly feedback reports on metrics selected by their individual practices (Fig. 46.1 provides an example). Examples of process metrics include train-of-four measurement after neuromuscular blockade reversal and treatment for glucose levels >200 mg/dL. Outcome measures include postoperative acute kidney injury and postoperative nausea and vomiting. MPOG reports not only provide information but also a

VI

Below is your new MPOG Quality performance report. For a case-by-case breakdown of each measure's result, click on the graph's label and you will be taken to our reporting website (login required).

If you have any questions, please read our FAQ or send them to QIChampion@example.org. Thank you for your participation in MPOG Quality.

Sincerely,
The MPOG Team

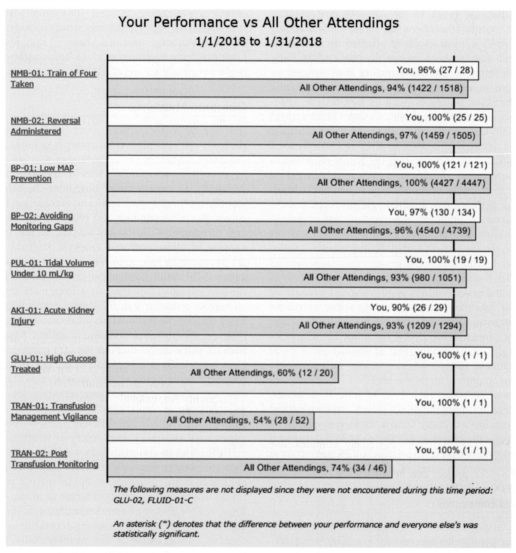

Fig. 46.1 Example of a feedback report generated by the MPOG data registry.

comparison to other practitioners and a link to allow the provider to review specific cases that passed or failed the measure. This last aspect is particularly important, as it allows providers to better integrate measure performance into their daily workflow and counters arguments that collected data are not accurate.

Outcome reporting initially seems straightforward and gives individuals or institutions a benchmark for measuring future performance. But accurately comparing outcomes between individuals or institutions requires some way to adjust for patient conditions unrelated to the anesthesia or surgical (or hospital) care. This "risk adjustment" can be extremely difficult, as different adjustment algorithms may produce different results,[33] algorithms may be vulnerable to "gaming" via favorable patient selection or inclusion of comorbidities,[34] the accuracy of data may be suspect,[3] and the adjustment algorithm itself may not be consistent from year to year.

Current evidence is mixed with regard to whether outcome reporting improves outcomes. Two recent studies[35,36] suggest that knowing one's outcomes may not by itself drive improvement. In addition, should a "bright spot" institution with unusually good outcomes be recognized, identifying and disseminating lessons from that institution would likely involve developing a set of process measures, which (as the SCIP program demonstrates) may only have limited effectiveness if not properly contextualized. Nevertheless, the use of both process and outcome measures is key to quality improvement. Without some method for measuring the incidence of targeted processes or outcomes, it is difficult to know whether interventions are effective. Yet as SCIP and other large-scale quality reporting programs suggest, measurement alone is inadequate. Current experience indicates that neither process nor outcome measurement automatically leads to improved quality and that truly improving performance in any domain requires sustained, focused effort.

TOOLS FOR IMPROVING LOCAL OUTCOMES

In addition to empiric observation and large database approaches, improvements in quality and safety at the individual hospital level occur continuously and may be driven by individuals, departments, or hospitals. This section discusses tools used at the organizational level for quality improvement.

Structured Quality Improvement Approaches: FADE, PDSA, and DMAIC

Because clinical care can be extremely complex and multifaceted, knowing where or how to begin a quality improvement project can be difficult. The acronyms FADE, PDSA, and DMAIC refer to commonly used blueprints for initiating and executing a quality improvement project. Although the letters are different, all three apply the same basic model: evaluate, implement, measure.

FADE stands for focus/analyze/develop/execute-evaluate. As the words suggest, one should first focus on the process to be improved, analyze data to establish root causes and baseline performance, use the data to develop an action plan, then execute the plan and evaluate the result.

PDSA stands for plan/do/study/act. As one might imagine, the general gist of a PDSA is similar to FADE. DMAIC stands for define/measure/analyze/improve/control, which has a similar meaning.

Because identifying, intervening, and assessing the outcome are core aspects of the anesthesia skill set, anesthesiologists are likely familiar with the general structure of a FADE or PDSA quality improvement program. After

all, the everyday act of titrating an anesthetic requires that a situational assessment be made, the anesthetic level be adjusted, and the outcome reviewed. However, creating lasting change can be difficult. A common trap in developing a quality improvement program is to identify an imperfect step and apply a remedy to that specific step without understanding or addressing how that step came to be imperfect. A plan to improve delivery of blood products to the operating room, for example, may be ineffective if the process for ordering blood is not also addressed (also see Chapter 25). Another often-missed aspect of quality improvement is the implementation of a change without measuring the result of that change. If an intraoperative handoff tool is implemented, for example, but no improvement in handoff errors results, the reason for that discrepancy should be identified. Attention to such details will help optimize the results of any quality improvement project.

Regardless of the specific blueprint used to address a clinical performance issue, some method is needed to track performance over time to determine whether interventions are successful. A run chart is the most widely used method for doing so. Run charts depict performance on a specific metric (usually on the Y axis) and time (usually on the X axis) to graphically represent performance over time. Such charts are useful to identify patterns or trends in performance. A run chart might be used, for example, to better understand whether dental injuries during anesthesia are more likely in months when new anesthesia residents start clinical training. Control charts are run charts that include upper and lower performance limits/targets and can be helpful for visually estimating whether a process is "in control" or whether it needs adjustment. An example of a run chart is shown in Fig. 46.2. For anesthesia providers, an important addition to the run chart should be links to specific cases that passed or failed the measure, as merely knowing the trend in performance without understanding why that trend exists will not lead to improvement.

Multidisciplinary Process Improvement: Root Cause Analysis, "Never Events," and Failure Mode Effects Analysis

Root cause analysis (RCA) was developed by manufacturers in the 1950s to better understand industrial events. The goal is, as the title suggests, to identify the primary, or "root," cause of the problem under analysis. One of the first users of this technique was Toyota, who famously used the "5 whys" technique. By continually asking "why" during the investigation of a breakdown or undesired event, quality personnel can drill down layer by layer to hopefully uncover progressively more fundamental causes.

When applied in medicine, the root cause process begins with a multidisciplinary group assembled to

VI

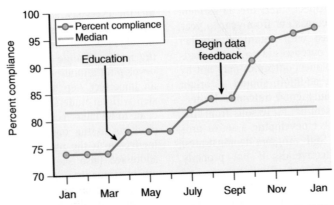

Fig. 46.2 Example of a run chart. The performance measure on the Y axis is compliance with timing of preoperative antibiotics. The X axis represents time in months. Arrows indicate the time of two interventions that were performed. (Figure from Varughese AM, Buck DW, Lane-Fall MB, et al. Quality improvement in anesthesia practice and patient safety. In Gropper M, ed. Miller's anesthesia, 9th ed. Elsevier, 2020: Figure 5.2, Amsterdam, NL.)

evaluate every step of the process that resulted in the event in question. Attention is focused strictly on system processes and not on individual provider behavior. A causal factor chart is often created in skeleton form, with details added as each specialty adds its expertise. Fig. 46.3 depicts a sample factor chart for an intraoperative transfusion reaction[37] (also see Chapter 25).

Although such charts are usually read from left to right, they may often be created from right to left, starting with the event and using logic and time information to add relevant causal factors. Note also that the blood bank, hospital engineering, preoperative nursing, anesthesia, and surgery are all involved in this particular event, underscoring the multidisciplinary nature of properly performed RCAs.

An RCA is mandated by The Joint Commission, a U.S.-based nonprofit organization that accredits health care organizations, whenever an accredited hospital experiences one of several prespecified types of adverse events. Such events are called "sentinel" because they expose a dangerous "gap" in care and signal the need for immediate investigation and response. A list of all Joint Commission–designated events can be accessed at their website (https://www.jointcommission.org/sentinel_event.aspx). Sentinel events relevant to the perioperative period are listed in Box 46.2.

The Joint Commission also explicitly defines events that do NOT require focused reporting and review. These include any near-miss, medication errors that do NOT result in death or functional loss, minor hemolysis, or death or functional loss after leaving against medical advice.

The Joint Commission requires (as a condition of accreditation) that hospitals respond to such events within 45 days by reporting them to the Joint Commission, performing an RCA, and developing an action plan to identify strategies the hospital intends to implement to reduce the risk of similar events in the future. Such a plan must include the action to be taken, who will implement, a timeline for implementation, and strategies for measuring the result and sustaining the changes. Although reporting to The Joint Commission is voluntary, identifying and responding to such events is a key component of accreditation visits.

Other patient safety organizations have suggested modifications to The Joint Commission list. The National Quality Forum (NQF), for example, endorses a large list

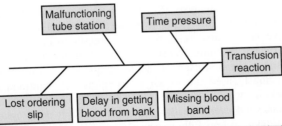

Fig. 46.3 Sample causal factor chart. (From Tung A. Sentinel events and how to learn from them. Int Anesthesiol Clin. 2014;52:53–68.)

> **Box 46.2   Sentinel Events Related to the Perioperative Period as Defined by The Joint Commission, 2015**
>
> - Hemolytic transfusion reaction
> - Invasive procedure on the wrong patient, wrong site, or wrong procedure
> - Prolonged fluoroscopy >1500 RADs
> - Fire; flame; or unanticipated smoke, heat, or flashes during an episode of patient care
> - Any intrapartum maternal death or severe morbidity
>
> *RADS,* Radiation absorbed dose units.

of "serious reportable events" (NQF: Serious Reportable Events: qualityforum.org). In addition to The Joint Commission events, the NQF list adds "intraoperative death in an ASA class I patient," death/disability from the irretrievable loss of an irreplaceable biologic specimen, or death from electric shock.

Although intuitively reasonable, the real-world effectiveness of RCA can be variable.[38] Adverse events and their investigations are often emotionally charged, and meetings to determine the cause can be limited by blame-oriented analysis (which leads to relatively weak "blame and train" remedies). Studies of action plans and implementations suggest that relatively few of these actively target true "root" causes.[39] Inadequate RCA may result from lack of time, inadequate resources, and even disagreement among reviewers with respect to "root" causes.[40] Even when appropriate action plans are created, insufficient resources may prevent effective implementation.

Nevertheless, when done properly, RCA can be tremendously useful in reducing the likelihood of adverse events. In addition to being a vehicle for local practice changes, The Joint Commission Sentinel Event program generates a series of sentinel event bulletins that warn clinicians of potential issues (https://www.jointcommission.org/resources/patient-safety-topics/sentinel-event/sentinel-event-alert-newsletters/). To date, this program has resulted in more than 50 events, including several relevant to anesthesia such as deaths resulting from concentrated potassium chloride solutions, ventilator-related deaths, medical gas mix-ups, transfusion errors, disruptive behavior, and magnetic resonance imaging accidents. These well-researched reports include case descriptions and analysis, including the Manufacturer and User Facility Device Experience (MAUDE) database (https://www.accessdata.fda.gov/scripts/cdrh/cfdocs/cfmaude/search.cfm).

A major drawback to the RCA process is its retrospective nature. By definition, process flaws in care delivery are not addressed until the event actually occurs and a patient is harmed. To prospectively identify process flaws, the failure mode effects analysis (FMEA) process has been adapted from industry to prospectively identify and neutralize areas of vulnerability.

An FMEA is a resource-intensive, comprehensive analysis of a specific process, with the goal of identifying all the potential ways that it can fail. A process to identify and record patient allergies, for example, might fail if the interviewer is unable to accurately identify allergies, if the documentation form is difficult to read or inaccessible, or if medications sound alike. Other sources for potential failure modes include sentinel event alerts, Institute for Safe Medication Practices information, and Food and Drug Administration (FDA) databases and advisories.

It is easy to see that an FMEA analysis of even a straightforward process can be extremely time consuming. In addition, once the relevant failure modes are identified,

quality champions may struggle to implement effective change, in part because no bad event has yet occurred. As a result, FMEA analyses should be reserved for large-volume, high-risk processes for which the risk of catastrophic failure is clear.

SUMMARY

Anesthesia providers should routinely strive for the safest and highest-quality care they can deliver. Although safety and quality are related concepts, safety is easier to measure and target because it focuses on adverse events. In contrast, quality is multidimensional and thus more difficult to measure and optimize, as many different outcomes may represent "quality." Because procedures and anesthetic strategies both evolve to meet changing needs, quality and safety in anesthesia are, by definition, a moving target.

Historically, anesthesiologists have led in patient safety by embracing pragmatic approaches to reducing adverse events. Among these are the empiric cataloging and describing of events to identify incidents and risk factors, a recognition that man–machine interface errors can contribute to adverse events, adoption of strategies from other similarly technical fields such as pin indexing to prevent gas source switch errors, and early specialty-wide agreement with respect to practice standards. Organized patient safety–focused organizations within the specialty have also contributed considerably to anesthesia safety by cataloguing, analyzing, and disseminating lessons learned from adverse events. These include the APSF and the ASA Closed Claims Project.

Although anesthesiologists have been focused on patient safety for decades, the tools to focus on care quality have only recently been developed. The availability of specialty registries, such as the STS Adult Cardiac Surgery Database, and of large surgical databases, such as NACOR and NSQIP, have allowed anesthesiologists to better explore how structural, process, and outcome measures are linked. Newer computerized databases such as MPOG offer greater case detail and provider-level feedback. Although no "magic bullet" strategy to quality improvement has yet emerged, process, structure, and outcome are all key elements in any comprehensive quality program.

Finally, multiple tools exist at the departmental and institutional levels for quality improvement. These include blueprints for local quality projects, nationally promulgated sentinel event programs, root cause, and failure mode analyses for adverse events.

Taken together, a wealth of quality and safety tools and approaches are available to anesthesia teams interested in patient safety. With the growth and maturation of large perioperative databases and the potential of electronic intraoperative records to shed light into the perioperative period, even more options will become available to improve both the safety and quality of anesthesia practice.[41]

VI

REFERENCES

1. Kohn KT, Corrigan JM, Donaldson MS. *Committee on Quality Health Care in America*. Washington, DC: Institute of Medicine: National Academy Press; 1999.

2. Lagasse RS. Anesthesia safety: Model or myth? A review of the published literature and analysis of current original data. *Anesthesiology*. 2002;97:1609–1617.

3. Brass P, Hellmich M, Kolodziej L, et al. Ultrasound guidance versus anatomical landmarks for internal jugular vein catheterization. *Cochrane Database Syst Rev*. 2015 Jan 9;1:CD006962.

4. Ament R, Papper EM, Rovenstine EA. Cardiac arrest during anesthesia; a review of cases. *Ann Surg*. 1951;134:220–227.

5. Beecher HK, Todd DP. A study of the deaths associated with anesthesia and surgery: Based on a study of 599, 548 anesthesias in ten institutions 1948-1952, inclusive. *Ann Surg*. 1954;140:2–35.

6. Kirmeier E, Eriksson LI, Lewald H, et al., POPULAR Contributors. Post-anaesthesia pulmonary complications after use of muscle relaxants (POPULAR): A multicentre, prospective observational study. *Lancet Respir Med*. 2019;7:129–140.

7. Ebert TJ, Muzi M. Sympathetic hyperactivity during desflurane anesthesia in healthy volunteers. A comparison with isoflurane. *Anesthesiology*. 1993;79:444–453.

8. Lienhart A, Auroy Y, Péquignot F et al. Survey of anesthesia-related mortality in France *Anesthesiology*. 2006;105:1087-1097.

9. Postoperative Visual Loss Study Group. Risk factors associated with ischemic optic neuropathy after spinal fusion surgery. *Anesthesiology*. 2012;116:15–24.

10. Pohl A, Cullen DJ. Cerebral ischemia during shoulder surgery in the upright position: A case series. *J Clin Anesth*. 2005;17:463–469.

11. Butwick AJ. Postpartum hemorrhage and low fibrinogen levels: The past, present and future. *Int J Obstet Anesth*. 2013;22:87–91.

12. Eichhorn JH, Cooper JB, Cullen DJ, et al. Standards for patient monitoring during anesthesia at Harvard Medical School. *JAMA*. 1986;256:1017–1020.

13. Eichhorn JH. Prevention of intraoperative anesthesia accidents and related severe injury through safety monitoring. *Anesthesiology*. 1989;70:572–577.

14. Lee LA, Domino KB. The Closed Claims Project. Has it influenced anesthetic practice and outcome?. *Anesthesiol Clin North America*. 2002;20:485–501.

15. Caplan RA, Posner KL, Ward RJ, et al. Adverse respiratory events in anesthesia: A Closed Claims analysis. *Anesthesiology*. 1990;72:828–833.

16. Dutton RP, Lee LA, Stephens LS, et al. Massive hemorrhage: A report from the anesthesia Closed Claims Project. *Anesthesiology*. 2014;121:450–458.

17. Caplan RA, Ward RJ, Posner K, et al. Unexpected cardiac arrest during spinal anesthesia: A Closed Claims analysis of predisposing factors. *Anesthesiology*. 1988;68:5–11.

18. Cheney FW, Domino KB, Caplan RA, et al. Nerve injury associated with anesthesia: A Closed Claims analysis. *Anesthesiology*. 1999;90:1062–1069.

19. Bhananker SM, Posner KL, Cheney FW, et al. Injury and liability associated with monitored anesthesia care: A Closed Claims analysis. *Anesthesiology*. 2006;104:228–234.

20. Lee LA, Caplan RA, Stephens LS, et al. Postoperative opioid-induced respiratory depression: A Closed Claims analysis. *Anesthesiology*. 2015;122:659–665.

21. Schulz CM, Burden A, Posner KL, Mincer SL, Steadman R, Wagner KJ, Domino KB. Frequency and Type of Situational Awareness Errors Contributing to Death and Brain Damage: A Closed Claims Analysis. *Anesthesiology*. 2017 Aug;127;2:326-337

22. Joffe AM, Aziz MF, Posner KL, Duggan LV, Mincer SL, Domino KB. Management of Difficult Tracheal Intubation: A Closed Claims Analysis. *Anesthesiology*. 2019 Oct;131;4:818-829.

23. Hawn MT, Vick CC, Richman J, et al. Surgical site infection prevention: Time to move beyond the Surgical Care Improvement Program. *Ann Surg*. 2011;254: 494–499.

24. Hawn MT, Richman JS, Vick CC, et al. Timing of surgical antibiotic prophylaxis and the risk of surgical site infection. *JAMA Surg*. 2013;148:649–657.

25. POISE Study GroupDevereaux PJ, Yang H, Yusuf S, et al. Effects of extended-release metoprolol succinate in patients undergoing non-cardiac surgery (POISE trial): A randomised controlled trial. *Lancet*. 2008;371:1839–1847.

26. Chen ZM, Pan HC, Chen YP. Early intravenous then oral metoprolol in 45,852 patients with acute myocardial infarction: Randomised placebo-controlled trial. *Lancet*. 2005;366:1622–1632.

27. Wachter RM, Flanders SA, Fee C, et al. Public reporting of antibiotic timing in patients with pneumonia: Lessons from a flawed performance measure. *Ann Intern Med*. 2008;149:29–32.

28. Kerlin MP, Small DS, Cooney E, et al. A randomized trial of nighttime physician staffing in an intensive care unit. *N Engl J Med*. 2013;368:2201–2209.

29. Wallace DJ, Angus DC, Barnato AE, et al. Nighttime intensivist staffing and mortality among critically ill patients. *N Engl J Med*. 2012;366:2093–2101.

30. Lilot M, Ehrenfeld JM, Lee C3, Harrington B, et al. Variability in practice and factors predictive of total crystalloid administration during abdominal surgery: Retrospective two-centre analysis. *Br J Anaesth*. 2015;114:767–776.

31. Fleischut PM, Eskreis-Winkler JM, Gaber-Baylis LK, et al. Variability in anesthetic care for total knee arthroplasty: An analysis from the Anesthesia Quality Institute. *Am J Med Qual*. 2015;30: 172–179.

32. Jacobs JP, Shahian DM, Prager RL, et al. Introduction to the STS National Database Series: Outcomes analysis, quality improvement, and patient safety. *Ann Thorac Surg*. 2015 Oct 31 [epub].

33. Shahian DM, Wolf RE, Iezzoni LI, et al. Variability in the measurement of hospital-wide mortality rates. *N Engl J Med*. 2010;363:2530–2539.

34. Cooper AL, Trivedi AN. Fitness memberships and favorable selection in Medicare Advantage plans. *N Engl J Med*. 2012;366:150–157.

35. Etzioni DA, Wasif N, Dueck AC, et al. Association of hospital participation in a surgical outcomes monitoring program with inpatient complications and mortality. *JAMA*. 2015;313:505–511.

36. Osborne NH, Nicholas LH, Ryan AM, et al. Association of hospital participation in a quality reporting program with surgical outcomes and expenditures for Medicare beneficiaries. *JAMA*. 2015;313:496–504.

37. Tung A. Sentinel events and how to learn from them. *Int Anesthesiol Clin*. 2014;52:53–68.

38. Wu AW, Lipshutz AK, Pronovost PJ. Effectiveness and efficiency of root cause analysis in medicine. *JAMA*. 2008;299:685–687.

39. Wallace LM, Spurgeon P, Adams S, et al. Survey evaluation of the National Patient Safety Agency's Root Cause Analysis training programme in England and Wales: Knowledge, beliefs and reported practices. *Qual Saf Health Care*. 2009;18:288–291.

40. Smits M, Janssen J, de Vet R, et al. Analysis of unintended events in hospitals: Inter-rater reliability of constructing causal trees and classifying root causes. *Int J Qual Health Care*. 2009;21:292–300.

41. Methangkool E, Cole DJ, Cannesson M. Progress in patient safety in anesthesia. *JAMA*. 2020;324(24):2485–2486. doi:10.1001/jama.2020.23205.

47 PALLIATIVE CARE

Ann Cai Shah, Sarah Gebauer

INTRODUCTION

Patients with serious illnesses often have an intense burden of symptoms that are poorly treated, such as pain, dyspnea, anxiety, and depression.[1] These patients also have frequent but often unsatisfying interactions with the health care team, often as a result of poor communication.[2] *Palliative care* is "an approach that improves the quality of life of patients and their families facing the problems associated with life-threatening illness, through the prevention and relief of suffering by means of early identification and impeccable assessment and treatment of pain and other problems, physical, psychosocial and spiritual."[3] *Palliative medicine* refers to the medical expertise provided within a palliative care team. Palliative care, with its emphasis on goal setting and symptom management, attempts to improve care for these patients and their families. Many palliative care skills can be used in a variety of settings, and concepts such as shared decision making and a biopsychosocial-spiritual approach should not be reserved only for seriously ill patients.

Modern palliative care started with the hospice movement in the 1960s and has spread to many health systems worldwide. In the United States at least two-thirds of hospitals have palliative care teams,[4] and hospice services are widely available. Despite their common roots, hospice and palliative care are not necessarily interchangeable terms. The meaning of *hospice* and the services offered vary by country, though hospices generally focus on later-stage illnesses. In the United States hospice refers to an insurance benefit for patients with a life expectancy of less than 6 months. *Palliative care* is a more inclusive term that is appropriate "at any age and any stage in a serious illness, and can be provided together with curative treatment."[5] In the past there was a perceived binary choice between aggressive curative treatment and then going onto hospice when those treatments failed. Palliative care now provides a more nuanced picture of the time before hospice, with patients receiving concurrent palliative and

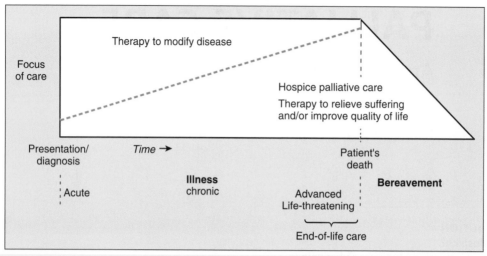

Fig. 47.1 The role of hospice and palliative care during illness and bereavement. (Redrawn from Ferris FD, Balfour HM, Bowen K, et al. A model to guide patient and family care: Based on nationally accepted principles and norms of practice. *J Pain Symptom Manage.* 2002;24:106–123.)

curative treatment with increasing palliative care support if the illness progresses, until hospice services are appropriate (Fig. 47.1).[6] For the purposes of this chapter, palliative care will encompass both palliative and hospice care unless otherwise specified.

Palliative care does not mean giving up, or even providing less aggressive care. It means talking to patients and families, eliciting their values and goals, and making medical recommendations and decisions based on those values and goals. This approach is sometimes referred to as *shared decision making.* It is not uncommon for the palliative care team to advocate for more aggressive treatment, either because it is in line with a patient's wishes and is reasonable medically or because aggressive treatment of specific medical problems can decrease a patient's symptom burden.

Palliative care teams generally approach symptom management by evaluating multiple aspects of a patient's condition, involving both physical and emotional pain. This concept acknowledges that part of the pain a patient feels may be, in part, the result of existential or spiritual suffering. This may take the form of a belief that the person's upcoming death is punishment from a higher power or that the person did not contribute enough to the world. Palliative care specialists attempt to determine what physical or psychosocial factors may be contributing to pain and use medications or the expertise of other team members such as chaplains, social workers, or art therapists to help alleviate a patient's symptoms in a broad sense.

Inpatient palliative care teams *reduce costs* while improving patient care. Medical advances and an aging population have led to an increase in the number of patients with serious illnesses. The beneficiaries using the most Medicare dollars include those in the last year

of life, even though many people say they do not want to die in a hospital. In 2017 benefits to the most costly 5% of members accounted for 41% of Medicare spending.[7] Not only is the care expensive, but patients and families often describe distressing symptoms, psychosocial needs that go unrecognized, and overall poor care.[8] Hospital costs decrease with palliative care consult services. For example, one study showed an average decrease in cost of $15,000 per patient, with similar duration of survival.[9] Cost reduction is not a primary goal of palliative care. Rather, patients who receive palliative care desire fewer interventions and resources. Importantly, palliative care teams do not increase in-hospital mortality rate.[10] In some situations palliative care may even *increase survival*. Patients with lung cancer, for example, lived at least 2 months longer compared with those receiving standard care in several studies.[11] The American Society of Clinical Oncology now recommends that patients with advanced cancer receive palliative care services early in the course of the illness.

What Is Hospice?

In the United States anesthesiologists should work closely with surgeon hospice generally refers to a set of benefits from Medicare or private insurers. More than 50% of all Medicare patient deaths in the United States occur on hospice.[12,13] Hospice care decreases patient symptom burden, increases patient and family satisfaction, and is associated with cost savings, especially for patients with longer durations of hospice use.[14] Hospice provides patients and families with the most help they can receive when caring for a person at home, including the services listed in Fig. 47.2. Contrary to some patients'

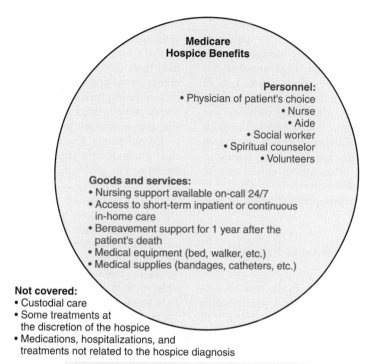

Medicare Hospice Benefits

Personnel:
• Physician of patient's choice
• Nurse
• Aide
• Social worker
• Spiritual counselor
• Volunteers

Goods and services:
• Nursing support available on-call 24/7
• Access to short-term inpatient or continuous in-home care
• Bereavement support for 1 year after the patient's death
• Medical equipment (bed, walker, etc.)
• Medical supplies (bandages, catheters, etc.)

Not covered:
• Custodial care
• Some treatments at the discretion of the hospice
• Medications, hospitalizations, and treatments not related to the hospice diagnosis

Fig. 47.2 Aspects of the Medicare hospice benefits.

beliefs, most hospice services are provided at home, and hospice does not pay for caregivers. The hospice nurses and staff teach and support the family in caring for a seriously ill, dying patient, but the families provide the bulk of the care. Some families may opt to have hospice services provided in a nursing home, though the "custodial care," or care of daily needs such as eating and bathing, provided by the nursing home will often not be covered by the patient's insurance. A few patients will qualify for services at an inpatient hospice facility because of specific intractable symptoms such as pain or vomiting, but usually not for the entire time they are receiving hospice (Fig. 47.3).

Hospice and Palliative Medicine Subspecialty

Hospice and palliative medicine is a board-certified subspecialty that requires a 1-year fellowship for certification. Physicians from 10 medical specialties, including anesthesiology, are eligible, and more than 120 anesthesiologists

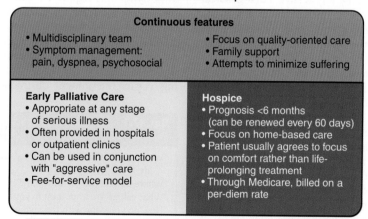

Palliative Care and Hospice

Continuous features
• Multidisciplinary team
• Symptom management: pain, dyspnea, psychosocial
• Focus on quality-oriented care
• Family support
• Attempts to minimize suffering

Early Palliative Care
• Appropriate at any stage of serious illness
• Often provided in hospitals or outpatient clinics
• Can be used in conjunction with "aggressive" care
• Fee-for-service model

Hospice
• Prognosis <6 months (can be renewed every 60 days)
• Focus on home-based care
• Patient usually agrees to focus on comfort rather than life-prolonging treatment
• Through Medicare, billed on a per-diem rate

Fig. 47.3 Features of palliative care and hospice in the United States.

VI

are board certified in hospice and palliative medicine.[15] Board-certified physicians provide specialist palliative care, which includes refractory symptom management and difficult family meetings.[16] Although most anesthesiologists will not go on to be palliative care physicians, all anesthesiologists should have a familiarity with primary palliative care. This includes goals-of-care conversations and perioperative advance directives, in addition to skills in symptom management for seriously ill patients related to issues commonly seen in anesthesiology practice.[17] These skills are important, as anesthesiologists may be the first provider to have these conversations, whether in an intensive care unit (ICU), perioperative arena, or pain management clinic.

Anesthesiologists' Contribution to Palliative Care

Anesthesiologists offer specific skills in the care of seriously ill patients in addition to standard perioperative care. Many elderly (also see Chapter 35) and seriously ill people have surgery,[18] pain issues (also see Chapter 44), or critical illness (also see Chapter 41). Anesthesiologists may interact with palliative and hospice care patients in these settings. Anesthesiologists have expertise in the management of symptoms such as pain and nausea, which are frequent complaints of palliative care patients. Crucially, they also possess insight about the risks to the patient for the entire perioperative course and can add valuable information to conversations with patients and families about goals of care. Pain medicine (also see Chapter 44) and critical care anesthesiologists (also see Chapter 41) offer advanced skills and knowledge that can be invaluable in a palliative care patient's care.

WHAT DO PALLIATIVE CARE TEAMS DO?

Palliative care is an interdisciplinary field involving multiple professionals, including physicians, nurses, social workers, chaplains, and others. Palliative care physicians are experts in symptom management and communication for seriously ill patients and their families. Palliative care nurses, including nurses who provide hospice care, practice symptom management, advanced communication skills, and assessment of the psychosocial and spiritual needs of a patient and family.[19] Social workers address the psychosocial needs of patients and families and may assist with complex discharge needs.[20] Chaplains assist patients and families in identifying and addressing spiritual distress related to serious illness and provide or facilitate appropriate spiritual or religious rituals.[21] Anesthesia pain experts may be involved in advanced pain (also see Chapters 40 and 44) management techniques, and anesthesia critical care specialists are often involved in complex goals-of-care discussions.

Palliative care teams assess and treat the patient's symptoms, discuss goals of care, and assess and treat the patient's and family's psychosocial issues. The palliative care team takes a biopsychosocial-spiritual approach to management and recognizes the interplay between these factors in improving overall patient care. Palliative care teams can either focus on a specific issue of concern to the team or perform a comprehensive assessment.

Consultations generally fall into two broad categories: goals-of-care consults and symptom management consults. For goals-of-care consults, palliative care specialists share information, get a sense of what a patient's goals and values are, and make medical recommendations based on those goals and values. For example, one patient's goal might be to stay out of the hospital and spend time with his or her dogs, and another's might be to live until the birth of a grandchild. Others may have goals like making amends with family members or being able to walk around the house without pain. Palliative care teams also perform an in-depth psychosocial assessment, with questions like those listed in Box 47.1. Talking with patients and families about their understanding of the medical issues, how they want to receive information, and how their home and spiritual lives contribute to their thinking about the medical situation can provide the primary teams with invaluable guidance. These conversations often include shared decision making and helping the patient and family determine a reasonable plan given the many complex factors in every patient's care. Including the patient and family in decision making does not mean offering or agreeing to a plan of care that the medical team believes is harmful or increases suffering, but rather helps create a shared treatment plan that incorporates meaningful goals of care.

Consultations for management of symptoms often focus on making the patient more comfortable and frequently involve management of pain or intractable nausea and vomiting. Symptoms that palliative care teams commonly address are listed in Box 47.2. A number of these symptoms require a sophisticated understanding of the patient's underlying pathophysiology. For example, patients with vomiting may have an abdominal tumor, medication effect, or opioid-induced constipation. Patients determined to have intraabdominal disease affecting the intestinal tract would need to be evaluated for ongoing versus intermittent obstruction and considered for

---

Box 47.1 Common Psychosocial Questions During Palliative Care Consults

"What role, if any, does religion or spirituality play in your life?"

"Where do you live? With whom?"

"What values are important in your life?"

"How do you cope with the changes that are happening?"

"What are your greatest concerns right now?"

Box 47.2 Commonly Assessed Symptoms During a Palliative Care Visit

Insomnia
Dyspnea
Fatigue
Pain
Anxiety
Depression
Nausea and vomiting
Constipation

---

treatment with octreotide or dexamethasone, and possibly a venting gastrotomy tube. Other symptoms close to the end of life, like terminal delirium, may require treatment with large doses of benzodiazepines or even phenobarbital. For patients whose symptoms do not respond to standard approaches, a palliative care consultation should be obtained.

Palliative Care in the Intensive Care Unit

Patients in the surgical ICU who stay more than 7 days have a mortality rate of more than 35%[22] and should receive a palliative care consultation.[23] Although some patients routinely stay in the ICU for specific nursing or monitoring needs after surgery, a significant proportion are treated for a worsening in their condition, and patients and families need to make difficult decisions about the treatment plan. Palliative care providers help patients and families determine goals of care, help resolve conflicts, and provide symptom management to patients in critical care units (Box 47.3).[24] Despite palliative care's perceived emphasis on comfort over cure, there is *no increased mortality rate* in patients in the ICU when palliative care teams are introduced (also see Chapter 41).

Communication among patients, families, and providers can be especially difficult in the surgical ICU. The common use of an "open-model" ICU in the surgical setting can make it difficult for providers and families to form a cohesive plan.[22] Additionally, what some authors have described as a "surgical covenant" between the surgeon and patient, in which the surgeon has "an

---

Box 47.3 Benefits Associated With Palliative Care in the ICU

- Decreased Time in the ICU
- Decreased hospital length of stay
- No increase in mortality rate
- Decreased family member PTSD and anxiety
- Decreased disagreements between families and providers
- Decreased disagreements among providers

ICU, Intensive care unit; *PTSD*, posttraumatic stress disorder.
From Aslakson R, Cheng J, Vollenweider D, et al. Evidence-based palliative care in the intensive care unit: A systematic review of interventions. *J Palliat Med.* 2014;17:219–235.

---

exaggerated sense of accountability for the patient's outcome," can further complicate the prognosis and make it difficult for all parties to agree on what constitutes a "good" outcome.[22] Though traditional surgical thinking viewed palliative care as being at odds with surgical goals, the current statement by the American College of Surgeons encourages integration of palliative care of surgical patients who have a range of conditions, not just those at the end of life.[22] Thus anesthesiologists should work closely with surgeons and palliative care specialists to ensure optimal care during periods of critical illness.

Withdrawal of Life Support

Many anesthesiologists may be involved in the withdrawal of life support for patients with poor prognoses whose families do not believe continued life-sustaining treatment is compatible with the patients' goals. For these patients, withdrawing life support is the ethical decision. It is important to note and clarify the distinction that family members may perceive when health care personnel discuss withdrawing life support (discontinuing a machine that keeps a patient alive artificially) and withdrawing care (discontinuing all concern about the patient's comfort and well-being). High-quality care and symptom management should be of utmost concern for all patients regardless of the treatment plan, and families should be reassured that the team will continue to care for the patient.

An important example arises in the context of withdrawing ventilator support. Many family members will prefer that the endotracheal tube be removed in addition to the ventilator being discontinued. It is crucial to prepare family members for the process of extubation of the trachea, including the expected coughing and secretions, and to have opioids and sedatives readily available to decrease any perceived discomfort during or after the extubation, such as shortness of breath. Anesthesiologists are experts in the rapid titration of fentanyl and midazolam, which are the most commonly used medications for withdrawal of mechanical ventilator support. A nurse or physician comfortable with administering these medications should be present during ventilator withdrawal in order to decrease signs of distress. Patients should not be paralyzed before ventilator withdrawal, as this would make it difficult or impossible to assess for proper titration of opioids and sedatives. Physicians overseeing withdrawal of life support should discontinue any unnecessary tubes and lines, contact the hospital chaplain for help accommodating spiritual care and religious rituals, and ensure family support.

Spirituality in Serious Illness

Serious illness and possible death often bring up spiritual issues like questioning the meaning of life or beliefs about what happens after death. Many patients say that

VI

religion is important in helping them adjust to, and cope with, the diagnosis of a terminal illness. Most physicians do not ask patients about their religious beliefs, though many patients and families describe their religion as being an important factor in their decisions about medical treatment and say they want to talk about this topic with their doctor.[25] A simple question like, "What role, if any, do religion or spirituality play in your life?" can help identify patients with unmet needs. There may also be religious rituals, such as the way a patient's body should be handled after death, that are important for the health care team to know. In addition to social workers, nurses, and physicians, chaplains may be particularly helpful in providing spiritual services to help cope with serious or terminal illnesses and are a critical part of the palliative care team.

PALLIATIVE CARE AND PAIN

Pain management is often an important aspect in the quality of a seriously ill person's life. As experts in pain management, anesthesiologists possess unique skills to contribute to this area. Many seriously ill patients have surgery and may have resulting acute-on-chronic pain (also see Chapter 44).

Use of Opioids at the End of Life

Opioids are commonly used to treat both pain and air hunger at the end of life and are an important component of symptom management. However, some health care professionals may have concerns about the effect of opioids on a patient's time to death and have apprehensions that the medications given are "killing" the patient. The ethical principle of double effect states that a physician can treat symptoms that may hasten death as a secondary effect, as long as the doctor's intention is to have a good outcome, like decreased pain and distress, rather than a bad outcome, like death.[26] Opioids should be administered to these patients in response to signs of pain or discomfort, rather than arbitrarily increased. Opioids do not shorten, and may even increase, the time to death in dying patients.[26] Thus the appropriate use of opioids at the end of life is indicated from both a medical and ethical standpoint. If, after discussion, a member of the health care team feels significant moral distress in such a situation, another team member should be assigned to the patient.

Cancer Pain

Cancer pain is the most recognized type of pain for patients with life-threatening illnesses. Most patients with cancer pain can be managed via the World Health Organization's Cancer Pain Stepladder,[27,28] but some will require the expertise of a pain medicine specialist. A variety of techniques to control cancer pain are available (see Chapter 44). Important factors to consider in cancer pain are the cause of the pain (such as tumor- or chemotherapy-related) and the natural history of cancer pain, which generally gets worse instead of better. The cause of cancer pain is often complex and can be caused by the tumor itself; edema around a tumor; or metastases in tissue, nerve, or bone; or it may be related to the cancer treatment itself, such as peripheral neuropathy or radiation-induced brachial plexopathy.[29] Treatment should be targeted to the cause of the pain when possible, and many patients may have pain from multiple sources. Given the complexities of cancer pain, adjunct medications are an important option (Table 47.1).

For some patients, chemotherapy, radiotherapy, or even surgery that aims to decrease the tumor burden may be pursued to decrease pain even when there is no anticipated increase in life expectancy.[29] Anesthesiologists may be asked to evaluate patients for techniques such as a celiac plexus block, which decreases pain scores but has mixed data regarding changes in opioid doses or the quality of life.[30] Bony pain may be caused by osteoblastic or osteolytic components, and approaches such as intrathecal catheters, hormonal therapy, bone-modifying agents, or radiotherapy may be helpful. There may also be psychological aspects related to grief, anxiety, or depression that exacerbate a patient's cancer pain. Addressing those issues often enhances the effects of treatments that target physical pain. Similarly, patients with pain that does not respond to traditional pain medications should be screened for spiritual or emotional pain, and these patients should be provided with resources and support to address their distress. Treatment of spiritual pain may involve social work, psychiatry, psychology, chaplaincy, integrative medicine, or other fields. With the increasing number of cancer survivors, physicians should be more aware of issues of long-term opioid dependence and addiction.

Noncancer Pain

Noncancer pain, or pain in patients without cancer, is a major and yet insufficiently studied issue for patients with serious illnesses. Patients with diagnoses other than cancer may have more difficulty achieving pain control because of lack of physician awareness that pain is associated with the patient's illness. Because anesthesiologists often provide much of the pain management expertise in a hospital, they should be aware of and knowledgeable about pain management in these seriously ill patients. Most patients with dementia have pain at the end of life, though the exact cause of the pain, such as ulcers or musculoskeletal pain, is unknown. Patients with chronic obstructive pulmonary disease (COPD) often have pain, though it is often not treated aggressively, possibly because of anesthesia providers being hesitant to provide

Table 47.1 Adjuvant Analgesic Agents in the Management of Cancer Pain by Conventional Use Category

Category	Examples	Comment
Multipurpose Analgesics		
Glucocorticoids	Dexamethasone, prednisone	Bone pain, neuropathic pain, lymphoedema pain, headache, bowel obstruction
Antidepressants		
Tricyclics	Desipramine, amitriptyline	Used for opioid-refractory neuropathic pain, first if comorbid depression; secondary amine compounds (e.g., desipramine) have fewer side effects and might be preferred
SNRIs	Duloxetine, milnacipran	Good evidence in some conditions, but overall less than for tricyclics; better side effect profile than tricyclics, however, and often tried first
SSRIs	Paroxetine, citalopram	Very scarce evidence, and if pain is the target, other subclasses are preferred
Other	Bupropion	Little evidence for effectiveness, but less sedating than other antidepressants, and often tried early when fatigue or somnolence is a problem
α_2-Adrenergic agonists	Tizanidine, clonidine	Seldom used systemically because of side effects, but tizanidine is preferred for a trial; clonidine is used in neuraxial analgesia
Cannabinoid	THC/cannabidiol, nabilone, THC	Good evidence in cancer pain for THC/cannabidiol; scarce evidence for other commercially available compounds
Topical Agents		
Anesthetic	Lidocaine patch, local anesthetic creams	
Capsaicin	8% patch; 0.25%, 0.75% creams	High-concentration patch indicated for postherpetic neuralgia
NSAIDs	Diclofenac and others	Evidence in focal musculoskeletal pains
Tricyclics	Doxepin cream	Used for itch; can be tried for pain
Others		Compounded creams with varied drugs tried empirically, but no evidence
Used for Neuropathic Pain		
Multipurpose drugs	As noted earlier	As noted earlier
Anticonvulsants		
Gabapentinoids	Gabapentin, pregabalin	Used first for opioid-refractory neuropathic pain unless comorbid depression; may be multipurpose in view of evidence in postsurgical pain; both drugs act at N-type calcium channel in CNS, but individuals vary in response to one or the other
Others	Oxcarbazepine, lamotrigine, topiramate, lacosamide, valproate, carbamazepine, phenytoin	Little evidence for all drugs listed; newer drugs preferred because of reduced side effect liability, but individual variation is great; all drugs considered for opioid-refractory neuropathic pain if antidepressants and gabapentinoids are ineffective
Sodium Channel Drugs		
Sodium channel blockers	Mexiletine, intravenous lidocaine	Good evidence for intravenous lidocaine
Sodium channel modulator	Lacosamide	New anticonvulsant with very scarce evidence of analgesic effects
GABA Agonists		
GABA$_A$ agonist	Clonazepam	Very scarce evidence, but used for neuropathic pain with anxiety
GABA$_B$ agonist	Baclofen	Evidence in trigeminal neuralgia is the basis for trials in other types of neuropathic pain

VI

(Continued)

Table 47.1 Adjuvant Analgesic Agents in the Management of Cancer Pain by Conventional Use Category—Cont'd

Category	Examples	Comment
N-methyl-D-aspartate inhibitors	Ketamine, memantine, others	Evidence scarce for ketamine, but positive experience with intravenous use in advanced illness or pain crisis; little evidence for oral drugs
Used for Bone Pain		
Bisphosphonates	Pamidronate, ibandronate, clodronate	Good evidence; like the NSAIDs or glucocorticoids, usually considered first-line treatment; also reduces other adverse skeletal-related events; concern about osteonecrosis of the jaw and renal insufficiency might restrict use
Calcitonin		Scarce evidence, but usually well tolerated
Radiopharmaceuticals	Strontium-89, samarium-153	Good evidence, but restricted use because of bone-marrow effects and need for expertise
Used for Bowel Obstruction		
Anticholinergic drugs	Hyoscine compounds, glycopyrronium (aka glycopyrrolate)	Along with a glucocorticoid, considered first-line adjuvant treatment for nonsurgical bowel obstruction
Somatostatin analog	Octreotide	Along with a glucocorticoid, considered first-line adjuvant treatment for nonsurgical bowel obstruction

CNS, Central nervous system; *GABA*, γ-aminobutyric acid; *NSAID*, nonsteroidal antiinflammatory drug; *SNRI*, selective noradrenaline reuptake inhibitor; *SSRI*, selective serotonin reuptake inhibitor; *THC*, tetrahydrocannabinol.
From Portenoy RK. Treatment of cancer pain. *Lancet*. 2011;377:2236–2247.

opioids to this patient population. However, opioids are considered an accepted part of the treatment of dyspnea for advanced lung disease, per the American College of Chest Physicians.[31] In this situation the COPD patient's pain may go untreated because of the physician's concern about respiratory depression, despite the evidence in favor of opioids in this patient population. As with all pain, ideally the cause of the pain should be identified, and the treatment should be matched with the cause.

CHALLENGES IN THE PALLIATIVE CARE PATIENT

Identifying Palliative Care and Hospice Patients

Knowing which patients are appropriate for palliative care or hospice consultation can be difficult and may depend on hospital or community norms. Seriously ill patients without clear treatment preferences or decision makers should have a palliative care consultation, as should patients whose care causes a conflict among staff members and those with refractory symptoms.[23]

Inpatient Palliative Care Consults

In general, patients with life-threatening diseases (i.e., metastatic cancer, cirrhosis, or chronic renal failure) or illnesses with a likely probability of death (i.e., multiorgan failure, major trauma, or sepsis) should be considered for a palliative care consultation.[23] Patients who are likely to die in the next year are good candidates for advance care planning. Also, patients with difficult-to-manage symptoms, like pain or nausea, or complex psychosocial or family issues often benefit from palliative care's interdisciplinary approach.

Hospice Consults

Hospice consultations should be sought for patients with a life expectancy of 6 months or less who are interested in focusing on symptom-related treatments rather than treatment with curative intent. Hospice services were initially designed primarily for cancer patients, who have relatively predictable courses in the last 6 months of life. However, cancer patients now make up less than half of hospice patients. Deciding which patients should receive hospice is more difficult for dementia, COPD, and congestive heart failure (CHF), which in combination compose the majority of hospice diagnoses, as these diseases lack good prognostic criteria.[12] Hospice referrals are often made very late in the course of illness, and the median time on hospice was only 18 days in 2018.[12] This means that a significant number of patients did not receive hospice services while they were eligible.

Hospice eligibility determinations are often straightforward, but at times can be a challenge even for hospice medical directors. Therefore there is room for medical interpretation in determining hospice eligibility, and some patients may qualify for enrollment with one hospice service but not with another.

Outpatient Palliative Care Consults

No clear criteria for outpatient palliative care referral exist. However, patients with complex symptoms, psychosocial issues, or advance care planning needs who are not eligible for hospice are often good candidates.[32] Outpatient palliative care clinics can help patients with advance care planning, such as creating advance directives, and serve as consultants for patients with difficult-to-manage symptoms like pain or nausea.

Prognosis

Inherent in many of the discussions about appropriateness of palliative care and hospice consultations, and the ability of anesthesiologists to discuss goals of care, is the concept of prognosis. Anesthesiologists need to have a general idea of prognosis in order to make appropriate medical recommendations.

Physician Estimate

Many clinical decisions are influenced by perceived prognosis, such as whether to withdraw ventilator support, give chemotherapy, and proceed with surgery. Despite its importance, prognosis continues to be extremely difficult to determine. Prognostic accuracy tends to be poor, and most physicians tend to overestimate prognosis by a factor of five, with estimates being worse the longer the physician knows the patient.[33] However, ICU physicians tend to be overly pessimistic about their patients' survival.[34] Nurses and physicians often disagree about the likelihood of a patient's survival and quality of life, with nurses tending to be more pessimistic.[35] One proposed approach is that of the "surprise question." A physician answering "no" to the question, "Would you be surprised if the patient died within the next 12 months?" is a relatively good predictor of patients who are likely to do so.[23] Although this question does not make the future easy to predict or provide clinicians with specifics about how long the patient will live, it can help frame some decisions, such as surgeries or treatments, and can help give families a better sense of what the health care team is thinking.

Disease Trajectories

It can be helpful for physicians to have and convey a concept of the patient's likely disease trajectory. Patients with most cancers follow a relatively predictable course, whereas those with COPD, for example, tend to have a long course of repeated hospitalizations and associated decline before death. These disease trajectories can be useful starting points for discussions with patients and families about what the future is likely to hold (Fig. 47.4).

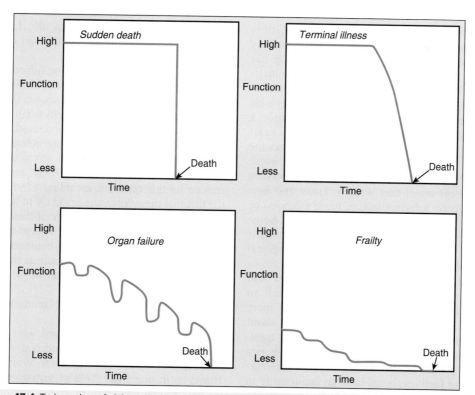

Fig. 47.4 Trajectories of dying. (Redrawn from Lunney JR, Lynn J, Hogan C. Profiles of older Medicare decedents. *J Am Geriatr Soc.* 2002;50:1108–1112.)

VI

Prognostic Tools

Multiple prognostic tools have been developed, particularly for critically ill patients,[36] and for patients with other specific conditions. These tools can synthesize broad information about the severity of a patient's disease into a single number or percentile that is easier for caregivers, patients, and families to understand. They can therefore be very useful but may not take into account all of a patient's comorbid conditions. In addition, these tools cannot predict which individual patients will live or die, which is the information that patients and families really want. Despite these limitations, prognostic calculators can be helpful in framing discussions with families about the patient's likely course.

Functional Status

Performance status generally correlates quite well with prognosis,[37] with a bedbound patient likely to have a much shorter life span than someone who is ambulatory. For example, a patient who is bedbound and recently stopped eating would likely have days to weeks, whereas a patient with a similar diagnosis who is up in a chair most of the day but needs help with bathing and dressing might have weeks to months.

Communication

An essential part of discussing medical issues with patients and families is ensuring understanding of a patient's medical issues. Although the medical team may take it for granted that a patient starting dialysis has failing kidneys, the patient and family may not automatically associate those two pieces of information. Additionally, different members of the health care team may give patients and families different messages. For example, a cardiologist may inform the family that a patient's heart is improving after a myocardial infarction, whereas the intensivist tells the family that he is becoming worse because of worsening pneumonia and sepsis. Querying patients about how much they want to know and how they prefer to receive information (i.e., broad overview or specific details) helps to guide these conversations. Some patients may not want to know anything about their illness and can designate a surrogate to receive medical information and make decisions on their behalf.

Asking what the patient and family have been told about the patient's condition can give the clinician an idea about what issues need to be discussed in more detail. "Checking in" with the patient and family about how they are reacting to this information by asking questions such as, "Is this a surprise for you?" can give them a chance to express their emotions related to new information. Patients and families should have an opportunity to ask questions, and a plan should be made for the patient's care and future meetings, if needed. When possible, family meetings should involve a representative from each specialty taking care of the patient, in addition to the patient or patient's surrogate and other family members requested by the patient or surrogate. Although it can be challenging to find a time for everyone in a patient's care team to meet, this investment generally leads to a more cohesive, thoughtful care plan for the patient.

Many physicians struggle with how to begin family meetings. Commonsense approaches include introducing the family and team members, giving a short explanation for the goals of the meeting, sitting down with the patient and family, and displaying empathy. A short meeting beforehand with the health care team members can be helpful. Sharing specialty-specific insights and getting a better sense of the decisions that will need to be made during the meeting are also helpful. Nurses, chaplains, social workers, and other professionals should be invited to attend as appropriate.

Occasionally, members of the health care team will disagree about a patient's prognosis, treatment plan, or a variety of other issues. This is expected[35] and should be addressed promptly and professionally and to the extent possible before the family meeting. Disagreements that are glossed over can quickly become adversarial and lead to poor patient care and confusion for the family. Many of the same skills in conflict resolution, negotiation, and facilitation that palliative care physicians use in family meetings can also be helpful in the setting of provider disagreement. By helping resolve any team conflicts, palliative care consultations can also help formulate a cohesive care plan and provide the best care possible.

Physician Tendencies in Addressing Difficult Topics

Most physicians never receive any training in how to discuss difficult topics with patients, yet they are expected to do so routinely. As a result, physicians at all levels of training often feel uncomfortable discussing difficult topics with patients. Recordings of physicians show that they tend to focus on technical detail, avoid emotional topics, and dominate conversations.[38] There are many possible reasons for this approach, including a lack of training and the fact that these behaviors are likely to be coping mechanisms. Physicians should be aware of these tendencies and make efforts to overcome them by using words that are understandable, acknowledging emotion, and allowing patients and families to speak. Ideally, patients and families should be speaking for at least half of the conversation.

Patient and Family Wishes About Communicating Prognosis

Because of the difficulty involved with accurately predicting an individual patient's survival, many physicians avoid giving any kind of estimate to avoid being wrong.[39] However, in one study 87% of surrogate decision makers wanted the physician to give a prognosis, even if it was uncertain.[40] When given a prognosis, though, surrogates tend to be overly optimistic, especially with worse prognoses.[41] Many practitioners choose to state clearly that any estimate is a guess and use ranges such as hours to days, days to weeks, or weeks to months to convey a general idea of the patient's life expectancy.

Frameworks for Communicating Difficult Information

Anesthesiologists in the ICU frequently need to communicate sensitive or difficult information about prognosis to patients and families, and it is often necessary in the perioperative or pain settings as well. Ensuring that patients understand their condition is an important part of informed consent for anesthesia. Most of the time, physicians will speak with families because many critically ill patients are unable to participate. Family–clinician communication in the ICU is often inadequate. In one study only half of families had an adequate understanding of the patient's prognosis, treatments, or diagnoses after a discussion with ICU physicians.[42]

There are several formal frameworks for communicating prognosis to patients and families. The SPIKES protocol[43] (Box 47.4), which includes asking for the patient's or family member's current understanding of the medical issues, responding with empathy, and agreeing on a follow-up plan, was originally described for breaking bad news, but the concepts apply in many instances.

Discussing Code Status

The palliative care framework functions in the setting of discussions about resuscitation orders as well. Ideally, discussions about code status should take place in the context of a larger conversation about a patient's overall condition and goals. For example, between 1 in 1400 and 1 in 1800 patients experiences a cardiac arrest in the operating room.[44] The survival rate in the immediate perioperative period for these patients is about 42%.[44] This survival rate is markedly better than that among cardiac arrests for all-hospital adult patients (26%) or out-of-hospital adults (10%),[45] which may be

an important part of a patient's decision regarding code status in the perioperative period.

Time-Limited Trials

A time-limited trial is "an agreement between clinicians and a patient/family to use certain medical therapies over a defined period to see if the patient improves or deteriorates according to agreed-on clinical outcomes."[46] A time-limited trial is a method of dealing with prognostic uncertainty and is a useful tool in family discussions. For example, the family of a patient with a COPD exacerbation and a do not resuscitate (DNR) order may desire a trial of bilevel positive airway pressure (BiPAP) for several days to evaluate whether the patient tolerates the intervention and has improved symptoms.[46] Before starting a time-limited trial of therapy, the medical team should take the following steps: (1) clarify the patient's medical issues and the risks and benefits of any proposed treatments, (2) decide on and discuss with the family a reasonable time frame for improvement and reevaluation, (3) implement the trial, and (4) reassess the patient at the end of the agreed-upon time frame. Time-limited trials will not work for every patient, especially those with rapid changes in their clinical conditions, but they can help patients, families, and providers determine a consensus plan when uncertainty or disagreement exists.

Identifying the Imminently Dying Patient

Anesthesiologists may care for dying patients in the ICU, and patients whose death process has not been identified may occasionally present to the operating room. Thus anesthesiologists should be able to recognize signs of the dying process in order to provide appropriate care for these patients. Additionally, anesthesiologists should be able to provide information for interested family members about what the dying process looks like. Unfortunately, there are few signs that are both sensitive and specific for impending death. Change of consciousness, dysphagia, and decreased oral intake are sensitive but not specific, for example.[47] Mandibular movement with breathing, peripheral cyanosis, and Cheyne-Stokes breathing are reasonably specific for patient death within 3 days but occur in less than 60% of patients.[47]

PERIOPERATIVE MANAGEMENT OF THE PALLIATIVE CARE PATIENT

A list of perioperative considerations is provided in Box 47.5.[48]

Advance Directives

Advance directives encompass a variety of legal documents such as living wills, Five Wishes, or state-specific advance directives, which describe a patient's wishes for

---

Box 47.4 A Framework for Breaking Bad News

Setting: Arrange for a quiet, private space large enough for all participants.

Perception: Assess understanding: *"What have the doctors told you about your wife's illness?"*

Invitation: Ask how much information is desired: *"Some people like all the details, others just like the big picture. What would you like?"*

Knowledge: Tell what you know. Use language that is easy to understand and avoid using complex medical phrases.

Empathy: Acknowledge emotions: *"I wish things were different."*

Sequelae: Agree on next steps: *"Let's meet tomorrow afternoon so I can update you on her condition."*

From Baile WF, Buckman R, Lenzi R, et al. SPIKES—A six-step protocol for delivering bad news: Application to the patient with cancer. *Oncologist.* 2000;5:302-311.

VI

Box 47.5 Perioperative Considerations for Palliative Care Patients

Preoperative Considerations

Look in chart for advance directive or documentation of code status

Determine whether the patient needs a surrogate and, if so, who that person is

If DNR or other limits on treatment are listed, clarify the patient's desires based on ASA guidelines:[46]

- Full attempt at resuscitation
- Limited attempt at resuscitation defined with regard to specific procedures
  - Patient or surrogate should be informed about which procedures are essential to providing anesthesia (i.e., an endotracheal tube) and which are not (i.e., chest compressions)
  - *Example:* Patient with extensive rib metastases declines chest compressions but desires other medications and procedures as appropriate
- Limited attempt at resuscitation defined with regard to the patient's goals and values
  - Patient or surrogate allows the medical team to decide which procedures are appropriate
  - *Example:* Patient wants to have issues that seem easily reversibly treated (i.e., respiratory depression in the PACU after accidental narcotic overdose) but does not want treatment that may lead to neurologic compromise (i.e., does not want prolonged CPR)

Document any changes in treatment limitation clearly in the chart:

- Include the people present during the discussion
- When the original advance directive will be reinstated

- Per ASA guidelines, "when the patient leaves the PACU or when the patient has recovered from the acute effects of anesthesia and surgery"

Discuss any changes in treatment limitation with the surgeon, nurse, or other appropriate parties

Ensure that the patient receives any scheduled pain medications preoperatively

Consider involving spiritual care to perform appropriate rituals if there is a high risk of death

Review past medications for agents like Adriamycin and bleomycin

Review records for sites of metastases, including lung or brain, that may affect physiology

Assess decision-making ability of patients with brain metastases or suspected cognitive impairment

Consider preoperative epidural placement for appropriate patients

Assess baseline functional status and general prognosis

Intraoperative Considerations

Take special care in positioning cachectic patients and those with poor skin integrity

Consider PONV prophylaxis for at-risk patients

Communicate any limitations in treatment to oncoming providers

Postoperative Considerations

Consider possibly increased postoperative pain requirements in context of baseline opioid use

Ensure availability of rescue antiemetic for at-risk patients

Communicate any limitations in treatment to PACU providers

ASA, American Society of Anesthesiologists; *CPR*, cardiopulmonary resuscitation; *DNR*, do not resuscitate; *PACU*, postanesthesia care unit; *PONV*, postoperative nausea and vomiting.

---

medical care. Many of these describe options such as artificial hydration and nutrition or life support if the patient has no hope of recovery. Although these documents can be useful as a guide, they rarely offer unambiguous guidance for the entirety of the wide range of clinical scenarios.[49] Many clinicians advocate for patients' naming a surrogate and for discussions about values and goals among the patient, surrogate, and health care team.[49] Patients who prepare advance directives are more likely to receive care that aligns with their preferences,[50] and many advance directives include the naming of a surrogate decision maker as part of the form.

Decision-Making Capacity

Many patients who are in the perioperative period or in the ICU may not have decision-making capacity because of an inability to communicate, medical issues, or medications.[51] Determining whether a patient has the capacity to make medical decisions can be difficult. In fact, identifying patient decision-making capacity[51] can change over time, so physicians must be cognizant that a patient who was

previously able to make decisions may have become delirious and unable to understand the risks of a procedure. The criteria used to decide whether a person has capacity are "the ability to communicate a choice, to understand the relevant information, to appreciate the medical consequences of the situation, and to reason about treatment choices."[51] Asking questions like, "Can you tell me what surgery we are doing and why?" and "Can you tell me the risks of the procedure?" can help clarify whether a patient has decision-making capacity. If the physician is uncertain whether a patient has decision-making capacity, a psychiatric consult may be appropriate. Deciding whether a patient has decisional capacity is a crucial step in the perioperative evaluation. Patients without decisional capacity cannot give informed consent for anesthesia, and a surrogate must be identified for the patient in most cases.

Surrogate Decision Makers

A surrogate decision maker is a person who makes medical decisions on the patient's behalf. Patients may name surrogate decision makers at any point. Patients with decisional capacity may either continue to make their own decisions or defer decisions to their surrogate. Some states have lists that order the priority of surrogates for patients who have not designated one. Surrogates' wishes may not always match those of the patient,[52] so communication about goals and values is crucial. Surrogates should make decisions in the patient's best interest and that are the surrogate's best guess as to what the patient would want, which is not necessarily what the surrogate would choose. Clarifying this distinction with questions like, "What do you think your father would say if he were able to sit with us and understand this information?" can be helpful.

How to Approach Perioperative DNR Conversations

Recommendations From the American Society of Anesthesiologists

About 15% of patients who present for surgery have a DNR order,[53] so all anesthesia providers should be well versed in discussing these important issues with patients and families. Additionally, almost 25% of surgical patients with DNR orders die within 30 days of surgery.[54] The American Society of Anesthesiologists (ASA) has published guidelines for care of patients with DNR orders and limitations on treatment.[55] For the purposes of this section, DNR will refer to both DNR orders and other limitations on treatment found in documents such as advance directives. The guidelines emphasize that the automatic and complete suspension of DNR orders (or other advance directives) may violate the patient's right to self-determination and that a discussion with the patient or surrogate before the procedure is essential. The ASA describes three outcomes for discussions for patients with a DNR order who present for surgery (Table 47.2). Importantly, a DNR order may be continued, completely suspended, or partially suspended in defined ways to meet patient preferences. An essential part of the ASA guidelines includes discussion and documentation regarding whether, and when, the original DNR order will be reinstated. According to the ASA, "this occurs when the patient leaves the postanesthesia care unit or when the patient has recovered from the side effects of anesthesia/procedure."[55] These discussions should always be clearly documented.

Recommendations From the American College of Surgeons and the Association of periOperative Registered Nurses

The similarities in recommendations among professional societies of anesthesiologists, surgeons, and nurses are striking (Table 47.3).[56,57] As with the ASA, they recommend a more tailored approach rather than automatic suspension. Despite this, 30% of physicians believe DNR orders should be automatically suspended during surgery, and a large majority of patients want to discuss perioperative changes in DNR orders with their physicians.[58] A study in 2012 demonstrated that only half of the surgeons discuss advance directives before surgery, and half would not take a patient to the operating room with limitations on treatment.[59]

Hospice Patients Who Present for Surgery

Hospice patients may decline hospice services at any point. There are cases in which surgery can reduce suffering, such as the surgical repair of an open fracture after trauma. Surgery for hospice patients should prompt a discussion of the risks and benefits of the procedure, in addition to the status of any orders for limitations on perioperative treatment.

Table 47.2 Scenarios for Patients With Perioperative Limitations on Treatment per the ASA

Full Attempt at Resuscitation	Limited Attempt at Resuscitation Defined With Regard to Specific Procedures	Limited Attempt at Resuscitation Defined With Regard to the Patient's Goals and Values
Full suspension of existing DNR. Any procedures may be used.	Specific procedures, for example, chest compressions, may not be used.	Anesthesiologist may use clinical judgment to determine which resuscitation procedures are appropriate.
	The anesthesiologist should inform the patient which procedures can, or cannot, reasonably be refused during an anesthetic.	Full resuscitation may be desired for events that are likely to be easily reversible, but not those likely to lead to an unwanted outcome.
A woman who was recently diagnosed with breast cancer decides to suspend her DNR during the surgery, saying, "I have two kids at home, and I want to live as long as I can for them."	A woman with breast cancer with extensive metastases to her ribs agrees to all interventions except chest compressions, saying, "Even if it worked, I don't want to be on a ventilator with shattered ribs."	A woman with breast cancer whose greatest fear is being unable to recognize her children says, "If you think you can fix the problem and I'll go back to being myself, please do that. If my brain is unlikely to recover, then please don't pursue more aggressive measures."

DNR, Do not resuscitate.
From American Society of Anesthesiologists (ASA). Ethical Guidelines for the Anesthesia Care of Patients with Do-Not-Resuscitate Orders or Other Directives That Limit Treatment. https://www.asahq.org/standards-and-guidelines/ethical-guidelines-for-the-anesthesia-care-of-patients-with-do-not-resuscitate-orders-or-other-directives-that-limit-treatment. Accessed May 26, 2021.

VI

Table 47.3 Comparison of Professional Society Statements Regarding Surgical Patients With DNR Orders

Topic	American Society of Anesthesiologists	American College of Surgeons	Association of periOperative Registered Nurses
Statement regarding automatic suspension of DNR orders for surgery	"Policies automatically suspending DNR orders or other directives that limit treatment prior to procedures involving anesthetic care may not sufficiently address a patient's rights to self-determination in a responsible and ethical manner"	"Policies that lead to either the automatic enforcement of all DNR orders or to disregarding or automatically cancelling such orders do not sufficiently support a patient's right to self-determination"	"Reconsideration of do-not-resuscitate or allow-natural-death orders is required and is an integral component of the care of patients undergoing surgery or other invasive procedures"
Guidelines for the care of surgical patients with DNR orders	"Prior to procedures requiring anesthetic care, any existing directives to limit the use of resuscitation procedures ... should, when possible, be reviewed with the patient or designated surrogate"[55]	"The best approach for these patients is a policy of 'required reconsideration' of the existing DNR orders ... [with] the patient or designated surrogate and the physicians who will be responsible for the patient's care"	"Health care providers should have a discussion with the patient or patient's surrogate about the risks, benefits, implications, and potential outcomes of anesthesia and surgery in relation to the do-not-resuscitate or allow-natural-death orders before initiating anesthesia, surgery, or other invasive procedures"

DNR, Do not resuscitate.
Data from the American Society of Anesthesiologists,[55] American College of Surgeons,[56] and Association of periOperative Registered Nurses.[57]

CONCLUSION

Palliative care is a new field that focuses on the relief of suffering in patients with life-limiting conditions. Anesthesiologists have many skills to offer palliative care patients, including skills in pain and symptom management and the care of the critically ill. Palliative care should not be reserved only for dying patients. Anesthesiologists should have a working knowledge of what palliative care and hospice offer, how the anesthetic care fits into the patient's overall course, and the legal and ethical issues surrounding perioperative limitations on treatment.

REFERENCES

1. Robinson J, Gott M, Ingleton C. Patient and family experiences of palliative care in hospital: What do we know? An integrative review. *Palliat Med.* 2014;28(1):18–33.
2. Nelson JE, Puntillo KA, Pronovost PJ, et al. In their own words: Patients and families define high-quality palliative care in the intensive care unit. *Crit Care Med.* 2010;38:808–818.
3. World Health Organization. Definition of Palliative Care. http://www.who.int/cancer/palliative/definition/en/. Accessed May 26, 2021.
4. Kelley AS, Morrison RS. Palliative care for the seriously ill. *N Engl J Med.* 2015;373(8):747–755. doi:10.1056/NEJMra1404684.
5. Center to Advance Palliative Care. About Palliative Care. http://www.capc.org/about/palliative-care/. Accessed May 26, 2021.
6. Ferris FD, Balfour HM, Bowen K, et al. A model to guide patient and family care: Based on nationally accepted principles and norms of practice. *J Pain Symptom Manage.* 2002;24:106–123.
7. Medicare Payment Advisory Commission. *A Data Book: Health Care Spending and the Medicare Program.* www.medpac.gov.
8. Meier DE. Increased access to palliative care and hospice services: Opportunities to improve value in health care. *Milbank Q.* 2011;89(3):343–380.
9. Jackman DM, Zhang Y, Dalby C, et al. Cost and survival analysis before and after implementation of Dana-Farber clinical pathways for patients with stage IV non-small-cell lung cancer. *J Oncol Pract.* 2017;13(4):e346–e352. doi:10.1200/JOP.2017.021741.
10. Scheunemann LP, McDevitt M, Carson SS, Hanson LC. Randomized, controlled trials of interventions to improve communication in intensive care: A systematic review. *Chest.* 2011;139:543–554.
11. Ambroggi M, Biasini C, Toscani I, et al. Can early palliative care with anticancer treatment improve overall survival and patient-related outcomes in advanced lung cancer patients? A review of the literature [published correction appears in Support Care Cancer. 2018 Jun 11]. *Support Care Cancer.* 2018;26(9):2945–2953. doi:10.1007/s00520-018-4184-3.
12. Rothenberg LR, Doberman D, Simon LE, et al. Patients surviving six months in hospice care: Who are they? *J Palliat Med.* 2014;17:899–905.
13. National Hospice and Palliative Care Organization (NHPCO). Facts and Figures: Hospice Care in America. Published August 20, 2020. https://www.nhpco.org/wp-content/uploads/NHPCO-Facts-Figures-2020-edition.pdf. Accessed May 26, 2021.
14. Kelley AS, Deb P, Du Q, et al. Hospice enrollment saves money for Medicare and improves care quality across a number of different lengths-of-stay. *Health Aff.* 2013;32:552–561.
15. American Board of Internal Medicine. Hospice and Palliative Medicine Policies. http://www.abim.org/certification/policies/imss/hospice.aspx. Accessed May 26, 2021.
16. Quill TE, Abernethy AP. Generalist plus specialist palliative care—Creating a more sustainable model. *N Engl J Med.* 2013;368:1173–1175.

17. Gebauer SL, Fine PG. Palliative medicine competencies for anesthesiologists. *J Clin Anesth.* 2014;26:429–431.

18. Kwok AC, Semel ME, Lipsitz SR, et al. The intensity and variation of surgical care at the end of life: A retrospective cohort study. *Lancet.* 2011;378:1408–1413.

19. Value of the Professional Nurse in Palliative Care. Hospice and Palliative Nurses Association. https://advancingexpertcare.org/position-statements. Accessed May 26, 2021.

20. National Association of Social Workers. The Certified Hospice and Palliative Social Worker. https://www.socialworkers.org/Careers/Credentials-Certifications/Apply-for-NASW-Social-Work-Credentials/Certified-Hospice-and-Palliative-Social-Worker. Accessed May 26, 2021.

21. Board of Chaplaincy Certification, Inc. Palliative Care Specialty Certification Competencies. http://bcci.professional-chaplains.org/content.asp?admin=Y&pl=45&sl=42&contentid=49. Accessed May 26, 2021.

22. Mosenthal AC, Weissman DE, Curtis JR, et al. Integrating palliative care in the surgical and trauma intensive care unit: A report from the Improving Palliative Care in the Intensive Care Unit (IPAL-ICU) Project Advisory Board and the Center to Advance Palliative Care. *Crit Care Med.* 2012;40:1199–1206.

23. Weissman DE, Meier DE. Identifying patients in need of a palliative care assessment in the hospital setting: A consensus report from the Center to Advance Palliative Care. *J Palliat Med.* 2011;14:17–23.

24. Aslakson R, Cheng J, Vollenweider D, et al. Evidence-based palliative care in the intensive care unit: A systematic review of interventions. *J Palliat Med.* 2014;17:219–235.

25. Phelps AC, Maciejewski PK, Nilsson M, et al. Religious coping and use of intensive life-prolonging care near death in patients with advanced cancer. *JAMA.* 2009;301:1140–1147.

26. Mazer MA, Alligood CM, Wu Q. The infusion of opioids during terminal withdrawal of mechanical ventilation in the medical intensive care unit. *J Pain Symptom Manage.* 2011;42:44–51.

27. Zech DF, Grond S, Lynch J, et al. Validation of World Health Organization Guidelines for cancer pain relief: A 10-year prospective study. *Pain.* 1995;63:65–76.

28. WHO Guidelines for the pharmacological and radiotherapeutic management of cancer pain in adults and adolescents. https://www.who.int/ncds/management/palliative-care/cancer-pain-guidelines/en/. Accessed May 26, 2021.

29. Portenoy RK. Treatment of cancer pain. *Lancet.* 2011;377:2236–2247.

30. Wong GY, Schroeder DR, Carns PE, et al. Effect of neurolytic celiac plexus block on pain relief, quality of life, and survival in patients with unresectable pancreatic cancer: A randomized controlled trial. *JAMA.* 2004;291:1092–1099.

31. Mahler DA, Selecky PA, Harrod CG, et al. American College of Chest Physicians consensus statement on the management of dyspnea in patients with advanced lung or heart disease. *Chest.* 2010;137(3):674–691. doi:10.1378/chest.09-1543.

32. Smith AK, Thai JN, Bakitas MA, et al. The diverse landscape of palliative care clinics. *J Palliat Med.* 2013;16(6):661–668.

33. Christakis NA, Lamont EB. Extent and determinants of error in doctors' prognoses in terminally ill patients: Prospective cohort study. *BMJ.* 2000;320:469–472.

34. Rocker G, Cook D, Sjokvist P, et al. Clinician predictions of intensive care unit mortality. *Crit Care Med.* 2004;32:1149–1154.

35. Frick S, Uehlinger DE, Zuercher Zenklusen RM. Medical futility: Predicting outcome of intensive care unit patients by nurses and doctors—A prospective comparative study. *Crit Care Med.* 2003;31(2):456–461.

36. Vincent JL, Moreno R. Clinical review: Scoring systems in the critically ill. *Crit Care.* 2010;14:207.

37. Olajide O, Hanson L, Usher BM, et al. Validation of the palliative performance scale in the acute tertiary care hospital setting. *J Palliat Med.* 2007;10:111–117.

38. Fine E, Reid MC, Shengelia R, Adelman RD. Directly observed patient-physician discussions in palliative and end-of-life care: A systematic review of the literature. *J Palliat Med.* 2010;13:595–603.

39. Ridley S, Fisher M. Uncertainty in end-of-life care. *Curr Opin Crit Care.* 2013;19:642–647.

40. Evans LR, Boyd EA, Malvar G, et al. Surrogate decision-makers' perspectives on discussing prognosis in the face of uncertainty. *Am J Respir Crit Care Med.* 2009;179:48–53.

41. Zier LS, Sottile PD, Hong SY, et al. Surrogate decision makers' interpretation of prognostic information: A mixed-methods study. *Ann Intern Med.* 2012;156:360–366.

42. Curtis JR, White DB. Practical guidance for evidence-based ICU family conferences. *Chest.* 2008;134:835–843.

43. Baile WF, Buckman R, Lenzi R, et al. SPIKES—A six-step protocol for delivering bad news: Application to the patient with cancer. *Oncologist.* 2000;5(4):302–311.

44. Nunnally ME, O'Connor MF, Kordylewski H, et al. The incidence and risk factors for perioperative cardiac arrest observed in the national anesthesia clinical outcomes registry. *Anesth Analg.* 2015;120:364–370.

45. Benjamin EJ, Muntner P, Alonso A, et al. Heart disease and stroke statistics—2019 update: A report from the American Heart Association. *Circulation.* 2019;139(10):e56–e528. Originally published January 31, 2019. https://doi.org/10.1161/CIR.0000000000000659.

46. Quill TE, Holloway R. Time-limited trials near the end of life. *JAMA.* 2011;306:1483–1484.

47. Hui D, dos Santos R, Chisholm G, et al. Clinical signs of impending death in cancer patients. *Oncologist.* 2014;19:681–687.

48. Ethical Guidelines for the Anesthesia Care of Patients with Do-Not-Resuscitate Orders or Other Directives That Limit Treatment. https://www.asahq.org/standards-and-guidelines/ethical-guidelines-for-the-anesthesia-care-of-patients-with-do-not-resuscitate-orders-or-other-directives-that-limit-treatment. Accessed May 26, 2021.

49. Sudore RL, Fried TR. Redefining the "planning" in advance care planning: Preparing for end-of-life decision making. *Ann Intern Med.* 2010;153:256–261.

50. Silveira MJ, Kim SY, Langa KM. Advance directives and outcomes of surrogate decision making before death. *N Engl J Med.* 2010;362:1211–1218.

51. Appelbaum PS. Clinical practice. Assessment of patients' competence to consent to treatment. *N Engl J Med.* 2007;357:1834–1840.

52. Shalowitz DI, Garrett-Mayer E, Wendler D. The accuracy of surrogate decision makers: A systematic review. *Arch Intern Med.* 2006;166:493–497.

53. Scott TH, Gavrin JR. Palliative surgery in the do-not-resuscitate patient: Ethics and practical suggestions for management. *Anesthesiol Clin.* 2012;30:1–12.

54. Kazaure H, Roman S, Sosa JA. High mortality in surgical patients with do-not-resuscitate orders: Analysis of 8256 patients. *Arch Surg.* 2011;146:922–928.

55. American Society of Anesthesiologists. Ethical Guidelines for the Anesthesia Care of Patients with Do-Not-Resuscitate Orders or Other Directives That Limit Treatment. Amended on October 16, 2013. http://www.asahq.org/223C/media/sites/asahq/files/public/resources/standards-guidelines/ethical-guidelines-for-the-anesthesia-care-of-patients.pdf/. Accessed May 26, 2021.

56. American College of Surgeons. Statement on Advance Directives by Patients. "Do Not Resuscitate" in the Operating Room. https://www.facs.org/about-acs/statements/19-advance-directives; 2014. Accessed May 26, 2021.

VI

57. Association of periOperative Registered Nurses. AORN Position Statement on Perioperative Care of Patients with Do-Not-Resuscitate or Allow-Natural-Death Orders. http://www.aorn.org/guidelines/clinical-resources/position-statements; 2014. Accessed May 26, 2021.

58. Burkle CM, Swetz KM, Armstrong MH, Keegan MT. Patient and doctor attitudes and beliefs concerning perioperative do not resuscitate orders: Anesthesiologists' growing compliance with patient autonomy and self determination guidelines. *BMC Anesthesiol.* 2013;13:2.

59. Redmann AJ, Brasel KJ, Alexander CG, Schwarze ML. Use of advance directives for high-risk operations: A national survey of surgeons. *Ann Surg.* 2012;255:418–423.

48 SLEEP MEDICINE AND ANESTHESIA

Joanna Bouez, Frances Chung, Mandeep Singh

INTRODUCTION

Human interest in sleep is as old as humanity itself, but the specialty of sleep medicine is less than 50 years old.[1] The characterization of sleep into periods based on electroencephalography (EEG) and the presence or absence of rapid eye movements (REMs) did not occur until the 1950s. Early developments in the field included the original description of sleep apnea and the development of all-night sleep studies incorporating EEG, respiratory, and cardiac measurements, known as *polysomnography (PSG)*.[1] More recently, additional research has elucidated the neurophysiologic mechanisms governing sleep and wakefulness. Anesthetic drugs modulate key components of sleep–wake neuronal circuits. This chapter will review basic sleep physiology, the differences between sleep and anesthesia states, functional neuroanatomy of sleep and arousal, and sleep-disordered breathing (SDB). The pathophysiology and perioperative management of obstructive sleep apnea (OSA) will be highlighted.

BASIC SLEEP PHYSIOLOGY

Sleep is defined as a state of decreased arousal that is actively generated by nuclei in the hypothalamus, brainstem, and basal forebrain. It is crucial for the maintenance of health.[2,3] Humans spend approximately one-third of their lives in sleep. Sleep is described to be under the control of two processes: a circadian clock (the circadian drive) that regulates the appropriate timing of sleep and wakefulness across the 24-hour day and a homeostatic process (the homoeostatic drive) that regulates sleep need and intensity according to the time spent awake or asleep.[4] The daily drive to sleep is modulated by the hypothalamic suprachiasmatic nuclei that coordinate circadian (24-hour) rhythm. The perceived sensation of sleepiness is the result of a circadian drive, process C (people tend to get sleepy according to their accustomed sleep times during a 24-hour cycle), along with a homeostatic drive, process S (sleep deprivation leads to increasing sleepiness).[5] These two sleep drives are additive, and temporal organization must be preserved to obtain a subjective experience of being refreshed and restful.[6] For example, patients with chronic insomnia often have difficulties because the two sleep drives are not aligned with each other (e.g., frequent afternoon naps would delay sleep onset later in the night).

Normal sleep exhibits a dynamic architecture and is a nonhomogeneous state that can be divided into non–rapid eye movement (NREM) and rapid eye movement (REM) sleep. These two states cycle at an ultradian (less than 24 hours) rhythm of approximately 90- to 120-minute intervals, consolidated in bouts of 6 to 8 hours.[3,6]

The American Academy of Sleep Medicine (AASM) has classified wakefulness and sleep into various stages based on characteristic EEG patterns.[7,8] *Wakefulness*, or *Stage W,* is characterized by beta activity with eyes open (low amplitude, 12–40 Hz) and alpha activity with eyes closed (low amplitude, 8–13 Hz). Non-REM sleep has three distinct stages, based on characteristic patterns on the EEG (Fig. 48.1). *Stage N1 sleep* is characterized by attenuation of alpha activity during wakefulness to a low-amplitude, mixed-frequency signal (4–7 Hz) and vertex sharp waves (prominent sharp waves lasting <0.5 second and maximal over the central EEG region). *Stage N2 sleep* is characterized by the presence of K-complexes (well-delineated, negative, sharp waves followed by a positive deflection, lasting 0.5 second) and sleep spindles (high-frequency bursts of 11 to 16 Hz, with tapering ends, distinct from the background rhythm and lasting ≥0.5 second). *Stage N3 sleep* is characterized by the presence of higher-amplitude (75 microvolts), lower-frequency (0.5–2 Hz) rhythms, also known as *delta waves,* accompanied by waxing and waning muscle tone, decreased body temperature, and

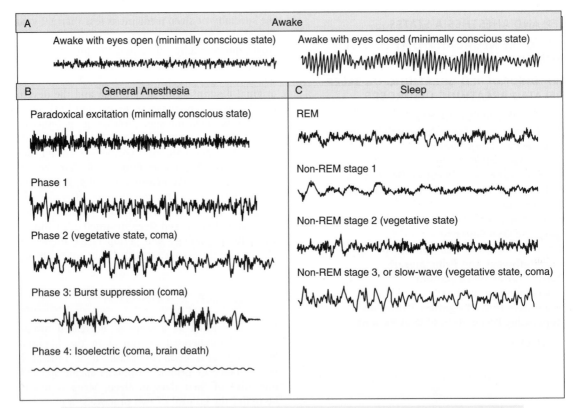

Fig. 48.1 Electroencephalographic patterns during awake state, general anesthesia, and sleep. Panel A shows the EEG patterns when the patient is awake, with eyes open (*left*) and the alpha rhythm (10 Hz) with eyes closed (*right*). Panel B shows the EEG patterns during the states of general anesthesia: paradoxical excitation, phases 1 and 2, burst suppression, and isoelectric tracing. Panel C shows the EEG patterns during the stages of sleep: rapid eye movement (REM) sleep, stage 1 non-REM sleep, stage 2 non-REM sleep, and stage 3 non-REM (slow wave) sleep. (EEG tracings during sleep from Watson C, Bagdoyan H, Lydic R. A neurochemical perspective on states of consciousness. In Hudetz AG, Pearce RA, eds. *Suppressing the Mind: Anesthetic Modulation of Memory and Consciousness,* New York, Springer/ Humana Press; 2010:33–80. Figure from Brown EN, Lydic R, Schiff ND. General anesthesia, sleep, and coma. *N Engl J Med.* 2010;363[27]:2638–2650.)

decreased heart rate.[3] *Stage R,* or *REM sleep,* is characterized by REMs, dreaming, irregular breathing and heart rate, and skeletal-muscle hypotonia.[2] In REM sleep the EEG shows active high-frequency, low-amplitude rhythms (see Fig. 48.1). This activated EEG pattern has given rise to descriptions of REM sleep as "active" or "paradoxical" sleep and to the NREM phase of sleep as "quiet" sleep.[9] Cognitive changes and vivid dreaming are well known to occur during REM sleep.[10]

GENERAL ANESTHESIA

General anesthesia could be described as a reversible drug-induced coma. Nevertheless, anesthesia providers refer to it as "sleep" to avoid disquieting patients when referring to unconsciousness induced by anesthetic drugs. The EEG patterns of general anesthesia–induced consciousness are described in three periods (see Fig. 48.1).

Before *induction,* the patient has a normal, active EEG with prominent alpha activity (10 Hz) when the eyes are closed. Small doses of hypnotic agents acting on the γ-aminobutyric acid type A (GABA$_A$) receptors induce a state of sedation in which the patient is calm and easily arousable, with the eyes generally closed. This is followed by a brief period of paradoxical excitation, characterized by an increase in beta activity on the EEG (13–25 Hz).

During the *maintenance* period, four distinct phases have been described.[11] *Phase 1,* a light state of general anesthesia, is characterized by a decrease in EEG beta activity (13–30 Hz) and an increase in EEG alpha activity (8–12 Hz) and delta activity (0–4 Hz). During *phase 2,* the intermediate state, beta activity decreases and alpha and delta activity increase, with so-called anteriorization—that is, an increase in alpha and delta activity in the anterior EEG leads relative to the posterior leads. The EEG in phase 2 resembles that seen in stage 3, non-REM (or slow wave) sleep. *Phase 3* is a deeper state, in which the EEG is characterized by flat periods interspersed with periods of alpha and beta activity (burst suppression). As this state of general anesthesia deepens, the time between the periods of alpha activity lengthens, and the amplitudes of the alpha and beta activity decrease. Surgery is usually performed during phases 2 and 3. In *phase 4* the most profound state of general anesthesia, the EEG is isoelectric (completely flat), indicated in conditions such as induced coma or neuroprotection during neurosurgery[11] (also see Chapter 30).

During *emergence* from general anesthesia, the EEG patterns proceed in approximately reverse order from phases 2 and 3 of the maintenance period to an active EEG that is consistent with a fully awake state. Anesthetic drugs induce unconsciousness by altering neurotransmission at multiple sites in the cerebral cortex, brainstem, and thalamus. Recent advances in spectral EEG analysis have allowed spatiotemporal characterization of the effects of various intravenous and inhalational anesthetics[12] (Figs. 48.2A and B).

OTHER AROUSAL STATES

Coma is characterized by a state of profound unresponsiveness, which could be drug-induced or a result of brain injury. EEG activity in comatose patients is variable and resembles the high-amplitude, low-frequency activity seen in patients under general anesthesia. The EEG patterns are also dependent on the severity and extent of brain suppression or injury (see Fig. 48.1).[3] The EEG patterns during recovery from coma—coma, vegetative state, and minimally conscious state—resemble the patterns during general anesthesia, sleep, and the awake state.[11]

SLEEP AND ANESTHESIA STATES

It is important to understand the similarities and differences between sleep and anesthesia states.[13] Sleep is a natural state of decreased arousal controlled by circadian and homeostatic drives. Anesthesia is a drug-induced state that is independent of these intrinsic rhythms. Sleep states are amenable to disruptive influences such as psychological and environmental factors. Anesthesia is immune to such influences. Sleep is a characteristically nonhomogeneous state with distinct stages, periodic arousals, and variable body postures, occurring in a cyclical pattern. Anesthesia is a more or less homogeneous state, the depth and duration of which are directly dependent on drug pharmacokinetics and pharmacodynamics. In the presence of significant sensory stimulation the sleep state becomes disrupted and the subject arouses. On the other hand, anesthesia results from suppression of arousals, rendering the subject insensate to bodily injury during surgery. Whereas sleep state reversal occurs spontaneously after restorative functions are completed, anesthesia state reversal requires voluntary stoppage of drug administration and effective drug elimination.

FUNCTIONAL NEUROANATOMY OF SLEEP AND AROUSAL PATHWAYS

Common neurophysiologic mechanisms and neural pathways engaged in sleep are activated by anesthetic drugs. This knowledge has provided new insights into the mechanisms of sedation and anesthesia.[11,14] Sedative drug requirements appear to decrease with both sleep deprivation and circadian rhythm disruption. In an animal model propofol anesthesia, in the absence of surgical stimulation, has been observed to have sleep-like restorative properties after a period of sleep deprivation.[15,16] However, isoflurane anesthesia did not demonstrate this

VI

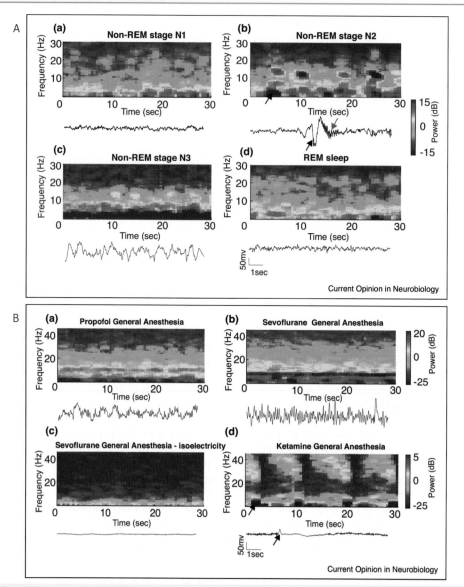

Fig. 48.2 Distinct EEG patterns during sleep and general anesthesia. (A-Sleep) Distinct EEG patterns during different sleep stages. Sleep stages have distinct EEG signatures that result from differences in the neural circuits that are involved in their generation and maintenance. The spectrogram, which is the decomposition of the EEG signal by frequency as a function of time, makes these differences clear. These signatures are also visible in the raw EEG signal (black traces represent the first 10 seconds of data shown in the spectrogram). (a) EEG slowing and the loss of the awake-state alpha oscillations are distinguishing features of N1 sleep. (b) Slow delta (0.1–4 Hz) oscillations, K-complexes (*black arrow* on spectrogram and raw EEG), and spindle oscillations (12–16 Hz, *red arrow* on spectrogram and raw EEG) are distinguishing features of N2 sleep. (c) The predominance of slow-delta oscillations is a distinguishing feature of N3 sleep. (d) Activated "saw-tooth" EEG without the awake-state alpha oscillations are distinguishing features of REM sleep. (B-General Anesthesia) Distinct EEG patterns during general anesthesia. Each anesthetic drug has a different EEG signature that results from differences in the neural circuits that are involved in state generation and maintenance. (a) Slow-delta (0.1–4 Hz) and alpha (8–12 Hz) oscillations are the predominant EEG signatures of propofol-general. This finding is consistent with the EEG signatures of other intravenous GABAA receptor anesthetics (e.g., benzodiazepines, etomidate) during general anesthesia. (b) Slow-delta oscillations, theta (4–8 Hz), and alpha oscillations are the predominant EEG signatures of sevoflurane-general anesthesia. This finding is consistent with the EEG signatures of other modern day derivatives of ether during general anesthesia (desflurane, isoflurane). The close similarities between the EEG signatures of propofol and modern derivatives of ether anesthesia have been suggested to result from enhancement of GABAA receptor spontaneous inhibitory inputs (IPSCs). (c) Isoelectricity is observed when high doses of anesthetics such as sevoflurane or propofol are administered. Significantly enhancement of IPSCs in cortical circuits is a mechanism to explain isoelectricity. (d) Gamma oscillations (30–45 Hz) that are interspersed with slow-delta (black arrow on spectrogram and raw EEG) oscillations are the predominant EEG signatures of general anesthesia maintained with the NMDA receptor antagonist ketamine. (From Akeju O, Brown EN. Neural oscillations demonstrate that general anesthesia and sedative states are neurophysiologically distinct from sleep. *Curr Opin Neurobiol.* 2017;44:178–185. Figs. 1 and 2.)

effect, suggesting differences in the neurophysiologic interface between sleep and anesthesia for inhaled anesthetics.[17]

Anesthesia-induced loss of consciousness results from interactions of anesthetics with the neural circuits regulating sleep and wakefulness states. Ascending activation of the cerebral cortex by subcortical center activity is important in the maintenance of wakefulness. Deactivation of thalamus activity has been observed in imaging studies for both the sleep and anesthesia states, suggesting that thalamic and extrathalamic pathways are involved in sleep state modulation.[18]

Sleep state modulation is regulated by two groups of neural centers: those that promote wakefulness and those that promote sleep[19,20] (Fig. 48.3). The wakefulness-promoting centers are the locus coeruleus (LC), dorsal raphe (DR), and tuberomammillary nucleus (TMN). The sleep-promoting center is primarily the hypothalamic ventrolateral preoptic nucleus (VLPO).[19,20] The preoptic area of the hypothalamus contains neurons active in both sleep and thermoregulation.[21] Discrete neurochemical mediators are involved in the sleep–wake transition[19] (see Fig. 48.3). The mutual inhibition between VLPO and LC acts to produce switchlike, *bistable states* of wakefulness

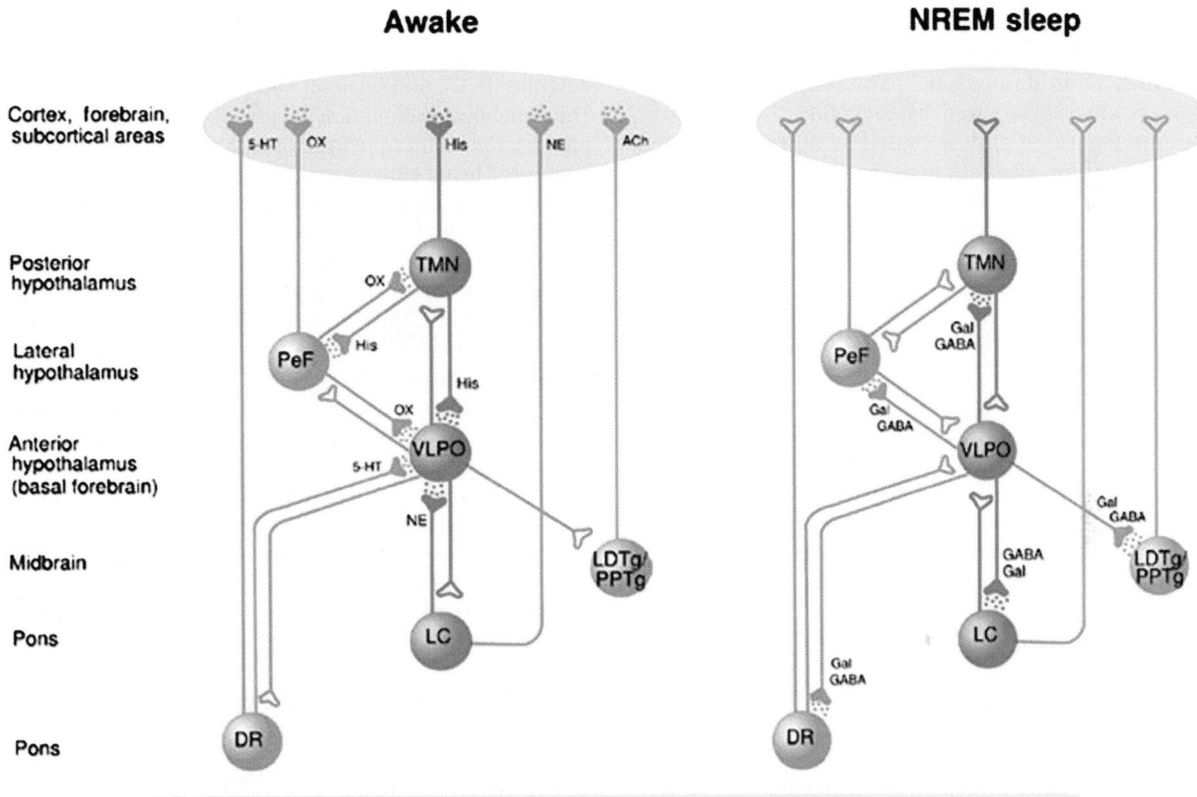

Fig. 48.3 Simplified NREM sleep-promoting pathway. During wakefulness, the LC is active and exerts an inhibitory influence on the hypothalamic VLPO. An inhibition of noradrenergic neurons in the LC, which accompanies endogenous NREM sleep, releases a tonic noradrenergic inhibition of the VLPO. The activated VLPO is believed to release GABA into the TMN, which inhibits its release of arousal-promoting histamine into the cortex and thus induces loss of consciousness. A number of pathways are involved in NREM sleep. The sleep-active VLPO projects to all the ascending monoaminergic, cholinergic, and orexinergic arousal nuclei (TMN, LC, DR, PPTg, LDTg, PeF), which project to the cortex, where they release arousal-promoting neurotransmitters to promote wakefulness. Therefore the activated VLPO exerts an inhibitory influence on key brainstem and thalamic centers, inhibiting the ascent of arousal-promoting pathways to the cortex through them. *5-HT*, serotonin; *Ach*, acetylcholine; *DR*, dorsal raphe nuclei; *GABA*, gamma-aminobutyric acid; *Gal*, galanin; *His*, histamine; *LC*, locus coeruleus; *LDTg*, laterodorsal tegmental nuclei; *NE*, norepinephrine; *NREM*, non–rapid eye movement; *OX*, orexin (hypocretin); *PeF*, perifornical area; *PPTg*, pedunculopontine tegmental nuclei; *TMN*, tuberomammillary nucleus; *VLPO*, ventrolateral preoptic nucleus. (From Nelson LE, Guo TZ, Lu J, et al. The sedative component of anesthesia is mediated by GABA(A) receptors in an endogenous sleep pathway. *Nat Neurosci*, 5[10]:979–984; with permission.)

and sleep at a certain threshold.[20] This effect is also seen with the use of anesthetic agents such as propofol and benzodiazepines acting on the same target receptors and neural pathways integral to sleep and wakefulness.

SLEEP-DISORDERED BREATHING OR SLEEP-RELATED BREATHING DISORDERS

SDB is characterized by abnormalities of respiratory patterns during sleep. The abnormal patterns of breathing are broadly grouped into OSA disorders, central sleep apnea (CSA) disorders, sleep-related hypoventilation disorders, and sleep-related hypoxemia disorder.[22] OSA disorders are characterized by complete or incomplete upper airway (UA) closure during sleep in the presence of respiratory effort during some portion of the event. CSA disorders are characterized by reduction (hypopnea) or cessation (apnea) of airflow caused by absent or reduced respiratory effort. Central apnea or hypopnea may occur in a cyclical, intermittent, or irregular (ataxic) fashion. We will primarily focus on OSA, as this is the most common entity encountered perioperatively.

OBSTRUCTIVE SLEEP APNEA

OSA is characterized by episodes of apnea or hypopnea during sleep, resulting in varying severity of hypoxemia and/or hypercapnia. The obstructive apnea or hypopnea is caused by repeated episodes of complete or partial closure of the pharynx, accompanied by hypoventilation and hypoxemia and terminated by EEG arousal.[23,24]

Pathophysiology of Upper Airway Collapse in Obstructive Sleep Apnea

UA collapsibility and patency are dependent on a continuous balance between collapsing and expanding forces influenced by sleep–wake arousal. Using polysomnographic data of important physiologic variables, important characteristic features of an obstructive apnea can be studied.[25] During wakefulness, the UA stability and patency are achieved by increased genioglossus muscle tone, which pulls the tongue forward.[24] During sleep, patients with OSA develop UA collapse because of a complex interaction of multiple factors such as loss of UA dilating muscle tone, impaired response to mechanoreceptors sensing intrapharyngeal pressures, ventilatory overshoot (high loop gain of the respiratory control system), and an increased arousal threshold.[24] Moreover, patients with OSA have a UA that is predisposed to collapse because of the presence of a smaller UA cross-sectional area and higher critical closure pressures than patients without OSA.[26] During NREM sleep and anesthesia, several factors contribute to UA collapse

and hypoventilation: reduction of wakeful cortical influences, reflex gain, and ventilatory drive.[13] These effects are greater during anesthesia, as the decrease in tonic and phasic muscle activity is profound and abolition of protective arousal response predisposes to prolonged obstruction and more severe oxygen desaturation.

Clinical Diagnostic Criteria

Classically, the gold standard for the definitive diagnosis of OSA requires an overnight PSG or sleep study. A laboratory-based sleep study is set up and analyzed by a registered sleep technologist using standard criteria.[8] All studies are performed using a uniform montage, including central, occipital, and frontal EEG; bilateral electro-oculogram (EOG), chin electromyogram (EMG), electrocardiogram (ECG), and bilateral anterior tibialis muscle EMG. Thoracoabdominal motion is usually monitored by respiratory inductance plethysmography (RIP), and airflow is monitored using either a nasal pressure transducer or nasal thermistor. Arterial oxygen saturation (Sao_2) is monitored by pulse oximetry. Body position and snoring are recorded manually. Fig. 48.4 provides an example of polysomnographic recording in a patient with OSA.

Based on the AASM recommendations, apneas and hypopneas are defined as a reduction in airflow from intranasal pressure of at least 90%, or between 50% and 90%, respectively, for at least 10 seconds accompanied by either a 3% to 4% drop in oxygen saturation or an EEG arousal.[7] Hypopneas are classified as obstructive if thoracoabdominal motion is out of phase or if airflow limitation is observed on the nasal pressure signal, whereas central hypopneas are classified where thoracoabdominal motion is in phase and there is no evidence of airflow limitation on the nasal pressure signal.[27] Mixed apneas are classified as events that begin as central for at least 10 seconds and end as obstructive, with a minimum of three obstructive efforts. Wherever applicable, ataxic breathing or Cheyne-Stokes type of respiration is also reported.[27-29]

The Apnea-Hypopnea Index (AHI) is defined as the average number of abnormal breathing events per hour of sleep. The criteria for OSA diagnosis, and its severity, is listed in Box 48.1.

Polysomnography and Portable Devices

Home sleep testing may be a viable alternative to standard PSG for the diagnosis of OSA in certain subsets of patients.[31,32]

The Portable Monitoring Task Force of the AASM has classified level 2 (full unattended PSG with seven or more channels), level 3 (devices limited to four to seven channels), and level 4 (one to two channels, including nocturnal oximetry) devices.[31] In particular, the level 2 portable PSG has been shown to have a diagnostic

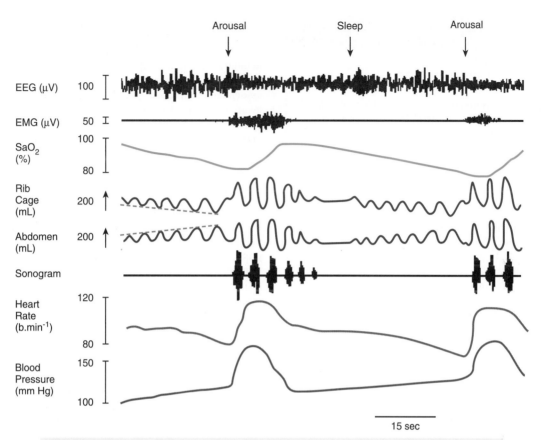

Fig. 48.4 Polysomnographic recordings of obstructive apnea in a patient with obstructive sleep apnea. Note that during the hypopnea, ribcage and abdominal motion are out of phase (i.e., moving in opposite directions), indicating upper airway obstruction. Upper airway obstruction leads to a drop in O_2 saturation. The ineffective breathing attempts continue until the patient awakes, as seen by the EEG arousal and pharyngeal obstruction is relieved. The resuscitative breath now leads to normalization of the oxygen saturation until the next obstructive event ensues. The surge in heart rate and blood pressure occurs along with the arousal, highlighting the activation of sympathetic stimulation in these patients and placing them at higher risk of long-term cardiovascular complications. The arrows indicate arousals from sleep and sleep onset as determined from the EEG and EMG traces. The sonogram indicates breathing sounds caused by snoring. *EEG,* Electroencephalogram; *EKG,* electrocardiogram; *EMG,* submental electromyogram; *Sao₂,* arterial oxygen saturation. (Modified with permission from Thompson SR, Ackermann U, Horner RL. Sleep as a teaching tool for integrating respiratory physiology and motor control. *Adv Physiol Educ,* 2001;25:101–116.)

accuracy similar to that of standard PSG,[33] whereas overnight oximetry is both sensitive and specific for detecting OSA in high-risk surgical patients.[34]

Preoperative overnight oximetry may be used as a screening test. The following findings predict postoperative adverse events: mean preoperative overnight saturation <93%, oxygen desaturation index >29 events per hour, and overnight duration of oxygen saturation <90% for >7% of total sleep time.[35] Portable devices may be considered when there is high pretest likelihood for moderate to severe OSA without other substantial comorbidities.[31] Proper standards must be followed for conducting the test and interpreting the results.[36]

Prevalence of OSA in the General and Surgical Populations

There is a wide variation in the reported prevalence of OSA because of substantial methodological heterogeneity (e.g., populations examined, periods of assessment, and how breathing events of OSA are defined).[37] The overall population prevalence of mild OSA ranged from 9% to 38%. OSA prevalence increases with advancing age and, in some elderly groups, was as high as 90% in men and 78% in women. The prevalence of moderate to severe OSA (AHI ≥15 events/hr) in the adult population ranges from 6% to 17%, being as high as 49% with increasing age and body mass index.[38] The risk factors

---

Box 48.1 Obstructive Sleep Apnea Diagnosis and Severity Based on Apnea-Hypopnea Index (AHI)

- Mild: 5–15 events per hour
- Moderate: ≥15–30 events per hour
- Severe ≥30 events per hour

AHI is defined as the average number of abnormal breathing events per hour of sleep. The clinical diagnosis of OSA requires either an AHI of 15 or more or AHI greater than or equal to 5, with symptoms such as excessive daytime sleepiness, unintentional sleep during wakefulness, unrefreshing sleep, loud snoring reported by a partner, or observed obstruction during sleep.[22,30,32]

---

for OSA are male sex, higher body mass index, and increasing age.[37] Nearly 80% of men and 93% of women with moderate to severe sleep apnea are undiagnosed in the community.[39] In one large case series 60% of surgical patients had undiagnosed moderate to severe OSA.[40]

OSA and Comorbid Conditions

OSA is associated with long-term cardiovascular morbidity, including myocardial ischemia, heart failure, hypertension, arrhythmias, cerebrovascular disease, metabolic syndrome, insulin resistance, gastroesophageal reflux,

and obesity (Box 48.2).[41] Craniofacial deformities (e.g., macroglossia, retrognathia, midfacial hypoplasia), endocrine disorders (e.g., hypothyroidism, Cushing disease), demographic (male, age above 50 years), and lifestyle factors (e.g., smoking, alcohol consumption) are closely associated with OSA.[41] Anesthesia providers should be aware of the possible coexistence of these medical conditions where further optimization and risk stratification may be indicated at the time of surgery. The symptoms and clinical features of OSA are listed in Box 48.2.

Surgery and OSA Severity

Several factors contribute to postoperative worsening of OSA. A prospective observational study evaluated patients undergoing elective surgery with portable PSG preoperatively and on postoperative nights 1 and 3.[37,38] Compared with the preoperative baseline, the AHI significantly increased on the first night, with peak increase occurring on the third night.[37,38] Preoperative AHI, age, and opioid dosage were significant predictors of postoperative AHI.[38] These findings are clinically significant for surgical patients, as they are not monitored as closely during the second and third postoperative days compared with the more frequent monitoring in the postanesthesia care unit (PACU) setting.

Box 48.2 Symptoms and Clinical Features of Obstructive Sleep Apnea (OSA)

Symptoms	Comorbid Conditions
Daytime sleepiness	Obesity
Loud snoring	Large neck circumference
Nonrestorative sleep	Craniofacial deformities (retrognathia, midfacial hypoplasia)
Witnessed apneas by bed partner	Crowded pharynx
Awakening with choking	Systemic hypertension
Insomnia with frequent brief nocturnal awakenings	Hypercapnia or high serum bicarbonate
Lack of concentration	Cardiovascular disease
Cognitive deficits	Cerebrovascular disease
Changes in mood	Cardiac dysrhythmia
Morning headaches	Metabolic syndrome
Sleep walking, confusional arousals (arousals from NREM sleep)	Pulmonary hypertension
Vivid, strange, or threatening dreams (arousals from REM sleep)	Obesity hypoventilation syndrome
Gastroesophageal reflux	Cor pulmonale
Nocturia	Polycythemia
Drowsy driving, and motor vehicle accidents	Floppy eyelid syndrome

Modified from Olson E, Chung F, Seet E. Surgical risk and the preoperative evaluation and management of adults with obstructive sleep apnea. In: Post TW, ed. *UpToDate.* https://www.uptodate.com/contents/surgical-risk-and-the-preoperative-evaluation-and-management-of-adults-with-obstructive-sleep-apnea. Accessed October 2021.
NREM, Non–rapid eye movement; *REM,* rapid eye movement

Another approach to analyzing life-threatening issues in patients with OSA is creation and analysis of a database of OSA-related critical events. The Society of Anesthesia and Sleep Medicine (SASM) partnered with the Anesthesia Closed Claims Project of the American Society of Anesthesiologists (ASA) to create an international registry of unexpected critical events in patients with OSA.[42] Over 60 patients with known or suspected OSA met inclusion criteria (adults, OSA diagnosed or suspected, event occurring within 30 days postoperatively). Most of the critical events occurred on the ward, and the majority occurred within 24 hours of anesthesia.[42] About 97% of patients received opioids within the 24 hours before the event, and two-thirds also received sedatives.[42] Death and brain damage were more likely to occur when the events were unwitnessed, with no supplemental oxygen, lack of respiratory monitoring, and coadministration of opioids and sedatives.

OSA and Perioperative Complications

OSA is a predictor of difficult intubation and impossible mask ventilation.[43,44] Difficult airway management is related to changes in UA anatomy with augmented collapsibility, impaired capability of UA dilator muscles to respond to airway obstruction, disparities in hypoxemia and hypercarbia arousal thresholds (waking up too easily to minor airway narrowing), and unstable ventilatory control.[45,46]

Patients with OSA are more likely to develop postoperative complications, especially those with undiagnosed OSA.[47,48] Respiratory complications include emergent reintubation, with absolute increases of 3% to 5% reported across a variety of surgery types.[49] A retrospective matched cohort analysis evaluated postoperative pulmonary and cardiovascular outcomes in over 4000 patients with OSA.[47] The risk of respiratory complications was approximately twofold higher for patients with diagnosed or undiagnosed OSA, with greatest risk in patients with severe OSA.[47] Another cohort study of over 50 hospitals in Michigan evaluated the impact of untreated OSA on cardiopulmonary complications after general and vascular surgery.[50] Patients with untreated OSA had more cardiopulmonary complications, including unplanned reintubations and myocardial infarction.[50] A large database review of patients who underwent orthopedic or general surgery identified over 100,000 patients with OSA and compared their perioperative pulmonary outcomes with a matched cohort without OSA.[51] Patients with OSA experienced a fivefold increase in intubation and mechanical ventilation after orthopedic surgery and a twofold increase after general surgery compared with controls.[51] Other pulmonary complications that were more likely in the OSA group included aspiration, acute respiratory distress syndrome (ARDS), and pulmonary embolism (only after orthopedic but not general surgical procedures).[51]

OSA is an independent risk factor for cardiovascular morbidity and mortality in the general population not undergoing surgery.[52–55] Several studies have clarified the impact of OSA on perioperative cardiovascular complications. OSA was independently associated with atrial fibrillation in a variety of elective surgeries.[49,56] A prospective study of over 1000 patients with unrecognized OSA undergoing major noncardiac surgery revealed significantly increased risk of postoperative cardiovascular events (a composite of myocardial injury, cardiac death, congestive heart failure, thromboembolism, atrial fibrillation and stroke) in those patients with severe OSA.[48] A retrospective matched cohort analysis evaluated postoperative cardiovascular outcomes in over 4000 patients with OSA. Patients with undiagnosed OSA were found to have a threefold higher risk of cardiovascular complications, primarily cardiac arrest and shock, compared with diagnosed OSA patients with a prescription of continuous positive airway pressure (CPAP) therapy.[47]

Clinical Pathways and Principles of Perioperative Management

Several authors have published recommendations for the perioperative management of patients with OSA.[57-59] As more studies in the field were conducted, specialty societies began issuing guidelines of their own. The Society for Ambulatory Anesthesia guidelines focused on patient selection for ambulatory surgery.[60] The ASA issued guidelines in 2006 and updated them in 2014.[61,62] In 2016 the SASM published guidelines for preoperative screening and assessment of adult patients with OSA.[63] (Box 48.3 provides an executive summary of these guidelines.)

Preoperative Assessment (Also See Chapter 13)

The following sections will follow the approach of the SASM guidelines on preoperative screening and assessment, which categorized patients into three groups: diagnosed and treated OSA; diagnosed OSA, partially treated, or untreated; and suspected OSA.

Patients With Diagnosed OSA

Fig. 48.5B provides an overview of the preoperative evaluation of a patient with OSA. The history and physical examination should focus on the nature and severity of OSA symptoms. Previous consultation with a sleep physician and sleep reports should be reviewed, if possible.

Patients with long-standing OSA may present with significant comorbidities, including morbid obesity, metabolic syndrome, uncontrolled or resistant hypertension, arrhythmias, cerebrovascular disease, and heart failure.[64] Preoperative assessment should rule out the presence of significant nocturnal hypoxemia, hypercarbia, polycythemia, and cor pulmonale. Obesity hypoventilation syndrome (OHS) and pulmonary hypertension should

VI

Box 48.3 Executive Summary of the Society of Anesthesia and Sleep Medicine (SASM) Guidelines on Preoperative Screening and Assessment of Adult Patients With OSA

- Patients with obstructive sleep apnea (OSA) undergoing procedures under anesthesia are at increased risk for perioperative complications compared with patients without the disease diagnosis. Identifying patients at high risk for OSA before surgery for targeted perioperative precautions and interventions may help to reduce perioperative patient complications.
- Screening tools help to risk-stratify patients with suspected OSA with reasonable accuracy. Practice groups should consider making OSA screening part of standard preanesthetic evaluation.
- There is insufficient evidence in the current literature to support canceling or delaying surgery for a formal diagnosis (laboratory or home polysomnography) in patients with suspected OSA unless there is evidence of an associated significant or uncontrolled systemic disease or additional problems with ventilation or gas exchange.
- The patient and the health care team should be aware that both diagnosed OSA (whether treated, partially treated, or untreated) and suspected OSA may be associated with increased postoperative morbidity.
- If available, consideration should be given to obtaining results of the sleep study and, where applicable, the patient's recommended positive airway pressure (PAP) setting before surgery.
- If resources allow, facilities should consider having PAP equipment for perioperative use or have patients bring their own PAP equipment with them to the surgical facility.

- Additional evaluation to allow preoperative cardiopulmonary optimization should be considered in patients with diagnosed, partially treated/untreated, and suspected OSA where there is indication of an associated significant or uncontrolled systemic disease or additional problems with ventilation or gas exchange such as (1) hypoventilation syndromes, (2) severe pulmonary hypertension, and (3) resting hypoxemia in the absence of other cardiopulmonary disease.
- Where management of comorbid conditions has been optimized, patients with diagnosed, partially treated/untreated OSA, or suspected OSA may proceed to surgery, provided strategies for mitigation of postoperative complications are implemented.
- The risks and benefits of the decision to proceed with or delay surgery include consultation and discussion with the surgeon and the patient.
- The use of PAP therapy in previously undiagnosed but suspected OSA patients should be considered case by case. Because of the lack of evidence from randomized controlled trials, we cannot recommend its routine use.
- Continued use of PAP therapy at previously prescribed settings is recommended during periods of sleep while hospitalized, both preoperatively and postoperatively. Adjustments may need to be made to the settings to account for perioperative changes such as facial swelling, upper airway edema, fluid shifts, pharmacotherapy, and respiratory function.

From Chung F, Memtsoudis SG, Ramachandran SK, et al. Society of Anesthesia and Sleep Medicine guidelines on preoperative screening and assessment of adult patients with obstructive sleep apnea. *Anesth Analg*. 2016;123(2):452–473.

---

be ruled out in OSA patients.[65,66] The likelihood of respiratory failure after surgery was more than 10-fold in patients with OHS with OSA compared with patients with OSA alone.[67] Serum bicarbonate level of 28 mmol/L or more can indicate metabolic compensation for chronic hypercapnia and is a useful screening tool for OHS.[68] A preoperative transthoracic echocardiography may be considered in patients suspected to have severe pulmonary hypertension, especially if intraoperative acute elevations in pulmonary arterial pressures are anticipated (e.g., high-risk or long-duration surgery).[69]

Patients with OSA may be using positive airway pressure (PAP) devices for treatment, such as CPAP, bilevel positive airway pressure (BPAP), and auto-titrating positive airway pressure (APAP) devices. APAP devices provide UA stability based on airflow measurements, fluctuations in pressure, or airway resistance based on internal algorithms. This approach has the potential to account for night-to-night variability of OSA severity.[70] It may be meaningful to review sleep study and compliance data from the PAP devices. Improvement in the AHI may indicate successful treatment of respiratory events at the current PAP setting.[63] For patients with known OSA who are nonadherent

or poorly adherent to PAP therapy, additional preoperative cardiopulmonary evaluation should be considered for uncontrolled systemic conditions or difficulty with ventilation or gas exchange. These conditions include hypoventilation syndromes, severe pulmonary hypertension, and resting hypoxemia not attributable to other cardiopulmonary disease.[63] The impact of CPAP on the postoperative course of patients with OSA is an active area of investigation. A 2015 metaanalysis of six studies and 904 patients found that perioperative CPAP significantly reduced the postoperative AHI from baseline preoperative AHI, along with a modest reduction in hospital length of stay.[71] A 2021 review identified 21 randomized controlled trials of perioperative CPAP, 4 of which involved patients with PSG-diagnosed OSA or a high suspicion of OSA.[72] Postoperative use of CPAP improves oxygenation and reduces the need for reintubation and mechanical ventilation.[72] However, none of the trials investigated the effect of CPAP exclusively in patients with experience of its use at home before surgery. The SASM guidelines strongly recommend that patients with OSA bring their PAP machine to the hospital and continue to wear it at appropriate times during their stay, both preoperatively and postoperatively.[63]

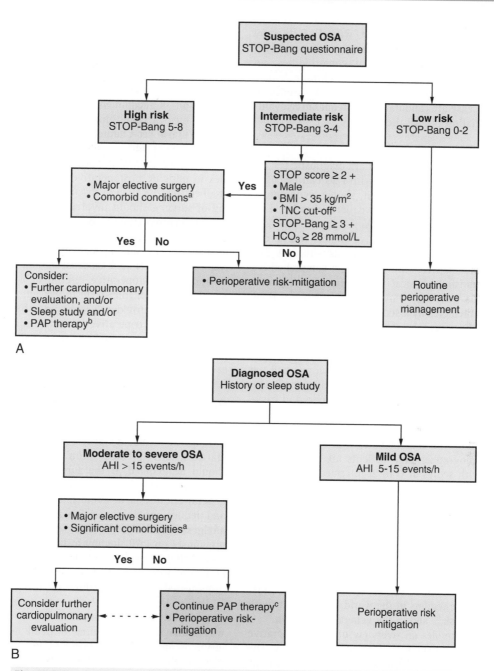

Fig. 48.5 Preoperative evaluation of a patient with known or suspected obstructive sleep apnea in the preadmission clinic. (A) Suspected OSA and (B) diagnosed OSA.
(A) [a]Per the 2016 SASM guidelines, further cardiopulmonary evaluation may be indicated in patients with uncontrolled systemic disease or additional problems with ventilation or gas exchange, such as hypoventilation syndromes, severe pulmonary hypertension, and resting hypoxemia in the absence of other cardiopulmonary disease. [b]Positive airway pressure (PAP) therapy includes continuous PAP, bilevel PAP, and auto-titrating PAP. [c]Neck circumference (NC) cut-offs 17 inches/43 cm in male, 16 inches/41 cm in female. (From Vasu TS, Doghramji K, Cavallazzi R, et al. Obstructive sleep apnea syndrome and postoperative complications: Clinical use of the STOP-BANG questionnaire. *Arch Otolaryngol Head Neck Surg.* 2010;136:1020–1024]. STOP-Bang—STOP-Bang questionnaire cut-off values. (B) [a]Significant comorbidities: heart failure, arrhythmias, uncontrolled hypertension, cerebrovascular disease, metabolic syndrome, obesity (body mass index >35 kg/m²), obesity hypoventilation syndrome, pulmonary hypertension. [c]Positive airway pressure (PAP) therapy: includes continuous PAP, bilevel PAP, and autotitrating PAP.

VI

Patients who are noncompliant with PAP therapy should be counseled to resume therapy preoperatively.[73] Moreover, patients with significant comorbidities, an elevated serum bicarbonate (indicating chronic hypercapnia), and preoperative hypoxemia in the absence of respiratory disease are candidates for preoperative evaluation and initiation of PAP therapy.[73]

Patients With Suspected OSA

An overnight PSG is the gold-standard diagnostic test for OSA. However, routine screening with PSG can be costly and resource intensive. As a result, simple, economical, and sensitive screening tests have been developed to detect patients with suspected OSA.

Preoperatively, the use of sensitive clinical criteria can identify and risk-stratify potential patients with OSA. The 2014 ASA Guidelines recommend using a comprehensive checklist comprising physical characteristics, symptoms, and complaints related to OSA.[61,62] The patient's perioperative risk is predicted by a scoring system based on OSA severity, invasiveness of the procedure, and expected postoperative opioid requirement.[62] Other screening tools that have been validated in surgical patients include the STOP-Bang questionnaire,[74] the Berlin Questionnaire,[75] and the Perioperative Sleep Apnea Prediction (P-SAP) score.[76]

The STOP-Bang questionnaire is a concise and easy-to-use screening tool for OSA consisting of eight easily administered questions (Box 48.4).[74,77] It is a self-administered screening tool that includes four "yes/no" questions and demographic data. Patients are deemed to be at low risk with scores of 0 to 2, intermediate risk with 3 to 4, and high risk of OSA with scores of 5 to 8.[74,77-79] The STOP-Bang questionnaire has a high sensitivity and a high negative predictive value for patients with moderate to severe OSA[74] (see Box 48.4). As the STOP-Bang score increases from 0–2 to 7–8, the probability of moderate to severe OSA increases from 18% to 60% and the probability of severe OSA rises from 4% to 38%.[80] The STOP-Bang questionnaire has been validated across different geographic regions in the world,[81] in patients with cardiovascular risk,[80] and in the general population.[82]

Fig. 48.5A provides an overview of the preoperative evaluation of a patient suspected of having OSA. The clinical evaluation should focus on pertinent symptoms and signs of OSA (see Box 48.2). History from the bed partner in the preoperative clinic is useful in the assessment of loud snoring and observed apneic episodes while asleep. In emergency situations the patient should proceed for surgery. Perioperative risk-mitigation strategies should be taken based on the clinical suspicion of OSA.[58,83]

For elective surgery, the 2016 SASM guidelines state that insufficient evidence exists to support canceling or delaying surgery to formally diagnose OSA in those patients identified as being at high risk of OSA preoperatively, unless there is evidence of uncontrolled

systemic disease or additional problems with ventilation or gas exchange such as hypoventilation syndromes, severe pulmonary hypertension, and resting hypoxemia in the absence of other cardiopulmonary disease[63] (see Box 48.3). In these patients additional cardiopulmonary evaluation is recommended to allow for optimization of the medical conditions and perioperative management[61,62] (also see Chapter 13).

After comorbid conditions have been optimized, patients may proceed to surgery after considering strategies to mitigate postoperative risk (described later). The preoperative risk/benefit discussion, which includes timing of surgery, should involve the patient, surgeon, and anesthesia provider[63] (see Box 48.3). If the patient's perioperative course suggests a higher likelihood of OSA (e.g., difficult airway management,[84] recurrent postoperative respiratory events such as desaturation, hypoventilation, or apnea[85]), postoperative referral to a sleep physician may be useful for long-term follow-up.

Table 48.1 provides a summary of the SASM 2016 guidelines on preoperative screening and assessment for adult patients with known or suspected OSA in the preadmission clinic setting, including levels of evidence for each recommendation.

Perioperative Risk Mitigation Strategies

Table 48.2 provides a summary of SASM guidelines for intraoperative management of adults with OSA. Preoperative sedative premedication in an unmonitored setting should be avoided. If the surgical procedure is appropriate, the use of regional anesthesia is preferred over general anesthesia to avoid manipulation of the airway and reduce the postoperative requirement for sedating analgesic medication[86] (also see Chapter 14). Patients previously on PAP therapy at home may continue using their PAP devices during procedures under mild to moderate sedation.[87] A secured airway is preferred to an unprotected one for procedures requiring deep sedation.[62]

For a general anesthetic, the anesthesia provider should anticipate a greater likelihood of difficult airway management, including difficult mask ventilation, laryngoscopy, and intubation.[88,89] Data on the placement of supraglottic airway devices are scarce, but available evidence does not suggest a difference between patients with and without OSA.[86] The ASA difficult airway management guidelines recommend the presence of skilled personnel and advanced airway equipment at the time of airway management.[90] Adequate preoxygenation; head elevated body position; and measures to decrease the risk of aspiration of gastric acid, such as preoperative proton pump inhibitors, antacids, and rapid-sequence induction with cricoid pressure, should be considered.

Pulmonary hypertension is a known complication of OSA and is more likely in patients with evidence of right heart failure and reduced exercise tolerance. For these

---

Box 48.4 STOP-Bang Questionnaire

Snoring?   Do you **Snore Loudly** (loud enough to be heard through closed doors or your bed partner elbows you for snoring at night)?

Tired?   Do you often feel **Tired, Fatigued, or Sleepy** during the daytime (such as falling asleep during driving)?

Observed?   Has anyone **Observed** you **Stop Breathing or Choking/Gasping** during your sleep?

Pressure?   Do you have or are being treated for **High Blood Pressure**?

Body mass index more than 35 kg/m^2?

Age older than 50 years old?

Neck size large (measured around Adams apple)? More than 40 cm?

Gender = Male?

Scoring criteria for general population
Low risk of OSA: Yes to 0–2 questions
Intermediate risk of OSA: Yes to 3–4 questions
High risk of OSA: Yes to 5–8 questions
The sensitivity of the STOP-Bang score ≥3 to detect moderate to severe OSA (AHI >15) and severe OSA (AHI >30) is 93% and 100%, respectively.
The corresponding negative predictive values are 90% and 100%.
Proprietary to University Health Network, www.stopbang.ca.

Table 48.1   Preoperative Evaluation of a Patient With Known or Suspected OSA in the Preadmission Clinic

Recommendations	Level of Evidence	Grade of Recommendation
3.1 Surgical patients with OSA who are adherent to PAP therapy		
3.1.1 The patient and the health care team should be aware that a diagnosis of OSA may be associated with increased postoperative morbidity.	Low	Strong
3.1.2 Consideration should be given to obtaining the results of the sleep study and the recommended PAP setting before surgery.	Low	Weak
3.1.3 Facilities should consider having PAP equipment available for perioperative use or have the patient bring their own PAP equipment to the surgical facility.	Low	Strong
3.1.4 Patients should continue to wear their PAP device at appropriate times during their stay in the hospital, both preoperatively and postoperatively.	Moderate	Strong
3.2 Surgical patients with OSA but who decline or are poorly adherent with PAP therapy		
3.2.1 The patient and the health care team should be aware that untreated OSA may be associated with increased postoperative morbidity.	Low	Strong
3.2.2 Consideration should be given to obtaining the results of the sleep study and the recommended PAP setting before surgery.	Low	Weak
3.2.3 Facilities should have PAP equipment for perioperative use or have the patient bring their own PAP equipment with them to the surgical facility.	Low	Strong
3.2.4 Additional evaluation for preoperative cardiopulmonary optimization should be considered in patients with known OSA who are nonadherent or poorly adherent with PAP therapy and have uncontrolled systemic conditions or additional problems with ventilation or gas exchange such as (1) hypoventilation syndromes, (2) severe pulmonary hypertension, and (3) resting hypoxemia in the absence of other cardiopulmonary disease.	Low	Weak
3.2.5 Untreated OSA patients with optimized comorbid conditions may proceed to surgery, provided strategies for mitigation of postoperative complications are implemented. The risks and benefits of the decision should include consultation with the surgeon and the patient.	Low	Weak
3.2.6 Patients should be encouraged to wear their PAP device at appropriate times during their stay in the hospital, both preoperatively and postoperatively.	Moderate	Strong

VI

(Continued)

Table 48.1   Preoperative Evaluation of a Patient With Known or Suspected OSA in the Preadmission Clinic—Cont'd

Recommendations	Level of Evidence	Grade of Recommendation
3.3 Surgical patients who have a high probability for OSA		
3.3.1 The patient and the health care team should be aware that a high probability of OSA may increase postoperative morbidity.	Low	Strong
3.3.2 Additional evaluation for preoperative cardiopulmonary optimization should be considered in patients who have a high probability of having OSA and have uncontrolled systemic conditions or additional problems with ventilation or gas exchange such as (1) hypoventilation syndromes, (2) severe pulmonary hypertension, and (3) resting hypoxemia in the absence of other cardiopulmonary disease.	Low	Weak
3.3.3 Patients who have a high probability of having OSA may proceed to surgery in the same manner as those with a confirmed diagnosis, provided strategies for mitigation of postoperative complications are implemented. Alternatively, they may be referred for further evaluation and treatment. The risks and benefits of the decision should include consultation with the surgeon and the patient.	Low	Weak
3.3.4 Patients should be advised to notify their primary medical provider that they were found to have a high probability of having OSA, thus allowing for appropriate referral for further evaluation.	Low	Weak

From Chung F, Memtsoudis SG, Ramachandran SK, et al. Society of Anesthesia and Sleep Medicine guidelines on preoperative screening and assessment of adult patients with obstructive sleep apnea. *Anesth Analg.* 2016;123(2):452–473, Table 9.
OSA, Obstructive sleep apnea; *PAP*, positive airway pressure.

Table 48.2   Society of Anesthesia and Sleep Medicine Guidelines on Intraoperative Management of Adult Patients With Obstructive Sleep Apnea

Recommendations	Level of Evidence	Grade of Recommendation
1 Airway management		
1.1 Known or suspected OSA should be considered an independent risk factor for difficult intubation, difficult mask ventilation, or a combination of both. Adequate difficult airway management precautions should be taken.	Moderate	Strong
2 Anesthetic medication in OSA		
2.1 Neuromuscular blocking agents		
2.1.1 Patients with OSA who received neuromuscular blocking agents may be at increased risk of effects of postoperative residual neuromuscular blockade, hypoxemia, or respiratory failure.	Low	Weak
2.1.2 Currently, there is insufficient evidence to suggest the preference of any neuromuscular blocking reversal agent to reduce the risks of postoperative respiratory complications in patients with OSA.	Low	NA
2.2 Opioids		
2.2.1 Patients with OSA may be at increased risk for adverse respiratory events from the use of opioid medication.	Low	Weak
2.2.2 The possibility of altered pain perception in patients with OSA should be considered.	Low	Weak
2.3 Propofol		
2.3.1 Patients with OSA may be at increased risk for adverse respiratory events from the use of propofol for procedural sedation.	Moderate	Strong
2.4 Inhalational agents		
2.4.1 There is a lack of evidence to assess residual effects of inhalational anesthetic agents in the population with OSA.	Moderate	No recommendation

Table 48.2 Society of Anesthesia and Sleep Medicine Guidelines on Intraoperative Management of Adult Patients With Obstructive Sleep Apnea—Cont'd

Recommendations	Level of Evidence	Grade of Recommendation
2.5 Ketamine		
2.5.1 There is a lack of evidence to assess residual effects of ketamine in the population with OSA.	Very low	No recommendation
2.6 Benzodiazepines		
2.6.1 Patients with OSA may be at increased risk for adverse respiratory events from intravenous benzodiazepine sedation. Intravenous benzodiazepine sedation should be used with caution.	Moderate	Weak
2.7 Alpha-2 agonists		
2.7.1 There is a lack of evidence to assess adverse effects of alpha-2 agonists in the population with OSA.	Low	No recommendation
3 Anesthesia technique		
3.1 When applicable, regional anesthesia is preferable over general anesthesia in patients with OSA.	Moderate	Strong

From Memtsoudis SG, Cozowicz C, Nagappa M, et al. Society of Anesthesia and Sleep Medicine guideline on intraoperative management of adult patients with obstructive sleep apnea. *Anesth Analg.* 2018;127(4):967–987, Table 48.2.
GRADE, Grading of Recommendations, Assessment, Development, and Evaluation; *OSA,* obstructive sleep apnea.

patients, care should be taken to prevent elevation of pulmonary artery pressures (e.g., avoiding hypercarbia, hypoxemia, hypothermia, and acidosis.)

For anesthetic drug choice, short-acting agents such as propofol and remifentanil should be used, and long-acting agents should be minimized. However, propofol has a relatively steep dose-response curve compared with other sedative/hypnotics; thus careful monitoring and titration are required to achieve the desired effect. Despite the lack of data on ketamine in the patient population with OSA, the potential advantages of ketamine over other sedatives include better preservation of UA and ventilatory function.[86] Intravenous benzodiazepine sedation may be associated with airway compromise in patients with OSA and should be used with caution.[86]

For postoperative analgesia, use of regional anesthesia techniques and multimodal analgesia are both strongly recommended to reduce opioid use and perioperative complications.[86] Opioid-induced respiratory depression includes alveolar hypoventilation, decreased level of consciousness, and UA obstruction.[91] Important components of OSA—sleep fragmentation and intermittent hypoxia—modulate pain behavior and increase sensitivity to opioid analgesics.[91] Nonopioid analgesics that can be used for multimodal analgesia include acetaminophen, nonsteroidal antiinflammatory drugs, partial opioid analgesics such as tramadol, anticonvulsants (pregabalin or gabapentin), corticosteroids such as dexamethasone, *N*-methyl-D-aspartate (NMDA) receptor antagonists, ketamine,[92] and the alpha-2 agonists clonidine and dexmedetomidine.[93]

Residual neuromuscular blockade is associated with significant postoperative respiratory complications.[86] It is unclear whether patients with OSA have a greater risk for postoperative respiratory complications caused by postoperative residual neuromuscular blockade compared with patients without OSA. Moreover, it is uncertain whether the type of reversal agent affects the risk of postoperative complications in patients with OSA.[86] However, even small degrees of residual neuromuscular blockade impair UA dilator muscle function. The following actions can minimize this risk in patients with OSA: minimize the use and dose of neuromuscular blocking agent (NMBA), monitor the level of neuromuscular blockade, and completely reverse NMBA before extubation.[86] Although neuromuscular blocking reversal agents can decrease postoperative residual paralysis and respiratory complications, current evidence does not favor any specific neuromuscular reversal agent with regard to outcome in patients with OSA[86] (also see Chapter 11).

Extubation should be performed in an awake, fully conscious patient with no neuromuscular blockade, who is able to obey commands and maintain a patent airway. Immediately after extubation, patients should be recovered in a semi-upright or lateral position instead of the supine position.[62]

Postoperative Disposition of OSA Patients

The postoperative disposition of the patient with OSA depends on the nature of the surgery, OSA severity, and requirement for postoperative parenteral opioids (Fig. 48.6).

VI

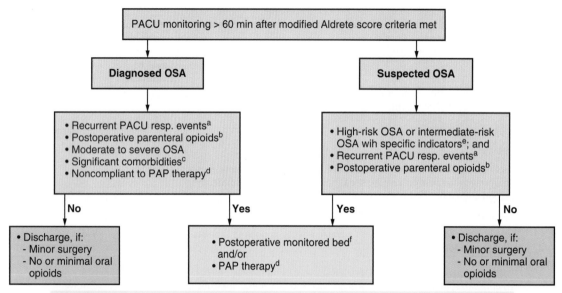

Fig. 48.6 Postoperative management of the patient with known or suspected obstructive sleep apnea after general anesthesia.

[a]Recurrent postanesthesia care unit (PACU) respiratory event: repeated occurrence of oxygen saturation less than 90%, or bradypnea less than 8 breaths/min, or apnea 10 seconds and longer, or pain-sedation mismatch (high pain and sedation scores concurrently).

[b]Postoperative parenteral opioid requirement more than the usual standard of care such as multiple routes, long-acting preparations, or high-dose infusions.

[c]Per the 2016 SASM guidelines, uncontrolled systemic disease or additional problems with ventilation or gas exchange such as hypoventilation syndromes, severe pulmonary hypertension, and resting hypoxemia in the absence of other cardiopulmonary disease.

[d]Positive airway pressure (PAP) therapy: includes continuous PAP, bilevel PAP, or auto-titrating PAP.

[e]Intermediate-risk and specific indicators include STOP score ≥ 2 + male or BMI >35 kg/m^2 or $\uparrow$NC cutoff (where NC: neck circumference cut-offs 17 inches/43 cm in male, 16 inches/41 cm in female) and STOP-Bang ≥ 3 + HCO$_3$ ≥ 28 mmol/L.

[f]Monitored bed: environment with continuous oximetry and the possibility of early medical intervention (e.g., intensive care unit, step-down unit, or remote pulse oximetry with telemetry in surgical ward).

A patient with severe OSA who underwent a major surgery and is receiving high-dose intravenous opioids is more likely to require continuous monitoring than another patient with suspected OSA undergoing a superficial cataract surgery under a local anesthetic with minimal opioid analgesic requirements. The anesthesia provider is responsible for the final decision, taking into account all patient-related, logistic, and circumstantial factors.

Based on the SASM guidelines and expert opinion[58,63,94] for perioperative management of patients with OSA, all patients with known or suspected OSA who have received general anesthesia should have extended monitoring in the PACU with continuous pulse oximetry. There are currently no evidence-based guidelines addressing the optimal length of monitoring required in the PACU, and some recommendations are difficult to adhere to, especially in the context of cost and resource management.[87] It is reasonable to observe a suspected or documented patient with OSA in the PACU for an additional 60 minutes in a quiet environment after the modified

Aldrete criteria for discharge have been met[58] (also see Chapter 39).

The occurrence of recurrent respiratory events in the PACU is another indication of continuous postoperative monitoring in a setting with continuous pulse oximetry and capability for early intervention (e.g., intensive care unit, step-down unit, or ward with pulse oximeter telemetry).[85] Recurrent PACU respiratory events are defined as (1) episodes of apnea for 10 seconds or more, (2) bradypnea fewer than 8 breaths per minute, (3) pain–sedation mismatch, or (4) repeated oxygen desaturation to less than 90%. Patients with suspected OSA (i.e., scored as high risk on screening questionnaires) and who develop recurrent PACU respiratory events postoperatively are at increased risk of postoperative respiratory complications.[85] Postoperative PAP therapy may be initiated on an empiric basis to abolish recurrent obstructive events associated with significant hypoxemia.[87] Patients with known OSA who are already on PAP devices should continue PAP therapy postoperatively.[73]

CONCLUSION

Understanding the similarities and differences between sleep and anesthesia has enhanced our learning of the neural pathways modulating arousal and their interactions with anesthetic medications. Common sleep disorders such as OSA are associated with multiple comorbid conditions and increased perioperative risk. Knowledge of appropriate diagnostic approaches, treatment options, and perioperative precautions is necessary for optimal patient care. Management guidelines from multiple specialty societies continue to evolve based on clinical research and expert opinion.

REFERENCES

1. Pelayo R, Dement WC. History of sleep physiology and medicine. In: Kryger MH, Roth T, Dement WC, eds., Principles and Practice of Sleep Medicine. Philadelphia: Elsevier, Inc; 2017. 6th ed.
2. McCarley RW. Neurobiology of REM and NREM sleep. *Sleep Med.* 2007;8(4):302–330.
3. Lydic R, Baghdoyan HA. Sleep, anesthesiology, and the neurobiology of arousal state control. *Anesthesiology.* 2005;103(6):1268–1295.
4. Borbély AA, Achermann P. Sleep homeostasis and models of sleep regulation. *J Biol Rhythms.* 1999;14(6):557–568.
5. Borbély AA. A two process model of sleep regulation. *Hum Neurobiol.* 1982;1(3):195–204.
6. Carskadon MA, Dement WC. Normal human sleep: An Overview. In: Kryger MH, Roth T, Dement WC, eds., Principles and Practice of Sleep Medicine. 6th ed. Philadelphia: Elsevier, Inc; 2017.
7. Berry RB, Budhiraja R, Gottlieb DJ, et al. Rules for scoring respiratory events in sleep: Update of the 2007 AASM Manual for the Scoring of Sleep and Associated Events. *J Clin Sleep Med.* 2012;8(5):597–619.
8. Iber C, Cheeson A, Quan S.F. AS. The AASM Manual for the Scoring of Sleep and Associated Events, Rules, Terminology and Techical Specifications. 2007.
9. Nofzinger EA. Functional neuroimaging of sleep disorders. *Curr Pharm Des.* 2008;14(32):3417–3429.
10. Stickgold R, Hobson JA, Fosse R, Fosse M. Sleep, learning, and dreams: Offline memory reprocessing. *Science.* 2001;294(5544):1052–1057.
11. Brown EN, Lydic R, Schiff ND. General anesthesia, sleep, and coma. *N Engl J Med.* 2010;363(27):2638–2650.
12. Purdon PL, Sampson A, Pavone KJ, Brown EN. Clinical electroencephalography for anesthesiologists: Part I: Background and basic signatures. *Anesthesiology.* 2015;123(4):937–960.
13. Hillman DR, Eastwood PR. Upper airway, obstructive sleep apnea, and anesthesia. *Sleep Med Clin.* 2015;8(1):23–28.
14. Allada R. An emerging link between general anesthesia and sleep. *Proc Natl Acad Sci U S A.* 2008;105(7):2257–2258.
15. Tung A, Lynch JP, Mendelson WB. Prolonged sedation with propofol in the rat does not result in sleep deprivation. *Anesth Analg.* 2001;92(5):1232–1236.
16. Tung A, Bergmann BM, Herrera S, Cao D, Mendelson WB. Recovery from sleep deprivation occurs during propofol anesthesia. *Anesthesiology.* 2004;100(6):1419–1426.
17. Mashour GA, Lipinski WJ, Matlen LB, et al. Isoflurane anesthesia does not satisfy the homeostatic need for rapid eye movement sleep. *Anesth Analg.* 2010 May 1;110(5):1283–1289. doi:10.1213/ANE.0b013e3181d3e861 PMID: 20418293; PMCID: PMC3767968.
18. Saper CB, Scammell TE, Lu J. Hypothalamic regulation of sleep and circadian rhythms. *Nature.* 2005;437(7063):1257–1263.
19. Vacas S, Kurien P, Maze M. Sleep and anesthesia—Common mechanisms of action. *Sleep Med Clin.* 2013 Mar;8(1):1–9. doi:10.1016/j.jsmc.2012.11.009 PMID: 28747855; PMCID: PMC5524381.
20. Harrison NL. General anesthesia research: Aroused from a deep sleep? *Nat Neurosci.* 2002;5(10):928–929.
21. Rothhaas R, Chung S. Role of the preoptic area in sleep and thermoregulation. *Front Neurosci.* 2021 Jul 1;15:664781. doi: 10.3389/fnins.2021.664781. PMID: 34276287; PMCID: PMC8280336.
22. American Academy of Sleep Medicine (AASM) 2014. *The International Classification of Sleep Disorders*–Third Edition (ICSD-3). www.aasmnet.org. Online version. Accessed on: May 30, 2015.
23. Subramani Y, Singh M, Wong J, Kushida CA, Malhotra A, Chung F. Understanding phenotypes of obstructive sleep apnea: Applications in anesthesia, surgery, and perioperative medicine. *Anesth Analg.* 2017;124(1):179–191.
24. Eckert DJ, White DP, Jordan AS, Malhotra A, Wellman A. Defining phenotypic causes of obstructive sleep apnea. Identification of novel therapeutic targets. *Am J Respir Crit Care Med.* 2013;188(8):996–1004.
25. Thompson SR, Ackermann U, Horner RL. Sleep as a teaching tool for integrating respiratory physiology and motor control. *Adv Physiol Educ.* 2001;25(1-4):101–116.
26. Isono S, Remmers JE, Tanaka A, Sho Y, Sato J, Nishino T. Anatomy of pharynx in patients with obstructive sleep apnea and in normal subjects. *J Appl Physiol.* 1997;82:1319–1326.
27. Yumino D, Bradley TD. Central sleep apnea and Cheyne-Stokes respiration. *Proc Am Thorac Soc.* 2008;5(2):226–236.
28. Farney RJ, Walker JM, Cloward TV, Rhondeau S. Sleep-disordered breathing associated with long-term opioid therapy. *Chest.* 2003;123(United States PT-Case Reports PT-Journal Article LG-English):632–639.
29. Berry RB, Brooks R, Garnaldo CE, Harding SM, Marcus CL and Vaughn BV for the American Academy of Sleep Medicine. The AASM Manual for the Scoring of Sleep and Associated Events: Rules, Terminology and Technical Specifiation, Version 2.0. www.aasmnet.org, Darien, IL: American Academy of Sleep Medicine.
30. Fleetham J, Ayas N, Bradley D, et al. Canadian Thoracic Society 2011 guideline update: Diagnosis and treatment of sleep disordered breathing. *Can Respir J.* 2011;18(1):25–47.
31. Collop NA, Anderson WM, Boehlecke B, et al. Clinical guidelines for the use of unattended portable monitors in the diagnosis of obstructive sleep apnea in adult patients. Portable Monitoring Task Force of the American Academy of Sleep Medicine. *J Clin Sleep Med.* 2007;3(1550-9389 (Print) LA-eng PT-Journal Article PT-Practice Guideline PT-Research Support, Non-U.S. Gov't SB-IM):737–747.
32. Collop NA. Home sleep testing: It is not about the test. *Chest.* 2010;138(2):245–246.
33. Chung F, Liao P, Sun Y, et al. Perioperative practical experiences in using a level 2 portable polysomnography. *Sleep Breath.* 2011;15(3):367–375.
34. Chung F, Liao P, Elsaid H, Islam S, Shapiro CM, Sun Y. Oxygen desaturation index from nocturnal oximetry: A sensitive and specific tool to detect sleep-disordered breathing in surgical patients. *Anesth Analg.* 2012;114(5):993–1000.
35. Chung F, Zhou L, Liao P. Parameters from preoperative overnight oximetry predict postoperative adverse events. *Minerva Anestesiol.* 2014;80(October):1084–1095.
36. Fleetham J, Ayas N, Bradley D, et al. Canadian Thoracic Society 2011 guideline update: Diagnosis and treatment of

VI

sleep disordered breathing. *Can Respir J.* 2011;18(1):25–47.

37. Chung F, Liao P, Yegneswaran B, Shapiro CM, Kang W. Postoperative changes in sleep-disordered breathing and sleep architecture in patients with obstructive sleep apnea. *Anesthesiology.* 2014;120(2):287–298.

38. Chung F, Liao P, Elsaid H, Shapiro CM, Kang W. Factors associated with postoperative exacerbation of sleep-disordered breathing. *Anesthesiology.* 2014;120(2):299–311.

39. Young T, Evans L, Finn L, Palta M. Estimation of the clinically diagnosed proportion of sleep apnea syndrome in middle-aged men and women. *Sleep.* 1997;20(9):705–706.

40. Singh M, Liao P, Kobah S, Wijeysundera DN, Shapiro C, Chung F. Proportion of surgical patients with undiagnosed obstructive sleep apnoea. *Br J Anaesth.* 2013;110(4):629–636.

41. Olson E, Chung F, Seet E. Surgical risk and the preoperative evaluation and management of adults with obstructive sleep apnea. In: Post TW, ed., UpToDate, Waltham: UpToDate. MA. (Accessed on October 01, 2015.).

42. Bolden N, Posner KL, Domino KB, et al. Postoperative critical events associated with obstructive sleep apnea: Results From the Society of Anesthesia and Sleep Medicine Obstructive Sleep Apnea Registry. *Anesth Analg.* 2020;131(4):1032–1041.

43. Seet E, Chung F, Wang CY, et al. Association of obstructive sleep apnea with difficult intubation: Prospective multicenter observational cohort study. *Anesth Analg.* 2021;133(1):196–204.

44. Seet E, Nagappa M, Wong DT. Airway management in surgical patients with obstructive sleep apnea. *Anesth Analg.* 2021;132(5):1321–1327.

45. Cozowicz C, Memtsoudis SG. Perioperative management of the patient with obstructive sleep apnea: A narrative review. *Anesth Analg.* 2021;132(5):1231–1243.

46. Altree TJ, Chung F, Chan MT V, Eckert DJ. Vulnerability to postoperative complications in obstructive sleep apnea: Importance of phenotypes. *Anesth Analg.* 2021;132(5):1328–1337.

47. Mutter TC, Chateau D, Moffatt M, Ramsey C, Roos LL, Kryger M. A matched cohort study of postoperative outcomes in obstructive sleep apnea: Could preoperative diagnosis and treatment prevent complications? *Anesthesiology.* 2014;121(4):707–718.

48. Chan MTV, Wang CY, Seet E, et al. Association of unrecognized obstructive sleep apnea with postoperative cardiovascular events in patients undergoing major noncardiac surgery. *JAMA.* 2019;321(18):1788–1798.

49. Mokhlesi B, Hovda MD, Vekhter B, Arora VM, Chung F, Meltzer DO. Sleep-disordered breathing and postoperative outcomes after elective surgery: Analysis of the nationwide inpatient sample. *Chest.* 2013;144(3):903–914.

50. Abdelsattar ZM, Hendren S, Wong SL, Campbell DA, Ramachandran SK. The impact of untreated obstructive sleep apnea on cardiopulmonary complications in general and vascular surgery: A cohort study. *Sleep.* 2015;38(8):1205–1210.

51. Memtsoudis S, Liu SS, Ma Y, et al. Perioperative pulmonary outcomes in patients with sleep apnea after noncardiac surgery. *Anesth Analg.* 2011;112(1):113–121.

52. Sánchez-de-la-Torre M, Campos-Rodriguez F, Barbé F. Obstructive sleep apnoea and cardiovascular disease. *Lancet Respir Med.* 2013;1(1):61–72.

53. Marshall NS, Wong KKH, Liu PY, Cullen SRJ, Knuiman MW, Grunstein RR. Sleep apnea as an independent risk factor for all-cause mortality: The Busselton Health Study. *Sleep.* 2008;31(8):1079–1085.

54. Gami AS, Olson EJ, Shen WK, et al. Obstructive sleep apnea and the risk of sudden cardiac death: A longitudinal study of 10,701 adults. *J Am Coll Cardiol.* 2013;62(7):610–616.

55. Marin JM, Carrizo SJ, Vicente E, Agusti AGN. Long-term cardiovascular outcomes in men with obstructive sleep apnoea-hypopnoea with or without treatment with continuous positive airway pressure: An observational study. *Lancet.* 2005;365(9464):1046–1053.

56. van Oosten EM, Hamilton A, Petsikas D, et al. Effect of preoperative obstructive sleep apnea on the frequency of atrial fibrillation after coronary artery bypass grafting. *Am J Cardiol.* 2014;113(6):919–923.

57. Adesanya AO, Lee W, Greilich NB, Joshi GP. Perioperative management of obstructive sleep apnea. *Chest.* 2010;138(6):1489–1498.

58. Seet E, Chung F. Management of sleep apnea in adults—Functional algorithms for the perioperative period: Continuing Professional Development. *Can J Anaesth.* 2010;57(9):849–864.

59. Porhomayon J, El-Solh A, Chhangani S, Nader ND. The management of surgical patients with obstructive sleep apnea. *Lung.* 2011;189(5):359–367.

60. Joshi GP, Ankichetty SP, Gan TJ, Chung F. Society for ambulatory anesthesia consensus statement on preoperative selection of adult patients with obstructive sleep apnea scheduled for ambulatory surgery. *Anesth Analg.* 2012;115(5):1060–1068.

61. Gross JB, Bachenberg KL, Benumof JL, et al. Practice guidelines for the perioperative management of patients with obstructive sleep apnea: A report by the American Society of Anesthesiologists Task Force on Perioperative Management of patients with obstructive sleep apnea. *Anesthesiology.* 2006;104(5):1081–1093 quiz 1117-1118.

62. American Society of Anesthesiologists Task Force on Perioperative Management of Patients With Obstructive Sleep Apnea. Practice guidelines for the perioperative management of patients with obstructive sleep apnea: An updated report by the American Society of Anesthesiologists Task Force on Perioperative Management of patients with obstructive sleep apnea. *Anesthesiology.* 2014;120(2):268–286.

63. Chung F, Memtsoudis SG, Ramachandran SK, et al. Society of Anesthesia and Sleep Medicine guidelines on preoperative screening and assessment of adult patients with obstructive sleep apnea. *Anesth Analg.* 2016;123(2):452–473.

64. Bradley TD, Floras JS. Obstructive sleep apnoea and its cardiovascular consequences. *Lancet.* 2009;373(9657):82–93.

65. Chau EH, Lam D, Wong J, Mokhlesi B, Chung F. Obesity hypoventilation syndrome: A review of epidemiology, pathophysiology, and perioperative considerations. *Anesthesiology.* 2012;117(1):188–205.

66. Bady E, Achkar A, Pascal S, Orvoen-Frija E, Laaban JP. Pulmonary arterial hypertension in patients with sleep apnoea syndrome. *Thorax.* 2000;55(11):934–939.

67. Kaw R, Bhateja P, Paz Y, Mar H, et al. Postoperative complications in patients with unrecognized obesity hypoventilation syndrome undergoing elective noncardiac surgery. *Chest.* 2015.

68. Balachandran JS, Masa JFC, Mokhlesi B. Obesity hypoventilation syndrome: Epidemiology and diagnosis. *Sleep Med Clin.* 2014;9(3):341–347.

69. Adesanya AO, Lee W, Greilich NB, Joshi GP. Perioperative management of obstructive sleep apnea. *Chest.* 2010;138(6):1489–1498.

70. Liao P, Luo Q, Elsaid H, Kang W, Shapiro CM, Chung F. Perioperative auto-titrated continuous positive airway pressure treatment in surgical patients with obstructive sleep apnea. *Anesthesiology.* 2013;119(4):837–847.

71. Nagappa M, Mokhlesi B, Wong J, Wong DT, Kaw R, Chung F. The effects of continuous positive airway pressure on postoperative outcomes in obstructive sleep apnea patients undergoing surgery. *Anesth Analg.* 2015;120(5):1013–1023.

72. Jonsson Fagerlund M, Franklin KA. Perioperative continuous positive airway pressure therapy: A review with emphasis on randomized controlled trials and obstructive sleep apnea. *Anesth Analg.* 2021;132(5):1306–1313.

73. Chung F, Nagappa M, Singh M, Mokhlesi B. CPAP in the perioperative setting: Evidence of support. *Chest.* 2015.

74. Chung F, Yegneswaran B, Liao P, et al. STOP questionnaire: A tool to screen patients for obstructive sleep apnea. *Anesthesiology.* 2008;108(5):812–821.

75. Netzer NC, Hoegel JJ, Loube D, et al. Prevalence of symptoms and risk of sleep apnea in primary care. *Chest.* 2003;124(4):1406–1414.

76. Ramachandran SK, Kheterpal S, Consens F, et al. Derivation and validation of a simple perioperative sleep apnea prediction score. *Anesth Analg.* 2010;110(4):1007–1015.

77. Chung F, Subramanyam R, Liao P, Sasaki E, Shapiro C, Sun Y. High STOP-Bang score indicates a high probability of obstructive sleep apnoea. *Br J Anaesth.* 2012;108(5):768–775.

78. Chung F, Abdullah HR, Liao P. STOP-Bang Questionnaire: A practical approach to screen for obstructive sleep apnea. *Chest.* September 2015.

79. Chung F, Yang Y, Brown R, Liao P. Alternative scoring models of STOP-Bang questionnaire improve specificity to detect undiagnosed obstructive sleep apnea. *J Clin Sleep Med.* 2014;10(9):951–958.

80. Hwang M, Zhang K, Nagappa M, Saripella A, Englesakis M, Chung F. Validation of the STOP-Bang questionnaire as a screening tool for obstructive sleep apnoea in patients with cardiovascular risk factors: a systematic review and meta-analysis. *BMJ Open Respir Res.* 2021;8(1):e000848.

81. Pivetta B, Chen L, Nagappa M, et al. Use and performance of the STOP-Bang Questionnaire for obstructive sleep apnea screening across geographic regions. *JAMA Netw Open.* 2021;4(3):e211009.

82. Chen L, Pivetta B, Nagappa M, et al. Validation of the STOP-Bang questionnaire for screening of obstructive sleep apnea in the general population and commercial drivers: A systematic review and meta-analysis. *Sleep Breath.* Jan 2021.

83. Olson E, Chung F, Seet E. Intraoperative management of adults with obstructive sleep apnea. In: Post TW, ed., UpToDate, Waltham: UpToDate, MA. (Accessed on October 01, 2015.).

84. Chung F, Yegneswaran B, Herrera F, Shenderey A, Shapiro CM. Patients with difficult intubation may need referral to sleep clinics. *Anesth Analg.* 2008 Sep;107(3):915–920. doi:10.1213/ane.0b013e31817bd36f PMID: 18713905.

85. Gali B, Whalen FX, Schroeder DR, Gay PC, Plevak DJ. Identification of patients at risk for postoperative respiratory complications using a preoperative obstructive sleep apnea screening tool and postanesthesia care assessment. *Anesthesiology.* 2009;110(4):869–877.

86. Memtsoudis SG, Cozowicz C, Nagappa M, et al. Society of Anesthesia and Sleep Medicine guideline on intraoperative management of adult patients with obstructive sleep apnea. *Anesth Analg.* 2018;127(4):967–987.

87. Sundar E, Chang J, Smetana GW. Perioperative screening for and management of patients with obstructive sleep apnea. *J Clin Outcomes Manag.* 2011;18(9):399–411.

88. Kheterpal S, Martin L, Shanks AM, Tremper KK. Prediction and outcomes of impossible mask ventilation: A review of 50,000 anesthetics. *Anesthesiology.* 2009;110(4):891–897.

89. Siyam MA, Benhamou D. Difficult endotracheal intubation in patients with sleep apnea syndrome. *Anesth Analg.* 2002;95:1098–1102.

90. Apfelbaum JL, Hagberg CA, Connis RT, et al. 2022 American Society of Anesthesiologists Practice guidelines for management of the difficult airway. *Anesthesiology.* 2022 Jan 1;136(1):31–81. doi:10.1097/ALN.0000000000004002 PMID: 34762729.

91. Lam KK, Kunder S, Wong J, Doufas AG, Chung F. Obstructive sleep apnea, pain, and opioids: Is the riddle solved? *Curr Opin Anaesthesiol.* 2015.

92. Eikermann M, Grosse-Sundrup M, Zaremba S, et al. Ketamine activates breathing and abolishes the coupling between loss of consciousness and upper airway dilator muscle dysfunction. *Anesthesiology.* 2012;116(1):35–46.

93. Ankichetty S, Wong J, Chung F. A systematic review of the effects of sedatives and anesthetics in patients with obstructive sleep apnea. *J Anaesthesiol Clin Pharmacol.* 2011;27(4):447–458.

94. Seet E, Han TL, Chung F. Perioperative clinical pathways to manage sleep-disordered breathing. *Sleep Med Clin.* 2013;8(1):105–120.

VI

49 ANESTHESIA AND ENVIRONMENTAL HEALTH

Hemra Cil, Seema Gandhi

HEALTH, HEALTH CARE, AND CLIMATE CHANGE

Climate change represents a defining challenge of our times, and tackling climate change could be the greatest global health opportunity of this century.[1] Climate change poses clear environmental, technologic, and economic challenges that affect food, water, and habitation, and therefore the health of the world's population.[2-4] Table 49.1 lists health issues related to climate change.

Although health care systems have responded to the growing health care needs and the catastrophes posed by climate change, health care itself is polluting and contributes to global warming. Health care is a large, socioeconomically vital sector that contributes significantly to national greenhouse gas (GHG) emissions, both directly from health care facilities and to a much greater extent indirectly from the production of energy, medical goods, and pharmaceuticals that support these facilities. A 2009 report estimated that U.S. health care contributed to 8% of the national GHG emissions.[5] Although many industries have taken actions to reduce emission of GHGs, for example, by producing less-polluting motor vehicles and using less-polluting fuels to produce heat and electricity, health care has been slow to respond. In 2013 an economic input-output life cycle assessment model showed a worsening trend and estimated that 10% of U.S. GHG emissions were attributable to health care.[6] Other national-level studies have shown significant contributions of health-care-sector GHG emissions compared with total GHG emissions: 7% in Australia,[7] 5% in the United Kingdom,[8] and 4% in Canada.[9]

The United States is the second-largest emitter of GHG globally, with 13% of global GHG emissions. China contributes the most, at 26% of global GHG emissions, and the European Union contributes the third most, at 7.5% of global GHG emissions.[10] If the U.S. health care sector were itself a country, it would rank 13th in the world for GHG emissions, ahead of the entire United Kingdom.[6]

Table 49.1 Global Health Issues Related to Climate Change

Climate Change	Health Risks
Increased frequency and intensity of extreme heat conditions	Increased risk of morbidity and mortality during heat waves, especially in urban settings and for manual workers outdoors
Increased variability in precipitation, increasing temperatures	Climate-induced reduction in local crop yields; food insecurity and undernutrition, especially in children
	Water- and vector-borne disease (e.g., malaria, dengue) more likely
Increased variability in precipitation; increased flood, fire, and drought risk	Greater risk of injury, disease, death
	Likely increase in diarrheal disease, with greater impact in children
Increased air pollution, reduced air quality	Increased risk of respiratory illnesses, cardiovascular disease

Health issues are more likely to affect vulnerable populations and increase the risk of social inequities.

Careful attention should be given to the current practice of health care, as it offers significant opportunities for environmental efficiency improvements that could decrease cost and resource utilization without compromising patient care.

ENVIRONMENTAL IMPACT OF ANESTHESIA GASES

Fifty percent of incoming solar energy is absorbed by the earth; the remainder is absorbed by the atmosphere and clouds or is reflected to space. GHGs, defined as gases that trap heat in the atmosphere,[11] contribute to global warming by absorbing the reflected heat and radiating it back to the earth's surface.[12] Anesthesia gases produce 5% of hospital GHG emissions.[13] The commonly used volatile anesthetics sevoflurane, desflurane, and isoflurane and the nonvolatile gas nitrous oxide (N_2O) are potent GHGs with high global warming potential (GWP). GWP is a measure of how much a given mass of GHG contributes to global warming over a specified time (typically 20 or 100 years, i.e., GWP_{20} or GWP_{100}); by definition, carbon dioxide (CO_2) has a GWP of 1.

The GWP of a GHG is primarily determined by two factors: (1) its atmospheric lifetime and (2) its radiative efficiency.[11] Because most halogenated anesthetic compounds other than halothane have similar radiative efficiencies, their GWPs depend primarily on their atmospheric lifetimes, which depends on how rapidly molecular bonds can be broken down by OH^- radicals. Table 49.2 lists the atmospheric lifetimes for inhaled anesthetics, in addition to their GWP_{100}, and a comparison to the GHG emission of driving a car.

A 2017 study analyzed the carbon footprint of the operating room (OR) across three health care systems in three different countries. Anesthetic gases and energy use were the largest sources of GHG emissions. In addition, preferential use of desflurane accounted for a 10-fold difference in carbon emissions from anesthesia gases between these hospitals[14] (Fig. 49.1).

N_2O is the third most significant GHG after CO_2 and methane.[11] It has the longest atmospheric lifetime of all inhaled anesthetics and a relatively high GWP_{100}.[15] Atmospheric N_2O originates primarily from agriculture, fuel combustion, wastewater management, and industrial processes. Anesthetic use is estimated to be responsible for 3% of global N_2O emissions.[12] However, this relatively small contribution should not be ignored, as it remains a significant source of ozone depletion caused by anesthesia.[16,17] Inhaled N_2O is still highly popular for labor analgesia outside the United States because it is inexpensive, easy to administer, and has a favorable safety profile for mother and child[18] (also see Chapter 33).

Even though the global amount of GHGs released each year from inhaled anesthetic administration is comparatively small (approximately 0.01% of total GHG emissions from fossil fuel combustion),[16] direct release of inhaled anesthetics is a major contributor to the environmental impact of anesthesia.[19] For individual anesthesia providers, the most effective climate change mitigation strategies are to avoid desflurane and N_2O, adopt low-flow and closed-circuit anesthesia, and familiarize themselves with techniques using regional and total intravenous anesthesia (TIVA).

OCCUPATIONAL HAZARDS OF INHALED ANESTHETICS

In addition to their environmental effects, inhaled anesthetic agents cause OR pollution and can increase health risks for providers in the OR. During induction of general anesthesia and before tracheal intubation, high fresh gas flow (FGF) rates are often used. This period represents the highest risk for spillage of waste anesthetic gases directly into the OR instead of the anesthesia workstation scavenging system (also see Chapter 15).

The potential health hazards of occupational exposure to waste anesthetic gases, including increased risk of spontaneous abortion, genetic damage, and cancer, were first noted in survey-based studies from the 1970s, an era in which scavenging of inhaled anesthetics was poor

Table 49.2 Atmospheric Lifetime, Global Warming Potential (GWP), and Driving Equivalent of Inhaled Anesthetic Agents

Gas	Lifetime[15,16] (years)	GWP$_{100}$ [15,52,c]	Driving Equivalent (miles/hr)[21,53,d] at Fresh Gas Flow			
			0.5 L/min[a]	1.0 L/min[a]	2 L/min[a]	5 L/min[a]
N$_2$O	114–121	265–298	29	57	112	282
Sevoflurane	1.1–2.2	130–216	–	4	8	19
Desflurane	10.8–14	1790–2540	93	190	378	939
Isoflurane	3.2–3.5	491–510	4	8	15	38
Halothane[b]	1.0	41				

[a]0.6 MAC-hour for N$_2$O and 1 MAC-hour for sevoflurane, desflurane, and isoflurane.
[b]Halothane is no longer commercially available in the United States but is available globally.
[c]GWP$_{100}$ is the global warming potential of a greenhouse gas over a 100-year period compared with CO$_2$. Desflurane has a GWP$_{100}$ of 2540, indicating that 1 kg of desflurane has the same global warming effect as 2540 kg of CO$_2$. The technical groups routinely reevaluate gases of concern in the context of changing atmospheric chemistry, a process that can take up to 5 years.
[d]The driving equivalent analogy provides a practical comparison to driving a typical passenger automobile, which emits approximately 400 g of CO$_2$ per mile. For example, administering desflurane at fresh gas flow of 1 L/min for 1 hour at 1 MAC produces the same GHG emission as driving a car for 190 miles.

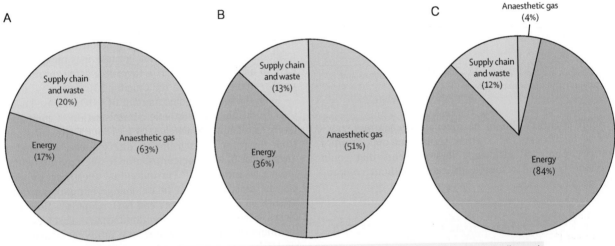

Fig. 49.1 Relative contributions of anesthetic gases, energy use, the supply chain, and waste disposal to the carbon footprint of operating rooms at (A) Vancouver General Hospital, (B) the University of Minnesota Medical Center, and (C) John Radcliffe Hospital, UK. (Adapted from MacNeill et al.,[14] with permission from Elsevier Ltd.)

by today's standards.[19] In 1977 the National Institute for Occupational Safety and Health (NIOSH) issued recommended exposure limits for both N$_2$O and halogenated agents, in addition to guidance on scavenging systems for waste anesthetic gases and ventilation system capacity in ORs and recovery rooms.[20] After implementation of waste anesthetic gas regulations from NIOSH (and similar regulations in other countries), more recent studies have found little to no increase in adverse effects associated with waste anesthesia gases when they are scavenged effectively.[19] However, these risks may remain for individuals chronically exposed to workplaces that do not

meet recommended guidelines for waste anesthetic gas exposure.

LOW-FLOW ANESTHESIA

Because inhaled anesthetics undergo very little in vivo metabolism, they are exhaled, scavenged, and vented into the atmosphere, largely unchanged, as medical waste gases.[21] Thus the ecologic impact is largely determined by the gas used and the FGF rate at which it is administered. Although there is no universal definition, low-flow anesthesia is most commonly defined as FGF <1 L/min and minimal flow anesthesia as FGF <0.5 L/min.[22,23] Essentially any technique in which the FGF is less than alveolar ventilation can be considered low-flow anesthesia.[24]

Table 49.3 lists advantages and disadvantages of low-flow anesthesia. The clinical use of low-flow anesthesia has been facilitated by newer anesthesia workstations, gas analyzers (for inspired/exhaled O_2, CO_2, and anesthetic agent), and CO_2 absorbents that do not produce compound A (also see Chapter 15).

The maintenance phase of anesthesia presents the best opportunity to reduce flows, but attention should also be given to the induction and emergence phases to minimize environmental contamination and decrease waste. Recommendations for low FGF management for all three phases of anesthesia are listed in Box 49.1.[25]

Some newer anesthesia workstations facilitate low-flow anesthesia by using automated gas controls and proprietary software algorithms to guide the administration of anesthetic agents and carrier gas.[25] An additional strategy to reduce waste of inhaled anesthetics is real-time decision support for intraoperative notification of excessive FGF.[26] Since 2018, the authors' institution (University of California San Francisco [UCSF]) has adopted this approach with their anesthesia information

| Box 49.1 | Recommendations for Managing Low Fresh Gas Flow (FGF) During Anesthesia[25] |

INDUCTION

1. Set FGF close to minute ventilation during mask ventilation
2. Increase FGF if measured FiO_2 and gas concentration lower than set level
3. During intubation, turn off the FGF, leave the vaporizer at its set point
4. Set FGF to half of the minute ventilation after intubation
5. Then watch measured anesthetic concentration after intubation
   Reduce FGF progressively based on gas concentration
   If needed, increase/decrease vaporizer setting to maintain desired concentration
6. Move to anesthesia maintenance management if there is no significant difference between exhaled and inspired anesthetic gas concentration

Maintenance

1. First, set total oxygen flow (mL/min):
   Patient's estimated oxygen consumption (5 mL/kg/min)
   Add 200 mL/min if sidestream gas analyzer sample gas does not return to the circuit
   Add 100 mL/min for potential leaks
2. Decrease total oxygen flow in 50-mL/min increments until FiO_2 begins to decrease
3. Monitor exhaled anesthetic gas concentration to maintain desired MAC level
4. Monitor FiO_2

Emergence

1. Maintain low FGF until the vaporizer is off

FiO_2, Fraction of inspired oxygen.

Table 49.3 Advantages and Disadvantages of Low-Flow Anesthesia

Advantages	Disadvantages
Environmental	Slower inhaled anesthesia induction
Decreased anesthetic gas consumption	Slower emergence from inhaled anesthesia
Decrease in waste anesthetic gas (greenhouse gases)	Reduced ability to rapidly change inspired anesthetic concentration
Decrease in operating room pollution	
Economic	Increased CO_2 absorbent consumption
Decreased cost of volatile anesthetic agents	Risk of hypercarbia (with exhausted CO_2 absorbent)
Physiologic	
Reduced respiratory heat loss	Requires ongoing adjustment of inspired oxygen concentration to prevent hypoxic gas mixture
Preservation of humidity of inspired gas, (helps to maintain mucociliary function)	

management system (Epic Systems, Verona, WI). This tool prompts providers to use lower FGF rates during the maintenance phase of general anesthesia; the set target for FGF is 1 L/min for sevoflurane and 0.7 L/min for desflurane or isoflurane. This best-practice advisory led to lower FGF rates, significantly reducing carbon emission and cost per case (Fig. 49.2).

CLOSED-CIRCUIT ANESTHESIA

The most extreme form of low-flow anesthesia is closed-circuit anesthesia. The first commercial closed anesthesia circuit was manufactured in 1925, after CO_2 absorbents were introduced into anesthesia practice; however, closed-circuit anesthesia was considered unsafe by many anesthesia providers because of the inability to measure inspired oxygen and inhalation agent concentrations.[27] Closed-circuit anesthesia is based on two key principles: (1) no gases are allowed to escape from the circuit and all exhaled gases are returned to the patient after elimination of CO_2, and (2) inhalational agents and carrier

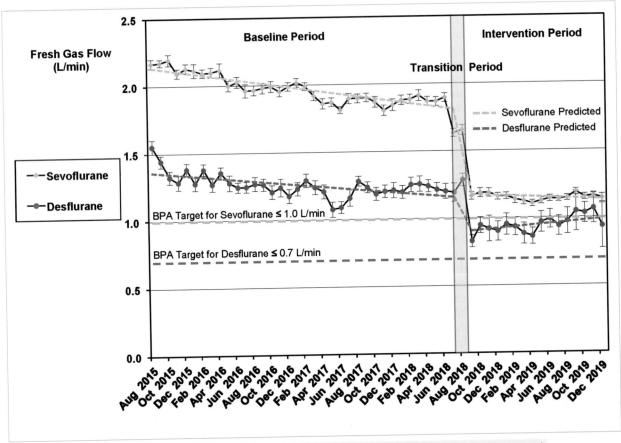

Fig. 49.2 Interrupted time series analysis showing the monthly mean FGF rates for sevoflurane and desflurane at University of California San Francisco. Horizontal dashed lines indicate the target FGF levels for each agent set by the Best Practice Advisory (BPA) (≤1.0 L/min for sevoflurane and ≤0.7 L/min for desflurane) using a real-time decision support tool into the anesthesia information management system. The decrease in FGF at the beginning of the intervention period was statistically significant (P <0.0001). Bars indicate 95% confidence intervals.

gases (O_2 and N_2O or air) are added to the circuit only in amounts equal to those eliminated and consumed.[28]

Closed-circuit anesthesia can be accomplished in different ways. Traditionally, a liquid form of inhaled anesthetic is infused or injected, rather than vaporized, according to a prescribed algorithm. Because the vaporizer concentration is not high enough for rapid deepening of anesthesia during induction, many providers preferred to inject liquid inhalation agents into the expiratory limb of the circuit with a syringe pump at prescribed intervals according to Lowe's square-root-of-time model.[29] Some providers monitor and maintain inspired or expired anesthetic tensions with a gas monitor that returns analyzed gas to the breathing circuit.[28,30] In an alternative closed-circuit anesthesia technique anesthesia is induced with inhalation agents at a higher FGF rate. Once a steady

state has been established, the minimal FGF can be set at 250 mL/min based on the patient's predicted oxygen consumption (243 mL for a 70-kg patient).[28] During emergence from anesthesia, the injection or vaporization of liquid inhalation agents is stopped and the breathing circuit is flushed with oxygen.[28]

Because closed-circuit anesthesia is a form of low-flow anesthesia, the advantages and disadvantages are the same (see Table 49.3). Although closed-circuit anesthesia increases the use of CO_2 absorbents, it lowers the overall cost per case.[29,31] Although rarely used in the United States, closed-circuit anesthesia is attracting more interest because of its environmental and cost benefits. Outside of the United States, some companies provide automated closed-circuit anesthesia workstations, and regulatory approval is proceeding in the United States.[28]

CO$_2$ ABSORBENTS

CO$_2$ absorbents have been used in anesthesia practice since they were introduced in 1924. Traditional soda lime absorbent consists of 95% calcium hydroxide [Ca(OH)$_2$] and 5% sodium hydroxide and potassium hydroxide; the latter degrades sevoflurane to the nephrotoxic compound A, and the desiccated soda lime degrades desflurane, enflurane, and isoflurane to carbon monoxide (CO).[32] New-generation CO$_2$ absorbents such as the lithium hydroxide–based absorbent Litholyme and strong alkali-free absorbent AMSORB Plus do not contain strong bases (calcium hydroxide or potassium hydroxide). These absorbents do not interact chemically with sevoflurane, isoflurane, or desflurane and thus cannot produce compound A (also see Chapter 15).

Typically, the decision to replace the CO$_2$ absorbent canister is based on a change in indicator dye color (to purple) reflecting decreased pH and reduced capacity for CO$_2$ absorption. However, to maximize absorbent utilization and decrease cost, the anesthesia provider can wait until the inspired CO$_2$ reaches 5 mm Hg and then replace the absorbent canister.[25,29] Because new CO$_2$ absorbents are made of nonhazardous materials, they are suitable for landfill waste, and their use is consistent with a sustainable anesthesia strategy.

WASTE ANESTHETIC GAS SCAVENGING SYSTEMS

Waste anesthetic gas scavenging systems eliminate vented anesthetic gases, thereby decreasing OR pollution, but these gases are emitted to the atmosphere largely unmetabolized and unregulated, causing environmental pollution. Newer waste anesthetic gas scavenging systems can mitigate the environmental impact by using technologies that capture, recycle/reuse, or destroy anesthetic gases. Some commercially available new technologies are described next.

N$_2$O is a commonly used anesthetic during labor. In Sweden a special double mask for use in maternity wards allows delivery of N$_2$O and removal of the exhaled gas. The exhaled N$_2$O is subsequently destroyed by oxidation, catalytic reduction, or catalytic splitting.[18]

Anesthesia scavenging systems continuously entrain large air volumes and thereby dilute waste gases. Often, a large continuously operating vacuum pump is used to generate the necessary vacuum. One novel approach uses a low-flow scavenger interface with a one-way on-demand valve that reduces air entrainment and further reduces both energy consumption and cost by reducing the vacuum pump's duty cycle.[33]

A Canadian manufacturer produces two types of portable canisters to capture (adsorb) anesthetic gases. They can be installed in-line with the anesthesia workstation exhaust in the OR or integrated into a central waste gas scavenging system. Used canisters are processed in the company's facility to recycle the captured waste gases. The canisters are approved for use with its branded desflurane in Canada but are not yet available in the United States.[34]

ENVIRONMENTAL IMPACT OF PROPOFOL

Total intravenous anesthesia (TIVA) refers to the administration of intravenous agents, most frequently propofol, to induce and maintain general anesthesia without inhaled anesthetics. The environmental impact of propofol can be determined by a life cycle assessment analyzing its entire production chain, including drug synthesis; transportation to the hospital; plastic syringes, tubing, and intravenous pumps for administration; and incineration of unused drug. The GHG impact of propofol is smaller than that of inhaled anesthetics and stems mainly from the electricity required for the syringe pump and not from drug production or direct release to the environment.[35] Using anesthetic techniques that avoid inhalation anesthesia, such as intravenous anesthesia, neuraxial, or peripheral nerve blocks, causes the least harm to the climate. Nevertheless, propofol is not biodegradable; even a small amount can cause long-term environmental contamination from improper disposal in landfills, dumping into wastewater drains, or human excretion.[35]

DRUG WASTE

Drug waste has been linked to unnecessary health care costs and negative environmental impact.[36,37] The cost of anesthetic drugs accounts for 5% to 15% of a hospital's pharmacy budget and approximately 4% of the cost of a single surgical procedure.[38] Although propofol has a lesser impact on GHG emissions than inhalation agents, up to 50% of propofol in an operating suite can go unused, making it the costliest among the commonly wasted drugs.[36] Because propofol is nonbiodegradable and accumulates in fat, it should be disposed of by incineration at >1000°C for more than 2 seconds. Improper disposal can have deleterious effects on aquatic wildlife and terrestrial ecosystems.[37] Propofol waste can be reduced by using smaller vials (20 mL instead of 50 to 100 mL).[36]

Drugs prepared in anticipation of emergencies go unused 50% of the time, and neuromuscular blocking drugs prepared by the anesthesia provider are unused in 30% of cases.[39] In a 2016 study preventable drug waste was calculated for the 10 most commonly used anesthetic drugs (excluding propofol): succinylcholine, vecuronium, rocuronium, ephedrine, phenylephrine, atropine, glycopyrrolate, lidocaine, ondansetron, and dexamethasone.

VI

The preventable waste of these noncontrolled medications was $3.90 per case.[40] Although this cost may seem trivial compared with that of a surgical procedure, it would amount to hundreds of thousands of dollars per year at a single medical center with a large surgical volume.

Several measures can be established to avoid drug waste, such as leaving emergency drugs/equipment unopened but easily available, drawing the minimal number of drugs, choosing smaller vials whenever possible, and having prefilled syringes available in the OR.[41]

Prefilled syringes are safe, accurate, and often prepared by a pharmacy or drug companies in accordance with U.S. Pharmacopeia (USP) guidelines. The use of prefilled syringes may reduce drug and dosing errors and decrease drug costs.[40] The most commonly available prefilled syringes include epinephrine, atropine, glycopyrrolate, phenylephrine, lidocaine, succinylcholine, rocuronium, and calcium.

ENVIRONMENTAL IMPACT OF OPERATING ROOM PRACTICES

Waste

The OR generates 20% to 30% of total hospital waste,[42] and anesthesia generates 25% of total OR waste, of which 60% could be recycled.[43] There are two types of waste: (1) noncontaminated solid waste and (2) regulated medical waste, such as infectious material, sharps, and certain medications. The treatment and decontamination of regulated medical waste to enable safe handling and disposal are energy-intensive and expensive. Appropriate classification of waste in the OR and recycling of paper, glass, and several types of plastics may reduce the requirement for this energy-intensive process.[42] Therefore, failure to segregate regulated medical waste from other types of waste increases environmental impact and costs.[42]

Reusable versus Single-Use Equipment

Environmental impact must also be considered in the selection and purchasing of medical equipment. The environmental benefits of reusable medical equipment, compared with single-use equipment, have been repeatedly demonstrated. Life cycle assessments of the laryngoscope and laryngeal mask airway (LMA; a supraglottic airway device that is available in reusable and single-use versions) have shown that reusables have a lesser environmental impact than single-use items.[44,45] For laryngoscopes, a single-use blade generates 5 to 6 times more CO_2 and a single-use handle 16 to 18 times more CO_2 than the reusable alternative.[44] The life cycle assessment of single-use versus reusable LMAs strongly favors reusable devices. Single-use LMAs have a greater negative

environmental impact because of the production of polymers, packaging, and waste management. A disadvantage of a reusable LMA is that more labor is required for washing and sterilization.[45]

Reprocessing allows for safe reuse of certain single-use devices to decrease waste, costs, and emissions while adhering to infection control guidelines.[46] This Food and Drug Administration (FDA)–approved process involves collecting, testing, packaging, and sterilizing single-use devices to meet the same standards as the original equipment manufacturer. Currently, many medical devices are approved for reprocessing, including invasive devices such as surgical trocars, staplers, and angiography catheters, and noninvasive devices, such as blood pressure cuffs, sequential compression device sleeves, and patient transfer mattresses.

Reusable versus Single-Use Textiles

The costs of reusable and single-use surgical textiles are similar.[47] However, single-use textiles consume 200% to 300% more energy and 250% to 330% more water and generate 200% to 300% more CO_2 and sevenfold more waste than reusable textiles, despite the environmental costs, including greater water use for cleaning, disinfection, and sterilization. Selection of reusable rather than single-use gowns reduces energy consumption by 64%, GHG emission by 66%, water consumption by 83%, and solid waste generation by 84%.[48]

Reusable Breathing Circuits

Reusable anesthesia breathing circuits with single-use airway filters can be safely used for up to 7 days without increasing bacterial/viral contamination risk, resulting in lower costs and less energy and water use. However, the recommended frequency of anesthesia breathing circuit change varies from country to country: from daily in the U.K., to weekly in Germany, and after each patient in the United States.[49,50] For example, in a U.S. center where 50 patients undergo surgery every weekday, anesthesia circuits are changed between every case, which leads to use and disposal of approximately 13,000 plastic anesthesia breathing circuits annually in landfills. Using reusable breathing circuits with single-use airway filters may decrease this waste, in addition to the carbon footprint and cost of circuits.

Energy Efficiency

Health care facilities provide round-the-clock care requiring energy-intensive equipment and systems. In the United States health care facilities use more energy than any sector besides food service.[51] Energy consumption is the second-largest source of GHG in the OR and is 3 to 6 times higher per square foot than in the hospital

Table 49.4 Strategies to Reduce Energy Waste in the Operating Room

Strategy	Description
HVAC occupancy-based approach	Reduce unnecessary airflow to unused space[14] (e.g., by reducing the frequency of room air exchanges in an empty OR from the normal setting of 20 times per hour to a lower number to maintain positive pressure).
HVAC maintenance	HVAC systems should be regularly maintained and inspected for seal leaks.
HVAC system choice	Ensure that HVAC systems are of the proper size; upgrade current systems to energy-efficient motors, optimizing airflow, and avoiding excessive air conditioning.
Energy use	Turn off energy-intensive systems and equipment such as lights, anesthesia machine scavenging, computers, surgical equipment, and fluoroscopy machines when they are not in use.
Energy source	Change medical center energy sources from coal and natural gas to renewables such as wind and solar power to decrease the carbon footprint.[54]
Lighting	Use LED bulbs to decrease energy consumption and generate less heat, which will reduce the amount of energy required for cooling.
OR waste	Recycle and appropriately classify waste in the OR to reduce medical waste that requires energy-intensive processing for safe handling and disposal.

HVAC, Heating, ventilation, air conditioning; *LED,* light-emitting diode; *OR,* operating room.

as a whole.[14] Heating, ventilation, and air conditioning (HVAC) are responsible for 90% to 99% of OR energy consumption.[14] However, effective, energy-efficient technologies and practices may reduce OR energy consumption without affecting patient care (Table 49.4).

SUMMARY

Climate change is a health issue. Health professionals worldwide, including anesthesia providers, must show strong leadership in tackling climate change. This leadership should include education and advocacy starting at institutional and local levels. At a personal level, anesthesia providers can update their practices to reflect current evidence. Strategies for mitigating the environmental impact of anesthesia practice and incorporating the topics discussed in this chapter are shown in Fig. 49.3. Resources for sustainable anesthesia practice are listed in Table 49.5.

Table 49.5 Resources for Sustainable Anesthesia Practice

Resource	Description
Dartmouth-Hitchcock Eco-Health Footprint Calculator[55]	Tool designed for health care institutions to comprehensively measure GHG production from their activities.
U.S. Environmental Protection Agency (EPA)[56]	Overview of greenhouse gases, including sources of GHG emissions, and carbon footprint and GHG equivalency calculators.
American Society of Anesthesiologists Greening the Operating Room and Perioperative Arena: Environmental Sustainability for Anesthesia Practice[57]	Document produced by the American Society of Anesthesiologists Task Force on Environmental Sustainability Committee on Equipment and Facilities. Revised January 2017. Addresses many issues related to environmental sustainability and anesthesia practice.
U.K. National Health Services—Greener NHS[58]	Description of the U.K. National Health Service program to reduce the impact of climate change on public health and the environment.
Yale Gassing Greener App[59]	For anesthesia providers to build sustainable practices.

VI

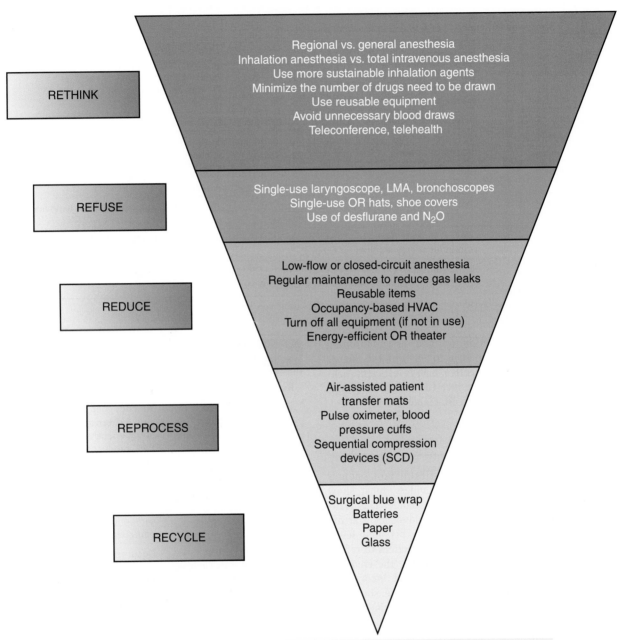

Fig. 49.3 Toolkit for individual anesthesia providers to mitigate the environmental impact of anesthesia practices.

REFERENCES

1. Wang H, Horton R. Tackling climate change: The greatest opportunity for global health. *Lancet.* 2015;386:1798–1799.

2. Roa L, Velin L, Tudravu J, et al. Climate change: Challenges and opportunities to scale up surgical, obstetric, and anaesthesia care globally. *Lancet Planet Health.* 2020;4:e538–e543.

3. IPCC. Climate Change 2014: Impacts, Adaptation, and Vulnerability. Summaries, Frequently Asked Questions, and Cross-Chapter Boxes. A Contribution of Working Group II to the Fifth Assessment Report of the Intergovernmental Panel on Climate Change. In: Field CB, Barros VR, Dokken DJ, et al. eds *World Meteorological Organization.* Geneva; 2014.

4. UNICEF: Unless we act now: The impact of climate change on children. https://sustainabledevelopment.un.org/content/documents/2161unicef.pdf. Accessed January 23, 2021.

5. Chung JW, Meltzer DO. Estimate of the carbon footprint of the US health care sector. *JAMA.* 2009;302:1970–1972.

6. Eckelman MJ, Sherman J. Environmental impacts of the U.S. health care system and effects on public health. *PLoS One.* 2016;11:e0157014.

7. Malik A, Lenzen M, McAlister S, et al. The carbon footprint of Australian health care. *Lancet Planet Health.* 2018;2:e27–e35.

8. National Health Service (NHS). https://www.england.nhs.uk/2020/01/greener-nhs-campaign-to-tackle-climate-health-emergency/ Accessed March 5, 2021.

9. Eckelman MJ, Sherman JD, MacNeill AJ. Life cycle environmental emissions and health damages from the Canadian healthcare system: An economic-environmental-epidemiological analysis. *PLOS Med.* 2018;15:e1002623.

10. World Resources Institute. The world's top 10 emitters. https://www.wri.org/insights/interactive-chart-shows-changes-worlds-top-10-emitters Accessed September 30, 2021. Based on 2018 data from https://www.climatewatchdata.org/.

11. U.S. Environmental Health Agency. Greenhouse gas emissions. https://www.epa.gov/ghgemissions. Accessed December 30, 2020.

12. Ishizawa Y. Special article: General anesthetic gases and the global environment. *Anesth Analg.* 2011;112:213–217.

13. Charlesworth M, Swinton F. Anaesthetic gases, climate change, and sustainable practice. *Lancet Planet Health.* 2017;1:e216–e217.

14. MacNeill AJ, Lillywhite R, Brown CJ. The impact of surgery on global climate: A carbon footprinting study of operating theatres in three health systems. *Lancet Planet Health.* 2017;1:e381–e388.

15. Myhre G, Shindell D, Bréon FM, et al. Anthropogenic and natural radiative forcing. *Climate Change 2013: The Physical Science Basis. Contribution of Working Group I to the Fifth Assessment Report of the Intergovernmental Panel on Climate Change.* Cambridge and New York: Cambridge University Press; 2013.

16. Sulbaek Andersen MP, Nielsen OJ, Wallington TJ, et al. Medical intelligence article: Assessing the impact on global climate from general anesthetic gases. *Anesth Analg.* 2012;114:1081–1085.

17. Ravishankara AR, Daniel JS, Portmann RW. Nitrous oxide (N_2O): The dominant ozone-depleting substance emitted in the 21st century. *Science.* 2009;326:123–125.

18. Ek M, Tjus K. Destruction of medical N_2O in Sweden. In: Liu G, ed. *Greenhouse Gases. Capturing, Utilization and Reduction.* London: IntechOpen; 2012.

19. Varughese S, Ahmed R. Environmental and occupational considerations of anesthesia: A narrative review and update. *Anesth Analg.* 2021;133(4):826–835.

20. National Institute for Occupational Safety and Health (NIOSH) Publication No 2007-151: Waste Anesthetic Gases, Occupational Hazards in Hospitals. https://www.cdc.gov/niosh/docs/2007-151/pdfs/2007-151.pdf?id=10.26616/NIOSHPUB2007151. Accessed December 9, 2020.

21. Ryan SM, Nielsen CJ. Global warming potential of inhaled anesthetics: Application to clinical use. *Anesth Analg.* 2010;11:92–98.

22. Baxter AD. Low and minimal flow inhalational anaesthesia. *Can J Anaesth.* 1997;44:643–652.

23. Baum JA. *Low Flow Anaesthesia: The Theory and Practice of Low Flow, Minimal Flow and Closed System Anaesthesia.* Oxford: Butterworth-Heinemann; 2001. 2nd ed.

24. Baker AB. Back to basics—A simplified non-mathematical approach to low flow techniques in anaesthesia. *Anaesth Intensive Care.* 1994;22:394–395.

25. Feldman JM. Managing fresh gas flow to reduce environmental contamination. *Anesth Analg.* 2012;114:1093–1101.

26. Nair BG, Peterson GN, Neradilek MB, Newman SF, Huang EY, Schwid HA. Reducing wastage of inhalation anesthetics using real-time decision support to notify of excessive fresh gas flow. *Anesthesiology.* 2013;118(4):874–884. doi:10.1097/ALN.0b013e3182829de0.

27. Schober P, Loer SA. Closed system anaesthesia—Historical aspects and recent developments. *Eur J Anaesthesiol.* 2006;23:914–920.

28. Philip JH. Closed-circuit anesthesia. In: Ehrenwerth J, Eisenkraft J, Berry J, eds. *Anesthesia Equipment: Principles and Applications.* Philadelphia: Elsevier; 2020. 3rd ed.

29. Feldman JM, Lo C, Hendrickx J. Estimating the impact of carbon dioxide absorbent performance differences on absorbent cost during low-flow anesthesia. *Anesth Analg.* 2020;13:374–381.

30. Lowe HJ, Ernst EA. *The Quantitative Practice of Anesthesia: Use of Closed Circuit:* Baltimore: Williams & Wilkins; 1981.

31. Feldman JM, Hendrickx J, Kennedy RR. Carbon dioxide absorption during inhalation anesthesia: A modern practice. *Anesth Analg.* 2020. doi:10.1213/ANE.0000000000005137.

32. Neumann MA, Laster MJ, Weiskopf RB, Gong DH, Dudziak R, Förster Eger E. The elimination of sodium and potassium hydroxides from desiccated soda lime diminishes degradation of desflurane to carbon monoxide and sevoflurane to compound A but does not compromise carbon dioxide absorption. *Anesth Analg.* 1999;89:768–773. doi:10.1213/00000539-199909000-00046.

33. Barwise JA, Lancaster LJ, Michaels D, et al. An initial evaluation of a novel anesthetic scavenging interface. *Anesth Analg.* 2011;113:1064–1067.

34. Blue Zone Technology, Toronto, ON, Canada. Deltasorb and Centralsorb Anesthetic Collection Service. https://www.blue-zone.ca. Accessed November 21, 2020.

35. Sherman J, Le C, Lamers V, et al. Life cycle greenhouse gas emissions of anesthetic drugs. *Anesth Analg.* 2012;114:1086–1090.

36. Mankes RF. Propofol wastage in anesthesia. *Anesth Analg.* 2012;114:1091–1092.

37. Gilbert N. Drug waste harms fish. *Nature.* 2011;476:265.

38. Allan BTW, Smith I. Cost considerations in the use of anaesthetic drugs. *Curr Opinion Anesthesiol.* 2002;15:227–232.

39. Dee H. Drug and material wastage in anesthesia care. *J Health Sci.* 2012;6:4–8.

40. Atcheson CL, Spivack J, Williams R, et al. Preventable drug waste among anesthesia providers: opportunities for efficiency. *J Clin Anesth.* 2016;30:24–32.

41. Sherman J, McGain F. Environmental sustainability in anesthesia: Pollution prevention and patient safety. *Adv Anesthes.* 2016;34:47–61.

42. Aggarwal S, Axelrod D, Bell C, et al. Greening the operating room and perioperative arena: Environmental sustainability for anesthesia practice. American Society of Anesthesiologists. https://www.asahq.org/about-asa/governance-and-committees/asa-committees/com-

VI

mittee-on-equipment-and-facilities/
environmental-sustainability/greening-
the-operating-room#appendB. Accessed
December 1, 2020.

43. McGain E, Hendel SA, Story DA. An
audit of potentially recyclable waste
from anaesthetic practice. *Anaesth
Intensive Care.* 2009;37:820–823.

44. Sherman JD, LAt Raibley, Eckelman
MJ. Life cycle assessment and costing methods for device procurement:
comparing reusable and single-use disposable laryngoscopes. *Anesth Analg.*
2018;127:434–443.

45. Eckelman M, Mosher M, Gonzalez A,
et al. Comparative life cycle assessment of disposable and reusable laryngeal mask airways. *Anesth Analg.*
2012;114:1067–1072.

46. Kwakye G, Pronovost PJ, Makary MA.
Commentary: A call to go green in
health care by reprocessing medical
equipment. *Acad Med.* 2010;85:398–
400.

47. Overcash M. A comparison of reusable
and disposable perioperative textiles:
Sustainability state-of-the-art 2012.
Anesth Analg. 2012;114:1055–1066.

48. Vozzola E, Overcash M. Griffing E: An
environmental analysis of reusable and
disposable surgical gowns. *AORN J.*
2020;111:315–325.

49. McGain F, Algie CM, O'Toole J, et al.
The microbiological and sustainability
effects of washing anaesthesia breathing circuits less frequently. *Anaesthesia.*
2014;69:337–342.

50. Dubler S, Zimmermann S, Fischer M,
et al. Bacterial and viral contamination
of breathing circuits after extended use–
An aspect of patient safety? *Acta Anaesthesiol Scand.* 2016;60:1251–1260.

51. Energy Information Administration:
2012 Commercial Buildings Energy Consumption Survey: Energy Usage Summary. http://www.eia.gov/consumption/
commercial/reports/2012/energyusage.
Accessed January 21, 2021.

52. Sulbaek Andersen MP, Nielsen OJ,
Karpichev B, et al. Atmospheric chemistry of isoflurane, desflurane, and sevoflurane: Kinetics and mechanisms of
reactions with chlorine atoms and OH
radicals and global warming potentials.
J Phys Chem A. 2012;116:5806–5820.

53. Sherman JD, Berkow L. Scaling up
Inhaled anesthetic practice improvement:
The role of environmental sustainability
metrics. *Anesth Analg.* 2019;128:1060–
1062.

54. Watts N, Amann M, Arnell N, et al. The
2019 report of The Lancet Countdown
on health and climate change: Ensuring
that the health of a child born today
is not defined by a changing climate.
Lancet. 2019;394:1836–1878.

55. Dartmouth-Hitchcock Eco-Health Footprint Calculator. https://sites.google.
com/site/dhmccalculator/home Last
Accessed October 3, 2021.

56. U.S. Environmental Protection Agency
(EPA). https://www.epa.gov/ghgemis-
sions/overview-greenhouse-gases Last
Accessed October 3, 2021.

57. American Society of Anesthesiologists
Greening the Operating Room and
Perioperative Arena. https://www.
asahq.org/about-asa/governance-
and-committees/asa-committees/com-
mittee-on-equipment-and-facilities/
environmental-sustainability/greening-
the-operating-room-complete. Last
Accessed October 3, 2021.

58. UK National Health Services (NHS)–
Greener NHS. https://www.england.nhs.
uk/greenernhs/Last Accessed October 3,
2021.

59. Yale Gassing Greener App. https://apps.
apple.com/us/app/yale-gassing-greener/
id1152700062 Accessed October 3, 2021.

INDEX

Note: Page numbers followed by "*b*," "*f*," and "*t*" indicate boxes, figures, and tables, respectively.

P

PAC. *See* Pulmonary artery catheter (PAC)
PACE technique. *See* Probe, Alert, Challenge, Emergency Action (PACE) technique
Packed red blood cells (PRBCs), 448
  transfusion of, 619
PaCO₂. *See* Arterial carbon dioxide tension (PaCO₂)
PACU. *See* Postanesthesia care unit (PACU)
Paddle electrodes, proper placement, 813*f*, 813
Pain
  acute. *See* Acute pain
  analgesic delivery systems, 720
  burns, trauma and, 787
  chronic. *See* Chronic pain
  leg, 797*t*–798*t*
  lower back, 797*t*–798*t*
  management of, 718
    in palliative care, 844
  neurobiology, 718
  neuropathic, 800
    complex regional pain syndrome, 800
    peripheral neuropathy, 800
  nociception, 717–718
    modulation of, 718
  perioperative recovery, multimodal approach, 720
  preventive analgesia, 719
  systemic local anesthetics for, 156
  TNS, relationship, 154
  in total knee replacements, 572–573
Pain relief
  μ-agonists opioids and, 130
  opioid analgesics and, 131
Palliative care, 839, 840*f*
  anesthesiologists' contribution to, 842
  cancer pain and, 844, 845*t*–846*t*
  communication and, 848
    difficult information, frameworks for, 849*b*, 849
    patient and family, prognosis and, 848
    physician tendencies in addressing difficult topics, 848
  end of life, use of opioids at, 844
  hospice, 840, 841*f*
  Hospice and Palliative Medicine subspecialty, 841
  identification of, and hospice patients, 846
    hospice consults, 846
    inpatient, 846
    outpatient, 847
  in intensive care unit, 843*b*, 843
  noncancer pain and, 844

nurses and, 842
and pain, 844
patient, challenges in, 846
perioperative management, 849, 850*b*
  advance directives and, 849
  decision-making capacity and, 850
  perioperative DNR conversations and, 851
  surrogate decision makers and, 850
physicians, 842
prognosis and, 847
  disease trajectories and, 847, 847*f*
  functional status and, 848
  physician estimate and, 847
  prognostic tools and, 848
specialists, 840
spirituality in serious illness, 843
teams, 842, 842*b*–843*b*
withdrawal of life support in, 843
Palliative medicine, 839
Pancreas transplantation, 668
Pancuronium
  chemical structure of, 164*f*
  as long-acting nondepolarizing neuromuscular blocking drugs, 171
  nondepolarizing NMBDs in, 165
PaO₂/FiO₂ (P/F) ratio, 411
PAP. *See* Pulmonary artery pressure
Para-aminobenzoic acid, metabolites, relationship, 153
"Paradoxical" sleep, 857
Paraganglioma, 527
  perioperative considerations, 527
Paramagnetic oxygen analysis, 242
Paramedian approach
  in epidural anesthesia, 308
  in spinal anesthesia, 303, 304*f*
Paraplegia, 311
Parasternal long-axis view
  cardiac ultrasound, 385
  image appearance and structures visualized, 386, 388*f*
  image interpretation, 386, 389*b*, 389*f*
  patient positioning, 385
  probe position and manipulation, 385–386, 387*f*
Parasternal short-axis view
  cardiac ultrasound, 386
  image appearance and structures visualized, 386, 388*f*
  image interpretation, 386, 390*b*, 390*f*
  patient positioning, 386
  probe position and manipulation, 386, 387*f*
Parasympathetic nerves (stimulation), effector organs (responses), 75*t*

Parasympathetic nervous system (PNS), 55, 69, 72, 644–646
  cranial nerves, origin of, 72
Parathyroid disease, 525
Parathyroid surgery, 557
Parkinson disease, 198
Parotid surgery, 557
Partial agonists, 42
Partial pressure, 235
  of inhaled anesthetic, 84–87, 102
Partition coefficients, of inhaled anesthetics, 85, 87*f*
Patent ductus arteriosus, 630
Patient-controlled analgesia (PCA), 216, 721
  delivery systems, usage (guidelines), 722*t*
  opioids and, 137
Patient factors
  epidural block height and, 305
  spinal block height and, 299
Patient positioning
  and associated risks, 336
  general, 337
    lateral decubitus, 340, 341*f*
    lithotomy, 339, 340*f*
    prone, 342, 342*f*
    sitting, 343*f*, 344
    supine, 337, 338*f*
  physiologic aspects of, 336
  for robotic surgery, 345
Patient safety, 19–20
Patient safety-focused programs, in anesthesia care, 831
Patient suction, anesthesia workstation, 249
Patients
  blood management, 449
  challenges, in palliative care, 846
  follow-up, 15
  head, elevation, 266
PAWP. *See* Pulmonary artery wedge pressure; Pulmonary artery wedge pressure (PAWP)
PCA. *See* Patient-controlled analgesia (PCA)
PCWP. *See* Pulmonary capillary wedge pressure (PCWP)
PDSA (Plan/Do/Study/Act), as quality improvement project, 835
Peak expiratory flow (PEF) rate, 478–479
Peak inspiratory pressure (PIP), 355–356
Pediatric advanced cardiovascular life support
  airway, 820
  defibrillation, 820
  drugs, 822
Pediatric advanced life support, 820
  circulation, 820, 822*f*